Davis's Laboratory and Diagnostic Test Handbook

D1025976

Marie S. Jaffe, RN, MS
(Deceased)
Former Faculty
University of Texas, El Paso
College of Nursing and Allied Health
El Paso, Texas

Barbara F. McVan, RN
Independent Nursing Consultant
Lansdale, Pennsylvania

 F.A. DAVIS COMPANY · Philadelphia

F. A. Davis Company
1915 Arch Street
Philadelphia, PA 19103

Printed in the United States of America

Last digit indicates print number: 10 9 8 7 6 5 4

Nursing Acquisitions Editor: Joanne P. DaCunha, RN, MSN
Production Editors: Glenn L. Fechner, Nancee A. Morelli
Cover Designer: Louis J. Forgione

As new scientific information becomes available through basic and clinical research, recommended treatments and drug therapies undergo changes. The authors and publisher have done everything possible to make this book accurate, up to date, and in accord with accepted standards at the time of publication. The authors, editors, and publisher are not responsible for errors or omissions or for consequences from application of the book, and make no warranty, expressed or implied, in regard to the contents of the book. Any practice described in this book should be applied by the reader in accordance with professional standards of care used in regard to the unique circumstances that may apply in each situation. The reader is advised always to check product information (package inserts) for changes and new information regarding dose and contraindications before administering any drug. Caution is especially urged when using new or infrequently ordered drugs.

Library of Congress Cataloging in Publication Data
Davis's laboratory and diagnostic test handbook / [edited by] Marie
  Jaffe, Barbara F. McVan.
      p.   cm.
    Includes index.
    ISBN 0-8036-0088-7 (soft cover)
    1. Diagnosis, Laboratory—Handbooks, manuals, etc.
    2. Diagnosis—Handbooks, manuals, etc.   I. Jaffe, Marie S.
  II. McVan, Barbara.
    [DNLM: 1. Diagnostic Tests,   Routine—handbooks.   WB 39
D265 1997]
    RB38.2.D38   1997
    616.07'56—dc21
    DNLM/DLC
    for Library of Congress   96-45650
                                                                CIP

Publisher's Note

During the development of this book, we were deeply saddened when we received word that Marie Jaffe had passed away. Marie was a very dynamic person who loved nursing and was so willing to share her knowledge and enthusiasm with her peers. She was instrumental in conceptualizing and refining the framework for this book. Her tireless attention to detail kept the book moving along despite many hurdles. Throughout the remainder of the work on this book, Marie's cheery phone calls and her sharing of ideas were sadly missed. She left a wonderful legacy of knowledge and love to all who knew her.

Joanne P. DaCunha, RN, MSN
Nursing Editor

Contributors

Kathleen M. Blade RN, MS
Junior Level Faculty
St. Joseph Hospital School of Nursing
North Providence, Rhode Island

Karen C. Johnson-Brennan, RN, EdD
Professor and Associate Director
School of Nursing
San Francisco State University
San Francisco, California

Bonita M. Cavanaugh, PhD, RN
Director, School of Nursing
University of Colorado
Denver, Colorado

Suzanne Chubinski, RN, BSN, MA
Assistant Professor of Health Sciences
Indiana University-Purdue University Fort Wayne
Fort Wayne, Indiana

Tita de la Cruz, RN, EdD
Associate Professor
Gwynedd Mercy College
Gwynedd Valley, Pennsylvania

Susan T. Eisenhower, RN, MSN
Nursing Instructor
Reading Hospital
School of Nursing
West Reading, Pennsylvania

Christabel A. Kaitell, RN, SCM, MPH
Assistant Professor
School of Nursing, Faculty of Health Sciences
University of Ottawa
Ottawa, Ontario, Canada

Gail Kelly, RN, MA
Consultant and Instructor
L.A. Wilson School of Nursing
Northport, New York

Deborah A. Raines, RN-C, PhD
Assistant Professor
Virginia Commonwealth University
School of Nursing
Richmond, Virgina

Judith A. Redman, RN, BScN, MEd
Clinical Instructor
University of Ottawa
Ottawa, Ontario, Canada

Barbara Rexilius, RN, MSN
Director of Nursing
Chair of Health Related Careers
North Country Community College
Saranac Lake, New York

Beverly A. Tscheschlog, RN
Nursing Consultant
Ottsville, Pennsylvania

Table of Contents

How to Use This Book, xi
Laboratory and Diagnostic Tests in Alphabetical Order, 1
Appendices, 1323

APPENDIX 1
Collection Procedures, 1325

Venous
Arterial
Urine

APPENDIX 2
Types of Vacuumized Tubes Used for Blood Tests, 1345

APPENDIX 3
Universal Precautions: OSHA Bloodborne Pathogens Standard, 1348

APPENDIX 4
Reference Values, 1362

For Laboratory Tests on Blood, 1362

For Laboratory Tests on Urine, 1383

APPENDIX 5
Profile Groups, 1390

SMA-4
SMA-6
SMA-12
SMAC CHEM 20

APPENDIX 6
Organ Function Tests, 1391

Cardiovascular System
Pulmonary System
Neurologic System
Hematologic System
Endocrine System
Renal-Urologic System
Musculoskeletal System
Hepatobiliary-Gastrointestinal Systems
Reproductive System
Immune and Autoimmune Conditions
Tumors

Indices, 1399
Index, 1401
The Disorder and Condition Index, 1416

How to Use This Book

Davis's Manual of Laboratory and Diagnostic Tests is a comprehensive, portable reference of laboratory and diagnostic tests that provides nurses with the information they need to understand why a test is done, how it is performed, and what results to expect.

Organization of the Book

This text is organized in an easy-to-use alphabetical format. To eliminate repetition, procedural steps for collecting specimens and general information of concern for all tests are detailed in Appendix 1. Only those steps unique to a specific test are discussed in each test monograph.

Organization of Monographs

Classification and *Type of Test*

Indications state why the test may be performed.

Reference Values, including SI Units, help the reader evaluate test results. It is essential to remember, however, that each laboratory has its own set of Reference Values or standards that may differ from those listed here.

Abnormal Values identify what disorders or conditions cause the test result.

Interfering Factors help determine if the valid results can be obtained if the test is performed.

Nursing Implications are organized by the nursing process, a framework used by most nursing schools.

> ***Assessment*** alerts the nurse to client information that may affect the results of the test.

Possible Nursing Diagnoses define problems or client needs that require a nursing intervention or management. A specific nursing diagnosis cannot be applied universally to any disease state, nor, particularly, to a specific laboratory or diagnostic test. However, the authors have selected those that could be related to potential problems that may be evident when the test is being performed and may affect the way you may proceed with the test. Also included are diagnoses for potential problems that may occur during or after the procedure and as clients deal with a perceived threat to their health. They are meant to be guideposts, ensuring more positive outcomes by directing the nurse to anticipate areas of concern.

Implementation provides the information the nurse needs to either assist with or perform the procedure. The steps of the procedure are highlighted in color.

Evaluation provides important information to consider when analyzing the test results.

Client/Caregiver Teaching, both *Pretest* and *Posttest,* is organized in one place to make planning easier.

Appendices

In addition to an appendix of detailed procedures

Types of Collection Tubes
OSHA Guidelines
Blood and Urine Values Chart
Profile Groups list the tests included in the combination tests, such as SMA.
Organ Function Tests help the nurse determine which tests may be performed to diagnose a particular disorder.

Two Indexes

- *The Index* helps the nurse find tests quickly if they are known by names other than the one listed in alphabetical order.
- *The Disorder and Condition Index* allows the nurse to identify all the tests in the book that show an abnormal result for a specific disorder or condition.

Laboratory and Diagnostic Test Monographs

Acetylcholine Receptor Antibody (AChR)

Classification: Immunology

Type of Test: Serum

This assay test determines the presence of the AChR antibody. When present, this antibody blocks acetylcholine from binding to receptor sites on the muscle membrane and destroys acetylcholine receptor sites interfering with neuromuscular transmission and causing muscle weakness.

Two test methods are available, the modulating, or binding, assay and a blocking antibody assay. Because these tests are about 90 percent accurate in diagnosis of myasthenia gravis (MG), they are replacing the Tensilon test.

Indications

- Confirm the presence, but not the severity, of MG
- Differentiate between generalized and ocular forms of MG, and the remission stage of the disease.
- Monitor effectiveness of immunosuppressive therapy for MG

Reference Values

- ≤ 0.03 nmol/L or negative

Abnormal Values

- Positive AChR
  Myasthenia gravis: 0.05 nmol/L indicates generalized MG; 0.11 nmol/L indicates ocular MG; and 0.67 nmol/L indicates remission
  Thymoma
  Amyotrophic lateral sclerosis
- Negative AChR
  Thymectomy
  Immunosuppressive therapy

Interfering Factors

- Antibodies and muscle relaxants (metacurine, succinylcholine) can produce false-positive results.
- False-positives may result in patients with amyotrophic lateral sclerosis who have been treated with cobra venom.

Nursing Implications

Assessment

- Obtain history of known or suspected MG as well as current drug therapy.

Possible Nursing Diagnoses

Anxiety related to perceived threat to health status
Aspiration, risk for, related to impaired swallowing
Physical mobility, impaired, related to neuromuscular impairment
Fatigue related to altered body chemistry

Implementation

- Put on gloves. Using aseptic technique, perform a venipuncture and collect 7 mL of blood in a red-top tube. Keep sample at room temperature.
- Note any recent immunosuppressive drug therapy on laboratory requisition slip. Send to laboratory immediately.

Evaluation

- Note results in relation to related tests and clinical presentation.

Client/Caregiver Teaching

Pretest

- Inform client that no special preparation is needed.

Acid Phosphatase (ACP), Prostatic Acid Phosphatase (PAP)

Classification: Chemistry

Type of Test: Serum

This test measures the blood level of acid phosphatase (ACP), an enzyme found mainly in the prostate gland, red blood cells (RBCs), and platelets, as well as in bone, spleen, liver, and kidney tissue. Two isoenzymes (prostate and RBC-platelet fractions) are diagnostically significant for prostate disorders and lymphoproliferative disorders. The tumor-marker test prostate-specific antigen (PSA) has replaced or served as an adjunct to this test for the diagnosis of prostate cancer.

Indications

- Investigate or evaluate an enlarged prostate gland, especially if prostatic carcinoma is suspected
- Evaluate the effectiveness of treatment for prostatic cancer (recurrence following prostatectomy). Levels will decrease if treatment is effective. Rising levels are associated with a poor prognosis
- Assist with differential diagnosis of other disorders associated with elevated prostatic ACP levels or with elevated RBC-platelet ACP, such as leukemia

Reference Values

	SI Units
0.1–5.0 U/dL (King-Armstrong)	0.2–8.8 IU/L
0.1–0.8 U/dL (Bessey-Lowry)	1.7–13.4 IU/L
0.5–2.0 U/dL (Bodansky)	2.7–10.7 IU/L

Abnormal Values

- Elevated prostatic ACP
  Prostatic cancer

- Elevated RBC-platelet ACP
    - Gaucher's disease
    - Niemann-Pick disease
    - Hemolytic anemia
    - Sickle cell crisis
    - Thrombocytosis
    - Acute myelogenous leukemia
    - Renal insufficiency
    - Liver disease
    - Metastatic bone cancer
    - Paget's disease
    - Osteogenesis imperfecta
    - Hyperparathyroidism
    - Multiple myeloma
- Decreased prostatic ACP
    - Estrogen therapy
    - Down syndrome

Interfering Factors

- Prostatic massage, rectal examination, or urinary catheriza-tion within 48 hours of the test can cause elevated levels.
- Androgen administration in females and clofibrate in either sex can produce elevated levels.
- Ingestion of alcohol, fluorides, oxalates, and phosphates can result in decreased levels.

Nursing Implications

Assessment

- Obtain a history of known or suspected prostatic disorders and related test results.
- Note any medications that can interfere with test results that were taken in the last 24 hours.
- Note any recent procedures that can interfere with test results.

Possible Nursing Diagnoses

Anxiety related to perceived threat to health status
Urinary elimination, altered, related to anatomical obstruction
Sexual dysfunction related to altered body function, drugs, or radiation

Implementation

- Put on gloves. Using aseptic technique, perform a venipunc-ture and collect 5 mL of blood in a red-top tube.
- Handle specimen gently to prevent hemolysis and transport

to laboratory immediately, as results can be altered within 1 hour.

Evaluation

- Note results in relation to prostate-specific antigen (PSA), if performed, or other organ function tests, if pathology is suspected.

Client/Caregiver Teaching

Pretest

- Instruct patient to withhold medications that may interfere with test results for 12 to 24 hours before the test, as ordered by the physician.

Posttest

- Remove adhesive bandage.
- Resume any medications withheld before the test.

Acid Phosphatase (ACP), Vaginal Swab

Classification: Cytology

Type of Test: Vaginal swab

This test measures the levels of acid phosphatase (ACP) in vaginal secretions. Normally, the levels are low in vaginal secretions but high in prostate gland secretions, including semen. Presence of high levels in vaginal secretions is strongly supportive of recent sexual intercourse. This test does not depend on the presence of sperm for a positive result.

Indications

- Investigate alleged or suspected rape
- Investigate sexual assault in homicide cases

Reference Values

<5	Normal vaginal secretions
<7	Inconclusive
7–50	Strongly suggestive of sexual intercourse within last 36 hours
>50	Confirms recent sexual intercourse

Interfering Factors

- Delay in collecting the specimen for 12 or more hours following rape will not be likely to reveal positive results.
- Bathing or douching following the rape can cause negative results.
- If the male had a vasectomy or is unable to ejaculate, results will also be negative.

> ### ▶ NURSING ALERT
>
> - Collect specimen as soon as possible following the rape. Best samples are collected within 5 hours after intercourse.
> - Follow all institution protocols for handling specimens.

Nursing Implications

Assessment

- Obtain a brief recall of the event by the client, including the time.

Possible Nursing Diagnoses

Anxiety related to threat to self-concept, interpersonal transmission of disease, or situational crisis

Rape-trauma syndrome (acute phase) related to actual or attempted sexual attack without consent

Implementation

- Display sensitivity to feelings of guilt or embarrassment about the event and the procedure; provide additional support during vaginal procedure.
- Handle the client's clothing carefully in suspected rape cases, because additional specimens can be obtained from stains. Stains can be tested for semen many months following the event.
- Assemble the equipment, including vaginal speculum, swabs, gloves, saline, syringes for lavage, slides, and container with 95% ethanol or sterile container for swabs.

- Have client void and inform not to wipe following urination.
- Place in lithotomy position and drape for privacy.
- Insert vaginal speculum and secure in place.
- Gently saturate the swab(s) with material from the vaginal walls and place in a sterile container. Ensure that the packaging of the specimen, the placement of the specimen in a container, and the transport of the specimen to the laboratory all comply with institutional and legal protocols.
- Properly identify the specimen and immediately transport to the laboratory. Supervise transport according to institutional protocol to maintain the chain of evidence. Have a witness sign the request form.
- Administer ordered spermicidal douche after the specimen has been collected.
- At the conclusion of the procedure, return the patient to a position of comfort and allow to rest.

Evaluation

- Remain with the client and monitor response to procedure.

Client/Caregiver Teaching

Pretest

- Explain that the procedure is performed by the physician or nurse but that a witness or law enforcement officer may need to be present.

Posttest

- Instruct the client in the use of prescribed medication to prevent pregnancy.
- Refer the client to counseling services, if appropriate.

Acoustic Admittance Tests

Classification: Sensory organ function

Type of Test: Auditory perception

This test measures the flow of sound into the ear (admittance) and resistance to that flow (impedance). The two tests usually performed include tympanometry and acoustic reflex testing. Tympanometry, which uses a sound source and microphone, measures the impedance of the middle ear to acoustic energy and is useful for evaluating effusions or eustachian-tube abnormalities. Acoustic reflex testing measures the admittance change caused by reflex contraction of the stapedius muscle to evaluate the VII (facial) and VIII (acoustic) cranial nerve function. These tests are very useful in evaluating hearing loss in children and older adults who are not able to cooperate with hearing tests that require active participation.

Indications

- Diagnose middle-ear pathology, as evidenced by changes in the shape, amplitude, and pressure readings on the tympanogram.
- Determine tympanic membrane abnormalities, as evidenced by large changes in admittance.
- Determine or confirm type of lesion in conductive hearing loss; this is suggested when the middle ear absorbs less sound and reflects more sound in tympanometry.
- Determine eustachian-tube dysfunction, as evidenced by pressure and amplitude changes and air-pressure fluctuations with respirations recorded in tympanometry.
- Determine ossicular chain discontinuity or fusion causing conductive hearing loss, as evidenced by changes in admittance.
- Diagnose VIIth nerve paralysis, as evidenced by compliance changes produced by reflex contraction of the stapedius muscle.
- Differentiate between cochlear lesions or abnormalities of the cochlear apparatus (sensory) and VIII nerve brain-stem lesions (neural); the latter cause sensorineural hearing loss by decreasing or distorting the transmission of information to the brain, as evidenced by reflex adaptation or decay in the acoustic reflex test.
- Differentiate between VIII nerve and peripheral brain-stem lesions caused by intra-axial brain-stem lesions; the latter are evidenced by ipsilateral and brain-stem determinations and changes in reflex magnitude.
- Differentiate between sensory and neural hearing loss, as evidenced by the presence or absence of reflex adaptation or decay below 2000 Hz
- Determine or confirm the presence of pseudohypacusis, as evidenced by confirming voluntary thresholds.

Reference Values

- *Tympanometry:* Smooth and symmetric tympanogram with middle-ear pressure range of about 100 daPa

- *Acoustic reflexes:* Transbrain-stem reflex threshold of tones of 70–100 dB; ipsilateral thresholds of 3–12 dB lower; reflex decay no more than half of the baseline over 10 seconds.

Abnormal Values

- Sensory or conductive hearing loss
- Middle-ear or eustachian-tube abnormalities (infection, tumor, effusion)
- Lesions of the cochlear apparatus, facial or auditory nerves

Interfering Factors

- Incorrectly placed, clogged, or moved probe
- Failure to obtain and maintain a seal of the probe in the ear canal during the test
- Equipment artifacts that produce inaccurate measurement of the admittance reflex stimuli
- Client movement, talking, or swallowing

NURSING ALERT

- Contraindicated in recent surgical procedures on the middle ear to treat chronic otitis media or correct anatomical abnormalities

Nursing Implications

Assessment

- Obtain a history of known or suspected hearing loss, including type and cause; ear conditions with treatment regimens; ear surgery; and other tests and procedures to assess and diagnose auditory deficit

Possible Nursing Diagnoses

Sensory-perceptual alteration (auditory) related to altered sensory reception, transmission, or integration
Anxiety related to perceived threat to health status
Communication, impaired, verbal, related to hearing loss

Implementation

- Place the client in a sitting position in a quiet room. A child can be held on the lap of the caretaker.
- Perform an otoscopy examination to ensure that the external ear canal is clear of any obstruction. The appropriate probe cuff is selected to fit the size and shape of the ear canal.
- Insert the calibrated probe tip into the ear canal with the

dominant hand while the nondominant hand pulls the ear upward and backward (adult) or downward (child). The probe tip is equipped with a microphone. The probe is sealed to maintain a negative pressure of 200 daPa; silicone putty is used to ensure the seal if needed to prevent possible leaks that would cause inaccurate threshold results.

- The calibrated probe contains an admittance meter, electronic tone generator (sound source), and air-pressure manometer and pump used in the delivery of sound and air-pressure stimuli. The probe tone level and meter sensitivity is set, and air pressure is delivered to perform tympanometry. At least six measurements are taken to measure extensive admittance changes.

- Perform the acoustic reflex by introducing a pure tone of 500–4000 Hz to one ear using the probe. This stimulus causes a bilateral reflex activation. Changes in admittance in the ear receiving the stimulus (ipsilateral) or in the opposite ear (transbrain stem) are measured and recorded. The reflex thresholds are determined by the introduction of the sound stimuli in increases of 10 dB at a time, then a decrease of 10 dB when the first reflex occurs, followed by increases of 5 dB at a time, with recordings made at the lowest level of stimulus that a reflex is noted.

- Measure the reflex decay in the opposite ear at 500–1000 Hz by introducing the sound stimulus at 10 dB for 10 seconds above the reflex threshold. The reflex magnitude at 5 or 10 seconds is compared with the baseline taken at 1 second to determine reflex decay. Abnormal reflex decay is determined if the reflex magnitude decreases to less than half of the baseline.

- Remove probe from the ear canal. Gently cleanse and dry the canal.

Evaluation

- Note test results in relation to the client's symptoms and other tests performed.

Client/Caregiver Teaching

Pretest

- Inform the client that the tests are performed by the audiologist or physician in a quiet room and that each test takes less than 5 minutes to complete.
- Ask the client to remain very still during the test and refrain from any movements of the face, mouth, and head regardless of the sounds heard.

- Inform the client that the tests do not do any harm to the ears when the air and sound stimuli are introduced.

Posttest

- If abnormality is detected, support the client and inform about future diagnostic tests, for example, evoked response audiometry or electrocochleography.

Activated Clotting Time (ACT)

Classification: Hematology

Type of Test: Blood

This test measures the blood's clotting ability. It is more sensitive to the effects of heparin and factor VIII deficiency than the whole-blood clotting time and is commonly performed during procedures that require extracorporeal circulation, such as cardiopulmonary circulation, hemodialysis, or extracorporeal membrane oxygenation (ECMO).

Indications

- Investigate suspected clotting disorders
- Investigate suspected factor deficiencies (except factor VII)
- Monitor the effect of heparin
- Monitor the effect of protamine sulfate in heparin neutralization

Reference Values

- 94 to 120 seconds in the nonanticoagulated client.
- During cardiopulmonary bypass, heparin is titrated to maintain ACT at 400 to 600 seconds; during ECMO, the heparin is titrated to maintain ACT at 220 to 260 seconds.

Abnormal Values

- Increased levels indicate:
  Circulating anticoagulants (heparin)
  Afibrinogenemia
  Factor deficiencies
  Hemophilia
  Hemorrhagic disease of newborn

Interfering Factors

- Normal levels vary by laboratory and activator lot number.
- Capillary specimens yield invalid results.
- Contamination from a line or vascular access device (VAD) containing heparin may alter results.

Nursing Implications

Assessment

- Obtain a history of cardiovascular system, known or suspected blood disorders, medication regimen, diagnostic tests, and results.
- Observe the patient for signs of bleeding.

Possible Nursing Diagnoses

Injury, risk for, related to altered clotting factors
Protection, altered, related to abnormal blood profiles
Anxiety related to perceived threat to health status

Implementation

- Put on gloves. Using aseptic technique, perform a venipuncture and collect the 5 to 10 mL blood in a blue-top tube. Discard tube, leaving needle in place.
- Remove tourniquet and attach gray-top Celite tube (contact activator). Fill with 2 mL of blood. Begin timing as tube fills; after 60 seconds, tilt the tube on side. Tilt on side every 5 to 10 seconds until clot is seen. Stop timming when first clot is seen.
- If the blood was withdrawn from a VAD, discard the first sample of blood and follow the procedure above. Then flush the device following the facility's protocol.
- If the client has a continuous infusion, stop the infusion before the sample is drawn. Remember to restart after blood samples drawn.
- Send specimen to laboratory immediately.

Evaluation

■ Compare the value with previous results and time of last heparin dose. Observe the patient for signs of bleeding if indicated.

Client/Caregiver Teaching

Pretest

■ Inform the patient that two blood samples will be taken and that the first one will be discarded.

Activated Partial Thromboplastin Time (aPTT), Partial Thromboplastin Time (PTT)

Classification: Hematology (hemostasis)

Type of Test: Plasma

This coagulation test evaluates the function of the intrinsic pathways (factors XII, XI, IX, and VIII) and common pathways (factors V, X, II, I, XIII) of the coagulation sequence, specifically the intrinsic thromboplastin system. It represents the time required for a firm fibrin clot to form after phospholipid reagents similar to thromboplastin reagent are added to the specimen. The PTT is abnormal in 90 percent of clients with coagulation disorders and is useful in monitoring the inactivation of factor II effect of heparin therapy. The aPTT has additional activators, making this test faster and more reliably reproducible than the PTT.

Indications

■ Evaluate response to anticoagulant therapy with heparin or coumarin derivatives
■ Detect congenital deficiencies in clotting factors such as hemophilia A (factor VIII) and hemophilia B (factor IX)

- Identify possible cause of abnormal bleeding such as epistaxis, easy bruising, bleeding gums, hematuria, and menorrhagia
- Identify individuals who may be prone to bleeding during surgical, obstetrical, dental, or invasive diagnostic procedures
- Monitor hemostatic effects of conditions such as liver disease, protein deficiency, and fat malabsorption

Reference Values

	PTT	aPTT
Newborn	<90 sec	
Infants/children	24–40 sec	
Adult	60–70 sec	30–40 sec
Critical value	>70 sec	

During heparin therapy values should be 1.5 to 2.5 times the control. Critical values would be >20 seconds above the control or 2.5 times greater than the control. Values <53 seconds indicate inadequate heparinization.

Abnormal Values

- Prolonged levels indicate:
  Coagulation-factor deficiencies
  Circulating products of fibrin and fibrinogen degradation
  Polycythemia
  Severe liver disease
  Vitamin K deficiency
  Disseminated intravascular coagulation (DIC)
  Von Willebrand's disease
  Drugs, including heparin, salicylates, and coumarin

Interfering Factors

- Anticoagulant therapy with heparin or coumarin derivatives will alter the aPTT.
- Drugs such as antihistamines, ascorbic acid, chlorpromazine, and salicylates may cause prolonged PTT.
- Traumatic venipunctures can lead to erroneous results from activation of the coagulation sequence.
- Excessive agitation that causes sample hemolysis can prolong the aPTT.

Nursing Implications

Assessment

- Obtain history of bleeding disorders. If client is receiving anticoagulant therapy, note time and amount of last dose.

Possible Nursing Diagnoses

Protection, altered, related to abnormal blood profiles
Injury, risk for, related to altered clotting factors
Anxiety related to perceived threat to health status

Implementation

- Put on gloves. Using aseptic technique, perform a venipuncture, collect 1 to 2 mL and discard; then collect and fill a light blue-top tube with the blood sample.
- Avoid traumatic venipuncture and excessive agitation of the sample.

Evaluation

- Note test results in relation to other tests performed, the time of the last dose of heparin, and the client's symptoms.

Client/Caregiver Teaching

Posttest

- Tell the client to report bleeding from any areas of skin or mucous membranes.
- Inform the client of the importance of periodic laboratory testing while taking an anticoagulant.

Adrenocorticotropic Hormone (ACTH), Corticotropin

Classification: Chemistry

Type of Test: Plasma

This test measures the level of ACTH, the anterior pituitary gland hormone that stimulates adrenal cortex secretion of glucocorticoids, androgens, and, to a lesser degree, mineralocorticoids. Secretion of this hormone is closely linked to melanocyte-stimulating hormone and is thought to stimulate pancreatic beta cells and the release of growth hormone. ACTH release is stimulated by hypothalamic-releasing factor. Cortisol test results are evaluated together, as they each control the other's concentrations and any change in one causes a change in the other.

ACTH levels exhibit a diurnal variation, peaking between 6 and 8 AM and reaching its lowest point between 6 and 11 PM. Evening levels are generally one-half to two-thirds lower than morning levels.

Indications

- Determine adrenocortical dysfunction
- Differentiate between increased ACTH release with decreased cortisol levels and decreased ACTH release with increased cortisol levels
- Determine adequacy of control-replacement therapy in congenital adrenal hyperplasia conditions

Reference Values

Type of Test	Values	SI Units
BioScience Labs Mayo Clinic	<80 pg/mL at 8 AM <120 pg/mL at 6–8 AM <50 pg/mL at 8–11 PM	<80 ng/L <120 ng/L in AM <50 ng/L in PM

Normal results vary according to the laboratory performing the test.

Abnormal Values

- Elevated ACTH (>200 pg/L)
    Primary adrenocortical hypofunction (Addison's disease)
    Idiopathic destruction of adrenal cortex
    Pituitary adenomas
    Nonendocrine malignant tumors, such as oat cell carcinoma
    Cushing's syndrome
- Decreased ACTH (<50 pg/L)
    Secondary hypoadrenalism
    Adrenal cortical hyperplasia or tumors
    Panhypopituitarism
    Hypothalamic dysfunction
    Drugs, including adrenal corticosteroids, estrogens, calcium gluconate, amphetamines, spironalactone, and ethanol

Interfering Factors

- Certain drugs can lead to decreased levels (see Abnormal Values).
- Physical or emotional stress, exercise, and elevated blood glucose levels can increase levels.
- Radioactive scan within 1 week of the test can affect results.

Nursing Implications

Assessment

- Obtain a focused history of complaints related to endocrine system and actual or suspected abnormalities of adrenal or pituitary function.
- Note compliance in withholding food for 12 hours and ingestion of low-carbohydrate diet for 48 hours before test.
- Note compliance in withholding of medications, especially steroids, that alter test results for 24 to 48 hours before test.
- Ensure that strenuous exercise has been avoided for 12 hours before the test and that 1 hour of bed rest is provided immediately before the test.

Possible Nursing Diagnoses

Anxiety related to perceived threat to health status
Coping, ineffective, individual, related to situation crisis
Body temperature, altered, risk for, related to illness affecting temperature regulation

Implementation

- Between 6 and 9 AM (peak secretion time), assemble supplies, including ice and a plastic bag.
- Put on gloves. Using aseptic technique, perform a venipuncture and collect 7 mL of blood in a plastic green- or lavender-top tube. Be sure to fill the tube.
- Label the specimen tubes and place them in ice in a plastic bag. Note the exact time that specimen was obtained on the laboratory requisition slip and attach it to the specimen.
- Send the specimen to the laboratory immediately as results can be altered within 15 minutes.
- When ACTH hypersecretion is suspected, obtain a second sample between 8 and 10 PM to determine if changes are the result of diurnal variation in ACTH levels.

Evaluation

- Note cortisol levels in relation to ACTH if adrenal or pituitary disorders are suspected.

Client/Caregiver Teaching

Pretest

- Inform the patient that more than one sample may be necessary to ensure accurate results and that the samples are obtained at specific times to determine high and low levels of the hormone.
- Instruct patient to eat a low-carbohydrate diet for 48 hours before test and then not to eat anything for 12 hours before the test.
- Instruct the patient not to take medications that interfere with test results for 24 to 48 hours before test, as ordered by the physician.
- Tell the patient to refrain from strenuous exercise for 12 hours before the test and to remain in bed 1 hour immediately before the test.

Posttest

- Resume food and fluid intake, medications, and usual activities withheld before the test.
- Inform the patient that ACTH suppression or stimulation testing may follow to confirm a diagnosis of hormonal dysfunction.

Alanine Aminotransferase (ALT), Alanine Transaminase, Glutamic-Pyruvic Transaminase (SGPT)

Classification: Chemistry

Type of Test: Serum

Alanine aminotransferase (ALT), formerly known as glutamic-pyruvic transaminase (SGPT), is an enzyme produced by the liver that acts as a catalyst in the transamination reaction necessary for amino acid production. ALT is found in liver cells in high concentrations and in moderate amounts in body fluids, heart, kidneys, and skeletal muscles. When liver damage occurs, serum levels of ALT rise to as much as 50 times normal, making this a very useful test in evaluating liver injury.

Indications

- Monitor liver disease or liver damage due to hepatotoxic drugs, as confirmed by elevated levels or a sudden drop following elevation in levels
- Monitor response to treatment for liver disease, with tissue repair indicated by gradually declining levels
- Compare serially with asparate aminotransferase (AST) levels to track the course of hepatitis
- Evaluate along with AST levels to determine degree of liver injury and confirm if hepatic damage is the cause of AST increase
- Differentiate etiology of jaundice, whether from liver pathology or from hemolytic disorders, which cause no increase in levels
- Routine screen by blood banks for hepatitis in donor blood samples; samples are rejected if levels exceed 1.5 times the upper limits of normal

Reference Values

	Values	*SI Units*
Infants	54 U/L or twice adult level	
Children	3–37 U/L	
Adults		4–36 U/L at 37°C
Women	5–35 U/mL	
Men	7–46 U/mL	

Reference values vary among laboratories and according to the method used for reporting results.

Abnormal Values

- Elevated levels (>300 U/L)
  Liver diseases and/or damage, such as hepatic cancer, hepatitis, or infectious mononucleosis

- Moderately elevated levels
  Biliary tract obstruction
  Recent cerebrovascular accident
  Muscle injury from intramuscular injections, trauma, infection, and seizures
  Muscular dystrophy
  Acute pancreatitis
  Intestinal injury
  Extensive muscle trauma
  Myocardial infarction
  Congestive heart failure
  Renal failure
  Hepatotoxic drugs, such as allopurinol, aspirin, antibiotics (oxacillin, ampicillin), narcotics, digitalis, captopril, heparin, barbiturates, and flurazepam

Interfering Factors

- Numerous drugs, including alcohol, can falsely elevate levels.
- Uremia and hemodialysis can cause falsely decreased levels.

Nursing Implications

Assessment

- Obtain a focused history of known or suspected liver disease, medication use, and related diagnostic tests.
- Note compliance with alcohol abstention for at least 24 hours before the study.
- Note compliance in withholding medications that alter test results for 12 hours before the test.

Possible Nursing Diagnoses

Fluid volume excess related to compromised regulatory mechanism

Pain related to inflammation or swelling of the liver or ischemia of myocardial tissue

Implementation

- Put on gloves. Using sterile technique, perform a venipuncture and collect 7 mL of blood in a red-top tube.
- Handle sample gently to avoid hemolysis and transport promptly to the laboratory. Specimen may be refrigerated.

Evaluation

- Note results of serum asparate aminotransferase (AST) levels and other liver function tests.

Client/Caregiver Teaching

Pretest

- Instruct patient to withhold medications that may interfere with test results for 12 hours and alcohol for 24 hours before the test, as ordered by the physician.

Posttest

- Resume medications withheld before the test.

Aldolase (ALS)

Classification: Chemistry

Type of Test: Serum

Aldolase, which is found throughout the body, is an enzyme that catalyzes glucose breakdown. Highest concentrations of this enzyme are found in skeletal and cardiac muscle, the liver, and the pancreas. When trauma or disease cause cellular breakdown of these muscles or organs, large amounts of this enzyme are released into the blood; therefore, measuring serum levels helps to determine the presence and, in some cases, the progress of disease.

Indications

- Permit early diagnosis of Duchenne's muscular dystrophy in those who have a family history of the disease
- Differentiate neuromuscular disorders from neurological disorders, such as multiple sclerosis or myasthenia gravis
- Perform a differential diagnosis of muscular and liver disorders
- Evaluate response of exposure to hepatoxic drugs or chemicals

Reference Values

	Sibley-Lehninger	*SI Units*
Newborns	4 X adult level @ 37°C	4 X adult level
Children	2 X adult level @ 37°C	2 X adult level
Adults	3.0–8.0 U/dL @ 37°C	22–59 mU/L @ 37°C

Abnormal Values

■ Pronounced elevated levels
    Duchenne's muscular dystrophy
    Limb girdle muscular dystrophy
    Polymyositis
    Dermatomyositis
    Trichinosis
    Severe crush injuries
    Gangrene
    Burns
    Surgical trauma
■ Moderately elevated levels
    Hepatitis
    Cirrhosis
    Use of hepatoxic drugs and chemicals such as insecticides, cortisone, narcotics, and antihelminthics
    Obstructive jaundice
    Neoplasms
    Leukemia
■ Mildly elevated levels
    Acute myocardial infarction (peak elevation occurs in 24 hours, with gradual return to normal within 1 week)
■ Decreased levels
    Late muscular dystrophy owing to loss of muscle cells
    Use of phenothiazines

Interfering Factors

■ A recent intramuscular injection can cause elevated levels.
■ Extensive delay in analyzing blood sample can affect results.

Nursing Implications

Assessment

■ Obtain history of neuromuscular disorders, related treatments, and complaints of muscle fatigue or loss of strength.

- Note use of any medications that can interfere with test results within the last 24 hours.

Possible Nursing Diagnoses

Anxiety related to perceived threat to health status
Physical mobility, impaired, related to neuromuscular impairment

Implementation

- Put on gloves. Using aseptic technique, perform a venipuncture and collect 5 mL of blood in a red-top tube.
- Handle sample gently to avoid hemolysis. Transport to the laboratory quickly. If the test cannot be performed within a few hours, freeze serum to avoid inaccurate results.

Evaluation

- Note increased levels in relation to increased levels of other enzymes, especially CPK, LD, and AST, and to clinical presentation.

Client/Caregiver Teaching

Pretest

- Instruct patient to withhold medications that may interfere with test results for 12 to 24 hours before the test, as ordered by the physician.

Posttest

- Resume any medications withheld before the test

Aldosterone

Classification: Chemistry

Type of Test: Plasma

Aldosterone is a mineralocorticoid secreted by the zona glomerulosa of the adrenal cortex in response to decreased serum sodium, decreased blood volume, and increased serum potassium. Aldosterone acts to increase sodium reabsorption in the renal tubules, resulting in potassium excretion and increased water retention, blood volume, and blood pressure. Serum aldosterone levels are influenced by a variety of factors, including sodium intake, certain medications, and activity. The results of this test must be evaluated in relation to 24-hour urine aldosterone levels or blood levels obtained at another time.

Indications

- Investigate suspected hyperaldosteronism, as indicated by elevated levels
- Investigate suspected hypoaldosteronism, as indicated by decreased levels
- Evaluate hypertension of unknown etiology

Reference Values

		SI Units
Adult, supine	3–10 ng/dL	0.14–1.9 nmol/L
Adult, standing		
Man	6–22 ng/dL	0.17–0.61 nmol/L
Woman (3 X higher if pregnant)	5–30 ng/dL	0.14–0.83 nmol/L

Abnormal Values

- Elevated aldosterone with decreased renin levels
    Primary hyperaldosteronism caused by benign adenomas or bilateral hyperplasia of the aldosterone-secreting zona glomerulosa cells
- Elevated aldosterone with elevated renin levels
    Secondary hyperaldosteronism caused by changes in blood volume and serum electrolytes, congestive heart failure, cirrhosis, nephrotic syndrome, chronic obstructive pulmonary disease, or renal artery stenosis
- Decreased aldosterone levels
    Hypoaldosteronism caused by diabetes mellitus or pregnancy-induced hypertension

Interfering Factors

- Upright body posture, stress, strenuous exercise, and late pregnancy can lead to increased levels.
- Therapy with diuretics, hydralazine diaoxzide, and nitroprusside can lead to elevated levels.
- Excessive licorice ingestion, propranolol, and fludrocortisone can decrease levels.

- Low-sodium diet can increase serum aldosterone and high sodium diet can decrease levels.
- Decreased serum sodium and elevated serum potassium increase aldosterone secretion.
- Elevated serum sodium and decreased serum potassium suppress aldosterone secretion.

Nursing Implications

Assessment

- Obtain a history of known or suspected fluid or electrolyte imbalance, hypertension, renal function or stage of pregnancy. Also note the amount of sodium ingested in the diet over the past 2 weeks.
- Note any medications that may interfere with test results.
- Note ingestion of licorice, which may interefere with test results.
- Determine that client has followed directions relating to rest, positioning, and activity before and during the test.

Possible Nursing Diagnoses

Fluid volume excess related to compromised regulatory mechanism, sodium levels

Fluid volume deficit related to compromised regulatory mechanism

Noncompliance related to lack of knowledge or inability to prepare for the test properly

Implementation

- Put on gloves. Using aseptic technique, perform a venipuncture and collect 5 mL of blood in a red-, green-, or lavender-top tube.
- Handle sample gently to avoid hemolysis and send to laboratory immediately.
- Indicate on the laboratory requisition slip if the patient was supine or sitting when the test was taken.
- Repeat the test in 2 to 4 hours if ordered.

Evaluation

- Compare test results with results from 24 hour urine tests for aldosterone, test results taken at another time, and clinical presentation.
- Note test results in relation to serum potassium, sodium, and renin levels. When aldosterone levels are elevated the renal tubules increase sodium absorption and excrete potassium, resulting in increased serum sodium and decreased potassium levels.

Client/Caregiver Teaching

Pretest

- As ordered by the physician, instruct the patient not to take medications that could interfere with the test results and to maintain a low-carbohydrate, normal-sodium diet for at least 2 weeks before the test.
- If the client is hospitalized, instruct not to get out of bed in the morning until the sample has been obtained. Explain that it may be necessary to obtain a second sample 2 to 4 hours after arising in the morning.
- Inform nonhospitalized clients how soon after getting up to arrive at the laboratory.

Posttest

- Resume normal diet, medications, and activities.
- Instruct patient to notify health-care provider of any signs and symptoms of dehydration and fluid overload related to elevated aldosterone levels.

Aldosterone Challenge Test

In normal individuals, increased sodium levels and blood volume suppress aldosterone secretion. However, this does not happen when a person has primary aldosteronism. This test challenges aldosterone secretion and measures the response to increase sodium. It is useful in differentiating between primary and secondary hyperaldosteronism.

If the aldosterone levels are properly controlled through negative feedback systems and the renin-angiotensin system, plasma aldosterone will be <50 percent of baseline level in response to the increased sodium load. An increase of >50 percent of aldosterone baseline level indicates primary aldosteronism.

Since large amounts of saline may exacerbate congestive heart failure and possibly increase the risk of uncontrolled hypertension in susceptible individuals, this test is contraindicated in individuals known to have these disorders.

Implementation

- Put on gloves. Using aseptic technique, perform a venipuncture and collect 5 mL of blood in a red-, green-, or lavender-top tube.
- Infuse 2 L normal saline solution over 2 to 4 hours depending on laboratory protocol.
- At the conclusion of the infusion, collect another 5 mL of blood in a red-, green-, or lavender-top tube.
- Handle all samples gently to avoid hemolysis and send to laboratory as they are collected. Include collection time and site on the laboratory request and tubes.

Aldosterone, Urine

Classification: Chemistry

Type of Test: Urine

This test measures the urinary excretion of aldosterone, a mineralocorticoid secreted by the zona glomerulosa of the adrenal cortex in response to decreased serum sodium, decreased blood volume, and increased serum potassium. Normally, aldosterone acts to increase sodium reabsorption in the renal tubules, resulting in potassium excretion, increased water retention, blood volume, and blood pressure. A 24-hour urine test is considered more reliable than a single plasma collection because blood levels of hormones tend to vary depending on time of day. Serum sodium, potassium, and renin levels should be obtained before this test.

Indications

- Diagnose suspected hyperaldosteronism, especially when plasma aldosterone levels are not definitive

Reference Values

	SI Units
2–26 µg/24 h	5.6–73 nmol/d

Abnormal Values

- Elevated aldosterone with decreased renin levels
  Primary hyperaldosteronism caused by benign adenomas or bilateral hyperplasia
- Elevated aldosterone with elevated renin levels
  Secondary hyperaldosteronism caused by congestive heart failure, cirrhosis, nephrotic syndrome, chronic obstructive pulmonary disease, or renal artery stenosis
- Decreased levels
  Hypoaldosteronism caused by Addison's disease, hypernatremia, hypokalemia, or diabetes mellitus
  Pregnancy-induced hypertension

Interfering Factors

- Radionuclide scan performed within 1 week of the test can cause inaccurate test results.
- Excessive licorice ingestion can cause decreased levels.
- Strenuous exercise can increase levels.
- Drugs such as methyldopa and fludrocortisone can cause decreased levels.
- Drugs such as steroids, diuretics that promote sodium excretion, oral contraceptives, and potassium can increase levels.
- Low-sodium diet can increase urinary aldosterone and high sodium diet can decrease levels. Low serum postassium increases levels.

Nursing Implications

Assessment

- Obtain a history of known or suspected fluid or electrolyte imbalance, hypertension, or renal function.
- Note any medications that can interfere with test results; it is recommended these drugs be withheld for up to 2 weeks before the test.
- Note ingestion of licorice within 2 weeks before the test.
- Determine whether client has ingested a diet with normal salt inclusion for 2 weeks before the test.

Possible Nursing Diagnoses

Fluid volume excess related to compromised regulatory mechanism, sodium or potassium levels

Fluid volume deficit related to compromised regulatory mechanism

Noncompliance related to lack of knowledge or inability to prepare for the test properly

Implementation

- Obtain the appropriate containers with preservative according to laboratory policy. Follow laboratory directions for any special care of the specimen, and maintain refrigeration of specimen during the entire collection time.
- Begin the test between 6 and 8 AM if possible; collect first voiding and discard. Record the time specimen was discarded as the beginning of the 24-hour test.
- The next morning, ask the client to void at the same time the collection was started and add this last voiding to the container.
- If an indwelling catheter is in place, replace tubing and container system with the preservative at the start of the collection time and keep container in ice during test time, or periodically empty the urine into a large container with the preservative that is kept in the refrigerator during the 24 hours; Ensure continued drainage and conclude the test the next morning at the same hour that the collection was begun.
- At the conclusion of the test, ensure that the label is properly completed and transport to the laboratory.

Evaluation

- Note test results in relation to serum potassium, sodium, and renin levels. When aldosterone levels are elevated the renal tubules increase sodium absorption and excrete potassium, resulting in increased serum sodium and decreased potassium levels.

Client/Caregiver Teaching

Pretest

- Tell the client to avoid excessive exercise and stress during the 24-hour urine collection.
- Inform the client that all urine for a 24-hour period must be saved; instruct client to avoid voiding in pan with defecation and to keep toilet tissue out of pan to prevent contamination of the specimen.
- Tell the client to withhold any medications that can interfere with test results for up to 2 weeks before the test, as ordered.
- Inform the client not to ingest licorice for 2 weeks before the test.
- Inform the client to ingest a diet with normal salt inclusion for 2 weeks before the test.

Posttest

■ Advise the client to resume medications and activity withheld before the test.

▲▲▲▲▲▲▲▲▲▲▲▲▲▲▲▲▲▲

Alkaline Phosphatase (ALP)

Classification: Chemistry

Type of Test: Serum

This test measures levels of alkaline phosphatase (ALP), an enzyme that is optimally active at a pH of 9. Highest concentrations are found in the liver, in the Kupffer's cells that line the biliary tract, and in bone, intestines, and placenta. Certain cancers produce small amounts of a distinctive form of ALP called the Regan enzyme. Additional sources of ALP are the proximal tubules of the kidneys, lactating mammary glands, and the granulocytes of circulating blood.

This test is most useful for determining the presence of liver or bone disease. Two isoenzymes, ALP_1, of liver origin, and ALP_2, of bone origin, help distinguish the source of serum elevations.

Indications

■ Evaluate signs and symptoms of various disorders associated with elevated ALP levels, such as biliary obstruction, hepatobiliary disease, and bone disease, including malignant processes.
■ Differentiate obstructive hepatobiliary tract disorders from hepatocellular disease; greater elevations of ALP are seen in the former.
■ Determine effects on bone metabolism in clients with known renal disease.
■ Determine bone growth or destruction in children with abnormal growth patterns.

Reference Values

		SI Units
Chemical inhibition		
Males	98–251 U/L	
Females < age 45 yrs	81–196 U/L	
Females > age 45 yrs	84–109 U/L	
Bessey-Lowry Method		
Adults	0.8–2.3 U/dL	13.3–38.3 IU/L
Bodansky Method		
Adults	2–4 U/dL	10.7–21.5 IU/L
King-Armstrong Method		
Adults	4–13 U/dL	28.4–92.3 IU/L
Adult isoenzyme levels		
Bone	24–146 U/L	
Intestine	0–22 U/L	
Liver	24–158 U/L	

Abnormal Results

- Pronounced elevations of ALP (≥5 × normal)
    - Advanced pregnancy
    - Biliary obstruction
    - Biliary atresia
    - Cirrhosis
    - Osteitis deformans
    - Osteogenic sarcoma
    - Hyperparathyroidism (primary, or secondary to chronic renal disease)
    - Paget's disease
- Moderate elevations of ALP (3–5 × normal)
    - Granulomatous or infiltrative liver diseases
    - Infectious mononucleosis
    - Metastatic tumors in bone
    - Metabolic bone diseases (rickets, osteomalacia)
    - Extrahepatic duct obstruction
- Mild elevations of ALP (up to 3 × normal)
    - Viral hepatitis
    - Chronic active hepatitis
    - Cirrhosis (alcoholic)
    - Healing fractures
    - Early pregnancy
    - Growing children
    - Large doses of vitamin D
    - Congestive heart failure

- Decreased ALP
    - Cretinism
    - Secondary growth retardation
    - Scurvy
    - Achondroplasia
    - Hypophosphatasia (rare)

Interfering Factors

- Many drugs, including intravenous albumin, methyldopa, allopurinol, antibiotics, and phenothiazines, may falsely elevate levels.
- Azathioprine, fluorides, and propranolol may falsely decrease levels.

Nursing Implications

Assessment

- Obtain history of known or suspected liver or bone disorders.
- Note any medications that alter ALP levels.
- Assess compliance with fasting 10 to 12 hours before the test, if required.

Possible Nursing Diagnoses

Anxiety related to perceived threat to health status

Physical mobility, impaired, related to musculoskeletal impairment

Implementation

- Put on gloves. Using aseptic technique, perform a venipuncture and collect 7 mL of blood in a red-top tube.
- Handle sample gently to avoid hemolysis and send promptly to the laboratory.

Evaluation

- Note results in relation to age of client and other enzyme test results, including ALT, LAP, and GGT.

Client/Caregiver Teaching

Pretest

- Tell the client to fast for at least 8 hours before the test.
- Tell client to withhold medications that interfere with test results, if ordered.

Posttest

- Resume food and fluid intake and medications withheld before the test.
- Inform client that results of isoenzymes can be obtained in 48 to 72 hours.

Allergen Skin Tests

Classification: Immunology

Type of Test: Skin scratch, skin patch, and intradermal injection

Three types of allergen skin tests—scratch test, patch test, or intradermal test—are performed to determine hypersensitivity to an unknown allergen. Results are obtained by exposing the individual to a potential allergen by scratching the skin and applying the suspected allergen, taping an allergen-impregnated filter paper, cotton square, or gauze square patch to the skin, or injecting the allergen under the skin. Individuals who are hypersensitive to the allergen will have changes to the skin surface, which are measured and evaluated. Suspected allergens that cause atopic disease and can be tested are inhaled allergens (dust, pollen, animal dander, grasses, and molds), food allergens (eggs, wheat, shellfish, and citrus fruits), injected allergens (horse serum and insect venom), and drugs (penicillin).

Indications

- Identify allergen causing hypersensitivity response

Reference Values

- Negative

Abnormal Values

Scratch test	Wheal or flare 0.5 cm or larger than control test area within 15 to 20 minutes of exposure to allergen
Patch test	Redness or edema at the site following removal of patch
Intradermal	Wheal 0.5 cm or larger than the control test area within 15 minutes of injection of test extract

Interfering Factors

- Improper technique
- Insufficient concentration of antigen administered
- Expired or contaminated antigen
- Use of corticosteroids or antihistamines before the test

> ### NURSING ALERT
>
> - Have emergency resuscitation equipment available in case of exaggerated response.

Nursing Implications

Assessment

- Obtain a history of suspected allergens and response to allergens and disease or conditions known to be caused by allergens. Note family history of allergens.
- Note any medications the client is taking especially those which interfere with hypersensitivity response.

Possible Nursing Diagnoses

Injury, risk for, related to biochemical regulatory function (immune response) or invasion of skin

Anxiety related to perceived threat to health status

Implementation

- Obtain the selected antigens in the proper concentrations and check the expiration dates.
- Select a site on the inner aspect of the forearm or scapular area of the back. Cleanse the area with alcohol or acetone swabs and allow to air-dry. Avoid using an area that has skin eruptions or inflammation.
- *Scratch test:* Remove the sterile lancet from the package with the dominant hand and hold the skin taut with the non-

dominant hand. For each allergen to be tested, make a 1-cm-long scratch through the epidermis without causing bleeding. Place a drop of concentrated antigen onto the scratch without touching the skin. Test each allergen about 2.5 cm apart. Make one scratch without applying antigen for a control.

- Alternately, place a drop of concentrated antigen on the skin and scratch the skin in the same way using a commercially prepared scarifier.
- *Patch test:* Remove the cover of each patch from the pad containing the antigen. Apply the patch by firmly pressing down on the adhesive area surrounding the pad. Leave the patch in place for 48 hours.
- *Intradermal test:* Administer the test extract, usually 0.02 mL of a 1/500 or 1/1000 concentration of antigen, intradermally. Use a different syringe for each antigen extract. Be sure extract is not injected into subcutaneous tissue since invalid results will occur. Each injection should be 2.5 cm apart. A control site is injected at the same time.
- Document sites of each test and the specific antigen administered.

Evaluation

- For scratch test, measure the skin response in 15 to 20 minutes.
- For patch test, evaluate response immediately after the patch is removed and again in 30 minutes. Sites may be re-evaluated again in 48 hours to determine delayed response.
- For intradermal test, evaluate the skin response in 15 minutes.

Client/Caregiver Teaching

Pretest

- Explain the purpose of the test. Tell the client that the test causes slight to moderate discomfort and takes about 15 to 30 minutes to complete, including reading the results, for scratch and patch tests.

Posttest

- Instruct client that redness and edema after a scratch or intradermal test should resolve within 24 hours.
- Have client notify physician if he or she experiences any allergic response symptoms. Topical corticosteroids may be ordered for side effects of a positive response after a patch test.

■ Instruct the client having intradermal patch tests to return in 48 hours for full evaluation of response.

Allergen-Specific IgE and Allergen-Specific IgE Antibody Radioallergosorbent Test (RAST)

Classification: Immunology

Type of Test: Serum

This test measures the immunoglobulin E (IgE) directed against specific allergens by radioimmunoassay (RIA), and the amount of IgE antibodies after exposure to specific antigens selected on the basis of a client's history. An antigen is bound to a substance and exposed to a specific IgE antibody in the client's blood sample. The IgE in the patient's serum forms a complex with those antigens to which the client is sensitive. It is also important to determine a total IgE level.

In some instances the radioallergosorbent test (RAST) has replaced skin tests and provocation procedures that are inconvenient, painful, and hazardous to the client.

Indications

■ Identify allergens causing hypersensitivity reactions such as asthma, hay fever, or dermatitis
■ Determine potential for systemic reactions to insect venom, drugs, or chemicals
■ Monitor response to desensitization procedures

Reference Values

IgE	<2% of total immunoglobulins
Newborn	<12 U/mL
Children	<10–116 U/mL depending on age
Adult	<41 U/mL
IgE antibody	
0	Negative
0–749 count	No activity according to RAST classifications

Abnormal Values

IgE	Positive
IgE antibody	
1	Borderline positive
750–1600 count	Borderline activity according to RAST classifications
1601–3600 count	Low positive
3601–8000 count	Moderate positive
8001–18,000 count	High positive
18,001–40,000 count	Very high positive according to RAST classifications
>40,000 count	Extremely high positive

Interfering Factors

- Radionuclide tests within 1 week of the test can alter results.
- Parasitic infections causing increased IgE can result in false-positive values.

Nursing Implications

Assessment

- Obtain a history of known or suspected conditions affecting protein levels, immunization within 6 months, blood or blood products within 6 weeks.
- Assess compliance with fasting 8 to 12 hours before the test (water is allowed).

Possible Nursing Diagnoses

Anxiety related to perceived threat to health status

Airway clearance, ineffective, related to tracheobronchial obstruction (allergic reaction)

Implementation

- Put on gloves. Using aseptic technique, perform a venipuncture and collect blood in a red-top tube.
- Indicate which allergy panel is desired on the laboratory request form; each panel usually consists of 5 to 6 antigens.
- Handle sample gently to avoid hemolysis and send promptly to the laboratory.

Evaluation

- Note test results in relation to skin-testing results, other tests performed, and the client's symptoms.
- If the RAST test is negative but total IgE is elevated, the allergy panel selected may not have included the allergans to which the client is sensitive.

Client/Caregiver Teaching

Pretest

- Inform the client to fast for 8 to 12 hours before the test.

Posttest

- Instruct the client to resume food intake withheld before the test.
- Tell the client that test results can take as long as 1 week and that these tests may avoid the need for skin testing.

Alpha-Fetoprotein (AFP)

Classification: Chemistry

Type of Test: Serum or Cord blood

This test measures alpha-fetoprotein (AFP) levels in the adult, pregnant woman, and newborn. AFP is the major serum protein in early fetal life, up to 10 weeks. (See amniocentesis and amniotic fluid analysis test for measurement of AFP levels in amniotic fluid.) After 10 weeks of gestation, levels af AFP can be detected in maternal blood, with peak levels occurring at 16 to 18 weeks. Elevated maternal levels on two tests taken 1 week apart suggest further investigation into fetal well-being by ultrasound or amniocentesis. Presence in excessive amounts is abnormal in adults and their measurements are most recently used as a tumor marker in the diagnosis of cancer.

Indications

- Routine prenatal screening at 13 to 16 weeks of pregnancy for fetal neural-tube defects and other disorders, as indicated by elevated levels in serum and amniotic fluid
- Investigate suspected intrauterine fetal death, as indicated by elevated levels
- Support diagnosis of embryonal gonadal teratoblastoma, hepatoblastoma, and testicular or ovarian carcinomas
- Diagnose primary hepatocellular carcinoma or metastatic lesions involving the liver, as indicated by highly elevated levels (30 to 50 percent of Americans with liver cancer do not have elevated AFP levels)
- Monitor response to treatment for hepatic carcinoma, with successful treatment indicated by an immediate drop in levels.
- Monitor for recurrence of hepatic carcinoma, with elevated levels occurring 1 to 6 months before the client becomes symptomatic.
- Investigate suspected hepatitis or cirrhosis as indicated by slightly to moderately elevated levels.

Reference Values

		SI units
Neonate	600,000 ng/mL	600,000 Ug/L
Infant and child	<30 ng/mL	<30 Ug/L
Adults	<10 ng/mL	<10 Ug/L
Pregnant woman		
2–4 months	<75–130 ng/mL	<75–130 Ug/L
4–6 months	<210–400 ng/mL	<210–400 Ug/L
6–9 months	<400–450 ng/mL	<400–450 Ug/L

Abnormal Values

- Elevated levels
    - Fetal neural-tube defects, such as anencephaly, spina bifida, myelomeningocele
    - Fetal distress
    - Fetal demise
    - Multiple pregnancy

- Decreased levels
    Down syndrome
- Slightly or moderately elevated levels (500 ng/mL)
    Hepatitis
    Cirrhosis
- Highly elevated levels (10,000–100,000 ng/mL)
    Hepatic carcinoma
    Metastatic lesions involving the liver

Interfering Factors

- Multiple fetuses can cause increased levels.
- Radionuclide scan within 2 weeks before the test causes inaccurate results.

Nursing Implications

Assessment

- Obtain history of known or suspected malignancy and weeks of gestation, if applicable.
- Assess if client had a radionuclide scan within 2 weeks of the test.

Possible Nursing Diagnoses

Anxiety related to perceived threat to health status
Self-esteem, situational low, related to failure at a life event

Implementation

- Put on gloves. Using aseptic technique, perform a venipuncture and collect 7 mL of blood in a red-top tube. (See Appendix I for cord-blood collection.)
- Handle sample gently to avoid hemolysis and send promptly to laboratory; note presence and weeks of pregnancy on laboratory request form.

Evaluation

- Monitor results with AFP levels for amniotic fluid analysis, if available.

Client/Caregiver Teaching

Posttest

- Inform the pregnant client that an ultrasound can be performed and AFP levels in amniotic fluid can be analyzed if

maternal blood levels are elevated in two samples obtained 1 week apart.
- Suggest genetic counseling, if applicable.

///

Alpha$_1$-Antitrypsin (α_1-AT)

Classification: Chemistry (protein)

Type of Test: Serum

Using protein immunoelectrophoresis, this test measures alpha$_1$-globulin produced by the liver. The function of alpha$_1$-globulin is inhibition of the proteolytic enzymes trypsin and plasmin, which are released by alveolar macrophages and by bacteria in the lungs.

Indications

- Confirm family history of alpha$_1$-antitrypsin deficiency
- Confirm the cause of early onset of emphysema in nonsmokers. Persons with this genetic disorder of alpha$_1$-antitrypsin deficiency develop severe, debilitating panacinar emphysema after age 30
- Confirm the cause of unexplained cirrhosis or jaundice, especially in children and young adults, which may be due to alpha$_1$-antitrypsin deficiency
- Confirm suspected chronic inflammatory disorder indicated by persistently elevated alpha$_1$-antitrypsin levels

Reference Values

		SI Units
Newborn	145–270 mg/dL	1.45–2.70 g/L
Adult	126–226 mg/dL	1.26–2.26 g/L

Abnormal Values

- Decreased alpha$_1$-antitrypsin
    Early onset emphysema and cirrhosis
    Nephrotic syndrome

Malnutrition
Congenital alpha$_1$-globulin deficiency
Newborn (transient)
■ Increased alpha$_1$-antitrypsin
Chronic inflammatory disorders
Necrosis
Pregnancy
Acute pulmonary infections
Hyaline membrane disease in infants
Hepatitis
Systemic lupus erythematosus
Rheumatoid arthritis
Drugs such as oral contraceptives and steroids

Interfering Factors

■ Oral contraceptives and steroids may falsely elevate values.
■ Failure to fast for 8 hours before the test could falsely elevate the levels.

Nursing Implications

Assessment

■ Obtain history of inflammatory or pulmonary disorders.
■ Ensure client has fasted for at least 8 hours before the test; water is not restricted.
■ Ensure that oral contraceptives and steroids have been withheld for 24 hours before the test, if ordered.

Possible Nursing Diagnoses

Airway clearance, ineffective, related to compromised pulmonary function with alpha$_1$-antitrypsin deficiency
Breathing pattern, ineffective, related to compromised pulmonary function with alpha$_1$-antitrypsin deficiency
Infection, risk for, related to stasis of pulmonary secretions

Implementation

■ Put on gloves. Using aseptic technique, perform a venipuncture and collect a 7-mL blood sample in a red-top tube.
■ Handle the sample gently to avoid hemolysis and send promptly to the laboratory.

Evaluation

■ Note results in relation to other test results and the client's symptoms.
■ If levels are <140 mg/dL, request phenotyping if not automatically performed.

Client/Caregiver Teaching

Pretest
- Instruct the client to fast for 8 hours before the test and to withhold oral contraceptives and steroids, if ordered.

Posttest
- Instruct the client to resume usual diet and medication.
- Instruct in deep breathing and pursed lip breathing to enhance breathing patterns, if appropriate.
- Instruct the client to refrain from smoking and avoid environmental pollutants and any contact with persons who have upper respiratory or other infections.

Amino Acid Screen, Blood

Classification: Chemistry

Type of Test: Blood

This qualitative screening test for amino acid inborn errors is generally performed on infants after an initial positive urine screening test. Certain congenital enzyme deficiencies interfere with normal amino acid metabolism and cause excessive accumulation or deficiencies. Reduced growth rates, mental retardation, or various unexplained symptoms can result.

Indications

- Detect inborn errors of amino acid metabolism

Reference Values

Normal findings are age-dependent; see levels below.

	Normal range (μmol/L)	
	---	---
Amino Acid	*Children (3 to 16 years)*	*Adults (>16 years)*
Alanine	200–450	230–510
Alpha-amino-*N*-butyric acid	8–37	15–41

	Normal range (μmol/L)	
Amino Acid	*Children* *(3 to 16 years)*	*Adults* *(>16 years)*
Arginine	44–120	45–130
Asparagine	8–37	24–79
Aspartic acid	0–26	0–6
Beta-Alanine	0–49	0–29
Citrulline	16–32	16–55
Cystine	19–47	30–65
Glutamic acid	32–140	18–98
Glutamine	420–730	390–650
Glycine	110–240	170–330
Histadine	68–120	26–120
Hydroxyproline	0–5	Not measured
Isoleucine	37–140	42–100
Leucine	70–170	66–170
Lysine	120–290	150–220
Methionine	13–30	16–30
Ornithine	44–90	27–80
Phenylalanine	26–86	41–68
Phosphoserine	0–12	0–12
Phosphoethanolamine	0–12	0–55
Proline	130–290	110–360
Serine	93–150	56–140
Taurine	11–120	45–130
Threonine	67–150	92–240
Tyrosine	26–110	45–74
Valine	160–350	150–310

Abnormal Values

- Increased total amino acids
     Reye's syndrome
     Acute or chronic renal failure
     Severe brain damage
     Eclampsia
     Diabetes with ketosis
     Fructose intolerance (hereditary)
     Malabsorption
     Aminoacidopathies
- Decreased total amino acids
     Adrenal cortical hyperfunction
     Hartnup disease
     Rheumatoid arthritis
     Huntington's chorea
     Malnutrition

Nephrotic syndrome
Phlebotomus fever

Interfering Factors

■ Failure to fast for 4 hours before the test may interfere with test results.

Nursing Implications

Assessment

■ Obtain a family history of genetic disorders that may have caused mental retardation, reduced growth rates, or unexplained symptoms.
■ Ensure that the infant has fasted for 4 hours before the test.

Possible Nursing Diagnoses

Communication, impaired, verbal, related to altered brain function
Physical mobility, impaired, related to neuromuscular/musculoskeletal impairment

Implementation

■ Put on gloves. Using aseptic technique, perform a heelstick, and collect 0.1 mL of blood in a heparinized capillary tube.
■ Handle sample gently and send promptly to the laboratory.

Evaluation

■ Note test results in relation to other tests performed and the client's symptoms.

Client/Caregiver Teaching

Pretest

■ Tell the caregiver that the infant must fast for 4 hours before the test.

Posttest

■ Tell the caregiver to resume the infant's food and fluid intake.

////////////////////////////////////

Amino Acids, Urine

Classification: Urinalysis

Type of Test: Urine, random

This test is the initial screening test for congenital defects and disorders of amino acid metabolism. The major genetic disorders include phenylketonuria, tyrosinuria, and alcaptouria, a defect in phenylananine-tyrosine conversion pathway. Renal aminoaciduria is also associated with conditions marked by defective tubular reabsorption from congenital disorders, such as hereditary fructose intolerance. Early diagnosis and treatment of certain aminoacidurias can prevent mental retardation, reduced growth rates, or various unexplained symptoms.

Indications

- Screen for inborn errors of amino acid metabolism

Reference Values

		SI Units
Total amino acids	200 mg/24 h	2 mmol/dL

Levels for specific amino acids

	Normal range (μmol/L)	
Amino Acid	*Children (3–16 years)*	*Adults (>16 years)*
Alanine	65–190	160–690
Alpha-aminoadipic acid	25–78	0–165
Alpha-amino-N-butyric acid	7–25	0–28
Arginine	10–25	13–64
Asparagine	15–40	34–100
Aspartic acid	10–26	14–89
Beta-alanine	0–42	0–93

Normal range (μmol/L)

Amino Acid	Children (3–16 years)	Adults (>16 years)
Beta-aminoisobutyric acid	25–96	10–235
Carnosine	34–220	16–125
Citrulline	0–13	0–11
Cystine	11–53	28–115
Glutamic acid	13–22	27–105
Glutamine	150–400	300–1040
Glycine	195–855	750–2400
Histadine	46–725	500–1500
Isoleucine	3–15	4–23
Leucine	9–23	20–77
Lysine	19–140	32–290
Methionine	7–20	5–30
1-Methylhistidine	41–300	68–855
3-Methylhistidine	42–135	64–320
Ornithine	3–16	5–70
Phenylalanine	20–61	36–90
Phosphoserine	16–34	28–95
Phosphoethanolamine	24–65	17–95
Serine	93–210	200–695
Taurine	62–970	267–1290
Threonine	25–100	80–320
Tyrosine	30–83	38–145
Valine	17–37	19–74

Abnormal Values

- Increased total amino acids

Osteomalacia	Multiple myeloma
Viral hepatitis	Hyperparathyroidism
Wilson's disease	Galactosemia
Hartnup disease	Cystinosis
Maple syrup urine disease	

Interfering Factors

- Improper specimen collection and testing can affect test results.
- Lack of protein intake can cause false-negative PKU results.

Nursing Implications

Assessment

- Obtain history of familial genetic disorders, medication regimen, and, if infant is breast-fed, any medications that the mother is taking.

Possible Nursing Diagnoses

Physical mobility, impaired, related to neuromuscular/musculoskeletal impairment

Fluid volume excess related to compromised regulatory mechanism

Pain related to inflammation or swelling of the liver or ischemia of myocardial tissue

Implementation

- Obtain the appropriate sized container for random specimen without preservative.
- If the test is performed on an infant, clean and dry the genital area, attach the collection device securely to prevent leakage, and observe for voiding. Remove collection device carefully from an infant to prevent skin irritation after specimen has been obtained. Transfer at least 20 mL of the collected urine into a specimen container.
- For dipstick method, place Phenistix or reagent pad into the urine specimen or on the diaper saturated with urine. Remove, compare to color chart for results, and record.
- If client is an adult or child, obtain at least 20 mL of a fresh random urine sample and transfer into specimen container. Send to the laboratory immediately.

Evaluation

- Note test results in relation to serum amino acid levels and other tests performed.

Client/Caregiver Teaching

Pretest

- Tell client to withhold drugs that may interfere with test results, if ordered. If the test is being performed on the breast-fed infant, the mother needs to withhold interfering drugs.
- Tell the client that there are no food or fluid restrictions before this test.

Posttest

- Tell the client or caregiver to resume medications withheld before the test.
- Tell the client of any further testing needed (blood test) based on results.
- Instruct caregiver in special dietary modifications to treat deficiency, or refer caregiver to a nutritionist.

Amniocentesis and Amniotic Fluid Analysis

Classification: Hematology, Microbiology
Chemistry, Cytology

Type of Test: Amniotic fluid

In amniocentesis, fluid is obtained by needle aspiration from the amniotic sac under the guidance of ultrasonography. This procedure is generally performed between the 14th and 16th week of gestation when there is sufficient amount of fluid for sampling and yet there is enough time for a safe therapeutic abortion to be performed, if desired by the client. It can also be performed between 26 and 35 weeks' gestation if fetal distress suspected.

Amniotic fluid is tested for genetic and neural-tube defects, hemolytic diseases of the newborn, fetal renal function, or maturity of the fetal liver.

Indications

- Evaluate fetus in families with a history of genetic disorders, such as Down syndrome, Tay-Sachs disease, chromosome or enzyme anomalies, or inherited hemoglobinopathies.
- Evaluate fetus in mothers with history of miscarriage or stillbirth.
- Determine fetal sex when the mother is a known carrier of a sex-linked abnormal gene that could be transmitted to male offspring, such as hemophilia or Duchenne's muscular dystrophy.
- Diagnose, in utero of metabolic disorders such as cystic fibrosis, diabetes mellitus, or other errors of lipid, carbohydrate, or amino acid metabolism.
- Evaluate suspected neural-tube defects, such as spina bifida or myelomeningocele, as indicated by elevated alpha-fetoprotein (AFP) and acetylcholinesterase levels.
- Evaluate known or suspected hemolytic disease involving the fetus in a Rh-sensitized pregnancy indicated by rising bilirubin levels, especially following the 30th week of gestation.
- Determine fetal maturity when preterm delivery is being con-

sidered. Fetal maturity is indicated by a lecithin-sphingomyelin (L/S) ratio of 2:1 or greater, positive shake test for surfactant, creatinine of >2.0 mg/dL, and a bilirubin density of <0.025 mg/dL (nonisoimmunized mother).

- Determine the presence of fetal distress in late-stage pregnancy.

Reference Values

		Early/Term	SI Units
Appearance/color		Clear	Clear
Volume	(early)	450–1200 mL	0.45–1.3 L
pH	(early)	7.12–7.38	7.12–7.38
	(term)	6.91–7.43	6.91–7.43
Osmolality	(early)	Same as serum	Same as serum
	(term)	230–270 mOsm/kg	230–270 mmol/kg
Carbon dioxide	(early)	33–55 mm Hg	4.4–7.3 kPa
	(term)	42–55 mm Hg	5.6–7.3 kPa
Albumin	(early)	0.39 g/dL	3.9 g/L
	(term)	0.19 g/dL	1.9 g/L
Total protein	(early)	0.60–0.24 g/dL	6.0–2.4 g/L
	(term)	0.19 g/dL	1.9 g/L
Bilirubin	(early)	<0.075 mg/dL	<1.3 Umol/L
	(term)	<0.025 mg/dL	<0.41 Umol/L
Chloride	(early)	02 mEq/L	16 mmol/L
	(term)	1–3 mEq/L lower	1–3 mmol/L lower
Sodium	(early)	133 mEq/L	133 mmol/L
	(term)	7–10 mEq/L lower	7–10 mmol/L lower
Creatinine	(early)	0.8–.1 mg/dL	71–97 Umol/L
	(term)	1.8–4.0 mg/dL	159–354 Umol/L
Estriol	(early)	<10 Ug/dL	<347 nmol/L
	(term)	>60 Ug/dL	>2081 nmol/L
Lecithin	(early)	<1:1	<1.1
Sphingomyelin	(term)	>2:1	>2.1
Urea	(early)	18.0–5.9 mg/dL	3.00–0.98 mmol/L
	(term)	30.3–11.4 mg/dL	5.04–1.90 mmol/L
Uric acid	(early)	3.72–0.96 mg/dL	221–57 Umol/L
	(term)	9.90–2.23 mg/dL	589–133 Umol/L
Alpha-fetoprotein	(early)	13–41 Ug/mL	
	(term)	0.2–3.0 Ug/mL	
Acetylcholinesterase		Absent	
Chromosome analysis		Normal karyotype	
Phosphatidyl glycerol (PG)		Present at about 36 weeks	
Phosphatidyl inositol (PI)		Peak amounts at 5 weeks before term	
Shake test		Positive	
Fern test		Positive	

Abnormal Values

- Yellow, green, red, or brown color
    Indicates presence of bilirubin, blood, meconium indicating fetal distress or death, hemolytic disease, growth retardation
- Elevated bilirubin levels
    Hemolytic disease
- Creatinine concentration >2.0
    At least 36 to 37 weeks of gestation
- L/S ratio <2:1 at term
    Fetal lung immaturity
- Elevated AFP levels
    Gestational age underestimated
    Open neural-tube defect
    Fetomaternal hemorrhage
    Omphalocele
    Congenital proteinuric nephropathies
    Sacrococcygeal teratoma
    Duodenal atresia
    Intrauterine death
    Esophageal atresia
    Tetralogy of Fallot
    Hydrocephaly
    Hydrops fetalis
    Twin pregnancy
    Turner's syndrome
    Cystic hygroma
    Cyclopia
    Microcephaly
    Gastroschisis
    Maternal cancer producing AFP
- Presence of acetylcholinesterase
    Neural-tube defect
- Abnormal karyotype
    Tay-Sachs disease
    Mental retardation
    Chromosome or enzyme anomalies
    Inherited hemoglobinopathies
- Abnormal PI levels
    Fetal lung immaturity
- Absence of PG after 36 weeks' gestation
    Possible respiratory distress syndrome (RDS)

Interfering Factors

- Failure to promptly deliver samples for chromosomal analysis to the laboratory performing the test, or improper incubation of the sample such that cells do not remain alive, will make karyotyping impossible to perform; sample should also be protected from light.

- AFP and acetylcholinesterase may be falsely elevated if the sample is contaminated with fetal blood.
- Bilirubin may be falsely elevated if maternal hemoglobin, or meconium are present in the sample; fetal acidosis may also lead to falsely elevated bilirubin levels.
- Bilirubin may be falsely decreased if the sample is exposed to light or if amniotic fluid volume is excessive.
- Contamination of the sample with blood or meconium, or complications in pregnancy, may yield inaccurate L/S ratios.

> **NURSING ALERT**

- Amniocentesis is contraindicated in women with a history of premature labor or incompetent cervix. It is also contraindicated in the presence of placenta previa or abruptio placenta.

Nursing Implications

Assessment

- Obtain maternal history, noting previous abnormalities in pregnancies or laboratory or diagnostic test results.
- Take and record maternal vital signs and fetal heart sounds and compare with the usual baseline.
- During the procedure, monitor for uterine contractions.

Possible Nursing Diagnoses

Anxiety related to perceived threat to health status
Injury, risk for, to fetus, related to invasive procedure
Grieving, anticipatory, related to perceived potential loss

Implementation

- Assemble the necessary equipment, including an amniocentesis tray with solution for skin preparation, local anesthetic, a 10 or 20 mL syringe, needles of various sizes (including a 22-gauge, 5-inch spinal needle), sterile drapes, sterile gloves, as well as special specimen collection tubes (either brown or foil-covered).
- Ensure client has a full bladder before the procedure if gestation is 20 weeks or less; have client void before procedure if gestation is 21 weeks or more.
- Assist the client to a supine position. Raise the head or legs

slightly to promote client comfort and to relax abdominal muscles. If the uterus is large, place a pillow or rolled blanket under the client's right side to prevent hypertension due to great-vessel compression.

- Note fetal position and pocket of amniotic fluid as determined by ultrasound and palpation.
- Cleanse suprapubic area with an antiseptic solution and protect with sterile drapes. A local anesthetic is injected. Explain that this may cause a stinging sensation.
- A 22-gauge, 5-inch spinal needle is inserted through the abdominal and uterine walls. Explain that a sensation of pressure may be felt when the needle is inserted. Explain to the client how to use focusing and controlled breathing for relaxation during the procedure. A sample of at least 10 mL of amniotic fluid is withdrawn.
- After the needle is withdrawn, apply slight pressure to the site. If there is no evidence of bleeding or other drainage, apply a sterile adhesive bandage to the site.
- Inject 5 mL of amniotic fluid into light-protected (foil-covered or amber) test tube to test for bilirubin; 10 mL of amniotic fluid is injected into a sterile, siliconized glass container or polystyrene container for culture and genetic and other studies (AFP).
- Pack specimens in cool, insulated container to maintain temperature of 2–5°C. Avoid freezing. Send specimens to the laboratory immediately.

Evaluation

- Note test results in relation to client's history and to other tests performed.

Client/Caregiver Teaching

Pretest

- Explain the purpose of the study and how the procedure is performed; inform the client that it is performed by a physician and takes 20 to 30 minutes to complete.
- Warn the client and spouse that normal results do not guarantee a normal fetus.
- Explain the necessity of remaining still during the procedure.

Posttest

- Explain that slight cramping can occur following the procedure.

- Tell the client to report fever, leaking amniotic fluid, vaginal bleeding, uterine contractions, or changes in fetal activity (either an increase or decrease) to physician.
- Inform the client that it may be 2 to 4 weeks before the results are available.
- Encourage family to seek counseling if concerned with pregnancy termination or genetic counseling if chromosomal abnormality is determined.

Ammonia (NH_3)

Classification: Chemistry

Type of Test: Plasma

Blood ammonia (NH_3) comes from two sources: deamination of amino acids during protein metabolism and degradation of proteins by colon bacteria. The liver converts ammonia in the portal blood to urea, which is excreted by the kidneys. When liver function is severely compromised, especially in situations when decreased hepatocellular function is combined with impaired portal blood flow, ammonia levels rise.

Indications

- Evaluate advanced liver disease or other disorders associated with altered serum ammonia levels (see Abnormal Values)
- Identify impending hepatic encephalopathy in clients with known liver disease
- Monitor the effectiveness of treatment for hepatic encephalopathy indicated by declining levels

Reference Values

		SI Units
Infants	90–150 μg/dL	64–107 μmol/L
Children	40–80 μg/dL	23–47 μmol/L
Adults	15–45 μg/dL	11–32 μmol/L

Values vary depending on the method and laboratory performing the test.

Abnormal Values

- Increased levels
  - Liver failure, late cirrhosis
  - GI hemorrhage
  - Late congestive heart failure
  - Azotemia
  - Hemolytic disease of the newborn
  - Chronic obstructive pulmonary disease
  - Leukemias
  - Reye's syndrome
  - Inborn enzyme deficiency
  - Excessive protein ingestion
  - Alkalosis
  - Drugs such as acetazolamide, ammonium salts, barbiturates, colistin, diuretics, heparin, methicillin, tetracycline, ethanol, morphine, and isoniazid
- Decreased levels
  - Renal failure
  - Hypertension
  - Drugs such as arginine, diphenhydramine, sodium or potassium salts, MAO inhibitors, and antibiotics (achromycin, kanamycin, neomycin)

Interfering Factors

- Failure to follow dietary restrictions
- Vigorous exercise before the test
- Numerous drugs (see Abnormal Values)

Nursing Implications

Assessment

- Obtain history of renal or hematologic disorders and gout.
- Ensure that client has fasted from food for at least 8 hours before the test; water is not restricted.
- Ensure that client has stopped smoking for 8 to 10 hours.
- Ensure that client has refrained from strenuous exercise and has avoided stress for several hours before the test.

Possible Nursing Diagnoses

Nutrition, altered, less than body requirements, related to ingestion of protein in presence of hepatic disease

Pain related to inflammation or swelling of the liver

Fluid volume deficit related to active loss

Fluid volume excess related to compromised regulatory function (renal)

Implementation

- Put on gloves. Using aseptic technique, perform a venipuncture and collect 10 mL of blood in a green-top tube. Place specimen in ice immediately upon collection according to laboratory policy.
- Handle the sample gently to avoid hemolysis. Send the sample to the laboratory for immediate analysis.

Evaluation

- Monitor renal and liver function tests in relation to ammonia levels.

Client/Caregiver Teaching

Pretest

- Tell the client to fast for 8 hours before the test; water is not restricted.
- Tell the client not to smoke for 8 to 10 hours before the test and to avoid strenuous activity and stress for several hours before the test.

Posttest

- Tell the client to resume usual pretest diet and activity.
- Instruct the client and caregiver on the importance of a low-protein diet to decrease ammonia level.
- Inform the client to report tremors or twitching of extremities and confusion or mental changes, which indicate rising ammonia in the presence of hepatic disease.

Amylase, Serum

Classification: Chemistry

Type of Test: Serum

This test measures amylase, a digestive enzyme that splits starch into disaccharides such as maltose. Although many cells have amylase activity (e.g., cells in the liver, small intestine, skeletal muscles, and fallopian tubes), circulating amylase is derived from the parotid glands and the pancreas. It is a sensitive indicator of pancreatic acinar cell damage and pancreatic obstruction.

Indications

- Diagnose early acute pancreatitis; serum amylase begins to rise within 6 to 24 hours after onset and returns to normal in 2 to 7 days.
- Detect blunt trauma or inadvertent surgical trauma to the pancreas. Serum levels are cleared by the kidney within 72 hours.
- Diagnose pancreatic duct obstruction, which causes serum levels to remain elevated.
- Differentiate between acute pancreatitis and other causes of abdominal pain that require surgery.
- Diagnose macroamylasemia, a disorder seen in alcoholism, malabsorption syndrome, and other digestive problems.

Reference Values

		SI Units
Adults	50–180 Somogyi U/dL	92–330 U/L
Older adults	20–160 Somogyi U/dL	

Values may vary according to the laboratory performing the test.

Abnormal Values

- Pronounced elevation (≥5 × normal)
    Acute pancreatitis
    Pancreatic pseudocyst
    Macroamylasemia
    Morphine administration
- Moderate elevation (3–5 × normal)
    Advanced carcinoma of the head of the pancreas
    Mumps
    Parotitis
    Perforated peptic ulcer (sometimes)
    Duodenal obstruction
- Mild elevation (<3 × normal)
    Chronic pancreatitis (nonadvanced)
    Renal failure
    Common bile duct obstruction
    Gastric resection

Drugs, including morphine, codeine, chlorothiazides, aspirin, pentazocine, corticosteroids, oral contraceptives, pancreozymin, and secretin
- Decreased values
  Presence of high blood glucose due to diabetes mellitus or intravenous glucose infusions
  Advanced chronic pancreatitis
  Advanced cystic fibrosis
  Hepatic disease
  Liver abscess
  Eclampsia
  Severe burns
  Cholecystitis

Interfering Factors

- Certain drugs may produce elevated or decreased levels (see Abnormal Values).
- Increased glucose or lipid levels can lead to falsely decreased amylase levels.

Nursing Implications

Assessment

- Obtain history of medication, previous gallbladder studies or surgery, and known pancreatic disorders.
- Ensure that any drugs that may alter test results have been withheld for 12 to 24 hours, and food for 2 hours before the test, as ordered by physician. Also ensure that the client has abstained from alcohol.

Possible Nursing Diagnoses

Pain related to inflammation or swelling of the pancreas
Anxiety related to perceived threat to health status
Infection, risk for, related to inadequate primary defenses

Implementation

- Put on gloves. Using aseptic technique, perform a venipuncture and collect 5 mL of blood in a red-top tube, 2 hours after a meal.
- Handle the sample gently to avoid hemolysis, and transport to the laboratory promptly.

Evaluation

- Note results in relation to urine amylase results and other pancreatic function studies.

Client/Caregiver Teaching

Pretest

- Tell the client not to eat for 2 hours before the test, to withhold medications that interfere with the test results, as ordered, and to abstain from alcohol.

Posttest

- Tell the client to resume usual medications and diet.
- Instruct the client to report abdominal pain to the physician if a pancreatic disorder is suspected.

Amylase, Urine

Classification: Urinalysis

Type of Test: Urine (timed)

A test to measure amylase, a digestive enzyme primarily produced by the pancreas and salivary glands, but also by the liver, small intestine, skeletal muscle, and fallopian tubes. This enzyme splits larger carbohydrate molecules (starch) into smaller units (disaccharides) for further action by intestinal enzymes. It is excreted into the urine following glomerular filtration. Serum and urine levels usually rise together (if renal function is adequate). In acute pancreatitis, serum amylase levels fall to normal in 2 to 3 days but urine levels remain elevated for 7 to 10 days.

Indications

- Perform a retrospective diagnosis of acute pancreatitis when serum amylase levels have returned to normal but urine levels remain elevated
- Diagnose chronic pancreatitis, as indicated by persistently elevated urinary amylase levels
- Monitor response to treatment for pancreatitis
- Assist in identifying the cause of "acute abdomen"
- Differentiate acute pancreatitis from perforated peptic ulcer (urinary amylase levels are higher in pancreatitis)

- Diagnose macroamylasemia, a disorder seen in alcoholism and malabsorption syndromes, indicated by elevated serum amylase and normal urinary amylase
- Confirm the diagnosis of salivary gland inflammation

Reference Values

		SI Units
Amylase	10–80 amylase U/h (Mayo clinic)	0–17 U/h
	35–260 Somogyi U/24 h (Somogyi)	6.5–48.1 U/h

Abnormal Values

- Elevated levels
    Acute pancreatitis
    Pancreatic pseudocyst
    Obstruction of the pancreatic duct (gallstones, tumor) or intestines or salivary duct
    Perforated peptic ulcer or duodenal ulcer
    Salivary gland inflammation or infection
    Acute injury of the spleen
    Gallbladder disease
    Macroamylasemia
    Trauma to pancreas or spleen
    Diabetic ketoacidosis
- Decreased levels
    Alcoholism
    Cachexia
    Cancer of the liver
    Chronic pancreatitis
    Cirrhosis
    Cystic fibrosis (advanced)
    Eclampsia
    Hepatic abscess
    Hepatitis
    Renal disease
    Drugs, including fluorides and glucose

Interfering Factors

- Medications that can falsely elevate amylase levels include morphine, codeine, meperidine, pentazocine, chlorothiazides, aspirin, corticosteroids, oral contraceptives, alcohol, indomethacin, urecholine, secretin, pancreozymin, bethanechol, and thiazide diuretics.

- Fluorides can decrease urine amylase levels.
- Heavy bacterial contamination of the specimen or blood can alter test results.
- Salivary amylase in the urine, caused by coughing or talking over the sample, can raise urine amylase levels.
- Incomplete specimen collection and improper specimen maintenance can lead to spurious results.

Nursing Implications

Assessment

- Obtain history of known or suspected pancreatic biliary disease, medications and treatments, diagnostic tests and procedures, and results.
- Ensure that the female client is not menstruating. If so, test needs to be rescheduled.
- Ensure proper fluid intake before and during test to promote hydration and specimen collection.

Possible Nursing Diagnoses

Pain related to inflammation or swelling of the pancreas
Anxiety related to perceived threat to health status
Infection, risk for, related to inadequate primary defenses

Implementation

- Obtain containers of appropriate size without preservatives for a 2-, 6-, 8-, 12- or 24-hour period. The sample must be kept refrigerated or on ice throughout the collection period unless the laboratory has added a preservative to the container.
- If an indwelling catheter is in place, replace tubing and container system at start of collection time. Clamp catheter tubing until next specimen is due, unless 24-hour specimen is to be collected. Place drainage bag on ice. Monitor to ensure that drainage continues.
- At the conclusion of the test, label the container(s) properly with start and completion times, collection times, and transport promptly to the laboratory.

Evaluation

- Note test results in relation to serum amylase.

Client/Caregiver Teaching

Pretest

- Instruct the client to avoid excessive exercise and stress during the collection of urine and to withhold medications that affect test results, as ordered.

- Inform the client that the sample must be kept refrigerated or on ice throughout the collection period unless the laboratory has added a preservative to the container.
- Tell the client to void all urine in a urinal or bedpan placed in the toilet for a specific time period and then either pour urine into the collection container or leave in the container for the nurse to add to the collection; instruct client to avoid voiding in pan with defecation and to keep toilet tissue out of pan to prevent contamination of the specimen.

Posttest

- Inform the client to resume medications and activity withheld before the test.
- Inform the client that test results take 2 days to report.

Androstenedione

Classification: Serology

Type of Test: Serum, plasma

This test measures androstenedione, a metabolite of dehydroepiandrosterone sulfate (DHEA-S), produced in the adrenal cortex and the ovaries and converted to testosterone in peripheral tissues and to estrone (an estrogen) by adipose tissue and the liver. In obesity and some other conditions, increased conversion of androstenedione to estrone may result in menstrual abnormalities.

In postmenopausal women and in children, estrone is the major source of estrogen. In postmenopausal women, androstenedione may cause renewed ovarian stimulation, bleeding, polycystic ovaries and endometriosis. In children, increased androstenedione production or increased conversion to estrone may induce premature sexual development. In men, feminizing signs such as gynecomastia may result from overproduction of androstenedione.

Indications

- Determine cause of gonadal dysfunction, menstrual or menopausal irregularities, and premature sexual development
- Evaluate androgen production in female hirsutism

Reference Values

Women		
Premenopausal	0.6–3 ng/ml	2–10 nmol/L
Postmenopausal	0.3–8 ng/ml	1–10 nmol/L
Men	0.9–1.7 ng/ml	3–6 nmol/L

Abnormal Values

- Increased levels
  Cushing's syndrome
  Ectopic ACTH-producing tumors
  Congenital adrenal hyperplasia (late onset)
  Ovarian stromal hyperplasia
  Ovarian, testicular, adrenal cortex tumors
  Stein-Leventhal syndrome
- Decreased levels
  Hypogonadism

Interfering Factors

- Scans involving radioactive dyes within 1 week of specimen collection will invalidate results.
- Use of steroids and pituitary hormones will affect test results.
- Failure to draw sample 1 week before or after menstrual period invalidates results.

Nursing Implications

Assessment

- Obtain history of menstrual irregularities in premenopausal women, premature sexual development in children, bleeding and endometriosis in postmenopausal women, male-pattern hair growth (hirsutism) in women; and gynecomastia and other feminizing signs in men.
- Obtain history of medications that may interfere with test results.
- Ascertain dates of menstrual period in premenopausal women.

Possible Nursing Diagnoses

Anxiety related to perceived threat to health status

Sexuality patterns, altered, related to illness or medical treatment

Body image disturbance related to change in structure/appearance

Infection, risk for, related to immunosuppressed inflammatory response

Implementation

- Put on gloves. Using aseptic technique, perform a venipuncture and collect a 10 mL sample in a red-top tube and a plasma sample in a green-top tube.
- Handle the sample gently to avoid hemolysis, and transport to the laboratory immediately.

Evaluation

- Note test results in relation to the client's symptoms and to other tests performed.

Client/Caregiver Teaching

Pretest

- Inform the premenopausal patient that the test should be done 1 week before or after her menstrual period and that it may need to be repeated.
- Instruct the client to withhold steroids or pituitary hormones, as ordered.

Posttest

- Tell the client to resume medication withheld before the test.

Angiography, Adrenal

Classification: Radiography

Type of Test: X-ray with contrast dye

This test is used to evaluate adrenal dysfunction. Angiography permits visualization of the arteries or veins of the adrenal glands after injection of an iodinated contrast medium using a catheter placed in the femoral artery for viewing the artery (arteriography) or femoral vein for viewing the veins (venography). After the catheter is in place, a blood sample may be taken from the vein of each gland to assess cortisol levels and determine the cause of Cushing's syndrome or the presence of pheochromocytoma.

Indications

- Investigate suspected benign or malignant adrenal tumor
- Diagnose adrenal hyperplasia
- Determine location of adrenal tumors

Reference Values

- Normal arteries and veins of adrenal glands

Abnormal Values

- Pheochromocytoma
- Adrenal adenoma
- Adrenal carcinoma
- Bilateral adrenal hyperplasia

Interfering Factors

- Inability to cooperate with the procedure and lie still when done under local anesthesia

> **NURSING ALERT**
>
> - The procedure is contraindicated in pregnancy, unless the benefits of performing the procedure greatly outweigh risks to the fetus.
> - If iodine is used, the procedure is contraindicated in the presence of allergy to iodine unless prophylactic medications are administered.
> - The test is contraindicated in presence of atherosclerosis.
> - Hemorrhage, embolism, thrombophlebitis, and infection may occur, depending on the vessel used.
> - Adrenal hemorrhage may occur from the pressure of the dye on the gland tissue leading to adrenal insufficiency in either procedure. In arteriography, severe hypertensive crisis may be precipitated if the client has a pheochromocytoma, leading to death. If a tumor is suspected, alpha- and beta-adrenergic blockers (phenoxybenzamine and propranolol) are administered for several days before the procedure to prevent this life-threatening complication.

Nursing Implications

Assessment

- Obtain a history of known hypersensitivity to iodine, seafood, or contrast dye from previous x-ray procedures, such as intravenous pyelogram (IVP).
- Determine if the client is pregnant.
- Determine if client has been taking anticoagulants. Anticoagulants are withheld or the dose reduced to prevent bleeding.
- Assess laboratory results of prothrombin and thromboplastin time if receiving anticoagulant therapy, and report prolonged time levels.
- Assess baseline vital signs and peripheral pulses.

Possible Nursing Diagnoses

Anxiety related to perceived threat to health status
Injury, risk for, related to exposure to contrast medium and insertion of intravascular catheter

Implementation

- Have client void before test.
- Provide the client with a gown without metallic closures and help the client put it on. Remove all metallic objects but allow the client to wear dentures and hearing aid.
- Have emergency cart readily accessible.
- If the client has a history of severe allergic reactions to various substances or drugs, administer ordered prophylactic steroids or antihistamines before the procedure.
- If the client is suspected of having a pheochromocytoma, administer propranolol and phenoxybenzamine as ordered to prevent a potentially fatal hypertensive episode.
- Mark the site of client's peripheral pulses with a pen before catheterization, permitting quicker assessment of the pulses after the procedure.
- Initiate an intravenous line to keep the vein open at a slow rate to provide access to administer emergency fluids and medications, if needed.
- Client is placed on x-ray table in a supine position. A sterile field is prepared by cleaning and draping the groin site. The site is anesthestized with a local injection and a catheter is inserted into the femoral artery (for arteriography) or femoral vein (for venography).
- For arteriography, the catheter is advanced into the aorta and then the inferior adrenal artery using the renal artery

under fluoroscopic visualization. For venography, the catheter is advanced into the adrenal vein under fluoroscopic visualization.

- Dye is injected into the catheter and x-ray films are taken for arteriographic studies and blood obtained for laboratory examination in venographic studies. After filming and blood samples are secured, the catheter is removed and a pressure dressing applied and taped in place at the insertion site.
- Apply pressure on the puncture site for 5 to 10 minutes or longer until bleeding has stopped.
- Assess vital signs every 15 minutes for 1 hour after the procedure and then every hour until client is stable.

Evaluation

- Assess neurologic status and vital signs every hour for 4 hours, then every 4 hours until client is stable. Assess extremities for signs of ischemia caused by a catheter induced thrombus.
- Observe the puncture site for hematoma or hemorrhage.
- Observe for a delayed allergic reaction to the contrast dye.
- Note test results in relation to other related tests and the client's symptoms. Particularly note results of adrenal hormone tests.

Client/Caregiver Teaching

Pretest

- Tell the client that the procedure is usually performed by an angiographer (radiologist) in the angiography room and will take 1 to 2 hours. Explain that the procedure will not be painful, but there may be moments of discomfort.
- Instruct client to discontinue anticoagulant therapy, as ordered.
- Inform the client that he or she may feel a warm flush when the dye is injected, and that he or she may also experience an urge to cough, a flushed sensation, nausea, or a salty taste about 5 minutes after the injection.
- Tell the client to remain still to ensure clear pictures.

Posttest

- Instruct client to maintain bedrest for 12 to 24 hours or as ordered.
- Instruct client to apply ice as needed to the puncture site to relieve discomfort and edema.

- Instruct client to restrict activities for a day.
- Instruct client to drink fluids to prevent dehydration caused by the diuretic action of the dye.
- Resume food and medications withheld before the test.

Angiography, Cerebral; Cerebral Angiogram

Classification: Radiography

Type of Test: X-ray with contrast dye

This test allows x-ray visualization of the cerebral vessels and the carotid and vertebral arteries after the intra-arterial injection of a contrast medium. Patterns of circulation, any interruptions to circulation, or changes in the vessel wall appearance can be viewed to help diagnose the presence of vascular abnormalities or lesions.

Indications

- Diagnose vascular disorders by assessing the changes in the size of the vessel lumina or vessel occlusion.
- Detect tumors; vessel displacement may indicate the position and type of tumor.
- Evaluate cerebral blood flow and determine the cause of increased intracranial pressure, such as hematoma, abscess, or cerebral edema.

Reference Values

- Normal structure and cerebral vasculature

Abnormal Values

- Cerebral aneurysm
- Atherosclerosis
- Vascular spasm
- Arterial fistulae

- Arteriovenous malformation
- Vascular tumor
- Nonvascular tumor
- Cerebral abscess
- Hematoma
- Cerebral edema
- Cerebral thrombosis

Interfering Factors

- Inability of client to cooperate
- Incorrect position of the client
- Incorrect size and type of catheter or needle lumen
- Incorrect amount and rate of injection of contrast medium into the vessel

NURSING ALERT

- This procedure is contraindicated in clients with allergies to shellfish or iodinated dye; atherosclerosis; renal, hepatic, or thyroid disease; or bleeding disorders; and in pregnant clients.
- Complications include hemorrhage, infection at the insertion site, or embolism caused by the inadvertent dislodgement of an atherosclerotic plaque. Other complications include cardiac dysrhythmias, which require continuous cardiac monitoring during the procedure, and possible reaction to the iodinated contrast material.

Nursing Implications

Assessment

- Obtain a history of known hypersensitivity to iodine, seafood, or contrast dye from previous x-ray procedures; a history of atherosclerosis; and a history of renal, hepatic, or thyroid disease or bleeding disorders.
- Determine if the client is pregnant.
- Ensure that the client has discontinued anticoagulant therapy before procedure.
- Ascertain that the client has refrained from eating solid foods after midnight on the day of the test.
- Obtain a baseline neurological assessment (eyes, speech, motor, strength).

Possible Nursing Diagnoses

Anxiety related to perceived threat to health status

Injury, risk for, related to exposure to contrast medium and insertion of arterial catheter

Communication, impaired, verbal, related to altered brain function

Physical mobility, impaired, related to neuromuscular impairment

Implementation

- Have emergency equipment readily accessible.
- If the client has a history of severe allergic reactions to various substances or drugs, administer ordered prophylactic steroids or antihistamines before the procedure.
- Mark the site of client's peripheral pulses with a pen before catheterization, permitting quicker assessment of the pulses after the procedure.
- Place the client in the supine position on a special radiographic table. Sedate the client usually with meperidine and atropine.
- Prepare the access site and drape appropriately. Access to the cerebral arteries is usually gained through the femoral artery, although the carotid or brachial arteries may be used. Needle and catheter placement is done by the physician and verified by fluoroscopy. Contrast medium is injected and the flow of blood through the cranial cavity is observed.
- A series of radiographs are taken in timed sequence to show the arterial and venous phases of the cerebral circulation. After the x-ray films are completed, the catheter is withdrawn.
- Apply pressure to the artery for at least 15 minutes. Apply a dry sterile or pressure dressing to the puncture site.

Evaluation

- Assess neurological status and vital signs every hour for 4 hours, then every 4 hours; also assess extremities for signs of ischemia caused by a catheter-induced thrombus.
- Monitor for absence of pulse distal to catheter insertion site.
- Observe the puncture site for hematoma or hemorrhage.
- Note test results in relation to other tests performed and the client's symptoms.

Client/Caregiver Teaching

Pretest

- Inform the client that the procedure is usually performed by an angiographer (radiologist), in the angiography room, and will take 1 hour. Explain that the procedure will not be painful, but there may be moments of discomfort.

- Instruct the client to discontinue anticoagulant therapy before the procedure, as ordered.
- Instruct the client not to eat solid foods after midnight on the day before the test.
- Tell the client to remove dentures, metallic objects, and valuables before the test.
- Inform the client that a warm flush may be felt when the dye is injected. The client must remain still, to ensure clear pictures; head movement during the procedure obscures the clarity of the radiographs.

Posttest

- Instruct the client to maintain bedrest as ordered, increase fluid intake to counteract diuretic effect of dye, and resume previous diet.
- Instruct the client to resume anticoagulant therapy, as ordered.

Angiography, Coronary; Cardiac Angiography

Classification: Radiography

Type of Test: X-ray with contrast dye

This test allows x-ray visualization of the heart, great vessels, and coronary arteries after cardiac catheterization is performed and contrast medium injected. The catheter can be inserted into either the right or left heart. Real-time views are displayed on a monitor and recorded on film. Patterns of circulation, any interruptions to circulation, or changes in vessel wall appearance can be viewed to help diagnose the presence of vascular abnormalities or lesions. Pulmonary artery abnormalities are seen with right heart views, and coronary artery and thoracic aorta abnormalities with left heart views.

Indications

- Detect narrowing of coronary vessels or abnormalities of the great vessels in patients with angina, consistent chest pain, syncope, abnormal ECG, hypercholesteremia with chest pain, and persistent chest pain after revascularization.

Reference Values

- Normal great vessels and coronary arteries

Abnormal Values

- Pulmonary artery abnormalities
- Coronary artery atherosclerosis and degree of obstruction
- Aortitis
- Aortic dissection
- Aneurysm
- Aortic atherosclerosis
- Tumor
- Trauma causing tears or other disruption
- Graft occlusion

Interfering Factors

- Inability of client to cooperate
- Incorrect position of client
- Incorrect amount and rate of injection of contrast medium into vessel

NURSING ALERT

- Contraindicated in the presence of known allergy to contrast medium without premedication for allergy.
- Complications of the procedure include bleeding, infection, thrombophlebitis, cardiac dysrhythmias, myocardial infarction, embolism (pulmonary or cerebral), or pneumothorax.
- The procedure must be terminated if chest pain, severe cardiac dysrhythmias, or signs of a cerebral vascular accident occur.

Nursing Implications

Assessment

- Obtain a history of allergy to iodine, seafood, contrast dyes, or local anesthetics.
- Take baseline vital signs and assess neurological status.
- Ensure that anticoagulant therapy has been discontinued before the procedure.
- Ensure that client has refrained from eating solid foods after midnight on the day of test.

Possible Nursing Diagnoses

Anxiety related to perceived threat to health status

Injury, risk for, related to exposure to contrast medium and insertion of intravascular catheter

Pain related to ischemia of myocardial tissue

Implementation

- Have emergency equipment readily available.
- If the client has a history of severe allergic reactions to various substances or drugs, administer ordered prophylactic steroids or antihistamines before the procedure.
- Put on gloves. Place client in supine position on a special radiographic table. Apply electrocardiography (ECG) leads for continuous cardiac monitoring and start an intravenous (IV) line with dextrose or saline at a keep-the-vein-open (KVO) rate. Sedate the client, as ordered.
- The physician will prepare the insertion site, inject a local anesthetic, and place the catheter into the right or left heart. The femoral or brachial artery is used for the left heart, and the femoral or anticubital vein for the right heart.
- Ask the client to breathe deeply to relieve nausea; to cough or breathe deeply to permit entry of the catheter into the pulmonary artery and to move the diaphragm in a downward position, allowing clearer visualization of the heart. Coughing also can correct some dysrhythmias.
- Assist in injection of iodinated contrast medium and in taking the rapid series of x-rays. The table may be tilted in various positions to facilitate different views of the heart.
- After the procedure is completed, the catheter is removed and a pressure dressing applied.

Evaluation

- Assess neurological status and vital signs every hour for 4 hours, then every 4 hours; also assess extremities for signs of ischemia caused by a catheter-induced thrombus.
- Monitor for absence of pulse distal to catheter insertion site.
- Observe the puncture site for hematoma or hemorrhage.
- Note test results in relation to other tests performed and the client's symptoms.

Client/Caregiver Teaching

Pretest

- Inform the client that the procedure is performed by a physician under local anesthesia in a special cardiac catheterization laboratory.

- Warn the client that he or she will feel a sting when the local anesthetic is injected, slight discomfort when the catheter is inserted, and a warm feeling when the dye is injected.
- Instruct client to withhold anticoagulants before the procedure, as ordered.

Posttest

- Instruct the client to maintain bedrest 8 to 12 hours, resume anticoagulant therapy, as ordered.
- Instruct the client to resume food and increase intake of fluids to counteract diuretic effect of dye.

Angiography, Digital Subtraction (DSA); Digital Venous Subtraction Angiography (DVSA); Digital Radiography

Classification: Radiography

Type of Test: X-ray with contrast dye

This test is a computerized, fluoroscopic radiology method of visualizing details of the vascular system following the intra-arterial injection of a contrast medium, usually in lower amounts than conventional filming. With this procedure, surrounding bone and soft-tissue images that inhibit visualization of the blood vessel to be evaluated are removed. With this technique, fluoroscopic images are taken before injection of contrast media and stored electronically on a videocassette. After injection, the images are retaken and the computer subtracts the preinjection images from the postinjection ones, removing all undesirable images and providing a high-contrast image of the arteries.

Indications

- Detect carotid and cerebral conditions causing blood-flow abnormalities

- Perform preoperative and postoperative evaluation of clients with obliterative disease or a central nervous system tumor.

Reference Values

- Normal carotid arteries, vertebral arteries, abdominal aorta and branches, renal arteries, and peripheral vessels

Abnormal Values

- Angiomas
- Aneurysms
- Tumors
- Thrombosis or embolism
- Arteriosclerosis
- Cerebrovascular accident (CVA)
- Aortic valvular stenosis
- Arterial occlusion
- Pheochromocytoma
- Carotid stenosis
- Hepatocellular carcinoma
- Nutcracker renal phenomenon
- Thoracic outlet syndrome
- Ulcerative plaques

Interfering Factors

- Inability of client to remain still; small amounts of movement, including swallowing and respirations, obscure results.
- Intracardiac or intra-arterial injection of contrast medium can effect results.

NURSING ALERT

- The procedure is contraindicated in clients with allergies to shellfish or iodinated dye; bleeding disorders, renal disorders, and unstable cardiac disorders; and in women who are pregnant.
- Complications of the procedure include hemorrhage, infection at the insertion site, or embolism caused by the inadvertent dislodgement of an atherosclerotic plaque.
- Other complications include cardiac dysrhythmias, which require continuous cardiac monitoring during the procedure, and possible reaction to the iodinated contrast material.

Nursing Implications

Assessment

- Obtain a history of known hypersensitivity to iodine, seafood, or contrast dye from previous x-ray procedures. Inform the radiologist of any suspected allergy to iodinated contrast.
- Take baseline vital signs and assess neurological status.
- Ensure that client has fasted before the test, usually 12 hours.
- Ensure that anticoagulant therapy has been discontinued before the procedure.

Possible Nursing Diagnoses

Anxiety related to perceived threat to health status

Injury, risk for, related to exposure to contrast medium and insertion of arterial catheter

Communication, impaired, verbal, related to altered brain function

Physical mobility, impaired, related to neuromuscular impairment

Pain related to tissue ischemia

Implementation

- Have emergency equipment readily accessible.
- If the client has a history of severe allergic reactions to various substances or drugs, administer ordered steroids or antihistamines before the procedure as a prophylactic measure.
- Place in supine position on an x-ray table. Administer sedation, if ordered. The selected vein is cleansed and covered with a sterile drape. A local anesthetic is administered by the physician.
- Venous or arterial catheterization is performed and iodine contrast media is injected at a controlled rate of 14 mL/s. Computer images are taken of arteries where the contrast media makes the blood vessels visible to radiography.
- The catheter is removed after the vessel being studied has been defined. Apply pressure to the artery for at least 15 minutes and then apply a pressure dressing to the puncture site.

Evaluation

- Monitor vital signs until they are stable.
- Note results in relation to other studies performed and to the client's symptoms.
- Observe arterial puncture site for hematoma, hemorrhage, or absence of pulse distal to insertion site.

Client/Caregiver Teaching

Pretest

- Inform the client that the procedure is usually performed by an angiographer in the angiography room and will take 45 minutes to complete.
- Warn the client that he or she may feel a sting when the local anesthetic is injected, slight discomfort when the catheter is inserted, and a warm flush when the dye is injected.
- Tell the client that remaining still is imperative to ensure clear pictures. Head movements during the procedure obscure the clarity of the radiographs.
- Instruct the client to discontinue anticoagulants (blood thinners) as ordered by the physician before the test.
- Instruct the client not to eat solid foods after midnight on the day of the test.
- Tell the client to remove dentures, metallic objects, and valuables before the test.

Posttest

- Instruct the client to resume anticoagulant therapy, as ordered.
- Instruct the client to maintain bedrest, as ordered, increase fluid intake to counteract diuretic effect of dye, and resume previous diet.

Angiography, Fluorescein

Classification: Radiography

Type of Test: X-ray with contrast dye

This test involves the color radiographic examination of the retinal vasculature following a rapid injection of a contrast medium known as sodium fluorescein. A special camera is used that allows for images to be taken in sequence and manipulated by a computer to provide views of abnormalities of the retinal vessels during filling and emptying of the dye.

Indications

- Detect possible vascular disorders affecting visual acuity
- Detect the presence of tumors, retinal edema, or inflammation, as evidenced by abnormal patterns of degree of fluorescence
- Diagnose past reduced flow or patency of the vascular circulation of the retina, as evidenced by neovascularization
- Diagnose presence of macular degeneration and any associated hemorrhaging
- Detect presence of microaneurysms caused by hypertensive retinopathy
- Detect arterial or venous occlusion evidenced by the reduced, delayed, or absent flow of the contrast medium through the vessels or possible vessel leakage of the medium
- Diagnose diabetic retinopathy resulting from long-term diabetes mellitus

Reference Values

- No leakage of dye from retinal blood vessels.
- Normal retina and retinal and choroidal vessels.
- No evidence of vascular abnormalities, such as hemorrhage, retinopathy, aneurysms, or obstructions caused by stenosis and resulting in collateral circulation.

Abnormal Values

- Diabetic retinopathy
- Aneurysm
- Macular degeneration
- Arteriovenous shunts
- Neovascularization
- Obstructive disorders of the arteries or veins that lead to collateral circulation

Interfering Factors

- Inability of client to cooperate in keeping eyes open for the test
- Presence of cataracts, which may interfere with fundal view
- Ineffective dilation of the pupils, which may impair clear imaging

> ◤ **NURSING ALERT**
>
> ■ This test is contraindicated in clients with a past history of hypersensitivity to radiographic dyes and in clients who are unable to keep their eyes open for the test.

Nursing Implications

Assessment

■ Obtain a history of known hypersensitivity to radiographic dyes.
■ Ensure that eye medications (particularly mydriatic eyedrops) have been withheld on the day of the procedure.

Possible Nursing Diagnoses

Anxiety related to perceived threat to health status

Injury, risk for, related to exposure to contrast medium and insertion of arterial catheter

Sensory-perceptual alterations, visual, related to retinal vascular abnormalities

Implementation

■ Have emergency equipment readily accessible.
■ Administer mydriatic eyedrops 15 to 30 minutes before the procedure, as ordered.
■ Insert an intermittent infusion device, if ordered, for subsequent injection of the contrast media or emergency drugs.
■ Seat the client in a chair that faces the camera. Administer eyedrops until dilation is achieved, usually every 5 minutes for 30 minutes. After the eyedrops are administered but before the dye is injected, color photographs are taken.
■ Ask the client to place the chin and forehead in position and immobilize the head. Ask that the client open the eyes wide and look straight ahead.
■ Fluorescein dye is then injected into the brachial vein using the intermittent infusion device, and a rapid sequence of photos are taken and repeated after the dye has reached the retinal vascular system. Follow-up photographs are taken in 20 to 30 minutes.
■ At the conclusion of the procedure, the intravenous needle is removed and an adhesive strip applied to the site.

Evaluation

■ Observe for hypersensitive reaction to the dye.
■ Note results in relation to client's symptoms and other tests performed.

Client/Caregiver Teaching

Pretest

- Inform the client that the procedure is usually performed by a physician in a special laboratory and takes about 1 hour to complete.
- Inform the client that when fluorescein dye is injected it may cause facial flushing or nausea.
- Instruct the glaucoma client not to use mydriatic drops the morning before the procedure.
- Instruct the client to remove dentures, metallic objects, and valuables before the test.
- Instruct the client on the importance of keeping eyes open for the test. Explain that the client will be exposed to bright lighting in the room and requested to fixate the eyes during the procedure.
- Explain that eyedrops will be instilled before the procedure and may cause a slight discomfort or burning sensation.

Posttest

- Inform the client that visual acuity and responses to light may change. Suggest that the client wear dark glasses after the test.
- Instruct the client to refrain from driving until the pupils return to normal (about 4 hours).
- Inform client that yellow discoloration of skin and urine is normally present for up to 2 days.
- Instruct the client to resume medications withheld before the test.

Angiography, Liver and Portal Vein

Classification: Radiography

Type of Test: X-ray with contrast dye

This test is performed to evaluate liver function and portal vein patency. Angiography allows visualization of the arteries or veins of the hepatic system after injection of an iodinated contrast medium. Either a direct approach or an indirect approach is used. The direct approach involves a transhepatic or transplenic insertion of a needle through the skin into the splenic or superior mesenteric vein; the indirect approach involves inserting a catheter through the femoral artery and advancing it through the superior mesenteric or gastric artery.

Hepatic arteriography helps determine the presence of tumors; portal venography assesses the patency and size of portal, splenic, and mesenteric veins.

Indications

- Diagnose malignant liver tumor when ultrasonography, computed tomography (CT) scanning, magnetic resonance imaging (MRI), or needle biopsy fail to provide a definitive diagnosis
- Determine location, number of nodes, and vascular invasion of a hepatic malignant tumor before surgery
- Determine advisability of arterial infusion of chemotherapy to treat a malignant tumor
- Determine the stage of cirrhosis of the liver, which is known to cause a reversal of portal venous blood flow
- Define and determine hepatic anatomy and blood flow before hepatic transplantation or a shunt placement
- Evaluate surgical placement of portosystemic shunt postoperatively
- Evaluate portal vein patency and size following hepatic transplantation
- Diagnose nodular hyperplasia or Budd-Chiari syndrome, which cause hepatic venous flow obstruction

- Evaluate tumors of the pancreas or other intra-abdominal masses before surgery to determine advisability of resection
- Diagnose suspected mesenteric venous thrombosis or varices of the colon or small bowel
- Determine portal vein pressure to diagnose portal hypertension as well as other liver diseases that produce venous obstruction
- Possibly evaluate liver trauma following injury

Reference Values

- Normal structure and patency of hepatic artery and portal vein

Abnormal Values

- Tumor
- Vascular obstruction

Interfering Factors

- Inability to cooperate with the procedure and lie still when done under local anesthesia

> ### NURSING ALERT
>
> - Contraindicated in pregnancy, unless benefits of performing the procedure greatly outweigh risks to the fetus
> - If iodine is used, contraindicated in presence of allergy to iodine unless prophylactic medications are administered
> - Contraindicated in presence of ascites or in presence of bleeding disorder or severely impaired liver or renal function

Nursing Implications

Assessment

- Obtain a history of known hypersensitivity to iodine, seafood, or contrast dye from previous x-ray procedures, such as intravenous pyelogram (IVP).
- Determine date of last menstrual period and possibility of pregnancy in premenopausal women.

- Determine if client has been taking anticoagulants. Anticoagulants are withheld or the dose reduced to prevent bleeding.
- Assess laboratory results of prothrombin and thromboplastin time if receiving anticoagulant therapy, and report prolonged time levels.

Possible Nursing Diagnoses

Anxiety related to perceived threat to health status

Injury, risk for, related to exposure to contrast medium and insertion of arterial catheter

Pain related to inflammation or swelling of the liver

Implementation

- Provide the client with a gown without metallic closures and help client put it on. Remove all metallic objects but allow the client to wear dentures and hearing aid.
- Have an emergency cart readily available.
- If the client has a history of severe allergic reactions to various substances or drugs, administer ordered prophylactic steroids or antihistamines before the procedure.
- If the client is suspected of having a pheochromocytoma, administer propranolol and phenoxybenzamine as ordered to prevent a potentially fatal hypertensive episode.
- Mark the site of client's peripheral pulses with a pen before catheterization, permitting quicker assessment of the pulses after the procedure.
- Initiate an intravenous line at a KVO rate to provide access to administer emergency fluids and medications, if needed.
- Client is placed on x-ray table in a supine position. A sterile field is prepared by cleansing and draping the site, usually the femoral for the indirect approach or upper right quadrant for the direct approach. The site is anesthetized with a local injection. Portal venous pressure can be taken if the direct approach is used once the transhepatic or transplenic needle has been placed and before x-ray filming is done. To obtain pressures, the catheter is placed in the hepatic vein until it occludes blood outflow from the vein. In the indirect approach the catheter is inserted into the femoral artery and advanced to the common hepatic artery via the superior mesenteric artery or gastric artery for arteriography or into the femoral vein and advanced into the major hepatic vein for venography. All catheter or needle placements are guided by fluoroscopic viewing. Once the catheter is properly placed, the contrast medium is injected. The amount of contrast medium used and the rate of infusion is based on the vessel and suspected liver abnormality.

- Injection rates of the dye depend on the flow rates within the vessels and the projected length of time needed for filming. Filming following dye injection is rapid for a few seconds and then slowed for about 30 seconds to include parenchymal and venous phases of hepatic arteriography and portography.
- Apply pressure on the puncture site for 5 to 10 minutes or longer until bleeding has stopped.

Evaluation

- Observe the puncture site for hematoma or hemorrhage.
- Assess neurological status and vital signs every hour for 4 hours, then every 4 hours until stable. Assess extremities for signs of ischemia caused by a catheter-induced thrombus.
- Observe for a delayed allergic reaction to the contrast dye.
- Note test results in relation to other related tests and the client's symptoms. Particularly note results of liver-function tests.

Client/Caregiver Teaching

Pretest

- Explain that the procedure is usually performed by an angiographer (radiologist) in the angiography room and will take 1 to 2 hours. Tell the client that the procedure will not be painful but there may be moments of discomfort.
- Inform the client that he or she may feel a warm flush when the dye is injected, and an urge to cough, a flushed sensation, nausea, or a salty taste about 5 minutes after the injection.
- Instruct the client to remain still to ensure clear pictures.

Posttest

- Instruct the client to maintain bedrest for 12 to 24 hours or as ordered.
- Instruct client to apply ice as needed to the puncture site to relieve discomfort and edema.
- Instruct client to drink fluids to prevent dehydration caused by the diuretic action of the dye, and resume food and medications withheld before the test.

Angiography, Lower Extremity

Classification: Radiography

Type of Test: X-ray with contrast dye

Angiography permits visualization of the arteries or veins to evaluate circulation of the leg and foot, after injection of an iodinated contrast medium. Catheterization or injection sites are chosen according to the areas or vessels to be examined. Abdominal aortography to evaluate aneurysms preoperatively and pelvic angiography to evaluate mesenteric circulation can also be performed with these studies. Digital subtraction angiography may also be performed for complete lower-extremity studies by filling in areas of special concern or to examine lower extremities separately in obese clients. If a thrombus is identified during the procedure, urokinase can be infused in an attempt to break down the clot and restore patency. This procedure may be done as an emergency if sudden or acute onset of occlusion occurs.

Indications

- Diagnose presence of a tumor compressing the arterial or venous system and causing obstruction
- Evaluate known or suspected deep-vein thrombosis of lower extremity
- Diagnose atherocclusive disease in clients with diabetes mellitus or peripheral arterial embolus
- Determine effect of thromboangitis obliterans on the small and medium-sized vessels of the extremity
- Determine cause of claudication or thrombosis such as popliteal entrapment syndrome, cystic adventitial disease, or atherosclerotic disease
- Evaluate arteriovenous malformation or other congenital abnormality
- Evaluate suspected vascular injury to extremity that disrupts or occludes arteries or veins
- Determine level of limb amputation caused by vascular occlusion following frostbite or electrical injury

- Identify and evaluate veins considered for use in bypass graft surgery
- Examine suspected venous valvular incompetence by descending venography in the presence of venous stasis symptoms
- Administer thrombolytic agents such as urokinase

Reference Values

- Normal structure and patency of leg and foot vascular system

Abnormal Values

- Aneurysm
- Vascular obstruction
- Vessel trauma
- Tumor
- Buerger's disease

Interfering Factors

- Inability to cooperate with the procedure and lie still during procedure
- Improper tourniquet or dye injection technique

> ### NURSING ALERT
>
> - Contraindicated in presence of allergy to iodine unless prophylactic medications are administered
> - Contraindicated in presence of edema of the extremity if access to the vessel is not possible; in presence of impaired renal function or bleeding disorder; or in poorly controlled hypertension

Nursing Implications

Assessment

- Obtain a history of known hypersensitivity to iodine, seafood, or contrast dye from previous x-ray procedures, such as IVP.
- Determine if client has been taking anticoagulants. Anticoagulants are withheld or the dose reduced to prevent bleeding.
- Assess laboratory results of prothrombin and thromboplastin time if receiving anticoagulant therapy, and report prolonged time levels.

Possible Nursing Diagnoses

Anxiety related to perceived threat to health status

Injury, risk for, related to exposure to contrast medium and insertion of arterial catheter

Pain related to tissue ischemia

Implementation

- Provide the client with a gown without metallic closures and help client to put it on. Remove all metallic objects, but allow the client to wear dentures and hearing aid.
- Have an emergency cart readily available.
- If the client has a history of severe allergic reactions to various substances or drugs, administer ordered prophylactic steroids or antihistamines before the procedure.
- If the client is suspected of having a pheochromocytoma, administer propranolol and phenoxybenzamine as ordered to prevent a potentially fatal hypertensive episode.
- Mark the site of the client's peripheral pulses with a pen before catheterization, permitting quicker assessment of the pulses after the procedure.
- Insert IV infusion line at a KVO rate to provide access to administer emergency fluids and medications, if needed.
- *Arterial studies:* The client is placed on the x-ray table in a supine position. The femoral arterial site is used for abdominal aortography and lower-extremity arteriography unless occlusive disease prevents its use. Alternative sites that can be used are the axillary or brachial artery. The site is anesthetized by local injection, and the catheter is advanced into the distal abdominal aorta under fluoroscopic guidance. A specified amount of contrast medium is injected at a calculated rate and period of time. Step-table filming is performed; this includes three films at the level of the pelvis, two films at the level of the thighs, four films at the level of the knees, and six films at the level of the calf. Further filming can be performed of the distal vessels of the ankle and foot in clients with diabetes mellitus, ulcers, or gangrene. The feet and legs can be warmed immediately before the filming to enhance distal vascular opacification. This is done by application of external heat, use of an occlusive cuff on the thigh, or intra-arterial injection of a vasodilator, such as tolazoline or dilute nitroglycerin.
- *Ascending phlebography or descending venography:* These tests can be performed for deep-vein thrombosis or venous incompetence. For lower-limb ascending phlebography, the client is placed on a tilting table in a supine position. The dorsum of the foot of the extremity to be examined is cleansed, and the table is tilted in a semi-upright position that allows for more complete filling of the vein. Weight bear-

ing is allowed on the foot not being examined to allow for optimal relaxation of the affected extremity. A superficial vein is catheterized, and the contrast medium is injected slowly following the preparation of the site. The flow is monitored by fluoroscopy. A tourniquet can be placed above the ankle and the knee to encourage the dye to flow into the deeper veins. Following the injection, spot films are taken in various views over the thigh, calf, knee, and also the foot, if a study of this area is desired.

- *Supine venography:* This test can be performed in clients who are not able to be maintained in the semi-upright position. This position requires that tourniquets be used and the contrast medium administered by continuous infusion rather than manual injection. In either position, a cutdown to expose a vein for cannulation can be performed if one cannot be used for a superficial injection of the dye.

- *Lower-limb descending venography:* The client is placed on the x-ray table in a supine position. The site used can be an arm vein or femoral vein from the side opposite the one to be examined. Following the preparation of the site, the vein is cannulated, and the contrast medium is injected. The dye can also be injected directly into the femoral vein of the side to be examined using a needle or catheter. After the dye is injected, the reflux of the dye is viewed by fluoroscopy and graded from 0 to 5, indicating the absence of reflux at the level of the ankle. The examination is done with the table tilted to the upright position or in the horizontal position, with the client performing the Valsalva maneuver.

- After the catheter is removed, apply pressure on the puncture site for 5 to 10 minutes or longer until bleeding has stopped.

Evaluation

- Observe the puncture site for hematoma or hemorrhage.
- Assess neurological status and vital signs every hour for 4 hours, then every 4 hours until stable. Assess extremities for signs of ischemia caused by a catheter-induced thrombus.
- Observe for a delayed allergic reaction to the contrast dye.
- Note test results in relation to other related tests and the client's symptoms. Particularly note results of adrenal hormone tests.

Client/Caregiver Teaching

Pretest

- Explain that the procedure is usually performed by an angiographer (radiologist) in the angiography room. Explain procedure will not be painful, but there may be moments of discomfort.

- Inform the client that he or she may feel a warm flush when the dye is injected, and an urge to cough, a flushed sensation, nausea, or a salty taste about 5 minutes after the injection.
- Instruct the client to remain still to ensure clear pictures.

Posttest

- Instruct client to maintain bedrest for 12 to 24 hours or as ordered.
- Instruct client to apply ice as needed to the puncture site to relieve discomfort and edema.
- Instruct client to drink fluids to prevent dehydration caused by the diuretic action of the dye and to resume food and medications withheld before the test.

Angiography, Lymph; Lymphangiography; Lymphangiogram

Classification: Radiography

Type of Test: X-ray with contrast dye

This test is an x-ray examination of the lymphatic flow and lymph node patterns after injection of dye into the lymph vessels of the hand or foot. Films are obtained of various parts of the abdomen and chest to determine abnormalities of the lymph channels or presence of displacement or collateral formation. The study takes 2 days to complete.

Indications

- Detect suspected lymphoma, tumor metastasis to lymph nodes, as evidenced by node size and filling defects.
- Determine stage of lymphoma to identify the extent of involvement; stages range from involvement of a single node (stage I) to diffuse metastasis, especially in Hodgkin's lymphoma (stage IV).

- Differentiate between a primary and secondary lymphedema in an extremity.
- Evaluate the effectiveness of therapy or progression of the disease.
- Evaluate nodal involvement before treatment regimen and possible surgical intervention.
- Diagnose testicular tumors, prostatic cancer, and cervical cancer in association with CT scanning procedures.

Reference Values

- Normal lymphatic vessels and nodes

Abnormal Values

- Hodgkin's lymphoma
- Testicular tumors
- Nodular lymphoma
- Cervical cancer
- Prostatic cancer

Interfering Factors

- Inability of client to cooperate
- Inability to cannulate lymphatic vessels

> **NURSING ALERT**
>
> - Contraindicated in clients with allergies to shellfish or iodinated dye, and in clients with cardiac, pulmonary, liver, or renal disease. Also, contraindicated in pregnancy unless benefits of performing the procedure outweigh the risk to the fetus.

Nursing Implications

Assessment

- Obtain a history of known hypersensitivity to iodine, seafood, or contrast dye from previous x-ray procedures.

Possible Nursing Diagnoses

Anxiety related to perceived threat to health status

Injury, risk for, related to exposure to contrast medium and insertion of arterial catheter

Implementation

- Have emergency equipment readily accessible.
- If the client has a history of severe allergic reactions to various substances or drugs, administer ordered steroids or antihistamines before the procedure as a prophylactic measure.
- Administer a mild sedative, as ordered.
- Place the client in supine position on an x-ray table. An oil-based dye is injected into several toes of each foot to stain the lymphatic vessels of the feet. Staining occurs within 15 to 20 minutes. (If the axillary nodes are to be visualized, injections are made in each hand.)
- About 30 minutes later, a local anesthetic is injected and small incisions are made on the dorsum of each foot (or the hand). After the vessels are cannulated, the contrast media is slowly infused with the aid of the infusion pump.
- The flow of the dye medium is monitored using fluoroscopy. When it reaches the level of the third or fourth vertebrae, the infusion is stopped.
- Radiographs are taken of the lymphatics in the leg, pelvic, abdominal, and chest area. A second set of films is taken in 24 hours.

Evaluation

- Note results in relation to other test results, particularly CT scanning procedures.
- Assess incisional site for signs of infection and the client for signs of fat embolism, such as dyspnea, pain, and hypotension.
- Monitor for delayed allergic response to the dye.

Client/Caregiver Teaching

Pretest

- Inform the client that the procedure, which is administered in a radiographic room, may take up to 3 hours and that the follow-up study in 24 hours will take about 30 minutes.
- Inform the client that the blue contrast dye will turn urine and stool blue for 48 hours and may cause the skin to have a bluish tinge for 24 to 48 hours.

Posttest

- Inform the client to elevate extremities for 24 hours to prevent swelling.

- Remind the client to return in 24 hours for more films.
- Inform the client that the dye can remain in the nodes for up to 1 year, allowing for follow-up x-rays to monitor progress.

Angiography, Mesenteric

Classification: Radiography

Type of Test: X-ray with contrast dye

This test involves the x-ray examination of the gastrointestinal vasculature after injection of a contrast medium to identify the source of acute bleeding that cannot be resolved by therapy or treated endoscopically. The contrast medium is injected through a catheter which is inserted through the artery and advanced into the aorta and the superior or inferior mesenteric or celiac artery. In addition to the diagnostic indications for the procedure, therapeutic arterial infusion of vasopressin may be employed to control gastric and colonic bleeding, as well as embolization with Gelfoam, which is effective in controlling bleeding from the gastric, colonic, and small intestine when other measures of treatment have failed.

Indications

- Identify bleeding site in the gastrointestinal (GI) tract before surgery or treatment
- Evaluate suspected aortoenteric fistula or intestinal angina
- Diagnose the presence of acute mesenteric ischemia, as evidenced by thrombus, embolus, or venous occlusion
- Determine the site and cause of gastrointestinal bleeding if other diagnostic studies or procedures have failed to reveal or treat and resolve the problem
- Evaluate the extent of suspected abdominal aortic aneurysm
- Treat GI hemorrhage by infusion of arterial vasopressin or arterial embolization
- Detect pancreatic cell tumors not diagnosed by other studies
- Detect type and extent of injury caused by trauma to the organs and major vessels

- Diagnose presence of colonic diverticula, angiodysplasia, Meckel's diverticulum, inflammatory bowel disease, which may be a source of existing or future bleeding
- Determine the status of mesenteric circulation, the condition of iliac or common femoral arteries before corrective surgery, and perform graft for abdominal aortic aneurysm

Reference Values

- Normal vascular structure and patency with no bleeding activity or ischemia in the vessels of the gastrointestinal organs

Abnormal Values

- Fistulae
- Intestinal angina
- Mesenteric ischemia
- Ulcerations
- Inflammatory lesions
- Diverticula
- Tumors
- Splenic and hepatic injury or rupture
- Pancreatic islet cell tumors

Interfering Factors

- Gas, feces, or barium in the GI tract, which may impair clear imaging
- Inability of the client to remain still during the procedure

NURSING ALERT

- Contraindicated in clients with allergy to iodine, unless prophylactic medications are administered. Also contraindicated in clients with bleeding or coagulation disorders, or in pregnant clients, unless the potential benefits of the procedure outweigh the risks to the fetus.

Nursing Implications

Assessment

- Obtain a history of known hypersensitivity to iodine, seafood, or contrast dye from previous x-ray procedures.
- Determine date of last menstrual period and possibility of pregnancy in premenopausal women.

- Ascertain that client has fluid and dietary restrictions.
- Ascertain that client has taken a cathartic, as ordered.
- Determine if client has been taking anticoagulants.
- Assess laboratory results of prothrombin and thromboplastin time if receiving anticoagulant therapy, and report prolonged time levels.

Possible Nursing Diagnoses

Anxiety related to perceived threat to health status
Injury, risk for, related to exposure to contrast medium and insertion of arterial catheter
Pain related to tissue ischemia

Implementation

- Have emergency equipment readily accessible.
- If the client has a history of severe allergic reactions to various substances or drugs, administer ordered prophylactic steroids or antihistamines before the procedure.
- Remove all metallic objects but allow the client to wear dentures and hearing aid.
- Administer a mild sedative, as ordered.
- Mark the site of client's peripheral pulses with a pen before catheterization, permitting quicker assessment of the pulses after the procedure.
- Start an IV line with dextrose or saline at KVO rate for administration of emergency drugs, if needed.
- Place the client in the supine position on an x-ray table. An abdominal flat plate may be taken at this time.
- Cleanse the puncture site, usually the femoral artery, and cover with a sterile drape.
- A local anesthetic is injected at the site and a small incision made or needle inserted into the femoral artery. The catheter is threaded into the abdominal aorta and mesenteric or celiac artery using fluoroscopy. The dye is injected for filming of the aortic structure and patency. Injection of the contrast medium is adjusted to match the blood flow of the aorta, celiac, and superior or inferior mesenteric artery, and a series of rapid films is taken. The filming may then be slowed for capillary and venous phases to complete the study.
- The catheter is removed and a pressure dressing is applied to the puncture site.

Evaluation

- Assess neurological status and vital signs every hour for 4 hours, then every 4 hours; also assess extremities for signs of ischemia caused by a catheter-induced thrombus.
- Monitor for absence of pulse distal to the catheter insertion site.

- Observe the insertion site for bleeding, inflammation, or hematoma.
- Note results in relation to other tests performed and to the client's symptoms.

Client/Caregiver Teaching

Pretest

- Inform the client that the procedure is usually performed by an angiographer in the angiography room and will take 1 to 3 hours to complete.
- Inform the client to withhold or reduce dosage of anticoagulants as ordered.
- Inform client to take only clear liquids for 24 hours and to fast for 8 hours before the test.
- Inform the client that a cathartic is necessary the day before the study, as ordered.
- Instruct client on the importance of lying still throughout the procedure.
- Inform the client that some pressure will be felt as the catheter is introduced into the vessel, and that there will be a feeling of warmth and palpitations when the dye is injected, but that this will only last about 30 seconds.
- Inform the client that for 5 minutes after the injection of the contrast medium, he or she will feel an urge to cough, a flushing sensation, nausea, or a salty taste.

Posttest

- Instruct the client to maintain bedrest for 8 to 12 hours after the procedure to allow for complete sealing of the arterial puncture. The extremity used should be extended and immobilized with a sandbag for 3 hours (arm) to 8 hours (leg).
- Instruct the client to resume previous diet and to increase fluid intake to counteract diuretic effect of dye.
- Advise the client to apply cold compresses to the punctured site for edema or pain, if ordered.

Angiography, Pulmonary; Pulmonary Angiogram

Classification: Radiography

Type of Test: X-ray with contrast dye

This test allows x-ray visualization of the pulmonary vasculature following the injection of an iodinated contrast medium into the pulmonary artery or a branch of this great vessel. It is the definitive test for pulmonary embolism, but it also useful for evaluating other types of pulmonary vascular abnormalities.

Indications

- Diagnose acute pulmonary embolism
- Detect tumors; aneurysms; congenital defects; vascular changes associated with emphysema, blebs, and bullae; and heart abnormality
- Evaluate pulmonary circulation
- Determine cause of recurrent or severe hemoptysis

Reference Values

- Normal pulmonary vasculature. Radiopaque iodine contrast medium should circulate symmetrically and without interruption through the pulmonary circulatory system.

Abnormal Values

- Pulmonary embolism (acute or chronic)
- Arterial hypoplasia or stenosis
- Arteriovenous malformations
- Aneurysms
- Pulmonary sequestration
- Tumors
- Inflammatory diseases
- Bleeding caused by tuberculosis, bronchiectasis, sarcoidosis, or aspergilloma

Interfering Factors

- Inability of client to cooperate
- Inability of client to lie motionless throughout the procedure
- Incorrect size and type of catheter or needle lumen
- Incorrect amount and rate of injection of contrast medium into the vessel

> **NURSING ALERT**
>
> - This test is contraindicated in clients with allergies to shellfish or iodinated dye, bleeding disorders, or in pregnant clients, unless the potential benefits of the procedure outweigh the risks.
> - Complications of these studies include cardiac dysrhythmias, which require continuous cardiac monitoring during the procedure, and possible reaction to the iodinated contrast material. Not as common are inadvertent myocardial perforation or arterial infarct.

Nursing Implications

Assessment

- Obtain a history of known hypersensitivity to iodine, seafood, or contrast dye from previous x-ray procedures. Also, obtain a history of ventricular dysrhythmias.
- Ascertain that client has discontinued anticoagulant therapy before the procedure. Assess recent coagulation times, as ordered.
- Ensure that client has fasted for 8 hours.

Possible Nursing Diagnoses

Anxiety related to perceived threat to health status

Injury, risk for, related to exposure to contrast medium and insertion of arterial catheter

Pain related to tissue ischemia

Gas exchange, impaired, related to ventilation-perfusion imbalance

Implementation

- Have emergency equipment readily accessible.
- If the client has a history of severe allergic reactions to various substances or drugs, administer ordered prophylactic steroids or antihistamines before the procedure.

- Mark the site of client's peripheral pulses with a pen before catheterization, permitting quicker assessment of the pulses after the procedure.
- Place electrocardiographic electrodes on client for cardiac monitoring. Establish baseline rhythm; determine if client has ventricular dysrhythmias.
- Establish intravenous fluid line for the injection of contrast medium or emergency drugs.
- Administer a mild sedative as ordered.
- Place the client in the supine position on an x-ray table. Cleanse the selected vein and cover with a sterile drape.
- A local anesthetic is injected at the site and a small incision made or needle inserted. The catheter is inserted into the femoral, brachial, or jugular vein and threaded into the inferior vena cava and the right side of the heart under fluoroscopy. From the right ventricle the catheter is threaded into the pulmonary artery and the dye injected. Serial films are taken during the injection of the dye to visualize the pulmonary circulation. Rapid sequence films with at least two views of each lung are obtained following the dye injection.
- The catheter is removed and a pressure dressing is applied over the puncture site.

Evaluation

- Assess neurological status and vital signs every hour for 4 hours, then every 4 hours; also assess extremities for signs of ischemia caused by a catheter-induced thrombus
- Observe the insertion site for bleeding, inflammation, or hematoma formation.
- Observe for a delayed allergic reaction to the contrast dye.
- Note results in relation to other tests performed and to the client's symptoms.

Client/Caregiver Teaching

Pretest

- Inform the client that the procedure will be performed by a physician and will take 1 hour. Explain that the procedure will not be painful but there may be moments of discomfort.
- Inform the client that a burning sensation and flush will be felt throughout the body during the injection of the dye. Also inform the client that for 5 minutes after the injection of the contrast medium, he or she may experience an urge to cough, flushing, nausea, or salty taste.
- Instruct client on the importance of lying motionless throughout the procedure.

- Instruct client to withhold anticoagulant medication or reduce dosage before the procedure, as ordered.
- Instruct client to fast for 8 hours before the test.
- Instruct client to remove dentures, metallic objects, and valuables before the test.

Posttest

- Instruct the client to resume ordered medications that were discontinued before the procedure.
- Instruct client to maintain bedrest for 8 to 12 hours following procedure, or as ordered, to resume previous diet, and to increase fluid intake to counteract diuretic effects of dye.
- Advise the client to apply cold compresses to the punctured site for edema or pain, if ordered.
- Advise the client to immediately report symptoms such as fast heart rate, difficulty breathing, skin rash, itching, or decreased urinary output.

Angiography, Renal; Renal Arteriography

Classification: Radiography

Type of Test: X-ray with contrast dye

This test allows x-ray visualization of the large and small arteries of the renal vasculature and parenchyma or the renal veins and their branches. A catheter is inserted into the femoral artery or vein and advanced through the iliac artery and aorta into the renal artery or the inferior vena cava into the renal vein. Contrast medium is then injected to enhance visualization.

Indications

- Detect renal tumors as evidenced by arterial supply, extent of venous invasion, and tumor vascularity
- Differentiate between renal tumors and renal cysts
- Detect nonmalignant tumors before surgical resection

- Evaluate renovascular hypertension as evidenced by atherosclerosis that causes narrowing or occlusion of arteries and renal insufficiency
- Diagnose renal artery stenosis as evidenced by vessel dilation, collateral vessels, or increased renovascular pressure
- Diagnose arterial occlusion as evidenced by a transection of the renal artery caused by trauma or a penetrating injury
- Evaluate tumor vascularity before surgery or embolization
- Evaluate the renal vascular system of prospective kidney donors before surgery
- Diagnose thrombosis, arteriovenous fistula, aneurysms, or emboli in renal vessels
- Evaluate postoperative renal transplantation for function or organ rejection
- Diagnose small kidney or absence of a kidney
- Evaluate renal function in chronic renal failure or end-stage renal disease or hydronephrosis
- Collect blood sample from renal vein for renin analysis

Reference Values

- Dye should circulate throughout the kidneys symmetrically and without interruption.
- Normal structure, function, and patency of renal vessels.
- No evidence of obstruction, variations in number and size of vessels and organs, malformations, cysts, or tumors.

Abnormal Values

- Renal tumors or cysts
- Arterial stenosis or infarction
- Arterial trauma
- Abscess or inflammation
- Aneurysms
- Arteriovenous abnormalities

Interfering Factors

- Barium, gas, or feces in the gastrointestinal tract, which may impair clear imaging
- Inability of the client to remain still during the procedure
- Failure to withhold sodium in diet or medications, which may interfere with accurate analysis of blood sample for renin in renal venography

> ◤ **NURSING ALERT**
>
> - This procedure is contraindicated in clients with allergies to shellfish or iodinated dye; bleeding disorders; end-stage renal failure; severe thrombosis of the inferior vena cava or renal vein; or in pregnancy, unless the benefits greatly outweigh the risks to the fetus.
> - Complications of the procedure include hemorrhage, infection at the insertion site, or embolism caused by the inadvertent dislodgement of an atherosclerotic plaque. Other complications include cardiac dysrhythmias and possible reaction to the contrast material.

Nursing Implications

Assessment

- Obtain a history of known hypersensitivity to iodine, seafood, or contrast dye from previous x-ray procedures.
- Ensure that client has fasted for 8 hours.
- Ensure that client has discontinued anticoagulant therapy before the procedure.

Possible Nursing Diagnoses

Anxiety related to perceived threat to health status
Injury, risk for, related to exposure to contrast medium and insertion of arterial catheter
Pain related to tissue ischemia
Fluid volume excess related to compromised regulatory function (renal)

Implementation

- Have emergency equipment readily accessible.
- If the client has a history of severe allergic reactions to various substances or drugs, administer ordered prophylactic steroids or antihistamines before the procedure.
- Mark the client's peripheral pulses with a pen before catheterization, thereby permitting quicker assessment of the pulses after the procedure.
- Start an IV line with dextrose or saline at a KVO rate for administration of emergency drugs, if needed.
- Administer a mild sedative, as ordered
- Place the client on the x-ray table in a supine position. The site is cleansed and draped to prepare the sterile field for the procedure. The site is anesthetized by local injection and the femoral artery or vein is punctured and the guide wire is inserted. The catheter is inserted over the guide wire and is

threaded up into the aorta and into the renal arteries under fluoroscopy (renal arteriography).
- The contrast medium is then injected and a series of rapid x-rays are taken during and after the filling of the vessels to be examined. Films may also be taken following injection of the dye for additional delayed studies or to monitor the venous phase of the procedure. At the conclusion of the study, the catheter is removed and site bandaged with a pressure dressing.

Evaluation

- Assess neurological status and vital signs every hour for 4 hours, then every 4 hours; also assess extremities for signs of ischemia caused by a catheter-induced thrombus.
- Monitor for absence of pulse distal to catheter insertion site.
- Observe the puncture site for hematoma or hemorrhage.
- Assess for delayed reaction to contrast dye; this usually occurs within the first 2 to 6 hours after the test.
- Note test results in relation to other studies performed and to the client's symptoms.

Client/Caregiver Teaching

Pretest

- Inform the client that the procedure is usually performed by an angiographer in the angiography room and will take about 1 hour to complete. Explain that the procedure will not be painful but there may be moments of discomfort.
- Instruct the client to discontinue anticoagulant therapy before the procedure, as ordered.
- Instruct the client not to eat solid foods after midnight on the day of the test.
- Instruct the client to remove dentures, jewelry, or metal objects before the procedure.
- Instruct the client of the importance of lying still throughout the procedure.
- Instruct the client that for 5 minutes after injection of the contrast dye, he or she may experience an urge to cough, a flushed sensation, nausea, or a salty taste.

Posttest

- Instruct the client to increase fluid intake after the test to counteract diuretic effects of dye and to resume food withheld before the test.
- Instruct the client to maintain bedrest for 8 to 12 hours as ordered to allow for complete sealing of the arterial puncture.

- Advise the client to apply cold compresses to the puncture site as needed to reduce discomfort or edema.
- Advise the client to immediately report symptoms of a delayed allergic reaction to the dye.

Angiography, Upper Extremity

Classification: Radiography

Type of Test: X-ray with contrast dye

This test permits visualization of the arteries or veins to evaluate circulation of the arm and hand. Catheterization or injection sites are chosen according to the areas or vessels to be examined. Low-osmolar agents and digital subtraction angiographic techniques have reduced the pain associated with the injection of the material used to perform this procedure.

Indications

- Diagnose Raynaud's phenomenon with or without a fixed vascular occlusion
- Determine unilateral or bilateral Raynaud's phenomenon in the diagnosis of an underlying arterial condition
- Differentiate between atherosclerosis and thromboangitis obliterans by the involvement of proximal or distal vessels, respectively
- Determine the extent of arterial involvement based on claudication
- Determine cause of embolization such as atherosclerosis or aneurysms
- Diagnose thoracic outlet syndrome by venous obstruction and thrombosis or aterial compression
- Diagnose arterial or venous insufficiency caused by repeated trauma events or other injuries such as thermal or electric shock to the extremity
- Determine treatment plan based on study findings for thrombolysis in arterial or venous thrombosis or balloon angioplasty for subclavian arterial stenosis

Reference Values

- Normal structure and patency of hand and arm vascular system

Abnormal Values

- Tumor
- Vascular obstruction
- Aneurysm
- Raynaud's phenomenon
- Thoracic outlet syndrome
- Vessel trauma

Interfering Factors

- Cold environmental temperature that affects the vascular tone and blood flow in the digits
- Vasospasms that affect the filling of the digital vessels with dye.
- Inability to cooperate with the procedure and lie still during procedure
- Improper tourniquet or dye injection technique

> **NURSING ALERT**
>
> - This procedure is contraindicated in the presence of allergy to iodine unless prophylactic medications are administered. It is also contraindicated in the presence of edema of the extremity.

Nursing Implications

Assessment

- Obtain a history of known hypersensitivity to iodine, seafood, or contrast dye from previous x-ray procedures, such as IVP.
- Determine if client has been taking anticoagulants.
- Assess laboratory results of prothrombin and thromboplastin time if receiving anticoagulant therapy, and report prolonged time levels.
- Assess baseline vital signs and peripheral pulses.

Possible Nursing Diagnoses

Anxiety related to perceived threat to health status

Injury, risk for, related to exposure to contrast medium and insertion of arterial catheter

Pain related to tissue ischemia

Implementation

- Have the client void before the test.
- Provide the client with a gown without metallic closures and help the client put the gown on. Remove all metallic objects, but allow the client to wear dentures and hearing aid.
- Have emergency equipment available.
- If the client has a history of severe allergic reactions to various substances or drugs, administer ordered prophylactic steroids or antihistamines before the procedure.
- If the client is suspected of having a pheochromocytoma, administer propranolol and phenoxybenzamine as ordered to prevent a potentially fatal hypertensive episode.
- Mark the site of the client's peripheral pulses with a pen before catheterization, permitting quicker assessment of the pulses after the procedure.
- Insert an intravenous infusion line at a KVO rate to provide access to administer emergency fluids and medications, if needed.
- The client is placed on the x-ray table in a supine position. The groin is cleansed and draped to prepare a sterile field for a femoral arterial catheterization. In cases of proximal disease or atherosclerosis, the axillary or brachial artery is prepared and used for cannulation. The site is anesthetized by local injection, and the catheter is inserted and advanced under fluoroscopy through the intrathoracic arteries, into the axillary artery for distal injection of the dye, and down into the distal brachial artery if the hand is to be studied. The dye is then injected and the filming is performed. Digital subtraction angiography can also be performed. To enhance filling of the vessels, spasms can be counteracted by the administration of tolazoline or phentolamine injected intra-arterially with immediate filming done. The extremity can be warmed with a heating pad combined with the injection to produce optimal vascular tone and blood flow for the best filming of hand angiography.
- After the catheter is removed, apply pressure on the puncture site for 5 to 10 minutes or longer until bleeding has stopped.

Evaluation

- Observe the puncture site for hematoma or hemorrhage.
- Assess neurological status and vital signs every hour for 4 hours, then every 4 hours until stable. Assess extremities for signs of ischemia caused by a catheter-induced thrombus.
- Observe for a delayed allergic reaction to the contrast dye.

■ Note test results in relation to other related tests and to the client's symptoms. Particularly note results of related tests.

Client/Caregiver Teaching

Pretest

■ Explain that the procedure is usually performed by an angiographer (radiologist) in the angiography room. Explain that the procedure will not be painful, but there may be moments of discomfort.
■ Inform client to withhold or reduce dosage of anticoagulants as ordered.
■ Inform the client that a warm flush may be felt when the dye is injected. The client may also experience an urge to cough, a flushed sensation, nausea, or a salty taste about 5 minutes after the injection.
■ Instruct the client to remain still to ensure clear pictures.

Posttest

■ Instruct client to maintain bedrest for 12 to 24 hours or as ordered.
■ Instruct client to apply ice as needed to the puncture site to relieve discomfort and edema.
■ Instruct client to drink fluids to prevent dehydration caused by the diuretic action of the dye, and resume food and medications withheld before the test.

Angiotensin-Converting Enzyme (ACE)

Classification: Serology

Type of Test: Serum

This test measures angiotensin-converting enzyme (ACE), which is found primarily in lung capillaries and, in lesser concentrations, in blood vessels and kidney tissue. ACE helps regulate arterial pressure by converting angiotensin I to angiotensin II, a powerful vasoconstrictor that stimulates the adrenal cortex to produce aldosterone. Elevated levels of ACE strongly correlated with pulmonary sarcoidosis reflect macrophage activity. Measurement of ACE is useful in evaluating the effectiveness of therapy and in confirming clinical status.

Indications

- Diagnose sarcoidosis, especially pulmonary
- Monitor response to sarcoidosis therapy
- Confirm Gaucher's disease or leprosy

Reference Values

Children	
< 1 yr	10.9–42.1 U/L
1–2 yr	9.4–36 U/L
3–4 yr	7.9–29.8 U/L
5–9 yr	9.6–35.4 U/L
10–12 yr	10–37 U/L
13–16 yr	9–33.4 U/L
17–19 yr	7.2–26.6 U/L
Adults > age 20	6.1–21.1 U/L

Abnormal Values

- Increased levels
    Cirrhosis (nonalcoholic)
    Gaucher's disease
    Histoplasmosis
    Hodgkin's disease
    Hyperthyroidism
    Leprosy
    Myeloma
    Non-Hodgkin's lymphoma
    Pulmonary embolus
    Pulmonary fibrosis (idiopathic)
    Sarcoidosis (active)
    Scleroderma
- Decreased levels
    Adult respiratory distress syndrome
    Coccidioidomycosis
    Diabetes mellitus
    Farmer's lung
    Hypothyroidism
    Severe illness
    Tuberculosis
    Drugs, including steroids

Interfering Factors

- Failure to fast before the test may cause significant lipemia, which may interfere with accurate test measurement.
- Failure to send sample to the laboratory immediately or to freeze it and place it on dry ice may cause enzyme degradation and yield artificially low ACE levels.

Nursing Implications

Assessment

- Obtain history of illness and symptoms, as well as current medication regimen.

Possible Nursing Diagnoses

Anxiety related to perceived threat to health status
Gas exchange, impaired, related to ventilation-perfusion imbalance

Implementation

- Put on gloves. Using aseptic technique, perform a venipuncture and collect 7 mL of blood in a clotted red-top or heparinized green-top tube.
- Handle sample gently to avoid hemolysis and send to the laboratory promptly.

Evaluation

- Note test results in relation to other related tests performed and to the client's symptoms.

Client/Caregiver Teaching

Pretest

- No fasting is required.

Anti-DNA Antibody

Classification: Immunology

Type of Test: Serum

This test measures the levels of the antibody to deoxyribonuclease (DNA) that correlate with disease activities. It is rarely found in individuals who do not have systemic lupus erythematosus (SLE) or related diseases but occurs in up to 80 percent of those who do. Levels can decrease with effective treatment of the disease.

Indications

- Diagnose and evaluate status of systemic lupus erythematosus (SLE) progression with increasing levels and remission with decreasing levels

Reference Values

Negative	<70 U
Borderline	70–200 U
Definite elevation	>25 U

Abnormal Values

- Increased levels
  - Systemic lupus erythematosus
  - Rheumatoid arthritis
  - Sclerosis (systemic)
  - SLE glomerulonephritis
  - Myasthenia gravis
  - Sjögren's syndrome

Interfering Factors

- Penicillin, procainamide, and hydralazine may cause a false-positive reaction.
- Scan using radioactive dye less than 1 week before the test can cause false results.

Nursing Implications

Assessment

- Obtain a history of known or suspected family history of autoimmune disorders and any drugs taken that affect the blood sample.

Possible Nursing Diagnoses

Anxiety related to perceived threat to health status

Physical mobility, impaired, related to neuromuscular/musculoskeletal impairment

Tissue perfusion, altered, peripheral, related to interruption of vascular flow

Implementation

- Put on gloves. Using aseptic technique, perform a venipuncture and collect 10 mL of blood in a red-, purple-, or gray-top tube, depending on laboratory.
- Handle sample gently and send to the laboratory promptly.

Evaluation

- Note test results in relation to the client's symptoms and to other test results.

Client/Caregiver Teaching

Pretest

- Instruct the client to withhold medications that interfere with test results, as ordered.

Posttest

- Instruct client to resume medications withheld before the test.

Anti-Insulin Antibody

Classification: Serology

Type of Test: Blood

This test detects insulin antibodies in the blood of a diabetic receiving insulin. The most common anti-insulin antibody is the immunoglobulin IgG, but IgA, IgM, IgD, and IgE have been reported. These antibodies usually do not cause clinical problems, but they may complicate insulin assay testing. It is thought that IgM immunoglobins participate in insulin resistance and IgE takes part in insulin allergy.

Indications

- Determine insulin allergy
- Confirm insulin resistance
- Determine if hypoglycemia is caused by insulin abuse

Reference Values

- Negative

Abnormal Values

- Elevated levels
  Insulin allergy or resistance
  Factitious hypoglycemia

Interfering Factors

- Radioactive tests within 1 week of the test may affect results.

Nursing Implications

Assessment

- Obtain history of endocrine system, known or suspected insulin allergy, medication regimen, diagnostic tests and results.

Possible Nursing Diagnosis

Anxiety related to perceived threat to health status

Implementation

- Put on gloves. Using aseptic technique, perform a venipuncture and collect 7 mL of blood in a red-top tube.

Evaluation

- If insulin antibodies are present, expect to perform C-peptide test. If this level is not increased, then endogenous insulin secretion has not increased.
- Monitor the client for signs of hyperglycemia and hypoglycemia.

Client/Caregiver Teaching

Pretest

- Inform the client that fasting is not required.

Posttest

- Reinforce instructions on medications and diabetes management.

Anti-Ro/Sjögren's Syndrome Antigen (SS-A)

Classification: Immunology

Type of Test: Blood

This immunodiffusion test diagnoses Sjögren's syndrome or Sjögren's with systemic lupus erthymatosus (SLE) by identifying the presense of anti-Ro/SS-A in blood. Anti-Ro/SS-A is an autoantibody to the RNA Ro antigen found in up to 70 percent of these patients and not present in the blood of persons without the disease.

Indications

- Diagnose systemic lupus erythematosus
- Diagnose Sjögren's syndrome
- Diagnose mixed connective tissue disorders

Reference Values

- Negative

Abnormal Values

- Positive levels
  Sjögren's syndrome
  Neonatal lupus
  ANA-negative SLE

Interfering Factors

- None

Nursing Implications

Assessment

- Obtain history of immune system, known or suspected connective tissue disorders, medication regimen, diagnostic tests and results.

Possible Nursing Diagnoses

Anxiety related to perceived threat to health status
Pain related to inflammatory process of connective tissues
Fatigue related to increased energy requirements and altered body chemistry

Implementation

- Put on gloves. Using aseptic technique perform a venipuncture and collect 7 mL of blood in a red-top tube.
- Send specimen to the laboratory immediately.

Evaluation

- Note results in relation to other related tests, particularly antinuclear antibodies.

Client/Caregiver Teaching

Pretest

- No fasting is required.

Antidiuretic Hormone (ADH)

Classification: Chemistry

Type of Test: Serum

This test is a quantitative analysis of antidiuretic hormone (ADH), also known as vasopressin. This hormone, which is formed by the hypothalamus and stored in the posterior pituitary gland, is released in response to increased serum osmolality or decreased blood volume. Although as little as a 1 percent change in serum osmolality will stimulate ADH secretion, blood volume must decrease by approximately 10 percent for ADH secretion to be induced. Psychogenic stimuli such as stress, pain, and anxiety may also stimulate ADH release, but the mechanism by which this occurs is unclear.

Indications

- Evaluate polyuria or altered serum osmolality of unknown etiology to identify possible alterations in ADH secretion as the cause
- Detect central nervous system trauma, surgery, or disease that may lead to impaired ADH secretion
- Differentiate neurogenic (central) diabetes insipidus from nephrogenic diabetes insipidus by decreased ADH levels in neurogenic diabetes insipidus or elevated levels in nephrogenic diabetes insipidus if normal feedback mechanisms are intact
- Diagnose known or suspected malignancy associated with syndrome of inappropriate ADH secretion (SIADH) such as oat cell lung cancer, thymoma, lymphoma, leukemia, and carcinoma of the pancreas, prostate gland, and intestine; the disorder is indicated by elevated ADH levels
- Diagnose known or suspected pulmonary conditions associated with SIADH, such as tuberculosis, pneumonia, and positive pressure mechanical ventilation; the disorder is indicated by elevated ADH levels

Reference Values

	SI Units
1.5 pg/mL	1.5 ng/L

Abnormal Values

- Increased ADH
  SIADH
  Disorders involving the central nervous system, thyroid gland, and adrenal gland
  Addison's disease
  Bronchogenic carcinoma
  Circulatory shock
  Cirrhosis of the liver
  Hypothyroidism
  Infectious hepatitis
  Severe hemorrhage
  Pain, stress, anxiety
  Drugs, including anesthetics, acetaminophen, carbamazepine, chlorothiazide, chlorpropamide, cyclophosphamide, estrogens, morphine sulfate, oxytocin citrate, oxytocin injection, barbiturates, cholinergic agents, clofibrate, nicotine, oral hypoglycemia agents, tricyclic antidepressants, thiazide diuretics, and cytotoxic agents
- Decreased ADH
  Pituitary diabetes insipidus
  Head trauma
  Metastatic cancer
  Neurohypophyseal or hypothalamic tumor
  Neurosurgical procedures
  Sarcoidosis
  Tuberculosis
  Syphilis
  Viral infection
  Drugs, including alcohol, phenytoin, beta-adrenergics, and morphine antagonists

Interfering Factors

- Drugs can lead to decreased or increased ADH secretion (See Abnormal Values).
- Pain, stress, and anxiety can lead to increased ADH secretion.

- Failure to follow dietary and exercise restrictions before the test can alter results.
- Failure to begin testing within 10 minutes of collection can result in inaccurate values.

Nursing Implications

Assessment

- Obtain history of endocrine system, infection, inflammation, and fluid imbalance.
- Assess medication history; ensure that any drugs that may alter test results have been withheld for 12 to 24 hours before the test, as ordered by the physician.
- Ensure that the client has not eaten and has avoided strenuous exercise for 12 hours before the test.

Possible Nursing Diagnoses

Anxiety related to perceived threat to health status
Fluid volume deficit related to failure of regulatory mechanisms
Pain related to inflammation or swelling of the liver

Implementation

- Put on gloves. Using aseptic technique, perform a venipuncture and collect 5 mL of blood in a plastic red-top tube. Plastic is used because contact with glass degrades presence of ADH.
- Handle the sample gently to avoid hemolysis and transport sample to the laboratory immediately.

Evaluation

- Note test results in relation to other tests performed and to the client's symptoms.

Client/Caregiver Teaching

Pretest

- Instruct the client to withhold any drugs that may alter test results for 12 to 24 hours before the test, as ordered by the physician.
- Instruct the client not to eat and to avoid strenuous exercise for 12 hours before the test.

Posttest

- Instruct the client to resume diet, activity, and medications withheld before the test.
- Instruct the client and caregiver to report changes in urinary output and urine characteristics to the physician.

Antinuclear Antibody (ANA)

Classification: Immunology (autoimmune)

Type of Test: Serum

This test measures titers of the antibodies that the body produces against DNA and nuclear material responsible for collagen vascular or immune-complex diseases. It has a high sensitivity for the diagnosis of systemic lupus erythematosus (SLE), and it is often used to screen for it.

Indications

- Diagnose SLE, as evidenced by a 95 percent sensitivity
- Evaluate suspected immune disorders such as rheumatoid arthritis, systemic sclerosis, polymyositis, Sjögren's syndrome, and mixed connective-tissue disease, as indicated by a 30 to 50 percent sensitivity

Reference Values

- Antinuclear antibodies (ANA) negative at <1:20 dilution

Abnormal Values

- Positive values
    Asbestosis
    Burns
    Dermatomyositis
    Hepatitis (chronic)
    Mixed connective-tissue disease
    Myasthenia gravis
    Polyarteritis nodosa
    Polymyositis
    Pulmonary fibrosis (idiopathic)
    Rheumatoid fever
    Rheumatoid arthritis
    Scleroderma
    Systemic lupus erythematosus (SLE)
    Sjögren's syndrome

Drugs such as acetazolamide, chlorothiazide, carbamaz-epine, ethosuximide, hydralazine, methyldopa, oral contraceptives, phenytoin, quinidine, reserpine, strep-tomycin, sulfonamides, tetracyclines, thiouracil, and tri-methadione, which can cause false-positive results due to a drug-induced SLE-syndrome

- Negative values
    Drugs such as corticosteroids, which can cause false-neg-ative results

Interfering Factors

- Hemolyzed blood sample will alter test results.
- False results can be obtained if client is receiving certain drugs (see Abnormal Values).

Nursing Implications

Assessment

- Obtain a family history of known or suspected autoimmune disorders.
- Ensure that the client has fasted for 8 hours before testing.
- Note drug therapy on the lab requisition.

Possible Nursing Diagnoses

Anxiety related to perceived threat to health status
Pain related to inflammatory process of connective tissues
Fatigue related to increased energy requirements and altered body chemistry
Physical mobility, impaired, related to musculoskeletal impairment

Implementation

- Put on gloves. Using aseptic technique, perform a venipunc-ture and collect 10 mL of blood in a red-top tube.
- Handle sample gently to avoid hemolysis and send to the laboratory promptly.

Evaluation

- Note test results in relation to lupus erythematosus cell test (LE prep), anti-DNA antibodies, and other studies performed and the client's symptoms.

Client/Caregiver Teaching

Pretest

- Instruct client to fast for 8 hours before test and to avoid drugs that may interfere with test results, as ordered.

Posttest

■ Tell the client to resume food and fluid intake and medications withheld before the test.

Antistreptolysin O Titer

Classification: Serology

Type of Test: Blood

Group A β-hemolytic streptococci secretes enzyme streptolysin O, which can destroy red blood cells. It acts as an antigen and stimulates the immune system to develop antistreptolysin O antibodies. These antibodies occur within 1 month after the onset of a streptococcal infection. Detection of the antibody over several weeks strongly suggests exposure to the organisms.

Indications

■ Confirm diagnosis of streptococcal infection
■ Monitor response to therapy in streptococcal illnesses
■ Differentiate between rheumatic fever and rheumatoid arthritis

Reference Values

Preschool children	<85 Todd U/mL
School-age children	<170 Todd U/mL
Adults	<85 Todd U/mL

Abnormal Values

■ Elevated levels
   Acute rheumatic fever caused by streptococcus infection
   Acute glomerulonephritis caused by streptococcus infection
   Acute poststreptococcal endocarditis

Interfering Factors

- Antibiotics and corticosteroid therapy may cause falsely decreased levels, since antibody response will be suppressed
- Elevated blood β-lipoproteins may result in falsely elevated levels

Nursing Implications

Assessment

- Obtain history of known or suspected exposure to streptococcal infections, joint or renal disease, medication regimen, and diagnostic tests and results.

Possible Nursing Diagnoses

Anxiety related to perceived threat to health status

Pain related to inflammatory process of connective tissues

Physical mobility, impaired, related to musculoskeletal impairment

Fluid volume excess related to failure of regulatory mechanisms

Implementation

- Put on gloves. Using aseptic technique, perform a venipuncture and collect 5 mL of blood in a red-top tube.
- Handle specimen gently to avoid hemolysis. Repeat the test in 10 days as indicated.

Evaluation

- Note test results in relation to other immunologic tests and clinical symptoms.

Client/Caregiver Teaching

Pretest

- No fasting is required.

Posttest

- Instruct client that repeat testing may be necessary to monitor response to therapy.

Antithrombin, Antithrombin III (AT-III)

Classification: Chemistry

Type of Test: Serum, Plasma

Antithrombin, formerly known as antithrombin III and heparin cofactor, is a naturally occurring protein that limits or restricts coagulation by inactivating thrombin (factor II) and other factors (X, XI, XII). Normally, antithrombin and thrombin achieve a balance that maintains hemostasis.

This test can be performed by functional assay, which determines antithrombin activity, and by immunologic assay, which measures antithrombin molecules using the antibody against antithrombin.

Indications

- Determine the cause of impaired coagulation, especially hypercoagulation
- Aid in the management of disseminated intravascular coagulation (DIC) or venous thrombotic disease

Reference Values

		SI Values
Plasma	>50% of control value	
Serum	15–35% lower than plasma values	
Immunologic method	20–30 mg/dL	200–300 mg/L
Functional method	80–120 mg/dL	800–1200 μ/L

Abnormal Values

- Increased levels
  Factor deficiency (V, VII)
  Hemophilia (A, B)
  Renal transplant
  Drugs, including anabolic steroids, androgens, bishydroxy-coumarin, oral contraceptives (containing progesterone), progesterone, and warfarin sodium

■ Decreased levels
    Arteriosclerosis
    Cardiovascular disease
    Cerebrovascular accident
    Cirrhosis
    Congenital deficiency
    Deep-vein thrombosis
    Disseminated intravascular coagulation
    Hepatic disease
    Hypercoagulation
    Malnutrition
    Nephrotic syndrome
    Postoperative condition
    Postpartum condition
    Pulmonary embolism
    Thromboembolism
    Drugs, including fibrinolytics, heparin calcium, heparin sodium, L-asparaginase, and estrogen-containing oral contraceptives

Interfering Factors

■ Hemolysis of specimens will affect results.

Nursing Implications

Assessment

■ Obtain history of known or suspected hemostatic dysfunction and medication regimen, especially anticoagulants, and other laboratory results, particularly factor assay.
■ Ensure client has not eaten for 10 to 12 hours before obtaining blood specimen.

Possible Nursing Diagnoses

Anxiety related to perceived threat to health status
Injury, risk for, related to altered clotting factors
Protection, altered, related to abnormal blood profiles
Pain related to altered tissue perfusion

Implementation

■ Put on gloves. Using aseptic technique, perform a venipuncture and collect 5 mL of blood in a red- or blue-top tube.
■ Handle sample gently to avoid hemolysis and send to the laboratory promptly.

Evaluation

■ Note test results in relation to other coagulation test results.

Client/Caregiver Teaching

Pretest

- Inform the client to fast (except for water) for 10 to 12 hours before the test.
- Tell the client to withhold medications that can interfere with test results, if ordered.

Posttest

- Tell the client to resume food and medications withheld before the test.
- Advise the client to report bleeding to the physician, if appropriate.

▲▲▲▲▲▲▲▲▲▲▲▲▲▲▲▲▲▲▲

Apolipoprotein A-1 (Apo A-1), Apoprotein-A (APO-A)

Classification: Chemistry

Type of Test: Plasma

This test measures apolipoprotein, which is the major protein component (70 percent) of high-density lipoprotein (HDL). It is essential for the transport of cholesterol for excretion by the liver and is synthesized in the liver and small intestine. The ratio of Apo A-1 to Apo B is considered to be a better determinant of the risk of coronary artery disease (CAD) from atherosclerosis than lipid or lipoprotein analyses.

Indications

- Identify those at risk for atherosclerosis and predict risk of coronary artery disease by determining the ratio of Apo A-1 to Apo B

Reference Values

		Ratio of A-1 to B
Women	94–172 mg/dL	0.76:3.23
Men	90–155 mg/dL	0.85:2.24

Abnormal Values

- Decreased level
  Myocardial infarction
  Coronary artery disease
  Angina pectoris

Interfering Factors

- Acute illness can cause false elevations.
- Alcohol ingestion within 24 hours of the test can alter test results.
- Specimen hemolysis can cause inaccurate results.

Nursing Implications

Assessment

- Obtain history of cardiac status, medication regimen, and laboratory test results.
- Ensure that the client has fasted for 12 to 14 hours and abstained from alcohol for 24 hours before the test.

Possible Nursing Diagnoses

Anxiety related to perceived threat to health status
Pain related to myocardial ischemia
Tissue perfusion, altered, cardiopulmonary, related to interruption of blood flow

Implementation

- Put on gloves. Using aseptic technique, perform a venipuncture and collect 7 mL of blood in a lavender-top tube containing EDTA.
- Handle sample gently to avoid hemolysis and send to the laboratory promptly.

Evaluation

- Note results in relation to the lipid panel and individual lipid tests, if performed.

Client/Caregiver Teaching

Pretest

- Tell the client to fast for 12 to 14 hours before the test.
- Tell the client to abstain from alcohol for 24 hours before the test.

Posttest

- Instruct the client to resume diet withheld before the test.

Apolipoprotein B, Plasma (Apo B), Apoprotein-B (APO-B)

Classification: Chemistry

Type of Test: Plasma

This test measures apolipoprotein B, which functions in cholesterol synthesis and is required for the secretion into plasma of intestinal and hepatic triglyceride-rich lipoproteins. A beta globulin, apolipoprotein B is the major protein component of low-density lipoprotein (LDL) and is also found in very low density lipoprotein (VLDL). The ratio of Apo A-1 to Apo B is thought to be more useful than LDL cholesterol for identifying persons at risk for coronary artery disease from atherosclerosis.

Indications

- Identify persons at risk for atherosclerosis and predict coronary heart disease by determining the ratio of apolipoprotein A-1 to apolipoprotein B

Reference Values

		Ratio of A-1 to B
Women	55–100 mg/dL	0.76:3.23
Men	45–110 mg/dL	0.85:2.24

Abnormal Values

- Increased levels
    Acute illness
    Angina pectoris
    Hyperlipemia (familial combined)
    Coronary artery disease
    Myocardial infarction

Interfering Factors

- Hemolyzed or lipemic specimens will affect results.
- Acute illness can falsely increase levels.
- Alcohol ingestion within 24 hours before the test can alter test results.

Nursing Implications

Assessment

- Assess client's health history, medication regimen, and laboratory test results.
- Ensure that the client has fasted for 12 to 14 hours and abstained from alcohol consumption for 24 hours before the test.

Possible Nursing Diagnoses

Anxiety related to perceived threat to health status
Pain related to myocardial ischemia or acute illness
Tissue perfusion, altered, cardiopulmonary, related to interruption of blood flow

Implementation

- Put on gloves. Using aseptic technique, perform a venipuncture and collect 7 mL blood in a lavender-top tube containing EDTA.
- Handle sample gently to avoid hemolysis and send to the laboratory promptly.

Evaluation

- Note test results in relation to the lipid panel and individual lipid tests, if performed. Also, calculate the ratio of Apo A-l to Apo B.

Client/Caregiver Teaching

Pretest

- Inform the client to fast for 12 to 14 hours before the test.
- Inform the client to abstain from alcohol for 24 hours before the test.

Posttest

- Inform the client to resume diet withheld before the test.

Arthrocentesis and Synovial Fluid Analysis

Classification: Hematology, microbiology
Chemistry, cytology

Type of Test: Synovial fluid analysis

Arthrocentesis is an invasive procedure involving insertion of a needle into the joint space. It is performed to remove synovial fluid secreted in small amounts ($\leq$3 mL) into the cavities of most joints. Synovial effusions are associated with disorders or injuries involving the joints. Samples for analysis are obtained by aspirating the fluid. The most commonly aspirated joint is the knee, although samples also can be obtained from the shoulder, hip, elbow, wrist, and ankle, if clinically indicated. Hematologic, cytologic, microbiologic, and chemistry examinations of the effusion are performed for complete analysis.

Indications

- Detect joint effusion
- Diagnose trauma, joint tumors, or hemophilic arthritis as indicated by an elevated red blood cell (RBC) count, elevated protein level, and possibly fat droplets if trauma is involved
- Diagnose joint effusion due to noninflammatory disorders, for example, osteoarthritis, degenerative joint disease as indicated by a white blood cell (WBC) count of <5,000/mm^3 with a normal differential and the presence of cartilage cells
- Diagnose rheumatoid arthritis as indicated by a white blood cell count of 2,000 to 100,000/mm^3 with an elevated neutrophil count (30 to 50 percent), presence of RA cells and possibly Rice bodies, cholesterol crystals if effusion is chronic, elevated protein level, decreased glucose level, moderately elevated lactate level (2 to 7.5 mmol/L), decreased pH, presence of rheumatoid factor (60 percent of cases), and decreased complement
- Diagnose systemic lupus erythematosus involving the joints as indicated by a white blood cell count of 2,000 to 100,000/mm^3 with an elevated neutrophil count (30 to 40 percent), presence of LE cells, elevated protein level, decreased glucose level (2 to 7.5 mmol/L), decreased pH, presence of an-

tinuclear antibodies (20 percent of cases), and decreased complement

- Diagnose acute bacterial arthritis as indicated by a white blood cell count of 10,000 to 200,000/mm^3 with a markedly elevated neutrophil count (as high as 90 percent), positive Gram stain (50 percent of cases), positive cultures (30 to 80 percent of cases), possibly presence of Rice bodies, decreased glucose, lactate level >7.5 mmol/L, pH <7.3, and complement levels paralleling those found in serum (may be elevated or decreased)

- Diagnose tuberculous arthritis as indicated by a white blood cell count of 2,000 to 100,000/mm^3 with an elevated neutrophil count (30 to 60 percent), possibly presence of Rice bodies, cholesterol crystals if effusion is chronic, positive AFB smear and culture in some cases (results are frequently negative), decreased glucose, elevated lactate levels, and decreased pH

- Diagnose joint effusion due to gout as indicated by a white blood cell count of 500 to 200,000/mm^3 with an elevated neutrophil count (approximately 70 percent), presence of MSU crystals, decreased glucose, elevated uric acid levels, and complement levels paralleling those of serum (may be elevated or decreased)

- Differentiate gout from pseudogout as indicated primarily by finding CPP crystals, which are associated with pseudogout (white blood cell count may not be as high)

Reference Values

Color	Colorless to pale yellow
Clarity	Clear
Viscosity	High
Red blood cells	None
White blood cells	<200/mm^3
Neutrophils	<25 percent
White cell morphology	No abnormal cells or inclusions
Crystals	None present
Gram stain and culture	No organisms present
AFB smear and culture	No acid-fast bacilli present
Protein	<3 g/dL
Glucose	<10 mg/dL of blood level
Uric acid	Parallels serum level
Lactate	5–20 mg/dL
pH	7.2–7.4
Antinuclear antibodies (ANA)	Parallel serum levels
Rheumatoid factor (RF)	Parallel serum levels
Complement	Parallel serum levels

Abnormal Values

- Trauma
- Joint tumors
- Hemophilic arthritis
- Osteoarthritis
- Degenerative joint disease
- Rheumatoid arthritis
- Lupus erythematosus
- Bacterial arthritis
- Tuberculous arthritis
- Gout

Interfering Factors

- Blood in the sample from traumatic arthrocentesis.
- Undetected hypoglycemia or hyperglycemia and/or failure to comply with dietary restrictions before the test.
- Contamination of the sample with pathogens.
- Improper handling of the specimen: refrigeration of the sample may result in an increase in monosodium urate (MS) crystals due to decreased solubility of uric acid; exposure of the sample to room air with a resultant loss of carbon dioxide and rise in pH encourages the formation of calcium pyrophosphate (CPP) crystals.

Nursing Implications

Assessment

- Obtain history of joint discomfort, pain, or other pertinent history. Assess history of hypersensitivity to iodine compounds and local anesthetics, abnormalities in laboratory results, and diagnostic findings.
- Ensure that anticoagulant medications and aspirin have been held, as ordered.
- Ensure that client has fasted for 6 to 12 hours before the procedure if glucose testing is to be done.

Possible Nursing Diagnoses

Anxiety related to perceived threat to health status

Physical mobility, impaired, related to musculoskeletal impairment

Pain related to joint inflammation, degeneration, or deformity

Implementation

- If client is extremely hirsute, shave area where the puncture is to be made.

- Assemble the necessary equipment, including an arthrocentesis tray with solution for skin preparation, local anesthetic, a 20-mL syringe, needles of various sizes, sterile drapes, sterile gloves, and specimen collection tubes and containers for the tests to be performed. For cell counts and differential, lavender-top tubes containing ethylenediaminetetraacetate (EDTA) are used. Green-top tubes containing heparin are used for certain immunological and chemistry tests. Samples for glucose are collected in either plain red-top tubes or gray-top tubes containing potassium oxalate. Plain sterile red-top tubes are recommended for microbiological testing and crystal examination.
- Help the client to the sitting or supine position, whichever will be used for the test, and instruct the client to remain still during the procedure. The skin or the injection site is cleansed with antiseptic solution using sterile technique, protected with sterile drapes, and infiltrated with local anesthetic that can cause a stinging sensation. Inform the client that some pain may be experienced as the aspirating needle is inserted into the joint space and as fluid is withdrawn.
- The physician inserts the needle and obtains at least 10 mL of synovial fluid for analysis. More fluid may be removed to reduce swelling. Manual pressure may be applied to facilitate fluid removal.
- If medication is to be injected into the joint, the syringe containing the sample is detached from the needle and replaced with the one containing the drug. The medication is injected with gentle pressure. The needle is then withdrawn and digital pressure is applied to the site for a few minutes. If there is no evidence of bleeding, a sterile dressing is applied to the site. An elastic bandage can be applied to the joint.
- Place samples of synovial fluid in the appropriate containers, label, and send to the laboratory immediately. Record any antibiotic therapy on the laboratory slip if bacterial culture and sensitivity tests are to be performed.

Evaluation

- Note results in relation to client's symptoms and other tests performed.
- Assess puncture site for bleeding, bruising, inflammation, and excessive drainage of synovial fluid approximately every 4 hours for 24 hours and daily thereafter for several days.

Client/Caregiver Teaching

Pretest

- Inform the client that the procedure is performed to remove fluid from around the joint and sent to the laboratory for analysis. It is performed by a specialized physician (possibly an orthopedic surgeon) and can take approximately 20 minutes to complete.

Posttest

- Tell the client to apply an ice pack to the site for 24 to 48 hours and administer ordered analgesics as needed.
- Instruct the client to avoid excessive use of the joint for several days to prevent pain and swelling.
- Instruct the client to report excessive pain, bleeding, or swelling to the physician immediately and to return for a follow-up visit as scheduled.
- Instruct the client or caregiver to handle linen and dispose of dressings cautiously, especially in suspected septic arthritis.

Arylsulfatase A (ARS-A), Urine

Classification: Urinalysis

Type of Test: Urine (timed)

A test to measure arylsulfatase-A, a lysosomal enzyme found in all body cells except red blood cells and acting primarily in the pancreas and liver, where it is responsible for detoxifying exogenous substances into ester sulfates. It is excreted into the urine following glomerular filtration. It rises in certain cancers.

Indications

- Confirm the presence of suspected bladder, colon, or rectal cancers
- Confirm suspected granulocytic leukemia

- Determine the presence of lipid storage diseases, such as mucolipidosis II and III, in those with a family history of the disease
- Determine the presence of metachromatic leukodystrophy

Reference Values

Children	>1 U/L
Men	1.4–19.3 U/L
Women	1.4–11 U/L

Abnormal Values

- Elevated levels
    Bladder cancer
    Colon or rectal cancer
    Granulocytic leukemia
    Genetic lyposomal disorder
- Decreased levels
    Metachromatic leukodystrophy

Interfering Factors

- Contamination of sample with blood, mucus, or feces may falsely elevate levels
- Abdominal surgery within 1 week of collection may falsely elevate levels.

Nursing Implications

Assessment

- Obtain history of known or suspected pancreatic biliary disease, medications, and treatments and diagnostic tests, procedures, and results.
- If the female client is menstruating, reschedule the test.
- Ensure proper fluid intake before and during test to promote hydration and specimen collection.

Possible Nursing Diagnoses

Anxiety related to perceived threat to health status
Infection, risk for, related to inadequate secondary defenses

Implementation

- Obtain containers of appropriate size without preservatives for a 2-, 6-, 8-, 12-, or 24-hour period. The sample must be kept refrigerated or on ice throughout the collection period unless the laboratory has added a preservative to the container.

- If an indwelling catheter is in place, replace tubing and container system at start of collection time, clamp catheter tubing until next specimen is due, unless 24-hour specimen is to be collected; place drainage bag on ice; monitor to ensure continued drainage.
- At the conclusion of the test, label the container(s) properly with start and completion collection times and transport to the laboratory promptly.

Evaluation

- Note test results in relation to serum amylase.

Client/Caregiver Teaching

Pretest

- Instruct client to avoid excessive exercise and stress during the collection of urine and withhold medications that affect test results, as ordered.
- Inform the client that the sample must be kept refrigerated or on ice throughout the collection period unless the laboratory has added a preservative to the container.
- Instruct the client to void all urine in a urinal or bedpan placed in the toilet for a specific time period and then either pour urine into the collection container or leave in the container for the nurse to add to the collection; instruct client to avoid voiding in pan with defecation and to keep toilet tissue out of pan to prevent contamination of the specimen.

Posttest

- Tell the client to resume medications and activity withheld before the test.
- Inform the client that test results take 2 days to report.

Aspartate Aminotransferase (AST), Glutamic-Oxaloacetic Transaminase (SGOT)

Classification: Chemistry (enzyme)

Type of Test: Serum

Formerly known as serum glutamic-oxaloacetic transaminase (SGOT), the aspartate aminotransferase (AST) test measures the level of the enzyme that catalyzes the reversible transfer of an amino between the amino acid, aspartate, and alphaketo-glutamic acid. AST exists in large amounts in both liver and myocardial cells and in smaller but significant amounts in skeletal muscles, kidneys, the pancreas, and the brain. Serum AST rises when there is cellular damage to the tissues in which the enzyme is found.

Indications

- Diagnose disorders or injuries involving the liver, myocardium, kidneys, pancreas, or brain: elevated levels indicating cellular damage to tissues in which AST is normally found.
- Diagnose myocardial infarction (MI): AST rises within 6 to 8 hours, peaks at 24 to 48 hours, and declines to normal within 72 to 96 hours
- Monitor response to therapy with potentially hepatotoxic or nephrotoxic drugs
- Monitor response to treatment for various disorders in which AST may be elevated, with tissue repair indicated by declining levels
- Compare serially with alanine aminotransferase (ALT) levels to track the course of hepatitis.

Reference Values

		SI Units
Newborns	16–72 U/L	16–72 U/L
Children		
6 mon	20–43 U/L	20–43 U/L
1 yr	16–35 U/L	16–35 U/L
5 yr	19–28 U/L	19–28 U/L
Adults		
Men	8–26 U/L	8–26 U/L
Women	8–20 U/L	8–20 U/L

Abnormal Values

- Pronounced elevation ($\geq$5 × normal)
    - Acute hepatocellular damage
    - Myocardial infarction
    - Shock
    - Acute pancreatitis
    - Infectious mononucleosis
- Moderate elevation (3–5 × normal)
    - Biliary tract obstruction
    - Cardiac arrhythmias
    - Congestive heart failure
    - Liver tumors
    - Chronic hepatitis
    - Muscular dystrophy
    - Dermatomyositis
- Slight elevation (2 to 3 × normal)
    - Pericarditis
    - Cirrhosis, fatty liver
    - Pulmonary infarction
    - Delirium tremens
    - Cerebrovascular accident
    - Hemolytic anemia

Interfering Factors

- Numerous drugs may falsely elevate levels, especially those known to be hepatotoxic or nephrotoxic. These may include antitubercular drugs, chlorpropamide, codeine, meperidine, methyldopa, morphine, phenazopyridine, acetaminophen in large doses, dicumarol, erythromycin, pyridoxine, salicylates, sulfonamides, vitamin A, and many others.

Nursing Implications

Assessment

- Obtain a history of systems affected by increases in this enzyme and known or suspected disorders.
- Ensure that medications that may alter test results have been withheld for 12 hours before the test.

Possible Nursing Diagnoses

Anxiety related to perceived threat to health status
Pain related to tissue ischemia or inflammation

Implementation

- Put on gloves. Using aseptic technique, perform a venipuncture and collect 7 mL of blood in a red-top tube.
- Handle the sample gently to avoid hemolysis and transport to the laboratory promptly. If repeated samples are needed, draw samples at the same time each day.

Evaluation

- Note results in relation to other tests performed, in particular the alanine aminotransferase (ALT) test if liver disease is suspected and creatine kinase (CPK) and lactic dehydrogenase (LDH) if myocardial infarction is suspected.

Client/Caregiver Teaching

Posttest

- Tell the client to resume medication withheld before the test.
- Instruct the client to report chest pain and changes in breathing pattern to the physician immediately.
- Instruct the client in dietary restrictions and inclusions ordered for cardiac or hepatic disorders.

Atrial Natriuretic Hormone (ANH), Atrial Natriuretic Factor (ANF)

Classification: Chemistry (hormone)

Type of Test: Plasma

This test measures atrial natriuretic factor, which is secreted from the cardiac atrium when expanded blood volume stretches the atrial tissue. This extremely potent hormone enhances salt and water excretions. It blocks aldosterone and resin secretion, angiotensin II, and vasopressin, resulting in a decrease in blood pressure and blood volume.

Indications

- Confirm congestive heart failure (CHF), as indicated by increased level
- Identify asymptomatic cardiac volume overload, as indicated by increased level

Reference Values

	SI Units
20–77 pg/mL	20–77 ng/L

Abnormal Values

- Increased levels
  Congestive heart failure
  Elevated cardiac filling pressure
  Paroxysmal atrial tachycardia
  Cardiac volume overload

Interfering Factors

- Drugs such as beta-blocking agents, calcium antagonists, cardiac glycosides, diuretics, and vasodilators can affect results.

Nursing Implications

Assessment

- Obtain history of cardiovascular condition and any current medications, especially those that can interfere with test results.
- Ensure that these medications have been withheld for 24 hours and that the client has fasted for 12 hours before obtaining blood sample, as ordered.

Possible Nursing Diagnoses

Anxiety related to perceived threat to health status

Tissue perfusion, altered, cardiopulmonary, related to ventilation-perfusion imbalance

Cardiac output, decreased, related to altered muscle contractility

Fluid volume excess related to reduced glomerular filtration rate

Implementation

- Put on gloves. Using aseptic technique, perform a venipuncture and collect the blood in a prechilled, purple-top tube.
- Handle sample gently to avoid hemolysis. Place on ice and send to the laboratory promptly for analysis.

Evaluation

- Note test results in relation to the client's symptoms and other related test results.

Client/Caregiver Teaching

Pretest

- Instruct the client to fast for 12 hours before the test and to withhold medications that interfere with test results, as ordered.

Posttest

- Inform the client to resume diet and medications withheld before the test.

Audiometry, Hearing Loss

Classification: Sensory organ function

Type of Test: Auditory perception

Hearing loss audiometry involves the quantitative testing for a hearing deficit using an electronic instrument called an audiometer that measures and records thresholds of hearing by air conduction and bone conduction tests. These results determine if the hearing loss is conductive, sensorineural, or a composite of both. An elevated air-conduction threshold with a normal bone-conduction threshold indicates a conductive hearing loss. An equally elevated threshold for both air and bone conduction indicates a sensorineural hearing loss. An elevated threshold of air conduction that is more than an elevated threshold of bone conduction indicates a composite of both types of hearing loss. A conductive hearing loss is caused by an abnormality in the external auditory canal or middle ear, a sensorineural hearing loss by an abnormality in the inner ear or of the VIII (auditory) nerve. Sensorineural hearing loss can be further differentiated clinically by sensory (cochlear) or neural (VIII nerve) lesions. Comparing and differentiating between conductive and sensorineural hearing loss can further be evaluated by performing hearing loss tuning-fork tests.

Indications

- Screen for hearing loss in infants and children and determine the need for a referral to an audiologist
- Determine the type and extent of hearing loss (conductive, as evidenced by a reduced air threshold and unchanged bone threshold, or sensorineural, as evidenced by a reduced air and bone threshold, or mixed, as evidenced by abnormal air and bone thresholds) and if further radiologic, audiologic, or vestibular procedures are needed to identify the cause
- Evaluate degree and extent of preoperative and postoperative hearing loss following stapedectomy in clients with otosclerosis
- Evaluate communication disabilities and plan for rehabilitation interventions

■ Determine the need for and type of hearing aid and evaluate its effectiveness

Reference Values

■ Normal pure tone average of 0–25 decibels (dB) for adults and 0–15 dB for children
■ Ability to detect 1 dB of increased intensity or loudness with the area of intelligible speech sounds anywhere between 0–70 dB

Abnormal Values

	Elevated Pure Tone Values
Mild loss	26–40 dB
Moderate loss	41–55 dB
Moderately severe loss	56–70 dB
Severe loss	71–90 dB
Profound loss	>91 dB

■ Causes of conductive hearing loss
    Otosclerosis
    Otitis media
    Obstruction of external canal
    Otitis externa
■ Causes of sensorineural hearing loss
    Congenital damage or malformations of the inner ear
    Tumor
    Trauma to the inner ear
    Vascular disorders
    Ototoxic drugs
    Serious infections

Interfering Factors

■ Obstruction of the ear canal by cerumen or other material or object will affect dB perception.
■ Noisy environment or extraneous movements can affect results.
■ Tinnitus or other sensations can cause abnormal responses.
■ Improper earphone fit or audiometer calibration can affect results.

■ Inability or refusal to cooperate or follow instructions can produce invalid responses.

Nursing Implications

Assessment

■ Obtain a history of known or suspected hearing loss and cause; use of a hearing aid; complaints of changes in auditory acuity; past auditory acuity testing, procedures, and results; and age of client.
■ Ensure that the external auditory canal is clear of impacted cerumen.
■ Ensure that client has been in an environment free of extremely loud noises for 16 hours before the test.

Possible Nursing Diagnoses

Anxiety related to perceived threat to health status
Sensory-perceptual alteration, auditory, related to altered sensory reception, transmission, or integration
Communication, impaired, verbal, related to hearing loss

Implementation

■ Perform otoscopy examination to ensure that the external ear canal is clear of any obstruction.
■ Test for closure of the canal by the pressure of earphones by compressing the tragus. Tendency for the canal to close (often the case in children and elderly clients) can be corrected by the careful insertion of a small stiff plastic tube into the anterior canal.
■ Place client in a sitting position in comfortable proximity to the audiometer in a soundproof room. The ear not being tested is masked to prevent crossover of test tones, and the earphones are positioned on the head and over the ear canals.
■ Start the test by providing a trial tone of 15 to 20 dB above the expected threshold to an ear for 1 second to familiarize the client with the sounds. Instruct the client to press the button each time a tone is heard, no matter how loudly or faintly it is perceived. The test results are plotted on a graph called an audiogram using symbols that indicate the ear tested and responses using earphones (air conduction) or oscillator (bone conduction).
■ *Air conduction:* Air conduction is tested first by starting at 1000 Hz and gradually decreasing the intensity 10 dB at a time until the client no longer presses the button, indicating that the tone is no longer heard. The intensity is then in-

creased 5 dB at a time until the tone is heard again. This is repeated until the same response is achieved two out of three times at the same level. The threshold is derived from the lowest decibel level that achieves a 50 percent response rate. The test is continued for each ear, testing the better ear first, with tones delivered at 1000 Hz, 2000 Hz, 4000 Hz, 8000 Hz, and again at 1000 Hz, 500 Hz, 250 Hz to determine a second threshold. Results are recorded on a graph called an audiogram. Averaging the air-conduction thresholds at the 500 Hz, 1000 Hz, and 2000 Hz levels reveals the degree of hearing loss.

- *Bone conduction:* Bone conduction is then tested using an oscillator placed on the mastoid process behind the ear(s) after removal of the earphones. The raised and lowered tones are delivered as in air conduction using 250 Hz, 500 Hz, 1000 Hz, 2000 Hz, and 4000 Hz to determine the thresholds. An analysis of threshold responses for air and bone conduction tones is done to determine the type of hearing loss (conductive, sensorineural, or mixed).
- A simpler test of hearing can be performed without the use of an audiometer, but it is not as accurate or comprehensive in determining the type and extent of hearing loss. It involves the use of a ticking watch or whispering at a specific distance from each ear. The ear not being tested is occluded with a finger and the tester stands at 15 feet from the client and whispers or speaks words toward the ear to be tested. If this is not heard, the tester moves closer to 10 or 5 feet from the client. The second ear is then tested in the same manner. The results are recorded as 15/15, 10/15, and so forth. The test using a ticking watch is similar, except that the watch is held next to the ear and moved away from the ear 1 foot at a time until the ticking is no longer heard. The test is repeated for the second ear and the results recorded at the distance when ticking is no longer heard.
- In the child between 6 months and 2 years of age, minimal response levels can be determined by behavioral responses to test tones. In the child 2 years of age and older, play audiometry that requires the child to perform a task or raise a hand in response to a specific tone is performed. In children 12 years of age and older, the child is asked to follow directions in identifying objects; response to speech of specific intensities can be used to evaluate hearing loss that is affected by speech frequencies.

Evaluation

- Note test results in relation to the client's symptoms.

Client/Caregiver Teaching

Pretest

- Inform the client and caregiver that the procedure is performed in a quiet room by the nurse or audiologist and will take about 20 minutes or less to complete, depending on the test. There is no pain associated with this procedure.
- Inform the client that there are no special restrictions required before the test.

Posttest

- Inform client or caregiver of the schedule for retesting and instruction in the use, cleansing, and storing of a hearing aid if one is used.
- Reinforce information given by audiologist and referral to a physician for further testing, treatment, or correction of hearing deficit.

Australia Antigen, Hepatitis B Surface Antigen

Classification: Serology

Type of Test: Serum

Hepatitis B antigen (HBsAg) is the earliest indicator of active infection, usually appearing within 4 to 12 weeks of infection or if the client is a carrier. It is the most frequent and easily performed test for diagnosing hepatitis B. Levels of the antigen rise before the onset of clinical symptoms and return to normal by the time jaundice disappears.

Indications

- Diagnose active hepatitis B, acute or chronic
- Screen blood donors or those at high risk
- Identify carriers of the disease; levels are persistently elevated

Reference Values

- Negative

Abnormal Values

- Elevated levels
  Hepatitis B
  Hemophilia
  Leukemia
  Hodgkin's disease
  Chronic hepatitis carrier

Interfering Factors

- Injection of radionucleotides within past week may falsely elevate results.

Nursing Implications

Assessment

- Obtain history of hepatobiliary system, known or suspected exposure to hepatitis, medication regimen, and diagnostic tests and results.
- Ensure that the client has not received radionucleotides within the past week.

Possible Nursing Diagnoses

Anxiety related to perceived threat to health status
Pain related to inflammation or swelling of the liver
Infection, risk for, related to immunosuppressed inflammatory response

Implementation

- Put on gloves. Using aseptic technique, perform a venipuncture and collect 5 to 7 mL of blood in a red-top tube.

Evaluation

- Note results in relation to other related tests, such as anti-HBC IgM and anti-HAV IgM
- Note and report positive results to physician, client, and local public health authorities.

Client/Caregiver Teaching

Posttest

- If results are positive, instruct client in importance of balanced diet, adequate fluid intake, and rest.

Bence Jones Protein

Classification: Immunology; Urinalysis
Type of Test: Urine

This test determines the presence in urine of monoclonal immunoglobulin light chains (Bence Jones proteins), proteins synthesized by malignant plasma cells in bone marrow. In multiple myeloma, these proteins are elevated in serum. The large amount of these serum proteins causes them to overflow through the glomerulus in quantities greater than what the renal tubules can absorb, and therefore they appear in the urine.

Indications

- Detect multiple myeloma

Reference Values

- Negative

Abnormal Values

- Multiple myeloma
- Amyloidosis
- Fanconi's syndrome (adult)
- Waldenström's macroglobulinemia

Interfering Factors

- Unrefrigerated or old specimen can cause false-negative results because heat-coagulable proteins decompose at room temperature.

- Chronic renal insufficiency, connective-tissue diseases, and other malignancies can falsely elevate results.
- Aspirin, cephaloridine, chlorpromazine, high doses of penicillin, promazine, and tolbutamide can cause false-positive results.
- Specimen contaminated with menstrual blood, semen, or prostatic secretions can cause false-positive results.

Nursing Implications

Assessment

- Obtain a history of clinical symptoms and hydration status.

Possible Nursing Diagnoses

Anxiety related to perceived threat to health status
Infection, risk for, related to immunosuppressed inflammatory response
Pain related to inflammatory process of connective tissues

Implementation

- Obtain the appropriate-sized container. Collect an early-morning, mid-stream specimen of at least 60 mL. Send specimen to laboratory promptly.

Evaluation

- Note test results in relation to other related tests.

Client/Caregiver Teaching

Pretest

- Teach client how to collect a specimen free of contaminants.
- Instruct client not to drink excessive amount of fluids before the specimen collection.
- Have the client refrigerate the specimen if it cannot be brought to the laboratory immediately.

Beta$_2$-Microglobulin

Classification: Hematology, Urinalysis

Type of Test: Blood, urine

Beta$_2$-microglobulin is an amino acid peptide component of lymphocyte human leukocyte antigen (HLA) complexes. It increases in inflammatory conditions, and when lymphocyte turnover increases, such as in lymphocytic leukemia or when T-lymphocyte helper (OKT4 cells) are attacked by human immunodeficiency virus (HIV).

Blood beta$_2$-microglobulin becomes elevated with malfunctioning glomeruli, but decreases with malfunctioning tubules because it is metabolized by the renal tubules. Conversely, urine beta$_2$-microglobulin decreases with malfunctioning glomeruli, but becomes elevated with malfunctioning tubules.

Indications

- Evaluate renal disease to differentiate glomerular from renal dysfunction
- Detect chronic lymphocytic leukemia, multiple myeloma, lung cancer, hepatoma, or breast cancer
- Detect HIV infection; levels do not correlate with stages of infection, however
- Detect aminoglycoside toxicity

Reference Values

		SI Units
Blood	<2 μg/mL	<170 nmol/L
Urine	<120 μg/24 h	<10 nmol/day

Abnormal Values

- Increased blood and urine levels
  Acquired immune deficiency syndrome (AIDS)
  Aminoglycoside toxicity

Breast cancer
Crohn's disease
Hepatitis
Hepatoma
Leukemia (chronic lymphocytic)
Lung cancer
Multiple myeloma
Poisoning with heavy metals, such as mercury or cadmium
Renal disease: glomerular (blood) and tubular (urine)
Sarcoidosis
Vasculitis

Interfering Factors

■ Radioactive dyes received within 1 week of blood and urine collection will invalidate results.

Nursing Implications

Assessment

■ Obtain history of illness and symptoms as well as recent diagnostic tests using radioactive dyes.

Possible Nursing Diagnoses

Anxiety related to perceived threat to health status
Infection, risk for, related to immunosuppressed inflammatory response
Pain related to inflammation or swelling of the liver
Grieving, anticipatory, related to perceived potential loss

Implementation

■ *Blood test:* Put on gloves. Using aseptic technique, perform a venipuncture and collect 10 mL of blood in a lavender-top tube containing EDTA.
■ Handle sample gently to avoid hemolysis and send promptly to laboratory.
■ *Urine test:* Obtain a clean 3-L urine collection container and toluene preservative. Discard first-morning urine specimen and indicate the starting time for the test. Instruct client to add all urine voided for a 24-hour period to the refrigerated container and to keep track of the amount of urine voided, if necessary. If an indwelling urinary catheter is in place, keep the drainage bag on ice and empty urine into collection bottle every hour.

- At the conclusion of the test, ensure proper labeling of specimen container, including the start and stop time, and send to the laboratory immediately.

Evaluation

- Note test results in relation to the client's symptoms and other tests performed, particularly the blood and urine beta$_2$-microglobulin.
- Compare urine quantity in the container with the record of urine output during the collection period. The test will need to be invalidated if the container contains less urine than was documented as output.

Client/Caregiver Teaching

Pretest

- Inform the client that there is no special preparation for the blood or urine test.
- Instruct client to save all urine voided for 24 hours, to urinate before defecating, and to avoid contaminating urine with stool or toilet tissue.

Bilirubin, Serum

Classification: Chemistry
Type of Test: Blood

This test measures the level of bilirubin, a degradation product of the pigmented heme portion of hemoglobin. Old, damaged, and abnormal erythrocytes are removed from the circulation by the spleen and, to some extent, by the liver and bone marrow. The heme component of the red blood cells is oxidized to bilirubin by the reticuloendothelial cells and released into the blood. The terms "indirect" and "direct," which are used to describe unconjugated (prehepatic) and conjugated (posthepatic) bilirubin, respectively, derive from the methods of testing for their presence in serum.

Indications

- Detect hemolytic disorders, including transfusion reaction, as indicated by elevated total and indirect bilirubin levels. (Hemolysis alone rarely causes indirect bilirubin levels higher than 4 or 5 mg/dL; if hemolysis is combined with impaired or immature liver function, levels may rise more dramatically.)
- Confirm observed jaundice with serum levels or indirect or direct bilirubin that reaches 2 to 4 mg/dL.
- Determine cause of jaundice, such as liver dysfunction, hepatitis, biliary obstruction, or carcinoma.

Reference Values

Total bilirubin	
Newborn	2–6 mg/dL
48 hours	6–7 mg/dL
5 days	4–12 mg/dL
1 month to adult	0.3–1.2 mg/dL
Indirect bilirubin	
(unconjugated, prehepatic)	
1 month to adult	0.3–1.1 mg/dL
Direct bilirubin	
(conjugated, posthepatic)	
1 month to adult	0.1–0.4 mg/dL

Abnormal Values

- Increased indirect (unconjugated) bilirubin
    Hemoglobinopathies, including spherocytosis
    G-6-PD deficiency
    Transfusion reaction
    Pernicious anemia
    Hemorrhage
    Hepatitis (all types)
    Gilbert disease
    Crigler-Najjar syndrome
    Neonatal hepatic immaturity
- Increased direct (conjugated) bilirubin
    Viral hepatitis
    Alcoholic hepatitis
    Cirrhosis
    Biliary cirrhosis
    Cholangitis (idiopathic, infectious)
    Biliary atresia

Gallstones

Carcinoma of gallbladder or head of pancreas

Bile duct stricture from inflammation or surgical mis-
adventure

Drugs, such as chlorpromazine

Interfering Factors

- Prolonged exposure of the client, as well as the blood sample, to sunlight and ultraviolet light, which reduce serum bilirubin levels.
- Failure to follow dietary restrictions before the test.
- Certain drugs may elevate bilirubin levels, including steroids,
sulfonamides, sulfonylureas, barbiturates, antineoplastic
agents, propylthiouracil, allopurinol, antibiotics, gallbladder
dyes, caffeine, theophylline, indomethacin, and any drugs
that are considered hepatotoxic.
- Hemolysis of sample.

Nursing Implications

Assessment

- Obtain history of hepatobiliary system, medication regimen,
diagnostic tests, and results.
- Ensure that client has fasted for 4 hours before the test and
withheld medication that could elevate levels.

Possible Nursing Diagnoses

Anxiety related to perceived threat to health status

Infection, risk for, related to immunosuppressed inflammatory
response

Pain related to inflammation or swelling of the liver

Fatigue related to decreased metabolic energy production

Implementation

- Put on gloves. Using aseptic technique, perform a venipuncture and obtain 5 mL of blood in a red-top tube.
- In infants, a capillary sample is obtained by heelstick.
- Handle sample gently to avoid hemolysis and send immediately to the laboratory.
- Do not expose the sample to sunlight for prolonged periods
(more than 1 hour), to ultraviolet light, or to fluorescent
lights.

Evaluation

■ Note result in relation to the client's symptoms and other test results, particularly urine bilirubin.

Client/Caregiver Teaching

Pretest

■ Instruct the client to fast for 4 hours before the test. Water is not restricted.
■ Instruct the client to withhold drugs that interfere with test results, as ordered.

Posttest

■ Tell the client to resume diet and medications withheld before the test.

Bilirubin, Urine

Classification: Chemistry, Urinalysis

Type of Test: Urine, random

A screening test performed to detect conjugated (direct) bilirubin in the urine (bilirubinuria). Bilirubin is the breakdown product of hemoglobin. Unconjugated bilirubin reaches the liver and is conjugated, which is normally absorbed by the bile ducts, stored in the gallbladder, and ultimately excreted as bile through the intestine. When obstructive or hepatic jaundice occurs, conjugated bilirubin enters the bloodstream rather than the gastrointestinal tract and is filtered and excreted by the kidneys. Bilirubinuria changes the color of urine to dark amber. This test is included in the routine urinalysis test.

Indications

■ Detect liver disease
■ Diagnose obstructive jaundice within the biliary tree

Reference Values

- Negative

Abnormal Values

- Positive value
  Cirrhosis
  Hepatitis (chronic, acute)
  Biliary obstruction
  Hepatic or biliary tract cancer
  Infectious mononucleosis
  Septicemia

Interfering Factors

- Salicylates can cause false-positive results with Icotest dip-stick or tablet; ascorbic acid and nitrites can cause false-negative results.
- Phenazopyridine and phenothiazines can cause false-positive N-Multistix results.
- Excessive exposure of urine sample to light and air can cause bilirubin degradation, leading to false-negative results.
- Bilirubin excretion is enhanced in alkalotic states, resulting in false-positives.
- Incorrect testing with dipstick and delayed testing by laboratory can result in false-negative results.

Nursing Implications

Assessment

- Obtain history of hepatobiliary system, medication regimen, and diagnostic tests and results.

Possible Nursing Diagnoses

Anxiety related to perceived threat to health status
Infection, risk for, related to immunosuppressed inflammatory response
Pain related to inflammation or swelling of the liver
Fatigue related to decreased metabolic energy production

Implementation

- Obtain the appropriate-sized clean container without preservative and place a 20-mL fresh random urine sample in the container.
- If bedside analysis is performed, follow package instructions carefully for the Icotest tablets or N-Multistix to obtain

immediate results. If specimen is sent to the laboratory, follow directions for any special care of the specimen during collection, such as refrigeration. Keep specimen protected from light.

- If an indwelling catheter is in place, empty a random sample of urine in collection container without the preservative.
- At the conclusion of the test, ensure that the label is properly completed and transport to the laboratory.

Evaluation

- Note result in relation to serum bilirubin tests in the presence of jaundice.

Client/Caregiver Teaching

Pretest

- Instruct the client to withhold medications that may interfere with test results.
- Instruct the bedridden client to void in a bedpan. Instruct client to avoid voiding in pan with defecation and to keep toilet tissue out of pan to prevent contamination of the specimen.
- Inform the client that results can be revealed immediately if the dipstick is used or in 24 hours if the specimen is sent to the laboratory.

Biopsy, Bladder

Classification: Histology

Type of Test: Excision and cell analysis

Bladder biopsy is the excision of a sample of suspicious bladder tissue that can be analyzed microscopically to determine the presence of cell morphology and tissue abnormalities. This test is used to confirm the diagnosis of cancer in a patient with unexplained hematuria. Bladder biopsy is obtained after surgical insertion of a cystoscope and bladder irrigation. Therapeutic procedures can be performed during the procedure, such as removal of small tumors or polyps.

Indications

- Suspected bladder malignancy
- Hematuria
- Recurrent changes in bladder cancer

Reference Values

- No abnormal cells or tissue

Abnormal Values

- Bladder cancer
- Bladder polyps

Interfering Factors

- None

NURSING ALERT

This procedure is contraindicated in
- Bleeding disorders, since instrumentation may lead to excessive bleeding from the lower urinary tract
- Acute cystitis or urethritis, since instrumentation could allow bacteria to enter the bloodstream and result in septicemia

Nursing Implications

Assessment

- Obtain history of urinary symptoms, medications, results of tests and procedures performed, and allergies.
- Assess hematological and blood clotting ability, including complete blood count (CBC), platelets, prothrombin time, partial thromboplastin time, clotting and bleeding time.

Possible Nursing Diagnoses

Anxiety related to perceived threat to health status
Urinary elimination, altered, related to obstruction
Grieving, anticipatory, related to perceived loss or threat of death

Implementation

- Position the client on examination table with legs in stirrups and draped. If a general or spinal anesthesia is used, it is administered before positioning on table.
- Cleanse the external genitalia with antiseptic solution. If a local anesthetic is used, it is instilled into the urethra and retained for 5 to 10 minutes. A penile clamp may be used for male clients to aid in retention of the anesthetic.
- The physician inserts a cystoscope and irrigates the bladder via an irrigation system attached to the scope. The irrigant is usually sterile water, unless an isotonic solution such as mannitol is used during transurethral resection procedures. The irrigation fluid aids in bladder visualization.
- When the suspicious area is found, the tissue sample is obtained by means of a cytology brush or biopsy forceps inserted through the scope. If polyps are present or the tumor is small and localized, it can be excised and fulgurated.
- Upon completion of examination and related procedures, the cystoscope is withdrawn.
- Place tissue samples in formalin solution and send to the laboratory.

Evaluation

- Observe for bleeding and infection.
- Note test results in relation to other related tests and clinical symptoms.

Client/Caregiver Teaching

Pretest

- Inform the client that the procedure is performed by a surgeon and usually takes about 30 minutes to complete.
- Explain that foods and fluids are restricted after midnight the day before the surgery.
- Inform the client that a general anesthetic will be administered.

Posttest

- Instruct the client to expect blood in the urine but to report excessive bleeding.
- Inform the client of a follow-up appointment.

////////////////////////////////

Biopsy, Bone

Classification: Histology

Type of Test: Excision and cell analysis

Biopsy is the excision of a sample of tissue that can be analyzed microscopically to determine the presence of cell morphology abnormalities and tissue abnormalities. This test is used to confirm the diagnosis of cancer when clinical symptoms or x-rays are suspicious. Bone biopsy is obtained after surgical incision to reveal the affected area.

Indications

- Suspected bone malignancy
- Abnormal x-rays

Reference Values

- No abnormal cells or tissue

Abnormal Values

- Multiple myeloma
- Osteosarcoma
- Ewing's sarcoma
- Osteoma

Interfering Factors

- None

NURSING ALERT

- This procedure is contraindicated in bleeding disorders.

Nursing Implications

Assessment

- Obtain clinical symptoms, medications, results of tests and procedures performed, and allergies.

- Assess hematological and blood clotting ability for those biopsies with risk of bleeding, include CBC (complete blood count), platelets, prothrombin time, partial thromboplastin time, clotting and bleeding time.

Possible Nursing Diagnoses

Anxiety related to perceived threat to health status
Physical mobility, impaired, related to musculoskeletal impairment
Grieving, anticipatory, related to perceived loss or threat of death

Implementation

- After surgical incision is complete, the surgeon locates the suspected lesion and removes sufficient tissue for analysis.
- Place tissue samples in formalin solution and send to the laboratory.

Evaluation

- Observe for bleeding and infection.
- Note test results in relation to other related tests and clinical symptoms.

Client/Caregiver Teaching

Pretest

- Inform the client that it is performed by a surgeon and usually takes about 30 minutes to complete.
- Explain that foods and fluids are restricted after midnight the day before the surgery.
- Inform the client that a general anesthetic will be administered.

Posttest

- Instruct the client in the care and assessment of the site.
- Inform the client of a follow-up appointment for removal of sutures, if indicated.

Biopsy, Breast

Classification: Histology

Type of Test: Excision and analysis

Breast biopsy is the excision of a sample of breast tissue that can be analyzed microscopically to determine the presence of cell morphology and tissue abnormalities. This test is used to confirm diagnosis of cancer when a breast lump is found or the results of mammogram or ultrasound are suspicious. Breast biopsy is obtained after surgical incision to reveal affected area or by using a needle to obtain the specimen.

Indications

- Suspected breast malignancy
- Palpable breast mass
- Abnormal mammogram or ultrasound of the breast

Reference Values

- No abnormal cells or tissue

Abnormal Values

- Adenofibroma
- Fibrocystic disease
- Malignant tumors

Interfering Factors

- None

NURSING ALERT

- This procedure is contraindicated in bleeding disorders.

Nursing Implications

Assessment

- Obtain history of clinical symptoms, medications, results of tests and procedures performed, and allergies.

- Assess hematological and blood-clotting ability, including CBC (complete blood count), platelets, prothrombin time, partial thromboplastin time, and clotting and bleeding time.

Possible Nursing Diagnoses

Anxiety related to perceived threat to health status
Body image disturbance related to change in appearance
Grieving, anticipatory, related to perceived loss or threat of death

Implementation

- Help client to the supine position after clothing above the waist is removed.
- *Open biopsy:* After anesthesia is delivered, the surgeon cleanses the site to prepare the sterile field. An incision is made, and the affected tissue is identified and removed.
- *Needle biopsy:* After cleansing with an antiseptic solution, the site is injected with a local anesthetic. A needle is inserted into the mass and the sample is aspirated with a syringe.
- Place a sterile dressing over the site when the excision is complete.
- Place tissue samples in formalin solution and send to the laboratory.

Evaluation

- Observe for bleeding and infection.
- Note test results in relation to other tests and clinical symptoms.

Client/Caregiver Teaching

Pretest

- Inform the client that the procedure is performed by a surgeon and usually takes about 30 minutes to complete.
- Explain that foods and fluids are restricted after midnight the day before the surgery.
- Inform the client that a general anesthetic will be administered.

Posttest

- Instruct the client in care and assessment of the site.
- Inform the client of a follow-up appointment for removal of sutures.

Biopsy, Cervical

Classification: Histology

Type of Test: Excision and analysis

Biopsy is the excision of a sample of tissue that can be analyzed microscopically to determine the presence of cell morphology abnormalities and tissue abnormalities. This test is used to confirm the diagnosis of cancer when screening tests are positive. Cervical biopsy is obtained using an instrument that punches into the tissue and returns a tissue sample.

Indications

- Suspected cervical malignancy
- Abnormal PAP smear, Schiller test, or colposcopy

Reference Values

- No abnormal cells or tissue

Abnormal Values

- Carcinoma in situ
- Cervical dysplasia
- Cervical polyps

Interfering Factors

- None

NURSING ALERT

This procedure is contraindicated
- If acute pelvic inflammatory disease or cervicitis is present
- In bleeding disorders

Nursing Implications

Assessment

- Obtain a history of clinical symptoms of the affected system, medications, results of tests and procedures performed, and allergies.
- Assess hematological and blood clotting ability for those biopsies with risk of bleeding, include CBC (complete blood count), platelets, prothrombin time, partial thromboplastin time, and clotting and bleeding time.

Possible Nursing Diagnoses

Anxiety related to perceived threat to health status

Sexuality patterns, altered, related to illness or medical treatment

Grieving, anticipatory, related to perceived loss or threat of death

Implementation

- Have client remove clothes below the waist.
- Position the client in a lithotomy position on a gynecologic examination table with feet in stirrups.
- Cleanse external genitalia with an antiseptic solution. The cervix is swabbed with 3% acetic acid and the colposcope is inserted. Biopsy forceps are inserted and tissue samples are obtained.
- Bleeding is controlled by cautery or silver nitrate application.
- Place tissue samples in formalin solution and send to the laboratory.

Evaluation

- Observe for bleeding.
- Note test results in relation to other tests and clinical symptoms.

Client/Caregiver Teaching

Pretest

- Inform the client that the procedure is performed by a surgeon and usually takes about 30 minutes to complete.
- Explain that foods and fluids are not usually restricted.
- Inform the client that a local anesthetic will be administered.
- Ensure that the client understands the procedure before signing the informed consent.

Posttest

- Instruct client to expect a gray-green vaginal discharge for several days, to avoid strenuous activity for 8 to 24 hours, to avoid douching or intercourse for 2 weeks or as instructed by the physician, and to report excess bleeding to the physician.
- Inform the client of a follow-up appointment, if indicated.

Biopsy, Chorionic Villus

Classification: Histology

Type of Test: Excision and analysis

Chorionic villus biopsy is the excision of a tissue sample from the villi in the chorion frondosum of an 8- to 12-week pregnancy uterus for microscopic analysis to determine cell morphology and tissue abnormalities. The chorionic villi are fingerlike projections that protect the embryo and anchor it to the uterine wall before the placenta develops. Because it is embryonic tissue, analysis provides very important information about the developing baby. This test is used to detect fetal abnormalities caused by many genetic and sex-linked disorders and to determine the sex of the baby. It is not useful in identifying neural-tube defects. Chorionic villus biopsy specimen is obtained using a catheter inserted through the cervix and into the area of the uterus where the embryo is located. Unlike amniocentesis, it is not necessary to puncture the amniotic sac to retrieve a specimen.

Indications

- Diagnose a possible or suspected genetic disorder, particularly if there is a family history of genetic disorder
- Determine presence of Down syndrome in pregnant women over age 35
- Determine sex of fetus in women who are carriers of sex-linked genetic disorders

Reference Values

- No chromosomal abnormalities

Abnormal Values

- Genetic disorders, such as Tay-Sachs, enzyme deficiencies, sickle-cell disease, or other hemoglobinopathies
- Chromosomal abnormalities, such as Down syndrome or Turner's syndrome

Interfering Factors

- History of incompetent cervix

Nursing Implications

Assessment

- Obtain family history of genetic disorders, results of tests and procedures performed.

Possible Nursing Diagnoses

Anxiety related to perceived threat to health status
Injury, risk for, to fetus, related to invasive procedure
Grieving, anticipatory, related to perceived potential outcome

Implementation

- Have client remove clothes below the waist.
- Position the client in a lithotomy position on a gynecologic examination table with feet in stirrups.
- The external genitalia are cleansed with an antiseptic solution. A vaginal speculum is inserted. A suction catheter is inserted through the cervical os to the biopsy site. Ultrasound is used to locate the site and direct the catheter. The catheter is connected to a 20-mL syringe, and approximately 10 cm of water suction is applied. Suction is maintained as the catheter is withdrawn so that cervical secretions are not introduced into the uterus.
- Tissue sample is flushed onto a Petri dish with a culture medium and sent immediately to the laboratory.

Evaluation

- Observe for excessive vaginal bleeding, infection, or signs of impending abortion.
- Note test results in relation to other tests.

Client/Caregiver Teaching

Pretest

- Explain the purpose of the test and the procedure involved. Tell the client that she will expereience slight to moderate discomfort and that deep breathing and relaxation can help.
- Inform the client that the test is performed by an obstetrician under sterile conditions and usually takes about 15 minutes to complete.
- Explain that food and fluids are not usually restricted.

Posttest

- Instruct the client to notify the physician if excessive bleeding or cramping occur.
- Inform the client that an ultrasound may be performed in 48 hours to ensure fetal viability.
- Instruct the client to expect a gray-green vaginal discharge for several days, to avoid strenuous activity for 8 to 24 hours, and to avoid douching or intercourse for 2 weeks or as instructed by the physician.

Biopsy, Intestinal

Classification: Histology

Type of Test: Excision and analysis

Intestinal biopsy is the excision of a tissue sample from the small intestine for microscopic analysis to determine the presence of cell morphology and tissue abnormalities. This test is used to confirm the diagnosis of cancer or intestinal disorders. Biopsy specimen is usually obtained during endoscopic examination.

Indications

- Confirm suspected intestinal malignancy
- Confirm suspicious findings during endoscopic visualization of the intestinal wall
- Diagnose various intestinal disorders, such as lactose and other enzyme deficiencies, celiac disease, and parasitic infections

Reference Values

- No abnormal cells or tissue

Abnormal Values

- Cancer
- Lactose deficiency
- Celiac disease
- Tropical sprue
- Parasitic infestation

Interfering Factors

- Barium swallow within 48 hours of small-intestine biopsy affects results.
- Inability of client to cooperate with endoscopic examination affects results.

NURSING ALERT

- This procedure is contraindicated in bleeding disorders and aortic arch aneurysm.

Nursing Implications

Assessment

- Obtain a history of clinical symptoms, medications, results of tests and procedures performed, and allergies.
- Assess hematologic status and blood clotting ability, including complete blood count, platelets, prothrombin time, partial thromboplastin time, and clotting and bleeding time.
- Ensure that the client has complied with food and fluid restrictions.

Possible Nursing Diagnoses

Anxiety related to perceived threat to health status
Injury, risk for, related to invasive procedure
Nutrition, altered, less than body requirements, related to inability to digest food and absorb nutrients

Implementation

- Administer ordered premedication.
- Position the client in a semireclining position.
- A local anesthetic is sprayed into the throat. A protective tooth guard and a bite block are placed in the mouth.

- The flexible endoscope is passed into and through the mouth, and the client is asked to swallow. Once the endoscope has passed into the esophagus, the client is helped into the left lateral position. A suction device is used to drain saliva.
- The esophagus, stomach, and duodenum are visually examined as the endoscope is passed through each section. A biopsy specimen can be taken from any suspicious sites.
- Tissue samples are obtained by inserting a cytology brush or biopsy forceps through the endoscope.
- When the examination and tissue retrieval are complete, the endoscope and suction device are withdrawn, and the tooth guard and bite block are removed.
- Place tissue samples in formalin solution and send to the laboratory.

Evaluation

- Note any chest pain, upper abdominal pain, pain on swallowing, difficulty breathing, or expectoration of blood. Report these to the physician immediately.
- Note test results in relation to other tests and clinical symptoms.

Client/Caregiver Teaching

Pretest

- Inform the client that the procedure is performed by a surgeon and usually takes about 60 minutes to complete.
- Explain that food and fluids are restricted for 6 to 8 hours before the test.
- Inform the client that a sedative will be administered to promote relaxation and reduce discomfort during the procedure.

Posttest

- Instruct the client not to eat or drink until the anesthesia has worn off.
- Have client maintain a side-lying position for 2 hours after the procedure to prevent aspiration of secretions.
- Instruct the client to immediately report any chest pain, upper abdominal pain, pain on swallowing, difficulty breathing, or expectoration of blood.

Biopsy, Kidney

Classification: Histology

Type of Test: Excision and analysis

Kidney, or renal, biopsy is the excision of a tissue sample from the kidney for microscopic analysis to determine the presence of cell morphology and tissue abnormalities. This test is used to confirm a diagnosis of cancer found on x-ray or ultrasound or to diagnose certain inflammatory or immunologic conditions. Biopsy specimen is usually obtained either percutaneously or after surgical incision.

Indications

- Confirm suspected renal malignancy
- Diagnose the cause of renal disease
- Monitor progression of nephrotic syndrome
- Determine extent of involvement in systemic lupus erythematosus or other immunologic disorders
- Monitor renal function after transplantation

Reference Values

- No abnormal cells or tissue

Abnormal Values

- Cancer
- Nephrotic syndrome
- Disseminated lupus erythematosus
- Amyloidosis infiltration
- Acute and chronic poststreptococcal glumerulonephritis
- Goodpasture's syndrome
- Renal vein thrombosis
- Pyelonephritis
- Immmunologic rejection of transplanted kidney

Interfering Factors

- Obesity and severe spinal deformity can make percutaneous biopsy impossible.

> ### ▶ NURSING ALERT
>
> - This procedure is contraindicated in bleeding disorders, advanced renal disease, uncontrolled hypertension, or solitary kidney (except transplanted kidney).
> - Percutaneous biopsy is contraindicated if the client is unable to remain still during the procedure.

Nursing Implications

Assessment

- Obtain a history of urinary symptoms, medications, results of tests and procedures performed, and allergies.
- Assess hematologic status and blood-clotting ability, including complete blood count, platelets, prothrombin time, partial thromboplastin time, and clotting and bleeding time.
- Ensure that client has complied with food and fluid restrictions.

Possible Nursing Diagnoses

Anxiety related to perceived threat to health status
Injury, risk for, related to invasive procedure
Infection, risk for, related to immunosuppressed inflammatory response
Fluid volume excess related to compromised regulatory mechanism

Implementation

- Administer ordered premedication.
- *Open biopsy:* After administration of anesthesia, surgical incision is made, suspicious areas are located, and tissue samples are collected.
- *Percutaneous needle biopsy:* Help the client to a prone position. After the site has been cleansed with antiseptic, a local anesthetic is injected and a sterile field is prepared. A sandbag may be placed under the abdomen to aid in moving the kidneys to the desired position. The client is instructed to take a deep breath and hold it while the needle is inserted under sterile conditions. As the needle enters the kidney, the client is instructed to exhale. The needle is rotated to obtain a plug of tissue, then removed. Manual pressure is applied for 5 to 20 minutes, and then a pressure dressing is applied.
- Place tissue samples in buffered saline solution and send to the laboratory.

Evaluation

■ Observe for hematuria. Small amounts of blood will be present in the urine for the first 24 hours.

■ Observe for bleeding, including hypotension, tachycardia, backache, flank pain, shoulder pain, or lightheadedness.

■ Monitor intake and output closely for 24 hours.

■ Note test results in relation to other tests and clinical symptoms.

Client/Caregiver Teaching

Pretest

■ Inform the client that the procedure is performed by a surgeon under sterile conditions and usually takes about 90 minutes to complete.

■ Explain that foods and fluids are restricted from midnight the day before the test.

■ Inform the client that a sedative will be administered to promote relaxation and reduce discomfort during percutaneous biopsy, and general anesthesia will be administered for open biopsy.

Posttest

■ Instruct the client in the care and assessment of the site.

■ After percutaneous biopsy, instruct the client to stay in bed lying on the affected side for at least 30 minutes with a pillow or sandbag under the site to prevent bleeding. The client will also need to remain on bedrest for 24 hours.

■ Instruct the client to increase fluid intake to 3000 mL during the first 24 hours after the procedure unless contraindicated by another medical condition.

■ Instruct the client to avoid strenuous activity, sports, and heavy lifting for 2 weeks after the procedure.

■ Instruct the client to report any burning on urination, hematuria, and discomfort in the kidney area, shoulders, or abdomen.

Biopsy, Liver

Classification: Histology

Type of Test: Excision and analysis

Liver biopsy is the excision of a tissue sample from the liver for microscopic analysis to determine the presence of cell morphology and tissue abnormalities. This test is used to confirm a diagnosis of cancer and to diagnose certain disorders of the hepatic parenchyma. Biopsy specimen is usually obtained either percutaneously or after surgical incision.

Indications

- Confirm suspected hepatic malignancy
- Confirm suspected hepatic parenchymal disease
- Diagnose the cause of persistently elevated liver enzymes, hepatomegaly, or jaundice

Reference Values

- No abnormal cells or tissue

Abnormal Values

- Cancer
- Benign tumor
- Cirrhosis
- Hepatic involvement with systemic lupus erythematosus, sarcoidosis, or amyloidosis
- Hepatitis
- Hemachromatosis
- Wilson's disease
- Reye's syndrome
- Galactosemia
- Cholesterol ester storage disease
- Parasitic infestations, such as malaria, visceral larva migrans, and amebiasis

Interfering Factors

■ Inability of the client to cooperate with needle biopsy.

> ### ▶ NURSING ALERT
>
> ■ This procedure is contraindicated in bleeding disorders, suspected vascular tumor of the liver, ascites that may obscure proper insertion site for needle biopsy, subdiaphragmatic or right-hemothoracic infection, or biliary tract infection.
>
> ■ Percutaneous biopsy is contraindicated if the client is unable to remain still during the procedure.

Nursing Implications

Assessment

■ Obtain a history of clinical symptoms, medications, results of tests and procedures performed, and allergies.
■ Assess hematologic status and blood-clotting ability, including complete blood count, platelets, prothrombin time, partial thromboplastin time, and clotting and bleeding time.
■ Ensure that client has complied with food and fluid restrictions.

Possible Nursing Diagnoses

Anxiety related to perceived threat to health status
Injury, risk for, related to invasive procedure
Pain related to inflammation or swelling of the liver
Fatigue related to increased energy requirements and altered body chemistry

Implementation

■ Administer ordered premedication.
■ *Open biopsy:* After administration of anesthesia, a surgical incision is made, suspicious areas are located, and tissue samples are collected.
■ *Percutaneous needle biopsy:* Help the client to a supine or left-lateral position with the right hand under the head. After the site has been cleansed with antiseptic, a local anesthetic is injected and a sterile field is prepared. The client is instructed to take a deep breath, exhale forcefully, and hold the breath while the needle is inserted under sterile conditions. The needle is rotated to obtain a core of liver

tissue and then removed. Once the needle is removed, the client may breathe. A pressure dressing is then applied.
- Place tissue samples in formalin solution and send to the laboratory.

Evaluation

- Observe for bleeding, hematoma formation, bile leakage, and inflammation.
- Note any pleuritic pain, persistent right-shoulder pain, or abdominal pain.
- Note test results in relation to other tests, particulary liver-function tests, and clinical symptoms.

Client/Caregiver Teaching

Pretest

- Inform the client that the procedure is performed by a surgeon under sterile conditions and usually takes about 90 minutes to complete. Needle biopsy should take about 15 minutes.
- Explain that food and fluids are restricted from midnight of the day before the test.
- Inform the client that a sedative will be administered to promote relaxation and reduce discomfort during percutaneous biopsy, and that general anesthesia will be administered for open biopsy.

Posttest

- Instruct the client in the care and assessment of the site.
- After percutaneous biopsy, instruct the client to stay in bed lying on the affected side for at least 2 hours with a pillow or rolled towel under the site to prevent bleeding. The client will also need to remain on bedrest for 24 hours.
- Instruct the client to avoid coughing or straining, as this may increase intra-abdominal pressure.

Biopsy, Lung

Classification: Histology

Type of Test: Excision and analysis

Lung biopsy is the excision of a tissue sample from the lung for microscopic analysis to determine the presence of cell morphology and tissue abnormalities. This test is used to confirm a diagnosis of cancer on x-ray, CT scan, or sputum analysis or to diagnose certain inflammatory or immunologic conditions. Biopsy specimen is obtained either percutaneously, during a bronchoscopy, or after thoracotomy.

Indications

- Confirm suspected lung malignancy
- Diagnose the cause of diffuse interstitial lung disease
- Determine extent of involvement in systemic lupus erythematosus or other immunologic disorders
- Diagnosis suspected lung infections

Reference Values

- No abnormal cells or tissue

Abnormal Values

- Cancer
- Diffuse interstitial lung disease such as fibrosis or pneumoconiosis
- Pulmonary involvement with systemic diseases, such as systemic lupus erythematosus, amyloidosis, and sarcoidosis
- Disorders such as histoplasmosis, blastomycosis, and *Pneumocystis carinii pneumoniae*
- Infections such as tuberculosis

Interfering Factors

- Inability of client to cooperate with bronchoscopic examination
- Inability of client to remain still during needle biopsy

> ### NURSING ALERT
>
> ■ This procedure is contraindicated in bleeding disorders, cor pulmonale, and hyperinflation of the lung.

Nursing Implications

Assessment

■ Obtain a history of respiratory symptoms, medications, results of tests and procedures performed, and allergies.
■ Assess hematologic status and blood-clotting ability, including, platelets, prothrombin time, partial thromboplastin time, and clotting and bleeding time.
■ Ensure that client has complied with food and fluid restrictions.

Possible Nursing Diagnoses

Anxiety related to perceived threat to health status
Injury, risk for, related to invasive procedure
Airway clearance, ineffective, related to compromised pulmonary function
Breathing pattern, ineffective, related to compromised pulmonary function
Infection, risk for, related to stasis of pulmonary secretions

Implementation

■ Administer ordered premedication.
■ *Needle biopsy:* Help client to a sitting position with arms on a pillow over a bed table. Site is cleansed with an antiseptic, injected with a local anesthetic, and draped with sterile towels. Instruct the client to remain still and avoid coughing during the procedure. The needle is inserted through the posterior chest wall into the intercostal space. The needle is rotated to obtain the sample and then withdrawn. Pressure is applied to the site, and a pressure dressing is applied.
■ *Bronchoscopy:* The client is positioned in relation to the type of anesthesia used. For general anesthesia, the client is placed in a supine position with the neck hyperextended. If local anesthesia is used, the client is seated and the tongue and oropharynx are sprayed and swabbed with anesthetic. The client is then helped to a supine or side-lying position, and the bronchoscope is inserted. After inspection, tissue samples are collected of suspicious sites by bronchial brush or biopsy forceps.

- *Open biopsies:* The client is prepared for a thoractomy under general anesthesia in the operating room. Tissue specimens are collected from suspicious sites. A chest tube is inserted following the procedure.
- Place tissue samples in formalin solution and send to the laboratory.

Evaluation

- Observe for hemoptysis, difficulty breathing, cough, air hunger, or absent breath sounds over affected area.
- Monitor chest-tube patency and drainage after a thoracotomy.
- Note test results in relation to other tests and clinical symptoms.

Client/Caregiver Teaching

Pretest

- Inform the client that the needle biopsy is performed by a surgeon under sterile conditions and usually takes about 30 minutes to complete. A bronchoscopy usually takes about 15 to 30 minutes.
- Explain that foods and fluids are restricted from midnight of the day before the test.
- Inform the client that a sedative will be administered before a needle biopsy or bronchoscopy to promote relaxation and reduce discomfort during the procedure.

Posttest

- Instruct the client not to eat or drink until the anesthesia has worn off.
- Have client remain in a semi-Fowler's position after bronchoscopy or needle biopsy to maximize ventilation.
- Instruct the client to use lozenges or gargle for throat discomfort.

Biopsy, Lymph Node

Classification: Histology

Type of Test: Excision and analysis

Lymph node biopsy is the excision of a tissue sample from one of many lymph nodes for microscopic analysis to determine the presence of cell morphology and tissue abnormalities. This test is used to confirm a diagnosis of cancer, to diagnose disorders causing systemic illness, or to stage metastatic cancer. Biopsy specimen is usually obtained either percutaneously or after surgical incision.

Indications

- Confirm suspected malignant involvement of the lymphatics
- Diagnose the cause of perisistent lymphadenopathy
- Confirm suspected fungal or parasitic infections of the lymphatics
- Determine the stage of metastatic cancer

Reference Values

- No abnormal cells or tissue

Abnormal Values

- Malignancy such as lymphomas and leukemias
- Metastatic disease
- Lymph involvement of systemic diseases such as systemic lupus erythematosus and sarcoidosis
- Parasitic infestation such as pneumoconiosis
- Fungal infection, such as cat scratch disease
- Chancroid
- Immunodeficiency
- Infectious mononucleosis
- Lymphangitis
- Lymphogranuloma venereum

Interfering Factors

- Inability of the client to cooperate with needle biopsy

Nursing Implications

Assessment

- Obtain a history of clinical symptoms of the affected system, medications, results of tests and procedures performed, and allergies.
- Assess hematologic status and blood-clotting ability including complete blood count, platelets, prothrombin time, partial thromboplastin time, and clotting and bleeding time.
- Note if the client has complied with food and fluid restrictions.

Possible Nursing Diagnoses

Anxiety related to perceived threat to health status
Activity intolerance related to reduced energy stores
Infection, risk for, related to inadequate secondary defenses
Pain related to inflammatory process of connective tissues

Implementation

- Administer ordered premedication.
- *Open biopsy:* After administration of local anesthesia (for surface nodes) or general anesthesia (for deeper nodes), a surgical incision is made and suspicious nodes are located, grasped with forceps, and removed. The site is closed and a dressing is applied.
- *Percutaneous needle biopsy:* Help the client to a position that exposes the affected node. After the site has been cleansed with antiseptic, a local anesthetic is injected and a sterile field is prepared. The node is grasped with the fingers, and a needle with syringe attached is inserted directly into the node. The node is aspirated to collect the specimen. A sterile dressing is then applied.
- Place tissue samples in normal saline solution and send to the laboratory.

Evaluation

- Observe for bleeding.
- Note test results in relation to other tests and clinical symptoms.

Client/Caregiver Teaching

Pretest

- Inform the client that the procedure is performed by a surgeon under sterile conditions and usually takes about 30 minutes to complete. Needle biopsy should take about 15 minutes.
- Explain that food and fluids are restricted from midnight of the day before the test.
- Inform the client that a sedative will be administered to promote relaxation and reduce discomfort during percutaneous biopsy and a general anesthesia will be administered for open biopsy.

Posttest

- Instruct the client in the care and assessment of the site.

Biopsy, Muscle

Classification: Histology

Type of Test: Excision and analysis

Muscle biopsy is the excision of a tissue sample from one of many muscles for microscopic analysis to determine the presence of cell morphology and tissue abnormalities. This test is used to confirm a diagnosis of neuropathy or myopathy and diagnose infestation. Biopsy specimen is usually obtained from the deltoid or gastrocnemius muscle after a surgical incision.

Indications

- Diagnose Duchenne's muscular dystrophy
- Diagnose the cause of neuropathy or myopathy

- Confirm suspected fungal or parasitic infections of the muscle

Reference Values

- No abnormal cells or tissue

Abnormal Values

- Duchenne's muscular dystrophy
- Amyotrophic lateral sclerosis
- Alcoholic myopathy
- Myasthenia gravis
- Myotonia congenita
- Polymyalgia rheumatica
- Polymyositis
- Parasitic infestation
- Fungal infection

Interfering Factors

- If electromyography is performed before muscle biopsy, residual inflammation may result, leading to false-positive biopsy results.

> ### NURSING ALERT
>
> - This procedure is contraindicated in bleeding disorders.

Nursing Implications

Assessment

- Obtain a history of clinical symptoms, medications, results of tests and procedures performed, and allergies.
- Assess hematologic status and blood-clotting ability, including complete blood count, platelets, prothrombin time, partial thromboplastin time, and clotting and bleeding time.
- Note if the client has complied with food and fluid restrictions.

Possible Nursing Diagnoses

Anxiety related to perceived threat to health status
Physical mobility, impaired, related to neuromuscular/musculoskeletal impairment
Activity intolerance related to reduced energy stores
Activity intolerance related to progressive disease

Implementation

- Administer ordered premedication.
- Help the client to a supine position (for deltoid biopsy) or prone position (for gastrocnemius biopsy).
- Cleanse the site with antiseptic solution and drape with sterile drapes. After infiltration with a local anesthetic, a small incision is made over the muscle and a small bit of muscle is grasped with a forceps. The area is closed with sutures or like material and a sterile dressing is applied.
- Place tissue samples in normal saline solution and send to the laboratory.

Evaluation

- Observe for bleeding.
- Note test results in relation to other tests and clinical symptoms.

Client/Caregiver Teaching

Pretest

- Inform the client that the procedure is performed by a surgeon under sterile conditions and usually takes about 15 minutes to complete.
- Explain that food and fluids are not usually restricted.
- Inform the client that a sedative will be administered to promote relaxation and reduce discomfort during the procedure.

Posttest

- Instruct the client in the care and assessment of the site.
- Inform the client that the site will be sore and tender and movement will be difficult for several days.

Biopsy, Prostate

Classification: Histology
Type of Test: Excision and analysis

Prostate biopsy is the excision of a tissue sample from the prostate gland for microscopic analysis to determine the presence of cell morphology and tissue abnormalities. This test is used to confirm a diagnosis of prostate cancer. Biopsy specimen can be obtained in one of three ways: transurethral, transrectal, and perineal. The disadvantage of the transurethral approach is that malignant cells may not be included in the biopsy specimen if they are not located close enough to the urethra.

Indications

- Diagnose prostate cancer
- Diagnose prostatic hypertrophy of unknown causes

Reference Values

- No abnormal cells or tissue

Abnormal Values

- Prostate cancer
- Benign prostatic hypertrophy
- Prostatitis

Interfering Factors

- None

NURSING ALERT

- This procedure is contraindicated in bleeding disorders.

Nursing Implications

Assessment

- Obtain a history of urinary symptoms, medications, results of tests and procedures performed, and allergies.
- Assess hematologic status and blood-clotting ability, including complete blood count, platelets, prothrombin time, partial thromboplastin time, and clotting and bleeding time.
- Ensure that client has complied with food and fluid restrictions.

Possible Nursing Diagnoses

Anxiety related to perceived threat to health status

Sexuality patterns, altered, related to illness or medical treatment

Body image disturbance related to change in structure/appearance

Infection, risk for, related to immunosuppressed inflammatory response

Implementation

- Administer ordered enemas. For perineal or transurethral approach, usually one enema is ordered. For transrectal approach, saline enemas are ordered until returns are clear.
- Administer ordered premedication.
- *Transurethral approach:* Help the client into a prone position on a urologic examination table with legs in a stirrup. The external genitalia are cleansed with antiseptic solution, and a local anesthetic is inserted into the urethra. The endoscope is inserted, the prostate gland is visualized, and tissue is removed with a cutting loop.
- *Transrectal approach:* Help the client into the Sims position. A rectal examination is performed to locate potentially malignant nodules. A biopsy needle is passed along the examining finger and the stylet is removed. The biopsy needle is inserted through the needle guide and rotated to obtain a sample.
- *Perineal approach:* Help the client into the lithotomy or jackknife position. The client is draped, the perineum is cleansed with antiseptic solution, and local anesthetic is injected. A small incision is made and the sample is obtained by biopsy needle or biopsy punch. Samples are taken from several locations. Digital pressure is applied, and a sterile dressing is applied.

- Place tissue samples in formalin solution and send to the laboratory.

Evaluation

- Observe for bleeding.
- Monitor intake and output for 24 hours.
- Note test results in relation to other tests and clinical symptoms.

Client/Caregiver Teaching

Pretest

- Inform the client that the procedure is performed by a surgeon under sterile conditions and usually takes about 30 minutes to complete.
- Explain that food and fluids are not usually restricted.
- Inform the client that a sedative will be administered to promote relaxation and reduce discomfort during procedure.

Posttest

- Instruct the client in the care and assessment of the site.
- Have the client report any rectal pain or bleeding, blood in the urine, or fever.

Biopsy, Skin

Classification: Histology

Type of Test: Excision and analysis

Skin biopsy is the excision of a tissue sample from suspicious skin lesions for microscopic analysis to determine the presence of cell morphology and tissue abnormalities. This test is used to confirm the diagnosis of malignant or benign skin lesions. Biopsy specimen can be obtained in one of four ways: currettage, shaving, excision, or punch.

Indications

- Diagnose skin cancer
- Diagnose benign skin lesions

Reference Values

- No abnormal cells or tissue

Abnormal Values

- Basal cell carcinoma
- Squamous cell carcinoma
- Malignant melanoma
- Cysts
- Seborrheic keratosis
- Warts
- Pigmented nevi
- Keloids
- Dermatofibroma
- Neurofibroma
- Skin involvement in systemic lupus erythematosus, discoid lupus erythematosus, and scleroderma
- Pemphigus
- Dermatitis

Interfering Factors

- None

Nursing Implications

Assessment

- Obtain a history of clinical symptoms, medications, results of tests and procedures performed, and allergies.

Possible Nursing Diagnoses

Infection, risk for, related to altered integrity of the skin
Body image disturbance related to change in structure/ appearance

Implementation

- Assist the client to a position of comfort. Biopsy site is cleansed with an antiseptic solution, local anesthetic is applied, and the area is draped with sterile towels.
- *Curretage:* The skin is scraped with a currette until adequate tissue samples are obtained.
- *Shaving or excision:* A scalpel is used to remove a portion of the lesion that protrudes above the epidermis. If the lesion is to be excised, the incision is made as wide and deep as needed to ensure that the entire lesion is removed.

Bleeding is controlled with external pressure to the site. Large wounds are closed with sutures. An adhesive bandage strip is applied when excision is complete.

- *Punch biopsy:* A small, round punch about 4 to 6 mm in diameter is rotated into the skin to the desired depth. The cylinder of skin is pulled upward with a forceps and separated at its base with a scalpel or scissors. If needed, sutures are applied. A sterile dressing is applied over the site.
- Place tissue samples in formalin solution and send to the laboratory.

Evaluation

- Observe for bleeding.
- Note test results in relation to other tests and clinical symptoms.

Client/Caregiver Teaching

Pretest

- Inform the client that the procedure is performed by a surgeon under sterile conditions and usually takes about 30 minutes to complete.
- Explain that food and fluids are not usually restricted.

Posttest

- Instruct the client in the care and assessment of the site.
- Have the client report any bleeding, redness, edema, or pain at the site.
- Instruct the client to return for suture removal as indicated.

Biopsy, Thyroid

Classification: Histology

Type of Test: Excision and analysis

Thyroid biopsy is the excision of a tissue sample from skin lesions for microscopic analysis to determine the presence of cell morphology and tissue abnormalities. This test is used to confirm a diagnosis of cancer or the cause of persisitent thyroid symptoms. Biopsy specimen can be obtained by needle aspiration or surgical incision.

Indications

- Diagnose thyroid cancer or benign cysts or tumors
- Diagnose enlargement of the thyroid gland
- Determine cause of hyperthyroidism
- Determine cause of inflammatory thyroid disease

Reference Values

- No abnormal cells or tissue

Abnormal Values

- Thryoid cancer
- Benign thyroid cyst
- Hashimoto's thyroiditis
- Granulomatous thyroiditis
- Nontoxic nodular goiter

Interfering Factors

- None

Nursing Implications

Assessment

- Obtain a history of clinical symptoms, medications, results of tests and procedures performed, and allergies.
- Ensure that client has complied with the food and fluid restrictions.

Possible Nursing Diagnoses

Anxiety related to perceived threat to health status

Swallowing, impaired, related to mechanical obstruction

Communication, impaired, verbal, related to discomfort after procedure

Implementation

- Administer ordered sedation.
- Help the client to a position of comfort. Cleanse the biopsy site with an antiseptic solution, apply local anesthetic, and drape the area with sterile towels.

- *Open biopsy:* After administration of general anesthesia, a surgical incision is made, suspicious areas are located, and tissue samples are collected.
- *Needle biopsy:* Help the client to a supine position with a small pillow or sandbag under the shoulders. The area is cleansed with an antiseptic solution, injected with a local anesthetic, and draped with sterile drapes. Instruct the client not to swallow as the anesthetic is injected. The biopsy needle is inserted and a sample is obtained. Pressure is applied to the site, and a sterile dressing is applied.
- Place tissue samples in formalin solution and send to the laboratory.

Evaluation

- Observe for bleeding.
- Note test results in relation to other tests and clinical symptoms.

Client/Caregiver Teaching

Pretest

- Inform the client that the open biopsy is performed by a surgeon under sterile conditions and usually takes about 30 minutes to complete. Needle biopsy takes about 15 minutes.
- Explain that food and fluids are not usually restricted for a needle biopsy but are restricted for 6 to 8 hours before the surgery.

Posttest

- Instruct the client in the care and assessment of the site.
- Have the client report any bleeding, redness, edema, or pain at the site.
- Instruct the client to return for suture removal as indicated.

Bleeding Time

Classification: Hematology

Type of Test: Serum

Bleeding time measures the duration of bleeding after a standardized skin incision to evaluate platelet function. In response to the incision, the vessel will contract and platelets will adhere to the vessel wall in an attempt to stop the bleeding. The amount of time this takes reflects platelet function.

Indications

- Detect presence of bleeding disorders, particularly in those with a family history of disorders such as von Willebrand's disease
- Determine the cause of clinical signs of bleeding, such as epistaxis, easy bruising, bleeding gums, hematuria, and menorrhagia
- Investigate cause of thrombocytopenia
- Determine the cause of platelet dysfunction
- Determine the effects of diseases and of drugs known to affect bleeding time

Reference Values

Duke method	1–3 min
Ivy method	3–6 min
Ivy critical value	>15 min
Template method	3–6 min

Abnormal Values

- Prolonged bleeding
  Platelet count below 10,000 per mm^3
  Platelet dysfunction (prolonged bleeding with platelet count above 10,000 per mm^3)
  von Willebrand's disease
  Hemophilia
  Hypersplenism

Leukemia
Aplastic anemia
Disseminated intravascular coagulation
Connective-tissue diseases
Hypothyroidism
Hepatic cirrhosis
Severe liver disease
Severe renal disease
Hodgkin's disease, multiple myeloma
Measles
Mumps
Scurvy
Bernard-Soulier syndrome (hereditary giant platelet syndrome)
Use of some drugs, including aspirin and other salicylates, alcohol, anticoagulants, high molecular weight dextran, mithramycin, streptokinase, alteplase, sulfonamides, and thiazide diuretics

Interfering Factors

- Ingestion of drugs affecting platelet function within 7 days of the test can alter results (see Abnormal Values).
- Inaccurate size of incision can affect results.
- Improper technique: excessive pressure with filter paper interferes with formation of platelet plug.

> ### NURSING ALERT
>
> - This procedure is contraindicated in severe bleeding disorders, skin infection, edema of the extremity, or platelet count <50,000 per mm^3.

Nursing Implications

Assessment

- Determine client's hemostasis status, including bleeding from any site or known or suspected family history of bleeding disorders.
- Assess skin for coldness, edema, infection, or rash.
- Determine ingestion of drugs that may affect platelet count in the last 7 days.

Possible Nursing Diagnoses

Injury, risk for, related to altered clotting factors
Protection, altered, related to abnormal blood profiles
Anxiety related to perceived threat to health status
Pain related to tissue ischemia or inflammation

Implementation

- Select a site for the puncture. Obtain a stopwatch to time the test.
- Cleanse the site with an antiseptic and allow to dry.
- *Duke method:* Make an incision 3-mm deep with a sterile lancet on the earlobe.
- *Ivy methods:* Apply a blood pressure cuff above the elbow. Inflate it to 40 mm Hg. Make two incisions 3-mm deep on the volar surface of the forearm with sterile lancets.
- *Template method:* Apply a blood pressure cuff above the elbow. Inflate it to 40 mm Hg. Make two incisions 1-mm deep by 9-mm long on the volar surface of the forearm with sterile lancets using the standardized template as a guide.
- After the skin is pierced, remove the oozing blood at 15-second intervals by touching the filter paper to the drop of blood without touching the wound. As platelets accumulate, the bleeding slows and the oozing drop of blood becomes smaller. The end point occurs when there is no fluid left to produce a spot on the filter paper.
- Discontinue the test and apply pressure to the site if bleeding persists longer than 10 minutes.
- Apply a sterile pressure dressing to the incision site.
- Apply ice to the site if persistent bleeding occurs.

Evaluation

- Observe incision sites every 5 minutes for evidence of bleeding. Clients with clotting disorders may rebleed for up to 30 minutes after initial bleeding has stopped. If this occurs, apply direct pressure to the site.
- Assess site in 24 hours for evidence of infection.
- Assess for excessive bruising of the site where the blood pressure cuff was applied after the Ivy or Template methods.
- Note results of test in relation to other tests.

Client/Caregiver Teaching

Pretest

- Instruct patient to avoid using drugs that may interfere with test results for 7 days before the test.

Posttest

- Have the client remove dressing 24 hours after the test.
- Have the client notify the physician if evidence of infection is present.
- Resume any medications discontinued before the test.

▰▰▰▰▰▰▰▰▰▰▰▰▰▰▰▰▰

Blood Gases, Arterial (ABG)

Classification: Chemistry

Type of Test: Arterial blood

Using a sample of arterial blood, this test not only measures the specific levels of actual blood gases but also determines the client's overall acid-base balance. Components include pH, Pao_2, $Paco_2$, HCO_3, O_2 saturation, and base excess.

- The pH, or power of hydrogen, reflects the number of hydrogen ions in the body and is influenced by the amount of carbon dioxide in the blood. The body demands that the pH remain constant, so the kidneys and lungs compensate by preserving the ratio of acid to base. Any change in ratio of bicarbonate (HCO_3) will cause a reciprocal change in uptake and release of free hydrogen.
- The Pao_2 indicates the partial pressure of oxygen in the blood.
- The $Paco_2$ is the partial pressure of carbon dioxide in the blood.
- O_2 saturation indicates the amount of oxygen the blood could carry if all the hemoglobin were fully saturated with oxygen.
- Base excess indicates the difference between client bicarbonate level and normal serum levels.
- Anion gap is the difference between electrolytes, measured cations, and measured anions. It determines unmeasured anions and cations in the serum. It is calculated by measuring the sum of $(Na + K) - (Cl + HCO_3)$. Metabolic acidosis with normal anion gap may occur in those with diarrhea, fistulas, hyperalimentation, or renal tubular acidosis.

Indications

- Determine need and evaluate effectiveness of mechanical ventilation
- Evaluate response to weaning from mechanical ventilation
- Evaluate effectiveness of cardiac output in clients with myocardial infarction or shock
- Determine need for oxygen therapy
- Diagnose respiratory failure, which is defined as a PaO_2 of $\leq$ 50 mm Hg and a $PaCO_2$ of $\geq$ 50 mm Hg
- Determine acid-base balance, type of imbalance, and degree of compensation
- Determine cause of metabolic acidosis (anion gap)

Reference Values

		SI Units
pH		
Newborn	7.32–7.49	7.32–7.49
Adult	7.35–7.45	7.35–7.45
PaO_2		
Newborn	60–70 mm Hg	8–9.4 kPa
Adult	75–100 mm Hg	10–13.3 kPa
$PaCO_2$	35–45 mm Hg	4.7–6 kPa
HCO_3		
Newborn	20–26 mEq/L	20–26 mmol/L
Adult	22–26 mEq/L	22–26 mmol/L
O_2 saturation	96–100%	0.96–1.00
Base excess	+ 1 to − 2	+ 1 to − 2
Anion gap	10–18 mEq/L	10–18 mmol/L

Abnormal Values

- Increased pH
    - Metabolic or respiratory alkalosis
    - Alkali ingestion
    - Cushing's disease
    - Excessive vomiting
    - High altitude
    - Salicylate intoxication
    - Intestinal obstruction (pyloric or duodenal)
- Decreased pH
    - Metabolic or respiratory acidosis
    - Addison's disease
    - Cardiac disease

Asthma
Arrhythmias
Pulmonary diseases or disorders
Sepsis

- Increased PaO_2
  Hyperbaric oxygenation
  Hyperventilation
- Decreased PaO_2
  Acute or chronic pulmonary disease
  Shock
  Cardiac disorders
  Arrhythmias
  Metabolic acidosis
  Respiratory alkalosis
  Diabetes mellitus
  Drugs, including acetazolamide, methicillin, nitrofurantoin, tetracycline, and triamterene
- Increased $PaCO_2$
  Respiratory acidosis
  Metabolic alkalosis
  Cardiac disorders
  Near drowning
  Respiratory disorders, including pneumothorax, pneumonia, pleural effusion and failure
- Decreased $PaCO_2$
  Arrhythmias
  Hyperventilation
  Metabolic acidosis
  Respiratory alkalosis
  High altitude
  Diabetic ketoacidosis
  Salicylate intoxication
- Increased HCO_3
  Anoxia
  Metabolic alkalosis
  Respiratory acidosis
- Decreased HCO_3
  Hypocapnia
  Metabolic acidosis
  Respiratory alkalosis
- Increased O_2 saturation
  Hyperbaric oxygenation
- Decreased O_2 saturation
  Anoxia
  Adult respiratory distress syndrome
  Atelectasis
  Carbon monoxide poisoning

Hyaline membrane disease

Near drowning

Respiratory disorders, including pleural effusion, pneumonia, pneumothorax, infection and failure

Sarcoidosis

Status epilepticus

Cardiac disorders, including valvular and septal defects

■ Increased base excess

Metabolic alkalosis

■ Decreased base excess

Metabolic acidosis

■ Increased anion gap

Lactic acidosis

Metabolic acidosis

Drugs, including salicylates, diuretics, penicillin, corticosteroids, and antihypertensives

■ Decreased anion gap

High electrolyte values (sodium, calcium, magnesium)

Drugs, including lithium, diuretics, and chlorpropamide

Interfering Factors

■ Fever may falsely elevate PaO_2 and $PaCO_2$; hypothermia may decrease levels.
■ Suctioning of respiratory passages within 20 to 30 minutes may alter results.
■ Excess heparin in sample will decrease pH and $PaCO_2$.
■ Air bubbles in sample may alter results.
■ Exposure of sample to room temperature >2 minutes may alter test results.

Nursing Implications

Assessment

■ Obtain a history of respiratory and cardiac systems, suspected or known thyroid cardiopulmonary or acid-base disorders, and results of tests and procedures performed.
■ Perform Allen test if sample is to be obtained by radial artery puncture.

Possible Nursing Diagnoses

Anxiety related to perceived threat to health status

Airway clearance, ineffective, related to presence of obstruction or secretions

Tissue perfusion, altered, cardiopulmonary, related to ventilation-perfusion imbalance

- Breathing pattern, ineffective, related to pain, decreased energy, or fatigue

Implementation

- Obtain a blood-gas collection kit. If prepackaged kits are not available, obtain 3-mL syringe, heparin (100 u/mL), 20- or 21-gauge needles, povidone-iodine or alcohol swabs, gauze pads, and tape. Fill a plastic cup or bag with ice.
- Put on gloves. Using aseptic technique, perform an arterial puncture and collect 2 to 3 mL of blood in a heparinized syringe.
- Expel any air from the syringe, and place it on ice.
- If the client is receiving oxygen, include the percentage on the requisition slip and transport to the laboratory immediately.
- Calculate anion gap using recently obtained electrolyte values of sodium, potassium, chloride, and bicarbonate according to the formula above.

Evaluation

- Note results in relation to the client's symptoms and other tests performed.

Client/Caregiver Teaching

Pretest

- Instruct the client to withhold drugs that interfere with test results, as ordered.
- Advise the client to rest for 30 minutes before the test.

Posttest

- Inform the client or caregiver that the test may be repeated until cardiopulmonary function or acid-base balance is stabilized.

Blood Typing ABO Group, Rh Factor, and Cross-match Compatibility

Classification: Immunohematologic

Type of Test: Blood

Blood typing is a series of tests that include the ABO and Rh blood-group system performed to detect surface antigens on red blood cells (RBC) by an agglutination test and compatibility tests to determine antibodies against these antigens. The major antigens in the ABO system are A and B, although AB and O are also common phenotypes. The client with A antigens has type A blood; the client with B antigens has type B blood. The client with both A and B antigens has type AB blood (universal recipient); the client with neither A nor B antigens has type O blood (universal donor). Blood type is genetically determined. After 6 months of age, individuals have serum antibodies that react with the A or B antigen absent from their own red blood cells. These are called anti-A and anti-B antibodies.

In ABO blood typing, the client's red blood cells are mixed with anti-A and anti-B sera, a process known as "forward grouping." The process is then reversed and the client's serum is mixed with type A and B cells ("reverse grouping").

Only blood with the same ABO and Rh group can be infused because the anti-A and anti-B antibodies are strong agglutinins that cause a rapid, complement-mediated destruction of incompatible cells. To prevent this, indirect Coombs' test is performed on both blood samples for antibodies. Then the antibody is identified by testing with various known antigens to determine antigen-antibody reactions. The samples from both are then combined and tested for antigen-antibody reaction that can result in a transfusion-reaction.

The test is also performed in pregnant women to identify the risk of hemolytic disease of the newborn. Although most of the anti-A and anti-B activity resides in the IgM class of immunoglobulins, some activity rests with IgG. Anti-A and anti-B antibodies of the IgG class coat the red blood cells without immediately affecting their viability and can readily cross the placenta, resulting in hemolytic disease of the newborn. Individuals with type O blood frequently have more IgG anti-A and anti-B, thus ABO hemolytic disease of the newborn affects infants of type O mothers almost exclusively.

Major antigens of the Rh system are D (or Rh_O), C, E, c, and e. Individuals whose red blood cells possess D antigen are called Rh-positive; those who lack D antigen are called Rh-negative, no matter what other Rh antigens are present. Individuals who are Rh-negative produce anti-D antibodies when exposed to Rh-positive cells by either transfusions or pregnancy. These anti-D antibodies cross the placenta to the fetus and can cause hemolytic disease of the newborn or transfusion reactions if Rh-positive blood is administered.

Indications

- Identify the client's ABO and Rh blood type, especially before procedure in which blood loss is a threat or replacement may be needed
- Identify donor ABO and Rh blood type for stored blood
- Determine ABO and Rh compatibility of donor's and recipient's bloods before transfusion
- Identify maternal and infant ABO and Rh blood types, to predict risk of hemolytic disease of the newborn
- Determine anti-D antibody titer after sensitization by pregnancy with an Rh-positive fetus
- Determine the need for immunosuppressive therapy (e.g., with Rhogam) when an Rh-negative woman has delivered or aborted an Rh-positive fetus

Reference Values

- ABO system: A, B, AB, or O specific to person
- Rh system: positive or negative specific to person
- Cross-matching: compatibility between donor and recipient

Abnormal Values

- Incompatibility indicated by clumping (agglutination) of red blood cells

Interfering Factors

- Recent administration of dextran, blood, blood products, or IV contrast media causes cellular aggregation resembling agglutination in ABO typing.
- Drugs, including levodopa, methyldopa, and nethyldopate hydrochloride, cause a false-positive in Rh typing.

Nursing Implications

Assessment

■ Obtain a history of pregnancy, known or anticipated need for transfusion, related diagnostic tests performed, any medications that can interfere with test results, and blood transfusion within the previous 3 months.

Possible Nursing Diagnosis

Anxiety related to perceived threat to health status

Implementation

■ Put on gloves. Using aseptic technique, perform a venipuncture and collect 10 mL of blood in a red-top tube for ABO and Rh typing and 10 to 15 mL of blood in lavender-top tubes for cross-matching.
■ Handle sample very gently to avoid hemolysis.

NURSING ALERT

Although correct client identification is important for test specimens, it is crucial when blood is collected for typing and cross-matching. Therefore, additional requirements are necessary, including

■ Verifying name, Social Security and hospital number, date, and blood bank number, on requisition and specimen labels
■ Completing and applying wrist band on arm with the same information
■ Placing labels with the same information and blood bank number on blood sample tubes

Evaluation

■ Note results of tests for typing and compatibility if done to prepare for transfusion.
■ If acute fluid volume loss (hemorrhage) occurs, initiate IV fluids (lactated ringers) until typing and cross-matching testing is completed (can take 1 hour to complete).

Client/Caregiver Teaching

Posttest

■ Inform client of blood and Rh type, and advise the client to record the information on a card or other document that he or she normally carries.

- Inform women who are Rh-negative to tell their physician if they become pregnant or need a transfusion.

Blood Urea Nitrogen (BUN)

Classification: Chemistry

Type of Test: Serum

Urea is a nonprotein nitrogen compound formed in the liver from ammonia as an end product of protein metabolism. Urea diffuses freely into both extracellular and intracellular fluid and is ultimately excreted by the kidneys. Blood urea levels reflect the balance between production and excretion of urea. Blood urea nitrogen (BUN) analysis involves the measurement of urea nitrogen and indicates the liver's ability to metabolize proteins and the kidneys' ability to excrete urea. Urea concentration can be calculated by multiplying the BUN result by 2.14.

Indications

- Evaluate renal function
- Evaluate liver function
- Evaluate hydration
- Monitor effects of drugs known to be nephrotoxic or hepatotoxic

Reference Values

		SI Units
Newborns	4–18 mg/dL	1.4–6.4 mmol/L
Children	5–18 mg/dL	1.8–6.4 mmol/L
Adults	5–20 mg/dL	1.8–7.1 mmol/L
Older adults	8–21 mg/dL	2.9–7.5 mmol/L
Critical value	>100 mg/dL	>35.7 mmol/L

Abnormal Values

- Increased BUN
    Congestive heart failure
    Shock

Hypovolemia
Urinary tract obstruction
Renal disease
Starvation
Infection
Myocardial infarction
Diabetes mellitus
Burns
GI bleeding (excessive blood protein in the GI tract)
Advanced pregnancy
Nephrotoxic agents
Excessive protein ingestion
Neoplasms
Addison's disease
Gout
Pancreatitis
Tissue necrosis
Advanced age
Certain drugs, including aspirin, acetaminophen, chemo-
therapeutic agents, antibiotics (amphotericin B, ceph-
alosporins, aminoglycosides), thiazide diuretics, in-
domethacin, morphine, codeine, sulfonamides,
methyldopa, propranolol, guanethidine, pargyline, lith-
ium carbonate, dextran, and sulfonylureas
- Decreased BUN
Inadequate dietary protein
Severe liver disease
Water overload
Nephrotic syndrome
Pregnancy
Amyloidosis
Malabsorption syndromes
Certain drugs, including IV dextrose, phenothiazines, and
thymol

Interfering Factors

- Therapy with drugs known to alter BUN levels (see Abnormal
Values)
- High protein intake can elevate BUN levels.

Nursing Implications

Assessment

- Obtain a history of known or suspected renal or hepatic dysfunction, signs and symptoms of fluid imbalance, or diet high
in protein.

■ Note if client has fasted for 8 hours before the test, if required by the laboratory.

Possible Nursing Diagnoses

Anxiety related to perceived threat to health status
Pain related to tissue ischemia or inflammation
Fluid volume excess related to compromised regulatory mechanism
Fluid volume deficit, risk for, related to active loss

Implementation

■ Put on gloves. Using aseptic technique, perform a venipuncture and collect 7 mL of blood in either a gray- or red-top tube.
■ Handle the sample gently to avoid hemolysis and send to the laboratory promptly.

Evaluation

■ Monitor intake and output for fluid imbalance in renal dysfunction and dehydration.
■ Compare with creatinine-level increases in renal dysfunction.

Client/Caregiver Teaching

Pretest

■ Instruct the client to fast for 8 hours before the test, if required by the laboratory.

Bone Marrow Aspiration and Analysis, Bone Marrow Biopsy

Classification: Hematology

Type of Test: Bone marrow

This test involves the removal of a small sample of bone marrow by aspiration, needle biopsy, or open surgical biopsy for a complete hematologic analysis. The marrow is evaluated for morphology and examination of erythrocytes and granulocytes in all stages of maturation; megakaryocytes, lymphocytes, and plasma cells; bone marrow iron stores; and ratios of myeloid to erythroid (M:E). Sudan B and periodic acid–Schiff (PAS) stains can be performed for microscopic examination to differentiate the different types of leukemia.

Indications

- Evaluate abnormal results of complete blood count or white blood cell (WBC) count with differential showing increased numbers of leukocyte precursors
- Monitor effects of exposure to bone marrow depressants
- Monitor bone marrow response to chemotherapy or radiation therapy
- Evaluate hepatomegaly or splenomegaly
- Identify bone marrow hyperplasia or hypoplasia
- Determine marrow differential (proportion of the various types of cells present in the marrow) and the M:E ratio

Interfering Factors

- Recent blood transfusions: iron, liver, or cytotoxic agents may alter test results.

Reference Values

- Iron stain: 2+ for hemosiderin
- Sudan B stain: Negative
- Periodic acid–Schiff (PAS): Negative

Cell Type (%)	Adults	Infants	Children
Undifferentiated	0–0.1	—	—
Reticulocytes	0.5–2.0	—	—
Granulocytes	6.0–12.0	3.6	12.9
Neutrophils (total)	56.5	32.4	57.1
Myeloblasts	0.3–5.0	0.62	1.2
Megaloblasts	0	0	0
Promyelocytes	1.0–8.0	0.76	1.4
Myelocytes	4.2–15.0	2.5	18.4
Neutrophilic	5.0–19.0	—	—
Eosinophilic	0.5–3.0	—	—
Basophilic	0–0.5	—	—
Bands (stabs)	9.5–15.3	14.1	0
Lymphocytes	2.7–24.0	49.0	16.0
Monocytes	0.3–2.7	—	—
Eosinophils	0.5–3.0	2.6	3.6
Basophils	0–0.2	0.07	0.06

(*continued*)

Cell Type (%)	Adults	Infants	Children
Plasma cells	0.3–1.5	0.02	0.4
Megakaryocytes	0.03–0.5	0.05	0.1
Normoblasts (total)	25.6	8.0	23.1
Basophilic	1.4–4.0	0.34	1.7
Polychromatophilic	6.0–29.0	6.9	18.2
Orthochromic	3.6–21.0	0.54	2.7
Pronormoblasts	0.2–4.0	0.1	0.5
M:E ratio	6:1–2:1	4.4:1	2.9:1

Abnormal Values

- Increased reticulocytes
    Compensated RBC loss
    Response to vitamin B_{12} therapy
- Decreased reticulocytes
    Aplastic crisis of sickle-cell disease or hereditary sphero-
    cytosa
- Increased neutrophils (total)
    Myeloid (chronic) leukemias
    Acute myeloblastic leukemia
- Decreased neutrophils (total)
    Aplastic anemia
    Leukemias (monocytic and lymphoblastic)
- Increased lymphocytes
    Viral infections
    Lymphatic leukemia
    Lymphosarcoma
    Lymphomas
    Mononucleosis
    Aplastic anemia
- Increased granulocytes
    Myelocytic leukemia
    Infections
- Increased plasma cells
    Cancer
    Ulcerative colitis
    Connective-tissue disorders
    Syphilis
    Infections
    Cirrhosis of the liver
    Hypersensitivity reactions
    Macroglobulinemia
    Radiation therapy

- Increased megakaryocytes
    Old age
    Myeloid leukemia
    Hemorrhage
    Polycythemia vera
    Megakaryocytic myelosis
    Infections
    Pneumonia
    Thrombocytopenia
- Decreased megakaryocytes
    Pernicious aplastic anemia
    Agranulocytosis
    Thrombocytopenia purpura
    Cirrhosis of the liver
    Radiation therapy
- Increased myeloid-erythroid (M:E) ratio
    Bone marrow failure
    Myeloid leukemia
    Infections
    Leukemia reactions
- Decreased myeloid-erythroid (M:E) ratio
    Anemias
    Posthemorrhage hematopoiesis
    Hepatic disease
    Polycythemia vera
- Increased normoblasts
    Polycythemia vera
    Anemias
    Chronic blood loss
- Decreased normoblasts
    Folic acid or vitamin B_{12} deficiency
    Aplastic anemia
    Hemolytic anemia
- Increased eosinophils
    Bone marrow cancer
    Lymphadenoma
    Myeloid leukemia

NURSING ALERT

- This procedure is contraindicated in clients with known coagulation defects, unless the importance of the information obtained outweighs the risks involved in performing the test.

Nursing Implications

Assessment

- Obtain a history of known or suspected conditions affecting hematologic status, results of tests and procedures performed, recent blood transfusions, drug therapy that includes iron or liver preparations or cytotoxic agents.

Possible Nursing Diagnoses

Anxiety related to perceived threat to health status
Injury, risk for, related to invasive procedure and immunosuppressed inflammatory response
Injury, risk for, related to altered clotting factors
Protection, altered, related to abnormal blood profiles

Implementation

- Provide a hospital gown if necessary for access to the biopsy site.
- Administer premedication prescribed for pain or anxiety.
- Help client to the desired position depending on the site to be used. In young children, the most frequently chosen site is the proximal tibia. Vertebral bodies T10 through L4 are preferred in older children. In adults, the sternum or iliac crests are the preferred sites.
- The client is placed in the prone, sitting, or side-lying position for the vertebral bodies; the side-lying position for iliac crest or tibial sites; or the supine position for the sternum.
- *Needle aspiration:* Prepare skin with an antiseptic solution and drape the site. The physician will anesthetize the site, preferably with procaine, then insert a needle with stylet into the marrow. The stylet is removed, a syringe attached, and an aliquot of 0.5 mL of marrow withdrawn. The needle is removed and pressure applied to the site. The aspirate is applied to slides and, when dry, fixative is applied.
- *Needle biopsy:* Local anesthetic is introduced deeply enough to include the periosteum. A cutting biopsy needle is introduced through a small skin incision and bored into the marrow cavity. A core needle is introduced through the cutting needle and a plug of marrow is removed. The needles are withdrawn and the specimen is placed in a preservative solution. Pressure is applied to the site for 5 to 10 minutes, and a dressing is applied.

Evaluation

- Note results in relation to other tests and the client's clinical presentation.

Client/Caregiver Teaching

Pretest

- Explain that the test is done at the bedside by a physician and requires about 20 minutes.
- Explain that discomfort of the puncture will be minimized with local anesthetics or systemic analgesics and that the site may remain tender for several weeks.
- For children, provide equipment and a doll with which to role-play a simulated procedure.
- Inform the client that bedrest for 10 to 30 minutes (depending on the site) is required after the procedure.

Posttest

- Advise the client or caregiver to keep ice on the site and not to remove the bandage for 24 hours.
- Instruct the client to report any signs of infections or excessive bleeding immediately.

Bronchoscopy

Classification: Endoscopy

Type of Test: Direct visualization

This procedure provides direct visualization of the larynx, trachea, and bronchial tree by means of either a rigid or a flexible bronchoscope. Its purposes are both diagnostic and therapeutic.

The rigid bronchoscope is designed to allow for visualization of the larger airways, including the lobar, segmental, and subsegmental bronchi, while maintaining effective gas exchange. Rigid bronchoscopy is preferred when large volumes of blood or secretions need to be aspirated, when foreign bodies are to be removed, when large-sized biopsy specimens are to be obtained, and for most bronchoscopies in children.

The flexible fiberoptic bronchoscope has a smaller lumen and is designed to allow for visualization of all segments of the bronchial tree. The accessory lumen of the bronchoscope is used for tissue biopsy, bronchial washings, instillation of anesthetic agents and medications, and to obtain specimens with brushes for cytologic examination. In general, fiberoptic bronchoscopy is less traumatic to the surrounding tissues than the larger rigid bronchoscopes. It is performed under local anesthesia, and client tolerance of the procedure is better than for rigid bronchoscopy.

Indications

- Determine etiology of persistent cough, hemoptysis, hoarseness, unexplained chest x-ray abnormalities, abnormal cytological findings in sputum
- Evaluate respiratory distress and tachypnea in an infant to rule out tracheoesophageal fistula or other congenital anomaly
- Detect and stage bronchogenic cancer
- Treat lung cancer through instillation of chemotherapeutic agents, implantation of radioisotopes, or laser palliative therapy
- Identify hemorrhagic and inflammatory changes in Kaposi's sarcoma
- Diagnose lung infections and inflammation
- Remove foreign body
- Determine extent of smoke-inhalation or other traumatic injury
- Evaluate airway patency; aspirate deep or retained secretions
- Identify bleeding sites and remove clots within the tracheobronchial tree
- Evaluate possible airway obstruction in clients with known or suspected sleep apnea
- Intubate clients with cervical spine injuries or massive upper-airway edema
- Evaluate endotracheal tube placement or possible adverse sequelae

Reference Values

- Normal larynx, trachea, bronchi, bronchioles, and alveoli

Abnormal Values

- Inflammation
- Abscess
- Tumors
- Foreign bodies
- Bronchial stenosis
- Bronchial diverticulum
- Interstitial pulmonary disease
- Bronchogenic cancer
- Tuberculosis

- Tuberculosis, coccidioidomycosis, histoplasmosis, blastomycosis, phycomycosis
- Opportunistic lung infections such as Pneumocystitis, Nocardia, or cytomegalovirus (CMV)

Interfering Factors

- Failure to follow dietary and fluid restrictions before the procedure
- Inability to cooperate with the procedure if it is to be done under local anesthesia

NURSING ALERT

This procedure is contraindicated in
- Bleeding disorders, especially those associated with uremia and cytotoxic chemotherapy
- Hypoxemic or hypercapnic states that require continuous oxygen administration
- Pulmonary hypertension
- Cardiac conditions or dysrhythmias
- Disorders that limit extension of the neck
- Severe obstructive tracheal conditions
- Presence of or potential for respiratory failure; introduction of the bronchoscope alone may cause a 10 to 20 mm Hg drop in Pao_2

Nursing Implications

Assessment

- Obtain a history of allergies or sensitivities to anesthetics, analgesics, and antibiotics and known or suspected pulmonary disorder.
- Determine previous abnormalities in laboratory test results, particularly hematologic or coagulation tests.
- Ensure that dietary and fluid restrictions were followed; no food or fluids for 6 to 8 hours before the procedure.

Possible Nursing Diagnoses

Anxiety related to perceived threat to health status
Airway clearance, ineffective, related to presence of obstruction or secretions
Tissue perfusion, altered, cardiopulmonary, related to ventilation-perfusion imbalance
Breathing pattern, ineffective, related to pain, decreased energy, or fatigue

Implementation

- Keep resuscitation equipment on hand in the case of respiratory impairment or laryngospasm following the procedure.
- Avoid using morphine sulfate in those with asthma or other pulmonary disease. It can further exacerbate bronchospasms and respiratory impairment.
- Have client remove dentures, contact lenses, eye glasses, and jewelry. Notify physician of permanent crown on teeth. Help client to disrobe and provide a hospital gown.
- Provide mouth care to reduce oral bacterial flora.
- *Rigid bronchoscopy:* In this procedure the client is placed in the supine position and a general anesthesia is administered. The client's neck is hyperextended, and the lightly lubricated bronchoscope is inserted orally and passed through the glottis. The client's head is turned or repositioned to aid visualization of various segments.
- After inspection, the bronchial brush, suction catheter, biopsy forceps, laser and electrocautery devices are introduced to obtain specimens for cytologic or microbiologic study or for therapeutic procedures.
- If a bronchial washing is performed, small amounts of solution are instilled into the airways and removed. These specimens are placed in labeled containers and sent to the laboratory promptly.
- After the procedure, the bronchoscope is removed and the client is placed in a side-lying position with the head slightly elevated.
- *Fiberoptic bronchoscopy:* In this procedure the client is placed in a sitting position and the tongue and oropharynx is sprayed or swabbed with local anesthetic. When loss of sensation is adequate, the client is placed in a supine position. The fiberoptic scope can be introduced through the nose, the mouth, an endotracheal tube, a tracheostomy tube, or a rigid bronchoscope. Most common insertion is the nose. Clients with copious secretions or massive hemoptysis, or in whom airway complications are more likely, may be intubated before the bronchoscopy. Additional local anesthetic is applied through the scope as it approaches the vocal cords and the carina, eliminating reflexes in these sensitive areas. The fiberoptic approach allows for visualization of airway segments without having to move the client's head through various positions.
- After inspection, specimens may be obtained for cytologic and microbiologic study. All specimens are placed in appropriate containers, labeled properly, and promptly sent to the laboratory.

■ After the procedure, the bronchoscope is removed. Clients who had local anesthesia are placed in a semi-Fowler's position to recover.

Evaluation

■ Note results in relation to other tests performed and the client's symptoms.

Client/Caregiver Teaching

Pretest

■ Inform the client that the procedure is generally performed in an endoscopy suite by a physician under local anesthesia and takes approximately 30 to 45 minutes.
■ Instruct the client to withhold food and fluids for 6 hours before the test.

Posttest

■ Instruct the client not to attempt to swallow saliva until the gag reflex has returned, but to expectorate saliva into an emesis basin.
■ Emphasize that any excessive bleeding, difficulty breathing, changes in sputum, or pain must be reported to the physician immediately.

Capillary Fragility, Rumpel-Leede Capillary Fragility Test, Tourniquet Test

Classification: Hematology

Type of Test: Skin

This test measures the ability of capillaries to resist rupturing under pressure. Capillary rupture suggests vessel weakness and possibly platelet dysfunction. Capillary breakdown can cause hemorrhage at any site, but most occur in the skin. Petechiae development after tourniquet or blood pressure cuff application lead to the alternate name of tourniquet test.

Indications

■ Evaluate history of "easy bruising" or development of petechiae

Reference Values

Less than 10 petechiae (excluding those which may have been present before the test) in a 2-inch circle is considered normal. Results may also be reported according to the scale below, with grade 1 indicating a normal or negative result.

Grade	Petechiae per 2-in circle
1	0–10
2	10–20
3	20–50
4	>50

Abnormal Values

■ Strongly positive (grade 4)
  Glanzmann's disease
  Idiopathic thrombocytopenic purpura
  Scurvy
  Thrombocytopenia due to acute infectious disease
  Aplastic anemia
  Leukemia
  Chronic renal disease
■ Moderately positive (grade 3)
  Hepatic cirrhosis
■ Slightly positive (grade 2)
  Decreased estrogen levels
  Dysproteinemia
  Polycythemia vera
  Allergic and senile purpuras
  Deficiency of vitamin K, factor VII, fibrinogen, or prothrombin
  von Willebrand's disease

Interfering Factors

■ Repeating the test on the same extremity within 1 week will yield inaccurate results.
■ Improper application of blood pressure cuff and inflation time will affect results.

> ## ◤ NURSING ALERT
>
> This procedure is contraindicated in clients known to have or suspected of having
> - Disseminated intravascular coagulation (DIC)
> - Platelet count <50,000/mm^3
> - Severe bleeding disorders
> - Anticoagulant therapy (or has taken aspirin within 7 days)
> - Senile skin changes
>
> This test is also contraindicated in
> - Clients with an edematous arm or very cold arm
> - If female client has a mastectomy
> - If client has an A-V fistula on that side

Nursing Implications

Assessment

- Obtain a personal and family history of known or suspected hematologic disorders, abnormal bleeding, or abnormal laboratory results, such as increased or decreased platelet count or coagulation studies.
- Ensure that client is not taking anticoagulants or has not taken aspirin or aspirin-containing products within 7 days of the test.
- Inspect the client's forearms and select a site that is as free as possible of petechiae.

Possible Nursing Diagnoses

Anxiety related to perceived threat to health status
Injury, risk for, related to altered clotting factors
Protection, altered, related to abnormal blood profiles

Implementation

- Measure an area 2 inches in diameter; circle the site lightly with a felt-tipped marker if necessary for reference. If petechiae are present in the site to be measured, note and record the number.
- Apply a blood pressure cuff to the arm and inflate to 100 mm Hg. Maintain pressure for 5 minutes. Remove blood pressure cuff, count the petechiae, and record the number.

Evaluation

- Note test results in relation to platelet count and other tests performed.

Client/Caregiver Teaching

Pretest

- Inform the client of the purpose of the test and that the tightness of the cuff may be uncomfortable but not painful.

Posttest

- Instruct the client to avoid traumas to the skin and mucous membranes if values are abnormal and to report any bleeding from any area to the physician.

C-Peptide

Classification: Blood chemistry

Type of Test: Serum

C-peptide is a biologically inactive peptide formed when beta cells of the pancreas convert proinsulin to insulin. Serum levels of C-peptide usually correlate with insulin levels and provide a reliable indication of how well the beta cells secrete insulin. Release of C-peptide is not affected by exogenous insulin administration, while serum insulin levels are elevated.

Indications

- Detect suspected excessive insulin administration: C-peptide levels do not increase with serum insulin levels
- Determine beta cell function when insulin antibodies preclude accurate measurement of serum insulin production
- Diagnose insulinoma
- Determine factitious cause of hypoglycemia: Serum levels of insulin will be elevated and C-peptide will be decreased

Reference Values

	SI Units
0.9–4.2 ng/mL	0.9–4.2 mg/L

Abnormal Values

- Increased values
  Islet cell tumor
  Endogenous hyperinsulinism
  Certain drugs, including oral hypoglycemics and sulfo-
      nylureas
- Decreased values
  Diabetes mellitus
  Hypoglycemia coinciding with elevated insulin levels

Interfering Factors

- Hepatic dysfunction causes elevated levels.
- Renal failure increases serum levels.
- C-peptide and intrinsic insulin levels do not always correlate
  in the obese.

Nursing Implications

Assessment

- Obtain a history of endocrine system, suspected or known
  insulin abnormality, and results of tests and procedures
  performed.
- Ensure that client has fasted for 8 to 12 hours before the test.
- Assess medication history and ensure that any drugs that may
  alter test results have been withheld for 12 to 24 hours before
  the test, as ordered.

Possible Nursing Diagnoses

Anxiety related to perceived threat to health status
Nutrition, altered, less than body requirements, related to in-
    ability to utilize nutrients
Therapeutic management, individual, ineffective related to
    [specify]

Implementation

- Put on gloves. Using aseptic technique perform a venipuncture and collect 7 mL of blood in a red-top tube for insulin

and C-peptide. Draw a 5-mL sample for glucose in a gray-top tube.

■ Handle sample gently to avoid hemolysis.

■ Pack the sample for insulin in ice. Label the samples and transport to the laboratory immediately.

Evaluation

■ Note test results in association with insulin levels.

Client/Caregiver Teaching

Pretest

■ Instruct the client to fast for 8 to 12 hours before the test.

Posttest

■ Instruct the client to resume diet and medications withheld before the test.

■ Instruct the client and caregiver to report signs and symptoms of hypoglycemia or hyperglycemia.

C-Reactive Protein (CRP)

Classification: Immunology

Type of Test: Serum

This abnormal glycoprotein is produced by the liver in response to acute inflammation. It is a nonspecific immunoassay test that determines the presence but not the cause of the inflammation. However, early detection of inflammation allows for prompt treatment. It disappears from the serum rapidly once inflammation has subsided.

Indications

■ Detect the presence or exacerbation of inflammatory processes

■ Monitor response to therapy for autoimmune disorders such as rheumatoid arthritis

Reference Values

- <0.8 mg/dL

Abnormal Values

- Increased values
    Rheumatic fever
    Rheumatoid arthritis
    Acute bacterial infections
    Inflammatory bowel disease
    Systemic lupus erythematosus
    Pregnancy (second half)
    Drugs, including oral contraceptives

Interfering Factors

- Falsely elevated levels may occur with presence of an intra-uterine device or overnight refrigeration of the specimen.
- Nonsteroidal anti-inflammatory drugs, salicylates, and steroids may cause false-negative results because of suppression of inflammation.

Nursing Implications

Assessment

- Obtain a history of immune system, suspected or known inflammatory disorders, and results of tests and procedures performed.
- Assess medication history and ensure that any drugs that may alter test results have been withheld for 12 to 24 hours before the test, as ordered.

Possible Nursing Diagnoses

Pain related to inflammatory process of connective tissues
Anxiety related to perceived threat to health status
Injury, risk for, related to immune response

Implementation

- Put on gloves. Using aseptic technique, perform a venipuncture and collect 7 mL of blood in a red-top tube.

Evaluation

- Note test results in relation to other diagnostic tests and the client's symptoms.

Client/Caregiver Teaching

Pretest

- Instruct the client to withhold medications that interfere with test results.

Posttest

- Instruct the client to resume medications withheld before the test.

Calcitonin, Thyrocalcitonin (hCT)

Classification: Chemistry

Type of Test: Plasma

This radioimmunoassay test measures levels of calcitonin, also called thyrocalcitonin (hCT), secreted by the parafollicular or C cells of the thyroid gland in response to elevated serum calcium levels. Although calcitonin's role is not completely understood, it is believed to antagonize parahormone and vitamin D effects, to inhibit osteoclasts that reabsorb bone so that calcium continues to be laid down and not reabsorbed into the blood, and to increase renal clearance of magnesium and inhibit tubular reabsorption of phosphates. The net result is that calcitonin decreases serum calcium levels. Some laboratories recommend pentagastrin (Peptavlon) provocative or the calcium infusion provocative test for diagnosis of medullary thyroid cancer.

Indications

- Diagnosis of medullary thyroid cancer
- Evaluate altered serum calcium levels
- Diagnose hyperparathyroidism

Reference Values

		SI Units
Basal		
Men	≤19 pg/mL	≤19 ng/L
Women	≤14 pg/mL	≤14 ng/L
Pentagastrin provocative test		
Men	≤110 pg/mL	≤110 ng/L
Women	≤30 pg/mL	≤30 ng/L
Calcium provocative test		
Men	≤190 pg/mL	≤190 ng/L
Women	≤130 pg/mL	≤130 ng/L

Abnormal Values

- Elevated levels
  Thyroiditis
  Medullary thyroid cancer
  Breast, lung, and pancreatic cancer
  Primary and secondary hyperparathyroidism
  Chronic renal failure
  Zollinger-Ellison syndrome
  C-cell hyperplasia

Interfering Factors

- Failure to fast from food for 8 hours before the test may alter results.

> **NURSING ALERT**
>
> - Some laboratories recommend that the pentagastrin test not be done in clients who have high basal calcitonin levels or who are hypocalcemic.

Nursing Implications

Assessment

- Obtain a history of known or suspected thyroid disorders and the results of and tests performed.
- Ensure that client has fasted from food for at least 8 hours before the test.

Possible Nursing Diagnoses

Anxiety related to perceived threat to health status

Swallowing, impaired, related to mechanical obstruction

Fluid volume excess related to compromised regulatory mechanism

Implementation

- Put on gloves. Using aseptic technique, perform a venipuncture and collect 10 mL of blood in a green-top or a chilled red-top tube.
- *Pentagastrin provocative test:* Draw a baseline blood sample, and then infuse pentagastrin 0.5 mcg/kg IV over 5 to 10 seconds. Obtain three blood samples, at 90 seconds, 2 minutes, and 5 minutes postinfusion.
- *Calcium provocative test:* Draw a baseline blood sample, and then infuse calcium 2.4 mg/kg IV over 5 to 10 seconds. Obtain two blood samples, at 5 minutes and 10 minutes postinfusion.
- Handle the sample gently to avoid hemolysis and transport to the laboratory promptly.

Evaluation

- Note results of other tests (serum calcium, parathyroid) in relation to any elevations in levels of calcitonin.

Client/Caregiver Teaching

Pretest

- Instruct the client to fast from food for 8 hours before the test. Sips of water will not affect test results.

Posttest

- Instruct the client to resume diet withheld before test.

Cancer Antigen 125 (CA-125)

Classification: Immunology

Type of Test: Blood

This qualitative test measures the amount of cancer antigen 125 (CA-125) in the blood. This glycoprotein is present in normal endometrial tissue and appears in the blood when natural endometrial protective barriers are destroyed, such as with cancer or endometriosis. Persistently rising levels indicate a poor prognosis, but absence of the tumor marker does not rule out tumor presence. Levels may also rise with pancreatic, liver, colon, breast, and lung cancers.

This test is 80 percent reliable and is most useful to monitor for treatment response. It is not useful as a screening test.

Indications

- Diagnose ovarian cancer
- Monitor response to treatment of ovarian cancer

Reference Values

	SI Units
<35 U/mL	<35 kU/L

Abnormal Values

- Positive levels
  Ovarian cancer
  Endometriosis
  Menses
  Breast cancer
  Liver cancer
  Endometrial cancer
  Lung cancer
  Colon cancer

Pancreatic cancer
Acute pancreatitis
Pelvic inflammatory disease
Peritonitis
First-trimester pregnancy
Ovarian abscess
Lymphoma

Interfering Factors

- Antineoplastic therapy can decrease levels.

Nursing Implications

Assessment

- Obtain a history of known or suspected disorders, medication regimen, and results of diagnostic tests performed.

Possible Nursing Diagnoses

Anxiety related to perceived threat to health status
Grieving, anticipatory, related to perceived potential loss
Body image disturbance related to potential change in structure/appearance

Implementation

- Put on gloves. Using aseptic technique, perform a venipuncture and collect 5 mL of blood in a red-top tube.
- Send specimen to laboratory immediately.

Evaluation

- Note test results in relation to other diagnostic tests and clinical symptoms.

Client/Caregiver Teaching

Pretest

- No fasting is required.

Carcinoembryonic Antigen (CEA)

Classification: Immunoassay

Type of Test: Serum or plasma

This test measures carcinoembryonic antigen (CEA), a glyco-protein produced only during early fetal life and rapid multi-plication of epithelial cells, especially those of the digestive system. It also appears in the blood of chronic smokers. Al-though the test is not diagnostic for any specific disease and is not useful as a cancer-screening test, it is useful for monitoring response to antineoplastic therapy in breast and gastrointesti-nal cancer.

Indications

- Monitor response to treatment of breast and gastrointestinal cancers
- Diagnose colon, pancreas, lung, or other cancers
- Determine stage of colorectal cancers and test for recurrence

Reference Values

		SI Units
Nonsmoker	<2.5 ng/mL	<2.5 μg/L
Smoker	<5.0 ng/mL	<5.0 μg/L

Abnormal Values

- Elevated levels
    Colorectal, pulmonary, gastric, pancreatic, breast, head or neck, esophageal, ovarian, or prostate cancer
    Recent radiation therapy
    Leukemia
    Lymphoma
    Sarcoma
    Benign tumors, including benign breast disease

Pulmonary emphysema
Bacterial pneumonia
Alcoholic cirrhosis
Alcoholic pancreatitis
Ulcerative colitis
Regional ileitis
Gastric ulcer
Colorectal polyps
Diverticulitis
Chronic ischemic heart disease
Hypothyroidism
Acute renal failure
Chronic tobacco smoking
Trauma
Medications, including antineoplastic and hepatotoxic agents

Interfering Factors

- Levels may be elevated in smokers who do not have malignancies.
- If radioimmunoassay method is used, radionuclide scans within 2 weeks before the test can invalidate test results.

Nursing Implications

Assessment

- Obtain a history of known or suspected cancer and any current medications.
- Determine if client smokes; smokers may have false elevations.

Possible Nursing Diagnoses

Anxiety related to perceived threat to health status
Body image disturbance related to change in appearance
Grieving, anticipatory, related to perceived loss or threat of death

Implementation

- Put on gloves. Using aseptic technique, perform a venipuncture and collect 7 mL of blood in a red-top tube.
- Handle sample gently to avoid hemolysis and send promptly to laboratory.

Evaluation

- Note results in relation to other tests performed and the client's symptoms.
- Note levels in relation to responses to treatment protocol.

Client/Caregiver Teaching

Posttest

- To monitor response to therapy, inform the client that the test can be repeated monthly.
- Provide support and instruct in importance of continuing scheduled therapy or follow-up visits.

Catecholamines, Plasma

Classification: Chemistry
Type of Test: Plasma

This test measures epinephrine, norepinephrine, and dopamine, the catecholamines produced by the adrenal medulla and found in sympathetic nerve endings and the brain. Catecholamines prepare the body for the fight-or-flight stress response and help regulate metabolism. Catecholamine levels are affected by diurnal variations and fluctuate in response to stress, postural changes, diet, smoking, drugs, and temperature—all which must be somewhat controlled when the test is performed to validate results. Because of the diurnal variation, this test is not as reliable as a 24-hour urine test for these substances.

Indications

- Identify cause of hypertension, such as pheochromocytoma
- Diagnosis of paragangliomas

Reference Values

		SI Units
Epinephrine and norepinephrine	150–650 pg/mL	86–3843 pmol/L
Epinephrine		
Supine	0–110 pg/mL	0–599 pmol/L
Standing	0–140 pg/mL	0–762 pmol/L
Norepinephrine		
Supine	70–750 pg/mL	381–4083 pmol/L
Standing	200–1700 pg/mL	1088–9256 pmol/L
Dopamine	<30 pg/mL	0–163 pmol/L

Abnormal Values

- Elevated levels
    Ganglioneuroblastoma
    Ganglioneuroma
    Neuroblastoma
    Pheochromocytoma
    Shock
    Hyperthyroidism
    Strenuous exercise
    Certain drugs, including dopamine, levophed, sympa-thomimetics, tricyclic antidepressants, alpha-methyl-dopa, hydralazine, quinidine, isoproterenol, epineph-rine, and ethanol
- Decreased levels
    Parkinson's disease
    Anorexia nervosa
    Autonomic nervous system dysfunction
    Drugs, including barbiturates, ganglionic and adrenergic blocking agents, guanethidine, and reserpine

Interfering Factors

- Stress, hypoglycemia, hyperthyroidism, strenuous exercise, smoking, and drugs can produce elevated plasma catecholamines.
- Diets high in amines can produce elevated plasma cate-cholamine levels, although this effect is more likely to be seen in relation to certain urinary metabolites.

Nursing Implications

Assessment

- Obtain a history of the endocrine system, known or suspected disorders, and results of tests and procedures.
- Ensure client has followed a normal sodium diet for 3 days, has fasted from food and fluids for 10 to 12 hours before the test, has abstained from smoking tobacco for 24 hours, has not consumed foods high in amines for 48 hours, has withheld medications as instructed, and has avoided strenuous exercise and rested for 1 hour before the test.

Possible Nursing Diagnoses

Anxiety related to perceived threat to health status
Physical mobility, impaired, related to neuromuscular impairment

Implementation

- If more than one sample is to be obtained, an intermittent infusion device should be inserted before the test to avoid the stress of repeated venipunctures.
- Put on gloves. Using aseptic technique, obtain a blood sample from the infusion device and discard. Collect a second specimen in a chilled lavender- or green-top tube between 6 and 8 AM.
- Handle sample gently to avoid hemolysis. Pack it on ice and promptly send to the laboratory.
- Ask the client to stand for 10 minutes. Obtain a second sample and handle as before.
- Remember to note the time(s) of collection and position of the client on the laboratory request forms.

Evaluation

- Note results in relation to 24-hour urinary vanillylmandelic acid (VMA) results and metanephrines.
- Assess client for increased pulse and blood pressure, hyperglycemia, shakiness, and palpitation associated with increased values.

Client/Caregiver Teaching

Pretest

- Instruct the client to fast for 10 to 12 hours before the test; to abstain from smoking for 24 hours; to avoid foods high in amines, including bananas, avocados, beer, cheese (aged),

chocolate, cocoa, coffee, fava beans, grains, tea, vanilla, walnuts, and Chianti wine; avoid self-prescribed medications for 2 weeks, especially cold and allergy medications.
- Inform the client that an intermittent infusion device may be inserted before the test because the stress of repeated venipuncture may increase catecholamine levels.
- Inform the client that he or she may be asked to keep warm and to rest for 45 to 60 minutes before the test.

Posttest

- Instruct the client to resume diet, medication, and activity withheld before the test.
- Instruct client in the collection of urine for testing, if ordered.
- Inform the client that it may take 1 week or more to get test results.

Catecholamines, Urine

Classification: Urinalysis

Type of Test: Urine (random or 24-hour)

This test uses spectrophotofluorometry to measure urine levels of the major catecholamines: epinephrine, norepinephrine, and dopamine. Catecholamines, which are produced by the adrenal medulla and found in sympathetic nerve endings and the brain, prepare the body for the fight-or-flight stress response and help regulate metabolism. Levels are affected by diurnal variations and fluctuate in response to stress, postural changes, diet, smoking, drugs, and temperature—all which must be somewhat controlled when the test is performed to validate results. The 24-hour specimen is preferred for this test because catecholamine secretion varies diurnally in response to environmental factors. However, a random specimen is helpful in evaluating an acute hypertensive episode.

Indications

- Evaluate hypertension of unknown etiology
- Aid in diagnosis of pheochromocytoma

- Evaluate acute hypertensive episode (random urine specimen)
- Aid in the diagnosis of neuroblastoma, ganglioneuroma, or dysautonomia

Reference Values

		SI Units
Total free catecholamines		
Random urine	0–18 µg/dL	0–103 nmol/dL
24-hour urine	4–126 µg/24 h	24–745 nmol/24 h
Critical level	200 µg/dL	1180 nmol/24 h
Epinephrine	<10 µg/24 h	55 nmol/24 h
Critical level	50 µg/24 h	295 nmol/24 h
Norepinephrine	<100 g/24 h	591 nmol/24 h
Metanephrines	0.1–1.6 mg/24 h	0.5–8.7 µmol/24 h
Dopamine	65–400 µg/24 h	384–2364 nmol/24 h

Abnormal Values

- Elevated levels
  Pheochromocytoma
  Ganglioneuroma
  Neuroblastoma
- Decreased levels
  Anorexia nervosa
  Dysautonomia, as indicated by orthostatic hypotension

Interfering Factors

- Failure to collect all urine and store 24-hour specimen properly will result in a falsely low result.
- Anxiety and strenuous exercise throughout collection period will affect results.
- Hypoglycemia can cause falsely elevated results.
- Foods that can cause falsely elevated levels include beer, wines, cheese, walnuts, and coffee, chocolate, vanilla, and bananas.
- For medications that affect the test results see Medications That Affect Test Results, at the end of this section.

Nursing Implications

Assessment

- Obtain a history of known or suspected tumors, neurologic status, and results of tests performed.

- Ensure that medications affecting the tests have been withheld.
- Ensure that client has not ingested any foods that may affect test results within the past 7 days.

Possible Nursing Diagnoses

Anxiety related to perceived threat to health status

Physical mobility, impaired, related to neuromuscular impairment

Body image disturbance related to psychosocial influences

Implementation

- *Random sample:* Obtain a clean container and ask client to collect at least 50 mL of urine.
- *24-hour specimen:* Obtain a clean 3-liter container with preservative (hydrochloric acid). Instruct the client to void and discard sample. The time the discard sample is obtained is the time the collection begins. All urine excreted during the 24-hour period must be saved.
- Instruct the client to maintain refrigeration of the specimen or place on ice during time of collection. If a urinary catheter is in place, keep drainage bag on ice and instruct the client or caregiver to periodically empty drainage bag into specimen container.
- Instruct the client to void the following day at the exact time the test was begun and to add this specimen to the container.
- Label the container properly, including the start and end date and times. Transport the specimen to the laboratory promptly.

Evaluation

- Compare findings with vanillylmandelic acid (VMA) and homovanillic acid (HVA) levels. Elevated HVA levels rule out pheochromocytoma because this tumor primarily secretes epinephrine. Elevated catecholamines without hypertension suggests neuroblastoma or ganglioneuroma.

Client/Caregiver Teaching

Pretest

- Instruct the client to avoid foods and medications that interfere with test results and to avoid stressful situations during the collection period.
- Instruct the bedridden client to void all urine in a bedpan and then either pour urine into the collection container or

leave in the container for the nurse to add to the collection; place a sign in the bathroom as a reminder to save all urine.

- Instruct the client to avoid voiding in pan with defecation and to keep toilet tissue out of pan to prevent contamination of the specimen; also inform client not to void directly into container, because the preservative is a strong acid.

Posttest

- Advise client to resume medications and activity withheld before the test.

Medications That Affect Test Results

Below is a list of medications that may elevate or decrease urine catecholamine levels. Phenothiazines, erythromycin, and methenamine compounds, including mandelamine, may elevate or decrease levels.

Elevated Urine Catecholamine Levels	Decreased Urine Catecholamine Levels
Aminophylline	Clonidine
B-complex vitamins	Guanethidine
Caffeine	Iodine-containing contrast
Chloral hydrate	media
Ethanol	Reserpine
Insulin	
Isoproterenol	
Levodopa	
Methyldopa	
Monoamine oxidase (MAO) inhibitors	
Nitroglycerin	
Quinidine	
Quinine	
Tetracycline	
Tricyclic antidepressants	

Catheterization, Pulmonary Artery

Classification: Catheterization

Type of Test: Invasive

Pulmonary artery catheterization provides information about the pumping ability of the heart by measuring pulmonary artery pressures and pulmonary artery wedge pressure. It is done in the acutely ill patient to monitor left atrial and ventricular end-diastolic pressure, cardiac output, and central venous pressure and is the most rapid and reliable determinant of ventricular failure. Pressure measurements are obtained using a pulmonary artery catheter that is inserted into a peripheral vein and advanced into the pulmonary artery. Once inserted, the catheter can remain in place and pressures can be monitored to ensure that even early stages of ventricular failure can be identified for prompt treatment.

Indications

- Monitor acutely ill clients with sudden respiratory or multi-system failure
- Determine right or left ventricular impairments, failure, or defects
- Determine pulmonary hypertension, edema, embolus, and pulmonary vascular resistance
- Monitor high-risk clients (those with angina, cardiopulmonary disease, or potential fluid shifts) during the pre-, intra-, and postoperative period
- Monitor effects of inotropic drugs, fluid infusions, and respiratory therapy

Reference Values

Right atrial (RA) pressure	3–11 mm Hg
Central venous pressure (CVP)	2.7–12 cm H_2O
Right ventricular systolic pressure	20–30 mm Hg
Right ventricular end-diastolic pressure	< 5 mm Hg
Pulmonary artery end-diastolic pressure (PAEDP)	8–15 mm Hg

Pulmonary artery (PAP) pressure	<20 mm Hg
Pulmonary artery wedge pressure (PAWP) or pulmonary capillary wedge pressure (PCWP)	6–12 mm Hg
Cardiac output	4–12 mm Hg
Cardiac index	5–8 L/min

Abnormal Values

- Multisystem failure
- Pulmonary diseases
- Right and left ventricular cardiac impairments or failure
- Atrial or ventricular septal defects
- Hypovolemia (low pressures) or hypervolemia (elevated pressures)

Interfering Factors

- Improper placement or catheter position
- Obstructed catheter
- Mechanical ventilation, which can alter pressure readings as intrathoracic pressure is increased
- Improper functioning of monitoring or recording equipment: air or clot in system, waveform or transducer damage, balloon overinflation, leaks from loose connections, or incorrect stopcock or monitor calibration

NURSING ALERT

- Possible complications of this procedure include perforation of the heart or vasculature, pulmonary embolus, and arrhythmias
- The client requires close monitoring, so this procedure is usually performed in a critical care unit.

Nursing Implications

Assessment

- Obtain a history of cardiovascular and pulmonary system, medications, results of tests and procedures performed, and baseline vital signs.
- Monitor pressures and waveforms routinely. In acutely ill patients, measurements may be recorded as often as every 15 minutes.

Possible Nursing Diagnoses

Injury, risk for, related to insertion of intravascular catheter
Gas exchange, impaired, related to ventilation-perfusion imbalance
Fluid volume excess related to compromised organ function
Fluid volume deficit related to compromised organ function

Implementation

- Have emergency equipment readily accessible.
- If not already in place, start an intravenous line for administration of emergency fluids or drugs, as needed.
- Place the client in a supine position in bed with selected site exposed.
- After the site is cleansed, a local anesthetic is injected. The catheter is inspected for defects, then inserted into a peripheral vein into the superior vena cava and right atrium. The balloon is partially inflated to allow it to move with the blood flow through the tricuspid valve into the right ventricle and pulmonary artery until it becomes wedged in a smaller distal pulmonary artery.
- Waveforms are recorded as the catheter is advanced to note any tachycardia caused by catheter irritation. Waveforms vary depending on the location of the catheter tip.
- PAP is obtained while the catheter is in the pulmonary artery. The catheter is advanced into one of the smaller arteries and inflated with 1 mL of air to obtain the PAWP. After PAWP is obtained, the balloon is deflated to prevent tissue necrosis and moved back to the pulmonary artery. Cardiac output can be measured with the catheter in the pulmonary artery, not in the wedged position.
- After x-ray verification of placement, the catheter is sutured to the skin.
- Monitor the client's vital signs, pressure measurements, and electrocardiogram, as ordered or depending on the clincal status of the patient.
- Flush the catheter with normal saline solution and recalibrate after each PAWP reading.

Evaluation

- Note test results in relation to client's symptoms and other tests performed.
- Note and report changes in ECG and vital signs, signs of pulmonary emboli, or infarct.
- Once the catheter is removed, observe the puncture site for hematoma, hemorrhage, and absence of pulses distal to the catheter insertion site.

Client/Caregiver Teaching

Pretest

- Explain the purpose of the procedure. Inform the client that it is performed by a physician at the bedside and takes 30 minutes to complete.
- Explain that the procedure is not painful, but that the client may experience discomfort from injection of local anesthetic at the insertion site.
- Inform the client that the catheter will be sutured and bandaged in place and will remain for 3 to 4 days or longer, depending on the clinical status of the patient.

Posttest

- Inform the client and caregiver of the need for possible further testing to evaluate and determine need for change in therapy.

Cerebrospinal Fluid Analysis, CSF Analysis

Classification: Chemistry, microbiology

Type of Test: Invasive (lumbar puncture)

Cerebral spinal fluid circulates in the subarachnoid space and acts to protect the brain and spinal cord from injury and to transport products of cellular metabolism and neurosecretion. Analysis of this fluid can aid in diagnosing cancer, infections, bleeding, and degenerative and autoimmune diseases of the brain and spinal cord. Specimens for analysis and immunofixation are most frequently obtained by lumbar puncture and sometimes by ventricular or cisternal puncture. Lumbar puncture can also have therapeutic uses, including injection of drugs and anesthesia.

Indications

- Detect obstruction of CSF circulation from hemorrhage, tumor, or edema

- Diagnose neurosyphilis and chronic CNS infections
- Diagnose and differentiate subarachnoid or intracranial hemorrhage
- Diagnose and differentiate viral or bacterial meningitis or encephalitis
- Confirm diagnosis of diseases such as multiple sclerosis, autoimmune diseases, or degenerative brain disease

Reference Values

See Cerebrospinal Fluid Findings, at the end of this section.

Abnormal Values

See Cerebrospinal Fluid Findings for findings and implications.

Interfering Factors

- Failure to collect the specimen properly can result in contamination from the skin and localized bleeding from the puncture site into the specimen.
- Failure to label the vials.
- Delayed analysis can cause false results from cell lysis.

NURSING ALERT

- This procedure is contraindicated if infection is present at the needle insertion site.
- It may also be contraindicated in degenerative joint disease, in clients with coagulation defects, or an uncooperative client.
- Use with extreme caution in clients with increased intracranial pressure because too rapid removal of fluid can result in herniation.

Nursing Implications

Assessment

- Obtain a history of neurological symptoms, medication regimen, and the results of other tests performed.
- Assess if the client has an allergy to local anesthetics and inform the physician accordingly.

Possible Nursing Diagnoses

Anxiety related to perceived threat to health status

Physical mobility, impaired, related to neurologic impairment

Communication, impaired, verbal, related to altered brain function

Sensory-perceptual alterations [specify] related to altered sensory transmission or integration

Implementation

- If an immunofixation test is to be performed, collect a 7-mL blood sample. Then within 2 hours obtain 3 mL of cerebrospinal fluid (CSF) by lumbar puncture in a sterile tube without additives.
- To perform a lumbar puncture, position the client in the knee-chest position at the side of the bed. Provide pillows to support the spine or for the client to grasp. The sitting position is an alternative. In this position, the client must bend neck and chest to knees.
- Prepare the site, usually between L3 and L4, with povidone iodine and drape the area.
- A physician injects a local anesthetic. Using sterile technique, the physician inserts the spinal needle through the spinous processes of the vertebrae and into the subarachnoid space. The stylet is removed. CSF will drip from the needle if it is placed properly.
- Attach the stopcock and manometer and measure initial pressure.
- If the initial pressure is elevated, the physician may perform Queckenstedt's test. To perform this test, apply pressure to the jugular vein for about 10 seconds. CSF pressure usually rises from 15 to 40 cm of water in response to the occulsion and then rapidly returns to normal within 10 seconds after the pressure is released. Sluggish response may indicate CSF obstruction.
- Obtain up to 4 vials of spinal fluid in separate tubes and label them numerically.
- A final pressure reading is taken and the needle is removed. Clean the puncture site with an antiseptic solution and apply a small adhesive bandage.
- Label samples and transport specimens to the laboratory promptly.
- Position the client flat, although some physicians allow 30-degree elevation. Maintain this position for up to 8 hours.
- Encourage client to drink fluids to replace lost CSF and reduce risk of headache.

Evaluation

- Monitor for changes in CNS status, headache, and inability to void.
- Assess insertion site for leakage of spinal fluid.
- Note test results in relation to the client's symptoms and to other tests performed.

Client/Caregiver Teaching

Pretest

- Inform the client the procedure will be performed by a physician and take about 20 minutes.
- Inform the client that the position required may be awkward but that someone will assist. Stress the importance of remaining still and breathing normally throughout the procedure.
- Inform the client that a stinging sensation may be felt as the local anesthetic is injected. Tell the client to report any pain or other sensations that may require repositioning of the spinal needle.

Posttest

- Inform the client that to avoid a headache, it is necessary to lie flat for 8 hours or with the head elevated no more than a 30-degree angle.
- Encourage increased fluid intake to replace what was lost in the samples.

Cerebrospinal Fluid Findings

Test	Reference Value	Abnormal Finding	Implication
Color	Clear	Cloudy	Elevated WBCs
		Yellow	Elevated protein
		Pink-red	Presence of RBCs
Pressure	Children: 50–100 mm H_2O	Increased	Increased ICP from hemorrhage, tumor or edema
	Adults: 75–200 mm H_2O	Decreased	Subarachnoid obstruction above puncture site

Cerebrospinal Fluid Findings (Continued)

Test	Reference Value	Abnormal Finding	Implication
Cell count	Children: 0–5 WBCs; up to 20 small lymphocytes per mm^3	Increased WBCs	Meningitis, acute infection, tumor, abscess, infarction, demyelinating disease
	Adults: 0–3 WBCs; up to 5 small lymphocytes per mm^3 No RBCs or granulocytes	RBCs	Hemorrhage or traumatic lumbar puncture
Total proteins	Infants: 30–100 mg/dL Children: 14–45 mg/dL	Increase	Hemorrhage, trauma, polyneuritis, RBC in sample, tumors
	Adults: 15–45 mg/dL or 1% of serum level	Decrease	Increased CSF production
Glucose	Infants: 20–40 mg/dL	Increase	Hyperglycemia
	Children: 35–75 mg/dL	Decrease	
	Adults: 40–80 mg/dL or less than 50–80% of blood glucose		Hypoglycemia, infection, mumps, postsubarachnoid hemorrhage, tumor (slight decrease)
Chloride	118–132 mEq/L	Decrease	Acute bacterial or syphilitic meningitis, suspected tuberculosis meningitis
Lactic acid	10–20 mg/dL	Increased	Brain abscess, infarction, trauma, intracranial hemorrhage, meningitis, multiple sclerosis, seizure disorders

(*continued*)

Cerebrospinal Fluid Findings *(Continued)*

Test	Reference Value	Abnormal Finding	Implication
Myelin basic protein	<4 ng/mL	Increased	Cerebral infarcts, acute multiple sclerosis, and other demyelinating diseases
Oligoclonal bands	Negative	Positive	Guillain-Barré syndrome, multiple sclerosis, neurosyphilis, encephalitis, CNS lesions, and vasculitis
Gamma globulin	3–13% of total protein	Increased	Multiple sclerosis, neurosyphilis, subacute sclerosing leukoencephalitis
IgG	<8.4 mg/dL	Increased	Guillain-Barré syndrome, encephalitis, multiple sclerosis, neurosyphilis, CNS lupus
Culture	Negative	Positive	CNS infection caused by mycobacteria or fungus
Fluorescent treponemal antibody (FTA)	Negative	Positive	Neurosyphilis

Ceruloplasmin (Cp)

Classification: Chemistry (protein)

Type of Test: Serum

Measurement by electrophoresis of ceruloplasmin (Cp), an alpha$_2$ globulin produced in the liver that binds copper for transport in the blood after it is absorbed from the gastrointestinal tract. Deposits of copper in body tissues, such as the brain, liver, corneas, and kidneys, results from a decreased production of this globulin.

Indications

- Diagnosis of Wilson's disease
- Determine genetic predisposition to Wilson's disease
- Diagnosis of Menkes's (kinky hair) syndrome
- Monitor client response to total parenteral nutrition (TPN) (hyperalimentation)

Reference Values

		SI Units
Newborns	1–30 mg/dL	0.06–1.99 μmol/L
Infants (6–12 mo)	15–50 mg/dL	0.99–3.31 μmol/L
Children (1–12 yr)	30–65 mg/dL	1.99–4.30 μmol/L
Adults	14–40 mg/dL	0.93–2.65 μmol/L

Abnormal Values

- Increased levels
    Acute infections
    Hepatitis
    Hodgkin's disease
    Hyperthyroidism
    Hypocupremia from TPN
    Pregnancy
    Cancer of the bone, lung, stomach
    Myocardial infarction

Rheumatoid arthritis

Drugs, including oral contraceptives, estrogens, and phenytoin

■ Decreased levels

Wilson's disease

Malabsorption syndromes

Long-term total parenteral nutrition

Menkes's (kinky hair) syndrome

Nephrosis

Severe liver disease

Interfering Factors

■ Results are not reliable in infants under 3 months of age.
■ Medications such as estrogen, methadone, and phenytoin can increase levels.

Nursing Implications

Assessment

■ Obtain a history of infections, pancreatic and liver disorders, and drug use that may influence ceruloplasmin levels.

Possible Nursing Diagnoses

Anxiety related to perceived threat to health status
Pain related to tissue ischemia or inflammation
Fluid volume excess related to decreased glomerular filtration

Implementation

■ Put on gloves. Using aseptic technique, perform a venipuncture and collect 7 mL of blood in a clotted red-top tube. Place the sample on ice immediately.
■ Handle the sample gently to avoid hemolysis and send to the laboratory promptly.

Evaluation

■ Assess eye for color change and skin for jaundice with increased ceruloplasmin levels. Kayser-Fleischer rings (green-gold rings) in the corneas and a liver biopsy showing more than 250 μg of copper per gram confirms Wilson's disease.

Client/Caregiver Teaching

Posttest

■ Inform the client of the need for follow-up medical care and genetic counseling.

Chlamydia Antibodies

Classification: Serology
Type of Test: Serum

This test measures the amount of IgG antibodies to *Chlamydia trachomatis* infection, the most common sexually transmitted disease. Testing is usually done at the time of suspected acute infection and then again in 3 weeks during convalescence to confirm the infection. Because it is a nonspecific antigen-antibody study, it can only detect previous exposure to the virus. This test is frequently used to screen donors before organ transplantation.

Indications

- Determine previous exposure to chlamydia
- Monitor the course of prolonged chlamydial infection

Reference Values

- Titer <1:10

Abnormal Values

- A fourfold or greater rise in titer between acute and convalescent serums indicates recent chlamydia infection.

Interfering Factors

- Immune disorders, immunosuppressive therapy, antibiotic therapy, or serious illness may cause false-negative results.
- Transfusion of whole blood or fractions within 2 months before the test may cause false-positive results.

Nursing Implications

Assessment

- Obtain a history of known or suspected exposure to chlamydia, medication regimen, and results of recent diagnostic tests.

Possible Nursing Diagnoses

Anxiety related to perceived threat to health status
Pain related to physical injuring agents
Urinary elimination, altered, related to urinary tract infection

Implementation

- Put on gloves. Using aseptic technique, perform a venipuncture and collect 1 mL of blood in a red-top tube.
- Handle sample gently to avoid hemolysis and send to the laboratory promptly.

Evaluation

- Note results of other related tests. Compare resuts of convalescent serum to that of acute serum for definitive results.

Client/Caregiver Teaching

Posttest

- Instruct the client that repeat testing may be necessary to confirm infection and monitor response to therapy.

Chlamydial Tests

Classification: Microbiology

Type of Test: Serum, eye, and cervical substance analysis

Chlamydia trachomatis is a microorganism responsible for urethritis, cervicitis, eye infections in the adult, and conjunctivitis in the neonate traumatized during birth. It is responsible for the most common sexually transmitted disease. A new strain of chlamydia, *C. pneumoniae,* is associated with respiratory infections in children and adults. It is diagnosed by culture of the suspicious area.

The chlamydia titer is performed on serum to detect exposure to *C. trachomatis, C. psittaci,* and *C. pneumoniae.* Specimens are taken in the acute stage of illness and again during the convalescent stage to confirm the diagnosis.

Indications

- Identify and confirm chlamydial eye or cervical infection by culture in adults
- Determine serum titers to indicate exposure or confirmation of lymphogranuloma venereum, psittacosis, or trachoma eye diseases by presence of chlamydia organism antibodies.
- Determine neonatal infection of the conjunctiva or respiratory tract

Reference Values

Culture	Negative for *C. trachomatis, C. psittaci, C. pneumoniae*
Titer	
Normal	<1:16 titer
Previous exposure	>1:16 titer

Abnormal Values

Culture	Positive for *C. trachomatis, C. psittaci, C. pneumoniae*
Titer	
Newborn	1:32 titer for *C. pneumonia*
	1:16 titer for *C. psittaci*
Adult	1:640 titer in chlamydial disease
	1:64 titer for lymphogranuloma venereum or psittacosis

Interfering Factors

- Pretest antimicrobial therapy, which will delay or inhibit growth of pathogens and cause a false-negative result
- Douching before cervical culture
- Culture not performed within 1 hour of collection
- Improper collection technique, hemolysis of the specimen, or inadequate amount of material to be tested

Nursing Implications

Assessment

- Obtain a history regarding exposure to the organism, including sexual practices or recent birth, and signs and symptoms of eye, genital, or lung infection.
- Note any antimicrobial therapy administered before the test.

Possible Nursing Diagnoses

Anxiety related to perceived threat to health status
Pain related to physical injuring agents

Implementation

- *Eye culture:* Cleanse around the eye to remove any drainage. Gently pull down on the lower lid and swab or scrape inside the lower lid conjunctiva. Place the swab in a tube of medium supplied by the laboratory to culture for chlamydia. Have the parent hold the child to obtain the specimen.
- *Urethral culture* (males only): Place client in a lithotomy position. Put on gloves. Insert a sterile swab into the urethra 2 to 4 inches and then rotate it. Place swab in the special collecting tube, break the swab shaft at the score marking, and replace the cap.
- *Cervical culture* (females only): Place client in a lithotomy position. Put on gloves. Insert a speculum and wipe the endocervix with a large swab. Dispose of the swab. Insert a second swab into the endocervical canal until the tip is no longer visible and rotate it for 5 to 10 seconds. Withdraw the swab without touching the vaginal surfaces and place in the collection kit's transport tube. Break the swab shaft at the score mark, and replace the cap.
- *Blood sample:* Put on gloves. Using aseptic technique, obtain a 5-mL blood sample and place in a red-top tube.
- Transport specimen to the laboratory immediately.

Evaluation

- Note test results in relation to the client's symptoms and other test results.

Client/Caregiver Teaching

Pretest

- Inform the client that there is no special preparation for this test unless a cervical culture is to be performed. For a cervical culture, inform the client not to douche before the test.

Posttest

- Inform the client that it may take 6 days to get a report on the culture.
- Inform the client having a serum titer that an additional sample may be required in about 2 to 3 weeks.
- Instruct and emphasize importance of compliance with antimicrobial medication regimen.

- Inform infected patients that their sex partners should be tested for the microorganism and subsequent treatment.
- Inform caregivers of infected newborns to wash hands after each contact with the child.

Cholangiography, Percutaneous Transhepatic (PTHC)

Classification: Radiography

Type of Test: Indirect visualization with contrast medium

The percutaneous transhepatic cholangiogram (PTHC) allows for visualization of the intrahepatic, extrahepatic, and biliary ducts as well as the gallbladder. With the aid of fluoroscopy, an iodinated contrast medium is administered through a long, fine needle inserted through the liver and into the bile duct outlining any strictures or obstructions. Fluoroscopic examination of the ducts is performed on spot films taken in various positions.

Indications

- Evaluate persistent upper right abdominal pain after cholecystectomy
- Differentiate between obstructive and nonobstructive jaundice
- Determine cause, location, and extent of obstruction of the ducts
- Diagnose biliary sclerosis or sclerosing cholangitis
- Perform liver biopsy, if ducts are salient, when hepatitis or cirrhosis of liver is suspected as the cause of jaundice

Reference Values

- Normal biliary ducts (cystic, hepatic, and common bile)

Abnormal Values

■ Dilated biliary ducts, indicating obstruction caused by cysts, stones (cholelithiasis), or strictures
■ Biliary tract carcinoma
■ Pancreatic carcinoma

Interfering Factors

■ Client is unable to remain still during procedure.
■ Obesity or gas overlying the biliary ducts can affect visualization.
■ Barium in the gastrointestinal tract or metal objects within field can impair clear imaging.
■ Failure to follow dietary restrictions before procedure.

> **NURSING ALERT**
>
> This procedure is contraindicated in
> ■ Pregnancy, unless benefits outweigh risk to the fetus
> ■ Persons with cholangitis, severe ascites, uncontrolled coagulopathy, or iodine allergy
> ■ Clients who are uncooperative or poor surgical risks

Nursing Implications

Assessment

■ Obtain a history of known or suspected gallbladder disease, pregnancies, bleeding abnormalities and hypersensitivity to iodine, shellfish, contrast medium, and anesthesia.
■ Obtain baseline bleeding, prothrombin, and clotting times, platelet count, complete blood count, blood typing and cross-matching.
■ Ensure that client has followed a fat-free diet for 24 hours before procedure and has had nothing to eat or drink for 8 hours before the procedure.
■ Ensure that a laxative has been given the evening before the procedure and an enema the day of the study, if ordered.

Possible Nursing Diagnoses

Anxiety related to perceived threat to health status
Grieving, anticipatory, related to perceived potential loss
Pain related to obstructive process

Implementation

- Administer antibiotics 24 to 72 hours before the procedure, if ordered.
- Administer a sedative and analgesic before the study for anxiety and pain control.
- Client is secured in a supine position with straps in place on the fluoroscopy tilt-table; the upper right abdomen is exposed and cleansed with povidone-iodine solution and surgically draped; the insertion site is injected with lidocaine for local anesthesia.
- A long, fine, flexible needle is inserted at the site and advanced in a smooth motion into the liver under fluoroscopy. The client is requested to hold the breath during needle insertion. When the needle attains its desired position in the bile duct, the stylet is removed and a syringe and tubing are connected to the needle. Once needle placement in the duct is confirmed by the flow of bile, the contrast dye is injected.
- The outline of the biliary ducts is then visualized through fluoroscopy, and spot x-rays with the client in various positions on the tilt-table are taken. The needle is then removed, and a dry, sterile dressing is applied to the puncture site.
- A sandbag may to placed over the insertion site to apply pressure and prevent bleeding.

Evaluation

- Check the insertion site frequently for bleeding.
- Note the test results in relation to other tests performed and the client's symptoms.

Client/Caregiver Teaching

Pretest

- Instruct the client to follow a fat-free diet for 24 hours and to have nothing to eat or drink for 8 hours before the procedure.
- Inform the client that the test is done by a physician in the radiology department and takes approximately 30 to 60 minutes; some discomfort is experienced during injection of the dye.

Posttest

- Advise the client to increase fluid intake to assist in excretion of the dye.
- Instruct the client to report any signs of bleeding, drainage from puncture site, and abdominal discomfort.
- Inform the client to resume previous diet in 5 to 8 hours.

- Instruct the client regarding bedrest, positioning, and activity restrictions.
- Instruct the client in antibiotic administration following study.
- Instruct the client to keep the dressing in place for at least 24 hours.

Cholangiography, Postoperative (T tube)

Classification: Radiography

Type of Test: Indirect visualization with contrast medium

This fluoroscopic and radiographic examination of the biliary tract involves the injection of a contrast medium (Hypaque) through the T tube inserted during surgery. T-tube cholangiography is performed 7 to 10 days after cholecystectomy to assess the patency of the common bile duct and detect any remaining calculi. It can also be performed during surgery following placement of the T tube to ensure that all stones have been removed. T-tube placement can also be performed after liver transplant, since biliary duct obstruction or anastomotic leakage is possible. This test should be performed before any gastrointestinal studies using barium and after any studies involving the measurement of iodinated compounds.

Indications

- Detect obstruction of the biliary ducts after surgery
- Evaluate biliary duct patency before T-tube removal

Reference Values

- Normal size of biliary ducts with contrast medium filling of the ductal system

Abnormal Values

- Filling defects, dilation, or shadows within the biliary ducts indicate calculi or neoplasm.
- Appearance of channels of contrast medium outside of the biliary ducts indicates a fistula.

Interfering Factors

- Air bubbles resembling calculi may be seen if there is inadvertent injection of air.
- Presence of barium in the gastrointestinal tract can impair clear visualization.

> ### NURSING ALERT
>
> This procedure is contraindicated in
> - Clients with hypersensitivity to iodine, seafood, or contrast medium and in postoperative wound sepsis
> - Pregnancy, unless the benefits of performing the procedure greatly outweigh the risks to the fetus

Nursing Implications

Assessment

- Obtain a history of gallbladder disease and hypersensitivity to iodine, shellfish, or contrast medium.
- Ensure client has fasted for 4 to 6 hours.
- Ensure cleansing enema is administered the morning of the procedure, if ordered, and results noted.

Possible Nursing Diagnoses

Anxiety related to perceived threat to health status
Grieving, anticipatory, related to perceived potential loss
Pain related to recent surgical procedure

Implementation

- Clamp T tube 24 hours before and during procedure, if ordered, to help prevent air bubbles from entering the ducts
- The client is placed in a supine position on the x-ray table and the area around the T tube is draped; the end of the T tube is cleansed with 70% alcohol; if T tube site is inflamed and painful, a local anesthetic (Xylocaine 2%) may be injected around the site. A needle attached to a tubing is in-

serted into the open end of the T tube and the clamp is removed.

- A radiographic contrast medium is instilled and fluoroscopy is performed to visualize dye moving through the duct system. Inform the client that although the procedure is not painful he or she may experience a bloating sensation in the upper right quadrant as the contrast dye is injected. The tube is again clamped and films taken of the right upper quadrant in prone, side-lying, and erect positions. An additional film can be taken 15 minutes later to visualize passage of the medium into the duodenum.
- The T tube is removed if findings are normal; a dry, sterile dressing is applied to the site.
- If retained calculi are identified, the T tube is left in place for 4 to 6 weeks until the tract surrounding the T tube is healed in order to perform a percutaneous removal.

Evaluation

- Note results in relation to other tests and client's symptoms.

Client/Caregiver Teaching

Pretest

- Instruct the client to fast for 4 to 6 hours before the procedure.
- Inform the client that the procedure is done by a physician in the radiology department and usually takes about 30 minutes.

Posttest

- Inform the client or caregiver to report any adverse signs or any signs of leakage or drainage from the T tube site.
- Advise the client to resume previous diet, if ordered.

Cholangiopancreatography, Endoscopic Retrograde (ERCP)

Classification: Endoscopy

Type of Test: Direct visualization

This study allows direct visualization of the pancreatic and biliary ducts with a flexible endoscope and, following injection of dye, with x-rays. It allows the physician to view the pancreatic, hepatic, and common bile ducts and the ampulla of Vater. During the endoscopy, specimens of suspicious tissue can be taken for histologic analysis, and manometry pressure readings can be obtained from the bile and pancreatic ducts. It is used to diagnose and follow up on pancreatic disease.

Indications

- Diagnose jaundice of unknown etiology to differentiate biliary tract obstruction from liver disease
- Identify obstruction caused by calculi, cysts, ducts, strictures, stenosis, and anatomic abnormalities
- Retrieve calculi from the distal common bile duct and release of strictures
- Perform therapeutic procedure such as sphincterotomy and placement of biliary drains or collect specimen for cytology

Reference Values

- Normal appearance of the duodenal papilla
- Patent common bile and pancreatic ducts

Abnormal Values

- Sclerosing cholangitis
- Pancreatitis
- Pancreatic fibrosis
- Duodenal papilla tumors
- Pancreatic cancer

Interfering Factors

- Inability of the client to cooperate with the procedure; general anesthesia can be used in this instance.
- Failure to follow dietary restrictions before the procedure.
- Previous surgery involving the stomach or duodenum can make locating the duodenal papilla difficult.
- Barium remaining in the stomach or bowel.

> **NURSING ALERT**
>
> This procedure is contraindicated in
> - Patients with unstable cardiopulmonary status; blood coagulation defects; or cholangitis unless the client received antibiotic therapy before the test
> - Patients with a large Zenker's diverticulum involving the esophagus

Nursing Implications

Assessment

- Obtain a history of allergies or sensitivities to anesthetics, analgesics, antibiotics, or iodine; known or suspected gastrointestinal disorders; and treatment regimen.
- Ensure food and fluids have been withheld for 8 to 12 hours before the procedure.

Possible Nursing Diagnoses

Anxiety related to perceived threat to health status
Grieving, anticipatory, related to perceived potential loss
Pain related to obstructive process

Implementation

- Obtain an informed consent.
- Adminster ordered sedative.
- Insert an intravenous line for administration of drugs, as needed.
- The client is placed on an x-ray table in the supine position and flat plate of the abdomen taken to check for any residual contrast media from previous studies.
- The oropharynx is sprayed or swabbed with a topical local anesthetic.
- The client is assisted to the left lateral position with left arm behind the back and right hand at the side with the neck slightly flexed. A protective guard is inserted into the mouth to cover the teeth. A bite block can also be inserted to maintain adequate opening of the mouth.

- The endoscope is passed through the mouth with a dental suction device in place to drain secretions. A side-viewing, flexible, fiberoptic endoscope is passed into the duodenum and a small cannula is inserted into the duodenal papilla (ampulla of Vater).
- The client is then placed in the prone position. The duodenal papilla visualized and cannulated with a catheter. Occasionally the client can be turned slightly to the right side to aid in visualization of the papilla.
- Intravenous glucagon or anticholinergics can be administered to minimize duodenal spasm and facilitate visualization of the ampulla of Vater.
- ERCP manometry can be done at this time to measure the pressure in the bile duct, pancreatic duct, and sphincter of Oddi at the papilla area via the catheter as it is placed in the area before the dye is injected.
- Once the catheter is in place, dye is injected into the pancreatic and biliary ducts via the catheter and fluoroscopic films are taken. Specimens for cytologic analysis and biopsies can be obtained during the procedure.
- Place specimens in appropriate containers, label them properly, and send them to the laboratory promptly.

Evaluation

- Note test results in relation to client's symptoms and other tests performed.

Client/Caregiver Teaching

Pretest

- Instruct the client to withhold food and fluids for 8 to 12 hours before the procedure.
- Inform the client that the procedure is generally performed in an endoscopy suite by a physician and takes 30 to 60 minutes to complete.
- Inform the client that a flushed feeling is experienced when contrast medicine is injected.

Posttest

- Tell the client to expect some throat soreness and possible hoarseness. Advise the client to use warm gargles, lozenges, or ice packs to the neck to alleviate throat discomfort.
- Inform the client that any belching, bloating, or flatulence is the result of air insufflation. Emphasize that any severe pain, fever, difficulty breathing, or expectoration of blood must be reported to physician immediately.

Cholesterol (Total)

Classification: Chemistry

Type of Test: Serum

This test measures circulating cholesterol and cholesterol esters. Cholesterol is a lipid needed to form cell membranes and a component of the materials that render the skin waterproof. It also helps form bile salts, adrenal cortical steroids, estrogens, and androgens. Cholesterol is obtained from the diet (exogenous cholesterol) or is synthesized in the body (endogenous cholesterol). Although most body cells can form some cholesterol, most is produced by the liver and intestinal mucosa.

Indications

- Determine risk of cardiovascular disease
- Investigate in light of family history of hypercholesterolemia and cardiovascular disease
- Aid diagnosis of nephrotic syndrome, hepatic disease, pancreatitis, and thyroid disorders
- Evaluate response to dietary/drug therapy for hypercholesterolemia

Reference Values

		SI Units
Newborn	45–100 mg/dL	1.16–2.59 mmol/L
Children	120–220 mg/dL	3.10–5.68 mmol/L
Adults		
<25 yr	125–200 mg/dL	3.27–5.20 mmol/L
25–40 yrs	140–225 mg/dL	3.69–5.85 mmol/L
40–50 yrs	160–245 mg/dL	4.37–6.35 mmol/L
>65 yrs	170–265 mg/dL	4.71–6.85 mmol/L

Values vary according to laboratory performing the test, age, sex, race, dietary pattern, and physical activity.

Abnormal Values

- Elevated levels

  Familial
  hyperlipoproteinemia
  Atherosclerosis
  Obstructive jaundice

  Hypertension
  Myocardial
  infarction
  Xanthomatosis

Hypothyroidism (primary)   Pregnancy
Nephrosis   Oophorectomy
Drugs, such as antidiabetic agents, ascorbic acid (falsely
elevated), androgens, bile salts, bromides (falsely elevated), catecholamine, chlorpromazine (falsely elevated), corticosteroids, iodides (falsely elevated), oral
contraceptives, phenothiazines, salicylates, vitamins A
and D (excessive)

■ Decreased levels
Malabsorption syndromes   Cushing's syndrome
Liver disease   Pernicious anemia
Hyperthyroidism   Carcinomatosis
Drugs, such as ACTH, cholestyramine, clofibrate, colchicine, colestipol, estrogen, dextrothyroxin, Dilantin, glucagon, Haldol, heparin, kanamycin, neomycin, nitrates,
nitrites (falsely decreased), PAS, propylthiouracil
(falsely decreased)

Interfering Factors

■ Ingestion of alcohol 24 hours and food 12 hours before the
test can falsely elevate levels.
■ Ingestion of drugs that alter cholesterol levels within 12 hr of
test, unless test is done to evaluate such effects.
■ Positioning can affect results; lower levels are obtained if
specimen is from a client who has been supine for 20 min.

Nursing Implications

Assessment

■ Obtain a history of cardiovascular status and risk for heart
disease, test, and procedure performed and results.
■ Ensure that client abstained from alcohol ingestion for 24
hours before the test, had a low-fat evening meal, and had
nothing to eat for 12 to 14 hours before the test.
■ Determine if client withheld drugs that may alter cholesterol
levels for 12 hours before the test.

Possible Nursing Diagnoses

Therapeutic management, individual, ineffective, related to
[specify]
Nutrition, altered, more than body requirements, related to increased intake of fats or excessive endogenous production
Injury, risk for, related to presence of excessive serum
cholesterol

Implementation

■ Put on gloves. Using aseptic technique, perform a venipuncture and collect 7 mL of blood in a red-top tube.

■ Send sample to the laboratory promptly; cholesterol is not stable at room temperature.

Evaluation

■ Note results in relation to other lipid results, including lipoprotein and cholesterol fractionation.

Client/Caregiver Teaching

Pretest

■ Instruct client not to eat food for 12 to 14 hr before test and to withhold medications that could interfere with results, unless study is being done to evaluate response.

Posttest

■ Instruct the client that the desirable blood cholesterol level is <200 mg/dL; levels of 200 to 240 mg/dL are considered borderline; and levels >250 mg/dL signify a definite high risk for cardiovascular disease, and treatment is required.
■ Instruct in dietary management of hypercholesterolemia to control or reduce cholesterol level.
■ Instruct the client to resume diet and medication withheld before the test, as ordered.
■ Inform the client that additional tests (lipoprotein and cholesterol fractionation) will be performed following abnormally high results of the test.

Cholesterol Fractionation

Cholesterol content can be broken down into high-density lipoproteins (HDL) and low-density lipoproteins (LDL) fractions. The HDL level is measured after selectively precipitating it and measuring its cholesterol. LDL is calculated using total cholesterol, total triglycerides, and HDL cholesterol levels. Below is a list of reference levels for HDL and LDL.

Age	HDL Cholesterol	LDL Cholesterol
<age 25 yr	32–57 mg/dL	73–138 mg/dL
age 25–40 yr	32–60 mg/dL	90–180 mg/dL
age 40–50 yr	33–60 mg/dL	100–185 mg/dL
age 50–65 yr	34–70 mg/dL	105–190 mg/dL
>age 65 yr	35–75 mg/dL	105–200 mg/dL

HDL levels are lower in men than in women and are inversely proportional to triglyceride levels. Much has been written about using HDL and LDL levels to predict cardiovascular risk. Studies such as the Framingham Heart Study suggest that high HDL level with a low LDL is predictive of less cardiovascular risk while high LDL level with low HDL level is considered a risk factor for cardiovascular disease.

Clotting Time (CT), Lee-White Clotting Time

Classification: Hematology

Type of Test: Blood

This test, which has largely been replaced by partial thromboplastin time (PTT) to monitor heparin therapy, measures the time it takes blood to clot in a test tube. It reflects the time for the interaction of all of the factors involved to form a clot. It is the least accurate of coagulation tests. Because of its low sensitivity, coagulation problems of mild to moderate severity will not be apparent.

Indications

- Evaluate response to heparin therapy, with an adequate anticoagulation indicated by clotting time of about 15 to 20 minutes
- Evaluate signs of abnormal bleeding such as epistaxis, easy bruising, bleeding gums, hematuria, and menorrhagia
- Evaluate suspected congenital coagulation defect that involves the intrinsic coagulation pathway

Reference Values

- Plain tube: 5 to 15 minutes

Abnormal Values

- Prolonged time
  Deficiency of coagulation factors VIII, IX, XI, XII
  Afibrinogenemia or hypofibrinogenemia
  Drugs such as heparin, warfarin, and dicumarol

Interfering Factors

- Heparin administration prolongs the blood-clotting time.
- Traumatic venipuncture or tube mishandling can lead to inaccurate or decreased time for clotting.

Nursing Implications

Assessment

- Obtain a personal and family history of known or suspected hematologic disorders, abnormal bleeding, or abnormal laboratory coagulation studies.
- Note if the client has received heparin up to 3 hours before the test. Note time and amount of last dose.

Possible Nursing Diagnoses

Injury, risk for, related to altered clotting factors
Protection, altered, related to abnormal blood profiles
Anxiety related to perceived threat to health status

Implementation

- Put on gloves. Using aseptic technique, perform a venipuncture and collect 3 mL of blood in a plastic syringe and then discard. Attach a new syringe to the venipuncture needle, and withdraw an additional 3 mL of blood. Place 1 mL in each of three test tubes.
- Begin timing with a stopwatch after the third tube is filled. Timing is completed when all tubes contain firm clots (third tube is clotted), and the interval is recorded as the clotting time.

Evaluation

- Note results in relation to other coagulation tests performed, including test for occult blood in body secretions and excretions.

Client/Caregiver Teaching

Posttest

- Instruct the client or caregiver to report bleeding from skin or mucosa to physician.

Clot Retraction

Classification: Hematology (hemostasis)

Type of Test: Blood

This test measures the adequacy of platelet function by measuring the speed and extent of clot retraction. Normally, when blood clots in a test tube, it retracts away from the side walls of the tube. Platelets play a major role in the clot retraction process. When platelets are decreased or function is impaired, scant serum and a soft, plump, poorly demarcated clot occurs in the tube.

Indications

- Evaluate the adequacy of platelet function
- Evaluate thrombocytopenia of unknown etiology
- Investigate suspected antiplatelet antibodies due to immune disorders of drug-antibody reactions
- Investigate suspected abnormalities of fibrinogen or fibrinolytic activity

Reference Values

- A normal clot, gently separated from the side of the test tube and incubated at 37°C, shrinks to about half of its original size within an hour. The result is a firm, cylindrical fibrin clot that contains red blood cells and is sharply demarcated from the clear serum. Complete clot retraction can take 6 to 24 hours.

Abnormal Values

- Decreased time and clot size
    Anemia (aplastic)
    DIC
    Factor XIII deficiency
    Fibrinogen deficiency
    Glanzmann's thrombasthenia
    Hodgkin's disease
    Leukemia

Multiple myeloma
Polycythemia or hemoconcentration
Thrombocytopenic purpura

Interfering Factors

- Rough handling of the sample alters clot formation.
- Use of wrong tube for blood collection.

Nursing Implications

Assessment

- Obtain a personal and family history of known or suspected hematologic disorders, abnormal bleeding, or abnormal laboratory results, such as increased or decreased platelet count or coagulation studies.

Possible Nursing Diagnoses

Injury, risk for, related to altered clotting factors
Protection, altered, related to abnormal blood profiles
Anxiety related to perceived threat to health status
Infection, risk for, related to immunosuppressed inflammatory response

Implementation

- Put on gloves. Using aseptic technique, perform a venipuncture and collect a 5-mL sample and discard it. Attach another syringe and obtain 5 mL of blood in a plain-top tube placed in a 37°C (98.6°F) water bath.
- The clotting is observed in 2, 6, 12, and 24 hours, and degree of retraction from walls of tube is recorded as the time taken to begin to clot, partially clot, and completely clot. The time it takes for these to occur and the volume and content of serum are also recorded.

Evaluation

- Note results in relation to other platelet and coagulation study results, for example, the hematocrit, fibrinogen level, and platelet count.

Client/Caregiver Teaching

Posttest

- Encourage client to keep follow-up appointment with physician.
- Have client report any excessive bleeding.

Coagulation Factor Assays

Classification: Hematology

Type of Test: Blood

A coagulation assay performed to measure specific coagulation factors if the prothrombin time (PT) or partial thromboplastin time (PTT/aPTT) is abnormal but the nature of the factor deficiency is unknown. The assays are used to discriminate between mild, moderate, and severe deficiencies and to follow the course of acquired factor inhibitors. Factor assays require specialized techniques not available in many laboratories.

Indications

- Assess prolonged PT or PTT of unknown etiology
- Monitor the effects of disorders and drugs known to lead to deficiencies in clotting factors

Reference Values

		SI Units
Factor I (Fibrinogen)	200–400 mg/dL	2.0–4.0 g/L
Factor II (Prothrombin)	50–150%	
Factor III (Thromboplastin)	30–45 s	30–45 s
Factor IV (Calcium)	9–11 mg/dL	0.09–0.11 g/L
Factor V (Accelerator globulin)	50–150%	
Factor VII (Proconvertin)	50–150%	
Factor VIII (Antihemophilic factor)	50–150%	
Factor IX (Christmas factor)	50–150%	
Factor X (Stuart-Prower factor)	50–150%	

(continued)

	SI Units
Factor XI (Thromboplastin antecedent)	50–150%
Factor XII (Hageman factor)	50–150%
Factor XIII (Fibrin stabilizing factor)	Dissolution of a formed clot within 24 h

Normal values for all factors vary among laboratories.

Abnormal Values

- Decreased levels
    Factor I: Liver disease, disseminated intravascular coagulation (DIC), hypofibrinogenemia
    Factor II: Liver disease, vitamin K deficiency
    Factor III: Thrombocytopenia
    Factor IV: Malnutrition, hypocalcemia, hyperphosphatemia
    Factor V: Leukemia, liver disease, DIC, surgery
    Factor VII: Antibiotic therapy, hepatitis, liver cancer, newborn hemorrhagic disease, vitamin K deficiency
    Factor VIII: DIC, fibrinolysis, hemophilia A, von Willebrand's disease
    Factor IX: Hemophilia B, hepatic disease, vitamin K deficiency, anticoagulants, nephrotic syndrome
    Factor X: Hepatic disease, vitamin K deficiency, DIC, newborn hemorrhagic disease, anticoagulants
    Factor XI: Hepatic disease, hemophilia C, vitamin K deficiency, congenital heart disease, anticoagulants
    Factor XII: Hepatic disease, nephrotic syndrome, normal pregnancy
    Factor XIII: Multiple myeloma, hepatic disease, agammaglobulinemia, lead poisoning, elevated fibrinogen levels

Interfering Factors

- Anticoagulants can cause false negative results. Oral contraceptives may cause abnormally high levels of factors II, VII, IX, and X.
- Traumatic venipunctures and excessive agitation of the sample can alter test results.

Nursing Implications

Assessment

- Obtain a history of hematologic system, known or suspected bleeding disorders, diagnostic tests and results, and current medications. If client is receiving anticoagulant therapy, note time and amount of last dose.

Possible Nursing Diagnoses

Injury, risk for, related to altered clotting factors
Protection, altered, related to abnormal blood profiles
Anxiety related to perceived threat to health status

Implementation

- Put on gloves. Using aseptic technique, perform a venipuncture, and collect 7 mL of blood in a light blue-top tube; for factor VIII assays, collect the sample in a red-top tube.
- As ordered in some laboratories, obtain a 2-mL blood sample and discard. Then, attach a second syringe, draw 5 mL of venous blood, and place in blue-top tube.
- Avoid traumatic venipunctures and excessive agitation of the sample and send sample to the laboratory immediately.

Evaluation

- If the PT is prolonged but the PTT is normal, factors of the extrinsic pathway are evaluated (i.e., factors II, V, VII, and X). If the PTT is prolonged but the PT is normal, factors of the intrinsic pathway are evaluated (i.e., factors VIII, IX, XI, XII).
- Observe client for excessive bleeding.

Client/Caregiver Teaching

Posttest

- Instruct the client to report bleeding from skin or mucous membrane sites.

Cold Agglutinin Titer

Classification: Immunology

Type of Test: Serum

Cold agglutinins are antibodies that cause clumping or agglutination of red blood cells at cold temperatures in individuals with certain diseases and infected by organisms, particularly *Mycoplasma pneumoniae*. The titer is the highest dilution of serum that will show a specific antigen-antibody reaction.

Indications

- Confirm primary atypical pneumonia, influenza, or pulmonary embolus
- Provide additional diagnostic support for cold agglutinin disease associated with viral infections or lymphoreticular cancers

Reference Values

- <1:16; may be higher in the elderly

Abnormal Values

- Elevated levels
  Mycoplasma pneumoniae (peaks 3 to 4 weeks after infection)
  Viral pneumonia
  Primary atypical pneumonia
  Influenza
  Cirrhosis
  Lymphatic leukemia
  Multiple myeloma
  Hemolytic anemia
  Infectious mononucleosis
  Pulmonary embolus
  Malaria
  Cytomegalovirus

Interfering Factors

- Antibiotic use may decrease antibody production.
- Refrigeration of the sample before serum is separated from RBCs may falsely depress titers.

Nursing Implications

Assessment

- Obtain a history of exposure to infectious diseases, respiratory symptoms, and current medications, particularly antibiotics that can interfere with test results.

Possible Nursing Diagnoses

Infection, risk for, related to immunosuppressed inflammatory response or excess pulmonary secretions

Gas exchange, impaired, related to ventilation-perfusion imbalance

Airway clearance, ineffective, related to compromised pulmonary function

Breathing pattern, ineffective, related to compromised pulmonary function

Implementation

- Put on gloves. Using aseptic technique, perform a venipuncture and collect 7 to 10 mL of blood in a red-top tube.
- Handle the specimen gently to avoid hemolysis. Transport to laboratory immediately. Indicate on laboratory requisition slip if client receiving antibiotics.

Evaluation

- Note test results in relation to other tests performed, in particular the white blood cell count.

Client/Caregiver Teaching

Pretest

- Inform the client that no special preparation is necessary.

Posttest

- Inform the client that the test may be repeated to monitor response to therapy.

Cold Stimulation

Classification: Vascular study

Type of Test: Noninvasive vascular test

This peripheral vascular procedure is performed to diagnose Raynaud's syndrome, a functional abnormality resulting in intense vasospasm of the small arteries and arterioles of the fingers. These vasospasms cause ischemia, which changes the skin color from pallor to cyanosis, starting at the fingertips and traveling to the distal portion of the phalanges. Tingling, numbness, and a cold sensation are experienced by the client. Following ischemia, hyperemia occurs, with a change in skin color to red, and the client experiences a throbbing sensation.

Indications

- Diagnose Raynaud's syndrome, as revealed by the inability of digits to return to pretest temperature within a specific length of time, usually 20 minutes

Reference Values

- Normal temperature and skin color of fingers and toes following exposure to cold temperatures

Abnormal Values

- Raynaud's disease (primary), cause unknown
- Raynaud's phenomenon (secondary), resulting from occupational trauma or arterial occlusive disease in association with a collagen disease such as scleroderma or lupus erythematosus

Interfering Factors

- Extreme environmental temperatures may cause false results.

> ### ▶ NURSING ALERT
>
> ■ This procedure is contraindicated in clients with infected or gangrenous digits.

Nursing Implications

Assessment

■ Obtain a history of vascular disease, of known or suspected collagen disease, effects of temperature and stress on digital blood flow, previous tests and results.
■ Determine if the client is a smoker.

Possible Nursing Diagnoses

Tissue integrity, impaired, related to peripheral vascular alterations

Tissue perfusion, altered, peripheral, related to reduced arterial blood flow

Thermoregulation, ineffective, related to disturbance in arterial blood flow

Implementation

■ Place the client in a sitting position in a room with optimal temperature control.
■ Attach a thermistor to each finger above the nail area. Make sure the tape is not too tight because it can restrict circulation. Record the baseline temperature.
■ Submerge the client's hand in ice water for 20 seconds.
■ Remove the client's hands from the ice water and immediately measure the temperature. Record temperature every 5 minutes until baseline temperature is attained. If more than 20 minutes passes and baseline temperature has not been reached, the client has Raynaud's syndrome.

Evaluation

■ Note test results in relation to other tests performed and the client's symptoms.

Client/Caregiver Teaching

Pretest

■ Inform the client that the procedure is performed by a physician or technician and takes about 30 minutes to complete.

- Inform the client that there are no food or fluid restrictions.
- Inform the client that slight discomfort may be experienced when the hands are immersed in the ice water, and when the digits rewarm, a throbbing feeling may be experienced.

Posttest

- Inform the client not to smoke because it causes vaso-constriction.
- Instruct the client on care of hands and feet in clients with Raynaud's syndrome.

Colonoscopy

Classification: Endoscopy

Type of Test: Direct visualization

This procedure allows inspection of the mucosa of the entire colon and terminal ileum using a flexible fiberoptic colono-scope inserted through the anus and advanced to the terminal ileum. During the procedure, tissue samples can be obtained for cytology and some therapeutic procedures can be performed, such as excision of small tumors or polyps and coagulation of bleeding sites.

Indications

- Determine cause of lower gastrointestinal disorders, especially when barium enema and proctosigmoidoscopy are inconclusive
- Determine source of rectal bleeding and perform hemostasis by coagulation
- Removal of foreign bodies and sclerosing strictures by laser
- Confirm diagnosis of colon cancer and inflammatory bowel disease
- Follow up on previously diagnosed and treated colon cancer
- Diagnose Hirschsprung's disease
- Reduce volvulus and intussusception in children

Reference Values

- Normal intestinal mucosa

Abnormal Values

- Abnormal tissue, such as tumors, polyps; abnormal conditions such as bleeding, bowel infection, or inflammation; foreign bodies; anatomical deviations such as diverticula and vascular abnormalities

Interfering Factors

- Inability to cooperate with procedure
- Strictures or other abnormalities preventing passage of scope
- Impaired visualization caused by severe gastrointestinal bleeding or inadequate bowel preparation or by residual barium from a barium enema

NURSING ALERT

- This procedure is contraindicated in bowel perforation, acute peritonitis, acute colitis, ischemic bowel necrosis, recent bowel surgery, advanced pregnancy, severe cardiac or pulmonary disease, recent myocardial infarction, known or suspected pulmonary embolus, large abdominal aortic or iliac aneurysm, and severe bleeding or coagulation abnormality.
- Avoid using bowel preparations that include laxatives or enemas in pregnant clients or clients with inflammatory bowel disease, unless specifically directed by physician.

Nursing Implications

Assessment

- Obtain a gastrointestinal history noting any information relating to bowel, anal, rectal, or coagulation disorders and use of drugs that affect bleeding, such as aspirin and other salicylates.
- Determine previous abnormalities in laboratory test results, particularly hematologic or coagulation tests.
- Note intake of oral iron preparations 1 week before the study, as these cause black, sticky feces that are difficult to remove with bowel preparation.

- Ensure that diet has been restricted to clear liquids for 48 hours before beginning oral bowel preparation.
- Ensure that ordered laxative has been administered late in the afternoon of the day before the procedure.

Possible Nursing Diagnoses

Diarrhea related to stress and anxiety or bowel irritation from procedure
Constipation related to inadequate fluid or bulk intake
Injury, risk for, related to postcolonoscopy distention syndrome, bleeding, or colon perforation
Anxiety related to perceived threat to health status

Implementation

- Two hours before the procedure, administer warm tap water or saline enemas until returns are clear, as ordered. Or administer 1 liter of saline as a colonic irrigation or give 1 liter of balanced electrolyte solution orally or by nasogastric tube 1 hour before the procedure.
- Administer ordered sedation.
- Insert a keep-vein-open IV line for administration of needed drugs.
- Client is placed in left lateral position and draped for privacy with buttocks exposed. The physician performs visual inspection of perianal area and digital rectal examination.
- Client is requested to bear down as if having a bowel movement as the fiberoptic tube is inserted through the rectum. The scope is advanced through the sigmoid. The client's position is changed to supine to facilitate passage into the transverse colon. Air is insufflated through the tube during passage to aid in visualization.
- Client is requested to take deep breaths to aid in movement of the scope downward through the ascending colon to the cecum and into the terminal portion of the ileum.
- Photographs are obtained for future reference; tissue biopsies and cultures are obtained; and foreign bodies or polyps removed. All samples are placed in appropriate containers, labeled, and sent to laboratory.

Evaluation

- Monitor for any rectal bleeding.
- Note results in relation to other tests and the client's symptoms.

Client/Caregiver Teaching

Pretest

- Instruct the client to maintain a clear liquid diet for 48 hours before the test.
- Inform the client that the procedure is generally performed in an endoscopy suite by a physician and takes 30 to 60 minutes to complete.
- Inform the client that it is important that the bowel be thoroughly cleaned so that the physician can visualize the colon and that the client will have to take laxatives and receive enemas before the test.

Posttest

- Instruct the client to resume food and fluid intake and activity 2 hours after the procedure or when the effects of sedation wear off.
- Emphasize that any chest pain, abdominal pain, or problems breathing must be reported to the physician immediately
- Instruct the client to expect slight rectal bleeding for up to 2 days following removal of polyps or biopsies, but that heavy rectal bleeding must be reported to the physician immediately.
- Encourage client to drink plenty of fluids to replace those lost during the preparation for the test.

Color Perception Test

Classification: Organ function study

Type of Test: Vision

Color perception tests are performed to determine the acuity of color discrimination. The most common test uses pseudo-isochromatic plates with numbers or letters buried in a maze of dots. Misreading of the numbers or letters indicates color-perception deficiency and may indicate color blindness, a genetic dysfunction, or retinal pathology.

Indications

- Detect deficiencies in color perception
- Investigate suspected retinal pathology affecting the cones
- Investigate because of a family history of color visual deficit

Reference Values

- Normal visual color discrimination. No difficulty in identification of color combinations.

Abnormal Values

- Identification of some but not all colors

Interfering Factors

- Inability of client to read
- Poor visual acuity or lighting
- Failure of client to wear corrective lenses
- Inability of client to participate in test
- Damaged or discolored plates

Nursing Implications

Assessment

- Obtain a history of known or suspected color visual impairment in client or family.
- Determine if the client uses corrective lenses and ask about the importance of color discrimination in work.

Possible Nursing Diagnosis

Sensory-perceptual alteration (visual) related to altered sensory reception, transmission, or integration

Implementation

- Occlude one eye and hold test booklet 12 to 14 inches in front of the exposed eye.
- Ask the client to identify the numbers or letters buried in the maze of dots or to trace the objects with a pointed object.
- Repeat on the other eye.

Evaluation

- Note results in relation to other retinal studies, if performed, and the impact of the results on the client's lifestyle.

Client/Caregiver Teaching

Pretest

- Instruct the client to bring corrective glasses or contact lenses to the test.
- Inform the client that the test is painless and should take 5 to 10 minutes to complete.

Colposcopy

Classification: Endoscopy

Type of Test: Direct visualization

In this procedure, the vagina and cervix are viewed using a special binocular microscope and light system that magnifies the mucosal surfaces. It is usually performed after suspicious Pap test results or when suspected lesions cannot be fully visualized by the naked eye. The procedure is useful in diagnosing cervical cancer because it provides the best view of the suspicious lesion, ensuring that the most representative area of the lesion is obtained for cytologic analysis to confirm malignant changes. Photographs (cervicography) can also be taken of the cervix.

Indications

- Evaluate the cervix after abnormal Papanicolaou (Pap) smear
- Evaluate vaginal lesions
- Monitor women whose mothers took diethylstilbestrol during pregnancy
- Localize the area from which cervical biopsy samples should be obtained, since such areas may not be visible to the naked eye

Reference Values

- Normal appearance of the vagina and cervix
- No abnormal cells or tissues

Abnormal Values

- Cervical intraepithelial neoplasia
- Invasive carcinoma
- Inflammatory changes
- Atrophic changes
- Cervical erosion
- Leukoplakia

Interfering Factors

- Inability of the client to cooperate with the procedure
- Failure to adequately cleanse the cervix of secretions and medications
- Scarring of the cervix

> **NURSING ALERT**
>
> - This procedure is contraindicated in bleeding disorders, especially if cervical biopsy specimens are to be obtained or in women who are currently menstruating.

Nursing Implications

Assessment

- Obtain a history of blood-clotting abnormalities
- Determine the date of the last menstrual period in premenopausal women; the procedure should not be done when the client is menstruating and is best performed 1 week after menses ends.

Possible Nursing Diagnoses

Anxiety related to threat to health status

Body image disturbance related to potential change in structure

Grieving, anticipatory, related to perceived loss or threat of death

Implementation

- Position the client in the lithotomy position on the examining table and drape. Cleanse the external genitalia with an antiseptic solution.
- If a Pap smear is performed, the vaginal speculum is inserted, using water as a lubricant.
- The cervix is swabbed with 3% acetic acid to remove mucus or any cream medication and improve the contrast between tissue types. The scope is positioned at the speculum and is focused on the cervix. The area is then examined carefully using light and magnification. Photographs can be taken for future reference.
- Tissues that appear abnormal or atypical are biopsied using a forceps inserted through the speculum. Bleeding, which is not uncommon following cervical biopsy, may be controlled by cautery, suturing, or application of silver nitrate or ferric subsulfate to the site.
- The vagina is rinsed with sterile saline or water to remove the acetic acid and prevent burning following the procedure. If bleeding persists, a tampon may be inserted by the physician following removal of the speculum.
- Samples are placed in appropriate containers with special preservative solution, properly labeled, and taken to the laboratory promptly.

Evaluation

- Note results in relation to other test results and the client's symptoms.

Client/Caregiver Teaching

Pretest

- Inform the client that the procedure is generally performed in a physician's office by a physician or nurse practitioner and takes approximately 10 to 15 minutes.
- Inform the client that if a biopsy is performed, slight discomfort and a minimal amount of bleeding will be experienced.

Posttest

- Inform the client to remove the vaginal tampon within 8 to 24 hours if one was inserted; after that time, wear pads if there is bleeding or drainage.
- Inform the client that if a biopsy was performed a gray-green discharge may persist for a few days to a few weeks.

- Advise the client to avoid strenuous exercise 8 to 24 hours following the procedure; douching and intercourse should be avoided for about 2 weeks or as directed by the practitioner.
- Emphasize that excessive vaginal bleeding or abnormal vaginal discharge, abdominal pain and fever must be reported to the physician immediately.

Complete Blood Count

Classification: Hematology
Type of Test: Blood

A complete blood count is a basic screening test that includes several tests that evaluate the cellular components of the blood. Probably the most widely ordered test, test results provide the enumeration of the cellular elements of the blood, evaluation of red cell indices, and determination of cell morphology by means of stained smears. These values can provide valuable diagnostic information regarding the overall health of the client and the client's response to the pathology and treatment.

Indications

- As part of a complete physical examination, especially upon admission to a health care facility or before surgery
- Detect hematologic disorder, neoplasm, or immunologic abnormality
- Determine presence of hereditary hematologic abnormality
- Detect local or systemic, acute or chronic infection
- Monitor effects of physical or emotional stress
- Monitor response to drug therapy and evaluate undesired reactions to drugs that may cause blood dyscrasias
- Monitor progression of nonhematologic disorders such as chronic obstructive pulmonary disease, malabsorption syndromes, cancer, and renal disease

Reference Values

Normal Reference Values for Complete Blood Count

	Newborn	Child	Adult Male	Adult Female
Red blood cells (RBC)	4.8–7.1 million/mm^3	4.5–4.8 million/mm^3	4.6–6.2 million/mm^3	4.2–5.4 million/mm^3
Hematocrit	44–64%	35–41%	40–54%	38–47%
Hemoglobin	12–24 g/dL	11–16 g/dL	13.5–18 g/dL	12–16 g/dL
Red cell indices				
MCV	96–108 mm^3	82–91 mm^3	80–94 mm^3	81–99 mm^3
MCH	32–34 pg	27–31 pg	27–31 pg	27–31 pg
MCHC	32–33%	32–36%	32–36%	32–36%
Stained red cell examination	Normochronic and normocytic	Normochronic and normocytic	Normochronic and normocytic	Normochronic and normocytic
Differential WBC				
Neutrophils	45% by 1 week	60% after age 2	54–74% (3000–7500/mm^3)	54–74% (3000–7500/mm^3)
Bands			3–8% (150–700/mm^3)	3–8% (150–700/mm^3)
Eosinophils		0–3%	1–4% (50–400/mm^3)	1–4% (50–400/mm^3)
Basophils		1–3%	0–1% (25–100/mm^3)	0–1% (25–100/mm^3)
Monocytes		4–9%	2–8% (100–500/mm^3)	2–8% (100–500/mm^3)
Lymphocytes	41% by 1 week	59% after age 2	25–40% (1500–4500/mm^3)	25–40% (1500–4500/mm^3)
T lymphocytes			60–80% of lymphocytes	60–80% of lymphocytes
B lymphocytes			10–20% of lymphocytes	10–20% of lymphocytes
Platelets	140,000–300,000/mm^3	150,000–450,000/mm^3	150,000–450,000/mm^3	150,000–450,000/mm^3

Abnormal Values

See individual test listings for specific abnormal values.

■ Blood dyscrasias from the following drugs

Acetaminophen and combination drugs containing acetaminophen
Acetophenazine maleate
Aminosalicylic acid
Amphotericin B
Antineoplastic agents
Arsenicals
Carbamazepine
Chloramphenicol
Chloroquine
Ethosuximide
Furazolidone
Haloperidol
Hydantoin derivatives
Hydralazine
Hydroxychloroquine
Indomethacin
Isoniazid
MAO inhibitors
Mefenamic acid
Mepacrine
Mephenoxalone
Mercurial diuretics
Metaxalone
Methyldopa
Nitrites
Nitrofurantoin
Novobiocin
Oleandomycin
Oxyphenbutazone
Paramethadione
Primethadione
Penicillamine
Penicillins
Phenacemide
Phenobarbital
Phenylbutazone
Phytonadione
Primaquine
Primidone
Pyrazolone derivatives
Pyrimethamine
Rifampin
Radioisotopes
Spectinomycin
Sulfonamides
Sulfones
Sulfonylureas
Tetracyclines
Thiazide diuretics
Thiocyanates
Tripelennamine
Troleandomycin
Valproic acid
Vitamin A

Interfering Factors

■ Failure to fill the tube sufficiently to yield proper blood and anticoagulant ratio in the specimen.

■ Obtaining a sample from an extremity that has an IV line in place yields hemodilution of the sample and false results.

■ Leaving the tourniquet in place longer than 60 seconds can affect test results.

■ Drugs such as the ones listed under *Abnormal Values* can affect results.

Nursing Implications

Assessment

- Obtain a history of hematologic disorders, medication regimen, and exposure to infectious diseases.

Possible Nursing Diagnoses

Injury, risk for, related to altered clotting factors
Protection, altered, related to abnormal blood profiles
Infection, risk for, related to inadequate primary defenses

Implementation

- Put on gloves. Using aseptic technique, perform a venipuncture and collect 5 to 7 mL of blood in a lavender-top tube.
- A capillary sample may be obtained in infants and children, as well as in adults for whom venipuncture may not be feasible.

Evaluation

- Note test results in relation to other tests performed and the client's symptoms.

Client/Caregiver Teaching

Pretest

- Inform the client that there is no special preparation before this test.

Computed Tomography (CT), Abdomen; Computerized Axial Tomography (CAT); Computerized Transaxial Tomography (CTT)

Classification: Radiography

Type of Test: Indirect visualization

Computed tomography (CT) scanning is a noninvasive procedure that becomes invasive when a contrast medium is used. It uses multiple x-ray beams with a special scanning machine to produce cross-sectional views in a three-dimensional fashion by detecting and recording differences in tissue density. These measurements are sent to a computer that produces a digital view of the anatomy, enabling the radiologist to look at "slices" of certain anatomical views of the liver, biliary tract, pancreas, kidneys, spleen, intestines, and vascular system. Differentiations can be made between solid, cystic, inflammatory, or vascular lesions as well as suspected hematomas or aneurysms. Repeated visualization after injection of contrast medium can be done to produce enhanced views. Images can be recorded on photographic or x-ray film.

Indications

- Detect abnormalities of the abdominal organs
- Diagnose and locate benign and cancerous tumors and metastasis to other organs

Reference Values

- Normal size and contour of abdominal organs and vascular system

Abnormal Values

- Primary and metastatic neoplasms
- Hepatic abscess or cyst

- Hematomas
- Abdominal aortic aneurysm
- Pancreatic pseudocyst
- Splenic laceration
- Abdominal abscess
- Hemoperitoneum
- Dilatation of the common hepatic duct, common bile duct, or gallbladder

Interfering Factors

- Inability of the client to remain still during the procedure may produce artifact.
- Incorrect positioning of the client can give poor visualization of area to be viewed.
- Metallic objects within the examination field such as jewelry, watches, or belts can produce unclear images.
- Extreme obesity can impair clear imaging.
- Presence of feces, gas, or barium in the gastrointestinal tract can hinder adequate imaging.

NURSING ALERT

- This procedure is contraindicated in pregnancy, especially during first trimester, unless the benefits of x-ray diagnosis far outweigh the possible risks to the fetus.
- It is also contraindicated in clients with allergies to shellfish or iodinated dye (if dye is to be used); in clients with unstable medical status; in extreme cases of claustrophobia unless sedation is given before the study; and in clients with severe renal or hepatic disease.
- Take special precautions with children to avoid excess exposure to x-rays.

Nursing Implications

Assessment

- Determine previous abnormalities in laboratory test results and diagnostic findings.
- Determine date of last menstrual period and possibility of pregnancy in premenopausal women.
- Obtain any history of disease of the abdominal organs.
- Obtain history of known sensitivity to iodine, shellfish, or contrast dye from previous x-ray procedure.

- Ensure barium studies have been performed more than 4 days before the scan.
- Ensure that the client has fasted after midnight of the night before the test.

Possible Nursing Diagnoses

Anxiety related to perceived threat to health status
Grieving, anticipatory, related to perceived potential loss
Fluid volume deficit related to active loss
Infection, risk for, related to exposure to contrast medium

Implementation

- Place the client in the supine position on flat table and ask the client to lie very still during the procedure as movement will cause blurring of the pictures. Make sure jewelry, watch, and belt have been removed.
- Administer enema to free gastrointestinal tract from barium, as ordered.
- Administer a sedative to a child under 3 years of age or an uncooperative adult, as ordered.
- Administer an antianxiety agent if claustrophobia is problematic for the client, as ordered.
- Move table into the scanner and instruct the client to remain still. The scanner will make loud noises as it rotates around the body. The client may be asked to take deep breaths to facilitate visualization. A series of pictures are taken. These images are reconstructed by a computer and reviewed.
- Administer a contrast medium, as ordered. A second series of films are then taken.

Evaluation

- Note test results in relation to other studies performed and the client's symptoms.
- Observe for delayed allergic reactions to contrast medium, including urticaria, headache, nausea, or vomiting.

Client/Caregiver Teaching

Pretest

- Inform the client that the procedure is performed to detect the cause of clinical symptoms. Explain that the procedure is performed in the radiology department by a technician and a physician. Inform the client that the scan can take 30 to 90 minutes to complete.
- Inform the client that intravenous iodinated contrast medium may be given before the imaging or that images are taken

first and then the medium is injected in order to enhance any unusual findings.

■ Inform the client to expect nausea, a feeling of warmth, a salty or metallic taste, or a transient headache after injection of the contrast medium. Instruct the client to take slow deep breaths if this occurs.

■ Instruct client to fast after midnight of the day before the test.

Posttest

■ Tell the client to resume normal activity and diet, unless otherwise indicated.

■ Tell the client to increase fluid intake to eliminate the contrast medium, if used.

■ In clients with impaired renal function, instruct the client or caregiver to note changes in urinary output following the administration of iodinated contrast medium.

Computed Tomography (CT), Biliary Tract and Liver; Computerized Axial Tomography (CAT); Computerized Transaxial Tomography (CTT)

Classification: Radiography

Type of Test: Indirect visualization

Computed tomography (CT) scanning is a noninvasive procedure that becomes invasive when a contrast medium is used. It uses multiple x-ray beams with a special scanning machine to produce cross-sectional views in a three-dimensional fashion by detecting and recording differences in tissue density. These measurements are sent to a computer that produces a digital view of the anatomy, enabling the radiologist to look at "slices" of certain anatomical views of the liver and biliary tract regions. Differentiations can be made between solid, cystic, inflammatory, or vascular lesions, as well as suspected hematomas. Repeated visualization after injection of contrast medium can be done to produce enhanced views. Images can be recorded on photographic or x-ray film.

Indications

- Detect liver abnormalities such as abscesses (intrahepatic, subhepatic, and subphrenic), cysts, cirrhosis with ascites and fatty liver, and intrahepatic tumors and hematomas
- Detect dilatation or obstruction of the biliary ducts with or without calcification or gallstones
- Distinguish between obstructive and nonobstructive jaundice
- Diagnose and locate benign and cancerous tumors and metastasis to other organs

Reference Values

- Normal size and contour of liver and biliary ducts

Abnormal Values

- Primary and metastatic neoplasms
- Hepatic abscess or cyst
- Hematomas
- Jaundice (obstructive or nonobstructive)
- Dilatation of the common hepatic duct, common bile duct, or gallbladder

Interfering Factors

- Inability of the client to remain still during the procedure may produce artifact.
- Incorrect positioning of the client can give poor visualization of area to be viewed.
- Metallic objects within the examination field, such as jewelry, watches, or belts, can produce unclear images.
- Extreme obesity can impair clear imaging.
- Presence of feces, gas, or barium in the gastrointestinal tract can hinder adequate imaging.

> ### NURSING ALERT
>
> - This procedure is contraindicated in pregnancy, especially during the first trimester, unless the benefits of x-ray diagnosis far outweigh the possible risks to the fetus.
> - It is also contraindicated in clients with allergies to shellfish or iodinated dye (if dye is to be used); in clients with unstable medical status; in extreme cases of claustrophobia unless sedation is given before the study; and in clients with severe renal or hepatic disease.
> - Take special precautions with children to avoid excess exposure to x-rays.

Nursing Implications

Assessment

- Determine previous abnormalities in laboratory test results (especially BUN and creatinine if dye is to be used) and diagnostic findings.
- Determine date of last menstrual period and possibility of pregnancy in premenopausal women.
- Obtain any history of hepatobiliary or gastrointestinal disease or findings.
- Obtain history of known sensitivity to iodine, shellfish, or contrast dye from previous x-ray procedure.
- Ensure barium studies have been performed more than 4 days before the scan of liver or biliary tract.
- Ensure that the client has fasted since midnight of the day before the test.

Possible Nursing Diagnoses

Anxiety related to perceived threat to health status
Injury, risk for, related to exposure to contrast medium
Pain related to inflammation or swelling of the liver
Grieving, anticipatory, related to perceived potential loss

Implementation

- Place the client in the supine position on flat table and ask the client to lie very still during the procedure, as movement will cause blurring of the pictures. Make sure jewelry, watch, and belt have been removed.
- Administer enema to free gastrointestinal tract from barium, as ordered.

- Administer a sedative to a child under 3 years of age or to an uncooperative adult, as ordered.
- Administer an antianxiety agent, as ordered, if claustrophobia is a problem for the client.
- Move the table into the scanner and instruct the client to remain still. The scanner will make loud noises when rotating around the body. The client may be asked to take deep breaths to facilitate visualization. A series of pictures are taken. These images are reconstructed by a computer and reviewed.
- Administer a contrast medium, if ordered. A second series of films are then taken.

Evaluation

- Note test results in relation to other studies performed and the client's symptoms.
- Observe for delayed allergic reactions, including urticaria, headache, nausea, or vomiting, if contrast medium was used.

Client/Caregiver Teaching

Pretest

- Inform the client that the procedure is performed to detect biliary tract and liver disease. Explain that the procedure is performed in a special radiology department by a technician and a physician. Inform the client that the scan can take 30 to 90 minutes to complete.
- Inform the client that intravenous iodinated contrast medium may be given before the imaging or that images are taken first and then the medium is injected to enhance any unusual findings.
- Instruct the client to expect nausea, a feeling of warmth, a salty or metallic taste, or a transient headache following injection. Instruct the client to take slow deep breaths if this occurs.
- Instruct client to fast after midnight of the day before the test.

Posttest

- Instruct the client to resume normal activity and diet, unless otherwise indicated.
- Instruct the client to increase fluid intake to eliminate the contrast medium, if used.
- Instruct the client or caregiver to note change in urinary output following iodinated contrast medium administration in clients with impaired renal function.

Computed Tomography (CT), Cranial; Computerized Axial Tomography (CAT); Computerized Transaxial Tomography (CTT)

Classification: Radiography

Type of Test: Indirect visualization

Computerized tomography (CT) is a nonnuclear, noninvasive procedure performed to assist in diagnosing abnormalities of the head, brain tissue, cerebrospinal fluid, and blood circulation. It becomes an invasive procedure if a contrast medium is used for image enhancement when pathology causing destruction of the blood-brain barrier is suspected. It uses multiple x-ray beams with a special scanning machine to produce cross-sectional views in a three-dimensional fashion by detecting and recording differences in tissue density. These measurements are sent to a computer that produces a digital view of the anatomy, enabling the radiologist to look at "slices" of bone (appearing white), brain matter (appearing gray), and circulating cerebrospinal fluid (appearing black). Images can be recorded on photographic or x-ray film.

Indications

- Diagnose multiple sclerosis, as evidenced by sclerotic plaques as small as 3 to 4 mm in diameter
- Determine cause of increased intracranial pressure (ICP)
- Diagnose intracranial benign and cancerous tumors and cyst formation, as evidenced by changes in tissue densities; white indicates increased density and darker areas indicating decreased density
- Determine size and location of a lesion causing a stroke, such as an infarct or hemorrhage
- Detect ventricular enlargement or displacement by cerebrospinal fluid increases and type of hemorrhage in infants and children experiencing signs and symptoms of intracranial

trauma or congenital conditions such as hydrocephalus and arteriovenous malformations
- Differentiate between cerebral infarction and hemorrhage
- Detect presence of brain infection or an inflammatory condition, such as abscess or necrosis, as evidenced by decreased density
- Differentiate among hematoma locations following trauma (for example, subdural, epidural, and cerebral), and determine the extent of edema resulting from injury, as evidenced by higher blood densities as compared with normal tissue
- Evaluate effectiveness of treatment and course of a disease
- Diagnose abnormalities of the middle ear ossicles, auditory nerve, and optic nerve

Reference Values

- Normal size, shape, and position of intracranial contents

Abnormal Values

- Tumor
- Hemorrhage
- Aneurysm
- Cerebral infarction
- Infection
- Ventricular or tissue displacement or enlargement
- Congenital abnormalities
- Hematomas (epidural, subdural, or intracerebral)
- Cysts
- Abscess
- Cerebral edema
- Cerebral atrophy
- Hydrocephaly
- Arteriovenous malformations
- Increased intracranial pressure or trauma
- Sclerotic plaques suggesting multiple sclerosis

Interfering Factors

- Inability of client to maintain head in an immobilized position during the procedure may produce artifact.
- Incorrect positioning of the client may give poor visualization of the area to be viewed.
- Metallic objects within the examination field, such as jewelry, hairpins, hearing aid, or dental or eye prostheses, can produce unclear images.

> ### NURSING ALERT
>
> - This procedure is contraindicated in pregnancy, especially during first trimester, unless the benefits of x-ray diagnosis far outweigh the possible risks to the fetus.
> - It is also contraindicated in clients with allergies to shellfish or iodinated dye (if contrast medium is to be used); in clients with unstable medical status; and in extreme claustrophobia unless sedation is given before the study.
> - Take precautions with children to avoid excess exposure to x-rays.

Nursing Implications

Assessment

- Obtain a history of known or suspected neurologic disorders, last menstrual date and possible pregnancy in women of childbearing age, known sensitivity to iodine or previous dyes used in procedures, results of laboratory tests and other diagnostic procedures, especially BUN and creatinine, if a contrast dye is used.
- Note if food and fluids have been withheld for 4 hours before the study if a contrast medium is to be used.

Possible Nursing Diagnoses

Anxiety related to perceived threat to health status

Injury, risk for, related to exposure to contrast medium

Communication, impaired, verbal, related to altered brain function

Physical mobility, impaired, related to neuromuscular impairment

Sensory-perceptual alteration [specify] related to altered sensory transmission or integration

Implementation

- Administer an ordered sedative to a child under 3 years of age or to an uncooperative or claustrophobic adult if needed.
- Administer an antihistamine and steroid, as ordered, for clients with known allergies to contrast medium.
- Place the client on a flat table in supine position with the head on an apparatus that fits into a frame that revolves around the head and from one side to another.

- Move table into the scanner and instruct the client to remain still. The scanner will make loud noises as it rotates around the head. The client may be asked to take deep breaths to facilitate visualization. A series of pictures are taken. These images are reconstructed by a computer and reviewed.
- Administer a contrast medium, if ordered. A second series of films are then taken.

Evaluation

- Note test results in relation to other studies performed and the client's symptoms.
- Note any reactions to the contrast medium such as rash, urticaria, changes in breathing pattern, headache, nausea, or vomiting.

Client/Caregiver Teaching

Pretest

- Inform the client of the purpose of the study, how the procedure is performed, and the possible administration of a contrast medium to obtain better views of the head.
- Inform the client that the procedure is performed in the radiology department by a technician and physician and takes 30 to 60 minutes to complete.
- If a contrast medium is to be used, tell the client to fast for 4 hours before the test. Also, inform the client that all metal objects (for example, jewelry, hairpins, hearing aid, or dental or eye prostheses) must be removed before the test.
- Instruct the client to expect nausea, a feeling of warmth, a salty or metallic taste, or a transient headache following injection of the contrast medium. Instruct the client to take slow deep breaths if this occurs.

Posttest

- Advise the client to drink additional fluids to assist in elimination of the dye.
- Instruct the client to resume food and fluid intake if withheld before the study.

Computed Tomography (CT), Orbital; Computerized Axial Tomography (CAT); Computerized Transaxial Tomography (CTT)

Classification: Radiography

Type of Test: Indirect visualization

Computed tomography (CT) scanning is a noninvasive procedure unless a contrast medium is used. It uses multiple x-ray beams with a special scanning machine to produce cross-sectional views in a three-dimensional fashion by detecting and recording differences in tissue density. These measurements are sent to a computer that produces a digital view of the anatomy, enabling the radiologist to look at "slices" of certain anatomical views of the orbital structures, including the ocular muscle, optic nerve, and bone structure. Contrast enhancement can give important information regarding circulation through abnormal ocular tissues. Images can be recorded on photographic or x-ray film.

Indications

- Detect eye and orbit disease
- Determine cause of unilateral exophthalmus
- Diagnose abnormalities of the optic nerve
- Evaluate orbital bone fractures
- Evaluate circulatory disorders, hemangiomas, or hematomas

Reference Values

- Normal size, shape, and position of orbital structures
- Clearly defined optic nerve and medial and lateral rectus muscles
- Optic canals of equal size

Abnormal Values

- Tumors invading the orbital space, including intracranial, intraorbital, extraorbital (lymphomas and metastatic carcinomas), and encapsulated tumors (benign hemangiomas and meningiomas)
- Unilateral exophthalmus
- Space-occupying lesions in the orbit or paranasal sinuses
- Circulatory disorders such as hemangioma or subdural hematoma

Interfering Factors

- Inability of the client to maintain head in an immobilized position during the procedure can produce artifact.
- Incorrect positioning of the client can give poor visualization of area to be viewed.
- Metallic objects within the examination field, such as jewelry, or eye prostheses, can produce unclear images.

> ### NURSING ALERT
>
> - This procedure is contraindicated in pregnancy, especially during first trimester, unless the benefits of x-ray diagnosis far outweigh the possible risks to the fetus.
> - It is also contraindicated in clients with allergies to shellfish or iodinated dye (if dye is to be used); in clients with unstable medical status; and in extreme cases of claustrophobia unless sedation is given before the study.
> - Take special precautions with children to avoid excess exposure to x-rays.

Nursing Implications

Assessment

- Determine previous abnormalities in laboratory test results, especially BUN and creatinine if dye is to be used, and diagnostic findings.
- Determine date of last menstrual period and possibility of pregnancy in premenopausal women.
- Obtain pertinent history related to trauma or disease processes of the orbital area.
- Obtain history of known sensitivity to iodine, shellfish, or contrast dye from previous x-ray procedure.
- Ensure that the client has fasted for 4 hours before the test if contrast medium is to be used.

Possible Nursing Diagnoses

Anxiety related to perceived threat to health status

Injury, risk for, related to exposure to contrast medium

Sensory-perceptual alteration, visual, related to altered sensory transmission or integration

Body image disturbance related to change in structure/ appearance

Implementation

- Place the client in supine position on flat table. Ask the client to lie very still during the procedure, as movement will produce unclear images. Head will be immobilized during the procedure. Make sure jewelry and eye prosthesis have been removed.
- Administer sedative to a child under 3 years of age or to an uncooperative adult, as ordered.
- Administer antianxiety agent, as ordered, if claustrophobia is a problem for the client.
- Move table into the scanner and instruct the client to remain still. The scanner will make loud noises as it rotates around body. The client may be asked to take deep breaths to facilitate visualization. A series of pictures are taken. These images are reconstructed by a computer and reviewed.
- Administer a contrast medium, if ordered. A second series of films are then taken.

Evaluation

- Note test results in relation to other studies performed and the client's symptoms.
- Observe the client for delayed allergic reactions, including, urticaria, headache, nausea, or vomiting, if contrast enhancement was used.

Client/Caregiver Teaching

Pretest

- Inform the client that the test permits assessment of the tissues and bones around the eyes.
- Explain that the procedure is performed in a special radiology department by a technician and a physician.
- Inform the client that intravenous iodinated contrast medium can be injected after the first series of x-rays, with a second series of scans following.
- Instruct the client to expect nausea, a feeling of warmth, a salty or metallic taste, or a transient headache following injection. Instruct the client to take slow deep breaths if this occurs.

Posttest

- Instruct the client to resume normal activity and diet, unless otherwise indicated.
- Instruct the client to increase fluid intake to help eliminate the contrast medium, if used.
- Instruct the client or caregiver to note changes in urinary output following iodinated contrast medium administration in clients with impaired renal function.

Computed Tomography (CT), Pancreatic; Computerized Axial Tomography (CAT); Computerized Transaxial Tomography (CTT)

Classification: Radiography

Type of Test: Indirect visualization

Computed tomography (CT) scanning is a noninvasive procedure unless a contrast medium is used. It uses multiple x-ray beams in conjunction with a special scanning machine to produce cross-sectional views with three-dimensional images by detecting and recording differences in tissue density. These measurements are sent to a computer that produces a digital view of anatomy, enabling the radiologist to look at "slices" of anatomical views of the pancreas. Intravenous or oral contrast medium can accentuate the difference in tissue density. Images can be recorded on photographic or x-ray film.

Indications

- Diagnose benign or cancerous tumors or metastasis to the pancreas
- Evaluate pancreatic abnormalities, for example, bleeding, pancreatitis, pseudocyst, or abscesses
- Detect dilatation or obstruction of the pancreatic ducts

- Evaluate effectiveness of medical or surgical regimen
- Differentiate between pancreatic disorders and disorders of the retroperitoneum

Reference Values

- Normal size and contour of the pancreas gland, which lies obliquely in the upper abdomen

Abnormal Values

- Acute or chronic pancreatitis
- Pancreatic carcinoma
- Pancreatic tumor
- Pancreatic abscess
- Pseudocyst
- Obstruction of pancreatic ducts

Interfering Factors

- Inability of the client to remain still during the procedure may produce artifact.
- Incorrect positioning of the client can give poor visualization of area to be viewed.
- Metallic objects within the examination field, such as jewelry, watches, or belts, can produce unclear images.
- Extreme obesity can impair clear imaging.
- Presence of barium in the gastrointestinal tract can hinder adequate imaging.
- Excessive peristaltic movement during scanning can produce artifact.

NURSING ALERT

- This procedure is contraindicated in pregnancy, especially during first trimester, unless the benefits of x-ray diagnosis far outweigh the possible risks to the fetus.
- It is contraindicated in clients with allergies to shellfish or iodinated dye (if dye is to be used); in clients with unstable medical status; in extreme cases of claustrophobia unless sedation is given before the study; and in clients with severe renal disease (if contrast dye is to be used).
- Take precautions with children to avoid excess exposure to x-rays.

Nursing Implications

Assessment

- Determine previous abnormalities in laboratory test results, especially BUN and creatinine if dye is to be used, and diagnostic findings.
- Determine date of last menstrual period and possibility of pregnancy in premenopausal women.
- Obtain pertinent history related to trauma or disease processes of the orbital area.
- Obtain history of known sensitivity to iodine, shellfish, or contrast dye from previous x-ray procedure.
- Ensure that barium studies have been performed more than 4 days before the pancreatic scan.

Possible Nursing Diagnoses

Pain related to inflammation or swelling of the pancreas
Anxiety related to perceived threat to health status
Infection, risk for, related to inadequate primary defenses
Injury, risk for, related to exposure to contrast medium

Implementation

- Place the client in a supine position on a flat table. Ask the client to lie very still during the procedure, as movement will produce unclear images. Make sure jewelry, watches, and belts have been removed.
- Administer sedative to a child under 3 years of age or to an uncooperative adult, as ordered.
- Administer antianxiety agent as ordered, if claustrophobia is a problem for the client.
- Move table into the scanner and instruct the client to remain still. The scanner will make loud noises as it rotates around the body. The client may be asked to take deep breaths to facilitate visualization. A series of pictures are taken. These images are reconstructed by a computer and reviewed.
- Administer a contrast medium, if ordered. A second series of films are then taken.

Evaluation

- Note test results in relation to other tests performed and the client's symptoms.
- Observe for delayed allergic reactions, for example, urticaria, headache, nausea, or vomiting, if contrast medium is used.

Client/Caregiver Teaching

Pretest

- Inform the client that the test permits the pancreas to be viewed and abnormalities identified.

- Explain that the procedure is performed in a special radiology department by a technician and a physician and takes about 30 minutes.
- Inform the client that intravenous iodinated contrast medium can be injected after the first series of x-rays, with a second series of scans following.
- Instruct the client to expect nausea, a feeling of warmth, a salty or metallic taste, or a transient headache following injection. Instruct the client to take slow deep breaths if this occurs.

Posttest

- Instruct the client to resume normal activity and diet, unless otherwise indicated.
- Instruct the client to increase fluid intake to eliminate the contrast medium, if used.
- Instruct the client or caregiver to note change in urinary output following iodinated contrast medium administration in clients with impaired renal function.

Computed Tomography (CT), Pelvic; Computerized Axial Tomography (CAT); Computerized Transaxial Tomography (CTT)

Classification: Radiography

Type of Test: Indirect visualization

Computed tomography (CT) scanning is a noninvasive procedure that becomes invasive when a contrast medium is used. It uses multiple x-ray beams with a special scanning machine to produce cross-sectional views in a three-dimensional fashion by detecting and recording differences in tissue density. These measurements are sent to a computer that produces a digital view of the anatomy, enabling the radiologist to look at "slices" of certain anatomical views of the ovaries, uterus, fallopian tubes, and bladder. Differentiations can be made between solid, cystic, inflammatory, or vascular lesions, as well as suspected hematomas. Repeated visualization after injection of contrast medium can be done to produce enhanced views. Images can be recorded on photographic or x-ray film.

Indications

- Detect abnormalities of the pelvic organs
- Diagnose and locate benign and cancerous tumors and metastasis to other organs

Reference Values

- Normal size and contour of pelvic organs and vascular system

Abnormal Values

- Primary and metastatic neoplasms
- Ovarian cyst or abscess
- Hydrosalpinx
- Fibroid tumors
- Ectopic pregnancy
- Bladder calculi

Interfering Factors

- Inability of the client to remain still during the procedure may produce artifact.
- Incorrect positioning of the client can give poor visualization of area to be viewed.
- Metallic objects within the examination field, such as jewelry, watches, or belts, can produce unclear images.
- Extreme obesity can impair clear imaging.
- Presence of feces, gas, or barium in the gastrointestinal tract can hinder adequate imaging.

> ### NURSING ALERT
>
> - This procedure is contraindicated in pregnancy, especially during first trimester, unless the benefits of x-ray diagnosis far outweigh the possible risks to the fetus.
> - It is also contraindicated in clients with allergies to shellfish or iodinated dye (if dye is to be used); in clients with unstable medical status; in extreme cases of claustrophobia unless sedation is given before the

study; and in clients with severe renal or hepatic disease.
- Take special precautions with children to avoid excess exposure to x-rays.

Nursing Implications

Assessment

- Determine previous abnormalities in laboratory test results and diagnostic findings.
- Determine date of last menstrual period and possibility of pregnancy in premenopausal women.
- Obtain any history of disease of the pelvic organs.
- Obtain history of known sensitivity to iodine, shellfish, or contrast dye from previous x-ray procedure.
- Ensure that barium studies have been performed more than 4 days before the scan.
- Ensure that the client has fasted since midnight of the day before the test.

Possible Nursing Diagnoses

Pain related to inflammation or swelling of ovary or fallopian tube

Anxiety related to perceived threat to health status

Injury, risk for, related to exposure to contrast medium

Body image disturbance related to change in structure/ appearance

Grieving, anticipatory, related to perceived potential loss

Implementation

- Place the client in the supine position on a flat table and ask the client to lie very still during the procedure, as movement will cause blurring of the pictures. Make sure jewelry, watch, and belt have been removed.
- Administer enema to free gastrointestinal tract from barium, as ordered.
- Administer a sedative to a child under 3 years of age or to an uncooperative adult, as ordered.
- Administer an antianxiety agent, as ordered, if claustrophobia is a problem for the client.
- Move the table into the scanner and instruct the client to remain still. The scanner will make loud noises as it rotates around body. The client may be asked to take deep breaths to facilitate visualization. A series of pictures are taken.

These images are reconstructed by a computer and reviewed.

- Administer a contrast medium, if ordered. A second series of films are then taken.

Evaluation

- Note test results in relation to other studies performed and the client's symptoms.
- Observe for delayed allergic reactions, including urticaria, headache, nausea, or vomiting, if contrast medium was used.

Client/Caregiver Teaching

Pretest

- Inform the client that the procedure is performed to detect the cause of clinical symptoms. Explain that the procedure is performed in a special radiology department by a technician and a physician. Inform the client that the scan can take 30 to 90 minutes to complete.
- Inform the client that intravenous iodinated contrast medium may be given before the imaging or that images may be taken first and then the medium injected to enhance any unusual findings.
- Instruct the client to expect nausea, a feeling of warmth, a salty or metallic taste, or a transient headache following injection. Instruct the client to take slow deep breaths if this occurs.
- Instruct client to fast after midnight of the day before the test.

Posttest

- Instruct the client to resume normal activity and diet, unless otherwise indicated.
- Instruct the client to increase fluid intake to eliminate the contrast medium, if used.
- Instruct the client or caregiver to note change in urinary output following iodinated contrast medium administration in clients with impaired renal function.

Computed Tomography (CT), Renal; Computerized Axial Tomography (CAT); Computerized Transaxial Tomography (CTT)

Classification: Radiography

Type of Test: Indirect visualization

Computed tomography (CT) scanning is a noninvasive procedure that becomes invasive when a contrast medium is used. It uses multiple x-ray beams with a special scanning machine to produce cross-sectional views in a three-dimensional fashion by detecting and recording differences in tissue density. These measurements are sent to a computer that produces a digital view of the anatomy, enabling the radiologist to look at "slices" of certain anatomical views of the kidneys and surrounding organs, specifically the adrenal gland. Differentiations can be made between solid, cystic, inflammatory, or vascular lesions, as well as suspected hematomas. Repeated visualization after injection of contrast medium can be done to produce enhanced views. Images can be recorded on photographic or x-ray film.

Indications

- Diagnose malignant and benign tumors or metastasis to kidneys
- Detect urinary calculi or obstruction
- Diagnose perirenal hematomas and abscesses and assist in localizing for drainage
- Diagnose congenital anomalies such as polycystic kidney disease, horseshoe kidney, absence of one kidney, or kidney displacement
- Detect abnormal fluid accumulation around kidneys
- Determine kidney size and location in relation to the bladder in posttransplant clients
- Detect bleeding or hyperplasia of the adrenal glands

- Determine presence and type of adrenal tumor such as benign adenoma, cancer, or pheochromocytoma
- Evaluate spread of a tumor or invasion of nearby retroperitoneal organs

Reference Values

- Normal size, shape, and position of kidneys

Abnormal Values

- Renal cysts
- Renal masses
- Renal cell carcinoma
- Renal calculi
- Congenital anomalies, such as polycystic kidney disease, horseshoe kidney, absence of one kidney, or kidney displacement
- Perirenal abscesses and hematomas
- Adrenal tumors

Interfering Factors

- Inability of the client to remain still during the procedure may produce artifact.
- Incorrect positioning of the client can give poor visualization of area to be viewed.
- Metallic objects within the examination field, such as jewelry, watches, or belts, can produce unclear images.
- Presence of barium in the gastrointestinal tract can impair clear imaging.
- Extreme obesity can impair clear imaging.

NURSING ALERT

- This procedure is contraindicated in pregnancy, especially during first trimester, unless the benefits of x-ray diagnosis far outweigh the possible risks to the fetus.
- It is also contraindicated in clients with allergies to shellfish or iodinated dye (if dye is to be used); in clients with unstable medical status; in extreme cases of claustrophobia unless sedation is given before the study; and in clients with severe renal disease (if contrast dye is to be used).
- Take special precautions with children to avoid excess exposure to x-rays.

Nursing Implications

Assessment

■ Determine previous abnormalities in laboratory test results, especially BUN and creatinine if dye is to be used, and diagnostic findings.

■ Determine date of last menstrual period and possibility of pregnancy in premenopausal women.

■ Obtain pertinent history related to trauma or disease processes of the renal area.

■ Obtain history of known sensitivity to iodine, shellfish, or contrast dye from previous x-ray procedure.

■ Ensure that barium studies have been performed more than 4 days before the scan.

Possible Nursing Diagnoses

Anxiety related to perceived threat to health status
Injury, risk for, related to exposure to contrast medium
Grieving, anticipatory, related to perceived potential loss
Fluid volume excess related to compromised regulatory mechanism or decreased glomerular filtration

Implementation

■ Place the client in the supine position on a flat table and ask the client to lie very still during the procedure, as movement will cause blurring of the pictures. Make sure jewelry, watch, and belt have been removed.

■ Administer a sedative to a child under 3 years of age or to an uncooperative adult, as ordered.

■ Administer an antianxiety agent, as ordered, if claustrophobia is a problem for the client.

■ Move the table into the scanner and instruct the client to remain still. The scanner will make loud noises as it rotates around body. The client may be asked to take deep breaths to facilitate visualization. A series of pictures are taken. These images are reconstructed by a computer and reviewed.

■ Administer a contrast medium, if ordered. A second series of films are then taken.

Evaluation

■ Note test results in relation to the client's symptoms and other studies performed, in particular excretory urography.

■ Observe for delayed allergic reactions, including urticaria, headache, nausea, or vomiting, if contrast medium was used.

Client/Caregiver Teaching

Pretest

- Inform the client that the test permits assessment of the kidneys and adrenal glands. Explain that the procedure is performed in a special radiology department by a technician and a physician and takes about 30 to 90 minutes to complete.
- Inform the client that intravenous iodinated contrast medium may be given before the imaging or that images may be taken first and then the medium injected to enhance any unusual findings.
- Instruct the client to expect nausea, a feeling of warmth, a salty or metallic taste, or a transient headache following injection. Instruct the client to take slow deep breaths if this occurs.

Posttest

- Instruct the client to resume normal activity and diet, unless otherwise indicated.
- Instruct the client to increase fluid intake to help eliminate the contrast medium, if used.
- Instruct the client or caregiver to note change in urinary output following iodinated contrast medium administration in clients with impaired renal function.

Computed Tomography (CT), Spinal; Computerized Axial Tomography (CAT); Computerized Transaxial Tomography (CTT)

Classification: Radiography

Type of Test: Indirect visualization

Computed tomography (CT) scanning of the spine, more versatile than conventional radiography, can easily detect and identify tumors and their types. It uses multiple x-ray beams with a special scanning machine to produce cross-sectional views in a three-dimensional fashion by detecting and recording differences in tissue density. These measurements are sent to a computer that produces a digital view of the anatomy, enabling the radiologist to look at "slices" of certain anatomical views of the spine and spinal cord. Two invasive procedures related to computed tomography of the spine are contrast enhancement and air CT. Contrast dye is given to enable the radiologist to visualize the spine and vasculature, highlighting even subtle differences in tissue density. Air CT intensifies contrast between subarachnoid space and surrounding tissue and is administered by removing a small amount of cerebral spinal fluid by lumbar puncture and injecting air. Images can be recorded on photographic or x-ray film.

Indications

- Diagnose tumors
- Diagnose paraspinal cysts
- Diagnose vascular malformations
- Diagnose congenital spinal anomalies, such as spina bifida, meningocele, and myelocele
- Diagnose herniated intervertebral disks
- Evaluate effects of spinal surgery or therapy

Reference Values

- Normal density, size, shape, and position of spinal structures

Abnormal Values

- Spinal tumors
- Herniated intervertebral disks
- Spondylosis (cervical or lumbar)
- Paraspinal cysts
- Vascular malformations
- Congenital spinal malformations, such as meningocele, myelocele, or spina bifida

Interfering Factors

- Inability of the client to remain in an immobilized position during the procedure can produce artifact.
- Incorrect positioning of the client can give poor visualization of the area to be viewed.
- Metallic objects within the examination field, such as jewelry or other radiopaque objects, can produce unclear images.

NURSING ALERT

- This procedure is contraindicated in pregnancy, especially during the first trimester, unless the benefits of x-ray diagnosis far outweigh the possible risks to the fetus.
- It is contraindicated in clients with allergies to shellfish or iodinated dye (if dye is to be used). It is also contraindicated in clients with unstable medical status; in extreme cases of claustrophobia unless sedation is given before the study; and in clients with severe renal disease (if contrast dye is to be used).
- Take precautions with children to avoid excess exposure to x-rays.

Nursing Implications

Assessment

- Determine previous abnormalities in laboratory test results, especially BUN and creatinine if dye is to be used, and diagnostic findings.

- Determine date of last menstrual period and possibility of pregnancy in premenopausal women.
- Obtain pertinent history related to trauma or disease processes of the spine.
- Obtain history of known sensitivity to iodine, shellfish, or contrast dye from previous x-ray procedure.
- Ensure that the client has fasted since midnight of the day before the test if contrast enhancement is to be used or as ordered.

Possible Nursing Diagnoses

Anxiety related to perceived threat to health status
Injury, risk for, related to exposure to contrast medium
Grieving, anticipatory, related to perceived potential loss
Physical mobility, impaired, related to neuromuscular impairment

Implementation

- Administer sedative to a child under 3 years of age or to an uncooperative adult, as ordered.
- Administer antianxiety agent, as ordered, if claustrophobia is present.
- Place the client in a supine position on a flat table. Ask the client to lie very still during the procedure, as movement will produce unclear images. Make sure jewelry, watches, and belts have been removed.
- Move table into the scanner and instruct the client to remain still. The scanner will make loud noises as it rotates around the head. The client may be asked to take deep breaths to facilitate visualization. A series of pictures are taken. These images are reconstructed by a computer and reviewed.
- Administer a contrast medium, if ordered. A second series of films are then taken.
- If air contrast is performed, the patient is removed from the scanner and a lumbar puncture is performed. A small amount of cerebrospinal fluid is removed and replaced with injected air. The client is placed back into the scanner and another series of films is taken.

Evaluation

- Monitor the client's vital signs and neurologic signs per institution policy until stable.
- If lumbar puncture was performed, keep patient in supine position for up to 8 hours. Assess for headache and leakage of spinal fluid.

- Observe for delayed allergic reactions, such as urticaria, headache, nausea, or vomiting, if contrast enhancement was used.
- Note test results in relation to other tests performed and the client's symptoms.

Client/Caregiver Teaching

Pretest

- Inform the client that the test permits assessment of the tissues and bones of the spine.
- Explain that procedure is performed in a special radiology department by a technician and a physician.
- Inform the client that intravenous iodinated contrast medium can be injected after the first series of x-rays, with a second series of scans following.
- Instruct the client to expect nausea, a feeling of warmth, a salty or metallic taste, or a transient headache following injection. Instruct the client to take slow deep breaths if this occurs.

Posttest

- Instruct the client to resume normal activity and diet, unless otherwise indicated.
- Instruct the client to remain lying down for up to 8 hours if lumbar puncture was performed.
- Instruct the client to increase fluid intake to help eliminate the contrast medium, if used.
- Instruct the client or caregiver to note changes in urinary output following iodinated contrast medium administration in clients with impaired renal function.

Computerized Tomography (CT), Thoracic; Computerized Axial Tomography (CAT); Computerized Transaxial Tomography (CTT)

Classification: Radiography

Type of Test: Indirect visualization

Thoracic computed tomography (CT) scanning, more detailed than chest x-ray, is a noninvasive procedure used to enhance certain anatomical views of the lungs, heart, and mediastinal structures. It uses multiple x-ray beams with a special scanning machine to produce cross-sectional views in a three-dimensional fashion by detecting and recording differences in tissue density. These measurements are sent to a computer that produces a digital view of the anatomy, enabling the radiologist to look at "slices" of certain anatomical views of the spine and spinal cord. Iodinated contrast medium is given IV for blood vessel evaluation or orally for esophageal evaluation, making this an invasive procedure. Images can be recorded on photographic or x-ray film. Cine scanning is used to produce moving images of the heart. Thoracic CT is used only for further evaluation of known lesions because of the high radiation levels.

Indications

- Diagnose primary and metastatic pulmonary, esophageal, or mediastinal tumors
- Differentiate benign tumors (granulomas) from malignancies
- Detect mediastinal and hilar lymphadenopathy
- Detect lymphomas, especially Hodgkin's disease
- Detect tumor extension of neck mass to thoracic area
- Differentiate tumors from tuberculosis (which appear as coin-sized calcified lesions)

- Detect bronchial abnormalities, such as stenosis, dilation, or tumor
- Detect aortic aneurysms
- Differentiate aortic aneurysms from tumors near the aorta
- Differentiate infectious from inflammatory processes (abscess, nodules, or pneumonitis)
- Determine blood, fluid, or fat accumulation in tissues, pleuritic space, or vessels
- Evaluate cardiac chambers and pulmonary vessels
- Monitor and evaluate effectiveness of medical or surgical therapeutic regimen

Reference Values

- Normal size, position, and shape of chest organ tissue and structures

Abnormal Values

- Aortic aneurysm
- Pleural effusion
- Chest lesions (benign, neoplastic tumors, or metastatic mediastinal lesions to ribs or spine)
- Cysts or abscesses
- Hodgkin's disease

Interfering Factors

- Inability of the client to remain immobilized during the procedure can produce artifact.
- Incorrect positioning of the client can give poor visualization of the area to be viewed.
- Metallic objects such as jewelry within the examination field can produce unclear images.

NURSING ALERT

- This procedure is contraindicated in pregnancy, especially during the first trimester, unless the benefits of x-ray diagnosis far outweigh the possible risks to the fetus.
- It is contraindicated in clients with allergies to shellfish or iodinated dye (if dye is to be used); in clients with unstable medical status; in extreme cases of claustrophobia unless sedation is given before the study; and

in clients with severe renal disease (if contrast dye is to be used).
- Take precautions with children to avoid excess exposure to x-rays.

Nursing Implications

Assessment

- Determine previous laboratory abnormalities, especially BUN and creatinine if dye is to be used, and prior diagnostic findings pertinent to thoracic diagnosis.
- Determine date of last menstrual period and possibility of pregnancy in premenopausal women.
- Obtain pertinent history of cardiac and pulmonary findings.
- Obtain history of known sensitivity to iodine, shellfish, or contrast dye from previous x-ray procedures.
- Ensure that the client has fasted overnight if contrast medium is to be used.

Possible Nursing Diagnoses

Anxiety related to perceived threat to health status
Injury, risk for, related to exposure to contrast medium
Grieving, anticipatory, related to perceived potential loss
Gas exchange, impaired, related to ventilation-perfusion imbalance

Implementation

- Administer sedative to a child under 3 years of age or to an uncooperative adult, as ordered.
- Administer antianxiety agent, as ordered, if claustrophobia is present.
- Place the client in a supine position on a flat table with foam wedges that will help maintain position and immobilization. Ask the client to lie very still during the procedure, as movement will produce unclear images. Make sure jewelry, watches, and belts have been removed.
- Move table into the scanner and instruct the client to remain still. The scanner will make loud noises as it rotates around the body. The client may be asked to take deep breaths to facilitate visualization. A series of pictures are taken. These images are reconstructed by a computer and reviewed.
- Administer a contrast medium, if ordered. A second series of films are then taken.

Evaluation

- Note test results in relation to other tests performed and the client's symptoms.
- Observe for delayed allergic reactions, such as urticaria, headache, nausea, or vomiting, if contrast enhancement was used.

Client/Caregiver Teaching

Pretest

- Inform the client that the test permits assessment of the chest. Explain that procedure is performed in a special radiology department by a technician and a physician.
- Inform the client that intravenous iodinated contrast medium can be injected after the first series of x-rays, with a second series of scans following.
- Instruct the client to expect nausea, a feeling of warmth, a salty or metallic taste, or a transient headache following injection. Instruct the client to take slow deep breaths if this occurs.

Posttest

- Instruct the client to resume normal activity and diet, unless otherwise indicated.
- Instruct the client to increase fluid intake to help eliminate the contrast medium if used.
- Instruct the client or caregiver to note change in urinary output following iodinated contrast medium administration in clients with impaired renal function.

Concentration Tests and Dilution Tests, Urine

Classification: Urinalysis

Type of Test: Urine

Concentration tests assess the ability of the renal tubules to appropriately absorb water and essential salts to ensure properly concentrated urine. The glomerular filtrate entering the renal tubules normally has a specific gravity of 1.010. If the renal tubules are damaged and cannot effectively reabsorb water and salt, the specific gravity of the excreted urine will remain at 1.010. Loss of tubular concentrating ability is one of the earliest indicators of renal disease and may occur before blood levels of urea and creatinine rise.

Urine concentration may be determined by measuring either the specific gravity or the osmolality of the sample. In some cases, a single early-morning specimen will suffice. In other situations, timed tests conducted over 12 to 24 hours may be necessary. Another approach is to measure both the serum and the urine osmolality and to compare the results

Measuring the osmolality of urine is considered more accurate than determining the specific gravity. Both the number and size of particles present influence the specific gravity of urine. In contrast, osmolality is affected only by the number of particles present.

Normally, the kidneys can concentrate urine to an osmolality of about three to four times that of plasma (normal plasma osmolality is 275 to 300 mOsm). If the client is overhydrated, the kidneys will excrete the excess water and produce urine with an osmolality as low as one-fourth or less that of plasma. Because factors such as fluid intake, diet (especially protein and salt intake), and exercise influence urine osmolality, it has been difficult to establish exact reference values. The possible range is from 50 to 1400 mOsm, with an average of 850 mOsm. As this is such a wide range, it is considered more reliable to measure serum and urine osmolalities and compare the two in terms of a ratio relationship.

Timed concentration tests are performed if early-morning samples indicate inadequate overnight urine-concentrating ability. In the Fishberg test, an attempt is made to maximally concentrate urine through fluid restriction. In the Mosenthal test, two consecutive 12-hour urine specimens are collected, one from approximately 8 AM to 8 PM and from 8 PM to 8 AM. If kidney function is normal, the specific gravity of the nighttime collection should be greater than that of the daytime collection.

It should be noted that tests of the kidney's ability to produce dilute urine are rarely done. These tests involve overhydrating the client and then observing for the appearance of dilute urine with low specific gravity and osmolality. The danger is that not all clients can tolerate the fluid load needed to produce the desired results.

Indications

- Concentration tests
    Detect renal tubular damage at an early stage as indicated by loss of tubular-concentrating ability

Detect disorders that impair renal concentrating ability, for example, diabetes insipidus

Differentiate psychogenic polydipsia from organic disease, as indicated by a normal response to timed concentration tests (Fishberg test)

Detect excessive or prolonged overhydration

- Dilution tests

    Evaluate renal tubular response to high fluid volume, as indicated by production of urine with low specific gravity and osmolality

Reference Values

- Specific gravity: 1.001–1.035 (usual range, 1.010–1.025)
- Osmolality: 50–1400 mOsm (usual range, 300–900 mOsm; average, 850 mOsm)
- Ratio of urine-to-serum osmolality: 1.2:1 to 3:1
- Fishberg test (standard): Specific gravity ≥1.026 on at least one sample
- Fishberg test (simplified): Specific gravity ≥1.022 on at least one sample
- Mosenthal test: Specific gravity ≥1.020, with at least a seven-point difference between the specific gravities of the daytime and nighttime samples

Abnormal Values

- Diabetes insipidus (central)
- Nephrogenic diabetes insipidus
- Prolonged overhydration
- Osmotic diuresis, especially due to uncontrolled diabetes mellitus
- Electrolyte imbalance, particularly hypokalemia, hypocalcemia, and hypercalcemia
- Hypoproteinemia
- Polycystic kidneys
- Chronic pyelonephritis
- Lithium and ethanol use
- Multiple myeloma
- Amyloidosis
- Sickle-cell disease or trait
- Psychogenic polydipsia
- Hydronephrosis

Interfering Factors

- Failure of the client to follow dietary and fluid restrictions will interfere with results.
- Clients who have been overhydrated for several days before the test may have falsely depressed concentration values; conversely, dehydrated clients or those with electrolyte imbalance may hold fluids and render results inaccurate.
- Administration of radiographic dyes within 7 days of the test can cause increased urine osmolality.
- Drugs such as diuretics increase urine volume and dilution and render the results inaccurate. Nephrotoxic drugs damage the renal epithelium and decrease renal concentrating ability.
- Baseline glucosuria invalidates the results.

> **NURSING ALERT**
>
> - Dilution tests should not be performed on clients who may have difficulty tolerating an increased fluid load, for example, clients with congestive heart failure.
> - Concentration tests can be contraindicated in persons with subnormal cardiac output because of the risk of depleting plasma volume.

Nursing Implications

Assessment

- Assess and record client's medical history and medications taken before the test.
- Ensure that proper fluid and dietary instructions have been followed before the test.
- Ensure that the client has withheld medications that interfere with test results.

Possible Nursing Diagnoses

Fluid volume excess related to active loss

Fluid volume deficit related to failure of regulatory mechanisms

Infection, risk for, related to immunosuppressed inflammatory response

Implementation

- *Specific gravity and urine osmolality test:* Provide a clean container and inform the client to obtain a random specimen (at least 15 mL) from the first-voided morning urine.

- *Fishberg test (standard version):* Inform the client that no fluids are to be taken from after breakfast one morning until the test is completed the following morning; solid (dry) foods are not restricted; the client empties the bladder at approximately 10 PM before retiring for the night and should remain in bed during the night. At 8 AM the client should provide a urine specimen, after 24 hours without fluids. Then the client should return to bed for 1 hour. A second specimen will be collected at 9 AM and the client may resume normal activity. A third specimen will be collected at 10 AM.
- *Fishberg test (simplified version):* Inform the client that no fluids should be taken from the time of the evening meal until the test is completed. The client should completely empty the bladder at approximately 10 PM before retiring for the night. Urine samples will be collected at 7 AM, 8 AM, and 9 AM after approximately 12 hours without fluids. (Note: Some laboratories require that the evening meal consist of a high-protein, low-salt diet with no more than 200 mL fluid.)
- *Mosenthal test:* Provide the client with two containers. Inform the client that two consecutive 12-hour urine collections will be obtained—one from 8 AM to 8 PM in one container and one from 8 PM to 8 AM in another container.
- *Dilution test:* Inform the client that it will be necessary to drink approximately 3 pints (1500 mL) of water in a half-hour period. The client will need to provide hourly urine specimens for 4 hours after ingestion of the water.

Evaluation

- Note results in relation to other tests performed and the client's symptoms.
- If dilution test is being performed, monitor client's response to the fluid load carefully. Note especially increased pulse rate or difficulty breathing.
- Compare quantity of urine with urinary output recorded for the collection; if specimen contains less than what was recorded as output, some urine may have been discarded, thus invalidating the test.

Client/Caregiver Teaching

Pretest

- Instruct the client in collection and provide appropriate container if specimen is to be obtained as an outpatient and brought to the laboratory.
- Inform the client that adherence to fluid and dietary restrictions is important for accurate test results.
- Instruct the client to avoid excessive exercise and stress dur-

ing the timed collection of urine and to withhold medications that interfere with test results, as ordered.

■ Instruct the client performing a dilution test to immediately report symptoms of fluid excess, for example, palpitations or shortness of breath.

Posttest

■ Instruct the client to resume medications and normal activity.

Contraction Stress Test (CST), Oxytocin Challenge Test (OCT)

Classification: Monitoring procedure

Type of Test: Indirect measurement

This noninvasive test measures the adequacy of the placenta to provide oxygen to the fetus during the stress of oxytocin-induced uterine contractions. Uterine contractions normally do produce a decrease in the placental blood flow, but with adequate placental reserve, the fetal heart rate is not affected. This study, done in the later stages of pregnancy (at least 34-week pregnancy), can predict that a fetus might be at risk for intrauterine hypoxia during labor. It involves infusion of oxytocin to stimulate uterine contractions and measures the fetal heart rate to assess placental adequacy. The test can be repeated weekly until the onset of labor and delivery if the fetus is at risk for intrauterine hypoxia.

Indications

■ Evaluate fetal risk for or effects of hypoxia and possible in utero or postpartum respiratory distress or death

■ Determine effects of maternal diabetes, hypertension with toxemia, on fetoplacental adequacy and fetal well-being

■ Evaluate a past history of stillbirth, postmaturity birth, intrauterine growth retardation, low estriol levels, and Rh-factor sensitization, indicating a possible high-risk pregnancy

- Evaluate a nonreactive result from a nonstress test to determine ability of fetus to withstand uterine contractions before labor begins
- Determine if cesarean birth would jeopardize the fetus
- Determine the need to terminate the pregnancy by labor induction and early birth when done in conjunction with other diagnostic procedures, such as ultrasonography or amniocentesis

Reference Values

- Negative result: fetal heart rate (FHR) within normal range, indicating fetus is not in jeopardy and can tolerate the stress of labor.

Abnormal Values

- Positive result: late deceleration in the FHR during 2 or more contractions, indicating inadequate oxygen supply and a risk of intrauterine fetal asphyxia.
- If the late decelerations are not consistent, the test is considered equivocal and repeated in 24 hours.

Interfering Factors

- Maternal hypotension can cause an inaccurate positive result.

NURSING ALERT

This procedure is contraindicated in women with
- Premature ruptured membranes, because the test can precipitate labor and early birth
- Multiple pregnancy, because the uterus is more susceptible to premature labor
- Previous transverse or classic cesarean birth or other surgical hysterotomy, because the induced contractions can rupture the uterus
- Previous premature labor, because this tendency might be repeated with this test
- Abnormalities such as abruptio placentae, because the placenta can separate from the uterus with uterine contractions
- Placenta previa, because the contractions can result in premature labor and a vaginal birth
- Pregnancy of less than 34 weeks' gestation

Nursing Implications

Assessment

- Obtain history of past pregnancies, known and suspected medical conditions, known and suspected risks to the fetus and mother, previous diagnostic tests and procedures, medical treatments for chronic disorders and those associated with the pregnancy.
- Assess and record baseline vital signs and fetal heart rate to use for comparison during and after the study.
- Assess compliance with food and fluid restrictions 4 to 8 hours before the study.
- Assess compliance with directions given for rest, positioning, and activity before and during the test.

Possible Nursing Diagnoses

Anxiety related to threat to health of fetus
Grieving, anticipatory, related to perceived potential loss

Implementation

- Have client empty her bladder.
- Place the client in a semi-Fowler's, slightly side-lying position on the examining table or bed and drape for privacy. Take the blood pressure every 10 minutes during the procedure, as a drop in the blood pressure can affect the placental blood flow and produce inaccurate results.
- Place the fetal monitor on the abdomen to monitor FHR and the tocodynamometer on the lower abdomen to monitor the contractions. A baseline recording is made of the fetal heart tones and uterine contractions. A continuous 20-minute monitoring and recording of the FHR and uterine movement is obtained.
- If no contractions occur, insert an IV infusion device and administer intravenous oxytocin (Pitocin) in the dilution and rate ordered by the physician. Regulate the flow rate using an infusion pump. The rate is increased until three contractions per minute are noted. The fetal heart rate and contractions are then monitored and recorded and the infusion discontinued to determine the FHR response to the stress of the contractions.
- Advise the client to use the deep-breathing exercises learned in childbirth class to control any discomfort from the contractions.
- Continue monitoring the fetal heart rate for 30 minutes (the time it takes to metabolize the oxytocin) as the uterine movements return to normal.

Evaluation

- Note results in relation to the client's history and symptoms and previous tests performed.
- If premature labor occurs, note frequency, strength, and continuation of contractions; prepare for first stage of labor or cesarean birth.

Client/Caregiver Teaching

Pretest

- Explain that procedure is performed near the delivery suite by a specially trained nurse with a physician in attendance and takes about 2 hours to complete.
- Instruct in the breathing and relaxation techniques that will be used during the study if the client has not attended childbirth class to allay the mild contractions that are induced to perform the test.
- Inform the client that mild contractions are the only discomfort experienced during the study.

Posttest

- Instruct the client to call the physician with any symptoms of labor or continued contractions.

Breast Stimulation Test

In clients who are more than 26 weeks pregnant, the breast stimulation test can be used for the contraction stress test. Oxytocin is released by stimulating the nipples instead of administering the drug intravenously. The stimulation creates nerve impulses to the hypothalamus, which causes the release of oxytocin into the bloodstream, resulting in uterine contractions. The same monitoring and recording are done when sufficient contractions have been obtained.

Coombs Antiglobulin, Direct (DAT); Direct Coombs; Direct IgG

Classification: Chemistry

Type of Test: Serum

This test detects antibody globulin (IgG), an autoantibody produced in certain disease states and by certain drugs. IgG coats the surface of red blood cells (RBCs) and can cause cellular damage and hemolytic anemia. When this test is performed, the red cells are taken directly from the sample, washed with saline to remove residual globulins, and mixed with antihuman globulin (AHG). If the AHG causes agglutination of the red blood cells, specific antiglobulins can be used to determine if the red cells are coated with IgG, complement, or both.

Indications

- Detect hemolytic anemia or hemolytic disease of the newborn
- Evaluate transfusion reaction
- Evaluate suspected drug sensitivity

Reference Values

- Negative (no agglutination)

Abnormal Values

- Positive (agglutination)
  Anemia (autoimmune hemolytic, drug-induced)
  Erythroblastosis fetalis
  Leukemia (chronic lymphocytic)
  Transfusion hemolytic reactions (blood incompatibility)
  Mycoplasma pneumonia
  Lymphomas
  Infectious mononucleosis
  Lupus erythematosus and other connective-tissue immune disorders

Metastatic carcinoma
Drugs (see Interfering Factors)

Interfering Factors

- Drugs that may cause positive reactions include:

Aldomet	Keflin	Rifampin
Alkeran	Levodopa	Streptomycin
Apresoline	Insulin	Sulfonamides
Cephalosporins	Penicillin	Tetracycline
Dilantin	Pronestyl	Thorazine
Isoniazid	Quinidine	

Nursing Implications

Assessment

- Obtain history of pregnancy status, past transfusion reactions, results of blood typing and cross-matching tests.
- Assess and note drugs currently being taken.

Possible Nursing Diagnoses

Anxiety related to perceived threat to health status or the health of fetus

Pain related to inflammatory process of connective tissues

Physical mobility, impaired, related to musculoskeletal impairment

Infection, risk for, related to immunosuppressed inflammatory response

Implementation

- Put on gloves. Using aseptic technique, perform a venipuncture and collect 7 mL of blood in a red- or lavender-top tube.
- For cord blood, collect the sample in a red- or lavender-top tube from the maternal segment of the cord after it has been cut and before the placenta has been delivered.
- Handle the sample gently to avoid hemolysis and transport to the laboratory immediately.

Evaluation

- Note test results in relation to blood-typing and cross-matching results.
- Note positive test results in cord blood of neonate; also assess newborn's bilirubin and hematocrit levels. Results may indicate the need for immediate exchange transfusion of fresh whole blood that has been typed and cross-matched with mother's serum.

Client/Caregiver Teaching

Posttest

- Inform the postpartum client of the implications of positive test results in cord blood.

Coombs Antiglobulin, Indirect (IAT); Indirect Coombs; Coombs Antibody Test

Classification: Chemistry

Type of Test: Serum

This test detects unexpected circulating antibodies in the client's serum before blood transfusion. It is performed by incubating the client's blood in the laboratory (in vitro) to allow any antibodies present every opportunity to attach to the red blood cells. The cells are then washed with saline to remove any unattached serum globulins, and antihuman globulin (AHG) is added. If the client's serum contains an antibody that reacts with and attaches to the donor red blood cells, the AHG will cause the antibody-coated cells to agglutinate—indicating an antigen-antibody reaction.

Indications

- Screen for antibodies before blood transfusions
- Determine antibody titers in Rh-negative women sensitized by an Rh-positive fetus
- Test for the weak Rh-variant antigen D''
- Detect other antibodies in maternal blood that can be potentially harmful to the fetus

Reference Values

- Negative (no agglutination)

Abnormal Values

- Positive (agglutination)
  Hemolytic anemia (drug-induced or autoimmune)
  Erythroblastosis fetalis
  Incompatible cross-match
  Maternal-fetal Rh incompatibility
  Leukemias
  Drugs, including levodopa, mefenamic acid, methyldopa, and methyldopate hydrochloride

Interfering Factors

- Recent administration of dextran, whole blood or fractions, or IV contrast media can result in a false-positive reaction.

Nursing Implications

Assessment

- Obtain history of previous transfusion reactions, pregnancy status of Rh-negative women, ABO, Rh typing and cross-matching tests and results.

Possible Nursing Diagnoses

Anxiety related to perceived threat to health status or the health of fetus

Infection, risk for, related to immunosuppressed inflammatory response

Injury, risk for, related to immune response

Implementation

- Put on gloves. Using aseptic technique, perform a venipuncture and collect 10 mL of blood in a red-top tube.
- Handle sample gently to avoid hemolysis. Note past transfusions on requisition; transport to the lab immediately.

Evaluation

- Note test result in relation to blood-typing and cross-matching test results.
- Positive test results in pregnant women after 28 weeks' gestation indicate the need for antibody identification testing.

Client/Caregiver Teaching

Posttest

- Inform pregnant women that negative tests during the first 12 weeks' gestation should be repeated at 28 weeks of pregnancy to determine presence of the antibody.

▲▲▲▲▲▲▲▲▲▲▲▲▲▲▲▲▲▲▲▲▲▲▲▲

Coproporphyrin, Urine (UCP)

Classification: Urinalysis

Type of Test: Urine (Random or 24-Hour)

Porphyrins are produced during the synthesis of heme, the iron-containing nonprotein portion of hemoglobin (see figure). If heme synthesis is deranged, these precursors accumulate and are excreted in the urine in excessive amounts. Those porphyrins for which urine can be tested include coproporphyrin.

Indications

- Diagnose obstructive jaundice (such as obstruction of the biliary tree) as indicated by presence of elevated coproporphyrins
- Differentiate etiology and type of porphyria

Reference Values

Random specimen	
Adults	0.045–0.30 μmol/L
24-hour specimen	
Children	0–0.12 μmol/24 h
	0–80 μg/24 h
Adults	0.075–0.24 μmol/24 h
	50–160 μg/24 h

Values may be slightly higher in men than in women.

Abnormal Values

- Increased values

Lead poisoning	pernicious,	Porphyria
Liver disease	sideroachrestic)	(congenital
Obstructive	Cirrhosis	erythropoietic)
jaundice	(alcoholic)	Porphyria cutanea
Exposure to toxic	Coproporphyria	tarda
chemicals	(erythropoietic)	Protoporphyria
Acute myocardial	Erythroid	(erythropoietic)
infarction	hyperplasia	Thyrotoxicosis
Acute	Exercise and fever	Vitamin
poliomyelitis	Hemochromatosis	deficiency
Anemia	Hodgkin's disease	
(hemolytic,	Leukemia	

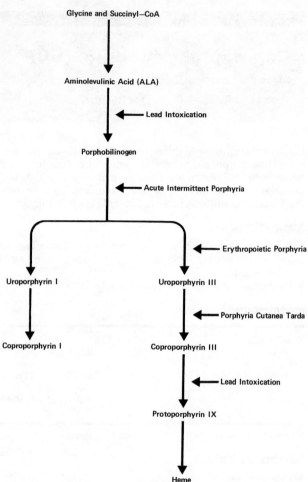

Pathway of heme formation, including stages affected by the major disorders of porphyrin metabolism. (From Strasinger, SK: Urinalysis and Body Fluids, ed 3. FA Davis, Philadelphia, 1994, p 125, with permission.)

Interfering Factors

- Drugs (chloral hydrate, chlordiazepoxide, chlorpropamide, meprobamate, and sulfonamides) may affect results.
- Phenothiazines may cause unreliable results.
- Failure to keep sample in dark surroundings (unexposed to light) can invalidate test results.

Nursing Implications

Assessment

- Assess and record medications client is taking, especially barbiturates, chloral hydrate, chlorpropamide, sulfonamides, meprobamate, and chlordiazepoxide. Ensure that these medications have been withheld 10 to 12 days before the test.
- Assess client's history for current pregnancy, menstruation, or oral contraceptive use; reschedule test if needed.

Possible Nursing Diagnoses

Anxiety related to perceived threat to health status or the health of fetus

Pain related to tissue ischemia or inflammation

Infection, risk for, related to immunosuppressed inflammatory response

Trauma, risk for, related to neuromuscular impairment resulting from high levels of lead in blood

Implementation

- Obtain the appropriate-sized light-resistant container with preservative according to laboratory policy. Follow laboratory directions for any special care of the specimen during collection; for example, refrigerate or place on ice, protect from light by covering with dark plastic or aluminum if light-resistant container is unavailable. Keep container tightly covered during the collection period.
- *24-hour urine sample:* Begin the test between 6 and 8 AM if possible; collect first voiding and discard. Record the time the specimen was discarded as the beginning of the 24-hour test. The next morning, ask the client to void at the same time the collection was started and add this last voiding to the container. If an indwelling catheter is in place, replace tubing and container system with the one containing preservative at the start of the collection, or empty the urine into a large light-resistant container with the preservative periodically during the 24 hours; monitor that continued drainage is ensured and conclude the test the next morning at the same hour the collection was begun. At the end of collection period, mix the specimen gently, transfer a 50-mL aliquot to a light-protected container, and cap tightly.
- *First morning-voided specimen:* Collect the entire first morning-voided urine specimen in a light-protected container. Transfer specimen to the laboratory within 1 hour.

Evaluation

- Note results in relation to the client's symptoms and other urine porphyrin levels, in particular uroporphyrin, protoporphyrin, delta-aminolevulinic acid (ALA), and porphobilinogen levels.
- Ensure that all urine for a 24-hour specimen has been collected by comparing urine quantity in specimen container with urinary output record for the test.

Client/Caregiver Teaching

Pretest

- Inform the client that this urine test detects abnormal hemoglobin formation. There are no food or fluid restrictions.
- Instruct the client to avoid excessive exercise and stress during the 24-hour collection of urine.
- Inform the client that all urine for a 24-hour period must be saved. Instruct client to avoid voiding in pan with defecation and to keep toilet tissue out of pan to prevent contamination of the specimen.
- Inform the client if providing a random sample that it must be fresh, must be kept unexposed to light, and must be sent to the laboratory immediately.

Posttest

- Instruct the client to resume medications and usual activity withheld before the test.

Corneal Staining

Classification: Sensory organ function

Type of Test: Visual acuity

This noninvasive procedure is performed to assist in diagnosing corneal or conjunctival abnormalities. The staining of the eye surface with fluorescein dye allows for a more detailed view of the anterior parts not ordinarily seen during slit-lamp examination. A special attachment is used on the slit lamp to enhance visualization.

Indications

- Detect minute abnormalities (depth and pattern of injuries) of the corneal surface
- Diagnose corneal injuries or damage, as evidenced by pre-determined staining patterns or colors

Reference Values

- Normal corneal surface

Abnormal Values

- Corneal scratches, abrasions, or ulcerations
- Keratitis

Interfering Factors

- Inability of the client to cooperate during the test

Nursing Implications

Assessment

- Obtain a history of known or suspected eye disorders or injuries; signs and symptoms of eye pain, irritation, or changes in visual acuity; and results of eye tests or procedures.

Possible Nursing Diagnoses

Anxiety related to perceived threat to health status
Pain related to corneal damage
Sensory-perceptual alteration (visual) related to altered sensory reception

Implementation

- Have client remove corrective lenses (glasses or contacts).
- Stain the eye surface with the fluorescein dye by touching the tip of a sterile fluorescein strip moistened with sterile saline to the lower conjunctival sac. Have client close the eye to spread the dye over the corneal surface.
- Seat the client in a chair with feet on the floor in a dimmed room with the chin on the rest apparatus and the forehead against the bar apparatus. Request client to remain still during the examination and look straight ahead while the eyes are examined with the slit lamp.

- The slit lamp is placed in front of the client's eyes in line with the examiner's eyes. The external and internal structures of the eyes are inspected with the special bright light and microscope of the slit lamp (see slit-lamp biomicroscopy). Defects are recorded depending on the amount of dye absorbed and the color that results: for example, green color for breaks, trauma, or chemical injury to the cornea.

Evaluation

- Note test results in relation to the client's symptoms and other tests performed.

Client/Caregiver Teaching

Pretest

- Explain the purpose of the procedure. Tell the client that the procedure is performed by a physician and takes about 15 minutes to complete. Explain that there is no pain associated with this procedure.

Posttest

- Inform the client that if some blurring of vision occurs, it will gradually disappear in less than 2 hours.

Cortisol

Classification: Chemistry

Type of Test: Plasma or serum

Cortisol (hydrocortisone) is the predominant glucocorticoid secreted in response to stimulation by adrenocorticotropin hormone (ACTH). Cortisol stimulates gluconeogenesis, mobilizes fats and proteins, antagonizes insulin, and suppresses inflammation. Measuring levels of cortisol in blood is the best indicator of adrenal function. Cortisol secretion varies diurnally, with highest levels occurring upon awakening and lowest levels late in the day. Bursts of cortisol excretion can occur at night.

Indications

- Detect adrenal hyperfunction (Cushing's syndrome)
- Detect adrenal hypofunction (Addison's disease)
- Monitor response to therapy with adrenal corticosteroids

Reference Values

	8 AM	*4 PM*
Children	15–25 μg/dL	5–10 μg/dL
Adults	9–24 μg/dL	3–12 μg/dL

Abnormal Values

- Elevated levels
    Cushing's syndrome
    Stress
    Hyperthyroidism
    Obesity
    Diabetic ketoacidosis
    Pregnancy
    Estrogen therapy or oral contraceptives
    Certain drugs, including lithium carbonate, methadone, and ethyl alcohol
- Decreased levels
    Addison's disease
    Certain drugs, including levodopa, barbituates, phenytoin, and androgens

Interfering Factors

- Test results will be affected by the time this test is done because cortisol levels vary diurnally, with highest levels seen upon awakening and lowest levels occurring late in the day.
- Stress and excessive physical activity can produce elevated levels.
- Drugs can increase or decrease levels (see Abnormal Values).

Nursing Implications

Assessment

- Obtain history of endocrine disorders and actual or suspected abnormalities of adrenal or pituitary function.

- Ensure that the client has not eaten for 8 to 12 hours before the test.
- Ensure that strenuous activity has been avoided for 12 hours before the test and that 1 hour of bedrest is provided immediately before the test.

Possible Nursing Diagnoses

Body image disturbance related to change in structure/appearance

Fatigue related to decreased metabolic energy production and altered body chemistry

Anxiety related to perceived threat to health status

Fluid volume excess related to cortisone levels

Implementation

- Put on gloves. Using aseptic technique, perform a venipuncture and collect 5 mL of blood in a red-top tube for serum level or lavender- or green-top tube for plasma levels at 8 AM after the client has slept.
- Repeat collection at 4 PM.
- Indicate collection time on the laboratory request form and send sample to laboratory promptly.

Evaluation

- Note cortisol levels in relation to ACTH levels, if available.

Client/Caregiver Teaching

Posttest

- Instruct the client to resume food and any activities withheld before the test.
- Provide information on corticosteroid therapy and effects of long-term therapy, as appropriate.

Adrenocorticotropic Hormone Stimulation Test

This test evaluates the response of the adrenal gland to the administration of cosyntropin, a synthetic hormone that produces the same corticosteroid stimulating effect as ACTH in healthy individuals.

To perform this test, have the client fast after midnight the day before the test. Collect 4 mL of blood in a plastic green- or lavender-top tube at 8 AM. Administer ordered dose of cosyntropin intravenously over 2 minutes. Obtain two additional 4-mL blood samples 30 minutes and 60 minutes after the injection.

In a normal response, serum cortisol levels increase more than 7 µg/dL above the baseline level. Decreased or absent response suggests adrenal insufficiency and hypopituitarism.

Cortisol-Free, Urine

Classification: Chemistry

Type of Test: Urine

Cortisol is secreted by the adrenal cortex in response to ACTH stimulation. It helps regulate fat, carbohydrate, and protein metabolism and promotes anti-inflammatory response, glyconeogenesis, and cell permeability. This test measures urine levels of the portion of cortisol not bound to the corticosteroid-binding globulin transcortin. Assays of free cortisol levels in a 24-hour urine specimen reflect cumulative secretion levels instead of diurnal variations.

Indications

■ Detect Cushing's syndrome

Reference Values

- 24 to 108 µg/24 hours or 60 to 300 nmol per day (SI units)

Abnormal Values

- Elevated levels
  Cushing's syndrome
  Benign or malignant adrenal tumors
  Medications, including adrenal corticosteroid therapy
  Stress

Interfering Factors

- Excessive stress and exercise during testing period may lead to falsely elevated results.
- Improper specimen collection and maintenance may affect results.
- Corticosteroid therapy and medications such as resperpine, phenothiazines, morphine, and amphetamines may elevate free cortisol levels.
- Levels are elevated during pregnancy.

Nursing Implications

Assessment

- Obtain history of adrenal disorders, current symptoms, medication regimen, diagnostic tests and results, and potential of pregnancy.
- Ensure that drugs that alter test results are withheld (see Interfering Factors).

Possible Nursing Diagnoses

Body image disturbance related to change in structure/appearance

Infection, risk for, related to immunosuppressed inflammatory response

Trauma, risk for fractures, related to demineralization of bones

Anxiety related to perceived threat to health status

Implementation

- Obtain a 3-liter container with preservative added. Perservative should keep urine at a pH of 4 to 4.5.
- Instruct the client to void and discard sample. The time the discard sample is obtained is the time the collection begins. All urine excreted during the 24-hour period must be saved.

■ Instruct the client to void the next day at the same time the collection was begun. Add this sample to the 24-hour collection and end the test. Transport container to laboratory promptly.

Evaluation

■ Compare the test results with the plasma cortisol and ACTH, urine 17-hydroxycorticosteroids, dexamethazone suppression test, tests taken at another time, and the client's clinical presentation.

Client/Caregiver Teaching

Pretest

■ Instruct the client to avoid stressful situations and excessive physical exercise during the collection period.
■ Advise the client to withhold medications that may interfere with the test.

Posttest

■ Instruct client to resume normal activities and any medications withheld before testing.

Coxsackie A or B Virus

Classification: Serology

Type of Test: Serum

The Coxsackie virus is a serotype of the enterovirus group and is divided into two groups: A and B. Coxsackie A includes 23 species and Coxsackie B includes 6 species that can be tested for heart, eyes, and respiratory diseases or meningitis. These viruses are formed in the alimentary tract and are easily transmitted via the fecal-oral route. They are commonly associated with epidemics in newborns, and assays on children are usually performed when an outbreak occurs. Early testing in the acute phase of a disease increases the possibility of a positive result.

Indications

- Diagnose viral infections caused by Coxsackie A or B virus

Reference Values

- Negative or no increase in titer

Abnormal Values

- Positive Coxsackie A virus
    Acute febrile respiratory disease
    Conjunctivitis (epidemic hemorrhagic)
    Viral carditis, myositis, and pericarditis
- Positive Coxsackie B virus
    Acute febrile respiratory disease
    Viral meningitis
    Viral carditis
    Epidemic pleurodynia
    Pericarditis
    Pleurisy

A 4-fold change in titer between the acute and convalescent phases (2 to 4 weeks later) is diagnostic of an active viral infection.

Interfering Factors

- Hemolysis of blood sample can cause inaccurate results.
- Paired samples not tested at the same time in the same laboratory can affect test results.
- Samples that are not frozen if not tested immediately will alter the results.
- Past Coxsackie A and B infections can cause an elevated acute-phase titer, resulting in a false-negative.

Nursing Implications

Assessment

- Obtain a history of suspected viral infection and current medication regimen.

Possible Nursing Diagnoses

Pain related to tissue inflammation
Body temperature, altered, risk for, related to illness affecting temperature regulation

Implementation

- Put on gloves. Using aseptic technique, perform a venipuncture and collect 8 to 10 mL (for children, 3 to 4 mL) of blood in a red-top tube.
- Collect sample 2 to 3 days after the onset of symptoms or 2 to 4 weeks after the acute-phase sample to determine acute and convalescence titers.
- Handle sample gently to avoid hemolysis and transport to the laboratory promptly.

Evaluation

- Note test results in relation to results of throat or fecal swabs for Coxsackie A or B and clinical symptoms.

Client/Caregiver Teaching

Posttest

- Advise client to return for a repeat test in 2 to 4 weeks or as ordered.

Cr-51 Platelet Survival Time

Classification: Hematology, Radionuclide

Type of Test: Blood

Platelet survival time measures the life span of circulating platelets to diagnose conditions involving vascular integrity and hemostasis. Platelets are formed in the bone marrow and have a normal life span of 9 days. Disappearance of the platelets from the circulating blood depends on their destruction by the reticuloendothelial system (RES). Within the few days of continuing platelet destruction, platelet production can increase 2 to 8 times.

To measure platelet survival time, a sample of the client's platelets is tagged with radioactive Cr-51 (chromium-51 chromate) or In-111 (indium-111 chloride). The tagged sample is reinjected into the client, and blood samples are periodically measured for radioactivity levels to determine the amount of time taken for the tagged platelets to disappear from the circulation. Scanning can also be performed to determine platelet disposition within the vascular system.

Indications

- Diagnosis of idiopathic thrombocytopenic purpura (ITP), as revealed by an extremely short survival time (minutes to hours)
- Evaluate known or suspected disorders associated with destruction of platelets (see Abnormal Values)
- Monitor drug therapy with drugs known to alter platelet survival
- Diagnose and localize deep venous thrombosis revealed by scanning

Reference Values

- Normal life span of platelets: 9 to 10 days
- Platelet turnover rate: 35,000/mm^3 per day
- Absence of concentration or uptake in a body area

Abnormal Values

- Increased uptake noted by scan
    Deep-vein thrombosis
    Embolus
- Decreased platelet survival time
    Idiopathic thrombocytopenic purpura
    Disseminated intravascular coagulation
    Crush injuries or surgical trauma
    Sepsis
    Vasculitis
    Hepatic cirrhosis
    Systemic lupus erythematosus
    Lymphomas
    Drugs such as heparin, quinine, sulfonamides, thiazides, gold salts, or digitoxin

Interfering Factors

- Administration of IV fluid or volume expanders before the test
- Drug therapy with agents known to alter survival time, unless performed to monitor therapy
- Large emboli that obstruct an artery and prevent other thrombi or emboli from being exposed to radionuclide

NURSING ALERT

- This test is contraindicated in pregnancy or lactation unless the benefits outweigh the risks.
- Use extreme caution in clients with suspected coagulation defects by avoiding excessive probing during venipuncture and not leaving the tourniquet on too long.

Nursing Implications

Assessment

- Obtain history of hematologic and vascular systems and use of medications.
- Assess platelet count and determine that it is above 20,000/mm^3, the critical level for this test to be performed.

Possible Nursing Diagnoses

Injury, risk for, related to altered clotting factors
Protection, altered, related to abnormal blood profiles
Anxiety related to perceived threat to health status
Tissue perfusion, altered, peripheral, related to occlusion

Implementation

- Put on gloves. Using aseptic technique, perform a venipuncture and collect 7 mL of blood in a lavender-top tube. The samples are centrifuged to remove the plasma. The remaining platelets are tagged.
- The tagged platelets are injected into the client.
- After 30 minutes, and again in 2 hours, collect a 7-mL sample of blood and place in a lavender-top tube.
- Perform a daily venipuncture and collect 7 mL of blood in a lavender-top tube for 7–8 days.
- Obtain a scan to determine platelet disposition and evaluation for thrombosis or embolus.

Evaluation

- Note test results in relation to other tests and the client's symptoms.
- Note excessive bleeding and institute measures to control, as needed.

Client/Caregiver Teaching

Pretest

- Inform the client that there is no special preparation for this test.

Posttest

- Inform the client of the need for repeat blood samples and when to expect the next collection.

▲▲▲▲▲▲▲▲▲▲▲▲▲▲▲▲▲▲▲▲▲▲

Cr-51 Red Cell Survival, Red Blood Cell Survival Time

Classification: Hematology, Radionuclide
Type of Test: Blood

Red blood cell survival time is measured by injecting radioactive Cr-51 to tag a sample of the client's red blood cells (RBCs). In the first part of the test, blood samples are periodically measured over a 4-week period after the injection for radioactivity levels to determine the amount of time taken for the tagged RBCs to disappear from the circulation. This provides a quantitative assessment of the degree of hemolysis occurring. The second part of the test consists of scanning the spleen, liver, and pericardium with a gamma camera to locate concentrations of radioactivity and sites of sequestration.

Indications

- Identify cause of anemia and sites of RBC destruction

Reference Values

- Normal life span of RBCs: 120 days, with normal loss of 0.8% per day
- Normal half-time of RBCs: 60 days
- Plasma radioactivity half-life: 2 hours

- Tagged Cr-51 red cell half-life: 25 to 35 days
- Gamma scan: Only slight spleen, liver, and bone marrow radioactivity
- Spleen-to-liver ratio: 1:1
- Spleen-to-pericardium ratio: 2:1 or less

Abnormal Values

- Increased survival time
  Thalassemia minor
  Primary or secondary polycythemia
  Chronic hypoxia
  Respiratory or cardiovascular disease
  High altitudes
  Hypoventilation syndromes
  Renal disorders that stimulate production of RBCs
- Decreased survival time
  Anemia (congenital nonspherocytic, idiopathic acquired hemolytic, megaloblastic of pregnancy, pernicious, sickle-cell)
  Elliptocytosis (with hemolysis)
  Hemoglobin C disease
  Hemoglobinuria (paroxysmal nocturnal)
  Hypersplenism
  Inherited erythrocyte enzyme disorders (G-6-PD, pyruvate kinase or pyrimidine-5'-nucleotidase deficiency)
  Leukemia (chronic lymphatic)
  Sickle-cell syndromes
  Spherocytosis (hereditary)
  Thalassemia syndrome
  Uremia
- Increased spleen-to-liver or spleen-to-pericardium ratio
  Hypersplenism
  Splenomegaly (differentiate from sequestration)

Interfering Factors

- Conditions that decrease red cell volume or the proportion of tagged to nontagged red cells, including frequent blood sampling, blood transfusions, chronic occult extravascular blood loss, and hemorrhage, will simulate decreased survival time.
- Increased white blood cell or platelet counts will falsely decrease RBC survival time.

> ▶ **NURSING ALERT**
>
> ■ This test is contraindicated in active bleeding, extended clotting times, lactation, and pregnancy, unless the benefits outweigh the risks.

Nursing Implications

Assessment

■ Obtain history of the hematologic system, chronic respiratory or cardiovascular diseases, and medication regimen.

Possible Nursing Diagnoses

Injury, risk for, related to altered clotting factors
Protection, altered, related to abnormal blood profiles
Anxiety related to perceived threat to health status
Infection, risk for, related to immunosuppressed inflammatory response

Implementation

■ Put on gloves. Using aseptic technique, collect a 10-mL venous blood sample. The sample is centrifuged to remove the plasma. The remaining cells are tagged with 100 μCi of Cr-51 (sodium chromate).
■ Administer tagged cells by intravenous injection.
■ After 30 minutes, collect a 6-mL venous blood sample in a purple-top tube to measure baseline volumes of blood and red cells.
■ After 24 hours, collect a 6-mL venous blood sample and place in a green-top tube. Send specimen to the laboratory for a same-day measurement of hematocrit and Cr-51 with a scintillation well counter.
■ Repeat every 1 to 3 days for 3 to 4 weeks. Each specimen is analyzed for counts per minute of the radionuclide and plotted on a graph to determine RBC survival half-time. The rate at which the labeled cells disappear indicates cell destruction progression.
■ After 4 weeks, collect a 6-mL venous blood sample in a purple-top tube for comparison measurement of blood and red cell volumes.
■ A scan of the spleen, liver, or pericardium is performed in conjunction with the sampling of the blood.

Evaluation

■ Note results in relation to other tests performed and the client's symptoms.

Client/Caregiver Teaching

Pretest

- Inform the client that there is no special preparation for this test.

Posttest

- Tell the client when to return for additional blood samples and testing.

Creatine Phosphokinase (CPK) and Isoenzymes, Creatine Kinase (CK) and Isoenzymes

Classification: Chemistry

Type of Test: Serum

Creatine phosphokinase (CPK), also called creatine kinase (CK), is an enzyme that exists almost exclusively in skeletal muscle, heart muscle, and, in smaller amounts, in the brain. This enzyme is important in intracellular storage and energy release. Three isoenzymes, based on primary location, have been identified by electrophoresis: brain CPK-BB, cardiac CPK-MB, and skeletal muscle CPK-MM.

When injury to these organs occur, the enzymes are released into the bloodstream and levels rise and then decrease in a predictable time frame. Measuring the serum levels can help determine both the extent and timing of the damage. Noting the presence of the specific isoenzyme helps determine the location of the tissue damage.

Indications

- Diagnose acute myocardial infarction and evaluate cardiac ischemia (CPK-MB)
- Detect musculoskeletal disorders that do not have a neurologic basis, such as dermatomyositis or Duchenne's muscular dystrophy

■ Determine success of coronary artery reperfusion following streptokinase infusion or percutaneous transluminal angioplasty, as evidenced by decrease in CPK-MB.

Reference Values

	Total CPK	*SI Units*
Women	25 to 140 U/L	0.42 to 2.3 μkat/L
Men	40 to 175 U/L	0.67 to 1.9 μkat/L
Isoenzymes		
CPK-BB (CPK$_1$)	Undetectable	
CPK-MB (CPK$_2$)	Undetectable to 7 U/L	
CPK-MM (CPK$_3$)	5–7 U/L	

Abnormal Values

■ Pronounced elevations ($\geq 5 \times$ normal)
  Early muscular dystrophy (CPK-MM)
  Acute myocardial infarction (CPK-MB)
  Severe angina (CPK-MB)
  Polymyositis (CPK-MM)
  Cardiac surgery or trauma (CPK-MM)
■ Moderate elevations (2–4 × normal)
  Vigorous exercise
  Deep intramuscular injections
  Surgical procedures affecting skeletal muscles
  Delirium tremens
  Seizures
  Dermatomyositis
  Alcoholic myopathy
  Hypothyroidism
  Pulmonary infarction
  Acute agitated psychosis
■ Mild elevations (2 × normal)
  Late pregnancy
  Women heterozygous for the gene causing Duchenne's muscular dystrophy (CPK-MM)
  Brain injury or surgery (CPK-BB)
■ Elevated levels
  Certain drugs, including anticoagulants, morphine, alcohol, furosemide, high-dose salicylates, amphotericin B, clofibrate, and certain anesthetics
■ Decreased levels
  Late muscular dystrophy

Interfering Factors

- Vigorous exercise, deep intramuscular injections, delirium tremens, invasive diagnostic procedures, and surgical procedures in which muscle is transected or compressed can produce elevated levels.
- Drugs can produce elevated levels (see Abnormal Values).
- Early pregnancy can cause decreased levels.

Nursing Implications

Assessment

- Obtain history of family members with Duchenne's muscular dystrophy and known or suspected cardiac disorders.
- Ensure that the client has withheld drugs, especially alcohol, that can alter test results 12 to 24 hours before the test.
- Ensure that the client did not receive any intramuscular injections and has avoided vigorous exercise 24 hours before the test.

Possible Nursing Diagnoses

Physical mobility, impaired, related to neuromuscular impairment

Pain related to tissue ischemia or inflammation

Anxiety related to perceived threat to health status

Implementation

- Put on gloves. Using aseptic technique, perform a venipuncture and collect 7 mL of blood in a red-top tube. Repeat test at designated times if serial testing is done.
- Handle sample gently and transport promptly to the laboratory, noting time of venipuncture on laboratory request form.

Evaluation

- Monitor results of total CPK and isoenzyme CPK-MB with lactic dehydrogenase (LDH) and isoenzymes and aspartate aminotransferase (AST) if myocardial infarction is known or suspected. CPK levels rise before AST and LDH levels rise.
- Acute myocardial infarction releases CPK into the serum within the first 48 hours; values return to normal in about 3 days. The isoenzyme CPK-MB appears in the first 6 to 24 hours and is usually gone in 72 hours.
- Expect the significant CPK elevations in early phases of muscular dystrophy, even before the clinical signs or symptoms appear. CPK elevation diminishes as the disease progresses and muscle mass decreases.
- Recurrent elevation of CPK suggests reinfarction or extension of ischemic damage.

Client/Caregiver Teaching

Pretest

- Inform the client that a number of venipunctures will be performed, usually daily for 3 days and then at 1 week.
- Have client refrain from using alcohol or other substances that can elevate levels prior to the test, if appropriate.

Posttest

- Instruct the client to resume medications and usual activities withheld before the test; inform client of any further medication restrictions if a series of tests is contemplated.
- As indicated, inform client when to return for the next scheduled test.

Creatinine

Classification: Chemistry

Type of Test: Serum or plasma

Serum creatinine is the end product of creatine metabolism. Creatine, although synthesized largely in the liver, is a nitrogen-containing compound found almost exclusively in skeletal muscle, where it reversibly combines with phosphate and functions as an energy source. This reaction (creatine + phosphate = phosphocreatine) repeats as energy is released and regenerated, but in the process small amounts of creatine are irreversibly converted to creatinine, which serves no useful function and circulates only for transportation to the kidneys. The amount of creatinine generated is proportional to the mass of skeletal muscle and level of muscular activity present. Daily generation of creatinine remains fairly constant unless crushing injury or degenerative diseases cause massive muscle damage. The kidneys excrete creatinine very efficiently. Creatinine is a more sensitive indicator of renal function than is blood urea nitrogen (BUN).

Indications

- Evaluate known or suspected renal function impairment
- Assess known or suspected disorder involving muscles in the absence of renal disease

Reference Values

Creatinine Level	SI Units	
Newborn	0.8–1.4 mg/dL	71–124 μmol/L
Infant	0.7–1.7 mg/dL	62–150 μmol/L
Children <6 yrs	0.3–0.6 mg/dL	27–54 μmol/L
Children >6 yrs	0.4–1.2 mg/dL	36–106 μmol/L
Adults		
Men	0.6–1.3 mg/dL	53–115 μmol/L
Women	0.5–1.0 mg/dL	44–88 μmol/L
Older adult	Reduced values related to reduced muscle mass associated with aging	

BUN-to-creatinine ratio: 10:1.
Higher BUN-to-creatinine ratio indicates renal dysfunction.

Abnormal Values

- Increased levels
  Renal disease, acute and chronic failure
  Prolonged shock
  Cancer
  Systemic lupus erythematosus
  Diabetic nephropathy
  Congestive heart failure
  Amyotrophic lateral sclerosis
  Diet high in beef, poultry, and fish (minimal effect)
  Acromegaly
  Gigantism
  Drugs such as antibiotics, ascorbic acid, L-dopa, methyl-dopa, and lithium carbonate
- Decreased levels
  Muscular dystrophy
  Diabetic ketoacidosis
  Drugs such as cefoxitin sodium, cimetidine, chlorpromazine, marijuana, thiazide diuretics, and vancomycin

Interfering Factors

- Therapy with drugs known to alter creatinine levels

Nursing Implications

Assessment

- Obtain history of renal or musculoskeletal disorders and results of tests and procedures performed.

- Ensure client has refrained from excessive exercise for 8 hours before the test.
- Ensure client has avoided excessive red meat intake for 24 hours before the test.

Possible Nursing Diagnoses

Anxiety related to perceived threat to health status
Body image disturbance related to change in appearance
Fluid volume excess related to compromised regulatory mechanism
Fluid volume deficit, risk for, related to active loss

Implementation

- Put on gloves. Using aseptic technique, perform a venipuncture and collect 7 mL of blood in a red-top tube.
- Send sample promptly to the laboratory.

Evaluation

- Note elevation in values in relation to age and presence of muscle disorders.
- Compare results to urinary creatinine and serum BUN results, if available.

Client/Caregiver Teaching

Posttest

- Instruct the client and caregiver to restrict protein and fluids if creatinine values are abnormally high or renal disease is present.

Creatinine, Urine

Classification: Chemistry

Type of Test: Urine

Creatinine, which is produced at a fairly constant rate within the body, is a sensitive indicator of glomerular function. This test measures urine creatinine levels. Urine creatinine is produced in amounts proportional to total skeletal muscle mass. Although this test is an effective indicator of renal function, the creatinine clearance test is more precise because it measures both urine and serum levels.

Indications

- Evaluate glomerular function
- Evaluate accuracy of a 24-hour urine collection, based on the constant level of creatinine excretion

Reference Values

		SI Units
Men	1.0–2.0 g/24 h	8.8–17.6 mmol/24 h
Women	0.8–1.8 g/24 h	7–15.8 mmol/24 h

Abnormal Values

- Decreased levels
    Urinary tract obstruction, e.g., from calculi
    Shock
    Chronic bilateral pyelonephritis
    Acute or chronic glomerulonephritis
    Polycystic kidney disease

Interfering Factors

- Failure to follow proper technique in collecting 24-hour specimen may invalidate test results.
- Drugs such as amphotericin B, corticosteroids, diuretics, gentamicin, tetracycline, and any nephrotoxic agents may affect urine creatinine levels.

Nursing Implications

Assessment

- Obtain a history of renal, genitourinary, or musculoskeletal disorders, results of tests performed, and medication regimen.

Possible Nursing Diagnoses

Fluid volume deficit, risk for, related to active loss
Anxiety related to perceived threat to health status
Fluid volume deficit, risk for, related to active loss

Implementation

- Obtain a 3-liter container without preservative.
- Instruct the client to void and discard sample. The time the discard sample is obtained is the time the collection begins. All urine excreted during the 24-hour period must be saved.
- Instruct the client to void the next day at the same time the collection was begun.
- Add this sample to the 24-hour collection and end the test.
- Transport container to laboratory promptly.

Evaluation

- Note test results in relation to other tests performed, particularly serum creatinine, if available.

Client/Caregiver Teaching

Pretest

- Instruct the client to withhold medications that interfere with test results, as ordered.
- Instruct the client in urine collection and provide appropriate container if specimen is to be obtained as an outpatient and brought to the laboratory.

Posttest

- Instruct the client to resume medications withheld before the test.

Creatinine Clearance, Urine

Classification: Chemistry

Type of Test: Urine (24-hour)

Creatinine is the ideal substance for determining renal clearance because a fairly constant quantity is produced within the body. Creatinine is the end product of creatine metabolism. Creatine resides almost exclusively in skeletal muscle where it participates in energy-requiring metabolic reactions. In these processes, a small amount of creatine is irreversibly converted to creatinine, which then circulates to the kidneys and is excreted. The amount of creatinine generated in an individual is proportional to the mass of skeletal muscle present and will remain fairly constant unless there is massive muscle damage due to crushing injury or degenerative muscle disease.

The creatinine clearance test measures both a blood sample and a urine sample to determine the rate that creatinine is being cleared from the blood by the kidneys; this accurately reflects the glomerular filtration rate. "Clearance" indicates the amount of blood cleared of creatinine in 1 minute and is independent of urine flow rate.

Indications

- Determine the extent of nephron damage in known renal disease (at least 50 percent of functioning nephrons must be lost before values will be decreased)
- Monitor effectiveness of treatment in renal disease
- Determine renal function before administering nephrotoxic drugs
- Evaluate glomerular filtration

Reference Values

		SI Units
Men	85–125 mL/min	
	20–26 mg/kg (24 h)	0.18–0.23 mmol/kg (24 h)
	1.0–2.0 g/24 h	8.8–17.6 mmol/24 h
Women	75–115 mL/min	
	14–22 mg/kg (24 h)	0.12–0.19 mmol/kg (24 h)
	0.8–1.8 g/24 h	7–15.8 mmol/24 h

Abnormal Values

- Increased values
  Renal disease
  Shock and hypovolemia
  Exposure to nephrotoxic drugs and chemicals
  Acute tubular necrosis
  Renal artery atherosclerosis
  Congestive heart failure
  Dehydration
  Glomerulonephritis
  Neoplasms (bilateral renal)
  Nephrosclerosis
  Renal artery obstruction
  Polycystic kidney disease

Pyelonephritis
Renal vein thrombosis
Tuberculosis
Certain drugs, including aminoglycosides, amphotericin B, ascorbic acid, barbiturates, capreomycin sulfate, car butamide, cefoxitin sodium, cephalothin sodium, chlorthalidone, clonidine, colistin sulfate, dextran, doxycycline hyclate, kanamycin, levodopa, methyldopa, methyldopate hydrochloride, para-aminohippurate, penicillins, phenacetin, and sulfobromophthalein

- Decreased values
Certain drugs, including barbiturates, anabolic steroids, androgens, thiazides, bromosulfophthalein, and phenolsulfonphthalein

Interfering Factors

- Incomplete urine collection may yield a falsely lowered value.
- Excessive ketones in urine may cause falsely lowered values.
- Failure to refrigerate specimen throughout urine collection period allows for decomposition of creatinine, causing falsely low results.
- Certain drugs can falsely elevate or lower values (see Abnormal Values).

Nursing Implications

Assessment

- Obtain history of renal disorders, results of tests performed, and medication regimen.
- Ensure that the client has avoided meat consumption and excessive exercise and stress for 24 hours before the test.

Possible Nursing Diagnoses

Anxiety related to perceived threat to health status
Fluid volume excess related to compromised regulatory mechanism
Fluid volume deficit, risk for, related to active loss
Pain related to tissue ischemia or inflammation
Tissue perfusion, altered, renal, related to decreased cellular exchange

Implementation

- Obtain a clean 3-liter container or 24-hour urine bag or bottle, with or without preservative, according to laboratory policy. Follow laboratory directions for any special care of the specimen during collection: refrigerate, place in ice, or protect from light by covering with dark plastic or aluminum.

- Begin the test between 6 and 8 AM if possible; collect first voiding and discard. Record the time specimen was discarded as the beginning of the 24-hour test.
- The next morning, ask the client to void at the same time the collection was started and add this last voiding to the container.
- If an indwelling catheter is in place, replace tubing and container system with the preservative and keep urine bag on ice, or empty the urine into a large container with the preservative every hour during the 24 hours; monitor to ensure continued drainage and conclude the test the next morning at the same hour the collection was begun.
- At the conclusion of the test, ensure that the label is properly completed and transport to the laboratory.

Evaluation

- Note test results in relation to other tests performed, in particular the BUN.

Client/Caregiver Teaching

Pretest

- Tell the client to avoid excessive exercise and stress during the 24-hour collection of urine.
- Instruct client to avoid excessive meat consumption before the test.
- Inform the client that all urine for a 24-hour period must be saved (2-, 6-, or 12-hour urine collections can also be done but a 24-hour is preferable).
- Instruct client to avoid voiding in pan with defecation and to keep toilet tissue out of pan to prevent contamination of the specimen.
- Instruct the client to withhold drugs that affect test results, if ordered.

Posttest

- Instruct client to resume medications and usual activity withheld before the test.

Cryoglobulin

Classification: Immunoelectrophoresis

Type of Test: Serum

This test detects the presence of cryoglobulins, abnormal serum proteins that cannot be detected by protein electrophoresis. The presence of cryoglobulins causes vascular problems because they precipitate in the blood vessels of the fingers when exposed to cold, causing Raynaud's phenomenom. They are usually associated with immunological disease.

The laboratory procedure is a two-step process. The serum sample is observed for cold precipitation after 72 hours of storage at 40°C. The sample is then rewarmed to confirm reversibility of the reaction.

Indications

- Detect cryobulinemia in clients with Raynaud-like symptoms
- Aid in diagnosis of neoplastic diseases, acute and chronic infections, and collagen diseases (see Abnormal Findings)
- Monitor course of collagen and rheumatic disorders

Reference Values

- Negative

Abnormal Values

- Positive type I cryoglobulin (>5 mg/mL)
    Chronic lymphocytic leukemia
    Lymphoma
    Multiple myeloma
    Waldenström's macroglobulinemia
- Positive type II cryoglobulin (>1 mg/mL)
    Lymphoma
    Multiple myeloma
    Rheumatoid arthritis
    Sjörgen's syndrome

- Positive type III cryoglobulin (>1 mg/mL with 50% <80 (μ/mL)
    Chronic infection
    Acute poststreptococcal glomerulonephritis
    Cirrhosis
    Endocarditis
    Infectious mononucleosis
    Polymyalgia rheumatica
    Rheumatoid arthritis
    Sarcoidosis
    Systemic lupus erythematosus

Interfering Factors

- Testing the sample prematurely (before total precipitation) may yield incorrect results.
- Recent fatty meal can increase turbidity of the blood.
- Failure to maintain sample at normal body temperature before centrifugation can affect results.

Nursing Implications

Assessment

- Obtain history of immunologic, neoplastic, or infectious disorders.
- Ensure that the client has fasted for 4 to 6 hours before the test.

Possible Nursing Diagnoses

Infection, risk for, related to immunosuppressed inflammatory response
Pain related to tissue inflammation
Fatigue related to decreased energy production and states of discomfort

Implementation

- Put on gloves. Using aseptic technique, perform a venipuncture and collect 10 mL of blood in a prewarmed red-top tube.
- Immediately transport the sample to the laboratory.

Evaluation

- Note test results in relation to other tests performed and the client's symptoms.

Client/Caregiver Teaching

Pretest

- Instruct the client to fast for 4 to 6 hours before the test.

Posttest

- Instruct the client to resume fluid and food intake.
- If the test is positive, tell the client to avoid cold temperatures.
- Tell the client to contact the physician immediately if pain increases in the distal extremities.

Cryofibrinogen

The presence of cryofibrinogen, a complex of protein fragments and fibrinogen, is abnormal and associated with positive cryoglobulin levels. Positive cryofibrinogen levels are also found in hemophilia, in acute familial Mediterranean fever, and in clients taking oral contraceptives. Heparin within 2 days of the test may cause a false-negative result. To perform this test, put on gloves and collect 5 mL of blood in a blue-, black-, or lavender-top tube (depending on the laboratory). Transport the sample to the laboratory immediately.

Culdoscopy

Classification: Endoscopy

Type of Test: Direct visualization

Culdoscopy permits visualization of the pelvic surfaces of the sigmoid colon and rectum, the pelvic ligaments, fallopian tubes, ovaries, and uterus using a culdoscope introduced through a small incision in the posterior vaginal fornix. Although it may be used in very obese women, this procedure has been largely replaced by laparoscopy.

Indications

- Diagnose pelvic masses of unknown etiology
- Help evaluate suspected ectopic pregnancy or tubal abnormalities
- Perform tubal ligation in obese clients

Reference Values

- Uterus, fallopian tubes, ovaries, and pelvic ligaments normal in appearance
- Pelvic surfaces of sigmoid colon and rectum normal in appearance

Abnormal Values

- Pelvic adhesions
- Tubal obstruction
- Ectopic pregnancy
- Pelvic inflammatory disease (PID)
- Pelvic mass
- Endometriosis

Interfering Factors

- Inability of the client to assume the knee-chest position
- Presence of pelvic adhesions, which can prevent adequate visualization

NURSING ALERT

- This test is contraindicated in acute infections involving the vulva or vagina, acute peritonitis, and pelvic masses that involve the cul-de-sac of Douglas.

Nursing Implications

Assessment

- Obtain a history of allergies or sensitivities to analgesics or anesthesia.
- Determine the date of the last menstrual period in premenopausal women.

- Ensure that food and fluids have been withheld for 6 to 8 hours before the procedure.
- Obtain baseline vital signs.

Possible Nursing Diagnoses

Anxiety related to perceived threat to health status

Pain related to inflammation or swelling of ovary or fallopian tube

Injury, risk for, related to invasive procedure

Grieving, anticipatory, related to perceived potential loss

Implementation

- Administer any ordered sedation.
- Position client on operating room table in a supported knee-chest position and drape. The table is tilted to shift the abdominal contents toward the diaphragm.
- If spinal anesthesia is used, it is administered before client assumes this position. If using local anesthesia, it is injected into posterior vaginal fornix either before or after knee-chest position is assumed.
- A vaginal speculum or retractor is inserted into vagina to provide visualization of posterior fornix, and a small incision is made in posterior vaginal wall. The culdoscope is inserted into the vagina and through the incision, and the pelvic organs are examined with a microscopic instrument.
- Upon completion of the examination and any therapeutic procedures, the scope is withdrawn. No sutures are required to close the incision.

Evaluation

- Note findings in relation to the client's symptoms.
- Monitor vital signs for changes from baseline according to institution policy.

Client/Caregiver Teaching

Pretest

- Inform the client that the procedure is generally performed in an operating room under local or spinal anesthesia by a physician and takes approximately 30 to 60 minutes.
- Instruct the client to withhold food and fluids for 6 to 8 hours before the procedure.

Posttest

- Tell the client to resume food and fluid intake and activity when the effects of sedation wear off.

- Instruct the client to avoid douching or intercourse for 2 weeks after the procedure or as otherwise directed by the physician.
- Inform the client that there may be a small amount or "spotting" for 1 to 2 days following the procedure, and a perineal pad can be worn.
- Emphasize that excessive vaginal bleeding, blood in the stool or urine, and fever should be reported to the physician immediately.

Culture, Anal; Genital

Classification: Microbiology

Type of Test: Specimen culture

Anal cultures are performed to isolate the organism responsible for sexually transmitted disease by inoculation of the material collected onto a medium of living cells.

Indications

- Diagnose sexually transmitted diseases
- Determine cause of genital itching or purulent drainage

Reference Values

- Negative culture for presence of pathogens

Abnormal Values

- Infections or carrier states caused by the following organisms:
    Chlamydia trachomatis
    Candida
    Mycoplasma
    Gardnerella vaginalis
    Neisseria gonorrhoeae
    Treponema pallidum (organism responsible for syphilis)
    Trichomonas
    Toxin-producing strains of *Staphylococcus aureus*

Interfering Factors

- Improper collection technique, contamination of specimen, or inadequate amount of material to be tested
- Pretest antimicrobial therapy, which will delay growth of pathogens
- Overgrowth by proteins or yeasts, which results in inaccurate identification of *Neisseria gonorrhoeae*

Nursing Implications

Assessment

- Obtain history of known or suspected infection, symptoms associated with sexually transmitted diseases, sexual practices, and recent administration of antimicrobial drug therapy.

Possible Nursing Diagnoses

Anxiety related to perceived threat to health status
Pain related to physical injuring agents
Skin/tissue integrity, impaired, related to invasion of pathogenic organisms

Implementation

- Place client in a lithotomy or side-lying position and drape for privacy. Observe universal precautions in collecting, handling, and transporting the specimens.
- Put on gloves. Insert the swab 1 inch into the anal canal and rotate, moving it from side to side to allow it to come in contact with the microorgansims. Remove the swab and place it in the appropriate transport medium. Repeat with a clean swab if the swab is pushed into feces. If genital culture, use new swab and collect drainage sample.
- Transport the specimen to the laboratory as soon as possible after collection. If the anticipated time between collection and inoculation into cell cultures exceeds 2 hours, keep specimen cold and transport as soon as possible. Do not freeze the specimen or allow it to dry.

Evaluation

- Note test results in relation to the client's symptoms and other test results.

Client/Caregiver Teaching

Pretest

■ Instruct female clients not to douche for 24 hours before a cervical or vaginal specimen is to be obtained.

Posttest

■ Inform the client that final results may take from 24 hours to 4 weeks, depending on test performed.
■ Advise the client to avoid sexual contact until test results are available.
■ Explain that treatment can begin after a positive culture is confirmed, except in clients who are experiencing symptoms or have had intercourse with someone diagnosed with gonorrhea.
■ Instruct in vaginal suppository and douche procedures and administration of topical medication to treat specific conditions, as indicated.
■ Inform the client that a repeat culture may be needed in 1 week following completion of anitmicrobial regimen.
■ Inform infected clients that all sexual partners must be tested for the microorganism.
■ Inform the client that positive culture findings for certain organisms must be reported to the local health department, who will question them regarding their sexual partners.

Culture, Blood

Classification: Microbiology

Type of Test: Blood

Blood culture involves the introduction of a specimen of blood into an artificial aerobic and anaerobic growth culture medium. The culture is incubated for a specific length of time, at a specific temperature, and under other conditions suitable for the growth of pathogenic microorganism. These pathogens enter the bloodstream from soft-tissue infection sites, contaminated IV lines, or invasive procedures (surgery, tooth extraction, cystoscopy).

A blood culture can also be done with an antimicrobial removal device (ARD). This involves putting the blood sample into a special vial that contains adsorbent resins which remove antibiotics from the blood sample before the culture is performed.

Indications

- Evaluate a sudden change in pulse and temperature with or without chills and diaphoresis
- Evaluate persistent, intermittent fever associated with a heart murmur
- Evaluate intermittent or continuous temperature elevation of unknown origin
- Evaluate suspected bacteremia following invasive procedures
- Identify the cause of shock in the postoperative period
- Determine presence of immunosuppression, which predisposes to invasion by microorganisms that rarely invade a healthy host
- Determine sepsis in the newborn as a result of prolonged labor, early rupture of membranes, maternal infection, or neonatal aspiration

Reference Values

- Negative; no growth of pathogens in a specific time span

Abnormal Values

- Bacteremia
- Septicemia: *Staphylococcus aureus, Escherichia coli, Aerobacter, Klebsiella;* in infants, *E. coli* and beta-hemolytic *Streptococcus*
- Typhoid fever
- Plague
- Malaria

Interfering Factors

- Pretest antimicrobial therapy, which will delay or inhibit growth of pathogens
- Contamination of the specimen by the skin's resident flora
- Inadequate amount of blood or number of blood specimens drawn for examination
- Specimens that are tested more than 1 hour after collection

Nursing Implications

Assessment

- Obtain history of fever of unknown origin, suspected bacterial or fungal infections, and antibiotic therapy.

Possible Nursing Diagnoses

Pain related to tissue inflammation

Body temperature, altered, risk for, related to illness affecting temperature regulation

Fluid volume deficit, risk for, related to marked increase in vascular compartment/massive vasodilatation

Cardiac output, decreased, related to decreased preload

Implementation

- Put on gloves. Using aseptic technique, collect 20 mL of blood (30 mL if an infection is suspected; 1 to 3 mL in an infant or young child) without allowing air to be aspirated into the syringe. Replace the needle with a new sterile needle on the syringe. Carefully clean the caps of two culture tubes with alcohol or iodine and remove them without touching the center of the cap. Inject half the blood into each bottle of aerobic and anaerobic media and gently mix with the culture media. The bottles should contain a 1:10 dilution of blood and media.
- For cultures to isolate parasites in blood, collect blood in a lavender-top tube or collect blood smears for microscopic examination.
- If the ARD container is used, the procedure is repeated at a different site immediately and in 3 hours or during a septic episode. Within 24 hours, as many as four cultures can be obtained to isolate the etiologic agent.
- Note the possible diagnosis on the laboratory slip and note any antibiotic therapy the client has received. All specimens should be sent to the laboratory within 1 hour.

Evaluation

- Note test results in relation to the client's symptoms and other test results, in particular the CBC and WBC differential. In infants, assess blood glucose levels and serum bilirubin.

Client/Caregiver Teaching

Posttest

- Inform the client that preliminary results should be available in 48 to 72 hours, but final results are not available for 1 to 2 weeks.

- Instruct the client in antimicrobial regimen.
- Instruct the client to report fever, chills, and other signs and symptoms of acute infection to the physician.

Culture, Duodenal and Gastric

Classification: Microbiology

Type of Test: Duodenal and gastric contents

Duodenal and gastric cultures are performed to isolate the organism responsible for upper gastrointestinal disease by inoculation of the material collected onto a medium of living cells to isolate the organism. This test involves aspiration and cultivation of any microbes present in duodenal and gastric contents. Specimens are often obtained after insertion of a nasogastric or nasoenteric tube but may also be obtained during endoscopy.

Indications

- Perform a rapid presumptive identification of bacteria (by Gram's stain) in neonatal septicemia
- Identify organisms causing infections which may result in duodenitis, cholecystitis, or cholangitis
- Detect peritonitis secondary to puncture or rupture of the stomach or duodenum
- Detect tuberculosis from the culture of swallowed sputum

Reference Values

- Duodenal contents culture normally contains small amounts of polymorphonuclear leukocytes and epithelial cells with no pathogens. The bacterial count usually is less than 100,000.
- Gastric contents cultures normally find no pathogenic mycobacteria growth during the culture period.

Abnormal Values

- Active tuberculosis, as indicated by identification of *Mycobacterium tuberculosis* in gastric contents
- Infection, as indicated by bacterial counts of 100,000 or more or the presence of pathogens in any number in duodenal contents cultures
- Presence of *Helicobacter pylori,* the organism associated with gastritis and peptic ulcer disease
- Inflammation of the biliary tract, as indicated by numerous polymorphonuclear leukocytes, copious mucous debris, and bile-stained epithelial cells in the bile fluid
- Inflammation of the pancreas, duodenum, or bile ducts, as indicated by many segmented neutrophils and exfoliated epithelial cells

Interfering Factors

- Failure of the client to observe a 12-hour fast; this can dilute the specimen, decreasing the bacterial count in duodenal contents.
- Improper collection technique can contaminate the specimen.

> **NURSING ALERT**
>
> - This test is contraindicated in acute cholecystitis, acute pancreatitis, aortic aneurysm, congestive heart failure, diverticula, esophageal varices, malignant neoplasm, myocardial infarction, pregnancy, recent severe gastric hemorrhage, and stenosis.

Nursing Implications

Assessment

- Obtain a history of gastrointestinal and respiratory disorders, medication regimen, and results of other tests performed.
- Ensure that the client has fasted for 12 hours before the test.

Possible Nursing Diagnoses

Pain related to tissue inflammation
Fluid volume deficit, risk for, related to active loss
Anxiety related to threat to health status

Implementation

- *Gastric contents culture:* Put on gloves. Perform a nasogastric intubation in the morning when the patient awakens, and obtain gastric washings using sterile distilled water to decrease risk of contamination with saprophytic mycobacteria. Place specimens in sterile containers. Clamp the tube and remove it quickly. Be sure to cap the specimen containers tightly. Note recent antibiotic therapy on the laboratory slip. Send to the laboratory immediately.

- *Duodenal contents culture:* Put on gloves. After nasoenteric tube is inserted, place the patient in a left lateral decubitus position, with feet elevated, to allow peristalsis to move the tube into the duodenum. The pH of a small amount of aspirated fluid determines tube position: If the tube is in the stomach, pH is <7; if the tube is in the duodenum, pH is >7. Correct position also can be confirmed by fluoroscopy. After the examiner aspirates duodenal contents, transfer the specimen to a sterile container. Send specimen to the laboratory immediately. Withdraw the tube slowly 6 to 8 inches every 10 minutes until it reaches the esophagus; then clamp it and remove it quickly. Notify the doctor if the tube cannot be withdrawn easily; never pull it forcefully.

Evaluation

- Note test results in relation to the client's symptoms and other test results.
- Observe the client carefully for signs of perforation from tube insertion, such as dysphagia, epigastric or shoulder pain, dyspnea, or fever.

Client/Caregiver Teaching

Pretest

- Instruct the client to restrict food and fluids for 12 hours before the test.
- Assure the client that following the examiner's instructions will minimize intubation discomfort.
- For gastric culture, explain that the test helps diagnose tuberculosis. Explain that it may be performed on three consecutive mornings. Instruct an ambulatory patient to remain in bed each morning until specimen collection has been completed, to prevent premature emptying of stomach contents.

Posttest

- Advise the client that test results may take 2 months because acid-fast bacteria generally grow slowly.
- After the aspiration of gastric culture, instruct the client to avoid blowing nose for at least 4 to 6 hours to prevent bleeding.
- Instruct the client to resume food and fluid intake.

Culture, Ear

Classification: Microbiology

Type of Test: Specimen culture

Ear cultures are performed to isolate the organism responsible for chronic infectious disease, local infections, or abscess in the ear by inoculation of the material collected onto a medium of living cells. Once the organism grows, it can be tested for sensitivity to various antibiotics so that the most effective treatment is ordered. This test involves obtaining a specimen from the outer ear or ear canal with a swab or Culturette. Optimally, the specimen should be obtained before antibiotic use; however, a broad-spectrum antibiotic may be prescribed.

Indications

- Identify organisms responsible for ear pain, drainage, or changes in hearing.
- Identify organisms responsible for outer-, middle-, or inner-ear infection.
- Determine antibiotic sensitivity of the organism.

Reference Values

- Culture contains no pathogens.

Abnormal Values

- Infection caused by *E. coli, Chlamydia* species, *Proteus species,* beta-hemolytic *Streptococcus, Staphylococcus aureus,*

Pseudomonas aeruginosa, Candida albicans, and *Aspergillus* species.

Interfering Factors

- Failure to collect adequate specimen
- Improper collection technique
- Antibiotic therapy before specimen collection

Nursing Implications

Assessment

- Obtain history of clinical symptoms, medication regimen, and results of other tests performed.

Possible Nursing Diagnosis

Pain related to tissue inflammation

Implementation

- Put on gloves. Cleanse the area surrounding the site with a swab containing cleaning solution to remove contaminating material or flora that have collected in the ear canal. If needed, remove any cerumen that has collected.
- Insert a Culturette swab into the external ear canal approximately ⅔ inch. Rotate the swab in the area containing the exudate. Carefully remove the swab, ensuring that it does not touch the sides of the canal or opening.
- Place the swab in the Culturette tube and squeeze the bottom, breaking the portion of the tube containing the medium. Ensure that the end of the swab is immersed in the medium.
- Label the container and send to the laboratory immediately.

Evaluation

- Note test results in relation to the client's symptoms and other test results.

Client/Caregiver Teaching

Pretest

- Inform the client or caregiver that the procedure will only take a few seconds. The client should not experience any pain from the procedure, unless an outer-ear infection causes the area to be extremely painful to the touch.

Posttest

- Advise the client that final test results may take 2 weeks, but antibiotic therapy may be started immediately.

Culture, Eye

Classification: Microbiology

Type of Test: Specimen culture

Eye cultures are performed to isolate the organism responsible for eye infections by inoculation of the material collected onto a medium of living cells. Once the organism grows, it can be tested for sensitivity to various antibiotics so that the most effective treatment can be ordered. This test usually involves obtaining a specimen of secretions from the eye with a swab or Culturette; however, scrapings from the cornea, or aspirate of intraocular fluid may also be used. Optimally, the specimen should be obtained before antibiotic use; however a broad-spectrum antibiotic may be prescribed.

Indications

- Identify organisms responsible for eye redness, drainage, or changes in vision
- Identify organisms responsible for eye infection
- Determine antibiotic sensitivity of the organism

Reference Values

- Culture contains no pathogens.

Abnormal Values

- Infection caused by *Hemophilus aegyptii, Neisseria gonorrhoeae, Chlamydia* species, adenovirus, or herpes virus.

Interfering Factors

- Failure to collect adequate specimen
- Improper collection technique
- Antibiotic therapy before specimen collection

Nursing Implications

Assessment

- Obtain history of clinical symptoms, medication regimen, and results of other tests performed.

Possible Nursing Diagnoses

Sensory/perceptual alterations, visual, related to infection
Infection, risk for transmission
Tissue integrity, impaired, related to invasion of pathogenic organism

Implementation

- Place the client in a sitting position with head tilted back.
- Put on gloves. Ask the client to look upward. Using a sterile swab, swipe the area of the inner canthus of the eye or the affected area of the eye and rotate the swab to collect an adequate sample.
- Remove the swab without touching surrounding areas.
- Place the specimen in the Culturette tube and squeeze the bottom of the tube to break the section containing the medium. Insert the swab into the medium completely.
- Label the container and send to the laboratory immediately.

Evaluation

- Note test results in relation to the client's symptoms and other test results.

Client/Caregiver Teaching

Pretest

- Inform the client or caregiver that the procedure will take only a few seconds. The client should not experience any pain from the procedure.

Posttest

- Advise the client that final test results may take 2 weeks, but that antibiotic therapy may be started immediately.

Culture, Gonorrhea

Classification: Microbiology

Type of Test: Specimen culture

This test uses Gram-stain examination to reveal the presence of *Neisseria gonorrhoeae,* the organism responsible for the sexually transmitted disease known as gonorrhea. This organism is a gram-negative diplococcus that is found in the genital tract, external genitalia, urethra, prostatic fluid, anorectal area if engaged in rectal sex, and pharyngeal area if engaged in oral sex. Men are the most likely to note the symptoms of the infection, which include discharge from the urethra, dysuria, and pharyngitis—symptoms that are most likely missed in the female.

Indications

- Detect gonorrhea in the presence of symptoms of purulent urethral drainage (urethritis), dysuria, pharyngitis, proctitis followed by sexual exposure to infected partner
- Detect gonorrhea in newborns of infected mothers

Reference Values

- Negative for *N. gonorrhoeae* in culture of vaginal, urethral, cervical, perineal, rectal, and pharyngeal exudates or prostatic fluid

Abnormal Values

- Positive for *N. gonorrhoeae*

Interfering Factors

- Pretest antimicrobial therapy, which will delay or inhibit growth of pathogens.
- Use of lubricants, disinfectants, and douching 24 hours before the test in females and voiding 1 hour before the test in males can reduce bacteria available for collection.
- Contamination of the specimen by the surrounding skin, mucosa, or feces.

- Improper collection technique or inadequate amount of material to be tested.
- Overgrowth by proteins or yeasts results in inaccurate identification of *N. gonorrhoeae*.
- Refrigeration will destroy the microorganism to be tested.

Nursing Implications

Assessment

- Obtain history of sexual practices if possible, symptoms of sexually transmitted diseases, and antimicrobial therapy administered before the test.
- Determine if the client complied with the instructions for preparing for the test: not douching for women and not voiding for men.

Possible Nursing Diagnoses

Infection, risk for transmission
Pain related to tissue irritation and inflammation
Skin/tissue integrity, impaired, related to invasion of pathogenic organisms

Implementation

- Place the female client in a lithotomy position and drape for privacy. Observe universal precautions, including the use of gloves in specimen collection, handling, transporting, and testing of body drainage materials.
- Cleanse the external genitalia and perineum from front to back with towelettes provided in culture kit. Using a Culturette swab, obtain sample of lesion or discharge from the urethra or vulva and place in the tube. Squeeze tube mix with medium.
- *To obtain a vaginal and endocervical culture,* insert a water-lubricated vaginal speculum, and gently apply pressure to the speculum to express exudate from the cervix. Insert the swab into the cervical orifice and rotate the swab to collect the secretions containing the microorganisms. Remove and place in the appropriate culture medium, depending on the suspected pathogen. Vaginal material can also be collected by moving the swab along the sides of the mucosa and then placing it in a tube of saline medium.
- *To obtain an anal culture,* insert the Culturette swab 1 inch into the anal canal; rotate and move from side to side to allow it to come in contact with the microorganisms. Then remove the swab, place it in the Culturette tube, and press to mix.

- *To obtain a urethral culture in men,* retract the foreskin, cleanse the penis, compress to express discharge from the urethra, and insert the swab into the urethral orifice to obtain a sample of the discharge. Remove and place the swab in the appropriate Culturette tube, squeeze bottom of tube to release medium, and immerse the end of the swab into it.
- Record source of specimen, age, sex, and antibiotic regimen on laboratory request form.
- Send specimen to the laboratory for immediate testing.

Evaluation

- Note test results in relation to client's symptoms and other test results.

Client/Caregiver Teaching

Pretest

- Instruct female clients to avoid douching for 24 hours and use of lubricants and disinfectants before the test.
- Instruct male clients not to void for at least 1 hour before the test.

Posttest

- Advise the client to avoid all sexual activities until test results are available. This can take 48 hours.
- Explain that treatment begins after a positive culture is confirmed, unless clients are experiencing symptoms or have had intercourse with someone diagnosed with gonorrhea.
- Inform the client that a repeat culture can be requested 1 week following completion of antibiotic regimen.
- Inform infected clients that all sexual partners must be tested for the microorganism.
- Inform the client that positive culture findings must be reported to the local health department and that the client will be questioned regarding sexual partners.

Culture, Herpesvirus (HSV-1, HSV-2)

Classification: Microbiology, cytology, serology

Type of Test: Culture specimen; serum

Cultures are made by inoculation of the material collected onto a medium of living cells to isolate the herpes simplex virus (HSV), which includes HSV-1 and HSV-2. HSV-1 affects the eyes, mouth, or respiratory tract, and HSV-2 affects the genital tract. If active infection is present at delivery of a newborn, the mortality of the neonate is severely compromised. Microscopic examination by cytology can confirm the presence of the virus.

Serological testing to determine antibodies for HSV-1 or HSV-2 can be performed on serum during acute and convalescent phases of the disease as a confirmation if the cultures have been found to be positive.

Indications

- Identify and differentiate the HSV-1 and HSV-2 by culture, cytology, or serology.
- Determine presence of active infection in near-term mothers. If negative, vaginal delivery is safe. If positive, cesarean delivery is needed.
- Determine cause of lesions of eyes, genitalia, and mouth.
- Determine HSV transmitted to infants as they pass through the genital tract during birth.

Reference Values

- Negative culture for presence of virus
- Negative antibody of <1:10 titer

Abnormal Values

- Postive culture
    Herpesvirus infection
    Genital herpes
    Vaginitis
    Meningitis
    Encephalitis

■ Positive titer
    Infection in past 7 days: 1:10–1:100
    Current infection: 1:100–1:500
    Latent infection: >1:500

Interfering Factors

■ Improper collection technique, contamination of specimen, or inadequate amount of material to be tested
■ Hemolysis of blood sample
■ Pretest antiviral therapy, which will delay growth of pathogens

Nursing Implications

Assessment

■ Obtain history of known or suspected viral infection and recent administration of antiviral drug therapy.
■ Note anticipated delivery date in pregnant women.

Possible Nursing Diagnoses

Pain related to tissue inflammation and open lesions
Infection, risk for secondary infection, related to break in skin integrity
Hyperthermia related to infectious process

Implementation

■ *Culture specimen from the lower eyelid or mouth:* Put on gloves. Swab or scrape affected area with a sterile Culturette swab or use a syringe and needle to aspirate material from a lesion. Place swab or fluid from lesion onto chilled viral medium. To prepare a slide for cytology, scrape the lesion and spread on the slide with a tongue depressor. Fix with alcohol and send to laboratory as soon as possible after collection.
■ *Culture specimen from urethra in males:* Place client in a supine position. Put on gloves. Insert a sterile swab into the urethral opening and rotate swab. Remove swab and place it in the Culturette tube. Squeeze the bottom of the tube to break the section containing the medium. Insert swab until it is fully immersed in the medium.
■ *Culture specimen of cervix:* Place client in lithotomy position. Put on gloves and insert a vaginal speculum. Insert the sterile swab of a Culturette tube into the vagina and swab

the cervix. Remove the swab, being careful not to touch the walls of the vagina. Squeeze the bottom of the tube to break the section containing the medium. Insert swab until it is fully immersed in the medium.

- *Blood specimen for serology:* Put on gloves and obtain 5 mL of blood in a red-top tube for antibody test and green-top tube for blood viral culture.
- Label the specimen and send to the laboratory immediately.
- If the anticipated time between collection and inoculation into cell cultures exceeds 2 hours, keep specimen cold and transport as soon as possible. Do not freeze the specimen or allow it to dry.

Evaluation

- Note test results in relation to the client's symptoms and other test results.

Client/Caregiver Teaching

Pretest

- Instruct female clients not to douche for 24 hours before the collection of a cervical or vaginal specimen.

Posttest

- Inform the client that results may take from 24 hours to 4 weeks depending on test performed.

Culture, Nasal; Throat

Classification: Microbiology

Type of Test: Culture specimen

This test involves collecting a specimen of material from the nose, nasopharynx, or throat so that the organism can be isolated and identified. It is used to determine causative organisms of symptomatic infections and carrier states. Once the organism grows, it can be tested for sensitivity to various antibiotics to determine the most effective treatment.

Indications

- Screen for carriers of *Staphylococcus aureus* or *Haemophilus influenzae* and to differentiate between these states and actual infection
- Diagnose upper respiratory viral infections causing bronchitis, pharyngitis, croup, and influenza
- Diagnose bacterial infections such as tonsillitis, diphtheria, thrush, gonorrhea, pertussis, or streptococcal throat infection
- Determine the cause of scarlet fever, rheumatic fever, and acute glomerulonephritis
- Determine effect of antimicrobial therapy specific to identified microorganism and sensitivity

Reference Values

- Negative, no growth of pathogens

Abnormal Values

Suspected infections or carrier states caused by *Staphylococcus aureus,* group A *Streptococcus, Neisseria gonorrhoeae, Corynebacterium diphtheriae, Bordetella pertussis, Candida albicans,* and *Haemophilus influenzae.* Disorders include:
- Upper respiratory viral infections causing bronchitis, pharyngitis, croup, and influenza
- Bacterial infections such as tonsillitis, diphtheria, thrush, gonorrhea, pertussis, or streptococcal throat infection
- Scarlet fever, rheumatic fever, and acute glomerulonephritis

Interfering Factors

- Pretest antimicrobial therapy, which will delay or inhibit the growth of pathogens
- Contamination of the specimen by the surrounding skin or mucosa
- Improper collection technique or inadequate amount of material to be tested
- Use of antiseptic mouthwashes, which may reduce amount of organisms available for culture

Nursing Implications

Assessment

- Obtain history of signs and symptoms of upper respiratory infectious process, past immunizations, and medications that can interfere with test results.

Possible Nursing Diagnoses

Hyperthermia related to infectious process
Infection, risk for transmission
Pain related to tissue inflammation

Implementation

- Place the client in a sitting position or, if a child, on the caregiver's lap with the head and body immobilized.
- *Nasal culture:* Put on gloves. Gently raise the tip of the nose, insert a sterile, flexible Culturette swab into the nares and rotate it in place against the sides. Then remove the swab and place it in the appropriate Culturette tube. Squeeze the end of the tube to break the section containing the medium and insert the swab fully into the medium. Repeat for other nares.
- *Nasopharyngeal culture:* Put on gloves. Gently raise the tip of the nose; insert a sterile, flexible swab along the bottom of the nares and into the back of the throat. Rotate the swab in place to obtain the secretions and then remove. Place the swab in the Culturette tube. Squeeze the end of the tube to break the section containing the medium and insert the swab fully into the medium.
- *Throat culture:* Put on gloves. Tilt the head slightly backward, depress the tongue with a tongue blade, and insert the swab through the mouth to the pharyngeal and tonsillar area without touching any part of the oral cavity. Rub the areas including any lesions, inflammation, or exudate with the swab. Remove the swab. Place the swab in the Culturette tube. Squeeze the end of the tube to break the section containing the medium and insert the swab fully into the medium.
- Transport the specimen to the laboratory for immediate testing.

Evaluation

- Note test results in relation to the client's symptoms and the results of other tests performed.

Client/Caregiver Teaching

Pretest

- Instruct the client not to use any antiseptic mouthwash before the test.

Posttest

- Resume the treatment regimen for signs and symptoms of upper respiratory infections.

- Instruct client to cover mouth and nose when coughing or sneezing, dispose of tissues carefully, and wash hands frequently.
- Instruct client and caregiver to use gargle, lozenges, and inhalants for comfort.

Culture, Skin

Classification: Microbiology

Type of Test: Specimen culture

Skin cultures are performed to isolate the organism responsible for skin infections by inoculation of the material collected onto a medium of living cells. Once the organism grows, it can be tested for sensitivity to various antimicrobials so that the most effective treatment is ordered. This test usually involves obtaining a specimen of exudates, skin or nail scrapings, or hair. Optimally, the specimen should be obtained before treatment. The method used to culture and grow the organism depends on the suspected infection.

Normally, the skin contains low amounts of many of the microorganisms that can cause infection. When present in large numbers, they can be pathogenic. This test determines both the specific organism and the number of colonies present.

Indications

- Identify organisms responsible for skin eruptions, drainage, or other evidence of infection
- Identify organisms responsible for nail infections or abnormalities
- Determine antimicrobial sensitivity of the organism

Reference Values

- Culture contains only normal quantities of microorganisms on the skin, hair, and nails.

Abnormal Values

Presence of large quantities of colonies of bacteria and fungi that may be normal flora on the skin. These organisms in large quantities can cause infection. They include:

- Skin

  Bacteroids
  Clostridium
  Corynebacterium
  Candida
  Pseudomonas
  Staphylococci
  group A *Streptococci*
  Trichophyton
  Epidermophyton
  Trichophyton
  Aspergillus

- Nails

  Candida
  Cephalosporium
  Epidermophyton
  Tricophyton

- Hair

  Blastomycoses
  Coccidioides
  Candida
  Trichophyton
  Microsporium

Interfering Factors

- Failure to collect adequate specimen
- Improper collection or storage technique
- Failure to transport specimen in a timely fashion

Nursing Implications

Assessment

- Obtain history of clinical symptoms, medication regimen, and results of other tests performed.

Possible Nursing Diagnoses

Infection, risk for secondary infection, related to break in skin integrity

Body image disturbance related to change in appearance

Anxiety related to perceived threat to health status

Implementation

- Place the client in a comfortable position and expose the affected area.
- Put on gloves. Gently clean the area with sterile saline solution or an alcohol sponge. Allow to air dry.
- *Skin culture:* Using a sterile scalpel, scrape the skin from several areas of the affected site. If indicated, select the dark, warm, moist areas of the folds of the skin where microogranisms are most likely to flourish. Place the scrapings in a petri dish or spread on a slide. Aspirate any fluid from a pustule or vesicle using a sterile needle and tuberculin syringe. Flush the exudate into a petri dish. If lesion is not fluid-filled, open the lesion with a sterile scalpel and swab the area with a sterile cotton-tipped swab. Place the swab in the appropriate container.
- *Nails:* Using a sterile scalpel, scrape the affected nail or clip the affected nail with sterile scissors. Place the specimen in a petri dish or clean envelope.
- *Hair:* Clip or pluck the hair with sterile forceps or scrape the hair shaft and root with a sterile scalpel. Place specimen in a petri dish.
- Label the container and send to the laboratory immediately.

Evaluation

- Note test results in relation to the client's symptoms and other test results.

Client/Caregiver Teaching

Pretest

- Inform the client or caregiver that it will take only a few seconds. The client should not experience any pain from the procedure.

Posttest

- Advise the client that final test results may take up to 72 hours, but that antibiotic therapy may be started immediately.

Culture, Sputum

Classification: Microbiology

Type of Test: Culture specimen

This test involves collecting a sputum specimen so that the organism can be isolated and identified. It determines both the type and the number of organisms present in the specimen and the antibiotics to which the organisms are susceptible. Routine culture will not identify mycoplasmas, respiratory viruses, and rickettsiae, organisms often responsible for pneumonia. Sputum collected by expectoration or suctioning with catheters and by bronchoscopy cannot be cultured for anaerobic organisms. Instead, transtracheal aspiration or lung biopsy must be used.

Gram staining, the first method used in analyzing the specimen, involves smearing a small amount of sputum on a slide and then exposing it to gentian or crystal violet, iodine, alcohol, and safranine, a red dye. This technique allows for rapid morphologic examination of the cells contained in the specimen and differentiates any bacteria present into either gram-positive organisms, which retain the iodine stain, or gram-negative organisms, which do not retain the iodine stain but can be counterstained with safranine.

Acid-fast stain involves an acid treatment of the specimen and decolorizes certain types of bacteria and allows for rapid morphologic identification of these organisms. It is a rapid way of identifying if the infection is caused by *Mycobacterium, Norcardia,* or *Actinomyces.*

Once the organism grows, it can be tested for sensitivity to various antibiotics to determine the most effective treatment.

Indications

- Diagnose respiratory infections, such as viral infections or Legionnaire's disease, as indicated by presence or absence of organisms in culture
- Diagnose tuberculosis (see also Culture and Smear, Acid-Fast Bacilli)
- Monitor response to treatment for respiratory infections, especially tuberculosis

- Identify antibiotics to which the cultured organism is sensitive
- Gram-stain indications

  Differentiation of sputum from upper respiratory tract secretions, the latter being indicated by excessive squamous cells or absence of polymorphonuclear leukocytes

  Determination of types of leukocytes present in sputum (e.g., neutrophils indicating infection and eosinophils seen in asthma)

  Differentiation of gram-positive from gram-negative bacteria in respiratory infections

  Identification of Curschmann's spirals, which are associated with asthma, acute bronchitis, bronchopneumonia, and lung cancer

Reference Values

- Normal respiratory flora include *Neisseria catarrhalis, Candida albicans,* diphtheroids, alpha-hemolytic *Streptococcus,* and some staphylococci. The presence of normal flora does not rule out infection.
- Gram-stain reference values: Normal sputum contains polymorphonuclear leukocytes, alveolar macrophages, and a few squamous epithelial cells.

Abnormal Values

- Bacterial pneumonia caused by *Streptococcus pneumoniae, Haemophilus influenzae,* staphylococci, and gram-negative bacilli.
- Other pathogens that can be identified include *Klebsiella pneumoniae, Haemophilus pertussis, Mycobacterium tuberculosis,* fungi such as *Candida* and *Aspergillus,* and *Corynebacterium diphtheria.*

Interfering Factors

- Improper specimen collection
- Delay in sending specimen to the laboratory

Nursing Implications

Assessment

- Obtain history of pulmonary problems such as chronic or acute cough, the amount and color of sputum expectorant, if any, and any other symptoms of illness experienced by client.

- Ensure oxygen has been administered 20 to 30 minutes before the procedure if specimen is to be obtained by tracheal suctioning.
- Ensure client has fasted 6 hours before the procedure if bronchoscopy is to be performed.

Possible Nursing Diagnoses

Hyperthermia related to infectious process
Infection, risk for transmission
Pain related to tissue inflammation
Airway clearance, ineffective, related to presence of secretions or obstructions

Implementation

- Assist in providing extra fluids, unless contraindicated, and proper humidification to decrease tenacious secretions.
- Assist with mouth care (rinsing mouth with water), if needed, before collection so as not to contaminate specimen by oral secretions.
- Provide sterile sputum containers.
- *Expectorated specimen:* Ask the client to sit upright, with assistance and support (such as with an overbed table) as needed. Ask the client to take two or three deep breaths and cough deeply. Any sputum raised should be expectorated directly into a sterile sputum container. A 10- to 15-mL specimen is adequate.
- If the client is unable to produce the desired amount of sputum, several strategies may be attempted. One approach is to have the client drink two glasses of water and then assume the positions for postural drainage of the upper and middle lung segments. Support for effective coughing may be provided by placing the hands or a pillow over the diaphragmatic area and applying slight pressure. Another approach is to place a vaporizer or other humidifying device at the bedside. After sufficient exposure to adequate humidification, postural drainage of the upper and middle lung segments may be repeated before attempting to obtain the specimen.
- Obtain an order for an expectorant and administer it along with additional water approximately 2 hours before attempting to obtain the specimen. In addition, chest percussion and postural drainage of all lung segments may be employed. If the client still is unable to raise sputum, the use of an ultrasonic nebulizer (''induced sputum'') may be necessary. This is usually done by a respiratory therapist.

- *Tracheal suctioning:* Obtain the necessary equipment, including a suction device, a suction kit, and a Lukens tube or in-line trap. Position the client with head elevated as high as tolerated. Put on sterile gloves, with the dominant hand maintained as sterile and the nondominant hand as clean. Using the sterile hand, attach the suction catheter to the rubber tubing of the Lukens tube or in-line trap. Then attach the suction tubing to the male adaptor of the trap with the clean hand. Lubricate the suction catheter with sterile saline.
- Tell nonintubated clients to protrude the tongue and take a deep breath as the suction catheter is passed through the nostril. When the catheter enters the trachea, a reflex cough will be stimulated; immediately advance the catheter into the trachea and apply suction. Maintain suction for approximately 10 seconds and never for more than 15 seconds. Then withdraw the catheter without applying suction. Separate the suction catheter and suction tubing from the trap, and place the rubber tubing over the male adaptor to seal the unit.
- For intubated clients or those with a tracheostomy, the procedure above is followed, except that the suction catheter is passed through the existing endotracheal or tracheostomy tube rather than through the nostril. The client should be hyperoxygenated before and after the procedure in accordance with usual protocols for suctioning such clients.
- Label the specimen, document any antimicrobial therapy, and send to the laboratory immediately.

Evaluation

- Note test results in relation to the client's symptoms and other test results.
- Observe the client's color and respiratory rate and administer supplemental oxygen, as necessary.

Client/Caregiver Teaching

Pretest

- Inform the client that the test helps identify organisms that cause respiratory tract infections and their sensitivity to certain antibiotics. Emphasize that sputum is not the same as saliva.
- Inform the client that three samples may be taken at the bedside, usually on three separate mornings, either by passing a small tube (tracheal catheter) and adding suction or by having the client expectorate sputum by coughing.

- Inform the client that increasing fluid intake before retiring for the night before the test aids in liquefying secretions and may make them easier to expectorate in the morning and that humidifying inspired air also helps to liquefy secretions.
- Instruct the client to brush the teeth or rinse the mouth before obtaining the specimen, to avoid excessive contamination of the specimen with organisms normally found in the mouth.
- Warn the client not to touch the lip or inside of the container with hands or mouth.

Posttest

- Instruct the client to perform mouth care after the specimen has been obtained. A cool beverage also may aid in relieving throat irritation due to coughing and suctioning.
- If bronchoscopy has been performed, inform the client to drink liquids only after gag reflex returns.
- Instruct the client to contact the physician immediately if difficulty in breathing or swallowing or bleeding occurs.

Culture, Stool

Classification: Microbiology

Type of Test: Specimen culture

Stool culture involves collecting a sample of feces so that organisms present can be isolated and identified. Certain bacteria and fungi are normally found in feces. However, when overgrowth of these organisms occur or pathologic organisms are present, diarrhea or other signs and symptoms of systemic infection occur. These symptoms are the result of damage to the intestinal tissue by the pathologic bacteria. Once the organism grows, it can be tested for sensitivity to various antimicrobials to determine the most effective treatment.

Indications

- Diagnose diarrhea of unknown etiology
- Identify pathogenic organisms causing GI disease and carrier states

Reference Values

- Normal flora including *Enterococcus, E. coli, Proteus, Pseudomonas, Staphylococcus aureus, Candida albicans,* bacteroids, and clostridia.

Abnormal Values

- Isolation of pathogens such as the following indicates bacterial infection:
  Salmonella
  Shigella
  Campylobacter
  Yersinia
  Vibrio
- Isolation of *Clostridium botulinum* suggests botulism, but the bacteria must also be isolated from the food.
- Isolation of *Staphylococcus aureus* or Candida may indicate infection or a carrier state.

Interfering Factors

- Therapy with antibiotics may decrease the type and the amount of bacteria.
- Excessive exposure of the sample to air or room temperature may damage bacteria so that they will not grow in the culture.
- Failure to transport the culture within 1 hour of collection or contamination of the sample with urine or blood may affect results.

Nursing Implications

Assessment

- Assess history of GI disorders, medication regimen (specifically, antimicrobial agents), travel to foreign countries, and recent dietary history.

Possible Nursing Diagnoses

Anxiety related to perceived threat to health status
Pain related to intestinal inflammation
Diarrhea related to bowel irritation or inflammation
Fluid volume deficit, risk for, related to excessive loss through
  diarrhea

Implementation

- Put on gloves. Collect a stool specimen directly into a clean container. If the client requires a bedpan, make sure it is clean and dry and use a tongue blade to transfer the specimen to the container. Make sure representative portions of the stool are sent for analysis.
- If collecting the specimen by rectal swab, insert the swab past the client's anal sphincter. Rotate the swab, withdraw it, and place in vial.
- Label the specimen and transport it to the laboratory within 1 hour of collection. Do not refrigerate.

Evaluation

- Note test results in relation to the client's symptoms and notify the physician if pathogens are detected.

Client/Caregiver Teaching

Pretest

- Inform the client that the test helps determine the cause of GI disorder.
- Inform the client that three specimens on consecutive days may be required.

Posttest

- Advise the client that final test results may take up to 72 hours but that antibiotic therapy may be started immediately.
- Inform the client that follow-up testing can be done to evaluate therapy.

Culture, Urine with Gram Stain

Classification: Microbiology

Type of Test: Specimen culture

This test involves collecting a urine specimen so that the organism can be isolated and identified. It determines both the type and the number of organisms present in the specimen and the antibiotics to which the organisms are susceptible. In addition to identifying the organism, this test quantifies the amount of colonies present in the sample. This helps determine the severity of the infection or contamination of the specimen. Urine can be collected by having the client collect a clean-catch specimen, with urinary catheterization or suprapubic aspiration. Once the organisms grow, they can be tested to determine sensitivity to various antibiotics to ensure an effective treatment plan.

Gram staining, the first method used in analyzing the specimen, involves staining an amount of urine on a slide with gentian or crystal violet, iodine, alcohol, and safranine, a red dye. This technique allows for rapid morphologic examination of the cells contained in the specimen and differentiates any bacteria present into either gram-positive organisms, which retain the iodine stain, or gram-negative organisms, which do not retain the iodine stain but can be counterstained with safranine. This assists in decision making for early, broad-spectrum antibiotic treatment.

Indications

- Diagnose suspected urinary tract infection (UTI)
- Determine sensitivity of antibiotics to specific organisms
- Monitor response to UTI treatment

Reference Values

- Negative; no growth

Abnormal Values

- Commonly found organisms are those normally found in the gastrointestinal tract, including *Escherichia coli,* enterococci, *Klebsiella, Proteus,* and *Pseudomonas.*
    Colony counts >100,000/mL, indicate urinary tract infection
    Colony counts <1000/mL, suggest contamination resulting from poor collection technique

Interfering Factors

- Antibiotic therapy initiated before specimen collection may produce false-negative results.
- Improper collection techniques may result in specimen contamination.

Nursing Implications

Assessment

- Obtain history of genitourinary system, current symptoms, medication regimen, diagnostic tests, and results.

Possible Nursing Diagnoses

Pain related to tissue inflammation and bladder spasms
Urinary elimination, altered, related to inflammation and irritation

Implementation

- Provide client with a clean-catch kit.
- *Clean-catch specimen:* Instruct the male patient to cleanse the meatus, void a small amount into the toilet, and then void directly into the specimen container. Instruct the female to cleanse the labia from front to back, then keep the labia separated while voiding a small amount into the toilet. Then void directly into specimen container.
- *Pediatric urine collector:* Put on gloves. Cleanse the genital area and allow to dry. Remove the covering of the adhesive strips on the collector or bag and apply over the area. Diaper the child. When specimen is obtained, place the entire collection container in a sterile urine container.
- *In-dwelling catheter:* Put on gloves. Empty drainage tube of urine. Cleanse specimen port with antiseptic swab, then aspirate 3 to 5 mL of urine with a 21-25 gauge needle and syringe. Place urine in sterile container.
- *Urinary catheterization:* Place female client in lithotomy position or male client in supine position. Using sterile technique, open the straight urinary catheterization kit and perform urinary catheterization. Place the returned urine in a sterile specimen container.
- *Suprapubic aspiration:* Place the client in a supine position. Cleanse area with antiseptic and drape with sterile drapes. Using sterile technique, insert needle and remove sterile sample. Place the returned sample in a sterile specimen container. Place a dry sterile dressing over the site.
- Label the specimen and send it to the laboratory within 30 minutes or refrigerate for up to 2 hours.

> **NURSING ALERT**
>
> - For the client with a urinary diversion, for example, an ileal conduit, perform the catheterization through the stoma. Do not collect urine from the pouch.

Evaluation

- Observe for signs of inflammation if the specimen is obtained by suprapubic aspiration
- Note results in relation to other tests performed, in particular the WBC count, and the client's symptoms.

Client/Caregiver Teaching

Pretest

- Hold antibiotics until after specimen has been collected.
- Instruct client on clean-catch procedure and provide necessary supplies.

Posttest

- Instruct client to begin antibiotic therapy, as prescribed.
- Instruct client on the proper technique for wiping the perineal area after a bowel movement.

Culture, Wound

Classification: Microbiology

Type of Test: Specimen culture

A wound culture involves collecting a specimen of wound exudates, drainage, or tissue so that the causative organism can be isolated and pathogens identified. Specimens can be obtained from superficial and deep wounds. Once the organisms grow, they can be tested to determine sensitivity to various antibiotics to ensure effective treatment plan.

Indications

- Determine if an infectious agent is the cause of wound redness, warmth, or edema with drainage at a site
- Detect presence of pus or other exudate in an open wound
- Detect abscess or deep-wound infectious process
- Determine presence of infectious agents in a stage 3 and stage 4 decubitus ulcer

- Determine effective antimicrobial therapy specific to identified microorganism and sensitivity

Reference Values

- Negative; no growth of pathogens

Abnormal Values

- Positive for both aerobic and anaerobic microorganisms identified in wound culture specimens. Common organisms include *Staphylococcus aureus,* group A *Streptococcus, Clostridium perfringens, Klebsiella, Proteus, Pseudomonas,* and *Mycobacterium* species, and the fungal infectious agents, *Candida albicans* and *Aspergillus* species.

Interfering Factors

- Pretest antimicrobial therapy will delay or inhibit the growth of pathogens.
- Testing specimens more than 1 hour after collection will interfere with results.
- A dried specimen cannot be effectively cultured for microorganisms.

Nursing Implications

Assessment

- Obtain a history of known or suspected wound infection, and note any medications (antimicrobials) that may interfere with test results.

Possible Nursing Diagnoses

Pain related to tissue inflammation and open wound
Infection, risk for secondary infection, related to break in skin integrity
Hyperthermia related to infectious process

Implementation

- Place the client in a comfortable position and drape the site to be cultured. Cleanse the area around the wound to remove flora indigenous to the skin.
- Place a Culturette swab in a superficial wound where the exudate is the most excessive without touching the wound edges. Place the swab soaked with the exudate in the tube, and squeeze the tube to allow for dispersion of the medium.

Use more than one swab and Culturette tube to obtain specimens from other areas in the wound.

- To obtain a deep-wound specimen, insert a sterile syringe and needle into the wound and aspirate the drainage. Following the aspiration, expel the air from the syringe and cover the needle with a rubber stopper or inject the material into a tube containing an anaerobic culture medium.
- Transport the specimen to the lab immediately for examination.

Evaluation

- Note test results in relation to other tests performed and the client's symptoms.

Client/Caregiver Teaching

Pretest

- Inform the client about the purpose of the test and the procedure for obtaining the specimen.
- Inform the client that some discomfort may be experienced.

Posttest

- Emphasize the importance of reporting continuing signs and symptoms of the infection and complying with antimicrobial regimen, if ordered.
- Instruct in wound care and nutritional requirements (protein, vitamin C) to promote wound healing.

Culture and Smear, Acid-Fast Bacillus (AFB)

Classification: Microbiology

Type of Test: Specimen culture

An acid-fast bacillus (AFB) smear is used for early detection of the tubercle organism and timely initiation of antituberculosis therapy. A sputum specimen is subjected to an acid treatment that decolorizes certain types of bacteria and allows for rapid morphologic identification of these organisms. It is a rapid way of identifying infections caused by *Mycobacterium, Norcardia,* or *Actinomyces.*

AFB cultures are used to confirm both positive and negative results of AFB smears. When the AFB organism is specified for detection on culture, the laboratory knows that several weeks may be needed for conclusive results. As noted, immunological methods may also be employed in diagnosing tuberculosis by sputum analysis. Sputum may be collected by expectoration, suctioning, bronchoscopy (see page 209), transtracheal aspiration (see page 386), or lung biopsy (see page 176).

Indications

- Diagnose pulmonary tuberculosis
- Monitor response to treatment for pulmonary tuberculosis
- Differentiate tuberculosis from carcinoma and bronchiectasis

Reference Values

- Negative for acid-fast bacillus

Abnormal Values

- Pulmonary tuberculosis
- *Norcardia* or *Actinomyces* infection.

Interfering Factors

- Improper specimen collection or delay in sending specimen to the laboratory can affect results.
- Antitubercular drug therapy can cause negative results because it inhibits growth of *M. tuberculosis.*
- High carbon dioxide atmosphere for growth can increase the number of positive cultures.
- Culture medium containing glycerin accelerates growth.

Nursing Implications

Assessment

- Obtain history of pulmonary problems such as chronic or acute cough, the amount and color of sputum expectorant, if any, and any other symptoms of illness experienced by client.

- Ensure oxygen has been administered 20 to 30 minutes before the procedure if the specimen is to be obtained by tracheal suctioning.
- Ensure client has fasted 6 hours before the procedure if bronchoscopy is to be performed.

Possible Nursing Diagnoses

Hyperthermia related to infectious process
Infection, risk for transmission
Pain related to tissue inflammation
Airway clearance, ineffective, related to presence of secretions or obstructions

Implementation

- Provide extra fluids, unless contraindicated, and proper humidification to liquefy tenacious secretions.
- Assist with mouth care (rinsing mouth with water), if needed, before collection so as not to contaminate specimen by oral secretions.
- Provide sterile sputum containers.
- *Expectorated specimen:* Ask the client to sit upright, with assistance and support (such as with an overbed table) as needed. Ask the client to take two or three deep breaths and cough deeply. Any sputum raised should be expectorated directly into a sterile sputum container. A 10- to 15-mL specimen is adequate.
- If the client is unable to produce the desired amount of sputum, several strategies may be attempted. One approach is to have the client drink two glasses of water and then assume the positions for postural drainage of the upper and middle lung segments. Support for effective coughing may be provided by placing the hands or a pillow over the diaphragmatic area and applying slight pressure. Another approach is to place a vaporizer or other humidifying device at the bedside. After sufficient exposure to adequate humidification, postural drainage of the upper and middle lung segments may be repeated before attempting to obtain the specimen.
- Obtain an order for an expectorant and administer it along with additional water approximately 2 hours before attempting to obtain the specimen. In addition, chest percussion and postural drainage of all lung segments may be employed. If the client still is unable to raise sputum, the use of an ultrasonic nebulizer (''induced sputum'') may be necessary. This is usually done by a respiratory therapist.

- *Tracheal suctioning:* Obtain the necessary equipment, including a suction device, a suction kit, and a Lukens tube or in-line trap. Position the client with head elevated as high as tolerated. Put on sterile gloves, with the dominant hand maintained as sterile and the nondominant hand as clean. Using the sterile hand, attach the suction catheter to the rubber tubing of the Lukens tube or in-line trap. Then attach the suction tubing to the male adaptor of the trap with the clean hand. Lubricate the suction catheter with sterile saline.
- Tell nonintubated clients to protrude the tongue and take a deep breath as the suction catheter is passed through the nostril. When the catheter enters the trachea, a reflex cough will be stimulated; immediately advance the catheter into the trachea and maintain suction for approximately 10 seconds and never for more than 15 seconds. Then withdraw the catheter without applying suction. Separate the suction catheter and suction tubing from the trap, and place the rubber tubing over the male adaptor to seal the unit.
- For intubated clients or those with a tracheostomy, the procedure above is followed, except that the suction catheter is passed through the existing endotracheal or tracheostomy tube rather than through the nostril. The client should be hyperoxygenated before and after the procedure in accordance with usual protocols for suctioning such clients. To obtain specimens by biopsy, bronchoscopy, or transtracheal aspiration, see entries.
- Label the specimen, document any antimicrobial therapy, and send to the laboratory immediately.

Evaluation

- Note test results in relation to the client's symptoms and other test results.
- Observe the client's color and respiratory rate and administer supplemental oxygen, as necessary.

Client/Caregiver Teaching

Pretest

- Inform the client that the test helps identify organisms that cause respiratory tract infections and their sensitivity to certain antibiotics. Emphasize that sputum is not the same as saliva.
- Inform the client that three samples may be taken at the bedside, usually on three separate mornings, either by passing a

small tube (tracheal catheter) and adding suction or by having the client expectorate sputum by coughing.

- Inform the client that increasing fluid intake before retiring for the night before the test aids in liquefying secretions and may make them easier to expectorate in the morning and that humidifying inspired air also helps to liquefy secretions.
- Instruct the client to brush the teeth or rinse the mouth before obtaining the specimen, to avoid excessive contamination of the specimen with organisms normally found in the mouth.
- Warn the client not to touch the lip or inside of the container with hands or mouth.

Posttest

- Instruct the client to perform mouth care after the specimen has been obtained. A cool beverage also may aid in relieving throat irritation due to coughing and suctioning.
- If bronchoscopy has been performed, inform the client to drink liquids only after gag reflex returns.
- Instruct the client to contact the physician immediately if difficulty in breathing or swallowing or bleeding occurs.

Cyclic Adenosine Monophosphate (cAMP)

Classification: Chemistry

Type of Test: Serum, urine

Cyclic adenosine monophosphate (cAMP) influences the rate of cellular protein synthesis and is formed by enzymatic action of adenylate cyclase on adenosine triphosphate. This test requires a serum sample and urine specimen taken at the same time.

Indications

- Diagnose hypoparathyroidism
- Differentiate hypoparathyroidism and pseudohypoparathyroidism

Reference Values

		SI Units
Serum	5.6–10.9 ng/mL	17–33 nmol/L
Urine		
Total	112–188 μg/L	340–570 nmol/L
Creatinine cAMP		3–5 μmol/g
Glomerular filtrate cAMP	6.6–15.5 μg/L	20–47 nmol/L
Glom filt nephrogenous cAMP	<9.9 μg/L	<30 nmol/L

Abnormal Values

- Increased serum cAMP
    Hyperparathyroidism
    Neoplastic disease combined with hypercalcemia
    Pseudohyperparathyroidism
- Decreased serum cAMP
    Hypoparathyroidism
    Pseudohypoparathyroidism
- Increased urinary cAMP
    Hyperthyroidism
    Neoplastic disease combined with hypercalcemia
    Pseudohyperparathyroidism
- Decreased urinary cAMP
    Hypoparathyroidism
    Pseudoparathyroidism

Interfering Factors

- Test results are not reliable in impaired renal function.
- Radioactive scans within 7 days of the test invalidate the results.
- Specimens sent to the laboratory more than 1 hour after collection should be rejected.

> **NURSING ALERT**
>
> - This procedure is contraindicated in clients with high serum calcium levels because parathyroid hormone will further increase blood levels.
> - It should be performed cautiously in those receiving digitalis or who have cardiac or renal disease.

Nursing Implications

Assessment

- Obtain a history of endocrine disorders, neoplastic disease, results of tests performed, and medication regimen.

Possible Nursing Diagnoses

Body temperature, altered, risk for, related to parathyroid dysfunction

Anxiety related to perceived threat to health status

Grieving, anticipatory, related to perceived potential loss

Implementation

- Perform a skin test to detect possible allergy to parathyroid hormone.
- Ask client to empty bladder.
- Put on gloves and, using aseptic technique, start an IV. Infuse parathyroid hormone IV over 15 minutes. Document the time of the start of the infusion as time zero.
- Using aseptic technique, obtain a 5-mL sample of blood in a red-top tube and send to the laboratory immediately.
- For some laboratories, a random urine specimen obtained at the same time as the serum sample is acceptable. Others require a 3- to 4-hour or a 24-hour urine specimen. Follow the respective guidelines for collection of these samples.
- Document the time the specimens were obtained on the laboratory requisition slip.

Evaluation

- Note test results in relation to other studies performed, particularly the serum calcium and serum phosphate levels.

Client/Caregiver Teaching

Pretest

- Inform the client that no special preparation is required.
- Instruct the client how to collect the urine specimen.

Posttest

- Instruct the client to notify the physician if signs of hypercalcemia, such as lethargy, anorexia, vomiting, abdominal cramps, and vertigo, are noted.

Cystometry (CMG)

Classification: Manometry

Type of Test: Urodynamic measurement

This noninvasive manometric study is performed to measure the bladder pressure in centimeters of water during the filling and emptying phases. It provides information about bladder structure and function that can lead to uninhibited bladder contractions, sensations of bladder fullness and need to void, and ability to inhibit voiding. These abnormalities cause incontinence and other impaired patterns of micturation. Cystometry can be performed with cystoscopy and sphincter electromyography.

Indications

- Determine cause of bladder dysfunction and pathology
- Evaluate signs and symptoms of urinary elimination pattern dysfunction
- Diagnose the type of incontinence: functional (involuntary and unpredictable), reflex (involuntary when a specific volume is reached), stress (weak pelvic muscles), total (continuous and unpredictable), urge (involuntary when urgency is sensed), psychological (dementia, confusion affecting awareness)
- Determine type of neurogenic bladder (motor or sensory)
- Evaluate the management of neurologic bladder before surgical intervention
- Evaluate the usefulness of drug therapy on the detrusor muscle function and tonicity and internal and external sphincter function
- Determine cause of urinary retention
- Detect congenital urinary abnormalities
- Determine the cause of recurrent urinary tract infections

Reference Values

- Normal sensory perception of bladder fullness, desire to void and ability to inhibit urination, and appropriate response to temperature (hot and cold)

- Normal bladder capacity: 350 to 750 mL for adult males and 250 to 550 mL for adult females
- Normal functioning bladder pressure: 8 to 15 cm H_2O
- Normal sensation of fullness: 40 to 100 cm H_2O or 300 to 500 mL
- Normal bladder pressure during voiding: 30 to 40 cm H_2O
- Normal detrusor pressure: <10 cm H_2O
- Normal urge to void: 150 to 450 mL
- Urethral pressure that is higher than bladder pressure to ensure continence
- Normal filling pattern
- Absence of residual urine

Abnormal Values

- Sensory or motor paralysis of bladder, flaccid bladder that fills without contracting, inability to perceive bladder fullness or initiate or maintain urination without applying external pressure, total loss of conscious sensation and vesical control, or uncontrollable micturation (incontinence)

Interfering Factors

- Inability to understand and carry out instructions during the procedure
- Movement during the procedure that can affect bladder reflexes
- Inability to void in a supine position or straining to void during the study
- High level of client anxiety or embarrassment
- Administration of drugs that affect bladder function such as muscle relaxants or antihistamines

▶ NURSING ALERT

- This procedure is contraindicated in acute urinary tract infection as the study can cause infection to spread to the kidneys.
- It is also contraindicated in urethral obstruction and in clients with cervical spinal cord lesions, who may exhibit autonomic dysreflexia as seen by bradycardia, flushing, hypertension, diaphoresis, and headache. Intravenous propantheline bromide (Pro-Banthine) can help to counteract this response.

Nursing Implications

Assessment

- Obtain history of signs and symptoms of impaired urinary function, known or suspected disorders leading to urinary dysfunction, previous tests and procedures done, medical and surgical therapeutic interventions performed, and medications that can affect the test results (antihistamines and muscle relaxants).

Possible Nursing Diagnoses

Pain related to urinary obstruction
Urinary elimination, altered, related to [specify]
Infection, risk for, related to invasive procedure

Implementation

- Place client in a supine or lithotomy position on the examining table or, if spinal cord injury is present, the client can remain on a stretcher in supine position and draped appropriately. Ask the client to void and lie still during the procedure. During the voiding, characteristics are assessed such as the time started, force and continuity of the stream, volume voided, and presence of dribbling, straining, or hesitancy.
- A urinary catheter is inserted into the bladder under sterile conditions and residual urine is measured and recorded. A test for sensory response to temperature is then done by instilling 30 mL of room-temperature sterile water followed by 30 mL of warm sterile water and sensations are assessed and recorded.
- Fluid is removed from the bladder and the catheter is connected to a cystometer that measures the pressure. Sterile normal saline or distilled water or carbon dioxide gas in controlled amounts is instilled into the bladder. When the client indicates the urge to void, the bladder is considered full and amounts and times are recorded. Pressure and volume readings are also recorded and graphed for response to heat, full bladder, urge to void, and ability to inhibit voiding. Client is requested to void without straining and pressures taken and recorded during this activity.
- Following completion of voiding, bladder is emptied of any other fluid and the catheter withdrawn unless further testing is planned.
- If further testing is done to determine if abnormal bladder function is caused by muscle incompetency or interruption in innervation, anticholinergic medication such as atropine

or cholinergic medication such as bethanechol (Urecholine) can be injected and the study repeated in 20 or 30 minutes.

Evaluation

■ Note test results in relation to client's symptoms and other tests performed.

Client/Caregiver Teaching

Pretest

■ Inform the client that the procedure is performed in a special urology room or in clinic setting by the physician and takes 30 to 45 minutes to complete. Also, inform the client that the only discomfort experienced is the insertion of the urethral catheter.
■ Instruct the client to report pain, sweating, nausea, headache, and urge to void during the study.
■ Explain that client cooperation with positioning and activity before and during the test is critical to accurate results.

Posttest

■ Advise the client to increase oral intake of fluids (125 mL per hour for 24 hours) after the procedure, unless contraindicated.
■ Instruct client to report any changes in voiding pattern or urine characteristics such as blood in the urine, cloudy and foul-smelling urine, inability to void or incontinence, dysuria, frequency, and urgency.
■ Inform the client that a warm tub bath can relieve discomfort at the urethral site.

Cystoscopy

Classification: Endoscopy

Type of Test: Direct visualization

This procedure provides direct visualization of the urethra, urinary bladder, and ureteral orifices—areas not usually able to be observed with x-ray procedures. Cystoscopes can be either rigid, containing an obturator and a telescope with a lens and light system, or flexible and fiberoptic. The procedure may be performed at the same time as or following ultrasonography, radiography or concurrently with urethroscopy or retrograde pyelography.

Indications

- Differentiate benign and cancerous lesions involving the bladder through tissue biopsy
- Evaluate the function of each kidney by obtaining urine samples via ureteral catheters
- Evaluate changes in urinary elimination patterns
- Determine source of hematuria of unknown etiology
- Determine possible source of persistent urinary tract infections
- Evaluate extent of prostatic hyperplasia and degree of obstruction
- Identify congenital anomalies such as duplicate ureters, ureteroceles, urethral or ureteral strictures, diverticula, and areas of inflammation or ulceration
- Remove renal calculi from the bladder or ureters
- Dilate strictures of the urethra or ureters
- Place ureteral catheters to drain urine from the renal pelvis or for retrograde pyelography
- Identify and remove polyps and small tumors (including fulguration) from the bladder
- Evacuate blood clots and perform fulguration of bleeding sites within the lower urinary tract
- Implant radioactive seeds into bladder tumors

Reference Values

- Normal urethra, bladder, and ureters

Abnormal Values

- Prostatic hypertrophy or hyperplasia
- Obstruction
- Inflammation or infection
- Renal calculi
- Polyps
- Tumors
- Urethral or ureteral stricture
- Urinary tract malformation

- This procedure is contraindicated in bleeding disorders since instrumentation may lead to excessive bleeding from the lower urinary tract, or in acute cystitis or urethritis since instrumentation could allow bacteria to enter the bloodstream, resulting in septicemia.

Nursing Implications

Assessment

- Obtain a history of genitourinary infections; bleeding disorders; and allergies or sensitivities to anesthetics, analgesics, and antibiotics.
- Determine the date of the last menstrual period in premenopausal women.
- Assess hematologic status and blood-clotting ability and urinalysis findings for abnormalities.
- Ensure that dietary and fluid restrictions are followed. For general or spinal anesthesia, withhold food and fluid for 8 hours before the procedure; for local anesthesia, allow clear liquids for only 8 hours before the procedure.

Possible Nursing Diagnoses

Pain related to tissue inflammation or irritation or obstruction
Urinary elimination, altered, related to [specify]
Infection, risk for, related to invasive procedure
Anxiety related to threat to health status

Implementation

- Administer ordered preoperative sedation.
- Position the client on the examination table with legs in stirrups and draped. If general or spinal anesthesia is to be used, it is administered before positioning on table.
- Cleanse external genitalia with antiseptic solution. If local anesthetic is used, it is instilled into the urethra and retained for 5 to 10 minutes. A penile clamp may be used for male clients to aid in retention of anesthetic.
- The physician will insert a cystoscope or a urethroscope to examine the urethra before cystoscopy. The urethroscope has a sheath that may be left in place and the cystoscope inserted through it, avoiding multiple instrumentations.
- After insertion of the cystoscope, a sample of residual urine may be obtained for culture or other analyses.
- The bladder is irrigated via an irrigation system attached to the scope. The irrigant is usually sterile water unless an isotonic solution such as mannitol is used during transure-

thral resection procedures. The irrigation fluid aids in bladder visualization.

- If a prostatic tumor is found, it may be biopsied by means of a cytology brush or biopsy forceps inserted through the scope. If the tumor is small and localized, it can be excised and fulgurated. This procedure is termed transurethral resection of the bladder (TURB). Polyps can also be identified and excised.
- Ulcers or bleeding sites can be fulgurated, using electrocautery. Renal calculi can be crushed and removed from the ureters and bladder. Ureteral catheters can be inserted via the scope to obtain urine samples from each kidney for comparative analysis and radiographic studies. Ureteral and urethral strictures can also be dilated during the procedure.
- Upon completion of examination and related procedures, the cystoscope is withdrawn.
- Place obtained specimens in proper containers, label properly, and send to laboratory promptly.

Evaluation

- Note results in relation to other test results and the client's symptoms.

Client/Caregiver Teaching

Pretest

- Inform the client that the procedure is generally performed under general, spinal, or local anesthesia by a physician in a special cystoscopy suite near or in the operating room department or in a physician's office and takes approximately 30 to 60 minutes.
- Depending on the type of anesthesia, inform the client to withhold food and fluids for varying lengths of time.
- If local anesthetic is used, inform the client that either a sensation of pressure, of having to void, or both may be felt.

Posttest

- Tell the client to resume food and fluid intake and activity when the effects of sedation wears off.
- Emphasize the need for adequate fluid intake (125 mL per hour for 24 hours) after the procedure.
- Inform the client that burning or discomfort on urination can be experienced for the first few voidings after the procedure and that the urine may be blood-tinged for the first and second voidings after the procedure.

■ Emphasize that any persistent flank or suprapubic pain, fever, chills, blood in urine, and any difficulty or change in urinary pattern that persists must be reported to the physician immediately.

Cytology, Sputum

Classification: Microbiology

Type of Test: Specimen analysis

Cytology is the study of the origin, structure, function, and pathology of cells. In clinical practice, cytological examinations are generally performed to detect cell changes resulting from neoplastic or inflammatory conditions.

Sputum specimens for cytological examination may be collected by expectoration alone, during bronchoscopy, or by expectoration following bronchoscopy. The method of reporting results of cytological examinations varies according to the laboratory performing the test. Terms used to report results include negative (no abnormal cells), inflammatory, benign atypical, suspect for neoplasm, and positive for neoplasm.

Sputum may be collected by expectoration, suctioning, bronchoscopy (see page 209), transtracheal aspiration (see page 386), or lung biopsy (see page 176).

Indications

■ Diagnose lung cancer
■ Screen cigarette smokers for metaplastic (nonmalignant) cellular changes
■ Screen clients with history of acute or chronic inflammatory or infectious lung disorders, which may lead to benign atypical or metaplastic cellular changes
■ Detect known or suspected viral disease involving the lung
■ Detect known or suspected fungal or parasitic infection involving the lung
■ Diagnose *Pneumocystis carinii* in persons with AIDS using bronchial washings

Reference Values

- Negative for abnormal cells, Curschmann's spirals, fungi, ova, and parasites

Abnormal Values

- Cellular changes from viral infections and lung diseases
- Neoplasms
- Infections caused by fungi, ova, or parasites
- Lipoid or aspiration pneumonia as seen by lipid droplets contained in macrophages

Interfering Factors

- Improper specimen collection
- Delay in sending specimen to the laboratory
- Improper technique used to obtain bronchial washing

> ### NURSING ALERT
>
> - Never suction longer than 15 seconds. If client becomes hypoxic or cyanotic, remove catheter immediately and administer oxygen. If client has asthma or chronic bronchitis, watch for aggravated bronchospasms with use of more than a 10% concentration of sodium chloride or acetylcysteine in an aerosol.

Nursing Implications

Assessment

- Obtain history of pulmonary problems such as chronic or acute cough, the amount and color of sputum expectorant, if any, and any other symptoms of illness experienced by client.
- Determine abnormalities in laboratory results and diagnostic findings.
- Ensure oxygen has been administered 20 to 30 minutes before the procedure if the specimen is to be obtained by tracheal suctioning.
- Ensure that the client has fasted 6 hours before the procedure if bronchoscopy is to be performed.

Possible Nursing Diagnoses

Airway clearance, ineffective, related to presence of secretions
   or obstructions
Anxiety related to threat to health status
Grieving, anticipatory, related to perceived potential loss

Implementation

- Provide extra fluids, unless contraindicated, and proper humidification to liquefy tenacious secretions.
- Assist with mouth care (rinsing mouth with water), if needed,
  before collection so as not to contaminate specimen by oral
  secretions.
- Provide sterile sputum containers.
- *Expectorated specimen:* Ask the client to sit upright, with
  assistance and support (such as with an overbed table) as
  needed. Ask the client to take two or three deep breaths
  and cough deeply. Any sputum raised should be expectorated directly into a sterile sputum container. A 10- to 15-
  mL specimen is adequate.
- If the client is unable to produce the desired amount of sputum, several strategies may be attempted. One approach is
  to have the client drink two glasses of water and then assume the positions for postural drainage of the upper and
  middle lung segments. Support for effective coughing may
  be provided by placing the hands or a pillow over the diaphragmatic area and applying slight pressure. Another approach is to place a vaporizer or other humidifying device at
  the bedside. After sufficient exposure to adequate humidification, postural drainage of the upper and middle lung segments may be repeated before attempting to obtain the
  specimen.
- Obtain an order for an expectorant and administer it along
  with additional water approximately 2 hours before attempting to obtain the specimen. In addition, chest percussion
  and postural drainage of all lung segments may be employed. If the client still is unable to raise sputum, the use
  of an ultrasonic nebulizer (''induced sputum'') may be necessary. This is usually done by a respiratory therapist.
- *Tracheal suctioning:* Obtain the necessary equipment, including a suction device, a suction kit, and a Lukens tube
  or in-line trap. Position the client with head elevated as high
  as tolerated. Put on sterile gloves, with the dominant hand
  maintained as sterile and the nondominant hand as clean.
  Using the sterile hand, attach the suction catheter to the
  rubber tubing of the Lukens tube or in-line trap. Then attach
  the suction tubing to the male adaptor of the trap with the

clean hand. Lubricate the suction catheter with sterile saline.

- Tell nonintubated clients to protrude the tongue and take a deep breath as the suction catheter is passed through the nostril. When the catheter enters the trachea, a reflex cough will be stimulated; immediately advance the catheter into the trachea and maintain suction for approximately 10 seconds and never for more than 15 seconds. Then withdraw the catheter without applying suction. Separate the suction catheter and suction tubing from the trap, and place the rubber tubing over the male adaptor to seal the unit.
- For intubated clients or those with a tracheostomy, the procedure above is followed, except that the suction catheter is passed through the existing endotracheal or tracheostomy tube rather than through the nostril. The client should be hyperoxygenated before and after the procedure in accordance with usual protocols for suctioning such clients. To obtain specimens by biopsy, bronchoscopy, or transtracheal aspiration, see specific entries.
- Label the specimen, document any antimicrobial therapy, and send to the laboratory immediately.

Evaluation

- Note test results in relation to the client's symptoms and other test results.
- Observe the client's color and respiratory rate and administer supplemental oxygen, as necessary.

Client/Caregiver Teaching

Pretest

- Inform the client that the test checks the sputum for origin, structure, function, and pathology of cells. Emphasize that sputum is not the same as saliva.
- Inform the client that increasing fluid intake before retiring the night before the test aids in liquefying secretions and may make them easier to expectorate in the morning, and that humidifying inspired air also helps to liquefy secretions.
- Instruct the client to brush the teeth or rinse the mouth before obtaining the specimen to avoid excessive contamination of the specimen with organisms normally found in the mouth.

Posttest

- Instruct the client to perform mouth care after the specimen has been obtained. A cool beverage also may aid in relieving throat irritation due to coughing and suctioning.

- Instruct the client to contact the physician immediately if bleeding or difficult breathing or swallowing occur.

D-Dimer

Classification: Hematology; chemistry

Type of Test: Plasma; spinal fluid

A D-dimer is an asymmetric carbon compound formed by two identical molecules. This fragment is formed after thrombin converts fibinogen to fibrin, factor XIIIa stabilizes it to a clot, and plasmin acts on cross-linked (clotted) fibrin. This test is specific for fibrinolysis because it validates the presence of fibrin degradation products, not fibrinogen degradation products. This test confirms the presence of disseminated intravascular coagulation.

Indications

- Diagnosis of disseminated intravascular coagulation (DIC)
- Differentiate subarachnoid hemorrhage from a traumatic lumbar puncture (spinal fluid only)

Reference Values

- Negative or <250 ng/mL or $250/\mu$g/L (SI units)

Abnormal Values

- Increased values
  DIC
  Pulmonary embolism
  Arterial or venous thrombosis
  Neoplastic disease
  Pregnancy (late and postpartum)
  Recent surgery (within 2 days)
  Subarachnoid hemorrhage (spinal fluid only)
  Secondary fibrinolysis

Interfering Factors

- High rheumatoid factor titers can cause a false-positive result.
- Increased CA-125 levels can cause a false-positive result.
- In infants less than 6 months old, a false-negative result can occur in spinal fluid analysis.

Nursing Implications

Assessment

- Obtain a history of hematologic diseases, recent surgery, and the results of other tests performed.

Possible Nursing Diagnoses

Protection, altered, related to abnormal blood clotting
Pain related to tissue ischemia
Tissue perfusion, altered [specify], related to occlusion of blood flow
Trauma/suffocation, risk for, related to altered level of consciousness

Implementation

- Put on gloves. Using aseptic technique, perform a venipuncture and obtain 5 mL of blood in a blue-top tube.
- For a spinal fluid, sample is collected during a lumbar puncture. See CSF analysis for details on the procedure. Place the sample in a plastic vial.
- Label specimen and send to laboratory immediately.

Evaluation

- Note test results in relation to other tests performed and the client's symptoms.

Client/Caregiver Teaching

Pretest

- Inform the client that no special preparation is required for this test.

D-Xylose Tolerance, D-Xylose Absorption Test

Classification: Chemistry

Type of Test: Blood; urine

This test measures the absorptive capacity of the small intestine. For this test, the client ingests pentose sugar (5 grams for children and 25 grams for adults), which is absorbed in the small intestine without pancreatic enzymes, metabolized in the liver, and excreted in the urine.

Indications

- Diagnose malabsorption syndromes

Reference Values

		SI Units
Children		
Serum (at 1 h)		
child <10 kg	≥15 mg/dL	1.0 mmol/L
child 10 kg to age 9 yr	≥20 mg/dL	1.3 mmol/L
Urine (at 5 h)	16%–33% of dose ingested	
Adults		
Serum (at 2 h)	30–52 mg/dL	2.0–3.47 mmol/L
Urine (at 5 h)	16% of dose ingested	

Abnormal Values

- Increased values
  Disaccharidase deficiency
  Hodgkin's disease
  Malabsorption
  Scleroderma
- Decreased values
  Amyloidosis
  Ascites
  Celiac disease

Cystic fibrosis
Diabetic neuropathic diarrhea
Regional enteritis (jejunum)
Severe congestive heart failure
Sprue
Whipple's disease

Interfering Factors

- Failure to adhere to dietary and activity restrictions affects absorption of D-xylose.
- Renal disease will decrease urinary output and vomiting decreases the amount of D-xylose available for absorption.
- Drugs, such as aspirin, atropine, and indomethacin will alter absorption or excretion of D-xylose.
- Inaccurate timing of sample collection will affect test results.

Nursing Implications

Assessment

- Obtain history of gastrointestinal or immunologic disorders, the results of other tests performed, and medication regimen.
- Ensure client has withheld medications that alter test results.
- Ensure that the client has fasted for 8 hours (4 hours for children) and that client has not consumed foods containing pentose such as fruit, jellies, jams, and pastries.

Possible Nursing Diagnoses

Diarrhea related to malabsorption syndrome or gastrointestinal dysfunction
Fluid volume excess related to compromised regulatory mechanism

Implementation

- Ask the client to void at 8 AM and discard sample.
- Put on gloves. Perform a venipuncture and obtain 10 mL of blood in a red-top tube and label as fasting sample.
- Give the client D-xylose (adults, 25 g; children, 5 g) dissolved in 8 oz of water. Ask the client to drink another full 8 oz of water. Record the time of ingestion.
- In 2 hours, using aseptic technique, collect a 10-mL blood sample in a red-top tube, or in a gray-top tube if the sample won't be tested immediately in the adult client. For the child, obtain the sample in 1 hour. Occasionally, a 5-hour sample will be required.
- Collect all the urine excreted in 5 hours unless a 24-hour

sample is requested for the client with low or borderline creatinine levels. Refrigerate the urine sample.

- Label the samples carefully and make sure all drugs the client is taking are noted. Transport the sample to the laboratory promptly.

Evaluation

- Note test results in relation to other tests performed and the client's symptoms.

Client/Caregiver Teaching

Pretest

- Instruct the client to fast for 8 hours (a child for 4 hours).
- Instruct the client to remain in bed throughout the test because activity affects results.
- Inform the client that urine will be collected for 5 to 24 hours.
- Warn the client not to contaminate the urine specimen with toilet tissue or stool.
- If ordered, tell the client to withhold aspirin, indomethacin, or atropine.
- Warn the client that mild abdominal discomfort or diarrhea may result from D-xylose.

Posttest

- Instruct the client to resume diet and medications withheld before the test.

Delta-Aminolevulinic Acid, Urine (Delta ALA); Aminolevulinic Acid (ALA)

Classification: Urinalysis

Type of Test: Urine, 24-hour

This quantitative analysis of urine uses the colorimetric technique. Delta-aminolevulinic acid (delta ALA), a basic precursor for the porphyrins, is an enzyme needed for the normal conversion to porphobilinogen through the action of the enzyme

ALA-dehydrase during heme synthesis. In porphyrins and lead poisoning where there is impaired conversion, urine ALA levels rise before other chemical or hematologic changes occur.

Indications

- Screen for lead poisoning
- Diagnose porphyrias and certain hepatic disorders, such as hepatitis and hepatic carcinoma

Reference Values

		SI Units
9 mo–5 yr	0–0.66 mg/dL	0–0.09 μmol/L
6 yr–adult	1.5–7.5 mg/24 h	11–57 μmol/day

Abnormal Values

- Increased levels
  Hepatitis
  Hepatic carcinoma
  Lead poisoning
  Porphyrias

Interfering Factors

- Drugs that may cause increased ALA levels include penicillin, barbiturates, and griseofulvin since they cause porphyrins to accumulate in the liver.
- Vitamin E in therapeutic doses may lower urine ALA levels.
- Failure of the client to collect all the urine and store it properly may interfere with results.

Nursing Implications

Assessment

- Obtain history of suspected lead poisoning or liver disease as well as current medication regimen.
- Ensure client has withheld medications that would alter results, as ordered.

Possible Nursing Diagnoses

Trauma, risk for, related to neuromuscular impairment resulting from high levels of lead in blood
Pain related to inflammation or swelling of the liver
Anxiety related to threat to health status

Implementation

- Obtain a clean 3-liter, dark container with preservative (usually glacial acid).
- Instruct client to void and discard sample. The time the discard sample is obtained is the time the collection begins. All urine excreted during the 24-hour period must be saved.
- Instruct the client to maintain refrigeration of the specimen or place on ice during time of collection. If a urinary catheter is in place, keep drainage bag on ice and instruct the client or caregiver to periodically empty drainage bag into specimen container.
- Instruct the client to void the following day at the exact time the test was begun and to add this specimen to the container.
- Label the container properly, including the start and end date and times. Transport the specimen to the laboratory promptly.

Evaluation

- Note results in relation to other tests performed, in particular lead mobilization (urine) or liver enzymes.

Client/Caregiver Teaching

Pretest

- Inform the client that this test detects abnormal hemoglobin formation or, when lead poisoning is suspected, the presence of excessive lead in the body.
- Instruct the client to avoid medications that interfere with test results.
- Instruct the client to void all urine in a bedpan placed in the toilet and then either pour urine into the collection container or leave in the container for the nurse to add to the collection; place a sign in the bathroom as a reminder to save all urine.
- Instruct client to avoid voiding in pan with defecation and to keep toilet tissue out of pan to prevent contamination of the specimen; also inform client not to void directly into container, because the preservative could splash.

Posttest

- Advise client to resume medications withheld before the test.

Dexamethasone Suppression (DST)

Classification: Chemistry

Type of Test: Plasma and urine, timed

Dexamethasone is a glucocorticoid that suppresses adrenocorticotropic hormone (ACTH) and cortisol. Because ACTH secretion is dependent on plasma cortisol levels, as plasma cortisol levels increase, ACTH secretion is suppressed, and as cortisol levels decrease, ACTH secretion is stimulated. Normally, administration of dexamethasone results in suppression of ACTH and a 50 percent or more drop in plasma cortisol and urine cortisol (17-hydroxycorticosteroid [17-OHCS]) levels. The test can be completed overnight or over a 4-day period, with a high or low dose of dexamethasone administered.

Indications

- Diagnosis of Cushing's syndrome
- Aid in diagnosis of depression
- Differentiate between adrenal tumor and hyperplasia

Reference Values

		SI Units
Overnight test		
Low dose	<3 μg/dL	<0.08 μmol/L
Urine 17-OHCS	<4 mg/5 h	<11.0 μmol/5 h
High dose	<50% of baseline	<0.50 of baseline
Urine 17-OHCS	<50% of baseline/24 h	<50% of baseline/24 h
Standard test (6 days) cortisol		
Low dose	<5 μg/dL (day 4)	<138 nmol/L (day 4)
Urine 17-OHCS	<4.5 mg/24 h	<12.4 μmol/24 h
High dose	<10 μg/dL (day 6)	<276 nmol/L (day 6)
Urine 17-OHCS	<50% of baseline (day 6)	<0.50 of baseline (day 6)

Abnormal Values

- Increased levels (failure of suppression)
    Severe stress
    Adrenal hyperplasia (at high doses)
    Adrenal tumors
    Cushing's syndrome
    Lung cancer
    Pregnancy
    Depression
- Decreased levels
    Histoplasmosis
    Tuberculosis

Interfering Factors

- High stress or improper administration of oral dexamethasone can elevate levels.
- Radionuclide scan within previous 24 hours can elevate results.
- Acute illnesses, alcoholism, anorexia nervosa, dehydration, diabetes mellitus, malnutrition, and pregnancy can cause false-positive results.
- Drugs such as barbiturates, carbamazepine, estrogens, meprobamate, methyprylon, phenytoin, reserpine, rifampin, and tetracycline can cause false-positive results.
- Adrenal or pituitary hypofunction can cause false-negative results.
- Drugs such as benzodiazepines, corticosteroids, and amphetamine can cause false-negative results.

Nursing Implications

Assessment

- Obtain history of endocrine disorder (adrenal or pituitary) and any medications that may interfere with test results.
- Ensure that baseline plasma cortisol and urine 17-OHCS have been obtained 24 hours before the test and results have been documented.
- Ensure that food is withheld for 8 hours for overnight test.

Possible Nursing Diagnoses

Fatigue related to decreased metabolic energy production and altered body chemistry
Anxiety related to perceived threat to health status
Fluid volume excess related to increased cortisone levels

Implementation

- Put on gloves. Using aseptic technique, obtain 5 mL of blood in a red-top tube as a baseline plasma cortisol level. Also obtain a baseline urine 17-OHCS level.
- *Overnight test:* Administer dexamethasone 1 mg or 5 mg/kg orally at 11 PM. Collect a 5-hour urine specimen for 17-OHCS from 7 AM to 12 noon. Put on gloves. Using aseptic technique, perform a venipuncture and collect 5 mL of blood at 8 AM in a red-top tube; send blood sample to lab within 30 minutes. Send 5-hour urine for 17-OHCS to lab at 12 noon.
- *Low-dose test:* Administer dexamethasone 0.5 mg every 6 hours for 2 days (total 4 mg); obtain a plasma cortisol level at 8 AM, 4 PM, and 11 PM. Collect a 24-hour urine 17-OHCS on day 2. The high-dose test can follow if low-dose test results in no suppression.
- *High-dose test:* Administer dexamethasone 2 mg PO every 6 hours for 2 days (total 16 mg); obtain a plasma cortisol level at 8 AM, 4 PM, and 11 PM and a 24-hour urine for 17-OHCS after day 2.
- If an indwelling catheter is in place, discard all urine immediately before starting urine collection; label drainage bag denoting times of collection; empty urine from the drainage bag into the plastic urine collection container; label and send to lab immediately.

Evaluation

- Compare results of plasma cortisol and urine cortisol levels. Also note results in relation to ACTH levels.

Client/Caregiver Teaching

Pretest

- Inform the client that the test will involve collection of both blood and urine; reinforce the importance of saving all urine during the designated time period.
- Instruct the client to withhold food for 8 hours before the overnight test.
- Advise client to take dexamethasone with food and antacid to prevent stomach irritation.

Posttest

- Instruct the client to resume medications withheld before the test.

Diaphanography, Breast

Classification: Imaging

Type of Test: Breast visualization

In diaphanography, also known as transillumination of the breast, infrared light is directed through the breast using fiber-optic device. The light that is transmitted through the breast is photographed using infrared film. This test is less reliable than mammography, since it cannot distinguish malignancy from mastitis or hemorrhage. Rarely done in the United States, it is useful in young women with dense breast tissue or fibrocystic disease, or in women who refuse mammography.

Indications

- Detect breast cancer
- Evaluate mammary dysplasia
- Monitor scar tissue of mastectomy patients for disease recurrence
- Guide needle for cyst drainage or biopsy
- Evaluate silicon-injected or augmented breasts

Reference Values

- Normal breast tissue is translucent, reddish-yellow; blood vessels appear dark red to black.

Abnormal Values

- Bright spots indicate fluid-filled cysts or fatty tissue.
- Red spots indicate benign tumors.
- Dark brown or black spots may indicate cancerous tumors.

Interfering Factors

- False-positive results are associated with mastitis, hematoma, fibroadenoma, and papillomatosis.

Nursing Implications

Assessment

■ Obtain history of breast disease, known or suspected breast cancer, presence of breast implants, current medication regimen, diagnostic tests, and results.

Possible Nursing Diagnoses

Anxiety related to perceived threat to health status
Body image disturbance related to change in appearance
Grieving, anticipatory, related to perceived loss or threat of death

Implementation

■ Assist client to a position of comfort. Examiner will shine a beam on breasts, and computerized camera will convert the light into images.

Evaluation

■ Compare the results to test performed in the past and to the clinical presentation.

Client/Caregiver Teaching

Pretest

■ Reassure the client that there is no discomfort involved, or risk factors associated with the procedure.

Posttest

■ Encourage the client to return for follow-up testing, as ordered.

Dick Test

Classification: Infectious disease diagnostic

Type of Test: Skin test

This skin test detects an immunologic response to *Streptococcus pyogenes*, the causative agent for scarlet fever, to determine susceptibility to the disease.

Indications

- Determine susceptibility or resistance to scarlet fever
- Establish immunity to scarlet fever

Reference Values

- No reaction or slight pink streak at the test site, indicating immunity to scarlet fever

Abnormal Values

- Positive response or indication of erythema reveals insufficient antibody protection and susceptibility to scarlet fever.

Interfering Factors

- Improper intradermal injection technique or inaccurate timing or measurement in reading the reaction

Nursing Implications

Assessment

- Obtain a history of previous streptococcal, skin, or other type of infection.
- Obtain a history of allergies or sensitivities to antibiotics.

Possible Nursing Diagnoses

Infection, risk for, related to immunosuppressed inflammatory response

Hyperthermia related to infectious process

Implementation

- Cleanse the skin site on the lower anterior area of the forearm with alcohol or acetone swabs and allow to air-dry. Draw the diluted erythrogenic toxin preparation (0.1 mL) into a tuberculin syringe with a 26-gauge needle attached.
- Inject preparation intradermally and record the test site.
- Read the results in 18 to 24 hours; a positive result at the site is defined as an induration measured at 3 to 5 mm in diameter, accompanied by red erythema and sharply raised edges of the edematous area; induration of less than 1 mm with some redness is classified as a slight positive result.

Evaluation

- Note results in relation to the client's symptoms and other test results, for example, throat culture.

Client/Caregiver Teaching

Pretest

- Inform the client that the test is generally done by a nurse in a physician's office or health care setting and takes about 5 to 10 minutes.

Posttest

- Emphasize to the client that the injection site should not be scratched or rubbed until it is read.
- Emphasize the importance of returning in 18 to 24 hours to have test results read.
- Instruct the client on the importance of taking antibiotics, if ordered.

Drug Levels, Serum

Classification: Toxicology

Type of Test: Serum

Usually performed to test for therapeutic effectiveness of a specific drug, this test is also used to determine if the client is toxic. It is important to know the exact time of the specific drug's ingestion for best interpretation of serum drug levels. Peak levels are generally drawn within 30 to 60 minutes of drug administration or when a drug's steady state has been achieved. Trough levels are drawn immediately before the next dose is to be administered and determines the dosage of drug the client receives.

Indications

- Determine therapeutic levels of prescribed drugs
- Evaluate degree of compliance with therapeutic regimen
- Evaluate known or suspected overdose

Reference Values

- See table, Serum Drug Levels, for specific therapeutic levels.

Abnormal Values

- See table, Serum Drug Levels, for specific toxic levels.

Interfering Factors

- Collecting the blood sample before the drug's steady state has been reached results in decreased levels.
- Antacids, anticholinergics, and barbiturates decrease serum phenothiazine levels.
- Other anticonvulsants such as carbamazepine, phenytoin, phenobarbital, and primidone reduce serum concentration of valproic acid.
- Administration of other anticonvulsants such as phenytoin, phenobarbital, or primidone reduce carbamazepine concentration.
- Drugs such as phenobarbital, carbamazepine, cimetidine, erythromycin, propoxyphene, and valproic acid can cause false values in clients taking phenytoin.

- Drugs such as phenobarbital, phenytoin, primidone, cimetidine, erythromycin, propoxphene, isoniazid, fluoxetine, and calcium channel blocker can cause false values in clients taking carbamazepine.
- Serum ethanol levels are elevated in client's taking chloral hydrate.
- Serum levels of ethanol, isopropanol, and methanol can also be affected by tincture of iodine or alcohol at the puncture site.
- High serum ethanol can result when clients take ethanol and barbiturates together. Increased CNS depression will also result.
- Antacids, aminosalicylic acid, cholestyramine, colestipol, kaolin-pectin, neomycin, phenobarbital, phenytoin, and phenylbutazone can decrease serum digoxin and digitoxin levels.
- Quinidine, calcium channel blockers, and spironolactone can falsely elevate digoxin or digitoxin levels.

Nursing Implications

Assessment

- Obtain medication history, history of known or suspected overdose, and results of tests and procedures performed.

Possible Nursing Diagnosis

Poisoning, risk for, related to blood levels of drugs outside the therapeutic margin of safety

Implementation

- Put on gloves. Using aseptic technique perform a venipuncture and collect a sample of blood using the guidelines detailed in the table, Serum Drug Levels.
- Label the specimen with the client's name, the time specimen was drawn, the site, and the last dose of medication (if known).
- If the client is involved in a medicolegal case, collection, delivery, and transportation of specimen should be witnessed by a legally responsible person.

Evaluation

- Note test results and report critical values to physician.
- Compare the results with urine drug levels.

Client/Caregiver Teaching

Pretest

- Inform the client that there is no special preparation for this test.

Serum Drug Levels

Drug	Peak and Trough Levels	Therapeutic and Toxic Levels	Nursing Implications
Acetaminophen (Tylenol, Tempra, Datril, Liquiprin, Paracetamol, Panadol, Aceta)	*Peak:* 30 min–1 h *Trough:* 1–4 h	*Therapeutic:* 10–30 µg/mL *Toxic:* >150 µg/mL, 4 h after ingestion *Panic:* >200 µg/mL	Collect 3 mL venous blood in clotted red-top or lavender-top tube with EDTA.
Alcohol		*Intoxication:* >150 mg/dL *Coma:* 300 mg/dL *Panic:* 350–800 mg/dL	Cleanse site with povidone iodine solution. Alcohol affects results. Collect 5 mL venous blood in clotted red-top, black-top with sodium oxalate, lavender-top with EDTA, or green- or blue-top tubes. If sample is to be used for legal evidence, follow legal procedures for the state. Collection must be witnessed and laboratory requisition signed by witness.
Amikacin (Amikin)	*Peak:* IM 30 min; IV 15 min *Trough:* 1.9–2.8 h	*Therapeutic:* 20–25 µg/mL *Toxic:* 35 µg/mL	Collect 7 mL venous blood in clotted red-top tube.

Serum Drug Levels

Drug	Peak and Trough Levels	Therapeutic and Toxic Levels	Nursing Implications
Amiodarone (Cordarone)		*Therapeutic:* 0.5–2.5 µg/mL *Toxic:* >2.5 µg/mL	Collect 7 mL venous blood in EDTA-anticoagulated lavender-top tube before dose or 12 h after last dose.
Amitriptyline (Elavil)		*Therapeutic:* 100–250 ng/mL *Panic:* >500 ng/mL	Collect 7 mL venous blood in clotted red-top tube 12 h after last dose.
Amphetamines		*Therapeutic:* 20–120 ng/mL *Toxic:* >2 mg/L	Collect 5 mL venous blood in lavender-top tube.
Amphotericin B (Fungizone)	*Peak:* 60–120 min after IV *Trough:* 24 h	*Therapeutic:* 1–2 µg/mL	Collect 5 mL venous blood (from extremity that does not have amphotericin B infusing into it) in clotted red-top tube.

Carbamazepine (Tegretol)	*Peak:* 4 h *Trough:* adults, 10–30 h children, 8–19 h	*Therapeutic:* 2–10 µg/mL *Toxic:* 12 µg/mL *Panic:* >15 µg/mL	Collect 7 mL venous blood in heparinized green-top tube or lavender-top tube with EDTA before morning dose.
Chlordiazepoxide (Librium)	*Trough:* 5–30 h	*Therapeutic:* 700–100 ng/mL *Panic:* >5000 ng/mL	Collect 5 mL venous blood in heparinized green-top tube or lavender-top tube with EDTA.
Clonazepam (Klonopin)	*Peak:* 1–4 h *Trough:* 18–50 h	*Therapeutic:* 5–70 ng/mL *Toxic:* >70 ng/mL *Panic:* >80 ng/mL	Collect 5 mL venous blood in green-top heparinized tube or lavender-top tube with EDTA.
Cocaine		*Therapeutic:* 100–500 ng/mL *Panic:* (fatal) >1000 ng/mL	Collect 5–10 mL venous blood in green-top tube, heparinized, or lavender-top tube, EDTA. Specimen must be transported on ice; cocaine hydrolyzes in blood and must be processed by gas chromatography within 1 h.

Serum Drug Levels

Drug	Peak and Trough Levels	Therapeutic and Toxic Levels	Nursing Implications
Despiramine (Norpramin)		*Therapeutic:* 75–225 ng/mL *Toxic:* 450–1000 ng/mL	Collect 7 mL venous blood in a red-top tube. Handle gently to prevent hemolysis.
Diazepam (Valium)	*Peak:* 1–4 h *Trough:* 2–4 day	*Therapeutic:* 5–70 ng/mL *Toxic:* >70 ng/mL	Collect 5 mL venous blood in clotted red-top tube 2 h after therapeutic dose.
Digitalis glycosides, including digoxin (Lanoxin) and digitoxin (Crystodigin)	Digoxin *Peak:* 6–8 h orally; 4–6 h IM; 1–5 h IV Digitoxin *Peak:* 4–12 h	Digoxin *Therapeutic:* 0.5–2 ng/mL *Toxic* >3 ng/mL Digitoxin *Therapeutic:* 20–35 ng/mL *Toxic:* >40–45 ng/mL	Collect trough-level sample of 7 mL venous blood in a red-top tube just before administration of next dose (6–8 h after the last dose of digoxin; 4–10 h after last dose of digitoxin).

Drug			
Disopyramide (Norpace, DSP, Napamide, Rythmodan)	*Peak:* 2 h *Trough:* 4–10 h	*Therapeutic:* 2–4.5 μg/mL *Toxic:* >9 μg/mL	Collect 7 mL venous blood in marble-top tube 2–3 hours after oral dose for evaluation of peak; just before the next dose for trough. Expect elevated results in renal failure.
Doxepin (Sinequan)		*Therapeutic:* 100–275 ng/mL *Toxic:* 500 ng/mL	Collect 3 mL venous blood in lavender-top tube.
Ethosuximide (Zarontin)	*Peak:* 1 h *Trough:* adults, 40–60 h children, 30–50 h	*Therapeutic:* 40–80 μg/mL *Toxic:* 100 μg/mL	Collect 5 mL venous blood in heparinized green-top tube.
Flecainide (Tambocor)	*Trough:* 20 h	*Therapeutic:* 0.2–1.0 μg/mL *Toxic:* >1.0 μg/mL	Indicate on lab requisition if client is also taking propranolol or quinidine (which cause unreliable results when spectrofluorometric method used). Collect 7 mL venous blood in clotted red-, green-, or lavender-top tube just before next scheduled dose.

Serum Drug Levels

Drug	Peak and Trough Levels	Therapeutic and Toxic Levels	Nursing Implications
Flucytosine (Ancobon)	*Trough:* 3–6 h	*Therapeutic:* 25–100 µg/mL *Panic:* >125 µg/mL	Collect 5 mL venous blood in clotted red-top or heparinized green-top tube 2 h after oral administration for peak levels and immediately before oral administration for trough levels.
Gentamicin (Garamycin, Jenamicin)	*Trough:* IM, 1 h; IV, 30 min to 1 h	*Therapeutic:* Peak, 4–8 µg/mL Trough, <2 µg/mL *Toxic:* Peak, >12 µg/mL Trough, >2 µg/mL	Collect 7 mL venous blood in a clotted red-top tube just before next dose for trough level; draw peak specimen 30 min to 3 h after IV dose or 15–60 min after IM dose. Mechanical ventilation can decrease gentamicin levels. Toxicity is more likely to occur when other nephrotoxic drugs are administered during therapy.
Haloperidol (Haldol)		*Therapeutic:* 5–16 ng/mL *Toxic:* >25 ng/mL	Collect 7 mL of venous blood in a red-top tube. Refrigerate specimen.

Lidocaine	*Therapeutic:* 2–5 µg/mL *Toxic:* >6 µg/mL	Collect 7 mL of venous blood in a red-top tube. Dialysis or cardiopulmonary bypass decreases levels.
Lithium (Eskalith, Eskalith CR, Lithonate, Lithotabs)	*Trough:* 8–12 h after last dose *Therapeutic:* Trough, 0.8–1.2 mEq/L *Toxic:* >1.5 mEq/L	Collect 7 mL of venous blood in a red-top tube. No relationship between peak concentration and degree of toxicity exists.
Mephobarbital (Mebaral)	*Therapeutic:* 1–7 µg/mL *Toxic:* >14.9 µg/mL	Collect 7 mL of venous blood in a red-top tube.
Meprobamate (Equanil, Meprospan, Miltown, Probate)	*Peak:* 2 hours after dose *Therapeutic:* <10 µg/mL *Toxic:* >99 µg/mL	Collect 5 mL of venous blood in a red-top tube.
Methotrexate (Folex PFS, Rheumatrex)	*Therapeutic:* <0.1 µmol/L after 48 h	Collect 7 mL of venous blood in a red-top tube. Chloral hydrate, phenytoin, salicylates, sulfonamides, and tetracyclines displace methotrexate from the plasma proteins and increase toxicity risk.

Serum Drug Levels

Drug	Peak and Trough Levels	Therapeutic and Toxic Levels	Nursing Implications
Methsuximide (Celontin)		*Therapeutic:* <1 µg/mL	Collect 7 mL of venous blood in a red-top tube.
Methylphenidate (Ritalin)		*Therapeutic:* 0.01–0.04 µg/mL	Collect 7 mL of venous blood in a lavender-top tube.
Nortriptyline (Aventyl, Pamelor)		*Therapeutic:* 50–150 ng/mL *Toxic:* >500 ng/mL	Collect 7 mL of venous blood in a red-top tube (serum) or green-top tube (plasma). Roll green-top tube gently to mix heparin and blood. Increased levels caused by cimetidine, methylphenidate, oral contraceptives, and steroids. Decreased levels may be caused by barbiturates, chloral hydrate, nicotine, and phenobarbital.
Phenobarbital		*Therapeutic:* Adults, 20–40 µg/mL Children, 15–30 µg/mL *Toxic:* >54 µg/mL	Collect 5 mL of venous blood in green- or black-top tube. Draw specimen 1 h before next dose for ongoing monitoring. Peak levels occur 6–18 h after dose.

Phenothiazines, including chlorpromazine (Thorazine, Ormazine), thioridazine (Mellaril), trifluoperazine (Stelazine)	*Therapeutic:* Chlorpromazine, >50 ng/mL Thioridazine, 1.1–1.5 µg/mL Trifluoperazine, <10 ng/mL *Toxic:* Chlorpromazine and thioridazine, >1500 ng/mL Trifluoperazine, >50 ng/mL	Collect 7 mL of venous blood in a red-top tube. For therapeutic monitoring, obtain specimen within 1 h before the next dose and at least 3 h after last dose.
Phenytoin (Dilantin)	*Therapeutic:* Total, 10–20 µg/mL Free, 1–2 µg/mL *Toxic:* Total, >25 µg/mL Free, >2.5 µg/mL	Collect 5 mL of venous blood in a red-top tube. Allow 48 h to pass before measuring plasma level after a dosage change.
Primidone (Mysoline)	*Therapeutic:* Adults, 9–12.5 µg/mL Children < 5 yrs, 7–10 µg/mL *Toxic:* >14.9 µg/mL	Collect 5 mL of venous blood in a red-top tube just before next dose for trough levels. After oral dose, peak levels occur in 2–4 h.

Serum Drug Levels

Drug	Peak and Trough Levels	Therapeutic and Toxic Levels	Nursing Implications
Procainamide (Pronestyl)	*Peak:* 75–90 min after PO dose or immediately after a loading dose *Trough:* Just before next dose	*Therapeutic:* 4–8 µg/mL *Toxic:* >15.9 µg/mL	Collect 5 mL of venous blood in a red-top tube.
Propoxyphene (Darvon)	*Peak:* Hydrochloride, 2–5 h Napsylate, 3–4 h	*Therapeutic:* 0.2–0.5 µg/mL *Toxic:* >5 µg/mL	Collect 5 mL of venous blood in a red-top tube. A urine sample may be obtained at the same time as the serum sample.
Propranolol (Inderal)	*Peak:* 1–2 h after PO dose	*Therapeutic:* 50–100 ng/mL *Toxic:* >1000 ng/mL	Collect 7 mL of venous blood using a syringe. After removing the stopper from the red-top tube, inject the blood sample. Smoking decreases plasma concentrations of this drug.

Drug	Reference Values	Peak	Collection
Quinidine (Quinaglute, Cardioquin, Quinidex)	*Therapeutic:* 2–6 µg/mL *Toxic:* > 10 µg/mL	*Peak:* 1.5–2 h after PO dose	Collect 5 mL of venous blood in a red-top or green-top tube.
Salicylates (Aspirin, acetylsalicylic acid)	*Therapeutic:* 2–20 mg/dL *Toxic:* >50 mg/dL		Collect 7 mL of venous blood in a red-top tube. Serum half-life is 2–3 h in short-term use and 15–30 h in chronic use.
Theophylline (Aminophylline)	*Therapeutic:* Adults, 10–20 µg/mL Children, 5–20 µg/mL *Toxic:* 20 µg/mL	*Peak:* 1–3 h after PO dose	Collect 5 mL of venous blood in a red-top tube. The client's ingestion of xanthines (chocolate, cocoa, coffee, cola or tea) can elevate levels; also drugs including allopurinol, metoprolol, oral contraceptives, and propranolol.
Tobramycin (Nebcin)	*Therapeutic:* Trough, 1–2 µg/mL Peak, 4–8 µg/mL *Panic:* Trough, ≥2 µg/mL Peak, ≥8 µg/mL	*Peak:* IV, 30 min; IM, 30 min–3 h	Collect 5 mL of venous blood in a red-top tube.

Serum Drug Levels

Drug	Peak and Trough Levels	Therapeutic and Toxic Levels	Nursing Implications
Tocainide (Tonocard)		*Therapeutic:* 5–12 μg/mL *Toxic:* >15 μg/mL	Collect 7 mL of venous blood in a green-top tube.
Valproic acid (Depakene, Myproic Acid)	*Peak:* 1–3 h	*Therapeutic:* Peak, 100 μg/mL Trough, 40 μg/mL *Toxic:* >120 μg/mL	Collect 7 mL of venous blood in a red- or green-top tube. Other antiseizure medication may decrease valproic acid levels.
Vancomycin (Vancocin)	*Peak:* IV, 30 min	*Therapeutic:* Peak, 20–40 μg/mL Trough, 5–10 μg/mL *Panic:* Peak, ≥40 μg/mL Trough, ≥15 μg/mL	Collect 5 mL of venous blood in a red-top tube.

Drug Levels, Urine; Drug Abuse Survey

Classification: Toxicology

Type of Test: Urine

Done primarily to test for illicit drugs, alcohol, or other toxins, this test may be used as a screening technique or in an emergency situation to determine if an unconscious or impaired client has ingested these substances. Urine is preferred for drug screening because most drugs (except alcohol concentration) are readily detectable in urine. However, presence of drugs in urine does not adequately reflect level of impairment or the time of ingestion. Serum concentrations more accurately reflects overdose degree and provide a better guide for treatment.

Indications

- Identify drugs used and abused
- Determine possible drug abuse by perspective employees
- Identify drug use to enhance athletic ability
- Confirm drug overdose as cause of death

Reference Values

- See table, Urine Drug Levels, for specific values.

Abnormal Values

- See table, Urine Drug Levels, for specific values.

Interfering Factors

- High or low urine or blood pH or other abnormal constituents can affect results.
- Low specific gravity causing urine dilution may cause false-negative results.

Nursing Implications

Assessment

- Assess history of drug use or abuse, medication regimen including over-the-counter preparations.
- Ensure that the specimen collection is witnessed by a legally responsible person if drug abuse is suspected.

Possible Nursing Diagnosis

Poisoning, risk for, related to blood levels of drugs outside the therapeutic margin of safety

Implementation

- Obtain a random sample of 30 to 50 mL of urine in a clean container.
- Label and place specimen in a plastic bag and seal to avoid tampering.
- If the client is involved in a medicolegal case, collection, delivery, transportation of specimen should be witnessed by a legally responsible person.

Evaluation

- Note results and report positive results to the physician.

Client/Caregiver Teaching

Pretest

- Inform the client of the collection protocol and the possible implications of results.
- Inform the client that confirming tests will be performed if test is positive.

Posttest

- If positive result is confirmed, advise client to consider counseling.

Urine Drug Levels

Drug	Therapeutic and Toxic Levels	Nursing Implications
Alcohol or ethanol	Negative; lower level of detectability; 300 µg/mL	Consent form necessary if test for medicolegal purposes. Collect 30 mL random urine specimen.
Amphetamines, including amphetamine, dextroamphetamine (Dexedrine, Oxydess, Robese), methamphetamine (Desoxyn), phendimetrazine (Adipost, Anorex, Bontril, Obezine, Phendiet, Rexigen, Trimstat, X-Trozine)	*Therapeutic:* Amphetamine, 2–3 µg/mL Dextroamphetamine, 1–15 µg/mL Methamphetamine, 3–5 µg/mL Phendimetrazine, 5–30 µg/mL *Toxic:* Amphetamine, >30 µg/mL Dextroamphetamine, > 15 µg/mL Methamphetamine, > 40 µg/mL Phendimetrazine, > 50 µg/mL	Consent form necessary if test for medicolegal purposes. Collect 30 mL random urine specimen. Acidic urine increases rate of amphetamine excretion while alkaline urine decreases excretion. Drugs such as pseudoephedrine, phenylpropanolamine, and related compounds can cause false-positive results.

Urine Drug Levels

Drug	Therapeutic and Toxic Levels	Nursing Implications
Benzodiazepines, including chlorazepate, chlordiazepoxide, clonazepam, diazepam, flurazepam, lorazepam, medazepam, oxazepam, prazepam, temazepam, and triazolam	Negative; lower level of detectability; 300 ng/mL	Collect 30 mL of clean, voided urine. Refrigerate until tested. To determine therapeutic and toxic levels, a blood sample is needed.
Cannabinoids (marijuana)	Negative; lower level of detectability: 15 ng/mL	Collection, transportation, and processing must be performed with a witness if testing is done for medicolegal purposes. Collect 50-mL urine sample, seal in a plastic bag, label as legal evidence.
Cocaine or benzoylecgonine (major metabolite of cocaine)	Negative; lower level of detectability: 150 ng/mL	Collect 25 mL of urine, seal in plastic bag, and label as legal evidence. After moderate cocaine use, urine remains positive for 2–3 days; with heavy use, it may remain positive for up to 1 week.

Heroin	Negative	Collect a 50-mL random urine sample. Refrigerate sample. Collection, transportation, and processing must be performed with a witness if testing is done for medicolegal purposes. False-positive results can result if the client ingested poppy seeds or cough syrup containing at least 20 mg of codeine. Heroin is rapidly metabolized to morphine and is eliminated from the system within 2 days.
Opiates	Negative; lower limit of detectability: 300 ng/mL	Consent form necessary if test is for medicolegal purposes. Collect 30 mL random urine specimen.
Phencyclidine (PCP)	Negative; lower limit of detectability: 25 ng/mL	Consent form necessary if test is for medicolegal purposes. Collection, transportation, and processing must be performed with a witness if testing is done for medicolegal purposes. Collect 30-mL random urine specimen.

Echocardiography

Classification: Ultrasonography

Type of Test: Indirect visualization

This noninvasive sound study uses high-frequency waves of various intensities to assist in diagnosing cardiovascular disorders. It records the echos created by the deflection of an ultrasonic beam off the cardiac structures and allows for visualization of size, shape, position, thickness, and movement of all four valves, the atria and the ventricles. This study can also determine blood-flow velocity during the movement of the transducer over the areas of the chest. Electrocardiography (ECG) and phonocardiography can be done simultaneously to correlate the findings with the cardiac cycle.

Included in the study are the M mode method, which produces a linear tracing of timed motions of the heart and its structures, and the two-dimensional method, which produces a cross-section of the structures of the heart and their relationship to one another and changes in the coronary vasculature.

Indications

- Diagnose or determine severity of valvular abnormalities
- Measure the size of the heart's chambers and determine if hypertrophic cardiomyopathy or congestive heart failure is present
- Diagnose and evaluate congenital heart disorders
- Diagnose atrial tumors (myxomas)
- Determine the presence of pericardial effusion
- Detect ventricular or atrial mural thrombi and evaluate cardiac wall motion following myocardial infarction
- Diagnose subaortic stenosis as evidenced by the displacement of the anterior atrial leaflet and a reduction in aortic valve flow depending on the obstruction
- Evaluate unexplained chest pain, electrocardiogram changes, and abnormal chest x-ray (enlarged cardiac silhouette)
- Evaluate or monitor prosthetic valve function

Reference Values

- Normal appearance of the size, position, structure, and movements of the heart valves visualized and recorded in a combination of ultrasound modes; normal heart muscle walls of both ventricles and left atrium with adequate blood filling. The established values for the measurement of heart activities obtained by the study may vary with physician and institution.

Abnormal Values

- Pulmonary hypertension
- Pulmonary valve abnormalities
- Mitral valve abnormalities
- Aortic valve abnormalities
- Pericardial effusion
- Ventricular or atrial mural thrombi
- Myxoma
- Coronary artery disease
- Congestive heart failure
- Cardiomyopathy
- Congenital heart defects

Interfering Factors

- Incorrect placement and movement of the transducer over the desired sites or lack of skill in performing the procedure.
- Client obesity, chest thickness, deformity, or other abnormality or trauma can affect the transmission of waves to and from the chest because of increased space between the heart and transducer.
- Presence of chronic obstructive pulmonary disease or use of mechanical ventilation, as this increases the air between the heart and chest wall (hyperinflation) that can attenuate the ultrasound waves.
- Dysrhythmias.
- Inability of the client to remain still during the procedure.

Nursing Implications

Assessment

- Obtain a history of previous cardiac tests and procedures, present cardiac conditions or abnormalities, and therapy received for cardiac condition.

Possible Nursing Diagnoses

Cardiac output, decreased, related to valvular dysfunction
Anxiety related to threat to health status or fear of death
Activity intolerance related to oxygen supply and demand
   imbalance

Implementation

- Place the client in a supine position on the examining table. Expose the chest and attach the electrocardiogram leads for simultaneous tracings, if desired.
- Apply conductive gel to the chest slightly to the left of the sternum. Place the transducer on the chest surface along the left sternal border, the subxiphoid area, suprasternal notch, and supraclavicular areas to obtain views and tracings of portions of the heart. Scan the areas by the systematic movement of the probe in a perpendicular position to direct the ultrasound waves to each part of the heart. These can be viewed immediately and recorded on moving graph paper (M mode) or videotape (two-dimensional).
- To obtain different views or information about heart function, position the client on the left side and sitting up or request that the client breathe slowly or hold breath during the procedure. Amyl nitrate (vasodilator) can be inhaled by the client to evaluate heart function changes.
- When the studies are completed, the leads and gel are removed from the chest.

Evaluation

- Note test results in relation to other tests performed and the client's symptoms.

Client/Caregiver Teaching

Pretest

- Inform the client that the procedure is performed by a technician in an ultrasound room or at the bedside and takes 30 to 45 minutes to complete. Results will be interpreted by a physician, who will discuss findings with the client.
- Inform the client that there are no food or fluid restrictions before the study and that there is no pain or risk of exposure to radiation or complications associated with this study.
- During the study, inform the client that cooperation is important and stress that lying quietly is important. Also warn client that he or she may be asked to inhale a drug, amyl nitrate, to test heart function and that any side effects (flushing, fast heart rate, and dizziness) will quickly subside.

Posttest

- Inform the client that the physician will discuss the findings of the study.
- Provide emotional support if needed while reinforcing information given by physician if more invasive procedures, such as angiography or angioplasty, are advised.

Echocardiography, Transesophageal

Classification: Ultrasonography

Type of Test: Indirect visualization

This noninvasive study is performed to assist in the diagnosis of cardiovascular disorders when the noninvasive echocardiography procedure is contraindicated or does not reveal the information necessary to confirm a diagnosis. This procedure is done with a small transducer attached to a gastroscope that is inserted into the esophagus. The transducer and the ultrasound instrument allows the beam to be directed to the back of the heart. The echoes are amplified and recorded on a screen for visualization and recorded on graph paper or videotape. The depth of the endoscope and movement of the transducer is controlled to obtain various images of the heart structures. This procedure is usually reserved for use during surgery or for those who are obese, suffer from trauma to the chest, or have a chest deformity (barrel chest) as a result of chronic obstructive pulmonary disease, any of which affect the transmission of the waves to and from the chest.

Indications

- Determine cardiac valve and chamber abnormalities when a conventional echocardiography does not produce clear image, for example, in obesity, trauma to or deformity of the chest wall, or lung hyperinflation associated with COPD
- Confirm diagnosis if conventional echocardiography does not correlate with other findings
- Monitor cardiac function during open-heart surgery

Reference Values

- Normal size, position, structures, and movement of the heart valves and heart muscle walls and chamber blood filling; no evidence of valvular stenosis or insufficiency, cardiac tumor, foreign bodies, or coronary artery disease

Abnormal Values

- Myocardial infarction
- Cardiac valve and chamber abnormalities

Interfering Factors

- Incorrect placement and manipulation of the transducer in the esophagus
- Inability of the client to remain still during the procedure

> ### NURSING ALERT
>
> - This procedure is contraindicated in infants and children; procedure should be postponed in clients with laryngospasm, dysrhythmias, or bleeding because of increased risk of complications.

Nursing Implications

Assessment

- Obtain a history of previous cardiac tests and procedures, present cardiac conditions or abnormalities, and therapy received for cardiac condition.
- Ensure that food and fluids have been restricted for 8 to 12 hours before the procedure.

Possible Nursing Diagnoses

Cardiac output, decreased, related to valvular dysfunction
Anxiety related to threat to health status or fear of death
Activity intolerance related to oxygen supply and demand imbalance

Implementation

- Spray or swab the client's throat with a local anesthetic and place device in the mouth to prevent biting of the endoscope.
- Place the client in a left side-lying position on the examining table. The pharyngeal area is anesthetized and the endo-

scope with the ultrasound device attached to its tip is inserted 30 to 50 cm to the posterior area of the heart, as in any esophagoscopy procedure.

- The client is requested to swallow as the scope is inserted. When the transducer is in place, the scope is manipulated by controls on the handle to obtain scanning that provides real-time images of the heart motion and recordings of the images for viewing. Actual scanning is usually limited to 15 minutes or until the desired number of image planes are obtained at different depths of the scope.
- When the studies are completed, the scope is removed and the client placed in a semi-Fowler's position to prevent aspiration until the gag reflex returns.

Evaluation

- Note test results in relation to other tests performed and the client's symptoms.

Client/Caregiver Teaching

Pretest

- Inform the client that the procedure is generally performed in a special laboratory room by a physician and that it takes about 1 hour to complete.
- Advise the client to withhold food and fluids for 8 to 12 hours before the procedure.
- Explain that some discomfort is experienced during the insertion of the scope.

Posttest

- Instruct client to treat throat discomfort with lozenges and warm gargles when the gag reflex returns.
- Inform the client that the physician will discuss the results of the study.

Electro-oculography (EOG)

Classification: Electrophysiologic study, sensory organ function

Type of Test: Visual perception

This ophthalmology study is performed to measure electrical potentials between the front of the eye and the retina. The study determines changes in the potentials in a dark and light environment with the eye at rest. Abnormalities are based on increases in electrical potentials in relation to increased light. The EOG study can be followed by fluorescein angiography to diagnose vascular disorders of the retina or done in conjunction with electroretinography to diagnose congenital disorders of the retina.

Indications

- Evaluate retinal functional status in retinitis pigmentosa when done in conjunction with electroretinography
- Diagnose retinopathy caused by antimalarial or other toxic drugs
- Evaluate retinal damage present in albinism or irideremia
- Diagnose congenital form of macular degeneration in younger clients

Reference Values

- Normal retinal function with an electrical potential of 1.80 to 2, depending on testing methods

Abnormal Values

- Retinitis pigmentosa
- Macular degeneration

Interfering Factors

- Improper placement of the electrodes around the eyes
- Inability to understand or cooperate with instructions for eye movement during the procedure

> ### ▶ NURSING ALERT
>
> - Perform electro-oculography (EOG) first if client is to receive both EOG and fluorescein angiography (FA).
> - If FA is performed first, wait at least 2 hours before performing electro-oculography.

Nursing Implications

Assessment

- Obtain history of known or suspected congenital or acquired eye disorders or diseases that predispose to eye abnormalities, signs and symptoms of eye condition, medication regimen, and previous tests and procedures.
- Determine whether electroretinography or fluorescein angiography is to be performed on the same day and the proper succession of the tests and waiting periods between them.
- Ensure no makeup is applied to face before study.

Possible Nursing Diagnoses

Sensory-perceptual alterations, visual, related to retinal abnormalities

Anxiety related to threat to health status

Implementation

- Place the client in a sitting position. Place electrodes to the skin at the inner and outer canthi of the eye. The electrodes receive the stimulus and the responses are recorded on a chart.
- The first recording is made of measurements of electrical potentials of the eye at rest and during specific movements in a dark room, then a light stimulus is provided and measurements of the eye potentials at rest and during the same movements are recorded. The normal recordings should reflect an increase in potentials between the front and back of the eye when light is applied, with increases proportional to increases in the light stimulus.

Evaluation

- Note results in relation to other tests performed and the client's symptoms.

Client/Caregiver Teaching

Pretest

- Inform the client that the procedure is performed in a special laboratory by a physician and evaluates the health of the retina in the eye and takes about 30 minutes.
- Instruct the client not to apply makeup the day of the test.

Posttest

- Inform the client that the physician will discuss the results. Also stress the importance of follow-up visits to evaluate retinal changes.
- Inform the client of aids to use to enhance visual perception, such as large-print materials.

Electrocardiography, Electrocardiogram (ECG)

Classification: Electrophysiologic study

Type of Test: Indirect measurement (cardiac activity)

A noninvasive study that measures the electrical currents or impulses that are generated by the heart during a cardiac cycle. The electrical activity is recorded in waveforms and complexes by an ECG, which are analyzed by time intervals and segments. Continuous tracing of cardiac cycle activities are captured as heart cells are electrically stimulated, causing depolarization and movement of the activity through the cells of the myocardium.

The ECG study is performed using 12 leads (electrodes) attached to the skin surface to obtain the total electrical activity of the heart. The different leads are the bipolar (standard limb leads I, II, III), the unipolar (augmented limb leads AVR, AVL, AVF), and the six chest precordial chest leads (V_1–V_6). Each lead records the electrical potential between the limbs or between the heart and the limbs.

The ECG machine records and marks the 12 leads on the strip in proper sequence, usually 6 inches of the strip for each lead. The tracings are recorded on graphic paper with vertical and horizontal lines for analysis and calculations of time measured by the vertical lines (1 mm apart and 0.04 seconds per line) and of voltage measured by the horizontal lines (1 mm apart and 0.5 mV per 5 squares). Pulse rate can be calculated from the ECG strip to obtain the beats per minute.

Indications

- Identify abnormal rhythms or dysrhythmias in adults and children to determine the cause, as evidenced by abnormal wave deflections
- Determine conduction defects or diseases, as evidenced by delay of electrical impulses with abnormal time duration and amplitude of PR waves and intervals recorded on the strip
- Diagnose and determine the site and extent of myocardial or pulmonary infarction and myocardial ischemia, as evidenced by abnormal ST wave, interval times, and amplitudes
- Determine hypertrophy of chambers of the heart (atrial and ventricular) or heart hypertrophy, as evidenced by P or R wave deflections
- Determine the position of the heart in the thoracic cavity
- Diagnose pericarditis and Wolff-Parkinson-White syndrome, as evidenced by ST-segment changes or shortened PR interval
- Determine electrolyte imbalances of potassium, calcium, and magnesium and possible effect on the heart, as evidenced by short or prolonged QT interval
- Evaluate and monitor the effect of drugs, such as digitalis, antiarrhythmic, or vasodilating agents
- Evaluate and monitor cardiac pacemaker function
- Monitor healing of myocardial infarction

Reference Values

- Normal heart rate according to age: range of 60–100/min in adults
- Normal, regular rhythm and wave deflections with normal measurement ranges of cycle components and height, depth, and duration of complexes as detailed below.
    P wave: 0.12 s or 3 small blocks with amplitude of 2.5 mm
    Q wave: <0.04 s
    R wave: range of 5–27 mm amplitude depending on lead
    T wave: range of 1–13 mm amplitude depending on lead
    QRS complex: 0.12 s or 3 small blocks
    PR interval: 0.2 s or 5 small blocks
    ST segment: 1 mm (see figure)

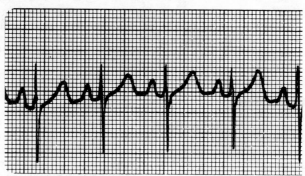

Lead II. (From Baldwin, et al. Davis's Manual of Critical Care Therapeutics, 1995, p 688, with permission.)

Abnormal Values

- Dysrhythmias
- Myocardial infarction or ischemia
- Pericarditis
- Atrial or ventricular hypertrophy
- Electrolyte imbalances
- Wolff-Parkinson-White syndrome

Interfering Factors

- Improper placement of electrodes or inadequate contact between skin and electrodes by insufficient conductive jelly or poor placement
- ECG machine malfunction or interference from electromagnetic waves in the vicinity
- Inability of client to remain still during the procedure; movement, muscle tremor, or twitching can affect accurate test recording
- Strenuous exercising before the procedure
- Increased client anxiety level with hyperventilations or deep respirations
- High intake of carbohydrates, electrolyte imbalances of potassium or calcium
- Cardiac cycle distortions caused by age and sex, especially if the client is an infant or adult female

- Obesity, ascites, and pregnancy
- Chest configuration and heart location in the chest if leads are not placed properly
- Medications such as barbiturates and digitalis preparations

---

NURSING ALERT

- If the ECG changes indicate severe ischemia or necrosis associated with myocardial infarction, immediate interventions should be carried out, such as the administration of oxygen, sedation, antiarrhythmics, vasodilators, and other medications to control coronary artery spasms and tachycardia.

Nursing Implications

Assessment

- Obtain history of cardiac disease and present cardiovascular status, cardiac medication regimen, and previous tests and procedures done.
- Ensure skin where electrodes will be placed is cleansed gently with an alcohol wipe.
- Assess for compliance with smoking restriction before the procedure.

Possible Nursing Diagnoses

Cardiac output, decreased, related to decreased myocardial contractility or dysrhythmias

Pain related to ischemia or inflammation

Anxiety related to threat to health status or fear of death

Activity intolerance related to oxygen supply and demand imbalance

Implementation

- Have client disrobe from waist up, remove hosiery, and put on a hospital gown.
- Place client in a supine position. Expose and appropriately drape the chest, arms, and legs and cleanse the electrode

placement sites with alcohol. Excessive hair on the skin can be shaved, if needed. Dry the skin sites and apply electrode paste to provide conduction between the skin and electrode.

- Apply the electrodes in the proper position using color-coding for placement sites (chest, right and left arm, and right and left leg). When placing the six unipolar chest leads (also called precordial leads or V leads) place V_1 at the fourth intercostal space at the border of the right sternum, V_2 at the fourth intercostal space at the border of the left sternum, V_3 between the V_2 and V_4, V_4 at the fifth intercostal space at the midclavicular line, V_5 at the level of V_4 horizontally and at the left axillary line, V_6 at the level of V_4 horizontally and at the left midaxillary line. The wires are connected to the matched electrodes and the ECG machine.
- Next place three limb bipolar leads (2 electrodes combined for each) on the arms and legs. Lead I is the combination of two arm electrodes, lead II is the combination of right arm and left leg electrodes, and lead III is the combination of left arm and left leg electrodes.
- Remind the client to lie still and refrain from tensing muscles following electrode placement. The machine is set and turned on after the electrodes, grounding, connections, and paper supply are checked.
- When test is complete remove the electrodes and clean the gel from the skin.

Evaluation

- Note results in relation to previous ECGs performed and serum electrolyte values.
- Note cardiac rhythm abnormalities on the strip; administer oxygen, vasodilators, antiarrhythmics if myocardial infarction, ischemia, life-threatening dysrhythmias or ventricular tachycardia are present.

Client/Caregiver Teaching

Pretest

- Explain that the electrocardiogram procedure is performed to assess the electrical impulses and activity of the heart and is completed within 15 minutes or less.

- Explain that the procedure is performed by a technician either at the bedside, a special laboratory room, or the physician's office, depending on client status, and that the results are interpreted by a physician.
- Inform the client that electric impulses from the heart are transmitted from the body and no electricity is delivered to the body and no discomfort is associated with this procedure.
- Instruct the client to lie very still in a relaxed position during the study and at rest for about 15 minutes before the study.

Posttest

- Instruct the client to immediately notify physician of chest pain, changes in pulse rate, or shortness of breath.
- Instruct the client or caregiver in the correct administration of heart medication and the side effects to report.

ECG Variations: Vectorcardiography (VCG), Apexcardiography, Signal-Averaged Electrocardiography

Vectorcardiography, another form of ECG, portrays a three-dimensional display of the heart's activity: the frontal, horizontal, and sagittal planes, as opposed to the two-dimensional display in the frontal and horizontal planes of the ECG. It is considered more sensitive and specific in diagnosing heart abnormalities and is frequently used to differentiate between causes of intraventricular conduction and ventricular hypertrophy. For vectorcardiography, conductive electrodes are applied to the anterior and posterior upper torso, the left lower extremity, and the forehead or nape of the neck. Findings are compared to the clients ECG.

Apexcardiography is a study performed with ECG or phonocardiography to record chest movements resulting from cardiac impulses and provides additional information in diagnosing ventricular abnormalities. After placing a transducer over the apex of the heart or the point of maximal impulse (PMI), the client is placed in the side-lying position and requested to breathe slowly, hold the breath, and perform hand gripping to determine effects of these activities on ventricular function. Changes are recorded as waveforms on the paper strip and identified as periods of systole and diastole. This test is used frequently to help identify heart sounds.

Signal-averaged electrocardiography, another electrophysiologic study, is performed to determine risk of ventricular dysrhythmias in clients with a myocardial infarction. Although the procedure is similar to ECG, the electrodes are placed on the abdomen and the anterior and posterior chest. The high-frequency, low-amplitude signals from the myocardium are converted into signals, which are compared to normal cardiac cycle signals, mainly the QRS complex. A number of heartbeats are averaged to obtain late potentials indicative of ventricular tachycardia, other ventricular abnormalities, or myocardial infarction.

Electrocardiography, Ambulatory; Ambulatory Monitoring; Holter Electrocardiography; Holter Monitoring

Classification: Electrophysiologic study

Type of Test: Indirect measurement (cardiac activity)

This noninvasive study is performed to record the cardiac activity on a continuous basis for 24 to 48 hours. The study includes the use of a portable device worn around the waist or over the shoulder that records cardiac electrical impulses on a magnetic tape. The recorder has a clock that allows for accurate time markings on the tape. When the client pushes a button indicating that symptoms (pain, palpitations, dyspnea, syncope) have occurred, an event marker is placed on the tape for later comparison with the cardiac activity.

Indications

- Detect dysrhythmias that occur during normal daily activities and correlate them with symptoms experienced by the client
- Evaluate the effectiveness of antiarrhythmic medications for dosage adjustment, if needed
- Monitor for ischemia and arrhythmias after myocardial infarction or cardiac surgery before changing rehabilitation and other therapy regimens
- Evaluate pacemaker function
- Evaluate chest pain

Reference Values

- Normal sinus rhythm

Abnormal Values

- Dysrhythmias such as premature ventricular contractions, bradyarrhythmias, tachyarrhythmias, conduction defects, brady-tachyarrhythmia syndrome
- Cardiomyopathy
- Mitral valve abnormality
- Palpitations

Interfering Factors

- Improper placement of the electrodes or movement of the electrodes
- Failure of the client to maintain a daily log of symptoms or to push the button to produce a mark on the strip when experiencing a symptom

NURSING ALERT

- This procedure is contraindicated in clients who are unable or unwilling to maintain the electrodes and ECG apparatus and the daily log of activities and symptoms.

Nursing Implications

Assessment

- Obtain history of cardiac disease and present cardiovascular status, cardiac medication regimen, and previous tests and procedures done.
- Ensure skin where electrodes will be placed is cleansed with an alcohol wipe.
- Assess for compliance with directions given regarding daily log and pressing button with pain or discomfort.

Possible Nursing Diagnoses

Cardiac output, decreased, related to decreased myocardial contractility, valvular dysfunction, or dysrhythmias

Pain related to ischemia or inflammation

Anxiety related to threat to health status or fear of death

Activity intolerance related to oxygen supply and demand imbalance

Implementation

- Place the client in a supine position. Expose the chest and cleanse the skin sites thoroughly with alcohol and rub until red in color. Shave excessive hair at sites. Apply electropaste to the skin sites to provide conduction between the skin and electrodes or apply disk electrodes that are prelubricated and disposable.
- Apply two electrodes on the manubrium (negative electrodes), one in the V_1 position (fourth intercostal space at the border of the right sternum), and one at V_5 position (level of fifth intercostal space at the midclavicular line, horizontally and at the left axillary line) positions (positive electrodes). A ground electrode is also placed and secured to the skin of the chest or abdomen.
- Following a check to ensure that the electrodes are secure, the electrode cable is attached to the monitor and the lead wires attached to the electrodes. The monitor is checked for paper supply and battery, the tape inserted, and the recorder turned on. All wires are taped to the chest and the belt or shoulder strap placed in the proper position.
- After the testing period, remove the chest electrodes and clean the sites.

Evaluation

- Note test results in relation to client symptoms. If available, compare the journal and tape recordings for changes during monitoring activities.

Client/Caregiver Teaching

Pretest

- Inform the client that the purpose of the procedure is to evaluate how the heart responds to normal activity or, if appropriate, to a medication regimen. Explain that no electricity is delivered to the body during this procedure and no discomfort is experienced during the monitoring.
- Inform the client that the ECG recorder is worn for 24 to 48 hours, at which time the client is to return to the laboratory with the log to have the monitor and strip removed for interpretation.
- Advise the client to avoid contact with electric devices that can affect the strip tracings (shavers, toothbrush, massager, blanket) and to avoid showers and tub bathing.
- Instruct the client to perform the normal activities and enter them in a log, such as walking, sleeping, climbing stairs, sexual activity, bowel or urinary elimination, cigarette smoking, emotional upsets, and medications.
- Instruct the client to wear loose-fitting clothing over the electrodes and not to disturb or disconnect the electrodes or wires.
- Advise the client to report a light signal on the monitor that indicates equipment malfunction or that an electrode has come off.

Electrocardiography, Exercise; Exercise Stress Test

Classification: Electrophysiologic study

Type of Test: Indirect measurement (cardiac activity under stress)

This noninvasive study is performed to measure cardiac function during physical stress. Exercise electrocardiography is primarily useful in determining the extent of coronary artery occlusion by the heart's ability to meet the need for additional oxygen in response to the stress of exercising in a safe environment. The client exercises to increase the heart rate to 80 to 90 percent of the maximal heart rate determined by age and sex, known as the target heart rate. The risks involved in the procedure are possible myocardial infarct and death in those experiencing frequent angina episodes prior to the test. Although useful, this procedure is not as accurate in diagnosing coronary artery disease as the nuclear scans, thallium-201 cardiac stress studies or technetium-99m labeled with red blood cells multigated cardiac stress studies.

Indications

- Evaluate suspected coronary artery disease (CAD) in the presence of chest pain and other symptoms
- Screen for CAD in the absence of pain and other symptoms in clients at risk
- Diagnose dysrhythmias during exercising, as evidenced by ECG changes
- Evaluate cardiac function following myocardial infarction or cardiac surgery in order to determine safe cardiac rehabilitation exercising and work limitations
- Determine hypertension as a result of exercising
- Detect peripheral arterial occlusive disease (intermittent claudication), as evidenced by leg pain or cramping during exercising
- Evaluate effectiveness of medication regimens, such as antianginals or antiarrhythmics

Reference Values

- Normal heart rate during physical exercise. Heart rate rises in direct proportion to the workload and metabolic oxygen demand as well as the systolic blood pressure. Normally maximal heart rate for adults is 150 to 200 beats per minute.

Abnormal Values

- Coronary artery disease
- Tachycardia
- Bradycardia
- Dysrhythmias
- Hypertension
- Peripheral arterial occlusive disease

Interfering Factors

- Improper electrode placement or ECG machine malfunction
- High food intake or smoking before testing
- Drugs, such as beta blockers, cardiac glycosides, calcium channel blockers, coronary vasodilators, and barbiturates
- Potassium or calcium imbalance

NURSING ALERT

This procedure is contraindicated in:
- Frequent angina episodes or presence of chest pain
- Following myocardial infarction, unless limitations are placed on testing activities
- Uncontrolled arrhythmias, dissecting aortic aneurysm, aortic valvular disease, inflammatory conditions of the cardiac muscles
- Clients with inability to walk or peddle because of motor disability or impaired lung function
- Congestive heart failure (severe), digitalis toxicity, heart blocks, and recent pulmonary embolism

Nursing Implications

Assessment

- Obtain history of cardiac disease and present cardiovascular status, cardiac medication regimen, and previous tests and procedures done
- Assess for chest pain within the prior 48 hours or attacks of angina several times a day; inform physician, as the stress test can be too risky and should be rescheduled in 4 to 6 weeks.
- Ensure that the client has abstained from food, fluids, and smoking for at least 4 hours before the test and that the client has discontinued specific medications that interfere with test results, as ordered.

Possible Nursing Diagnoses

Cardiac output, decreased, related to decreased myocardial contractility, valvular dysfunction, or dysrhythmias

Pain related to ischemia or inflammation

Anxiety related to threat to health status or fear of death

Activity intolerance related to oxygen supply and demand imbalance

Tissue perfusion, altered, peripheral, related to vascular occlusion

Implementation

- Clients are instructed to remove clothing from the waist up; women are given a hospital gown that opens in the front. Electrodes are placed in appropriate positions on the client, a blood pressure cuff connected to a monitoring device is applied, and the client's oxygen consumption is continuously monitored via a mouthpiece.
- Baseline ECG tracing and blood pressure readings are obtained. Client is requested to walk on a treadmill (most commonly used) or peddle a bicycle. As the stress is increased, client is requested to report any symptoms such as chest or leg pain, dyspnea, or fatigue. Stress is increased until the client's maximal heart rate level is reached.
- Tell the client to report symptoms such as dizziness, sweating, breathlessness, or nausea, which can be normal as speed is increased. The test is terminated if pain or fatigue is severe, maximum heart rate under stress is attained, signs of ischemia are present, maximum effort has been achieved, or dyspnea, hypertension (systolic blood pressure >250 mm Hg), tachycardia (>200 beats per minute minus person's age), new dysrhythmias, chest pain that begins or worsens, faintness, extreme dizziness, or confusion develops.
- Following the exercise period, a 3- to 10-minute rest period is given with the client in a sitting position. During this period the ECG, blood pressure, and heart rate monitoring is continued.

Evaluation

- Note results in relation to the client's symptoms and other test results.

Client/Caregiver Teaching

Pretest

- Inform the client that the procedure is performed in a special laboratory by a technician with a physician in attendance to interpret results. Explain that this procedure is performed to evaluate the heart's ability to respond to an increased workload and takes from 45 minutes to 90 minutes to complete.
- Assure client that the test has very few risks and that exercising can be terminated if extreme symptoms occur.

- Advise client to wear comfortable shoes and clothing for the exercise.

Posttest

- Instruct client to call physician to report any anginal pain or other discomforts experienced after the test.
- Instruct in special dietary intake and medication regimen, as needed.

Electrocardiography, His Bundle

Classification: Electrophysiologic study

Type of Test: Invasive measurement (cardiac activity)

Performed during cardiac catheterization, this test provides information on intra-atrial and intraventricular conduction, which is not provided by a regular ECG. During right heart catheterization, a bipolar or tripolar electrode catheter is slowly withdrawn from the right ventricle through the His bundle to the sinoatrial (SA) node. Impulses are measured as the catheter is withdrawn and the intervals are measured.

Indications

- Determine precise location of bundle branch block
- Evaluate bypass tract physiology
- Evaluate syncope and determine appropriateness of permanent pacemaker implantation
- Diagnose sick sinus syndrome and evaluate tachyarrhythmias
- Monitor effectiveness of antiarrhythmic drug therapy

Reference Values

- H-V interval: 35–55 msec
- A-H interval: 45–150 msec
- P-A interval: 20–40 msec

Abnormal Values

- Prolonged H-V interval
  His-Purkinje disease
- Prolonged A-H interval
  AV node disease
  Atrial pacing
  Recent myocardial infarction
- Prolonged P-A interval
  Atrial disease (acquired or surgically induced)
  Atrial pacing
- Prolonged sinus node recovery time
  Sick sinus syndrome
- Prolonged SA conduction time
  Sinus exit block
- Split or wide His bundle
  His bundle lesion

Interfering Factors

- Improper catheter position

NURSING ALERT

- This procedure is contraindicated in clients with coagulopathy, acute pulmonary embolism, allergy to contrast media, or extreme cardiomegaly.

Nursing Implications

Assessment

- Obtain a cardiac history, including signs and symptoms, results of other tests performed, and medication regimen.
- Ensure that the client fasted from foods and fluids for 6 hours before the test.

Possible Nursing Diagnoses

Cardiac output, decreased, related to dysrhythmias
Pain, risk for, related to ischemia
Anxiety related to threat to health status or fear of death
Activity intolerance related to oxygen supply and demand imbalance

Implementation

- Make sure emergency equipment and medications are available throughout the procedure.

- Place the client supine on an x-ray table and attach ECG leads.
- Prepare the catheter insertion site and drape for the surgical procedure. The physician will inject the insertion site with local anesthesia.
- As the catheter is inserted (fluoroscopy can be used to guide insertion) into the right ventricle, baseline information is recorded.
- Then the catheter is slowly withdrawn from the tricuspid area and readings are taken from each pole of the catheter. In some cases the heart is stimulated by a pacemaker, to induce a dysrhythmia while readings are taken.
- Catheters are removed and a pressure bandage applied to the catheter site.

Evaluation

- Note results in relation to the client's symptoms.
- Monitor vital signs according to institution policy.
- Monitor the catheter insertion site for bleeding.

Client/Caregiver Teaching

Pretest

- Inform the client that the procedure will be performed in a special laboratory by a physician and may take up to 3 hours.
- Instruct the client to fast from food and fluids for at least 6 hours before the test.
- Inform the client that feelings such as bugs crawling (as the catheter is advanced) may be noted; also fast heart rates and lightheadedness or dizziness may be experienced.

Posttest

- Inform the client that bed rest may be required for up to 12 hours after the test. The affected extremity should be immobilized with sandbags, as required, and ice applied, if ordered.
- Instruct the client to notify the physician of any bleeding from the insertion site, chest pain, or pain, redness, or swelling of the extremity used for the catheter insertion.
- Encourage increased fluid intake unless contraindicated.

Electroencephalography, Electroencephalogram (EEG)

Classification: Electrophysiologic study

Type of Test: Indirect measurement (cerebral activity)

This noninvasive study measures the brain's electrical activity and records it on graph paper. Electrodes placed at 8 to 16 sites (or pairs of sites) on the client's scalp record the brain's electrical activity and transmit the different frequencies and amplitudes to the electroencephalograph, which records the results in graph form on a moving paper strip.

Indications

- Diagnose seizure disorders and identify focus of seizure and seizure activity, as evidenced by abnormal spikes and waves recorded on the graph
- Diagnose intracranial cerebrovascular lesions such as hemorrhages and infarcts
- Determine presence of tumors or abscesses
- Confirm suspicion of increased intracranial pressure caused by trauma or disease
- Identify area of abnormality in dementia
- Evaluate sleeping disorders such as sleep apnea and narcolepsy
- Evaluate the effect of drug intoxication on the brain
- Detect cerebral ischemia during endarterectomy
- Confirm brain death

Reference Values

- Normal occurrences of alpha, beta, theta, and delta waves. Rhythms vary depending on the client's age.

Abnormal Values

- Glioblastoma and other brain tumors
- Encephalitis

- Seizure disorders
- Head injury
- Abscess
- Migraine headaches
- Psychosis
- Narcolepsy
- Sleep apnea

Interfering Factors

- Inability to remain still and refrain from moving facial muscles, mouth, head, or eyes during the study will alter brain waves.
- Drugs such as sedatives, anticonvulsants, antiaxolytics, and alcohol, or caffeine or other stimulants can affect results.
- Hypoglycemic or hypothermic states can cause alterations in wave patterns.
- Hair that is dirty, oily, or sprayed or treated with hair preparations can affect test results.

Nursing Implications

Assessment

- Obtain history and assessment of neurologic system, known or suspected seizure activity, intracranial abnormalities, and sleep disorders as well as previous tests and procedures done.
- Ensure caffeine-containing beverages have been withheld and that a meal has been ingested before the study.
- Ensure specific drugs that can interfere with test results have been withheld for 24 to 48 hours before the test, as ordered.
- Ensure client is able to relax; report any extreme anxiety or restlessness.
- Ensure hair is clean and free of gels, hairsprays, or lotions.

Possible Nursing Diagnoses

Pain related to altered cerebral blood flow
Trauma, risk for, related to altered level of consciousness
Tissue perfusion, cerebral, altered, related to obstruction of blood flow

Implementation

- Place the client in the supine position in bed or semi-Fowler's position on a recliner in a special room protected from any noise or electrical interferences that could affect the tracings.

Remind the client to relax and not move any muscles or parts of the face or head. The technician should be able to observe the client for movements or other interferences through a window into the test room.

- The electrodes are prepared and applied to the scalp. Electrodes are placed in as many as 16 locations over the frontal, temporal, parietal, and occipital areas and amplifier wires attached. An electrode is also attached to each ear lobe as grounders. At this time, a baseline recording can be made with the client at rest.
- As the test begins, recordings are made with the client at rest and eyes closed. Recordings are also made during a drowsy and sleep period depending on the client's clinical condition and symptoms. In certain instances, procedures are done to bring out abnormal patterns, such as hyperventilation for 3 minutes to produce a state of alkalosis, which could precipitate a seizure pattern or other abnormalities; stroboscopic light stimulation to record seizure activity produced by photic stimulation; sleep induction by administration of a sedative to detect abnormalities that occur only during sleep.
- Observations for seizure activity are carried out during the study and a description and time of the activity is noted by the technician.
- Remove electrodes from hair and remove paste by cleansing with acetone.

Evaluation

- Note results in relation to other studies and the client's symptoms.

Client/Caregiver Teaching

- Instruct client to limit sleep to 5 hours for an adult and 7 hours for a child the night before the study. Young infants and children should not be allowed to nap before the study.
- Explain that the procedure is performed in a special EEG or sleep laboratory by a technician trained to do the procedure and interpreted by a physician. Explain that this procedure is performed to evaluate the electrical activity of brain and takes from 1 to 2 hours to complete.
- Assure client that there is no discomfort during the test. However, if needle electrodes are used, a slight pinch may be felt. Also explain that electricity flows from the body and not into the body during the study. Inform the client that the test only reveals brain activity, not thoughts, feelings, or intelligence.

- Instruct the client to remain very still and relaxed and co-operate with the instructions given. Tell clients that they may be asked to alter their breathing pattern; follow simple commands such as opening or closing their eyes, blinking, or swallowing; be stimulated with bright lights; or given a drug to induce sleep during the study. A period in which the recording is stopped and movement is allowed during the test is provided about every 5 minutes.

Posttest

- Inform the client to resume medication regimen.
- Instruct the client to report any seizure activity.
- Provide support during or after diagnostic findings are revealed, especially if more invasive procedures such as cerebral angiography or a nuclear scan is necessary. Provide appropriate instruction.

Electrolytes, Serum: Calcium (Ca), Chloride (Cl), Sodium (Na), Potassium (K) Magnesium (Mg), Phosphorus (P), Bicarbonate (HCO₃)

Classification: Chemistry

Type of Test: Serum, plasma

Electrolytes dissociate into electrically charged ions when dissolved. Cations carry positive charges, while anions carry negative charges. Both affect the electrical and osmolar functioning of the body. Body fluids contain equal numbers of positive and negative charges, although the nature of the ions and mobility differ in the intracellular and extracellular fluid compartments. Electrolyte quantities and the balance among them in the body-fluid compartments are controlled by oxygen and carbon dioxide exchange in the lungs; absorption, secretion, and excretion of many substances by the kidneys; and secretion of regulatory hormones by the endocrine glands.

Calcium (Ca^{++}) is the most abundant cation in the body and participates in almost all vital processes. About half the total amount of calcium circulates as free ions that participate in blood coagulation, neuromuscular conduction, intracellular regulation, glandular secretion, and control of skeletal and cardiac-muscle contractility. The remaining calcium is bound to circulating proteins and plays no physiological role. Serum calcium measurement includes both ionized and protein-bound calcium. Calcium levels are largely regulated by the parathyroid glands and vitamin D.

Chloride (Cl^-) is the most abundant anion in extracellular fluid. Its most important function is in the maintenance of acid-base balance. It participates with sodium in the maintenance of water balance and aids in the regulation of osmotic pressure. It contributes to gastric acid (hydrochloric acid, HCl) for digestion and activation of enzymes.

Sodium (Na^{++}) is the most abundant cation in extracellular fluid and, together with its accompanying chloride and bicarbonate anions, accounts for 92 percent of serum osmolality. It plays a major role in maintaining homeostasis in a variety of ways, including maintaining osmotic pressure of extracellular fluid, regulating renal retention and excretion of water, maintaining acid-base balance, regulating potassium and chloride levels, stimulating neuromuscular reactions, and maintaining systemic blood pressure.

Potassium (K^+) is the most abundant intracellular cation. It is essential for the transmission of electrical impulses in cardiac and skeletal muscle. It also helps to maintain osmolality and electroneutrality of cells, functions in enzyme reactions that transform glucose into energy and amino acids into proteins, and participates in the maintenance of acid-base balance.

Phosphorus (P), the dominant intracellular anion, is measured in serum as phosphate (HPO_4^-). Results are reported as inorganic phosphorus. Phosphates are vital constituents of nucleic acids, intracellular energy storage compounds, intermediary compounds in carbohydrate metabolism, and various regulatory compounds, including those that modulate the dissociation of oxygen from hemoglobin. It aids in the regulation of calcium levels and functions as a buffer in maintaining acid-base balance. It contributes to the mineralization of bones and teeth, promotes renal tubular reabsorption of glucose, and aids in fat transport as a component of phospholipids. Phosphorus levels are largely regulated by the parathyroid glands and vitamin D and are reciprocal to the calcium level.

Magnesium (Mg^{++}) is most abundant in red blood cells and is an essential nutrient found in bone and muscle. It functions to control sodium, potassium, calcium, and phosphorus; the utilization of carbohydrate, lipid, and protein; and activation of enzyme systems that enable B vitamins to function. It is also essential for oxidative phosphorylation, nucleic acid synthesis, and blood clotting.

Bicarbonate (HCO_3^-) is the major extracellular buffer in the blood and functions to maintain acid-base balance. Normally, the ratio of bicarbonate to dissolved carbon dioxide (CO_2) is 20 to 1. If this ratio is altered, an acid-base imbalance occurs. Additional CO_2 will produce acidity (decreased pH) and loss of CO_2 will produce alkalinity (increased pH), while the same changes in bicarbonate will produce the opposite pH values. CO_2 levels are controlled by the lungs and bicarbonate levels are controlled by the kidneys.

Indications

This test is carried out as part of a routine screening in acute and critical illness or where there is a known or suspected disorder associated with fluid, electrolyte, or acid-base balance.

Calcium

- Evaluate effects of various disorders on calcium metabolism, especially diseases involving bone
- Detect parathyroid gland loss after thyroid or other neck surgery, as indicated by decreased levels
- Monitor effects of renal failure and various drugs on calcium level
- Evaluate cardiac dysrhythmias and coagulation disorders to determine if altered serum calcium level is a contributing problem
- Monitor treatment effectiveness for abnormal calcium levels, especially deficiencies

Chloride

- Help confirm a diagnosis of disorders associated with abnormal chloride levels
- Differentiate between types of acidosis (hyperchloremic versus anion gap)
- Monitor effectiveness of drug therapy on serum chloride levels

Sodium

- Determine whole-body stores of sodium, since ion is predominantly extracellular

- Estimate serum osmolality, which is usually 285 to 310 mOsm/kg, by using the following formula:

$$\text{Serum osmolality} = 2\ (\text{Na}^+) + \frac{\text{glucose}}{20} + \frac{\text{BUN}}{3}$$

- Monitor effectiveness of drug therapy, especially diuretics, on serum sodium levels

Potassium

- Assess known or suspected disorder associated with renal disease, glucose metabolism, trauma, and burns
- Evaluate cardiac dysrhythmias to determine if altered level is contributing to the problem, especially during digitalis therapy, which leads to ventricular irritability
- Evaluate effects of drug therapy, especially diuretics
- Evaluate response to treatment for abnormal potassium levels

Phosphorus

- Support diagnosis of disorders associated with altered phosphorus-phosphate levels
- Monitor effects of renal failure on phosphorus levels
- Help identify cause of growth abnormalities in children
- Monitor effectiveness of drug therapy on serum chloride levels

Magnesium

- Determine balance in renal failure and chronic alcoholism
- Evaluate cardiac dysrhythmias; decreased magnesium levels can lead to excessive ventricular irritability
- Evaluate known or suspected disorders associated with altered magnesium levels
- Monitor effects of various drugs on magnesium levels

Bicarbonate

- Support diagnosis of disorders associated with altered bicarbonate levels
- Evaluate effects of drug therapy on bicarbonate levels
- Determine the degree of compensation in acidotic and alkalotic states

Reference Values

		SI Units
Calcium		
Newborn	7.6–10.4 mg/dL	1.90–2.60 mmol/L
Infant	9.0–11.0 mg/dL	2.25–2.75 mmol/L
Child	8.8–10.8 mg/dL	2.20–2.70 mmol/L
Adult	8.6–10.0 mg/dL	2.15–2.50 mmol/L
Older adult	8.8–10.2 mg/dL	2.20–2.55 mmol/L
Chloride		
Newborn	98–113 mEq/L	98–113 mmol/L
Infant	95–110 mEq/L	95–110 mmol/L
Child	98–105 mEq/L	98–105 mmol/L
Adult	98–107 mEq/L	98–107 mmol/L
Sodium		
Newborn	133–146 mEq/L	133–146 mmol/L
Infant	139–146 mEq/L	139–146 mmol/L
Child	138–145 mEq/L	138–145 mmol/L
Adult	136–145 mEq/L	136–145 mmol/L
Potassium		
Newborn	3.7–5.9 mEq/L	3.7–5.9 mmol/L
Infant	4.1–5.3 mEq/L	4.1–5.3 mmol/L
Child	3.4–4.7 mEq/L	3.4–4.7 mmol/L
Adult	3.5–5.1 mEq/L	3.5–5.1 mmol/L
Critical values		
Newborn	<2.5 mEq/L	<2.5 mmol/L
	>8.1 mEq/L	>8.1 mmol/L
Adult	<2.5 mEq/L	<2.5 mmol/L
	>6.6 mEq/L	>6.6 mmol/L
Phosphorus		
Newborn	4.5–9.0 mg/dL	1.45–2.91 mmol/L
Infant	4.5–6.7 mg/dL	1.45–2.16 mmol/L
Child	4.5–5.5 mg/dL	1.45–1.78 mmol/L
Adult	2.7–4.5 mg/dL	0.87–1.45 mmol/L
Older adult	2.3–3.7 mg/dL	0.74–1.20 mmol/L
Magnesium		
Newborn	1.4–2.9 mEq/L	1.4–2.9 mmol/L
Child	1.6–2.6 mEq/L	1.6–2.6 mmol/L
Adult	1.5–2.5 mEq/L	1.5–2.5 mmol/L
	1.8–3.0 mg/dL	
Bicarbonate		
Arterial	21–28 mEq/L	21–28 mmol/L
Venous	22–29 mEq/L	22–29 mmol/L
Arterial whole blood		
Newborn	17–24 mEq/L	17–24 mmol/L
Infant	19–24 mEq/L	19–24 mmol/L
Child	16–23 mEq/L	16–23 mmol/L
Adult	22–26 mEq/L	22–26 mmol/L

Abnormal Values

Calcium

- Increased levels
  Acidosis
  Hyperparathyroidism
  Cancers (bone, leukemia, myeloma)
  Drugs, including thiazide diuretics, hormones, vitamin D, calcium
- Decreased levels
  Alkalosis
  Hypoparathyroidism
  Inadequate dietary intake of calcium, vitamin D
  Drugs, including barbiturates, anticonvulsants, acetazolamide, adrenocorticosteroids

Chloride

- Increased levels
  Acidosis
  Hyperkalemia, hypernatremia
  Dehydration
  Renal failure
  Drugs, including potassium chloride, acetazolamide, methyldopa, diazoxide, guanethidine
- Decreased levels
  Alkalosis
  Hypokalemia, hyponatremia
  GI loss from vomiting, diarrhea, nasogastric suction, fistula
  Diuresis
  Drugs, including ethacrynic acid, furosemide, thiazide diuretics, bicarbonate

Sodium

- Increased levels
  Hypovolemia
  Dehydration
  Diabetes insipidus
  Excessive salt ingestion
  Gastroenteritis
  Drugs, including adrenocorticosteroids, methyldopa, hydralazine, cough medication
- Decreased levels
  Addison's disease
  Renal disorder
  GI fluid loss from vomiting, diarrhea, nasogastric suction, ileus
  Diuresis
  Drugs, including lithium, vasopressin, diuretics

Potassium

- Increased levels
    Acidosis
    Insulin deficiency
    Addison's disease
    Acute renal failure
    Hypoaldosteronism
    Transfusion of old banked blood
    Drugs, including amphotericin-B, tetracycline, heparin, epinephrine, potassium-sparing diuretics, isoniazid, marijuana
- Decreased levels
    Alkalosis
    Chronic excessive licorice ingestion (from licorice root not licorice flavor)
    Excess insulin
    GI loss from vomiting, diarrhea, nasogastric suction, fistula
    Laxative abuse
    Cushing's syndrome
    Hyperaldosteronism
    Thyrotoxicosis
    Anorexia nervosa
    Diet deficient in meat and vegetables
    IV therapy with inadequate potassium supplementation
    Drugs, including furosemide, ethacrynic acid, thiazide diuretics, insulin, aspirin, prednisone, cortisone, gentamicin, lithium, and laxatives

Phosphorus

- Increased levels
    Diabetic ketoacidosis
    Renal failure
    Hypercalcemia
    Prolonged immobilization
    Bone growth or active bone formation
    Hyperthyroidism
    Sarcoidosis
    Drugs, including sodium phosphate, heparin, phenytoin, androgens
- Decreased levels
    Recovery phase of diabetic ketoacidosis
    Renal tubular acidosis
    Hypocalcemia
    Vitamin D deficiency
    Malnutrition
    Malabsorption syndromes

Alcoholism
Prolonged vomiting and diarrhea
Drugs, including acetazolamide, insulin, epinephrine, aluminum hydroxide

Magnesium

- Increased levels
  Addison's disease
  Adrenalectomy
  Renal failure
  Diabetic ketoacidosis
  Dehydration
  Hypothyroidism
  Hyperthyroidism
  Drugs, including antacids and laxatives containing magnesium, salicylates, lithium
- Decreased levels
  Hyperaldosteronism
  Hypokalemia
  Diabetic ketoacidosis
  Alcoholism
  Acute pancreatitis
  GI loss from vomiting, diarrhea, nasogastric suction, fistula
  Malabsorption syndromes
  Pregnancy-induced hypertension
  High phosphate diet
  Drugs, including thiazide diuretics, ethacrynic acid, calcium gluconate, amphotericin B, insulin, neomycin, aldosterone, ethanol

Bicarbonate

- Increased levels
  Metabolic alkalosis
  Respiratory acidosis (slightly elevated or normal)
  Chronic obstructive pulmonary disease (COPD)
  Hypoventilation
  Hypokalemia
  Cushing's syndrome
  Congestive heart failure
  Pulmonary edema
  Drugs, including aldosterone, ACTH, viomycin, thiazide diuretics
- Decreased levels
  Metabolic acidosis
  Respiratory alkalosis (slightly decreased or normal)
  Hyperventilation

Diarrhea
Dehydration
Severe malnutrition
Burns
Myocardial infarction
Acute ethanol intoxication
Salicylate toxicity
Renal disease
Hyperthyroidism
Drugs, including triamterene, acetazolamide, ammonium chloride, paraldehyde, sodium citrate

Interfering Factors

■ Calcium

Values are higher in children due to growth and active bone formation.

Numerous drugs may alter serum calcium levels (see Abnormal Values).

Increased or decreased serum protein levels.

■ Chloride

Elevated serum triglyceride levels and myeloma proteins may lead to falsely decreased levels.

Numerous drugs may alter serum sodium levels (see Abnormal Values).

■ Potassium

False elevations can occur with vigorous pumping of the hand during venipuncture, hemolysis of the sample, or high platelet counts during clotting.

False decreases are seen in anticoagulated samples left at room temperature.

Numerous drugs can alter potassium levels (see Abnormal Values).

■ Phosphorus

Phosphate levels are higher in children due to bone growth and active bone formation.

Values are higher at night than in the morning.

Numerous drugs can alter serum phosphate levels (see Abnormal Values).

Hemolysis of the sample may cause falsely elevated values resulting from release of phosphate from red blood cells.

■ Magnesium

Hemolysis of a sample leads to false elevated levels.

Numerous drugs can alter levels (see Abnormal Values).

■ Bicarbonate

Numerous drugs can alter levels (see Abnormal Values).

Nursing Implications

Assessment

- Obtain history of renal or pulmonary disorders, hormonal disorders, fluid deficits or excesses, and medication regimen.

Possible Nursing Diagnoses

Fluid volume excess related to excess sodium intake
Fluid volume deficit related to active loss
Injury, risk for, related to alteration in body chemistry

Implementation

- Put on gloves. Using aseptic technique, perform a venipuncture and collect 7 mL of blood in a red- or green-top tube.
- Handle the sample gently to avoid hemolysis. Label the sample and transport to the laboratory promptly.

Evaluation

- Note and report increased or decreased values and symptoms of fluid imbalance to physician.

Client/Caregiver Teaching

Pretest

- Instruct the client to withhold any medications that could alter test results, if ordered.
- Instruct the client in dietary inclusions or restrictions of food containing sodium, calcium, and potassium.

Posttest

- Tell the client to resume normal diet and any medications withheld before the study.

////////////////////////////////

Electrolytes, Urine

Classification: Chemistry

Type of Test: Urine study

Regulating electrolyte balance is one of the major functions of the kidneys. In normally functioning kidneys, urine levels increase when serum levels are high and decrease when levels are low to maintain homeostasis. Analyzing these urinary levels can provide important clues to the functioning of the kidneys and other major organs. Electrolytes most commonly measured in urine are sodium, chloride, potassium, calcium, phosphorus, and magnesium. Tests for electrolytes in urine usually involve 24-hour urine collections but can be performed on 12-hour or random specimens. With the exception of magnesium, electrolytes are more likely to be measured by serum determinations than by urinary measures of the substances.

Indications

- Evaluate known or suspected renal disease
- Evaluate known or suspected endocrine disorder
- Determine potential cause of renal calculi
- Evaluate malabsorption problem
- Determine magnesium imbalance

Reference Values

		SI Units
Sodium		
Newborn	14–40 mEq/24 h	14–40 mmol/24 h
Children	20–115 mEq/24 h	20–115 mmol/24 h
Adults	75–200 mEq/24 h	75–200 mmol/24 h
Chloride		
Children	15–115 mEq/24 h	15–115 mmol/24 h
Adults	110–250 mEq/24 h	110–250 mmol/24 h
Potassium		
Children	17–57 mEq/24 h	17–57 mmol/24 h
Adults	25–123 mEq/24 h	25–123 mmol/24 h

		SI Units
Calcium		
Quantitative: 24-h specimen		
Low-calcium diet	<150 mg/24 h	<3.75 mmol/24 h
Average-calcium diet	100–250 mg/24 h	2.5–6.2 mmol/24 h
High-calcium diet	250–300 mg/24 h	6.2–7.5 mmol/24 h
Random	<40 mg/dL	1.0 mmol/L
Qualitative		
Sulkowitch	0–+2 turbidity	
Phosphorus		
Adults	0.4–1.3 g/24 h	13–42 mmol/24 h
Restricted diet	<1.0 g/24 h	<32 mmol/24 h
Magnesium		
Adults	6.0–8.5 mEq/24 h	3.0–4.3 mmol/24 h

Abnormal Values

Sodium

- Increased levels
    Excessive salt intake
    Diuretic therapy
    Diabetic ketoacidosis
    Adrenocortical hypofunction
    Toxemia of pregnancy
    Hypokalemia
    Excessive licorice ingestion
    Salicylate toxicity
    Intrinsic renal failure
    Acute tubular necrosis
    Fever
    Dehydration
- Decreased levels
    Hyperaldosteronism
    Hemorrhage
    Diarrhea
    Congestive heart failure with inadequate renal perfusion
    Therapy with adrenal corticosteroids
    Acute renal failure
    Decreased salt intake

Chloride

- Increased levels
    Adrenocortical insufficiency (Addison's disease)
    Diabetic acidosis
    Salicylate toxicity

Salt-losing renal disease
Dehydration
Starvation
Hypernatremia
Diuretic therapy
- Decreased levels
    Congestive heart failure
    Excessive diaphoresis
    Diarrhea
    Gastric suctioning
    Low sodium intake

Potassium

- Increased levels
    Diabetic ketoacidosis
    Diuretic therapy
    Vomiting
    Diarrhea
    Dehydration
    Starvation
    Cushing's disease
    Salicylate intoxication
    Hyperkalemia
    Steroid therapy
- Decreased levels
    Renal failure
    Malabsorption syndrome
    Hypokalemia
    Aldosteronism
    Renal tubular acidosis

Calcium

- Increased levels
    Hyperparathyroidism
    Sarcoidosis
    Renal tubular acidosis
    Cancers of the lung, breast, and bone
    Multiple myeloma
    Metastatic cancer
    Paget's disease
    Osteoporosis
    Medications such as vitamin D, adrenal corticosteroids, calcitonin, androgens, antacids, and diuretics
- Decreased levels
    Hypoparathyroidism
    Nephrosis
    Acute nephritis

Chronic renal failure
Osteomalacia
Malabsorption and steatorrhea
Vitamin D deficiency
Medications such as thiazides
Viomycin
Oral contraceptives

Phosphorus

- Increased levels
  Hyperparathyroidism
  Renal tubular acidosis
  Multiple myeloma
  Sarcoidosis
  Excessive intake of vitamin D
  Paget's disease
  Diuretics
- Decreased levels
  Hypoparathyroidism
  Nephrosis
  Acute nephritis
  Chronic renal failure
  Osteomalacia
  Steatorrhea

Magnesium

- Increased levels
  Alcoholism
  Adrenocortical insufficiency (Addison's disease)
  Renal insufficiency
  Hypothyroidism
  Renal calculi
  Hyperparathyroidism
  Excessive ingestion of magnesium-containing antacids
  Medications such as thiazide diuretics, ethacrynic acid,
  and steroids
- Decreased levels
  Malabsorption syndromes
  Acute or chronic diarrhea
  Dehydration
  Hyperaldosteronism
  Diabetic acidosis
  Pancreatitis
  Advanced chronic renal disease
  Decreased dietary intake of magnesium
  Increased calcium intake
  Osteoporosis

Interfering Factors

- Dietary deficiency or excess of the electrolyte to be measured can lead to spurious results.
- Increased calcium intake may result in decreased magnesium excretion.
- Increased sodium and magnesium intake can cause increased calcium excretion.
- Diuretic therapy with excessive loss of electrolytes into the urine may falsely elevate results.
- Corticosteroids can lead to decreased sodium loss and increased calcium loss.
- Excessive ingestion of magnesium-containing antacids may lead to increased excretion of magnesium.
- All urine voided for the 24-hour period must be included to avoid a false low result.
- Random specimens for sodium are higher at morning than in the evening and for potassium are higher at night than in the morning.
- Certain medications and dietary intake influence specific electrolyte levels.

Nursing Implications

Assessment

- Assess and record client's history of symptoms of electrolyte imbalances and serum electrolyte levels, renal function, and any medications currently being used that may influence test results.

Possible Nursing Diagnoses

Fluid volume excess related to excess sodium intake
Fluid volume deficit related to active loss
Injury, risk for, related to alteration in body chemistry

Implementation

- Obtain the appropriate-sized containers without preservative according to laboratory policy. Follow laboratory directions for any special care of the specimen during collection, such as instructions to refrigerate, place in ice, or protect specimen from light by covering with dark plastic or aluminum. Instructions for specific ions may include the following:

    Sodium: Collect in container with preservatives; keep refrigerated.

    Chloride: Collect in container without preservative or refrigeration.

Potassium: Collect in container with preservative; keep refrigerated.

Calcium: Collect in container with preservative without refrigeration.

Phosphorus: Collect in container without preservative; keep refrigerated.

Magnesium: Collect in container without preservative; keep on ice.

- Begin the test between 6 and 8 A.M. if possible. Collect first voiding and discard. Record the time specimen was discarded as the beginning of the 24-hour test. The next morning, ask the client to void at the same time the collection was started and add this last voiding to the container.
- If an indwelling catheter is in place, replace tubing and container system at the start of the collection time. Keep the container system on ice or empty the urine into a large container periodically during the 24 hours; monitor to ensure continued drainage and conclude the test the next morning at the same hour the collection was begun.
- For a random test, obtain urine specimen in a special container from the lab and transport urine immediately to lab or keep refrigerated.
- Ensure that the specimen is properly labeled and transport to the laboratory. Include on the label the amount of urine and ingestion of any foods or medications that can affect test results.

Evaluation

- Note and compare serum electrolyte levels to urine electrolyte levels. Also evaluate in relation to urine osmolality.
- Monitor the client with suspected electrolyte imbalances for signs and symptoms related to increases or decreases in levels.

Client/Caregiver Teaching

Pretest

- Tell the client to avoid excessive exercise and stress during the 24-hour collection of urine.
- Inform the client that all urine for a 24-hour period must be saved. Tell the client to avoid voiding in the pan with defecation and to keep toilet tissue out of the pan to prevent contamination of the specimen; provide a nonmetallic urinal or bedpan.
- Instruct the client in collection and provide an appropriate container if the specimen is to be obtained on an outpatient basis and brought to the laboratory.

Posttest

- Resume medications, dietary restrictions, and activity withheld before the test.
- Tell the client to report any signs and symptoms that lead to electrolyte imbalance, such as dehydration, diarrhea, vomiting, or prolonged anorexia.
- Instruct the client in electrolyte replacement therapy and changes in dietary intake that affect electrolyte levels.

Electromyography, Electromyogram (EMG)

Classification: Electrophysiologic study

Type of Test: Invasive study

In this study, skeletal muscle activity is measured during rest, voluntary contraction, and electrical stimulation. Needle electrodes containing fine wires are inserted into muscles. The electrical potentials are amplified, displayed on a screen in waveforms, and recorded on a magnetic tape, all at the same time. Comparison and analysis of the amplitude, duration, number, and configuration of the muscle activity provides diagnostic information about the extent of nerve and muscle involvement in the detection of primary muscle diseases, including lower motor neuron, anterior horn cell, or neuromuscular junction diseases; defective transmission at the neuromuscular junction; and peripheral nerve damage or disease. (To test pelvic muscle function, see "Pelvic Floor Sphincter Electromyography.")

Responses of a relaxed muscle are electrically silent, but fibrillation and fasciculations can be detected in a relaxed denervated muscle. Muscle action potentials are detected with minimal or maximal muscle contractions. The differences in the size and numbers of activity potentials during voluntary contractions determine whether the muscle weakness is myogenic or neurogenic. Nerve conduction studies or electroneurography are commonly done in conjunction with electromyelography; the combination of the procedures is known as electromyoneurography.

Indications

- Diagnose primary muscle diseases affecting striated muscle fibers or cell membrane, such as muscular dystrophy or myasthenia gravis
- Diagnose secondary muscle disorders caused by polymyositis, sarcoidosis, hypocalcemia, thyroid toxicity, tetanus, and other disorders
- Diagnose neuromuscular disorders, such as peripheral neuropathy caused by diabetes or alcoholism, and locate the site of the abnormality
- Diagnose muscle disorders caused by diseases of the lower motor neuron involving the motor neuron on the anterior horn of the spinal cord, such as anterior poliomyelitis, amyotrophic lateral sclerosis, amyotonia, or spinal tumors
- Diagnose muscle disorders caused by diseases of the lower motor neuron involving the nerve root, such as Guillain-Barré syndrome, herniated disk, or spinal stenosis
- Differentiate between primary and secondary muscle disorders or neuropathy and myopathy
- Determine if a muscle abnormality is caused by the toxic effects of drugs (antibiotics, chemotherapy) or toxins (botulism, snake venom, heavy metals)
- Monitor and evaluate progression of myopathies or neuropathies, including confirmation of diagnosis of carpal tunnel syndrome

Reference Values

- Normal muscle electrical activity during rest and contraction states

Abnormal Values

- Evidence of neuromuscular disorders or primary muscle disease. Findings must be correlated with the client's history, clinical features, and results of other neurodiagnostic tests.

Interfering Factors

- Hemorrhage, edema, excessive subcutaneous fat, and pain can affect test results.
- Electrical activity decreases with age, and this affects accurate testing and results.
- Medications such as muscle relaxants, cholinergics, and anticholinergics can affect test results.
- Improper placement of surface or needle electrodes can affect test results.
- Inability of the client to remain still and cooperate with instructions during the study will affect accurate testing.

> ### NURSING ALERT
>
> - This procedure is contraindicated in clients receiving anticoagulant therapy or in clients with an infection near or at the sites of electrode placement.

Nursing Implications

Assessment

- Obtain history and assessment of neuromuscular and neurosensory status, disease, or conditions that affect muscle function, level of muscular function and range of motion, traumatic events, and previous tests and procedures done.
- Ensure that the client has refrained from smoking and caffeine-containing beverages for 3 hours before the test.
- Ensure that medications such as muscle relaxants, cholinergics, and anticholinergics have been withheld, as ordered.
- Assess for compliance with directions given for exercising during the test.

Possible Nursing Diagnoses

Physical mobility, impaired, related to neuromuscular impairment

Trauma, risk for, related to unstable or difficult ambulation

Anxiety related to perceived threat to health status

Implementation

- Administer mild analgesic (adult) or sedative (children), as ordered, to promote a restful state before the procedure.
- Place the client in a supine or sitting position depending on the location of the muscles to be tested. Ensure that the area or room is protected from noise or metallic interference that may affect the test results.
- An electrode is applied to the skin to ground the client. Twenty-four-gauge needles containing a fine wire electrode are inserted into the muscle. The electrical potentials of the muscle are amplified, displayed on a screen, and recorded on a magnetic tape. During the test, the muscle activity is tested while at rest, during incremental needle insertion, and during varying degrees of muscle contraction.
- Ask the client to alternate between a relaxed and a contracted muscle state, or perform progressive muscle contractions while the potentials are being measured.

Evaluation

- Note test results in relation to other tests performed and the client's symptoms.
- Monitor electrode sites for hematoma or inflammation.

Client/Caregiver Teaching

Pretest

- Explain that the procedure is performed in a special laboratory by a physician. Explain that this procedure is performed to evaluate the electrical activity of muscles and takes from 1 to 3 hours to complete.
- Inform the client that as many as 10 electrodes may be inserted. Warn the client that the procedure may be uncomfortable but that an analgesic or sedative will be administered.
- Tell the client to refrain from smoking and caffeine-containing beverages 3 hours before the test.
- Tell the client to remain very still and relaxed and cooperate with instructions given to contract muscles during the test.

Posttest

- If residual pain is noted after the procedure, instruct the client to apply warm compresses and take analgesics, as ordered.
- Tell the client to resume substances withheld before the test, as ordered.

Electromyography, Pelvic Floor Sphincter

Pelvic floor sphincter electromyography, also known as rectal electromyography, is performed to measure electrical activity of the external urinary sphincter. This test is often done in conjunction with cystometry and voiding urethrography as part of a full urodynamic study and is indicated to diagnose neuromuscular dysfunction and incontinence.

To perform this study ask the client to void immediately before the test. Then place the client in a supine position on the examining table and drape and expose the perineal area. Two skin electrodes are positioned slightly to the left and right of the perianal area and a grounding electrode is placed on the thigh. If needle electrodes are used, they are inserted into the muscle surrounding the urethra. Muscle activity signals are recorded as waves, which are interpreted for numbers and configurations in diagnosing urinary abnormalities.

An indwelling urinary catheter is inserted, and the bulbocavernosus reflex is tested: the client is instructed to cough while the catheter is being carefully tugged on. Then voluntary control is tested by requesting the client to contract and relax the muscle. Electrical activity is recorded during this period of relaxation with the bladder empty. The bladder is filled with sterile water at a rate of 100 mL per minute while the electrical activity during filling is recorded. The catheter is then removed and the client is placed in a position to void and requested to urinate and empty the full bladder. This voluntary urination is then recorded until completed. The complete test includes recordings of electrical signals before, during, and at the end of urination.

Inform the client that the test is performed in a special laboratory and takes about 30 minutes to complete. Assure the client that the pain is minimal during the catheter insertion. After the test, advise client to take a warm sitz bath and encourage fluids unless contraindicated.

Warn the client to expect hematuria after the first voiding in a female client tested with needle electrodes. Advise the client to report symptoms of urethral irritation such as dysuria, hematuria, and urinary frequency.

Electroneurography (ENG), Nerve Conduction Studies

Classification: Electrophysiologic study

Type of Test: Nerve function

This test, which is usually performed in conjunction with electromyography in a combined test called electromyoneurography, measures an impulse's conduction velocity. After a nerve is electrically stimulated proximally, the time for the impulse to travel to a second or distal site is measured. Because the conduction study of a nerve can vary from nerve to nerve, it is important to compare the results of the affected side to the contralateral side. The results of the stimulation are shown on an oscilloscope, but the actual velocity must be calculated by dividing the distance in meters between the stimulation point and the response point, by the time between the stimulus and response.

Indications

- Confirm diagnosis of peripheral nerve damage or trauma

Reference Values

- Variable depending on nerve being tested. For clients age 3 years and older, the maximum conduction velocity is 40 to 80 milliseconds; for infants and the elderly, the values are divided by 2.

Abnormal Values

- Carpal tunnel syndrome
- Diabetic neuropathy
- Guillain-Barré syndrome
- Muscular dystrophy
- Myasthenia gravis
- Tarsal tunnel syndrome
- Thoracic outlet syndrome

Interfering Factors

- Poor electrode conduction or failure to obtain contralateral value for comparison may affect interpretation.
- Clients in severe pain may have false results.

Nursing Implications

Assessment

- Obtain history of neuromuscular and neurosensory status, disease that affects the peripheral neurologic system, the results of previous tests and procedures.

Possible Nursing Diagnoses

Pain related to trauma or entrapment of peripheral nerve

Physical mobility, impaired, related to neurovascular impairment

Trauma, risk for, related to unstable or difficult ambulation

Implementation

- Place the client in a position that exposes the nerve to be tested.
- Shave the area to be stimulated if conduction problem is anticipated.
- Identify the point for electrical stimulation in the area innervated by the nerve being tested.
- Apply electrode gel and place a recording electrode at a known distance from the stimulation point. The distance between the stimulation point and the site of the recording electrode is measured in centimeters.
- The nerve is electrically stimulated and the time between nerve impulse and muscular contraction, measured in milliseconds (distal latency), is shown on the oscilloscope.
- The nerve is electrically stimulated in a similar fashion at a location proximal to the area of suspected injury or disease. The time required for the impulse to travel from the stimulation site to muscle contraction (total latency) is recorded in milliseconds.
- Calculate the conduction velocity. The conduction velocity is converted to meters per second and computed using the following equation:

$$\text{Conduction velocity (in meters per second)} = \frac{\text{distance (in meters)}}{\text{total latency} - \text{distal latency}}$$

- When the test is completed, remove the electrodes and conduction gel.

Evaluation

- Note results in relation to other tests performed and the client's symptoms.

Client/Caregiver Teaching

Pretest

- Inform the client that the test will be performed in a nerve conduction laboratory by a physiatrist or neurologist and takes about 15 minutes.
- Inform the client that the test is uncomfortable but that the electrical shock is brief.

Electronystagmography (ENG)

Classification: Electrophysiologic study

Type of Test: Eye movements

This noninvasive study is performed to indirectly measure direction and degree of nystagmus—the involuntary back-and-forth eye movement resulting from initiation of the oculovestibular reflex that maintains visual fixation when the head's position is changed. This study measures the electrical responses of and around the eye at rest and when stimulated to elicit nystagmus and provides a permanent recording of the results so they can be compared to normal values.

Indications

- Determine cause of dizziness, vertigo, tinnitus, or hearing loss
- Diagnose lesions of the brainstem and cerebellum
- Diagnose lesions of the end organ or vestibular branch of VIIIth cranial nerve
- Differentiate between nystagmus caused by the peripheral or central nervous systems
- Diagnose congenital disorders in infants

Reference Values

- Normal nystagmus response during turning of the head and oculovestibular reflex

Abnormal Values

- Evidence of hearing loss or lesions of the ocular or vestibular systems
- Lesions of the central nervous system
- Tumors
- Circulatory disorders
- Demyelinating diseases
- Lesions of the peripheral nervous system
- Middle ear disorders

- Ototoxicity from drugs or food allergies
- Head trauma
- Changes caused by advancing age

Interfering Factors

- Improper placement of electrodes around the eyes.
- Inability to understand or cooperate by refraining from blinking eyes.
- Visual impairment that prevents ability to cooperate.
- Drugs such as stimulants, sedatives, depressants, antivertigo drugs can cause inaccurate results by affecting cooperation with the test, suppressing nystagmus, or producing other eye movements.

NURSING ALERT

- This procedure is contraindicated in conditions such as a perforated eardrum if water caloric test is scheduled unless the procedure is modified by placing a fingercot in the canal.
- It is also contraindicated in clients with pacemakers because the test can interfere with pacemaker function and in neck disorders that prevent position changes of the head during the test.

Nursing Implications

Assessment

- Obtain history and assessment of neurologic system, symptoms or problems of tinnitus, hearing loss, vertigo, dizziness, ear pain or drainage, drug regimen, as well as previous tests and procedures done.
- Ensure that the client has refrained from alcohol, caffeine-containing beverages, and tobacco for 48 hours before testing.
- Ensure that medications such as stimulants, depressants, antianxiety agents, sedatives, or antivertigo drugs are withheld for at least 5 days before the test, as ordered.
- Ensure that the client is not wearing any makeup.

Possible Nursing Diagnoses

Physical mobility, impaired, related to alterations in nerve transmission

Sensory-perceptual alteration (auditory) related to altered sensory reception, transmission, or integration

Anxiety related to perceived threat to health status

Implementation

- Place the client in a supine or seated position in a darkened room. Remove cerumen from the ears. Cleanse and dry the skin at the electrode sites. Prepare five electrodes with paste.
- Position electrodes at the outer canthus of each eye to test horizontal nystagmus, above and below the eye center for vertical nystagmus, and a ground electrode at the center of the forehead. The electrodes pick up the potentials as the eyes move in a horizontal or vertical direction and a recorder amplifies the signals and charts them.
- Several tests can be performed to examine the nystagmus response to the different procedures:

    Gaze nystagmus test: The client is asked to close eyes and spontaneous eye movements are recorded while concentrating on a mental task: center gaze recorded by having client fix eyes on a center light, right gaze by moving the eyes to the right, and left gaze by moving the eyes to the left. A recording is made with eyes closed after each directional change; each gaze change and closed eyes periods are timed.

    Pendulum tracking test: Eye movements are recorded as the client tracks a pendulum or light movement with eyes open, with eyes closed, and looking straight ahead.

    Positional changes: The client is asked to change head position with eyes looking straight ahead and closed, then turning head to the right and return to center, turning head to the left and return to center; moving from a lying to a sitting position and a sitting to a lying position; while lying supine in both right and left side-lying position; with head hanging over the edge, moving from lying to sitting; and after sitting position and head hanging over the edge to the right and left positions

    Water caloric test: While in a supine position with the head elevated to a semi-Fowler's position, water of a specific temperature is instilled into the ear canals for 30 seconds. The irrigation return is collected in a basin placed under the ear. Recordings are made during the study as the client is asked to perform some mental tasks, to open and fix the eyes on an object, and then to close the eyes. Stimulation by different water temperatures can be done, with cold water in some instances, and the response recorded; air of different temperatures can also be introduced into each ear to obtain the same information.

■ The results of these tests are recorded on charts and are analyzed for abnormalities by comparing them to the established values. Results are noted as normal, borderline, or abnormal, indicating peripheral, central, or undetermined lesion.

Evaluation

■ Note test results in relation to other tests performed and client's symptoms.

Client/Caregiver Teaching

Pretest

■ Inform the client that the procedure is performed in a special laboratory by a physician, that it evaluates eye movements, and that it takes about 1 hour to complete.

■ Inform the client that there is some discomfort associated with some of the tests, and nausea and vomiting can occur.

■ Inform the client that instructions for activities to be performed during the test will be given.

Posttest

■ Tell the client to report continuing dizziness, nausea, or fatigue.

■ Advise the client to resume medications, as ordered.

Electroretinography (ERG)

Classification: Electrophysiologic study

Type of Test: Visual perception

This ophthalmologic study is performed to measure the electrical activity of the retina in response to a flash of light stimulus. A corneal contact lens with electrodes imbedded is placed on the eye and an electrode is placed on the client's forehead, and these electrodes record the changes in electrical activity.

The changes are displayed on a screen for viewing and evaluation. The study allows for diagnostic information in evaluating retinal function and viability in clients with opaque lens, corneal opacity, or vitreous body.

Indications

- Detect retinal detachment or degeneration in the presence of opacities of the ocular contents
- Diagnose retinal damage caused by drugs
- Evaluate the extent of color or night blindness
- Diagnose congenital disorders such as mucopolysaccharidosis
- Diagnose retinitis pigmentosa when performed with electro-oculography
- Detect retinopathy or vascular ischemia and other blood-vessel abnormalities
- Evaluate retinal status before surgery or other treatment

Reference Values

- Normal electrical responses to light (alpha and beta waveforms)

Abnormal Values

- Decreased response
   Acquired or inherited retinal conditions, for example, giant arteritis
   Siderosis
   Retinal detachment
   Opacities of the ocular media
   Night blindness usually resulting from vitamin A deficiency
   Mucopolysaccharidosis
   Color blindness
   Retinitis pigmentosa, when this is performed together with electro-oculography

Interfering Factors

- Client inability to remain still during the procedure unless a general anesthetic is administered. This applies especially to children.
- Improper placement of the electrode on the cornea.

Nursing Implications

Assessment

- Obtain a history of known or suspected congenital or acquired eye disorders or diseases that predispose to eye abnormalities, signs and symptoms of eye condition, and medications, as well as to the results of previous tests and procedures.

Possible Nursing Diagnoses

Sensory-perceptual alterations, visual, related to retinal vascular abnormalities

Anxiety related to perceived threat to health status

Injury, risk for, related to insertion of corneal lens for procedure

Implementation

- Administer eyedrops, as ordered. Place client in a supine or sitting position.
- Anesthetize the eyes and prop them open with a retractor. Place electrodes that have been saturated with saline on the cornea. These electrodes receive the light stimulus and record and display electrical changes on a screen.
- Recordings are made in ordinary room light, in a dark room with a flash of white light delivered after the eye has had a chance to accommodate to the dark, and a flash of a very bright light if vitreous opacity is present. Normal values are established depending on the intensity of the wavelengths of light that determines the expected electrical response (wavelengths are usually increased in proportion to the intensity).

Evaluation

- Note results in relation to the client's symptoms and other studies performed, such as electro-oculography.

Client/Caregiver Teaching

Pretest

- Explain that the procedure is performed in a special laboratory by a physician and evaluates the eyes' response to various light levels. The procedure takes about 1 hour to complete.
- Reassure client that little or no discomfort is felt during the test.

Posttest

- Warn the client not to rub the eyes for 1 hour after testing to prevent corneal abrasion.
- Inform the client that the effects of the anesthetic will disappear in about 20 minutes.
- Instruct the client to immediately report eye pain or changes in visual acuity.

Enzyme-Linked Immunosorbent Assay (ELISA)

Classification: Immunology

Type of Test: Serum

This test detects the antibodies that result from exposure to human immunodeficiency virus (HIV), the virus that causes acquired immunodeficiency syndrome (AIDS) and AIDS-related complex (ARC) disorders. The virus infects and destroys T-helper lymphocytes, affecting the body's ability to produce antibodies and decreasing cellular immune response. Antigens are detectable in the serum as early as 2 weeks after the virus has been acquired, and they remain for 2 to 4 months. In most cases, at this time antibodies can be detected; however, it may take 6 weeks to 12 months for antibodies to be detected.

Indications

- Diagnose HIV infection
- Screen blood intended for transfusion

Reference Values

- Negative for HIV antibody

Abnormal Values

- Indicative of HIV infection, HIV exposure, or AIDS-related complex
- Autoimmune disorders

Interfering Factors

- Negative results can occur if the test is performed early in the disease, before antibodies have formed.
- Negative results can occur in clients with advanced AIDS from severe immunologic depression resulting in absence of detectable antibodies.
- Children infected before birth can have inaccurate negative results.
- Inaccurate results can occur with the use of test kits that contain a protein medium to which the client has been exposed.

Nursing Implications

Assessment

- Obtain a history of known or suspected exposure to HIV, risk factors, immunological disorders, medication regimen, diagnostic tests and results.
- Assess skin for lesions and edema, and veins for sclerosis and past phlebitis, when selecting a venipuncture site.

Possible Nursing Diagnoses

Anxiety related to perceived threat to health status
Infection, risk for secondary, related to immunosuppressed inflammatory response
Infection, risk for transmission

Implementation

- Obtain an informed consent as required, and inform the client of the confidentiality and legal requirements regarding the test performance and test results. If the patient wants to remain anonymous, assign a number to the specimen and record it accurately.
- Put on gloves. Using aseptic technique, perform a venipuncture and collect 7 mL of blood in a red-top tube.

Evaluation

- If the test is positive two consecutive times, the Western Blot or immunofluorescence assay test is performed on the same sample.
- Note and report positive test results to the physician.

Client/Caregiver Teaching

Pretest

- Provide a supportive environment and allow the client to express concerns about the procedure.
- Emphasize confidentiality of the test and results.

Posttest

- Instruct client to not engage in unprotected intercourse, avoid donating blood or sharing needles, and notify sexual contacts, if positive.
- If only the ELISA test is positive, the client requires retesting in 6 months.
- Explain to the client that a positive result means exposure to and infection with HIV but does not indicate active AIDS. Symptoms may not be present.

Epstein-Barr Virus (EBV) Antibodies

Classification: Serology
Type of Test: Serum

This test detects the presence of heterophile antibodies to the Epstein-Barr virus. This virus is a B lymphocyte herpesvirus that causes infectious mononucleosis and is transmitted through direct contact with saliva of an infected person. Of the clients with Epstein virus infectious mononucleosis, 95 percent will have a positive result, 86 percent in the first week of illness.

Indications

- Diagnose Monospot-negative infectious mononucleosis
- Monitor the course of prolonged infectious mononucleosis
- Determine antibody status of immunocompromised clients with lymphoproliferative processes

Reference Values

- Negative or titer <1:56 heterophile antibodies

Abnormal Values

- Elevated levels
  Burkitt's lymphoma
  Chronic Epstein-Barr virus carrier state
  Infectious mononucleosis
  Hepatitis
  Lymphoproliferative processes in immunosuppressed clients

Interfering Factors

- Cytomegalovirus (CMV) in those with organ transplants will cause a positive result.
- Posttransfusion reactions will cause a temporary increase in EBV.

Nursing Implications

Assessment

- Obtain a history of known or suspected exposure to infectious mononucleosis, medication regimen, diagnostic tests and results.

Possible Nursing Diagnoses

Infection, risk for secondary, related to immunosuppressed inflammatory response

Fatigue related to decreased energy production and states of discomfort

Anxiety related to perceived threat to health status

Implementation

- Put on gloves. Using aseptic technique, perform a venipuncture and collect 5 mL of blood in a red-top tube.
- Handle the sample gently to avoid hemolysis.

Evaluation

- Note and report positive results to physician.

Client/Caregiver Teaching

Posttest

- If results are positive, instruct client in methods of preventing transmission.
- Tell client to contact the physician if symptoms persist.

Erythrocyte Distribution, Fetal-Maternal; Kleihauer-Betke or Fetal Hemoglobin Stain

Classification: Hematology

Type of Test: Serum

This test measures the number of fetal red blood cells (RBCs) in maternal circulation in order to calculate the Rh_o, or D, immune globulin dosage needed to prevent complications in subsequent pregnancies in an unsensitized Rh-negative mother.

During most normal deliveries, as well as in spontaneous abortions, some RBCs transfer from fetal to maternal circulation. Normally, the amount of blood transfer is minimal and not clinically significant. However, when a significant amount of blood from an Rh-positive fetus transfers to an Rh-negative mother, it can cause maternal immunization to the Rh_o (D) antigen and the development of anti-Rh-positive antibodies in maternal circulation. This maternal immunization subjects a subsequent Rh-positive fetus to potentially fatal hemolysis and erythroblastosis during a pregnancy.

Erythrocyte screening is recommended during the first prenatal visit and at 24, 28, 32, and 36 weeks' gestation for all Rh-negative mothers; and for all Rh-positive mothers with a history of cesarean birth, a jaundiced infant, a transfusion, stillbirth, or induced or spontaneous abortion.

Indications

- Detect and measure fetal-maternal blood transfer
- Determine amount of Rh_o (D) immune globulin needed to prevent maternal immunization to the Rh_o (D) antigen

Reference Values

- No fetal RBCs contained in maternal whole blood

Abnormal Values

- Presence of increased fetal RBC volume in maternal circulation

Interfering Factors

- Hemolysis caused by improper handling of the sample may cause inaccurate test results.
- Sample analysis 72 hours after sample collection can cause inaccurate results.
- Clients with elevated fetal hemoglobin from a hemoglobinopathy will have falsely elevated results.

Nursing Implications

Assessment

- Obtain history of previous pregnancy, cesarean section, stillbirth, jaundice infant, blood transfusion, spontaneous or elective abortion.

Possible Nursing Diagnoses

Anxiety related to perceived threat to health status and fetal well-being

Injury, risk for, fetal, related to abnormal maternal-fetal circulation

Implementation

- Put on gloves. Using aseptic technique, perform a venipuncture and collect at least 1 mL of blood in a lavender-top tube.
- Handle specimen gently to prevent hemolysis and keep it at room temperature. Send sample to the laboratory immediately.

Evaluation

- Note test results in relation to client's history.

Client/Caregiver Teaching

Pretest

- Inform the client that no special preparation is required for this test.

Posttest

- Inform the client that Rh_o (D) immune globulin dosage, if necessary, will depend on test results.
- Encourage the client to return for follow-up tests, as necessary.

Erythrocyte Fragility, Osmotic Fragility, Red Cell Fragility

Classification: Hematology

Type of Test: Blood

This test determines the ability of the red cell membrane to resist rupturing in an increasingly dilute saline solution. The spherocyte, an erythrocyte (red blood cell) that assumes a spherical shape and is common in certain hemolytic anemias, is particularly fragile when exposed to osmotic stress. Normal disc-shaped cells take on water and swell significantly before rupturing. The test is performed by exposing red cells to increasingly dilute saline solutions. The percentage of the solution at which the red cells swell and rupture is then noted.

Indications

- Confirm disorders that alter red cell fragility, including hereditary anemias
- Evaluate the extent of extrinsic damage to red cells from burns, inadvertent instillation of hypotonic intravenous fluids, microorganisms, and excessive exercise

Reference Values

- Normal erythrocytes will rupture in saline solutions of 0.30% to 0.45%. Red cell rupture in solutions of >0.50% saline indicates increased fragility. Lack of red cell rupture in solutions of <0.30% saline indicates decreased red cell fragility.

Abnormal Values

- Increased fragility
  Hereditary spherocytosis
  Hemolytic anemias
  Autoimmune anemias
  Burns
  Toxins (bacterial, chemical)
  Hypotonic infusions
  Transfusion with incompatible blood
  Mechanical trauma to red cells (prosthetic heart valves, disseminated intravascular coagulation, parasites)
  Enzyme deficiencies (PK, G-6-PD)
- Decreased fragility
  Iron-deficiency anemias
  Hereditary anemias (sickle cell, hemoglobin C, thalassemias)
  Liver diseases
  Polycythemia vera
  Splenectomy
  Obstructive jaundice

Interfering Factors

- None

Nursing Implications

Assessment

- Obtain family history of anemias and red cell abnormalities obtained from laboratory testing.

Possible Nursing Diagnoses

Tissue perfusion, altered [specify], related to oxygen supply/demand imbalance
Protection, altered, related to altered hematopoiesis
Infection, risk for secondary, related to immunosuppressed inflammatory response

Implementation

■ Put on gloves. Using aseptic technique, perform a venipuncture and collect 7 mL of blood in a green-top tube. A capillary sample may be obtained in infants and children, as well as in adults for whom a venipuncture may not be feasible.

Evaluation

■ Note results in relation to other tests performed, including a complete hematologic profile.

Client/Caregiver Teaching

Pretest

■ Inform the client that fasting is not required.

Erythrocyte Sedimentation Rate (ESR, Sed Rate)

Classification: Hematology

Type of Test: Blood

The basis of the ESR is the alteration of blood proteins by the inflammatory and necrotic processes. These processes causes the red cells to become heavier and settle at the bottom of a vertically held pipette drawn from a tube of whole venous blood. The test measures the time required for a columnlike formation of red cells to develop. Three different methods to test ESR are available: the Westergren (or modified Westergren) method, the Wintrobe method, and the zeta sedimentation ratio. Although nonspecific, the ESR is frequently the earliest indicator of widespread inflammatory reaction from infection or autoimmune disorders. Prolonged elevations are also present in malignant disease.

Indications

■ Diagnose acute inflammatory processes
■ Diagnose acute infection such as tuberculosis or tissue necrosis

- Diagnose and monitor temporal arteritis and polymyalgia rheumatica
- Monitor inflammatory and malignant disease
- Diagnose chronic infections
- Diagnose rheumatoid, anal, or autoimmune disorders

Reference Values

Westergren method	
Newborn	0–2 mm/h
Children	0–10 mm/h
Women	
<50 yr	0–20 mm/h
50–85 yr	<30 mm/h
>85 yr	<42 mm/h
Men	
<50 yr	0–15 mm/h
50–85 yr	<20 mm/h
>age 85 yr	<30 mm/h
Wintrobe method	
Women	0.36–0.45
Men	0.41–0.51
Zeta sedimentation ratio	41–54%

Abnormal Values

- Increased values
  Anemia
  Rheumatoid arthritis
  Cat scratch fever
  Carcinoma
  Collagen diseases, including systemic lupus erythematosus
  Crohn's disease
  Rheumatic fever
  Endocarditis
  Heavy-metal poisoning
  Macroglobulinemia
  Lymphosarcoma
  Multiple myeloma
  Nephritis
  Pregnancy
  Subacute bacterial endocarditis
  Acute myocardial infarction
  Temporal arteritis
  Toxemia
  Drugs, including Aldomet, dextran, fat emulsions, heparin, Pronestyl, theophylline, oral contraceptives, and vitamin A

- Decreased values
  Polycythemia
  Congestive heart failure
  Sickle-cell anemia
  Infectious mononucleosis
  Low plasma protein levels
  Poikilocytosis
  Drugs, including high-dose aspirin, cortisone, prednisone, corticotropin, and lecithin

Interfering Factors

- Prolonged tourniquet constriction around the arm may cause hemoconcentration and false-low values.
- Hemolysis or clotting of the sample invalidates results.
- *Westergren or modified Westergren method:* Heparin falsely increases the results; bubbles in the pipette or tilting the pipette more than 3° from vertical falsely increases the values.
- *Wintrobe method:* Overdilution with EDTA or inadequate duration or speed of the centrifuge causes unreliable results.

Nursing Implications

Assessment

- Obtain a history of infectious, autoimmune, or neoplastic diseases; hematologic disorders; results of other tests performed; and medication regimen.

Possible Nursing Diagnoses

Protection, altered, related to altered hematopoiesis
Hyperthermia related to infectious process
Anxiety related to perceived threat to health status

Implementation

- *Westergren method:* Put on gloves. Using aseptic technique, obtain 5 mL of blood in a blue-top tube. Gently roll the tube to mix the sample. In the laboratory, a pipette is filled to the 0 mark and placed vertically in a Westergren rack.
- *Modified Westergren method:* Put on gloves. Using aseptic technique, obtain 3 mL of blood in a lavender-top tube. In the laboratory, sodium citrate and sodium chloride are added to the sample; a pipette is filled to the 0 mark and placed vertically in a Westergren rack.
- *Wintrobe method:* Put on gloves. Using aseptic technique, obtain 7 mL of blood in a lavender-top tube. In the laboratory, transfer specimen to a 7 cm long Wintrobe capillary

tube. After replacing the tube's cap the sample is spun for 5 minutes.

- *Zeta sedimentation ratio:* Put on gloves and obtain 7 mL of blood in a lavender-top tube. Gently roll the tube (lavender top) to mix the sample. Fill the capillary tube with 100 μL of the venous blood sample and place in centrifuge for 45 seconds. Sample is read as Zetacrit and this value is divided by the client's true hematocrit and expressed as a percentage.
- Transport sample to the laboratory within 2 hours.

Evaluation

- Note test results in relation to other tests performed and the client's symptoms.

Client/Caregiver Teaching

Pretest

- Inform the client that no special preparation is required for this test.

Posttest

- Inform the client of the results and begin teaching about the disorder, if appropriate.

Esophagogastroduode- noscopy (EGD)

Classification: Endoscopy

Type of Test: Direct visualization

This test provides direct visualization of the upper GI tract mucosa, which includes the esophagus, stomach, and the upper portion of the duodenum, by means of a flexible fiberoptic endoscope. The standard flexible fiberoptic endoscope contains three channels that allow for passage of the instruments needed to perform therapeutic or diagnostic procedures, such as biopsies or cytology washings. This tube also allows for removal of foreign bodies by suction or by snare or forceps. Direct visualization yields greater diagnostic data than is possible through radiologic procedures such as an upper GI and is rapidly replacing it as the diagnostic procedure of choice.

Indications

- Diagnose upper GI inflammatory disease and benign or neoplastic tumors
- Evaluate extent of esophageal injury after ingestion of chemicals
- Diagnose gastric or duodenal ulcers
- Evaluate stomach or duodenum after surgical procedures

Reference Values

- Esophageal mucosa is normally yellow pink; about 9 inches from the incisor teeth, a pulsation indicates the location of the aortic arch. The gastric mucosa is orange-red and contains rugal folds. The proximal duodenum is reddish and contains a few longitudinal folds, while the distal duodenum has circular folds lined with villi.

Abnormal Values

- Acute and chronic gastric and duodenal ulcers
- Esophagitis or strictures
- Hiatal hernia
- Esophageal varices
- Mallory-Weiss tears
- Tumors (benign or malignant)
- Gastritis
- Diverticular disease
- Esophageal or pyloric stenosis
- Duodenitis

Interfering Factors

- Inability of client to cooperate with the procedure can affect results.
- Failure to follow dietary restrictions before the procedure.
- A barium swallow within the preceding 48 hours can hinder adequate visualization.
- Severe upper GI bleeding or the presence of blood or clots can interfere with visualization.

> ### NURSING ALERT
>
> - This procedure is contraindicated in clients with an unstable cardiac status, known aortic arch aneurysm, or large esophageal Zenker's diverticulum, esophageal varices, or known perforation.

Nursing Implications

Assessment

- Obtain a history of GI disorders and related symptoms, results of other tests and procedures, and medication regimen.
- Ensure that the client has fasted for 8 hours before the test.
- Ascertain that the client understands the procedure and risks before signing the informed consent.

Possible Nursing Diagnoses

Pain related to tissue inflammation
Nutrition, altered, less than body requirements, related to gastrointestinal dysfunction
Anxiety related to perceived threat to health status
Fluid volume deficit, risk for, related to active loss

Implementation

- As ordered, administer preprocedural sedation.
- Ask the client to sit up and spray the mouth and throat with local anesthetic. Provide an emesis basin for the increased saliva and encourage the client to spit out the saliva because the gag reflex may be impaired.
- Place the client in the left lateral position with the head bent forward.
- The examiner inserts the finger into the mouth and uses it to guide the endoscope to the back of the throat. The endoscope's tip is deflected with the left index finger and the scope advanced and visualization of the tract is started.
- Air is insufflated to distend the upper GI tract, as needed. Biopsies or any endoscopic surgery is performed.
- At the end of the procedure, excess air and secretions are aspirated through the scope and the endoscope is removed.
- Prepare and label the samples. Transfer them to the laboratory as soon as possible.

Evaluation

- Note the results in relation to the client's symptoms and other tests performed.

Client/Caregiver Teaching

Pretest

- Inform the client that the procedure will be performed by a specialized physician in the endoscopy laboratory and usually takes 20 to 30 minutes.
- Tell the client to fast after midnight or for 8 hours before the test.
- Inform the client that the procedure is not painful and that the throat will be anesthetized with a spray.
- Inform the client that dentures and eyewear will be removed before the test.
- Inform the client that he or she will not be able to speak during the procedure but that breathing will not be affected.

Posttest

- Inform the client that he or she may have a sore throat or hoarseness after the procedure.
- Inform the client that no fluids will be allowed until the gag reflex returns.
- Inform the client that belching, bloating, and gas may be experienced after the test.
- Tell the client to notify the physician immediately if bleeding, or extreme pain is noted.

Estradiol Receptor and Progesterone Receptor Assay

Classification: Cytology

Type of Test: Tissue analysis

Estradiol receptor assay is used to identify clients with a type of breast cancer that may be responsive to estrogen-deprivation therapy. Estradiol is an estrogen hormone. Tumors associated with a positive assay are more responsive to estrogen-deprivation therapy. This test is normally done in conjunction with progesterone receptor assays. Progesterone receptor assay also tests the tumor's responsiveness for this type of therapy. Progesterone-positive tumors seem to be associated with a better prognosis than progesterone-negative ones. In some cases, this test measures the potential tumor responsiveness to hormonal or antihormonal therapy.

Indications

- Identify clients with breast or other types of cancer that may respond to hormone or antihormone therapy
- Monitor responsiveness to hormone or antihormone therapy

Reference Values

- *Estrogen receptor assay:* negative, or ≤3 femtomoles (fmol)/ mg of protein
- *Progesterone receptor assay:* negative, or ≤10 fmol/mg of protein or negative

Abnormal Values

- Positive values
    Hormonal therapy
    Estrogen-positive breast tumors
    Progesterone-negative breast tumors

Interfering Factors

- Antiestrogen preparations (e.g., tamoxifen) ingested 2 months before tissue sampling will affect test results.
- Tissue specimens contaminated with formalin or failure to freeze the specimen adequately using liquid nitrogen, dry ice, or microtome will falsely decrease results.
- Failure to transport specimen to the lab immediately can result in degradation of receptor sites.
- Massive tumor necrosis or tumors with low cellular composition lower the assay result.

Nursing Implications

Assessment

- Ensure that the client has not received antiestrogen therapy within 2 months of the test.
- Ensure that the client understands the procedure and risks before signing the informed consent.

Possible Nursing Diagnoses

Anxiety related to threat to health status
Body image disturbance related to change in structure/
  appearance
Grieving, anticipatory, related to perceived potential loss

Implementation

- Administer preoperative sedation, as ordered.
- Assemble supplies and prepare client for surgical biopsy or resection. Supplies should include a waxed cardboard specimen container without preservatives.
- Using a needle biopsy or resection, the physician obtains a tissue specimen of at least 200 mg. The specimen is placed in a formalin-free container frozen immediately and transported to pathology laboratory immediately.

Evaluation

- Note test results: Most estrogen-positive tumors respond to therapy, while estrogen-negative tumors do not.

Client/Caregiver Teaching

Pretest

- Explain the purpose of the test and the procedure for obtaining the specimen. Tell client that some discomfort is experienced from the procedure.
- Inform the client that the excision is considered a surgical procedure and that the client will have to fast for 8 hours before the procedure.

Posttest

- Instruct the client in care and observation of the incision site.
- Instruct the client in hormone therapy, based on test results.

Estrogens, Serum: Estradiol (E_2) and Estriol (E_3)

Classification: Chemistry

Type of Test: Serum, plasma

This test measures the estrogens, the hormones that are secreted in large amounts by the ovaries and during pregnancy by the placenta. Small amounts are also secreted by the adrenal cortex and the testes. Only three types of estrogen are present in the blood in measurable amounts: estrone, estradiol, and estriol. Estrone (E_1) is the immediate precursor of estradiol (E_2), which is the most biologically potent. Estriol (E_3) is secreted in large amounts from the placenta during pregnancy from precursors produced by the fetal liver. Although total plasma estrogens are difficult to measure, radioimmunoassay is used to measure estradiol (E_2) and estriol (E_3).

Indications

- Evaluate fetal and placental abnormality
- Determine presence of gonadal dysfunction
- Evaluate estradiol in menstrual abnormalities, fertility problems, and estrogen-producing tumors in women and testicular or adrenal tumors and feminization disorders in men

Reference Values

		SI Units
Total estrogens		
Children	<25 pg/mL	>25 ng/L
Men	20–80 pg/mL	20–80 ng/L
Women		
Follicular phase	60–200 pg/mL	60–200 ng/L
Luteal phase	160–400 pg/mL	160–400 ng/L
Late phase	150–350 pg/mL	150–350 ng/L
Postmenopausal	<130 pg/mL	>130 ng/L
Estradiol (E_2)		
Children	<15 pg/mL	<55 pmol/L
Men	10–50 pg/mL	37–184 pmol/L

		SI Units
Women		
Follicular phase	20–150 pg/mL	73–551 pmol/L
Peak phase	150–750 pg/mL	551–2753 pmol/L
Luteal phase	30–450 pg/mL	110–1652 pmol/L
Postmenopausal	<20 pg/mL	<73 pmol/L
Estriol (E_3)		
Weeks of gestation		
28–30 w	38–140 ng/mL	132–486 nmol/L
31–35 w	30–260 ng/mL	121–902 nmol/L
36–38 w	48–570 ng/mL	167–1978 nmol/L
39–40 w	95–460 ng/mL	330–1596 nmol/L

Abnormal Values

- Elevated total estrogens
    - Ovarian tumor
    - Testicular tumor
    - Adrenal tumor or hyperplasia
    - Precocious puberty
    - Severe hepatic disease
    - Drugs such as digoxin and oral contraceptives
- Decreased total estrogens
    - Ovarian agenesis, such as Turner's syndrome
    - Primary or secondary hypogonadism
    - Adrenal or pituitary hypofunction
    - Stress
    - Anorexia nervosa
    - Menopause
- Elevated E_2 levels
    - Adrenal tumors
    - Testicular tumors
    - Feminization in children
    - Ovarian neoplasm
    - Cirrhosis
    - Hyperthyroidism
    - Gynecomastia
    - Klinefelter's syndrome
    - Drugs, including diazepam, clomiphene, antibiotics, hormones, meprobamate, hydrochlorothiazide
- Decreased E_2 levels
    - Primary and secondary hypogonadism
    - Amenorrhea

Ovarian disease
Pituitary dysfunction
Infertility
Menopause
Osteoporosis
Drugs such as oral contraceptives and megestrol
- Elevated E_3 levels
    Imminent birth
    Multiple pregnancy
    Precocious puberty
    Drugs such as oxytocin
- Decreased E_3 levels
    Down syndrome
    Impending toxemia of pregnancy
    Drugs such as penicillins

Interfering Factors

- Radionuclide scan within 48 hours will alter test results.
- Estradiol level of prepubertal children may not be accurate, and the test may need to be repeated.
- Numerous drugs may lead to increased and decreased levels (see Abnormal Values).

Nursing Implications

Assessment

- Obtain history of known or suspected diseases associated with sexuality or reproductive organs, pregnancy (in weeks), recent diagnostic testing, and results.
- Obtain medication history; ensure drugs altering estrogen levels have been withheld for 12 to 24 hours before the test, as ordered by physician.

Possible Nursing Diagnoses

Anxiety related to threat to health status
Grieving, anticipatory, related to perceived potential loss

Implementation

- Put on gloves. Using aseptic technique, perform venipuncture and collect 3 mL of blood in a red-top tube.
- Handle specimen gently to avoid hemolysis and transport it to the laboratory promptly.

Evaluation

- Note results in relation to age, sex, pregnancy and menopausal status and to associated levels of 24-hour urinary hormonal analyses.

Client/Caregiver Teaching

Posttest

- Tell the client to resume medications withheld before the test.

Estrogens, Urine: Total and Fractions

Classification: Hormone

Type of Test: Urine, timed

This test is a quantitative analysis of total estrogens and estrogen fractions (estrone, estradiol, and estriol) in urine over 24 hours. Estrone is the immediate precursor of estradiol, the most active of the endogenous estrogens. Estriol increases in urine as pregnancy advances and is a good indicator of placental function and fetal well-being.

Indications

- Diagnose suspected tumor of the ovary, testicle, or adrenal gland, as indicated by elevated total estrogens and fractions.
- Diagnose suspected ovarian failure, as indicated by decreased total estrogens and fractions.
- Detect placental and fetal problems, as indicated by estriol levels that fail to show a steady increase over several days or weeks. (A sharp decline over several days indicates impending fetal demise; consistently low levels may indicate fetal anomalies.)
- Detect maternal disorders of pregnancy, as indicated by estriol levels that fail to show a steady increase over several days or weeks.

Reference Values

	SI Units

Total

Children	<10 μg/24 h	1.13 mg/mol
Men	4–25 μg/24 h	0.45–2.60 mg/mol
Nonpregnant females		
Preovulatory phase	7–65 μg/24 h	0.79–7.35 mg/mol
Ovulatory phase	32–104 μg/24 h	3.62–11.75 mg/mol
Luteal phase	8–135 μg/24 h	0.90–15.26 mg/mol
Postmenopausal females	<20 μg/24 h	<2.26 mg/mol

Estrone (E_1)

Children	0.2–1 g/24 h	
Men	2.0–8.0 μg/24 h	0.8–3.3 mmol/mol
Nonpregnant females		
Early in cycle	2–39 μg/24 h	0.8–16.3 mmol/mol
Ovulation peak	11–46 μg/24 h	4.6–19.2 mmol/mol
Luteal phase	3–52 μg/24 h	1.2–21.7 mmol/mol
Postmenopausal females	0.8–7.1 g/24 h	

Estradiol (E_2)

Children	<5 μg/24 h	<2.1 μmol/mol
Men	1–4 μg/24 h	0.4–1.7 μmol/mol
Nonpregnant females		
Early in cycle	1–13 μg/24 h	0.4–5.4 μmol/mol
Luteal phase	4–20 μg/24 h	1.7–8.3 μmol/mol
Postmenopausal females	1–17 μg/24 h	.04–7.1 μmol/mol

Estriol (E_3)

Children	0.3–2.4 μg/24 h	1.04–8.33 nmol/24 h
Men	1.0–11.0 μg/24 h	3.5–38.2 nmol/24 h
Nonpregnant females		
Early in cycle	0–15 μg/24 h	0–52.0 nmol/24 h
Ovulation peak	13–54 μg/24 h	45.1–187.4 nmol/24 h
Luteal phase	8.0–60.0 μg/24 h	27.8–208.2 nmol/24 h
Postmenopausal females	0.6–6.8 μg/24 h	2.08–23.6 nmol/24 h
Pregnant females		
1st trimester	0–800 μg/24 h	0–2.776 nmol/24 h
2nd trimester	800–12,000 μg/24 h	2,776–41,640 nmol/24 h
3rd trimester	5,000–50,000 μg/24 h	17,350–173,500 nmol/24 h

Abnormal Values

- Increased levels
    Advancing and multiple pregnancy
    Ovarian, testicular, and adrenal tumors
    Drugs such as levodopa and spironolactone (in males), adrenal corticosteroids, tetracyclines, vitamins, ampicillin, phenothiazines
- Decreased levels
    Primary and secondary ovarian failure
    Turner's syndrome
    Hypopituitarism
    Adrenogenital syndrome
    Stein-Leventhal syndrome
    Anorexia nervosa
    Drugs such as oral contraceptives, probenecid, ampicillin, and neomycin
    Menopause
    Maternal complications of pregnancy (diabetes, hypertension)
    Placental insufficiency, impending fetal distress, fetal anomalies (e.g., anencephaly), and Rh isoimmunization

Interfering Factors

- Improper specimen collection and maintenance can affect results.
- Numerous drugs can alter test results (see Abnormal Values).

Nursing Implications

Assessment

- Obtain history of hormonal disorders, pregnancy status and trimester, and medication regimen.
- Ensure that the client has withheld medications that may interfere with the test results.

Possible Nursing Diagnoses

Anxiety related to threat to health status or fetal well-being
Grieving, anticipatory, related to perceived potential loss
Body image disturbance related to change in structure/appearance

Implementation

- Obtain the appropriate container for a 24-hour specimen from the laboratory for either a preservative or refrigerated specimen or place container on ice.
- Begin the test between 6 and 8 A.M. if possible. Collect first voiding and discard. Record the time specimen was discarded as the beginning of the 24-hour test.
- The next morning, request the client to void at the same time the collection was started and add this to the container.
- If an indwelling catheter is in place, place collection bag on ice at the start of the collection time, or empty the urine into a large container in the refrigerator periodically during the 24-hours; monitor that continued drainage is ensured and conclude the test the next morning at the same hour the collection was begun.
- At the conclusion of the test, ensure that the label is properly completed with start and completion times. Transport to the laboratory promptly.

Evaluation

- Note results and compare with serum estrogen levels, if available.

Client/Caregiver Teaching

Pretest

- Inform the client that all urine for a 24-hour period of time must be saved. Instruct client to avoid voiding in pan with defecation and to keep toilet tissue out of pan to prevent contamination of the specimen.

Posttest

- Tell the client to resume any medications withheld before the test.

Euglobulin Clot Lysis Time

Classification: Hematology

Type of Test: Blood

This coagulation test is performed to document excessive fibrinolytic activity. Euglobulins are proteins that precipitate from acidified dilute plasma, which prevent fibrin formation in the clotting process. When fibrinolytic process is overactive, clots break down quickly, resulting in a tendency to bleed. This test measures the time interval between a clot formation and lysis in the euglobulin plasma fraction.

Indications

- Diagnose suspected abnormal fibrinolytic activity, as indicated by lysis of the clot within 1 hour
- Differentiate between primary fibrinolysis, which has a rapid euglobulin lysis time, from disseminated intravascular coagulation (DIC), which usually presents with a normal euglobulin lysis time
- Monitor the effects of fibrinolytic therapy on normal coagulation

Reference Values

- Lysis in 2 to 4 hours
- *Critical time:* Complete lysis in 1 hour

Abnormal Values

- Decreased lysis time
    Fibrinolytic therapy with streptokinase or urokinase
    Prostatic cancer
    Severe liver disease
    Extensive vascular trauma or surgery
    Shock (hemorrhagic)

Interfering Factors

- Decreased fibrinogen levels (<100 mg/dL) can shorten lysis time.

- Traumatic venipunctures and excessive agitation of the sample can alter results.
- Failure to collect the blood in the proper tube can affect results.
- Vigorous exercise and use of steroids can increase fibrinolysis.

Nursing Implications

Assessment

- Obtain history of bleeding disorders and fibrinolytic therapy.
- Obtain history of medication use.

Possible Nursing Diagnoses

Injury, risk for, related to altered clotting factors
Protection, altered, related to abnormal blood profiles
Anxiety related to perceived threat to health status
Fluid volume deficit related to active loss

Implementation

- Put on gloves. Using aseptic technique, perform a venipuncture and collect 2 mL of blood and discard; then collect 10 mL of blood in each of a light blue-top tube and plain tube. Place tubes in ice and send to laboratory immediately.
- Avoid prolonged tourniquet constriction, tapping the vein, excessive pumping of the fist and excessive probing during venipuncture because it may alter results. Also, avoid excessive agitation because hemolysis can alter results.

Evaluation

- Note results in relation to other tests performed and the client's symptoms.

Client/Caregiver Teaching

Posttest

- Tell the client to report bleeding from any area of the skin and mucous membranes.

Evoked Brain Potentials, Evoked Potential Studies (EP Studies)

Classification: Electrophysiologic study

Type of Test: Indirect measurement

Evoked brain potentials, also known as evoked potential responses, are electrophysiologic studies performed to measure the brain's electrical responses when stimulated by various sensory stimuli or skin electrodes. Three response types are measured: the visual evoked response (VER), auditory brainstem response (ABR), and somatosensory response (SER). Another cognitive study, called event-related potential (ERP), can be performed to measure perceptomotor skills, mental function, and ability to discriminate sensory perceptions.

The stimuli activate the nerve tracts that connect the area stimulated (receptor area) with the cortical (visual and somatosensory) or midbrain (auditory) sensory area. A series of stimuli are given and electronically displayed in waveforms and recorded. Abnormalities are determined by a delay in time between the stimulus and the response, also known as an increased latency, and measured in milliseconds (msec). VER provides information about visual pathway function to identify lesions of the optic nerves and tracts; ABR provides information about auditory pathways to identify hearing loss and lesions of the brainstem; SER provides information about the somatosensory pathways to identify lesions at various levels of the central nervous system (spinal cord and brain); and ERP provides information about cognitive changes in the presence of neurologic disorders.

The studies are especially useful in clients with behavior problems and those unable to speak or respond to instructions during the test, since they do not require voluntary cooperation or participation in the activity. This allows for objective diagnostic information about visual or auditory disorders affecting infants and children and differentiating between organic brain and psychological disorder in adults.

Indications

VER (potentials)
- Diagnose neurologic disorders such as multiple sclerosis, Parkinson's disease, Huntington's chorea
- Diagnose cryptic or past retrobulbar neuritis
- Evaluate optic pathway lesions and visual cortex defects
- Diagnose lesions of the eye or optic nerves
- Evaluate binocularity in infants

ABR (potentials)
- Detect abnormalities or lesions in the brainstem or auditory nerve areas
- Screen or evaluate low-weight neonates, infants, children, and adults for auditory problems
- Early detection of brainstem tumors and acoustic neuromas

SER (potentials)
- Evaluate spinal cord and brain injury and function
- Diagnose sensorimotor neuropathies and cervical pathology
- Diagnose multiple sclerosis and Guillain-Barré syndrome
- Monitor sensory potentials to determine spinal cord function during a surgical procedure or medical regimen

ERP (potentials)
- Differentiate between organic brain disorder and cognitive function abnormality
- Diagnose suspected psychosis or dementia

Reference Values

- *VER and ABR:* Normal latency in recorded cortical and brainstem waveforms depending on age, sex, and stature.
- *ERP:* Normal recognition and attention span.
- *SER:* No loss of consciousness or presence of weakness.

Abnormal Values

VER (potentials)
- P100 latencies (extended) confined to one eye suggest a lesion anterior to the optic chiasm.
- Bilateral abnormal P100 latencies indicate multiple sclerosis, optic neuritis, retinopathies, spinocerebellar degeneration, sarcoidosis, Parkinson's disease, Huntington's chorea, and amblyopias.

ABR (potentials)
- Normal response at high intensities; wave V may occur slightly later and earlier wave distortions suggest cochlear lesion.
- Absent or late waves at high intensities; increased interval between waves I and V; possible decreased amplitude of wave V suggests retrocochlear lesion.

SER (potentials)
- Abnormal upper-limb latencies suggest cervical spondylosis or intracerebral lesions.
- Abnormal lower-limb latencies suggest peripheral nerve root disease such as Guillain-Barré syndrome, multiple sclerosis, transverse myelitis, or traumatic spinal cord injuries.

Interfering Factors

- Improper placement of electrodes.
- Inability of client to understand instructions or cooperate with requests made during the study.
- Client stress.
- Extremely poor visual acuity can hinder accurate determination of VER; severe hearing loss can interfere with accurate determination of ABR.

Nursing Implications

Assessment

- Obtain history and assessment of neurological system, known or suspected neurological conditions and traumatic incidents to head or spinal cord as well as previous tests and procedures done.
- Ensure that the client is able to relax; report any extreme anxiety or restlessness.
- Ensure that hair is clean and free from hair sprays or solutions.

Possible Nursing Diagnoses

Physical mobility, impaired, related to neuromuscular impairment

Sensory-perceptual alteration [specify] related to altered sensory reception, transmission, or integration

Confusion related to cerebral dysfunction

Anxiety related to perceived threat to health status

Implementation

- Shampoo the client's hair before the procedure and remove any jewelry or metallic objects above the neck.
- *Visual evoked potentials:* Place client in a comfortable position about 1 meter from the stimulation source. Attach electrodes to the occipital and vertex lobe areas and a reference electrode to the ear. A light-emitting stimulation or a checkerboard pattern is projected on a screen at a regulated speed. This procedure is done for each eye (with the opposite eye covered) as the client is asked to look at a dot on

the screen without any change in the gaze while the stimuli are delivered. A computer interprets the brain's responses to the stimuli and records them in waveforms.

- *Auditory evoked potentials:* Place the client in a comfortable position and position the electrodes on the scalp at the vertex lobe area and each earlobe. Earphones are placed on the client's ears and a clicking noise stimulus is delivered into one ear while a continuous tone is delivered to the opposite ear. The responses to the stimuli are recorded as waveforms for analysis.
- *Somatosensory evoked potentials:* Place the client in a comfortable position and position the electrodes at the nerve sites of the wrist, knee, and ankle and on the scalp at the sensory cortex of the hemisphere on the opposite side (the electrode that picks up the response and delivers it to the recorder). Additional electrodes can be positioned at the cervical or lumbar vertebrae for upper- or lower-limb stimulation. The rate at which the electric shock stimulus is delivered to the nerve electrodes and travels to the brain is measured and interpreted by a computer and recorded in waveforms for analysis. Both sides can be tested by switching the electrodes and repeating the procedure.
- *Event-related potentials:* Place the client in a sitting position in a chair in a quiet laboratory room. Earphones are placed on the client's ears and auditory cues are administered. The client is asked to push a button when the tones are recognized. Flashes of light are also used as visual cues, with the client pushing a button when cues are noted. Results are compared to evoked potential waveforms for correct responses or lack of responses.

Evaluation

- Note results in relation to other studies performed and the client's symptoms. Information from evoked potential studies are insufficient to confirm a specific diagnosis.

Client/Caregiver Teaching

Pretest

- Inform the client that the procedure is performed in a special EEG lab by a technician trained to do the procedure and interpreted by a physician.
- Tell the client that this procedure is performed to measure electrical activity in the nervous system and takes about 30 minutes to 2 hours to complete, depending on the test.
- Assure the client that there is no discomfort during the test and encourage relaxation.

Exophthalmometry

Classification: Sensory organ function

Type of Test: Visual perception

A noninvasive procedure done to measure the amount of forward displacement of the eyeball from its orbit. It is performed with an instrument called an exophthalmometer, a horizontal calibrated bar with movable carriers on both sides. The mirrors attached to the carrier are inclined at a 45° angle and reflect the scale reading and profile of the corneal apex.

Indications

- Measure the amount of forward protrusion of the eye
- Evaluate the progression or resolution of exophthalmos

Reference Values

- Normal measurement of orbital protrusion of 12 to 20 mm in each eye
- No evidence of inward or outward eye displacement in the orbital cavity

Abnormal Values

- Thyroid disease, Grave's disease
- Xanthomatosis
- Retinoblastoma
- Eye tumor
- Edema, trauma
- Inflammatory diseases such as periostitis or cellulitis
- Hypertrophy of the orbital bone

Interfering Factors

- Improper technique in measurement by the exophthalmometer
- Inability of the client to remain still and fixate the eyes

Nursing Implications

Assessment

- Obtain a history of thyroid, other systemic diseases, and eye conditions; results of other tests and procedures; and medication regimen, in particular, use of corticosteroids.

Possible Nursing Diagnoses

Body image disturbance related to change in structure/appearance

Anxiety related to perceived threat to health status

Implementation

- Have client remove corrective lenses (glasses or contacts).
- Place the client in a sitting position facing the examiner with the eyes at the same level as the examiner. The client is asked to remain very still and look straight ahead while the test is performed.
- The exophthalmometer is placed in front of the eyes across the face. It is a calibrated horizontal bar that is equipped with movable carriers on each side and holding mirrors that reflect the corneal apex and a scale of measurement readings. A baseline reading is made and recorded by placing the two carriers against the lateral margins of the ocular orbit and noting the scale readings in millimeters. The mirrors are then locked into this position by tightening the screws.
- The client is asked to fixate the right eye on the examiner's left eye and, with the use of the mirrors, the apex of the right cornea is superimposed on the scale and the degree of protrusion beyond the orbital rim is measured. The procedure is repeated with the left eye fixated on the examiner's right eye.

Evaluation

- Note the results in relation to other tests and the client's symptoms. Particularly note the serum thyroxine and triiodothyronine levels if hyperthyroidism is suspected.

Client/Caregiver Teaching

Pretest

- Inform the client that the procedure is performed in a specially equipped room by a physician and takes about 5 minutes to complete; explain that there is no pain associated with this procedure.

- Inform the client that there are no restrictions or special preparations before the test.

Posttest

- Tell the client to use moisturizing eyedrops and tape lids closed during sleep, if ordered.
- Advise client to comply with schedule for further eye testing.

Extractable Nuclear Antigen (ENA) Antibodies

Classification: Immunoassay (enzyme-linked)

Type of Test: Serum

This tests for antibodies to three antigens, including ribonucleoprotein (anti-RNP), Smith's (anti-Sm) antigen, and Sjögren's (anti-SS-A and anti-SS-B) antigen. To test the blood sample, sheep's red blood cells sensitized with extractable nuclear antigen (ENA) are incubated with the serum samples. If agglutination occurs, ENA antibodies are present. To differentiate the antigen, a double immunoassay is performed.

Indications

- Differentiate autoimmune disorders, such as systemic lupus erythematosus (SLE), progressive systemic sclerosis, rheumatic disorders, collagen vascular autoimmune disease, and Sjögren's disease and syndrome

Reference Values

- Negative

Abnormal Values

- Positive RNP autoantibodies
  SLE
  Progressive systemic sclerosis
  Rheumatic disorders

Collagen vascular disease
- Positive anti-Sm antibodies
   SLE
   Collagen vascular disease
- Positive SS-B antibodies
   Primary Sjögren's disease (50 percent have rheumatoid arthritis)
- Positive SS-A antibodies
   Possible Sjögren's syndrome (sometimes associated with SLE)

Interfering Factors

- Failure to send the blood sample to the laboratory promptly may affect results.

Nursing Implications

Assessment

- Obtain a history of immune system, known or suspected connective tissue disorders, medication regimen, and diagnostic tests and results.

Possible Nursing Diagnoses

Anxiety related to perceived threat to health status
Physical mobility, impaired, related to neuromuscular/musculoskeletal impairment
Tissue perfusion, altered, peripheral, related to interruption of vascular flow
Pain related to inflammatory process of connective tissues

Implementation

- Put on gloves; using aseptic technique, perform a venipuncture and collect 7 mL of blood in a red-top tube.
- Send the sample to the laboratory promptly.

Evaluation

- Note results in relation to other test results, such as anti-DNA, serum complement, and antinuclear antibody (ANA) tests.
- Clients with Sjögren's syndrome and rheumatoid arthritis have neither anti-SS-A nor anti-SS-B antibodies.
- SS-A and SS-B antibody is useful when a client with suspected SLE is antinuclear antibody (ANA) negative.

Client/Caregiver Teaching

Posttest

■ Inform the immunocompromised client to check the venipuncture site for infection and promptly report any change.

Fecal Analysis

Classification: Microbiology

Type of Test: Feces

Feces consist mainly of cellulose and other undigested foodstuffs, bacteria, and water (as much as 70 percent). Other substances normally found include epithelial cells shed from the gastrointestinal tract, small amounts of fats, bile pigments in the form of urobilinogen, gastrointestinal and pancreatic secretions, and electrolytes. The average adult excretes 100 to 300 g of fecal material per day, the residue of approximately 10 L of liquid material that enters the tract each day. The laboratory analysis of feces includes macroscopic examination (volume, odor, shape, color, consistency, mucus), microscopic examinations (leukocytes, epithelial cells, qualitative fats, meat fibers, and parasites), chemical tests for specific substances (occult blood, qualitative fats, trypsin, urobilinogen, bile, and an estimation of carbohydrate), and microbiologic tests. (See "Culture, Stool" and "Ova and Parasites Stool.")

Indications

■ Diagnose diarrhea of unknown etiology such as ulcerative colitis and bacterial infections, as indicated by the presence of leukocytes, or disorders resulting from toxins, as indicated by the absence of leukocytes
■ Confirm diagnosis of suspected inflammatory bowel disorder, as indicated by large numbers of epithelial cells
■ Confirm diagnosis of pseudomembranous enterocolitis following use of broad-spectrum antibiotic therapy
■ Confirm diagnosis of pancreatitis, as indicated by excessive fat (steatorrhea) with elevated triglycerides (neural fats)
■ Confirm diagnosis of malabsorption syndromes, as indicated

by steatorrhea, elevated fatty acids, normal triglycerides, and positive for carbohydrate utilization
- Detect altered protein digestion, as indicated by presence of meat fibers
- Detect intestinal parasitic infestation, as indicated by diarrhea of unknown origin
- Diagnose disorder associated with gastrointestinal bleeding or drug therapy that leads to bleeding
- Detect anemias, as indicated by decreased levels of urobilinogen and bile
- Detect liver and biliary tract disorders, as indicated by decreased levels
- Monitor effectiveness of therapy for intestinal malabsorption or pancreatic insufficiency

Reference Values

- *Normal fecal flora:* 96 to 99 percent anaerobes and 1 to 4 percent aerobes
- Negative for pathogens
- Negative for leukocytes
- Few to moderate epithelial cells
- *Fat (qualitative):* <60 normal-sized droplets per HPF
- *Triglycerides (neutral fats):* 1 to 5 percent
- *Fatty acids:* 5 to 15 percent
- Negative for meat fibers
- Negative for occult blood
- Trypsin 2+ to 4+
- Negative for carbohydrates (Clinitest)
- *Urobilinogen, random:* Negative
- *Urobilinogen, 24-hour:* 40 to 200 mg/24 h; 80 to 280 Ehrlich units/24 h
- Negative for bile (adults)
- Positive for bile (children)

Abnormal Values

- Positive for pathogens
  Parasitic infestations by *Ascaris lumbricoides, Diphyllobothrium latum, Taenia saginata,* and protozoan infestations by *Giardia lamblia*
  Bacterial infection with *Salmonella, Shigella, Yersinia,* and invasive *Escherichia coli*
- Positive for leukocytes
  Infections of the intestinal wall
- Excessive epithelial cells
  Inflammatory bowel disorders

- Elevated fat content
  Pancreatitis with elevated triglycerides
  Malabsorption
  Cystic fibrosis
- Elevated meat fibers
  Altered protein digestion
- Positive for occult blood
  Ulcers
  Gastritis
  Esophageal varices
  Esophagitis
  Mallory-Weiss tears
  Polyps
  Infectious diarrheas
  Inflammatory bowel disease
  Diverticular disease
  Tumors
  Hemorrhoids
  Anal fissure
- Positive carbohydrate levels
  Malabsorption syndromes
- Increased bile levels
  Hemolytic anemia
- Negative or decreased trypsin levels
  Pancreatic insufficiency in children
- Decreased urobilinogen levels
  Anemias
  Liver and biliary tract diseases
- Increased urobilinogen levels
  Hemolytic anemia

Interfering Factors

- Pretest antimicrobial therapy will delay growth of pathogens.
- Failure to collect an adequate amount of material for culture.
- Barium and mineral oil reduces bacterial growth.
- Ingestion of diet high in red meat, certain vegetables, and bananas can cause false-positive results for occult blood.
- A diet too high or low in fats or failure to follow prescribed diet can alter results of quantitative fat tests.
- Exposure of specimen to light can produce false-negative results for urobilinogen; exposure to air or room temperature can damage bacteria and prevent growth during culture.
- Ingestion of drugs such as aspirin, anticoagulants, corticosteroids, iron preparations, colchicine, and phenylbutazone can cause positive result for occult blood.

Nursing Implications

Assessment

- Obtain a history of known or suspected diarrhea, inflammatory bowel disorder, and therapy with drugs that lead to bleeding.

Possible Nursing Diagnoses

Diarrhea related to gastrointestinal dysfunction
Pain related to tissue inflammation or irritation
Anxiety related to perceived threat to health status

Implementation

- Collect a stool specimen in a half-pint, waterproof container with tight-fitting lid; if the patient is not ambulatory, collect in a clean, dry bedpan.
- Transfer the specimen using a tongue blade to the container and include any mucoid and bloody portions. Collect specimen from the first, middle, and last portion of feces.
- To collect specimen by rectal swab, insert the swab past the anal sphincter, rotate gently, and withdraw. Place the swab in the appropriate container. (For a viral test, consult with the laboratory for proper collection procedure.)
- Label the container with the date and time of collection and suspected cause of enteritis, noting any current or recent antibiotic therapy. Place the container in a leakproof bag and send it immediately to the laboratory.

Evaluation

- Note test results in relation to other tests performed and the client's symptoms.

Client/Caregiver Teaching

Pretest

- Tell the client to follow a normal diet for several days before the test. However, the client should avoid foods that interfere with test results (see Interfering Factors).
- Inform the client of the procedure for collecting a stool sample, including the importance of good hand-washing techniques. The client should place the sample in a tightly covered container.
- Tell the client not to use laxatives, enemas, or suppositories for 3 days before the test.

- Tell the client not to contaminate the specimen with urine or water.
- Stress the importance of transporting the sample to the laboratory promptly. The client should refrigerate the sample if it will be longer than 60 minutes.

Posttest

- Tell the client to resume normal diet after the test.

Fecal Fat

Classification: Specimen (quantitative) analysis

Type of Test: Feces

Fats are found in feces primarily in the form of triglycerides (neutral fats), fatty acids, and fatty acid salts. Through microscopic examination, the number and size of fat droplets can be determined and the type of fat identified. Malabsorption disorders and blockage of the pancreatic ducts by mucus, such as in cystic fibrosis, prevents the enzymes from reaching the duodenum and results in lack of fat digestion. Without digestion, the fats cannot be absorbed and steatorrhea results.

Indications

- Diagnose malabsorption or pancreatic insufficiency, as indicated by elevated fat levels
- Monitor effectiveness of therapy

Reference Values

- 2–7 g/24 h and <20 percent of total solids

Abnormal Values

- Increased values
    Amyloidosis
    Blind-loop syndrome
    Celiac disease
    Crohn's disease

Cystic fibrosis
Diverticulosis
Enteritis
Hepatobiliary disease
Lymphoma
Pancreatic disease
Short-bowel syndrome
Sprue
Whipple's disease
Zollinger-Ellison syndrome

Interfering Factors

- Failure to collect all stools will cause false-negative results.
- Ingestion of a diet too high or low in fats may alter results.
- Use of suppositories, oily lubricants, or mineral oil in the perineal area for 3 days before the test can alter the results.

Nursing Implications

Assessment

- Obtain a history of gastrointestinal disorders, results of tests performed, and medication regimen.
- Confirm that the client ingested a diet of 50 to 150 grams of fat per day for 3 days before the test.
- Confirm that the client has not used laxatives, enemas, or interfering drugs for 3 days before the test.

Possible Nursing Diagnoses

Diarrhea related to gastrointestinal dysfunction
Pain related to tissue inflammation or irritation
Anxiety related to perceived threat to health status
Nutrition, altered, less than body requirements, related to inability to digest food and absorb nutrients
Fluid volume deficit, risk for, related to active loss

Implementation

- Obtain a 500-mL clean plastic container or plastic bag, dry ice, and a toilet-mounted collection container to aid in collecting the stool, if available.
- Collect each stool and place it in the container during the 72-hour testing period. Keep container in dry ice or plastic bag in the freezer.
- When collection is complete, label the specimen and transport to the laboratory.

Evaluation

- Note test results in relation to other tests performed and the client's symptoms.

Client/Caregiver Teaching

Pretest

- Tell the client to ingest a diet containing 50 to 150 grams of fat per day for at least 3 days before the test.
- Inform the client not to use laxatives, enemas, or suppositories for 3 days before the test.
- Inform the client not to urinate in the stool container or put toilet paper in the container.
- Stress to the client or caregiver the importance of collecting all stools, including diarrhea.

Posttest

- Tell the client to resume normal diet after the test.

Febrile Agglutinins, Serum

Classification: Immunology

Type of Test: Blood

When the suspected infecting organism is difficult or dangerous to culture, serologic diagnosis is made by means of agglutination tests using antigens to specific organisms that cause the individual's antibodies to clump. This test may also be performed in conjunction with the blood culture.

Indications

- Determine possible cause of fever of unknown origin (FUO)
- Confirm diagnosis of typhus, Rocky Mountain spotted fever, or other disorder for which selected tests are specific
- Detect a suspected "carrier" state for typhoid
- Perform if blood or stool culture is positive for salmonella

Reference Values

Weil-Felix reaction (proteus antigen test)	< 1:80
Widal's test (O and H antigen tests)	< 1:160
Brucella agglutination test (slide agglutination test)	< 1:80
Tularemia agglutination test (tube dilution test)	< 1:40

Abnormal Values

- Weil-Felix reaction
  Positive in rickettsial infections such as Rocky Mountain spotted fever and typhus (murine, scrub, epidemic, and recrudescent)
- Widal's test
  Positive in salmonella infections such as typhoid and paratyphoid fevers
- Brucella agglutination test
  Positive in brucella infections: cattle, hog, goat (hosts may transmit infections to humans)
- Tularemia agglutination test
  Positive in tularemia, rabbit fever, and deer fly fever

Interfering Factors

- Vaccination, chronic exposure to infected animals, and cross-reactions with other antibodies may result in falsely elevated titers.
- Individuals who are immunosuppressed or receiving antibiotic therapy may have false-negative results.

Nursing Implications

Assessment

- Obtain a history of exposure to infectious diseases, results of other tests performed, and medication regimen.

Possible Nursing Diagnoses

Anxiety related to perceived threat to health status
Hyperthermia related to infectious process
Activity intolerance related to compromised respiratory status

Implementation

- Put on gloves. Using aseptic technique, obtain 7 mL of blood in a red-top tube.
- Handle the sample gently to avoid hemolysis and send to the laboratory immediately.

Evaluation

- Note test results in relation to other tests performed, particularly the blood culture, and the client's symptoms.

Client/Caregiver Teaching

Pretest

- Inform the client that no fasting is required for this test.

Posttest

- Inform the client that if not performed before another test, blood culture may be necessary.

▲▲▲▲▲▲▲▲▲▲▲▲▲▲▲▲▲▲▲▲▲

Ferric Chloride (FeCl$_3$)

Classification: Chemistry

Type of Test: Urine, random

Ferric chloride is a diagnostic test on urine that doesn't specifically diagnose any one disease but can be used to narrow down the suspected diagnosis of amino acid and metabolic disorders and use of certain drugs. The test produces highly variable color reactions in urine.

Indications

- Confirm known or suspected drug or alcohol ingestion
- Confirm diagnosis of phenylketonuria or other metabolic disorders

Reference Values

- Negative

Abnormal Values

Disease/Disorder	Color Indicator
Alcoholism	Red or reddish brown
Diabetes	Red or reddish brown
Histidinemia	Green or blue-green
Phenylketonuria	Blue or blue-green; fades to yellow
Starvation	Red or reddish brown

Drug	Color Indicator
Acetophenetidin	Red
Alcohol	Red to reddish brown
Aminosalicylic acid	Reddish brown
Antipyrines	Red
Cyanides	Red
Phenols	Violet
Phenothiazines	Purplish-pink
Salicylates	Purple

Interfering Factors

- Drugs such as levodopa, salicylates, phenazone, and phenothiazines can cause false-positives

Nursing Implications

Assessment

- Obtain a history of the purpose for test, known or suspected drug ingestions, and current medication regimen

Possible Nursing Diagnoses

Anxiety related to perceived threat to health status

Nutrition, altered, less than body requirements, related to inability to digest food and absorb nutrients

Trauma, risk for, related to ingestion of mind-altering substances

Implementation

- Obtain a clean plastic specimen container; instruct client to void into the container (an early-morning random specimen is needed). The test can also be performed on an infant by using a wet diaper.

- If client has an indwelling catheter, collect a fresh specimen from the drainage bag using aseptic technique.
- If testing specimen, add 10 percent $FeCl_3$ drops to 1 to 2 mL of urine; compare to color range provided.
- Send properly labeled specimen to the laboratory promptly if not performing immediately.

Evaluation

- Note results and report findings to physician. Also compare results to client's symptoms.

Client/Caregiver Teaching

Posttest

- Instruct client to resume medications, if withheld.
- Tell client that results can be revealed immediately if test drops are used or in 24 hours if sent to the laboratory.

Ferritin

Classification: Hematology

Type of Test: Serum

Ferritin is a protein that is naturally manufactured in the liver, spleen, and bone marrow and is produced by tumor cells and at sites of inflammation. The amount of ferritin in the circulation usually is proportional to the amount of storage iron (ferritin and hemosiderin) in body tissues. Levels vary according to age and sex.

Indications

- Determine cause and type of anemia of unknown etiology when used with serum iron and total iron-binding capacity
- Diagnose iron-deficiency anemia
- Support diagnosis of hemochromatosis or other disorders of iron metabolism and storage
- Monitor hematologic responses during pregnancy, when serum iron is usually decreased and ferritin may be decreased

Reference Values

		SI Units
Infant	50–200 ng/mL	50–200 µg/L
Newborn	25–200 ng/mL	25–200 µg/L
Children	7–140 ng/dL	7–140 µg/L
Men	20–250 ng/dL	20–250 µg/L
Women	10–120 ng/dL	10–120 µg/L
Crisis value (iron overload)	>220 ng/dL	>220 µg/L

Note: Average is 30 ng/dL.

Abnormal Values

- Increased levels
  Hemochromatosis or hemosiderosis
  Acute or chronic hepatocellular disease
  Hodgkin's disease
  Leukemia
  Acute or chronic infection
  Inflammatory diseases
  Breast cancer
  Chronic anemias (hemolytic, pernicious, megaloblastic)
- Decreased levels
  Iron deficiency anemia
  Hemodialysis

Interfering Factors

- Recent transfusion can elevate serum ferritin.
- Drugs, such as ethanol, iron salts, oral contraceptives can increase levels.
- Test should not be performed if client had a radioactive scan within 48 hours.
- Levels may be lower during menstruation.

Nursing Implications

Assessment

- Obtain a history of known or suspected anemia, cancer, hepatic disease, and inflammatory diseases.

Possible Nursing Diagnoses

Protection, altered, related to abnormal blood profiles
Anxiety related to perceived threat to health status
Infection, risk for secondary, related to immunosuppressed inflammatory response

Implementation

■ Put on gloves. Using aseptic technique, perform a venipuncture and collect 10 mL of blood in a red-top tube.

Evaluation

■ Note results and compare with results of iron studies, red blood cell count, hemoglobin, and reticulocyte count.

Client/Caregiver Teaching

Posttest

■ Instruct the client and caregiver in dietary inclusion of iron-rich foods.
■ Instruct the client in the administration of iron supplement, including side effects.

Fetal Monitoring, External: Nonstress Test

Classification: Fetal monitoring

Type of Test: Indirect fetal heart rate measurement

This noninvasive test involves the measurement of the antepartal fetal heart rate (FHR) during activity or movement that occurs without the stress of labor contractions. It is done to evaluate fetal viability and central and autonomic nervous system integrity and helps identify fetal risk for uterine asphyxia by the determination of its ability to respond with FHR accelerations during movement that occurs spontaneously or following stimulation by external manipulation or vibroacoustic methods. This test can also be performed in the early stages of labor to monitor contractions and fetal response.

During the test, the FHR is amplified and recorded on a strip by an external electronic fetal monitor situated on the mother's abdomen. FHR accelerations in a specific number and for a specific time period result in a reactive, nonreactive, or equivocal response. A reactive result is the detection of two or more accelerations consisting of 15 beats per minute and lasting at least 15 seconds each over a 10-minute period. An equivocal result involves the detection of one acceleration over the 10-minute period.

Indications

- Evaluate fetal health by determining the potential for or presence of fetal distress caused by intrauterine hypoxia, evidenced by quality of FHR acceleration responses during nonstress situations.
- Screen high-risk pregnancies to determine the need for a contraction stress test.

Reference Values

- *Fetal heart rate:* 120 to 160 bpm
- *Reactive response:* two or more accelerations during fetal movement, each acceleration with an FHR of 15 beats per minute lasting 15 seconds or more during a 10-minute period

Abnormal Values

- Fetal distress, as indicated by a nonreactive response. This response may be confirmed by the contraction stress test, which involves the administration of oxytocin to produce uterine contractions.

Interfering Factors

- Supine position can affect readings, as this can distress the fetus.
- Excessive movement by the mother or fetus can affect accuracy of results.
- Medications such as sedatives can reduce the activity of the fetus and produce inaccurate results.

Nursing Implications

Assessment

- Obtain an obstetric history, history of medical conditions such as diabetes mellitus, hypertension, expected date of delivery, and other diagnostic tests and procedures.
- Ensure that the client has eaten a full meal just before the study as sounds from an empty stomach can interfere with the sounds from the fetal heart rate (FHR) and fetal move-

ment can be increased by a higher glucose level in the mother.

Possible Nursing Diagnoses

Anxiety related to threat to health of fetus

Grieving, anticipatory, related to perceived potential loss

Coping, ineffective, individual, risk for, related to fear of fetal demise

Implementation

- Ask the client to void.
- Place the client in a semi-Fowler's or side-lying position and drape the exposed abdomen.
- Cover the transducer with conductive jelly and place it at the best site to hear fetal heart tones. The transducer is strapped to the abdomen with a stretchable band.
- Give the mother the marking button to press when she feels fetal movement. The FHR and fetal movements are each recorded on a strip, one graph line for the FHR and one for the movements to be viewed, and compared in determining accelerations. This monitoring is done until two fetal movements are detected within 20 minutes that last longer than 15 seconds each and increase the FHR by 15 beats per minute over the baseline.
- Failure to obtain these recordings for a time period of 20 minutes can be followed by external stimulation maneuvers to be done to encourage fetal movement. These maneuvers include rubbing or compressing the abdomen or producing a sound source with an artificial larynx placed on the abdomen. The client may also be giving a fruit juice to increase the glucose level and stimulate fetal movement. Nipple stimulation may also be used to stimulate uterine contractions and fetal movements.

Evaluation

- If the fetus is nonreactive, notify the physician and prepare the client for a contraction stress test, which involves the administration of oxytocin.

Client/Caregiver Teaching

Pretest

- Inform the client how the procedure is performed and that the procedure is generally performed in the obstetric department or physician's office by a nurse experienced in the type of monitoring with results interpreted by a physician.

Also tell her that the test will take 30 to 45 minutes to complete.
- Inform the client that no pain is associated with the procedure.
- Tell the client to eat a meal and void before the procedure.

Posttest

- Inform the client that weekly external fetal monitoring may be indicated for diabetes, hypertension, fetal growth retardation, and in pregnancy over 42 weeks' gestation.

Fetal Monitoring, Internal

Classification: Fetal monitoring

Type of Test: Direct uterine and fetal heart rate measurement

Performed during labor, this procedure directly monitors fetal heart rate (FHR) as an indication of fetal well-being and measures the frequency and strength of uterine contractions. It is not performed until the membranes have ruptured, the cervix is dilated >3 cm, the fetal head is lower than -2 station. It is usually only done when external monitoring isn't providing adequate data.

Indications

- Monitor fetal heart rate, including beat-to-beat variability
- Measure frequency and strength (pressure) of contractions
- Evaluate fetal health during labor

Reference Values

Fetal heart rate (FHR)	120–160 beats per minute
FHR variability	5–25 beats per minute
Maternal contractions and intrauterine pressure during labor	

First stage	<6 contractions every 10 min
	8–12 mmHg (baseline pressure)
	30–40 mmHg (contraction pressure)
Second stage	1 contraction every 2 min
	10–20 mmHg (baseline pressure)
	50–80 mmHg (contraction pressure)

Abnormal Values

- Bradycardia (FHR <120 bpm)
    Fetal heart block
    Hypoxia
    Malposition
- Tachycardia (FHR >160 bpm)
    Vagolytic drugs
    Early hypoxia
    Fetal infection
    Prematurity
- Late decelerations (FHR slows after contraction begins, lag time >20 s, recovery time >15 s)
    Fetal hypoxia
    Acidosis
    Uteroplacental insufficiency
- FHR <70 bpm for >60 s
    Fetal distress

Interfering Factors

- Drugs that affect sympathetic and parasympathetic nervous system may influence FHR.
- Maternal position may affect FHR; left side-lying promotes best oxygen delivery to fetus.

> **NURSING ALERT**
>
> - Contraindicated in active genital herpes
> - Contraindicated if uncertainty exists about the presenting fetal part

Nursing Implications

Assessment

- Obtain obstetrical history, pattern of FHR and contractions during present labor, and medication use.

Possible Nursing Diagnoses

Anxiety related to threat to health of fetus

Grieving, anticipatory, related to perceived potential loss

Coping, ineffective, individual, risk for, related to fear of fetal demise

Injury, risk for, to fetus, related to invasive procedure

Implementation

- Place the patient in a dorsal lithotomy position and prepare the perineal area.
- The physician or trained professional will locate the fetal scalp and then insert the plastic tube with the transducer into the cervix. The electrode is attached to the fetal scalp by rotating the tube clockwise. After checking the attachment, the tube is withdrawn and then the electrode wire is attached to the leg plate placed on the woman's leg. Attach the cable to the monitor.
- Next, the physician or trained professional fills the uterine catheter with sterile normal saline. The fluid-filled catheter and catheter guide are inserted 1 to 2 cm into the cervix, between the posterior cervix and the fetal head. The catheter is advanced until the black mark on the catheter lines up with the vulva. The guide is removed and the catheter is connected to the transducer.
- Prevent artifacts in pressure readings by flushing the transducer with sterile normal saline solution.
- After the delivery and the fetal scalp electrode is removed, an antibiotic solution is applied to the site.

NURSING ALERT

- If the FHR indicates fetal distress, turn the mother on her left side and administer oxygen. If these efforts fail to increase the heart rate, a cesarean birth may be necessary. Prepare the patient for removal of the electrode and the catheter before the cesarean.

Evaluation

- Watch the electrode site for signs of abscess.
- Monitor the mother for signs of intrauterine infection.

Client/Caregiver Teaching

Pretest

- Inform the client that she may feel mild discomfort when the electrode and uterine catheter are inserted. Deep breathing through her mouth and relaxation of abdominal muscles may minimize the discomfort.

■ Stress to the client that this test assesses fetal health. Encourage questions.

Posttest

■ Advise the client to notify the physician if she develops a fever, abdominal pain, or foul-smelling vaginal drainage.

Fetoscopy

Classification: Endoscopy

Type of Test: Direct visualization

Usually performed at 18 weeks' gestation when the placental vessels are of adequate size, this test uses a fiberoptic fetoscope with a light source and telescopic lens inserted through the abdomen into the uterus to visualize the fetus. Before the procedure, ultrasonography is done to identify the area of the fetus to be viewed and to aid insertion of the fetoscope.

Indications

■ Diagnose severe fetal malformations, for example, neural tube defect
■ Obtain fetal blood samples to detect congenital blood disorders
■ Obtain fetal skin biopsy to determine the presence of skin disorders

Reference Values

■ Absence of fetal distress, congenital malformation, or blood disorders

Abnormal Values

■ Neural-tube defects
■ Hemophilia
■ Sickle-cell anemia

Interfering Factors

- Inability of the client to cooperate with the procedure.
- Obesity may impair visualization.
- Abdominal or pelvic adhesions can affect insertion of the scope.

NURSING ALERT

- Contraindicated in patients with a history of multiple abdominal operations or peritonitis since dense adhesions may have resulted from them
- Contraindicated if there is acute infection involving the abdominal wall, since organisms may be introduced into the normally sterile peritoneal cavity
- Contraindicated in gestations of less than 18 weeks, since the fetal parts are not able to be identified and the blood vessels in the placental surface are not of appropriate size to secure blood samples

Nursing Implications

Assessment

- Obtain a history of allergies or sensitivities to anesthetics, analgesics, antibiotics, and gestational age.
- Assess and record baseline vital signs and fetal heart rate (FHR) for later comparison readings.

Possible Nursing Diagnoses

Anxiety related to threat to health of fetus
Grieving, anticipatory, related to perceived potential loss
Coping, ineffective, individual, risk for, related to fear of fetal demise
Injury, risk for, to fetus, related to invasive procedure

Implementation

- Ask client to void, then administer ordered premedication, usually meperidine, which crosses the placenta, quiets the fetus, and facilitates the procedure.
- Place the client in a supine position on the examining table and drape with the abdomen exposed. The insertion site is identified after ultrasonography locates the fetus and placenta, and local anesthetic is injected. The fetoscope, which is a very small telescopic instrument, is inserted through the incision made at the site and into the uterine cavity near

the placental site. Visualization of the fetus is done and accessory instruments are inserted to obtain blood samples from the vessels of the umbilical cord or skin samples from the fetus.

- After examination and collection of specimens, the scope is withdrawn. The skin incision is closed with a suture or sterile strip and a small dressing or adhesive strip applied.
- Administer RhoGAM to Rh-negative clients unless fetal blood is Rh negative.

Evaluation

- Monitor client and fetus for changes in blood pressure, pulse, uterine activity, fetal activity, vaginal bleeding, and leakage of amniotic fluid.

Client/Caregiver Teaching

Pretest

- Explain the purpose of the study and how the procedure is performed. Inform the client that the procedure is generally performed in an operating room by a physician under local anesthesia and takes approximately 1 to 2 hours.

Posttest

- Tell the client to avoid strenuous activity for 1 to 2 weeks following the procedure.
- Remind the client to keep her appointment for ultrasonography the following day to ensure the adequacy of the amniotic fluid and fetal viability.
- Tell the client to take prescribed prophylactic antibiotic to prevent infection of the amniotic fluid.
- Inform client that no discomfort should be experienced following the procedure.
- Tell the client to report any abdominal pain, vaginal bleeding or amniotic fluid loss, fever, redness or swelling of the incisional area to the physician immediately.

Fibrin Degradation Products (FDP), Fibrin Split Products (FSP), Fibrin Breakdown Products (FBP)

Classification: Hematology

Type of Test: Serum

This coagulation test is performed to evaluate fibrin split products (FSP) or fibrinogen degradation products (FDP) that interfere with normal coagulation and formation of the hemostatic platelet plug. After a fibrin clot has formed, the fibrinolytic system acts to prevent excessive clotting. In this system, plasmin digests fibrin. Fibrinogen also can be degraded if there is a disproportion among plasmin, fibrin, and fibrinogen. Seven substances result from this degradation which can indicate abnormal coagulation. Normally, FSPs are removed from the circulation by the liver and reticuloendothelial system.

Indications

- Diagnose suspected disseminated intravascular coagulation (DIC), as indicated by elevated FSP levels or positive results of protamine sulfate test (secondary fibrinolysin activity)
- Evaluate response to therapy with fibrinolytic drugs
- Monitor the effects on hemostasis by trauma, extensive surgery, obstetrical complications, and disorders such as liver or renal disease

Reference Values

- 2–10 μg/mL
- *Critical value:* >40 μg/mL

Abnormal Values

- Elevated FSP
  DIC
  Excessive bleeding

Liver disease
Various obstetrical complications, such as preeclampsia, abruptio placentae, intrauterine fetal death
Congenital heart disease
Leukemia
Thermal injury
Thromboembolic states
Renal disease
Transplant rejection
Postcardiothoracic surgery
Administration of heparin, fibrinolytic drugs such as streptokinase and urokinase, and large doses of barbiturates

Interfering Factors

- Drugs can produce elevated levels of FSP (see Abnormal Values).
- Traumatic venipunctures and excessive agitation of the sample can alter test results.

Nursing Implications

Assessment

- Obtain history of pregnancy complication, bleeding, or vascular disorder; results of tests performed; and current medication regimen, especially heparin and fibrinolytic drugs.

Possible Nursing Diagnoses

Injury, risk for, related to altered clotting factors
Protection, altered, related to abnormal blood profiles
Anxiety related to perceived threat to health status
Tissue perfusion, altered, related to occlusive disease

Implementation

- Put on gloves. Using aseptic technique, perform a venipuncture and collect 2 mL of blood in a red-top tube or in a special tube provided by the laboratory.
- Avoid traumatic venipunctures and excessive agitation of the sample and send sample to the laboratory promptly.

Evaluation

- Note results in relation to other tests performed and the client's symptoms.

Client/Caregiver Teaching

Posttest

- Tell the client to report bleeding from skin or mucous membranes.

Fibrinogen

Classification: Hematology

Type of Test: Plasma

A test performed to measure fibrinogen (factor I), which is converted to fibrin by thrombin in the common final pathway of the coagulation sequence. Fibrinogen is synthesized in the liver. It converts to fibrin and clots blood as it combines with platelets. In normal healthy individuals, the serum should contain no residual fibrinogen after clotting has occurred.

Indications

- Diagnose suspected disseminated intravascular coagulation (DIC), as indicated by decreased fibrinogen levels
- Evaluate congenital or acquired dysfibrinogenemias
- Monitor hemostasis in disorders associated with low fibrinogen levels or elevated levels that can predispose to excessive thrombosis

Reference Values

		SI Units
Newborns	>150 mg/dL	>1.5 g/L
Men	180–340 mg/dL	1.8–3.4 g/L
Women	190–420 mg/dL	1.9–4.2 g/L
Critical values	<100 mg/dL	

Abnormal Values

- Elevated levels
    Immune disorders of connective tissue
    Infections
    Glomerulonephritis
    Hepatitis
    Late pregnancy
    Oral contraceptive use
    Rheumatoid arthritis
    Cancer of the breast, stomach, or kidney
- Decreased levels
    DIC
    Leukemia, lymphoma, multiple myeloma
    Congenital fibrinogen deficiency (rare)
    Severe liver disease (cirrhosis)
    Dysfibrinogenemia
    Cancer of the prostate, lung, or pancreas
    Thrombocytopenic purpura
    Drugs, including phenobarbital, streptokinase

Interfering Factors

- Transfusions of whole blood, plasma, or fractions within 4 weeks of the test invalidate results.
- Traumatic venipuncture and excessive agitation of the sample can alter test results.

Nursing Implications

Assessment

- Obtain a history of bleeding disorders, chronic or acute medical conditions, diagnostic tests and results, and current medications, especially anticoagulants and oral contraceptives.
- Assess if the client has received blood products within the last 4 weeks.

Possible Nursing Diagnoses

Injury, risk for, related to altered clotting factors
Protection, altered, related to abnormal blood profiles
Anxiety related to perceived threat to health status

Implementation

- Put on gloves. Using aseptic technique, perform a venipuncture and collect 5 mL of blood in a light blue-top tube.

- Avoid excessive agitation of the sample and send to the laboratory immediately.

Evaluation

- Note results of other coagulation tests (PT, PTT, platelets) in association with factor I results, and observe the client for excessive or active bleeding.

Client/Caregiver Teaching

Pretest

- Inform the client that no food or fluid restrictions are required before the test.

Posttest

- Tell the client to report bruising, petechiae, and bleeding from mucous membranes.

Fibrinogen Uptake Test (FUT)

Classification: Nuclear medicine

Type of Test: Radionuclide imaging

This noninvasive test is performed to detect the presence of thrombus in the lower extremities. When thrombi form, large amounts of fibrinogen are present. After an injection of radionuclide-labeled fibrinogen (I-125), these thrombi and clots absorb the radionuclide, and their presence can be detected by a scanner (gamma-ray detector). This is a very accurate test for diagnosing deep-vein thrombosis.

Indications

- Monitor development and progression of deep-vein thromboses
- Screen for those at risk for thrombotic processes

Reference Values

- *Normal:* no areas of abnormal radionuclide concentration in deep veins of lower legs

Abnormal Values

- Positive values
  Thrombophlebitis
  Deep-vein thrombosis
  Thrombosis

Interfering Factors

- False-positive results may result with bacterial inflammation of the legs.
- False-negative results may occur when active clot formation ceases but thrombus remains.

Nursing Implications

Assessment

- Obtain a history of vascular system, known or suspected thromboses, medication regimen, and diagnostic tests and results.
- Obtain an allergy history, particularly to iodine or shellfish because radioactive tracer is iodine-based.

Possible Nursing Diagnoses

Injury, risk for, related to altered clotting factors
Anxiety related to perceived threat to health status
Tissue perfusion, altered, related to occlusive disease

Implementation

- Administer 10 drops of Lugol's solution to block thyroid uptake of the radioactive tracer, if prescribed by physician.
- Inject I-125–labeled fibrinogen intravenously. Multiple areas are marked and scans are obtained 10 minutes after the injection.
- After 24 hours, scans of the affected extremity are again obtained at predetermined intervals. The scans may be performed once daily for up to 1 week after the injection.

Evaluation

- Note results in relation to other studies performed.

Client/Caregiver Teaching

Pretest

- Inform the client that the test will be performed by a technician and take about 1 hour.
- Warn the client that the leg will be marked in multiple areas for the scanning process. The client should not wash off these markings.
- Caution breast-feeding mothers not to breast-feed infant for 24 to 48 hours after the radionuclide injection.

Fluorescent Rabies Antibody Test (FRA), Rabies Antibody Test

Classification: Serology

Type of Test: Blood

This test detects the presence of the rabies rhabdovirus in a human bitten by an infected animal. The potentially infected client's serum is examined by immunofluorescence to detect a serum antibody rise. It can be used to diagnose people who have never received a rabies vaccine or passive antibody. The disease is 99 percent fatal in clients whose symptoms begin before the treatment is begun. A vaccine can be administered to those at risk, such as veterinarians and zoo and kennel workers.

Indications

- Diagnose rabies in clients who have never received a rabies vaccine or passive antibody

Reference Values

- Negative or IFA $<1:16$

Abnormal Values

- Elevated levels indicate rabies

Nursing Implications

Assessment

- Assess the history of the animal bite, including the behavior of the animal and whether or not the animal was captured.

Possible Nursing Diagnoses

Infection, risk for, related to animal bite
Anxiety related to threat to health status

Implementation

- Put on gloves. Using aseptic technique, perform a venipuncture and collect 7 mL of blood in a red-top tube.
- Administer rabies immunoglobulin (Rig) after the bite. If vaccine is administered, give human diploid cell rabies vaccine in 1-mL doses IM five times. Give the first dose with the Rig and repeat at 3, 7, 14, and 28 days.

Evaluation

- Notify physician immediately of results.

Client/Caregiver Teaching

Pretest

- Inform the client that no food or fluid restriction is required before the test.

Posttest

- Inform the client of the importance of completing all five doses of the rabies vaccine series.

Fluorescent Treponemal Antibody Test (FTA-ABS)

Classification: Serology

Type of Test: Serum or CSF

This test provides the most sensitive detection of treponemal antibodies in all stages of syphilis. A serum sample is layered onto a slide fixed with *Treponema pallidum* organisms. If the antibody is present, it will attach to the organisms and can be identified by its reaction with fluorescein-labeled antiglobulin serum.

Indications

- Confirm the presence of treponemal antibodies in the serum or cerebrospinal fluid (CSF) to confirm tertiary syphilis
- Verify syphilis as the cause of positive venereal disease research laboratory (VDRL) and rapid plasma reagin (RPR) test results

Reference Values

- Negative

Abnormal Values

- Elevated levels
    Primary syphilis (80 to 90 percent of patients)
    Secondary syphilis (all patients)

Interfering Factors

- False-positive results may occasionally occur in the elderly and in those with systemic lupus erythematosus or other immune complex diseases, genital herpes, and pregnancy.
- Excessive chyle in the blood interferes with test results.
- Alcohol ingestion within 24 hours of the test can cause false-negative results.

Nursing Implications

Assessment

- Obtain a history of genitourinary symptoms, presence of skin lesions, and sexual contacts.
- Assess history for possible sources of false-positive or false-negative results.

Possible Nursing Diagnoses

Anxiety related to threat to health status
Infection, risk for transmission
Skin integrity, impaired, related to invasion by pathogenic organism

Implementation

- Put on gloves. Using aseptic technique perform a venipuncture and collect 7 mL of blood in a red-top tube.

Evaluation

- Notify the physician of positive results.

Client/Caregiver Teaching

Pretest

- Inform the client that food or fluid restriction is not required before the test.
- Tell the client to avoid alcohol ingestion for 24 hours before the test.

Posttest

- Tell the client to return for follow-up testing if findings are negative or borderline and syphilis has not been ruled out. (*T. pallidum* causes no immunological changes in the blood for 14 to 21 days after infection.)
- If the test is reactive, explain the disease process, the importance of proper treatment, and the need to find and treat all sexual contacts.
- Tell the client with early-stage syphilis to be retested at 3-month intervals to monitor declining reactivity.
- Inform the client that high levels may persist for years with or without treatment.

Fluoroscopy, Thoracic

Classification: Radiography

Type of Test: X-ray

This imaging technique allows a continuous stream of x-rays to pass through the client to a fluorescent viewing screen that is coated with calcium tungstate. Unlike with standard x-rays, movement can be visualized in the chest and diaphragm and subtle changes are better detected. Because this test delivers more radiation than standard x-rays, it is only used when it is necessary to visualize physiologic or pathologic motion of the thoracic contents.

Indications

- Assess diaphragmatic function
- Localize a lung mass
- Screen for coronary artery disease

Reference Values

- Symmetric pulmonary and diaphragmatic motion, with absence of calcifications in coronary arteries. Normal diaphragmatic excursions range from 2 to 4 cm.

Abnormal Values

- Decreased diaphragmatic function
- Bronchial obstructions and pulmonary disease
- Coronary artery disease

Interfering Factors

- Metallic objects interfere with quality of films.

NURSING ALERT

- This procedure is contraindicated in pregnancy.

Nursing Implications

Assessment

- Obtain a history of respiratory system, known or suspected pulmonary or coronary disease, current symptoms, medication regimen, and diagnostic tests and results.
- Ensure that the client has removed all jewelry and metal items.

Possible Nursing Diagnoses

Airway clearance, ineffective, related to compromised pulmonary function

Breathing pattern, ineffective, related to compromised pulmonary function

Anxiety related to threat to health status

Implementation

- If the client is intubated, make sure the the tube is not dislodged during positioning.
- The x-ray machine is positioned over the area to be visualized. When the x-rays are delivered the views are shown on a screen in real-time motion. As needed, help the client to turn in different positions. The films can be recorded on videotape and saved for future analysis and still films can be taken, as indicated. Special equipment may also be used to intensify images as needed.
- Help the client down from the x-ray table. Return jewelry and personal items.

Evaluation

- Note results in relation to client's symptoms and test findings.

Client/Caregiver Teaching

Pretest

- Inform the patient that the test is painless and that following instructions regarding deep-breathing and coughing is important.

Folic Acid, Folate, Folic Acids (RBCs)

Classification: Hematology

Type of Test: Serum; blood

Folic acid is a water-soluble vitamin that is stored in small amounts in the liver. It is needed for normal red blood cell and white blood cell function, normal DNA replication, and cell division. Normally functioning intestinal mucosa allow the absorption of folic acid. The test is often performed with serum B_{12} determinations.

Indications

- Diagnose megaloblastic anemia due to deficient folic acid intake or increased folate requirements, such as in pregnancy and hemolytic anemia
- Monitor response to disorders that may lead to folate deficiency or decreased absorption and storage
- Monitor effects of drugs that are folic acid antagonists, such as alcohol, anticonvulsants, antimalarials, and certain drugs used to treat leukemia
- Monitor effects of prolonged parenteral nutrition

Reference Values

Serum	3.5–25 mg/L
Red blood cells	
0–11 mo	74–995 ng/mL
1–11 yr	96–362 ng/mL
≥12 yr	180–600 ng/mL

Abnormal Values

- Elevated levels
   Excessive dietary intake of folic acid or folic acid supplements
   Pernicious anemia
- Decreased levels
   Folic acid anemia

Malnutrition
Pregnancy
Chronic alcoholism
Sprue
Cirrhosis
Uremia
Some neoplasms

Interfering Factors

- Hemolysis of blood sample falsely elevates results.
- Radioisotopes administered within 24 hours of the test can alter results.

Nursing Implications

Assessment

- Obtain a hematologic history and medication regimen.
- Assess if client fasted for 8 hours before the test and abstained from alcohol for 24 hours.

Possible Nursing Diagnoses

Tissue perfusion, altered [specify], related to oxygen supply/ demand imbalance

Nutrition, altered, less than body requirements, related to decreased intake

Anxiety related to perceived threat to health status

Implementation

- Put on gloves. Using aseptic technique, perform a venipuncture and collect 5 mL of blood in a red-top tube.

Evaluation

- Note test results in relation to other tests performed, tests for particularly B_{12}, and the client's symptoms.

Client/Caregiver Teaching

Pretest

- Tell the client to fast from food for 8 hours before the test and abstain from alcohol for 24 hours.
- If the client is receiving B_{12} injections, the sample must be obtained before the injection.
- Inform the client that the test cannot be performed if radioisotopes were administered within 24 hours before the test.

Posttest

- Tell the client to resume food, alcohol, and medications, as ordered.

Follicle-Stimulating Hormone (FSH)

Classification: Chemistry

Type of Test: Serum

This test measures follicle-stimulating hormone (FSH), which is secreted by the basophil cells of the adenohypophysis. In women, FSH promotes maturation of the graafian (germinal) follicle, causing estrogen secretion and allowing the ovum to mature. In men, FSH partially controls spermatogenesis, but the presence of testosterone is also necessary. GnRH secretion, which in turn stimulates FSH secretion, is stimulated by decreased estrogen and testosterone levels. FSH production is inhibited by rising estrogen and testosterone levels.

Indications

- Evaluate ambiguous sexual differentiation in infants
- Evaluate early sexual development in girls under age 9 or boys under age 10, with precocious puberty associated with elevated levels
- Evaluate failure of sexual maturation in adolescence
- Evaluate sexual dysfunction or changes in secondary sexual characteristics in men and women
- Evaluate pituitary or hypothalamic dysfunction
- Evaluate suspected disorders associated with elevated or decreased FSH levels (see Abnormal Values)

Reference Values

		SI Units
Children	5–10 mIU/mL	5–10 IU/L
Men	10–15 mIU/mL	10–15 IU/L
Women (menstruating)		
Early in cycle	5–25 mIU/mL	5–25 IU/L
Midcycle	20–30 mIU/mL	20–30 IU/L
Luteal phase	5–25 mIU/mL	5–25 IU/L
Women (menopausal)	40–250 mIU/mL	40–250 IU/L

Abnormal Values

- Increased FSH
    - Precocious puberty in children
    - Pituitary tumors
    - Polycystic ovary disease
    - Postviral orchitis
    - Adrenogenital syndrome in females
    - Turner's syndrome in females
    - Klinefelter's syndrome in males
    - Early acromegaly
    - Drugs such as clomiphene
- Decreased FSH
    - Anovulation in women
    - Aspermatogenesis in men
    - Hypothalamic lesions
    - Panhypopituitarism
    - Neoplasms of the testes
    - Excessive sex hormone production
    - Anorexia nervosa
    - Cirrhosis
    - Renal disease
    - Drugs containing estrogen, progesterone, and phenothiazines

Interfering Factors

- Radioactive scans performed within 1 week of the test can affect test results.
- In menstruating women, values vary in relation to the phase of the menstrual cycle.
- Values are higher in postmenopausal women.
- Administration of the drugs such as clomiphene can affect FSH levels.

Nursing Implications

Assessment

- Obtain a history of endocrine and reproductive systems, menstruation and date of last period, and results of diagnostic tests and procedures performed.
- Assess medication history and ensure that any drugs that may alter FSH levels have been withheld for 12 to 24 hours before the test, as ordered by physician.

Possible Nursing Diagnoses

Anxiety related to perceived threat to health status

Sexuality patterns, altered, related to illness or medical treatment

Body image disturbance related to change in structure/appearance

Grieving, anticipatory, related to perceived potential loss

Implementation

- Put on gloves. Using aseptic technique, perform a venipuncture and collect 7 mL of blood in a red- or lavender-top tube.
- If client is female, indicate the phase of her menstrual cycle on the laboratory slip.
- Handle the sample gently to avoid hemolysis and transport to the laboratory immediately.

Evaluation

- Note test results in relation to other tests of gonadal (luteinizing hormone) function.

Client/Caregiver Teaching

Posttest

- Tell the client to resume medications withheld before the test.
- Inform the client that serial tests can be performed to obtain more accurate results, as FSH levels are dependent on pituitary gland formation.

Free Fatty Acids (FFA)

Classification: Chemistry

Type of Test: Serum or plasma

This test measures free (nonesterified) fatty acids (FFA), which are substances that travel through the blood and combine with albumin. In this form, they are called nonesterified fatty acids (NEFA). Free fatty acids are essential components of lipoproteins and triglycerides and account for 2 to 5 percent of all lipids in the plasma. Synthesized within the cells or as a result of breakdown of lipoproteins or triglycerides, fatty acids are released from adipose tissue when stimulated by hormones, usually as a response to stress, anxiety, fasting, or malnutrition.

Indications

- Aid in diagnosis of diabetes mellitus
- Evaluate response to treatment for diabetes
- Diagnose suspected malnutrition
- Assess known or suspected disorder associated with excessive hormone production
- Evaluate response to therapy with drugs known to alter FFA levels

Reference Values

- Free fatty acids of 8 to 20 mg/dL or 80 to 200 mg/L (SI units)

Abnormal Values

- Increased levels
  - Acute alcohol intoxication
  - Starvation
  - Pheochromocytoma
  - Diabetes mellitus
  - Chronic hepatitis
  - Acute renal failure
  - Glycogen storage disease
  - Hypoglycemia
  - Hypothermia
  - Hormones such as adrenocorticotropic hormone, cortisone, epinephrine, norepinephrine, growth hormone, thyroid-stimulating hormone, and thyroxine
  - Drugs such as amphetamines, chlorpromazine, isoproterenol, reserpine, tolbutamide, caffeine, and nicotine
- Decreased levels
  - Drugs such as aspirin, clofibrate, glucose, insulin, neomycin, and streptozocin

Interfering Factors

- Ingestion of alcohol 24 hours before and food 12 hours before the test can falsely elevate levels.
- Ingestion of drugs known to alter cholesterol levels within 12 hours of the test and affect results. However, this test may be done specifically to evaluate these effects.

■ Delay in sending the sample to the laboratory can cause triglyceride breakdown and falsely elevate fatty acid levels.

Nursing Implications

Assessment

■ Obtain a history of cardiovascular status and risk for heart disease and the results of tests and procedures performed.
■ Assess client's compliance with abstention from alcohol for 24 hours and from food for at least 8 hours before the test; water is not restricted.
■ Assess compliance in withholding drugs known to affect FFA levels, as ordered. (This may not always be done if the therapeutic effect on FFA levels is being evaluated.)

Possible Nursing Diagnoses

Nutrition, altered, less than body requirements, related to insufficient intake
Fluid volume excess related to compromised regulatory mechanism or decreased glomerular filtration

Implementation

■ Put on gloves. Using aseptic technique, perform a venipuncture and collect 10 to 15 mL of blood in a red-top tube.
■ Send the blood collection to the laboratory immediately as serum triglycerides break down rapidly and increase fatty acid levels.

Evaluation

■ Note results in relation to glucose and ketone levels (diabetes mellitus) or lipid and lipoprotein electrophoresis (cardiovascular disease).
■ Note results in relation to recent weight gain or loss.

Client/Caregiver Teaching

Pretest

■ Inform client not to ingest alcohol for 24 hours and food for 8 hours before the test.
■ Tell the client to withhold drugs that affect test results, as ordered, unless test is performed to determine drug's effectiveness.
■ Encourage client to relax before the test, as the epinephrine secretions associated with stress elevate FFA levels.

Posttest

- Tell the client to resume diet and drugs withheld before the test.
- As necessary, instruct the client about appropriate dietary fat and carbohydrate intake.

Fructose Challenge Test

Classification: Chemistry

Type of Test: Blood

This test detects hereditary fructose intolerance, which can lead to renal and hematologic abnormalities by detecting a change of serum and urine values after administration of a body-weight adjusted dose of intravenous fructose. Fructose is a carbohydrate found in fruit and honey and is a product of sucrose hydrolysis. Hereditary fructose intolerance is an autosomal-recessive condition.

Indications

- Diagnosis of suspected hereditary fructose intolerance

Reference Values

- Stable serum glucose, phosphate, carbon dioxide, lactate, potassium, uric acid, and magnesium in the presence of intravenous fructose administration
- Stable urine phosphorus excretion, lactate, urate, alanine, and magnesium levels in the presence of intravenous administration

Abnormal Values

- Hereditary fructose intolerance, with a decrease in serum glucose, carbon dioxide, and phosphate and an increase in serum lactate, potassium, uric acid, and magnesium

Interfering Factors

- Abnormally low fructose levels may result if urine specimen is not tested when fresh.

Nursing Implications

Assessment

- Obtain a history of suspected hereditary fructose intolerance and assess diet for absence of sucrose and fructose for 3 weeks, and fasting for 8 hours before the test.

Possible Nursing Diagnoses

Anxiety related to perceived threat to health status

Nutrition, altered, less than body requirements, related to inability to digest food and absorb nutrients

Diarrhea related to metabolic disorder

Implementation

- Two hours before the test, insert an indwelling urinary catheter using sterile technique; obtain a 2-hour baseline urine sample.
- Put on gloves. Using aseptic technique, insert an intravenous line using 0.9 percent normal saline at a keep-open rate. Perform a venipuncture and collect 10 mL of blood in a red-top tube for baseline fructose, glucose, potassium, phosphate, lactate, magnesium, uric acid, and carbon dioxide values.
- Administer bolus of 20% solution of fructose (200 mg/kg body weight) over 1 minute for children and 2 minutes for adults.
- Perform venipuncture immediately after injection and after 5, 10, 15, 20, 30, 45, 60, 90, and 120 minutes in a red-top tube for tests above.
- Obtain 2-hour postinjection urine samples for urate, lactate, phosphorus, alanine, magnesium, and fructose.

Evaluation

- Notify the physician immediately of abnormal results.

Client/Caregiver Teaching

Pretest

- Inform client to consume a diet without sucrose and fructose for 3 weeks and to fast for 8 hours before the test.

Posttest

- Tell the client to resume fluid and food withheld for the test.
- Inform the client diagnosed with hereditary fructose intolerance that a normal life can be led with sucrose-free and fructose-free diet. Instruct the client and caregiver on the diet.

Fungal Antibody Tests

Classification: Immunology
Type of Test: Blood

Fungal antibody tests detect the presence of antibodies to specific fungi and monitor the infection's extent by determining the titer. Presence of antibodies suggest exposure to the fungi or active infection. Several assay techniques are used to determine the presence of the antibodies, including agglutination, complement fixation, immunodiffusion, indirect fluorescence, latex agglutination, and enzyme immunoassay.

Indications

- Diagnose fungal infection
- Evaluate persistent pulmonary symptoms after pneumonia
- Determine possible fungal etiology of acute meningitis
- Monitor fungal infection by changing titers
- Confirm previous exposure to fungus despite absence of clinical symptoms

Reference Values

Histoplasma capsulatum	Complement fixation titer <1:8
	Immunodiffusion test negative
Blastomyces dermatitidis	Complement fixation titer <1:8
	Immunodiffusion test negative

Coccidioides immitis	Complement fixation titer <1:2
	Immunodiffusion test negative
Aspergillus fumigatus	Complement fixation titer <1:8
	Immunodiffusion test negative
Cryptococcus neoformans	Agglutination negative
Sporothrix schenckii	Agglutination 1:40
Candida albicans	Latex agglutination test <1:8
Toxoplasma gondii	Indirect fluorescent antibody <1:16
Entamoeba histolytica	Indirect hemagglutination test <1:32

Abnormal Values

- Elevated levels
    Histoplasmosis
    Blastomycosis
    Coccidioidomycosis
    Candidiasis (skin, vaginal, nails, and mucous membranes)
    Cryptococcal meningitis
    Deep-tissue infection
    Aspergillosis
    Acute or chronic toxoplasmosis
    Amebic dysentery

Interfering Factors

- Recent fungal skin tests may alter results.
- Contaminated specimen from obtaining sample near fungal skin lesions may affect results.

Nursing Implications

Assessment

- Obtain a history of immune system, chronic disease, and suspected or known exposure to fungal diseases, medication regimen, diagnostic tests and results.
- Ensure that the client has fasted for 12 hours before the test.

Possible Nursing Diagnoses

Anxiety related to perceived threat to health status
Fluid volume deficit related to excessive diarrhea

Skin/tissue integrity, impairment, related to invasion and irritation from pathogenic organisms

Hyperthermia related to infectious process

Implementation

■ Put on gloves. Using aseptic technique, perform a venipuncture and collect 5 mL of blood in a red-top tube. Venipuncture should not be performed on or near the site of fungal skin infection.

Evaluation

■ Note and report positive results to physician.

Client/Caregiver Teaching

Pretest

■ Tell the client to fast from food and fluids for 12 hours before the test.

Posttest

■ Tell the client to resume food and fluids withheld before the test.

Gamma Glutamyl Transpeptidase (GGTP, GGT)

Classification: Chemistry

Type of Test: Serum

This test measures gamma glutamyl transpeptidase (GGT), an isoenzyme of alkaline phosphatase. It assists with the transfer of amino acids and peptides across cellular membranes. Hepatobiliary tissues and renal tubular and pancreatic epithelium contain large amounts of GGT. Other sources include the prostate gland, brain, and heart.

Indications

- Diagnose obstructive jaundice in neonates
- Evaluate elevated alkaline phosphatase of uncertain etiology with pronounced early rises in hepatic disease and modest elevation in cirrhosis and pancreatic or renal disease
- Evaluate and monitor client with known or suspected alcohol abuse; levels rise even after ingestion of small amounts of alcohol

Reference Values

		SI Units
Newborn	56–233 IU/L	56–233 U/L
Children (1–15 yr)	0–23 IU/L	0–23 U/L
Men		
18–50 yr	10–39 IU/L	10–39 U/L
>50 yr	10–48 IU/L	10–48 U/L
Women	6–29 IU/L	6–29 U/L

Abnormal Values

- Elevated GGT
   Hepatobiliary tract disorders
   Hepatocellular carcinoma
   Hepatocellular degeneration such as cirrhosis
   Hepatitis
   Pancreatic or renal cell damage or neoplasm
   Congestive heart failure
   Acute myocardial infarction (after 4 to 10 days)
   Hyperlipoproteinemia (type IV)
   Diabetes mellitus with hypertension
   Seizure disorders
   Significant alcohol ingestion

Interfering Factors

- Alcohol, barbiturates, and phenytoin can elevate GGT levels.
- Late pregnancy and oral contraceptives and clofibrate can cause lower GGT levels.

Nursing Implications

Assessment

- Obtain a history of known or suspected hepatic or pancreatic diseases, and results of tests and procedures performed.
- Assess client's intake of drugs or alcohol, which can elevate GGT, and note prior use on the laboratory slip and medication history for therapeutic medications that can alter test results.
- Ensure that the client has fasted from food for 8 hours before the test depending on laboratory procedure.
- Ensure that the client has abstained from alcohol for 2 to 3 weeks before the test if test is done to determine if the liver is the source of elevated alkaline phosphatase. (This restriction may not apply when the test is used to monitor compliance with alcohol-abstinence programs.)

Possible Nursing Diagnoses

Pain related to tissue inflammation
Infection, risk for, related to immunosuppressed inflammatory response
Trauma, risk for, related to altered level of consciousness
Anxiety related to perceived threat to health status

Implementation

- Put on gloves. Using aseptic technique, perform a venipuncture and collect 5 mL of blood in a red-top tube.
- Handle the sample gently to avoid hemolysis and transport to the laboratory promptly.

Evaluation

- Note results in relation to other test results and the client's symptoms.

Client/Caregiver Teaching

Pretest

- Tell the client to fast for 8 hours before the test; water is allowed. Client should avoid alcohol and drugs that affect levels.

Posttest

- Tell the client to resume usual diet.
- Encourage client in alcohol-abstinence program to continue therapy.

Gastric Acid Stimulation Test

Classification: Chemistry

Type of Test: Gastric secretions

This test is performed to determine the response to substances that are administered to induce increased gastric acid production, after determining the basal acidity. Substances used to induce gastric secretion include histamine, histalog, and pentagastrin. Pentagastrin is the usual drug of choice because it is without major side effects.

As with basal gastric acidity tests, samples obtained from gastric acid stimulation tests are examined for volume, pH, and amount of acid secreted. First, basal acid output (BAO) is determined. Maximal acid output (MAO) is also determined by adding the total milliequivalents of acid secreted in all samples after injection of the gastric acid stimulant. Peak acid output (PAO) also may be determined by adding the greatest acid output in two consecutive 15-minute samples. Finally, BAO and MAO are compared as a ratio, which normally ranges from 0.3 to 0.6. That is, the maximal output should be 1.5 to 3 times the basal output.

Indications

- Detect duodenal ulcer, as indicated by elevated BAO (5 to 7 mEq/h), and MAO (greater than 40 mEq/h). *Note:* Individuals with peptic ulcer disease who have stomach ulcers may have low to normal BAO and MAO.
- Detect Zollinger-Ellison syndrome, as indicated by elevated BAO, normal or elevated MAO (elevated MAO after gastric stimulation is frequently not seen in these individuals since gastric acid output is already at maximum levels), and high BAO:MAO ratio
- Detect pernicious anemia, as indicated by decreased or absent gastric acid output with BAO, MAO, and BAO:MAO ratio frequently at 0
- Detect gastric carcinoma, as indicated by decreased BAO (e.g., 1.0 mEq/h), decreased MAO (e.g., 4.0 mEq/h), and decreased BAO:MAO ratio (e.g., 0.25)

■ Evaluate effectiveness of vagotomy in the treatment of peptic ulcer disease, as indicated by absence of response to gastric stimulation with insulin (Hollander insulin test)

Reference Values

Volume	20–100 mL (usually 30–60 mL)
Basal acid output (BAO)	2–6 mEq/h (values vary with body weight; may be lower in women and elderly)
Maximal acid output (MAO) after stimulation tests	16–26 mEq/h or at least 1.5–3 times the BAO
BAO:MAO ratio	0.3–0.6 (usually <0.4)

Abnormal Values

■ Elevated levels
   Peptic ulcer disease
   Zollinger-Ellison disease
■ Decreased levels
   Pernicious anemia
   Gastric cancers
   Hypochromic anemia
   Nutritional megaloblastic anemia
   Rheumatoid arthritis
   Myxedema

Interfering Factors

■ Failure to follow dietary restrictions, resulting in stimulation of gastric secretions
■ Exposure to the sight, smell, or thought of food immediately before and during the test
■ Ingestion of drugs that may alter gastric secretions, including alcohol, histamine, nicotine, adrenocorticotropic steroids, insulin, parasympathetic agents, belladonna alkaloids, anticholinergic drugs, and histamine receptor antagonists, unless administered as part of the testing procedure

NURSING ALERT

■ Use of histamine diphosphate is contraindicated in clients with a history of asthma, paroxysmal hypertension, urticaria, or other allergic conditions.

Nursing Implications

Assessment

- Obtain a history of gastrointestinal disorders, medications in use, and results of other tests performed. Also note history of allergies.
- Assess for compliance with abstention from food after the evening meal the night before the test and from water for 1 hour before the test. Also determine if the client abstained from nicotine for 12 hours before the test.

Possible Nursing Diagnoses

Pain related to tissue inflammation and irritation
Anxiety related to perceived threat to health status
Protection, altered, related to abnormal blood profiles
Tissue perfusion, altered [specify], related to oxygen supply/
 demand imbalance

Implementation

- Put on gloves. Pass a lubricated nasogastric tube into the stomach and connect to a 50-mL syringe adapted for use with nasogastric tubes. Confirm placement of tube. Place client in a sitting position.
- Administer gastric stimulant subcutaneously.
- For pentagastrin and histamine tests, gastric samples are obtained at 15-minute intervals for 1 hour after injection; for histology, the samples are obtained at 15-minute intervals for 2 hours after injection.
- Place aspirated samples in labeled container, include time obtained, and send to laboratory.

Evaluation

- Monitor for side effects of drugs administered to induce gastric secretion (flushing, headache, nasal stuffiness, dizziness, faintness, and nausea).
- Note test results in relation to results of other tests performed and the client's symptoms.

Client/Caregiver Teaching

Pretest

- Explain the purpose of test and the procedure for obtaining the specimens.
- Tell the client that some discomfort is experienced from insertion of the nasogastric tube.
- Tell the client to fast from food after the evening meal the night before the test and not to drink water for 1 hour before

the test. Also, tell the client to abstain from nicotine for 12 hours before and during the test.

Posttest

■ Tell the client to resume food and fluids withheld before the test.

Gastrin

Classification: Chemistry

Type of Test: Serum

This test measures the hormone gastrin, which is secreted by the stomach and duodenum in response to vagal stimulation, the presence of food, alcohol, or calcium in the stomach and the alkalinity of secretions. Following its absorption into the circulation, gastrin returns to the stomach and acts as a stimulant for acid secretion, insulin, and pepsin and the intrinsic factor. Gastrin stimulation tests can be performed after a test meal or an IV infusion of calcium or secretin.

Indications

■ Diagnose Zollinger-Ellison syndrome (gastrinoma), as indicated by elevated levels (>500 pg/mL) and marked response to calcium challenge (620–66,000 pg/mL)
■ Aid in differential diagnosis of ulcers from other gastrointestinal peptic disorders
■ Support diagnosis of gastric carcinoma, pernicious anemia, or G-cell hyperplasia, as indicated by increased levels

Reference Values

		SI Units
Fasting		
Child	<10–125 pg/mL	<10–125 ng/L
Adult		
16–60 yr	25–90 pg/mL	25–90 ng/L
>60 yr	<100 pg/mL	<100 ng/L
Postprandial (1 h)	40 pg/mL	40 ng/L

Abnormal Values

- Elevated gastrin levels
  Zollinger-Ellison syndrome
  G-cell hyperplasia
  Gastric carcinoma
  Age-related changes in gastric acid secretion
  Gastric and duodenal ulcers
  Pernicious anemia
  Uremia
  Chronic gastritis
  Drugs, including calcium products, insulin, catecholamines, coffee, amino acids, histamine blockers, and hydrogen pump inhibitors
- Decreased gastrin levels
  Gastric hyperacidity
  Stress ulcers
  Vagotomy
  Hypothyroidism
  Drugs, including atropine sulfate, and antidepressants

Interfering Factors

- Protein ingestion and calcium infusion will elevate serum gastrin levels in some cases.
- Drugs can cause inaccurate increases or decreases (see Abnormal Values).

Nursing Implications

Assessment

- Obtain a history of gastrointestinal disorders and suspected peptic ulcer disease, noting any medications that may interfere with test results.
- Ensure that the client has fasted from food for 12 hours before the study.
- Withhold medications and alcohol for 12 to 24 hours, as ordered by physician.

Possible Nursing Diagnoses

Pain related to tissue inflammation and irritation
Anxiety related to perceived threat to health status
Protection, altered, related to abnormal blood profiles
Tissue perfusion, altered [specify], related to oxygen supply/ demand imbalance

Implementation

- Put on gloves. Using aseptic technique, perform a venipuncture and collect 5 to 7 mL of blood in a red-top tube.
- *Calcium stimulation test:* Administer calcium gluconate IV 5 mg/kg over 3 hours. Subsequent blood samples are taken every 30 minutes for 4 hours and compared to the baseline level.
- *Secretin test:* Pass a GI tube past the ligament of Treitz. Administer secretin 2 clinical units/kg by IV bolus. Obtain samples of GI fluid at 20-minute intervals.

Evaluation

- Note test results in relation to other tests performed and the client's symptoms.
- If levels are ≥500 pg/mL, indicating Zollinger-Ellison syndrome associated with peptic ulcer disease, assess bowel sounds.

Client/Caregiver Teaching

Pretest

- Tell the client to fast from food for 12 hours before the study.
- Tell the client to withhold medications, caffeine, and alcohol for 12 to 24 hours, as ordered.

Posttest

- Tell the client to resume medications and diet withheld before testing.

Globulin

Classification: Chemistry

Type of Test: Plasma

This test measures globulins, a group of proteins that are produced in the liver and lymphoid tissue. These proteins are divided according to mobility in electrophoresis and include alpha, beta, and gamma fractions. Their functions involve maintenance of acid-base balance, formation of antibodies, and transport of constituents in the blood (lipids, hormones, enzymes, and other substances). Test results reveal levels of total protein, alpha$_1$, alpha$_2$, beta, and gamma globulins that include IgA, IgD, IgE, IgG, IgM antibodies (see Immunoglobulin Assay Test). Globulin measurement is usually performed with total protein, albumin, and the albumin:globulin (A:G) ratio tests.

Indications

- Perform routine screening as part of a complete physical examination
- Monitor response to therapy with drugs that can alter serum protein levels
- Diagnose a variety of clinical disorders associated with abnormal specific globulin levels (see Abnormal Values)

Reference Values

	Total Proteins (%)	*SI Units*
Total globulin	2.3–3.5 g/dL (32–48%)	23–35 g/L
Alpha$_1$	0.1–0.4 g/dL (1–5%)	1–4 g/L
Alpha$_2$	0.4–1.0 g/dL (4.6–14%)	4–10 g/L
Beta	0.5–1.2 g/dL (7.3–15%)	5–12 g/L
Gamma	0.6–1.6 g/dL (8–21%)	6–16 g/L

Abnormal Values

Globulin	*Increased Levels*	*Decreased Levels*
Alpha$_1$	Pregnancy Burns Malignancies Acute inflammation Tissue necrosis	Genetic deficiency of alpha$_1$ antitrypsin Hepatitis Starvation
Alpha$_2$	Acute infections Dehydration Trauma, burns Allergies Advanced malignancies Rheumatic fever Rheumatoid arthritis Sarcoidosis Acute myocardial infarction Ulcerative colitis Nephrotic syndrome	Hemolytic/megaloblastic anemias Severe liver disease Malnutrition Malabsorption Neoplastic syndrome

Globulin	Increased Levels	Decreased Levels
Beta	Hypothyroidism Biliary cirrhosis Nephrotic syndrome Diabetes mellitus Hyperparathyroidism Cushing's disease Sarcoidosis Malignant hypertension Iron deficiency anemia Dehydration	Hypocholesterolemia Malabsorption Malnutrition Ulcerative colitis Lupus erythematosus
Gamma	Connective tissue diseases (such as SLE and rheumatoid arthritis) Dehydration Hodgkin's disease Leukemia Chronic active liver disease Crohn's disease Congestive heart failure Infections Drugs, such as tolinase, tubocurarine, and anticonvulsants	Nephrotic syndrome/ nephroses Cushing's syndrome Lymphocytic leukemia Lymphosarcoma Asthma Ulcerative colitis Malabsorption Drugs, such as BCG vaccine and methotrexate

Interfering Factors

- High serum lipid levels can cause abnormal results.
- Numerous drugs can alter protein levels: ACTH, corticosteroids, BSP, clofibrate, dextran, growth hormone, heparin, insulin, x-ray contrast media, thyroid preparations, tolbutamide, acetaminophen, azathioprine, cyclophosphamide, heroin, niacin, estrogen, Estinyl, Enovid, as well as those listed in Abnormal Values.

Nursing Implications

Assessment

- Obtain a history of known or suspected liver or other disorders affecting protein levels, especially those associated with hematologic and gastrointestinal systems.
- Note compliance with fasting 8 hours before the test and low-fat diet several days before test.

Possible Nursing Diagnoses

Anxiety related to perceived threat to health status

Nutrition, altered, less than body requirements, related to abnormal levels of protein, inability to absorb nutrients

Implementation

- Put on gloves. Using aseptic technique, perform a venipuncture and collect 7 mL of blood in a red-top tube.
- Handle sample gently to avoid hemolysis and send promptly to the laboratory; note administration of blood or blood products within 6 weeks of the test on laboratory request form.

Evaluation

- Monitor total protein and albumin levels in relation to globulins as the globulin level can be calculated by subtracting albumin from total protein. Also calculate the A:G ratio.
- Note results in relation to other tests performed and the client's symptoms.

Client/Caregiver Teaching

Pretest

- Tell the client to withhold food for 8 hours before the test and to eat a low-fat diet for several days before the test.
- Tell the client to withhold drugs that could interfere with test results, as ordered.

Posttest

- Tell the client to resume food and fluid intake and drugs withheld before the test.
- Instruct the client to report signs and symptoms of dehydration.

Glucagon

Classification: Chemistry

Type of Test: Plasma

This test measures quantitative serum glucagon levels by radio-immunoassay. Normally, glucagon is a hormone secreted in response to hypoglycemia by the alpha cells of the islets of Langerhans in the pancreas. It acts primarily on the liver to promote glucose production and control glucose storage. The coordinated release of insulin, glucagon, and somatostatin ensures an adequate fuel supply while maintaining stable blood sugar.

Indications

- Diagnose suspected glucagonoma (alpha islet-cell neoplastic tumor)
- Confirm glucagon deficiency
- Diagnose suspected renal failure or renal transplant rejection, since kidneys excrete glucagon

Reference Values

- 50–200 pg/mL or 30–210 ng/L (SI units)

Abnormal Values

- Elevated
  - Renal failure
  - Rejection of a transplanted kidney
  - Glucagonoma
  - Acute pancreatitis
  - Pheochromocytoma
  - Uncontrolled diabetes
  - Burns
- Decreased
  - Elevated blood glucose not associated with lack of insulin (food ingestion)
  - Chronic pancreatitis

Pancreatic cancer
Surgical resection of pancreas
Cystic fibrosis

Interfering Factors

- Trauma, infection, starvation, and excessive exercise may lead to elevated levels.
- Failure to follow dietary restrictions before the test may lead to falsely decreased levels.
- Atenolol, propranolol, and secretin may cause falsely decreased levels; insulin, nifedipine, danazol, glucocorticoids, gastrin, and some amino acids may cause falsely elevated levels.

Nursing Implications

Assessment

- Obtain a history of compliance with dietary restrictions, recent strenuous exercise, and use of medications.

Possible Nursing Diagnoses

Fluid volume excess related to compromised regulatory mechanism or decreased glomerular filtration
Infection, risk for secondary, related to immunosuppressed inflammatory response
Pain related to tissue inflammation
Anxiety related to perceived threat to health status

Implementation

- Put on gloves. Using aseptic technique, perform a venipuncture and collect at least 5 mL of blood in a lavender-top tube.

Evaluation

- Note results in relation to the client's symptoms and other test findings.

Client/Caregiver Teaching

Posttest

- Inform the client or caregiver to resume diet, exercise, and any medications withheld before the test.

Glucose, Fasting Blood Sugar (FBS), Random Glucose

Classification: Chemistry

Type of Test: Serum, whole blood

This test measures blood glucose levels following an 8- to 12-hour fast to determine overall glucose homeostasis. The body acquires most of its energy from oxidative metabolism of glucose. Glucose, a simple six-carbon sugar (monosaccharide), enters the diet as part of the sugars sucrose, lactose, and maltose and as the major constituent of the complex polysaccharides called dietary starch. It is necessary for body function. Excesses are stored in the liver or muscle as glycogen. Random testing for glucose can be performed at regular intervals throughout the day to monitor diet and medications in those with abnormal glucose metabolism.

Indications

- Screen for diabetes mellitus
- Identify hypoglycemia, as indicated by a fasting blood sugar as low as 40 mg/dL
- Determine insulin requirements

Reference Values

		SI Units
Fasting Blood Glucose		
Whole blood		
Newborn	34–68 mg/dL	1.9–3.8 mmol/L
Children	51–85 mg/dL	2.8–4.7 mmol/L
Adult	60–100 mg/dL	3.3–5.6 mmol/L

		SI Units
Fasting Blood Glucose		
Serum		
Newborn	40–80 mg/dL	2.2–4.4 mmol/L
Children	60–100 mg/dL	3.3–5.6 mmol/L
Adult	70–100 mg/dL	3.9–5.6 mmol/L
Critical values		
Newborn	<30 or >300 mg/dL	<1.6 or >16.5 mmol/L
Adult	<40 or >700 mg/dL	<2.2 or >38.6 mmol/L
Random Blood Glucose*		
Serum		
Newborn	40–80 mg/dL	2.2–4.4 mmol/L
Children	60–100 mg/dL	3.3–5.5 mmol/L
Adult	70–105 mg/dL	3.9–5.8 mmol/L
Critical values		
Newborn	<30 or >300 mg/dL	<1.6 or >16.5 mmol/L
Adult	<40 or >700 mg/dL	<2.2 or >38.6 mmol/L

*Varies with time of last meal.

Abnormal Values

- Persistent increased levels (hyperglycemia)
    Diabetes mellitus
    Hemochromatosis
    Cushing's syndrome
    Hyperthyroidism
    Acromegaly, gigantism
    Obesity
    Chronic pancreatitis
    Pancreatic adenoma
- Transient increased levels
    Pheochromocytoma
    Pregnancy (gestational diabetes)
    Severe liver disease
    Acute stress reaction
    Shock, trauma
    Seizures, eclampsia
    Drugs, including glucagon, adrenal corticosteroids, oral
        contraceptives, estrogens, thyroid hormones, anabolic
        steroids, thiazide diuretics, loop diuretics, propranolol,

antipsychotic drugs, hydantoins, clonidine, dextrothyroxine, and niacin

Hormones including glucagon, epinephrine, cortisol, ACTH, growth hormone, and thyroxine

- Persistent decreased levels (hypoglycemia)
  Insulinoma
  Addison's disease
  Hypopituitarism
  Galactosemia
  Ectopic insulin production from tumors (adrenal carcinoma, retroperitoneal sarcomas, pleural fibrous, mesotheliomas)
  Starvation
- Transient decreased levels
  Malabsorption syndrome
  Postgastrectomy "dumping syndrome"
  Acute alcohol ingestion
  Severe liver disease
  Severe glycogen storage diseases
  Stress-related catecholamine excess ("functional" hypoglycemia)
  Hereditary fructose intolerance
  Myxedema
  Drugs, including salicylates, antituberculosis agents, sulfonylureas, sulfonamides, insulin, ethanol, clofibrate, and MAO inhibitors
  Hormones, including insulin and somatostatin

Interfering Factors

- Elevated urea levels and uremia can lead to falsely elevated levels.
- Extremely elevated white blood counts can lead to falsely decreased values.
- Failure to follow dietary restrictions before the test can lead to falsely elevated values.
- Administration of insulin or oral hypoglycemic agents within 8 hours of a fasting blood glucose can lead to falsely decreased values.

Nursing Implications

Assessment

- Obtain a history of signs and symptoms of hypo- or hyperglycemia, known or suspected diabetes mellitus, and results of tests done.

■ Assess compliance in withholding food and fluid (except water), insulin, and oral hypoglycemia agents for approximately 8 to 12 hours before the test.

Possible Nursing Diagnoses

Anxiety related to threat to health status
Coping, ineffective, individual, related to [specify]
Infection, risk for, related to decreased circulation
Adjustment, impaired, risk for, related to need for lifestyle changes or threat to self-concept

Implementation

■ Put on gloves. Using aseptic technique, perform a venipuncture and collect 5 mL of blood in the morning or at other designated times of day in a gray- or red-top tube. A capillary sample may be obtained in infants and children, as well as in adults for whom venipuncture may not be feasible.
■ Handle the sample gently to avoid hemolysis and transport to the laboratory promptly.

Evaluation

■ Observe for signs of hypoglycemia or hyperglycemia, especially in those who are insulin-dependent.
■ Monitor and report levels that fall in the critical range.

Client/Caregiver Teaching

Pretest

■ Tell the client to withold food, insulin, or hypoglycemic agent for 8 hours before a fasting test.

Posttest

■ Tell the client or caregiver to resume usual diet and medications withheld before the test.
■ Tell the client to report signs and symptoms of hypoglycemia (weakness, confusion, diaphoresis, rapid pulse) or hyperglycemia (thirst, polyuria, hunger, lethargy).
■ Advise client and caregiver to attend classes for diabetes mellitus care, if appropriate.
■ Instruct the client and caregiver in the use of home-monitoring machines for glucose testing.

Glucose, 2-Hour Postprandial (PPBS)

Classification: Chemistry (carbohydrates)

Type of Test: Serum, whole blood

This test reflects the metabolic response to a carbohydrate challenge. It measures the blood glucose 2 hours after the client ingests a meal containing at least 100 g of carbohydrate. Normally, the blood sugar returns to the fasting level within 2 hours. Insulin and other medications are administered as usual before the test. This is a useful screening test for diabetes mellitus.

Indications

- Evaluate an abnormal fasting blood sugar
- Screen for diabetes mellitus, as indicated by a blood glucose level greater than the fasting level and especially by a 2-hour level greater than 200 mg/mL
- Identify postprandial hypoglycemia and differentiation of this state from fasting hypoglycemia, with fasting hypoglycemia almost always indicative of a pathological state
- Confirm known or suspected disorder associated with abnormal glucose metabolism
- Monitor metabolic response to drugs known to alter blood glucose levels

Reference Values

		SI Units
Blood		
Children	65–120 mg/dL	3.6–6.6 mmol/L
Adults	65–120 mg/dL	3.6–6.6 mmol/L
Older adults	65–140 mg/dL	3.6–7.7 mmol/L
Serum		
Children	65–150 mg/dL	3.6–8.3 mmol/L
Adults	65–140 mg/dL	3.6–7.7 mmol/L
Older adults	65–160 mg/dL	3.6–8.8 mmol/L

Clients with no family or personal history of diabetes can have an increase of 6 mg/dL every 10 years of life over age 30.

Abnormal Values

- Persistent increased levels (hyperglycemia)
  Diabetes mellitus
  Hemochromatosis
  Cushing's syndrome
  Hyperthyroidism
  Acromegaly, gigantism
  Obesity
  Chronic pancreatitis
  Pancreatic adenoma
- Transient increased levels
  Pheochromocytoma
  Pregnancy (gestational diabetes)
  Severe liver disease
  Acute stress reaction
  Shock, trauma
  Seizures, eclampsia
  Drugs: glucagon, adrenal corticosteroids, oral contraceptives, estrogens, thyroid hormones, anabolic steroids, thiazide diuretics, loop diuretics, propranolol, antipsychotic drugs, hydantoins, clonidine, dextrothyroxine, and niacin
  Hormones: glucagon, epinephrine, cortisol, ACTH, growth hormone, and thyroxine
- Persistent decreased levels (hypoglycemia)
  Insulinoma
  Addison's disease
  Hypopituitarism
  Galactosemia
  Ectopic insulin production from tumors (adrenal carcinoma, retroperitoneal sarcomas, pleural fibrous, mesotheliomas)
  Starvation
- Transient decreased levels
  Malabsorption syndrome
  Postgastrectomy "dumping syndrome"
  Acute alcohol ingestion
  Severe liver disease
  Severe glycogen storage diseases
  Stress-related catecholamine excess ("functional" hypoglycemia)
  Hereditary fructose intolerance
  Myxedema
  Drugs: salicylates, antituberculosis agents, sulfonylureas, sulfonamides, insulin, ethanol, clofibrate, and MAO inhibitors
  Hormones: insulin and somatostatin

Interfering Factors

- Failure to follow dietary instructions can alter test results.
- Smoking and drinking coffee during the 2-hour test period can lead to falsely elevated values.
- Strenuous exercise during the 2-hour test period can lead to falsely decreased values.

Nursing Implications

Assessment

- Obtain a history of past laboratory tests for glucose and results.
- Note compliance in ingesting a meal (usually breakfast) containing at least 100 g of carbohydrate 2 hours before the test.
- Note time medication was taken and ensure that the client has avoided smoking and strenuous exercise until the sample is obtained.

Possible Nursing Diagnoses

Anxiety related to threat to health status
Coping, ineffective, individual, related to [specify]
Infection, risk for, related to decreased circulation
Adjustment, impaired, risk for, related to need for lifestyle changes or threat to self-concept

Implementation

- Put on gloves. Using aseptic technique, perform a venipuncture and collect 5 mL of blood in a gray or red-top tube 2 hours after the carbohydrate challenge is ingested. A capillary sample may be obtained in children, as well as in adults for whom venipuncture may not be feasible.
- Handle the sample gently to avoid hemolysis and transport to the laboratory promptly.

Evaluation

- Note results of fasting glucose test, if performed before this test.

Client/Caregiver Teaching

Pretest

- Tell the client to fast overnight and to ingest a high-carbohydrate breakfast (including orange juice, milk, cereal with sugar, and toast) 2 hours before the blood sample is scheduled to be drawn. A high-carbohydrate drink may be given.

- Tell the client not to smoke and to avoid strenuous exercise after the meal.

Posttest

- Tell the client to resume usual diet and medications withheld before the test.
- Inform the client that additional testing may be required.

▲▲▲▲▲▲▲▲▲▲▲▲▲▲▲▲▲▲▲▲▲▲▲

Glucose, Urine

Classification: Chemistry

Type of Test: Urine

Normally, glucose is virtually absent from the urine. Although nearly all glucose passes into the glomerular filtrate, most of it is reabsorbed by the proximal renal tubules through active transport mechanisms. Usually there are enough carrier molecules to transport all of the glucose from the renal tubules back to the blood. However, if plasma glucose levels are very high and carrier mechanisms are overwhelmed, glucose will appear in the urine. The point at which a substance appears in the urine is called its renal threshold. The renal threshold for glucose ranges from 160 to 200 mg/dL, depending on the individual. That is, the blood sugar must rise to its renal threshold level before glucose will appear in the urine.

Disorders that may lead to elevated blood glucose levels, and thus to glycosuria, are listed in Abnormal Values. In addition, several drugs are known to elevate the blood sugar enough to produce glycosuria. These are also listed in Abnormal Values.

Indications

- Detect glycosuria
- Monitor control of diabetes mellitus

Reference Values

- Negative

Abnormal Values

Elevated levels indicate uncontrolled diabetes mellitus. Certain disorders and drugs may result in glycosuria.

- Glycosuria with high blood sugar
    Diabetes mellitus
    Gestational diabetes
    Acromegaly
    Cushing's syndrome
    Hyperthyroidism
    Pheochromocytoma
    Advanced cystic fibrosis
    Hemochromatosis
    Severe chronic pancreatitis
    Pancreatic carcinoma
    Hypothalamic dysfunction
    Brain tumor or hemorrhage
    Massive metabolic derangement
    Severe burns
    Uremia
    Advanced liver disease
    Sepsis
    Cardiogenic shock
    Glycogen storage disease
    Obesity
    Medication-induced hyperglycemia
    Adrenal corticosteroids
    ACTH
    Thiazide diuretics
    Oral contraceptives
    Excessive intravenous glucose
    Dextrothyroxine
- Glycosuria without high blood sugar
    Renal tubular dysfunction
    Fanconi's syndrome
    Galactosemia
    Cystinosis
    Lead poisoning
    Multiple myeloma
    Pregnancy (must be distinguished from gestational diabetes)
- Drugs that may produce false-positive glucosuria results
    Ascorbic acid
    Cephalosporins
    Chloral hydrate
    Levodopa
    Morphine

NegGram
PABA
Paraldehyde
Penicillins
Radiographic contrast media
Salicylates
Skelaxin
Streptomycin
Terramycin

Interfering Factors

- With Clinitest:

    Use of the wrong color chart: charts for the 2-drop and 5-drop methods are different and must be used with the appropriate test.

    False findings and possibly an explosion can occur if tablets are exposed to moisture and light.

    Use of discolored tablets invalidates test results.

    False-negative results can occur if radiographic contrast media is present in urine.

    Certain medications can produce false-positive results: aminosalicylic acid, ampicillin, ampicillin sodium, ascorbic acid, camphor, cephalosporins, chloral hydrate, chloramphenicol, chloroform, creatinine, formaldehyde, fructose, galactose, glycocyamine, glucuronic acid, homogentisic acid, isoniazid, levodopa, maltose, menthol, metolazone, nitrofurantoin, nitrofurantoin sodium, penicillin G benzathine, penicillin G potassium, pentose, phenol, salicylates, streptomycin sulfate, tetracyclines, turpentine, and uric acid.

- With Clinistix:

    Use of the wrong color chart: Reagent strips must be compared with color chart on bottle from which they were taken.

    Darkened strips or those exposed to prolonged moisture or air invalidate results.

    Certain medications can produce false-negative results: ascorbic acid, levodopa, methyldopa, methyldopate hydrochloride, phenazopyridine, and salicylates.

Nursing Implications

Assessment

- Obtain a history of diabetes, other endocrine disorder, medication regimen, and time when the last food or fluids were consumed.

Possible Nursing Diagnoses

Anxiety related to threat to health status
Coping, ineffective, individual, related to [specify]
Infection, risk for, related to decreased circulation
Therapeutic regimen, individual, ineffective management, related to [specify]

Implementation

- Ask client to completely empty bladder and then drink at least 8 ounces of fluid. Have client void at least 20 mL of urine into a clean plastic container 30 minutes later. If client has an indwelling catheter, obtain a fresh specimen.
- *Clinitest:* Obtain freshly voided urine sample (a fresh-voided postprandial specimen is recommended); add 5 drops of urine to a clean test tube and rinse dropper with water. Then add 10 drops of water to a test tube. Add one Clinitest tablet to this mixture. Observe color changes during the boiling phase. Handle tube with care. Glucose >2 g/dL causes a rapid color change to orange during boiling phase. If this occurs, repeat the test as above, using 2 drops instead of 5 drops of urine, and compare results to the Clinitest color chart for the 2-drop test. In 15 seconds after the boiling stops, agitate test tube; immediately compare mixture color to Clinitest color chart and record results per chart on tube.
- *Clinistix:* Obtain urine sample. Dip reagent strip into urine; ensure complete immersion of the test pad for 2 seconds. Slide the pad side of strip against the edge of container while removing it. Exactly 30 seconds after removal from the urine, compare the color of test pad to colors on bottle.

Client/Caregiver Teaching

Pretest

- Inform the client that the most accurate results are obtained if specimen is collected before meals when blood sugar should be at the lowest point; similarly, urine that has been accumulating in the bladder overnight can contain excessive amounts of glucose from increased concentration of urine and also from something eaten the previous evening.
- Inform the client for the Clinitest procedure to check the expiration date on the container and to discard any dark blue tablets; use only fresh tablets that are light blue with dark blue flecks.
- If using Clinitest, tell the client to avoid touching tablets to avoid burns and to wash affected area quickly if skin contact occurs.
- If using Clinistix, tell the client to keep the bottle tightly capped. Light exposure and moisture speed degradation of

Clinistix. Inspect strip before using; if strip is darkened, discard strip and bottle from which it was taken.

Posttest

- Tell the client to record the urine glucose test results and to notify the health care professional if the values are elevated.

Glucose Tolerance Tests: Oral (OGTT), Intravenous (IVGTT)

Classification: Chemistry

Type of Test: Serum, blood

This test measures glucose levels after administration of an oral or intravenous carbohydrate challenge. The oral glucose tolerance test (OGTT) is used for individuals who are able to eat and who are not known to have problems with gastrointestinal malabsorption. The intravenous glucose tolerance test (IVGTT) is performed for individuals who are unable to tolerate oral glucose. The test usually takes 3 hours, with specimens taken hourly, but if abnormal hypoglycemia or gastrointestinal malabsorption is suspected, it may be extended to 5 hours. The oral glucose tolerance test may be performed using blood samples only or with urine samples as well. If the test is normal, the urine will be negative for sugar throughout the test.

In cases when prediabetes or borderline diabetes is suspected, cortisone acetate is administered orally 8 hours and again 2 hours before the oral glucose load to produce an abnormal value of >165 mg/dL at the 2-hour interval, indicating the existence of diabetes mellitus.

Indications

- Evaluate abnormal fasting or postprandial blood glucose levels that are not clearly indicative of diabetes mellitus
- Identify impaired glucose metabolism without overt diabetes mellitus, which is characterized by a modest elevation in blood glucose after 2 hours and a normal level after 3 hours

- Evaluate glucose metabolism in women of childbearing age, especially those who are pregnant and have a history of previous fetal loss, birth of babies weighing 9 pounds or more, or positive family history for diabetes mellitus
- Support for diagnosing hyperthyroidism and alcoholic liver disease, which are characterized by a sharp rise in blood glucose followed by a decline to subnormal levels
- Identify true postprandial hypoglycemia (5-hour OGTT) due to excessive insulin response to a glucose load
- Provide support for diagnosing gastrointestinal malabsorption, which is characterized by peak glucose levels lower than what is normally expected and hypoglycemia in the latter hours of the test (5-hour OGTT)
- Identify abnormal renal tubular function if glycosuria occurs without hyperglycemia

Reference Values

OGTT times after carbohydrate challenge

		SI Units
Blood		
Fasting	70–150 mg/dL	3.9–5.8 mmol/L
½ h	150–160 mg/dL	8.3–8.8 mmol/L
1 h	160 mg/dL	8.8 mmol/L
2 h	115 mg/dL	6.6 mmol/L
3 h	70–150 mg/dL	3.9–5.8 mmol/L
Serum		
Fasting	70–105 mg/dL	3.9–5.8 mmol/L
30 min	150–160 mg/dL	8.3–8.8 mmol/L
1 h	160–170 mg/dL	8.8–9.4 mmol/L
2 h	120 mg/dL	6.6 mmol/L
3 h	70–105 mg/dL	3.9–5.8 mmol/L

IVGTT times after carbohydrate challenge

Blood		
Fasting	70–105 mg/dL	3.9–5.8 mmol/L
5 min	300–400 mg/dL	16.5–22.0 mmol/L
30 min	180–200 mg/dL	9.9–11.0 mmol/L
1 h	170 mg/dL	9.4 mmol/L
2 h	140 mg/dL	7.7 mmol/L
3 h	70–105 mg/dL	3.9–5.8 mmol/L

Children >6 yr: same as adult
Older adults: 10–30 mg/dL higher at each interval related to decline in glucose clearance with age

Abnormal Values

- Increased values (decreased OGTT)
    Diabetes mellitus (also IVGTT)
    Diabetic acidosis
    Pheochromocytomas (also IVGTT)
    Cystic fibrosis (also IVGTT)
    Forbes' disease (also IVGTT)
    Gigantism (also IVGTT)
    Hemochromatosis (also IVGTT)
    Hepatic damage (severe) (also IVGTT)
    Hyperlipidemia
    Central nervous system lesions (also IVGTT)
    Cirrhosis
    Myocardial or cerebral infarction
    Hyperthyroidism (also IVGTT)
    Louis-Bar syndrome (also IVGTT)
    Neoplasm (also IVGTT)
    Pregnancy
    Adrenal gland hyperfunction (Cushing's syndrome) (also IVGTT)
    Stress
    Burns
    Infections
    Exercise
    Extensive surgery or injury
    Acute myocardial infarction or congestive heart failure
    Uremia (also IVGTT)
    Von Gierke's disease (also IVGTT)
    Acute pancreatitis
    Chronic pancreatitis (also IVGTT)
    Acromegaly (also IVGTT)
    Certain drugs that may decrease OGTT and IVGTT values, including beta-adrenergic blockers, amphetamines, salicylates, antituberculosis agents, sulfonylureas, sulfonamides, insulin, ethanol, clofibrate, and MAO inhibitors
- Decreased values (increased OGTT)
    Hyperinsulinism
    Addison's disease
    Celiac disease
    Hypoparathyroidism
    Hypothyroidism
    Hypoglycemia reaction (insulin shock) (also IVGTT)
    Cancer of the stomach, liver, and lung
    Malnutrition
    Alcoholism
    Narcotic addiction (also IVGTT)
    Pancreatic islet cell hyperplasia (also IVGTT)

Sprue
Cirrhosis
Hepatic disease (also IVGTT)
Strenuous exercise
Adrenal gland insufficiency
Malabsorption
Certain drugs that may increase OGTT and IVGTT values, including glucagon, adrenal corticosteroids, oral contraceptives, estrogens, thyroid hormones, anabolic steroids, thiazide diuretics, loop diuretics, propranolol, antipsychotic drugs, hydantoins, clonidine, dextrothyroxine, and niacin

Interfering Factors

- Failure of client to ingest a diet with sufficient carbohydrate content (e.g., 150 g per day) for at least 3 days before the test can result in falsely decreased values.
- Impaired physical activity can lead to falsely increased values.
- Excessive physical activity before or during the test can lead to falsely decreased values.
- Smoking before or during the test can lead to falsely increased values.
- Ingestion of drugs known to alter blood glucose levels may lead to falsely increased or decreased values (see Abnormal Values).
- Infusions of total parenteral nutrition (TPN) during test can lead to falsely elevated results. IVGTT, solutions with less glucose should be infused for at least 3 hours before and during test.

> ### NURSING ALERT
>
> - Clients with fasting blood sugars of greater than 150 mg/dL or postprandial blood glucose levels of greater than 200 mg/dL should not receive the glucose load required for this test.

Nursing Implications

Assessment

- Obtain a history of endocrine system, known or suspected disorders, and results of glucose tests.
- Note compliance in eating a diet containing at least 150 g of carbohydrate per day for 3 days before the test.

■ Ascertain that client has withheld drugs that affect blood glucose levels and food after midnight before the test and refrained from smoking and strenuous exercise after midnight before the test and until the test is completed.

Possible Nursing Diagnoses

Anxiety related to threat to health status
Coping, ineffective, individual, related to [specify]
Adjustment, impaired, risk for, related to need for lifestyle changes or threat to self-concept

Implementation

■ Put on gloves. Using aseptic technique, perform venipuncture and collect 7 mL of blood in a gray-top tube for a fasting blood sugar.
■ If IVGTT is to be performed, insert a venous access device to administer the glucose and obtain the blood samples.
■ If ordered, ask the client for a second-voided (double-voided) urine sample.
■ Administer the glucose load orally or intravenously. This is a calculated dose, either 1.75 g/kg body weight or 75–100 g carbohydrate in 15 to 20 minutes (OGTT) or 50% glucose calculated according to body weight in 5 minutes (IVGTT). Several commercial preparations are available that are flavored for palatability.
■ Obtain blood and urine samples at 30-minute, 1-hour, 2-hour, and 3-hour intervals. If the test is extended to 5 hours, additional samples are collected at 4- and 5-hour intervals.

Evaluation

■ Note results in relation to fasting blood glucose, 2-hour postprandial blood glucose, and urine glucose levels.

Client/Caregiver Teaching

Pretest

■ Tell the client to eat a diet containing at least 150 g of carbohydrate per day for 3 days before the test; to withhold drugs that affect blood glucose levels and food after midnight the day before the test; and to refrain from smoking and strenuous exercise after midnight the day before the test and until the test is completed.
■ If a second-voided specimen is required, instruct the client to void a half-hour before the required specimen is due. Dis-

card this urine, then collect the second-voided specimen at the designated time. Advise the client that a second-voided urine specimen is necessary only at the beginning of the test.
■ Advise the client to drink one glass of water each time a urine sample is collected to ensure adequate urinary output for remaining specimens.

Posttest

■ Tell the client to resume usual diet, medications, and activity withheld before the test.

Growth Hormone (GH, hGH, STH, SH)

Classification: Chemistry

Type of Test: Serum

This test measures human growth hormone (hGH), also known as somatotropic hormone (STH, SH) or somatotropin. This hormone is secreted in episodic bursts by the anterior pituitary gland, usually during early sleep, and plays an integral role in growth from birth to puberty. GH promotes skeletal growth by stimulating hepatic production of proteins; it also affects lipid and glucose metabolism.

Indications

■ Evaluate growth retardation in children with decreased levels, indicative of pituitary etiology
■ Monitor response to treatment of growth retardation
■ Detect suspected disorder associated with decreased growth hormone
■ Diagnosis of gigantism in children with increased levels indicative of pituitary etiology
■ Diagnosis of acromegaly in adults, as indicated by elevated levels, and frequently attributed to acidophil or chromophobe tumors of the adenohypophysis

Reference Values

		SI Units
Newborns	15–40 ng/mL	660–1760 pmol/L
Children	0–20 ng/mL	0–880 pmol/L
Adults	0–10 ng/mL	0–440 pmol/L

Abnormal Values

- Increased levels
  Pituitary or hypothalamic tumor
  Gigantism in children
  Acromegaly in adults
  Hypoglycemia
  Anorexia nervosa, starvation
  Hyperpituitarism
  Drugs, including amphetamines, arginine, dopamine, levodopa, methyldopa, beta blockers, histamine, nicotinic acid, estrogens, glucagon, insulin, and oral contraceptives
- Decreased levels
  Congenital growth hormone deficiency
  Congenital pituitary hypoplasia
  Dwarfism
  Failure to thrive
  Growth hormone deficiency
  Pituitary tumors, lesions, or fibrosis
  Craniopharyngiomas
  Pituitary damage or trauma
  Hyperglycemia
  Tuberculosis meningitis
  Hypothalamic degeneration, lesion
  Hypopituitarism
  Drugs, including corticosteroids, chlorpromazine, glucose, or phenothiazines

Interfering Factors

- Hyperglycemia and therapy with drugs can cause falsely decreased levels (see Abnormal Values).
- Hypoglycemia, physical activity, stress, and a variety of drugs can cause falsely elevated levels (see Abnormal Values).
- Radioactive scan performed within 48 hours of the test can affect results.

Nursing Implications

Assessment

- Obtain a history of growth pattern, endocrine system disorders, and results of tests and procedures performed.
- Assess medication history; ensure that any drugs that may alter test results have been withheld for 12 hours before the test, as ordered by physician.
- Ensure that the client has fasted from food and has avoided strenuous exercise for 8 hours before the test.
- Ensure that the client has maintained bed rest for 1 hour before each sample is obtained, if recommended.

Possible Nursing Diagnoses

Body image disturbance related to change in structure/appearance

Coping, ineffective, individual, related to [specify]

Anxiety related to threat to health status

Implementation

- Put on gloves. Using aseptic technique, perform a venipuncture and collect 5 mL of blood in a red-top tube on two consecutive days between the hours of 6 and 8 A.M.
- Handle the sample gently to avoid hemolysis and transport to the laboratory immediately.

Evaluation

- Note test results in relation to other studies performed and the client's symptoms.

Client/Caregiver Teaching

Pretest

- Inform the client that the test will be performed on two consecutive days and to return to the laboratory between the hours of 6 and 8 A.M.

Posttest

- Tell the client to resume medications withheld before the tests.

Growth Hormone Stimulation Test

Classification: Chemistry

Type of Test: Serum

This test measures human growth hormone (hGH), following administration of substances that normally stimulate hGH secretion, such as arginine, insulin, and levodopa. Since growth hormone secretion by the anterior pituitary gland is episodic, obtaining a random specimen may not produce reliable results. In addition, growth hormone baseline levels are affected by many factors and have idiosyncratic responses to the different stimulants. Consequently, it may be necessary to perform two or three different stimulation tests before arriving at diagnostic conclusions.

Indications

- Evaluate low or undetectable serum GH levels, with GH deficiency or adult panhypopituitarism confirmed by no increase after administration of the stimulant.
- Confirm the diagnosis of acromegaly, as evidenced by reduced GH output after levodopa is administered as a stimulant.

Reference Values

		SI Units
Arginine		
Men	>10 ng/mL	>440 pmol/L
Women	>15 ng/mL	>660 pmol/L
Levodopa or insulin		
(above baseline level)	>7 ng/mL	>340 pmol/L

Abnormal Values

- Dwarfism in children
- Panhypopituitarism in adults

Interfering Factors

- Hyperglycemia and therapy with drugs such as adrenal, corticosteroids, and chlorpromazine can cause falsely decreased levels.
- Hypoglycemia, physical activity, stress, and a variety of drugs, such as amphetamines, arginine, dopamine, levodopa, methyldopa, beta blockers, histamine, nicotinic acid, estrogens can cause falsely elevated levels.

Nursing Implications

Assessment

- Obtain a history of growth pattern and previous growth hormone tests and results.
- Assess medication history and ensure that any drugs that may alter test results have been withheld for 12 hours before the test, as ordered by physician.
- Ensure that the client has fasted from food and has avoided strenuous exercise for 8 to 12 hours before the test.
- Assess weight, as dosage of the stimulant is determined by the client's weight.
- Ensure that the client has maintained bed rest for 1 hour before each sample is obtained, if recommended.

Possible Nursing Diagnoses

Body image disturbance related to change in structure/appearance

Coping, ineffective, individual, related to [specify]

Anxiety related to threat to health status

Implementation

- At about 8 A.M., put on gloves and insert an intermittent infusion device. Using aseptic technique, perform a venipuncture and obtain 6 mL of blood and place in a red-top tube.
- Administer the stimulant: levodopa orally or arginine and insulin intravenously in a saline infusion. If insulin is used to lower blood sugar, an ampule of 50% glucose solution should be on hand in the event that severe hypoglycemia occurs.
- After the stimulant is administered, obtain three 6-mL blood samples at 30-minute intervals using the intermittent infusion device. Place samples in red-top tubes.
- Handle all samples gently to avoid hemolysis and send to the laboratory immediately.

Evaluation

- Note results of hGH test as a basis for this more invasive procedure and also in relation to client's symptoms.

Client/Caregiver Teaching

Pretest

- Tell the client to fast from food and to avoid strenuous exercise for 8 to 12 hours before the test.
- Tell the client to withhold drugs that may affect results, as ordered, and maintain bed rest for 1 hour before the test.

Posttest

- Tell the client to resume diet, activity, and medications withheld before the test.

▲▲▲▲▲▲▲▲▲▲▲▲▲▲▲▲▲▲

Growth Hormone Suppression Test

Classification: Chemistry (Pituitary hormone)

Type of Test: Serum

This test evaluates excessive levels of human growth hormone (hGH) secreted by the anterior pituitary by measuring the secretory response to a loading dose of glucose. Administration of a loading dose of glucose should decrease serum GH levels within 1 to 2 hours. In individuals who are hypersecreting GH, a decrease in serum GH will not occur in response to hyperglycemia. This test may need to be repeated to confirm results.

Indications

- Evaluate elevated serum hGH levels
- Evaluate signs of hGH hypersecretion when serum hGH levels are within normal limits
- Confirm hGH hypersecretion, as indicated by decreased response to hGH suppression

Reference Values

	SI Units
<3 ng/dL	<132 pmol/L

Abnormal Values

- Acromegaly
- Gigantism

Interfering Factors

- Hyperglycemia and therapy with drugs such as adrenal corticosteroids and chlorpromazine may cause falsely decreased levels.
- Hypoglycemia, physical activity, stress, and a variety of drugs (e.g., amphetamines, arginine, dopamine, levodopa, methyldopa, beta blockers, histamine, nicotinic acid, estrogens) may cause falsely elevated levels.

Nursing Implications

Assessment

- Obtain a history of growth pattern and previous growth hormone test results.
- Assess medication history. Ensure that any drugs that may alter test results have been withheld for 12 hours before the test, as ordered by physician.
- Ensure that the client has fasted from food and has avoided strenuous exercise for 8 to 12 hours before the test.
- Ensure that the client has maintained bed rest for 1 hour before each sample is obtained, if recommended.

Possible Nursing Diagnoses

Body image disturbance related to change in structure/appearance

Coping, ineffective, individual, related to [specify]

Anxiety related to threat to health status

Implementation

- Put on gloves. Using aseptic technique, perform a venipuncture and collect 6 mL of blood in a red-top tube.
- Administer the glucose solution (usually 100 g) orally. If the client is unable to drink or retain the glucose solution, the

physician is notified. Intravenous glucose may be administered, if necessary, to perform the test.

- After 1 to 2 hours, depending on laboratory procedures, collect a second 6-mL blood sample in a red-top tube.
- Handle samples gently to avoid hemolysis and transport to the laboratory immediately.

Evaluation

- Note results in relation to growth hormone test.

Client/Caregiver Teaching

Pretest

- Tell the client to fast from food and avoid strenuous exercise for 8 to 12 hours before the test, to withhold medications that may interfere with test results for 12 hours, and to rest for 1 hour before drawing blood samples.

Posttest

- Tell the client to resume diet, activity, and medications withheld before the test.

Guthrie Test, Serum Phenylalanine Screening

Classification: Chemistry

Type of Test: Blood

This screening test helps detect elevated serum phenylalanine, which is a naturally occurring amino acid essential to growth and nitrogen balance. It detects abnormal phenylalanine levels through observation of the growth rate of the organism *Bacillus subtilis,* which needs phenylalanine to thrive. High serum phenylalanine levels result in mental retardation, neurological manifestations, light skin pigmentation, and eczema. With earlier hospital discharge after normal delivery, the caregiver must bring the infant to the laboratory for the test to be performed.

Indications

■ Routine screening test for phenylketonuria (PKU); testing is mandatory in most states

Reference Values

■ Negative; <2 mg/dL

Abnormal Values

■ Positive levels
   PKU, confirmation of diagnosis needed with further testing
   Galactosemia
   Hepatic disease
   Delayed development of certain enzyme systems

Interfering Factors

■ Performing the test before the infant has had 3 days of formula or breast milk causes false-negative results.

Nursing Implications

Assessment

■ Assess infant's heel for lesions, edema, and previous puncture sites.
■ Determine the number of days that the infant has had formula or breast milk.

Possible Nursing Diagnoses

Anxiety related to threat to health status
Adjustment, impaired, risk for, related to need for lifestyle changes or threat to self-concept
Nutrition, altered, less than body requirements, related to inability to digest food and absorb nutrients

Implementation

■ Put on gloves. Using aseptic technique, perform a heelstick until free flow of blood is obtained. Allow several drops of blood to collect on the filter paper.
■ Place sample in plastic bag labeled with baby's name, date of birth, and date of first feeding, and send to laboratory.

Evaluation

■ Notify physician immediately if test result is positive.

Client/Caregiver Teaching

Pretest

- Inform the caregiver of the importance of having the test performed after infant has had food formula or breast milk for 3 days.
- Inform caregiver that no fluid restrictions are required before the test.

Posttest

- Inform the caregiver that if screening test is positive, serum levels of phenylalanine and tyrosine will be measured to confirm the diagnosis. Elevated phenylalanine (>4 mg/dL) with decreased tyrosine (<0.6 mg/dL) and urinary excretion of phenylpyruvic acid, confirms the diagnosis.
- Inform the caregiver if the diagnosis is confirmed that early detection and treatment can prevent retardation.
- Teach the caregiver about the low-phenylalanine diet.

Ham Test, Acidified Serum Test

Classification: Hematology

Type of Test: Blood

Performed to test the stability of the red blood cell (RBC) membrane, the client's blood sample is mixed with its own serum and the serum of an ABO compatible donor. This combined sample is acidified and examined for lysis. The presence of lysis in client's serum is definitive for abnormality in RBC membrane. Because RBCs are sensitive to carbon dioxide, which increases during sleep and tends to increase plasma pH, hemolysis results and hemoglobin appears in the urine intermittently, especially during and after sleep.

Indications

- Diagnose paroxysmal nocturnal hemoglobinuria (PNH)
- Determine cause of undiagnosed hemolytic anemia and bone marrow aplasia

Reference Values

- Negative

Abnormal Values

- Hemolysis indicates PNH

Interfering Factors

- False-positive results may occur in leukemia, spherocytosis, aplastic anemia, and dyserythropoietic anemia.
- False-negative results may occur if the client received a transfusion of red blood cells within 3 weeks of test.
- Hemolysis of the sample invalidates the results.

Nursing Implications

Assessment

- Obtain a history of the hematologic and urinary systems and determine frequency of the client's symptoms.

Possible Nursing Diagnoses

Anxiety related to threat to health status
Protection, altered, related to abnormal blood profiles
Tissue perfusion, altered [specify], related to oxygen supply/ demand imbalance

Implementation

- Put on gloves. Using aseptic technique, perform a venipuncture and collect 7 mL of blood in a purple-top tube. (Some laboratories perform the stick because the sample requires defibrination immediately.)
- Handle the specimen gently to avoid hemolysis and transport to the laboratory promptly.

Evaluation

- Note test results in relation to other tests performed and the client's symptoms.

Client/Caregiver Teaching

Pretest

- Inform the client that there are no fluid or food restrictions before the test.

Haptoglobin (Hp)

Classification: Chemistry (protein)

Type of Test: Serum

This test measures haptoglobin (Hp), an alpha$_2$ (α_2) globulin produced in the liver that binds with free hemoglobin released by the hemolysis of red blood cells (RBCs). The new complex is quickly catabolized. If left unchecked, free hemoglobin in the plasma can cause renal damage; haptoglobin prevents it from accumulating. In conditions such as hemolytic anemia, so many hemolyzed red blood cells are available for binding that the liver cannot compensate by producing more fast enough, resulting in low serum levels.

Indications

- Evaluate known or suspected disorder characterized by excessive red blood cell hemolysis, as indicated by decreased levels
- Evaluate known or suspected chronic liver disease, as indicated by decreased levels
- Evaluate known or suspected disorders involving a diffuse inflammatory process or tissue destruction, as indicated by elevated levels

Reference Values

		SI Units
Newborn	0–30 mg/dL	0–0.3 g/L
Child	0–10 mg/dL	0–0.1 g/L
Adult	60–270 mg/dL	0.6–2.7 g/L

Abnormal Values

- Increased levels
  Inflammatory diseases, such as ulcerative colitis, arthritis, pyelonephritis

Disorders involving tissue destruction, such as cancers, burns, acute myocardial infarction

Steroid therapy

- Decreased levels

Acute and chronic hemolysis

Infectious mononucleosis

Severe hepatocellular disease

Transfusion reactions

Interfering Factors

- Steroid therapy can result in elevated levels.

Nursing Implications

Assessment

- Obtain a history of infectious processes, hepatic or hematologic disorders, and drugs that can influence haptoglobin levels.

Possible Nursing Diagnoses

Injury, risk for, related to hemolysis

Anxiety related to threat to health status

Protection, altered, related to abnormal blood profiles

Tissue perfusion, altered [specify], related to oxygen supply/demand imbalance

Implementation

- Put on gloves. Using aseptic technique, perform a venipuncture and collect a 7-mL blood sample in a red-top tube. Some laboratories require that the sample be placed in ice immediately upon collection.
- Handle the sample gently to avoid hemolysis and send the sample promptly to the laboratory.

Evaluation

- Note test results in relation to RBC and hemoglobin values.
- Monitor for change in respirations caused by decreased RBC levels resulting in hypoxia.

Client/Caregiver Teaching

Posttest

- Tell the client to report chills, fever, flushing, back pain, and fast heartbeat (signs of hemolysis) to the physician immediately.

Heinz Bodies Stain

Classification: Hematology

Type of Test: Blood

Heinz bodies are small, irregularly shaped bodies of denatured hemoglobin that have precipitated out of the cytoplasm of the RBCs and attached to the cell membrane. They can be visualized by phase microscopy or with stains, such as crystal violet or methylene blue. Presence of Heinz bodies in a specimen indicates an abnormal hemoglobin structure.

Indications

- Determine causes of hemolytic anemia

Reference Values

- Negative

Abnormal Values

- Elevated levels
  Presence of unstable hemoglobins
  Inherited RBC enzyme deficiency
  Drug-induced RBC injury
  Thalassemia
  G-6-PD deficiency if >40 percent of cells have 5 or more
    Heinz bodies
  Postsplenectomy

Interfering Factors

- Use of antimalarials, procarbazine, furazolidone, and sulfon-amides may interfere with results.
- Clotting or hemolysis of the sample invalidates results.

Nursing Implications

Assessment

- Obtain a history of suspected hemolytic anemia and medication regimen.

Possible Nursing Diagnoses

Injury, risk for, related to hemolysis
Anxiety related to threat to health status
Protection, altered, related to abnormal blood profiles
Tissue perfusion, altered [specify], related to oxygen supply/
   demand imbalance

Implementation

- Put on gloves. Using aseptic technique, perform a venipuncture and collect 3 mL of blood in a purple-top tube.
- Handle the specimen gently to avoid hemolysis and transport to the laboratory promptly.

Evaluation

- Note test results in relation to other tests performed and the client's symptoms.

Client/Caregiver Teaching

Pretest

- Inform the client that no fluid or food restriction is required before the test.

Hemagglutination Treponemal Test for Syphilis (HATTS)

Classification: Serology

Type of Test: Serum

In this test, the client's serum is treated and mixed with *Treponema pallidum*-sensitized red blood cells. After it has incubated, the sample is compared to a control sample. A positive result occurs when agglutination occurs in client's sample but not in the control sample. Even after treatment, clients previously infected with syphilis will have a positive test result.

Indications

- Confirm syphilis when nontreponemal antibody test is positive

Reference Values

- Titer <1:160

Abnormal Values

- Positive levels
  Active syphilis
  Other treponemal diseases, such as bejel, pinta, and yaws

Interfering Factors

- Infectious mononucleosis, systemic lupus erythematosus, and leprosy may cause false-positive results.
- AIDS may cause false-negative results.

Nursing Implications

Assessment

- Obtain a history of reproductive system disorders, known or suspected exposure to syphilis, medication regimen, diagnostic tests and results.
- Ascertain that the client has fasted for at least 8 hours before the test.

Possible Nursing Diagnoses

Infection, risk for transmission
Anxiety related to threat to health status
Skin/tissue integrity, impaired, related to invasion of pathogenic organisms

Implementation

- Put on gloves. Using aseptic technique, perform a venipuncture and collect 7 mL of blood in a red-top tube.
- Send the specimen to the laboratory promptly and refrigerate until tested.

Evaluation

- Note and report positive results to physician and the Centers for Disease Control and Prevention.

Client/Caregiver Teaching

Pretest

- Tell the client to fast overnight before the test.

Posttest

- Inform the client and caregiver to resume food and fluids.
- Inform the client that in the event of positive test result, all sexual contacts need to be notified.

Hematocrit (Hct)

Classification: Hematology

Type of Test: Blood

Blood consists of a fluid portion (plasma) and a solid portion that includes red blood cells, white blood cells, and platelets. The hematocrit, or the packed red cell volume, is the percentage of red blood cells in a volume of whole blood. For example, a hematocrit of 45 percent means that a 100-mL sample of blood contains 45 mL of packed red blood cells. While the hematocrit depends primarily on the number of red blood cells, the average size of the RBCs plays a role. Conditions that cause the RBCs to swell, such as when the serum sodium concentration is elevated, may increase the hematocrit. Hematocrit level is included in the complete blood count (CBC) and generally performed with a hemoglobin. These levels parallel each other and are the best determinant of the degree of anemia. Hematocrit is usually three times the hemoglobin unless the erythrocytes are abnormal in size and shape.

Indications

- Perform a routine screening as part of a complete blood count
- Monitor blood loss along with hemoglobin findings
- Evaluate known or suspected anemia and related treatment
- Monitor hematologic status in pregnancy, along with hemoglobin
- Monitor fluid imbalances or treatment for fluid imbalances

Reference Values

Infants	
Newborn	44–64%
1 mo	35–49%
6 mo	30–40%
Children (1–10 yr)	35–41%
Adults	
Men	40–54%
Women	38–47%

Abnormal Values

- Elevated values
  - Dehydration
  - Polycythemia
  - Blood loss
  - Hemoconcentration states
  - Acute pancreatitis
- Decreased values
  - Bone marrow hyperplasia
  - Burns
  - Anemia
  - Hemodilution
  - Cirrhosis
  - Congestive heart failure

Interfering Factors

- Abnormalities in the red blood cell size and extremely high white blood cell count may alter values.
- Elevated blood glucose or serum sodium levels may produce elevated levels because of swelling of the erythrocytes.
- Hemolysis of the sample may affect results.
- Having the tourniquet in place for longer than 1 minute can falsely increase level 2 to 5 percent.
- Improper technique such as using the improper anticoagulant, filling the tube inaccurately, mixing the sample with the anticoagulant, or collecting the sample from the same arm being used for IV fluids (hemodilution) affects results.

Nursing Implications

Assessment

- Obtain a history of hematologic status, any recent trauma, hematopoietic tests and results, and medication regimen.

Possible Nursing Diagnoses

Anxiety related to threat to health status

Protection, altered, related to abnormal blood profiles

Tissue perfusion, altered [specify], related to oxygen supply/demand imbalance

Fatigue related to oxygen supply/demand imbalance

Implementation

- Put on gloves. Using aseptic technique, perform a finger stick and fill two-thirds of a heparinized capillary tube with blood. Seal the end of the capillary tube with clay and send to the laboratory immediately.
- Alternatively, obtain 3 mL of blood in a lavender-top tube. Invert the tube 10 times to mix the sample with the anticoagulant in the tube.
- Handle the sample gently to avoid hemolysis and transport to the laboratory promptly.

Evaluation

- Note test results in relation to other tests performed, particularly hemoglobin, and the client's symptoms.

Client/Caregiver Teaching

Pretest

- Inform the client that there are no food or fluid restrictions before this test.

Hemoglobin (Hb)

Classification: Hematology

Type of Test: Blood

This test measures the amount of hemoglobin in the blood, the main intracellular protein of erythrocytes. It functions to carry oxygen to and remove carbon dioxide from the cells and as a buffer in the maintenance of acid-base balance. Each Hb molecule consists of heme and globulin, with approximately 250 million molecules in each red blood cell. Hemoglobin level is included in the complete blood count (CBC) and generally performed with a hematocrit. These levels parallel each other and are the best determinant of the degree of anemia. Hematocrit is usually three times the hemoglobin, unless the erythrocytes are abnormal in size and shape.

Indications

- Evaluate known or suspected anemia and related treatment, in combination with hematocrit
- Monitor blood loss and response to blood replacement, in combination with hematocrit
- Monitor hematologic status during pregnancy, in combination with hematocrit
- Perform routine diagnostic screen as part of a complete blood count (CBC)

Reference Values

		SI Units
Newborn	14–27 g/dL	9.6–15.5 mmol/L
<1 yr	10–15 g/dL	6.1–9.0 mmol/L
Children 1–10 yr	11–16 g/dL	5.8–9.6 mmol/L
Adults		
Men	14–18 g/dL	8.7–11.2 mmol/L
Women	12–16 g/dL	7.4–9.9 mmol/L
Pregnant women	10–15 g/dL	6.3–9.3 mmol/L
Critical values	<5 g/dL	<3.1 mmol/L
	>20 g/dL	>11.2 mmol/L

Ratio of hematocrit to hemoglobin is 3:1.

Abnormal Values

- Increased Hb levels
    Chronic obstructive pulmonary disease
    Congestive heart failure
    Congenital heart defect
    Polycythemia vera
    Thrombocytopenic purpura
    Hemoconcentration
    Dehydration
    Severe burns
    High altitudes
- Decreased Hb levels
    Anemias
    Acute or chronic hemorrhage

Hemoglobinopathies
Hemolytic disorders
Lymphomas
Carcinoma
Fluid retention
Nutritional deficit
Renal disease
Cirrhosis, fatty liver
Systemic lupus erythematosus
Thyroid disease
Pregnancy

Interfering Factors

- Improper collection technique such as prolonged use of the tourniquet, hemolysis of the sample, and delayed testing without refrigeration of the sample will affect results.
- Excessive exercise, anxiety, pain, dehydration, or sample obtained after certain procedures or treatments can lead to false increases.
- Drugs such as gentamicin and methyldopa can cause elevated erythrocyte count (RBC), resulting in increased Hb.
- Certain drugs can cause a reduction in circulating RBCs and decreased Hb: antibiotics, antineoplastics, anticonvulsants, sulfonamides, monoamine oxidase inhibitors, indomethacin, rifampin, aspirin, and others.

Nursing Implications

Assessment

- Obtain a history of known or suspected hematologic disorders and related treatments and assess for signs and symptoms resulting from changes in hematologic status.

Possible Nursing Diagnoses

Anxiety related to threat to health status
Infection, risk for, related to inadequate secondary defenses
Tissue perfusion, altered [specify], related to oxygen supply/demand imbalance
Fatigue related to oxygen supply/demand imbalance

Implementation

- Put on gloves. Using aseptic technique, perform a venipuncture and collect 7 mL of blood in a lavender-top tube. A capillary sample can be obtained in infants and children, as well as adults in whom venipuncture is not feasible.

- Handle specimen gently to avoid hemolysis and send to the laboratory.

Evaluation

- Note results in relation to other tests, particularly hematocrit and serum iron studies.
- Report critical values to the physician immediately and prepare for transfusion of whole blood or packed red cells, if ordered for decreased level, or for phlebotomy, if ordered for increased level.

Client/Caregiver Teaching

Pretest

- Inform the client that there are no food and fluid restrictions.

Hemoglobin, Glycosylated (GHB), Glycohemoglobin

Classification: Chemistry (carbohydrate)

Type of Test: Blood

A diagnostic test performed to monitor overall blood glucose control and provide information that can be missed by random blood and urine glucose tests. Throughout the red blood cell's life span (3 months), the hemoglobin molecule incorporates glucose onto its beta chain. Glycosylation is irreversible and occurs at a stable rate. The amount of glucose permanently bound to hemoglobin depends on the blood sugar level. The level of glycosylated hemoglobin, designated Hgb A_{1c}, reflects the average blood sugar over a period of several weeks. Insulin-dependent diabetics can have undetected periods of hyperglycemia alternating with postinsulin periods of normoglycemia or even hypoglycemia. High Hgb A_{1c} levels reflect inadequate diabetic control in the preceding 3 to 5 weeks. After normoglycemic levels are stabilized, Hgb A_{1c} levels return to normal in about 3 weeks.

Indications

- Monitor overall blood glucose control in clients with known diabetes, as evidenced by prolonged hyperglycemia, with levels of Hgb A_{1c} rising to as high as 18 to 20 percent; after normoglycemic levels are stabilized, Hgb A_{1c} levels return to normal in about 3 weeks.
- Monitor adequacy of insulin dosage for blood glucose control, especially that administered by automatic insulin pumps.
- Evaluate the diabetic client's degree of compliance with the prescribed therapeutic regimen.

Reference Values

Total GHB	5.5–8.8% of total Hb
Controlled diabetes	7.5–11.4%
Uncontrolled diabetes	>15%
Hbg A_{1a}	1.8%
Hbg A_{1b}	0.8%
Hbg A_{1c}	3.5–6.0%

Abnormal Values

- *Increased GHB:* hyperglycemia within last 5 weeks

Interfering Factors

- Individuals with hemolytic anemia and high levels of young red blood cells can have spuriously low levels.
- Elevated fetal hemoglobin, heparin therapy, and pregnancy can elevate levels.
- Anemia, acute or chronic blood loss, splenectomy, chronic renal failure, and thalassemia can decrease levels.

Nursing Implications

Assessment

- Obtain a history of diabetes management, diet compliance, any related test results, and medications taken.

Possible Nursing Diagnoses

Anxiety related to threat to health status
Coping, ineffective, individual, related to [specify]
Infection, risk for, related to decreased circulation

Therapeutic regimen, individual, ineffective management, related to [specify]

Adjustment, impaired, risk for, related to need for lifestyle changes or threat to self-concept

Implementation

- Put on gloves. Using aseptic technique, perform a venipuncture and collect 5 mL of blood in a lavender-, green-, or gray-top tube.
- Invert tube gently several times to adequately mix the sample and transport promptly to the laboratory.

Evaluation

- Compare results to related tests, clinical symptoms, and client history.

Client/Caregiver Teaching

Pretest

- Inform client that this test provides information regarding the adequacy of treatment over a long period of time. Changing dietary habits immediately before the test will not affect test results.

Hemoglobin, Unstable

Classification: Hematology
Type of Test: Blood

Unstable hemoglobin is a rare congenital abnormality in hemoglobin that causes it to precipitate faster then normal hemoglobin. After precipitation, it forms Heinz bodies, which attach to cell membrane and increase fragility of the red blood cell, leading to hemolysis. Unstable hemoglobin is detectable when exposed to isopropanol or when subjected to acid and heated to 50°C. Isopropanol test is more sensitive than the heat-labile test.

Indications

- Detect unstable hemoglobins

Reference Values

- *Heat-labile test:* negative
- *Isopropanol precipitation:* stable

Abnormal Values

- Increased levels
  Heinz body anemia
  Thalassemia

Interfering Factors

- High levels of Hgb F may cause a false-positive isopropanol test.
- Sulfanomides, antimalarials, nitrofurantoin, procarbazine, and furazolidine in infants may induce sample hemolysis.
- False-positive results may occur when specimens are tested more than a week after the blood is drawn.

Nursing Implications

Assessment

- Obtain a history of anemia, known or suspected hemoglobin abnormality, diagnostic tests, and results.
- Obtain a drug history. Ask specifically about drugs that may interfere with test results.

Possible Nursing Diagnoses

Anxiety related to threat to health status
Protection, altered, related to abnormal blood profiles
Tissue perfusion, altered [specify], related to oxygen supply/demand imbalance

Implementation

- Put on gloves. Using aseptic technique, perform a venipuncture and collect 7 mL of blood in a lavender-top tube.
- Invert the tube gently 6 to 10 times to mix the specimen. Handle sample carefully; to avoid hemolysis, do not shake.
- Label specimen and send to laboratory immediately. Test must be performed within 3 hours after collection.

Evaluation

- Note results in relation to other studies performed and clinical symptoms.

Client/Caregiver Teaching

Pretest

- Instruct the client and caregiver not to take drugs such as sulfonamides, nitrofurantoin, procarbazine, and furazolidone (in infants).

Posttest

- Advise the client to resume medications withheld before the test.

Hemoglobin and Blood, Urine

Classification: Urinalysis

Type of Test: Urine, random

Blood may be present in the urine as either red blood cells or hemoglobin. If enough is present, the urine will be pink-tinged to red to brownish black. The presence of red blood cells (hematuria) is relatively common. However, the presence of hemoglobin (hemoglobinuria) occurs much less frequently and is usually associated with any disorder that causes hemolysis of red blood cells. Normally the hemoglobin combines with haptoglobin, forming a complex that is too large to pass through the glomerular membrane. But if the amount of free hemoglobin exceeds the amount of haptoglobin, the hemoglobin passes through and is excreted in the urine.

Indications

- Detect excessive red blood cell hemolysis within the systemic circulation

- Diagnose hemolytic anemias
- Determine severe intravascular hemolysis from a transfusion reaction
- Determine bleeding in the urinary tract evidenced by the presence of red blood cells and hemoglobin

Reference Values

- Negative for random and dipstick

Abnormal Values

- Hemoglobinuria
  Autoimmune hemolytic anemia
  Trauma to red blood cells by prosthetic cardiac valves
  Trauma to muscles and blood vessels
  Malaria
  Burns
  Hemolytic anemia
  Paroxysmal nocturnal hemoglobinuria
  Transfusion reaction
  Fever or infectious diseases
  Drugs, including bacitracin, Coumadin, cyclophospha-
    mide, fenoprofen, gold salts, indomethacin, nitrofuran-
    toin, phenacetin, phenothiazines, phenylbutazone,
    polymyxin B, and quinine
- Hematuria
  Cystitis
  Pyelonephritis
  Renal calculi
  Tumors of the genitourinary tract
  Trauma to urinary tract
  Renal artery stenosis

Interfering Factors

- Contamination with menstrual blood can cause false-positive results.
- Ascorbic acid can cause false-negatives if tested with reagent strips.
- Bromides, copper, iodides, and oxidizing agents can cause false-positives.

Nursing Implications

Assessment

- Obtain a history of hematologic status, hematopoietic tests and results; assess any medications that the client is taking (see Abnormal Values and Interfering Factors). Discontinue medications as ordered before the test.
- Ensure that the test is not performed during client's menstrual period; reschedule test if need be.

Possible Nursing Diagnoses

Injury, risk for, related to hemolysis
Anxiety related to threat to health status
Protection, altered, related to abnormal blood profiles
Tissue perfusion, altered [specify], related to oxygen supply/ demand imbalance

Implementation

- Obtain the appropriate-sized sterile plastic container without preservative according to laboratory policy. Explain to the client that the procedure is to obtain a random 20-mL urine sample.
- If using a commercial urine dipstick, follow directions for timing and match with color chart.
- If sending sample to the laboratory, make sure it is properly labeled. Refrigerate specimen if not taken to laboratory immediately.
- If an indwelling catheter is in place, obtain random sample from the catheter and put into container to test by dipstick or send to laboratory.

Evaluation

- Compare results with red blood count.

Client/Caregiver Teaching

Posttest

- Tell the client to resume medications and activity withheld before the test.

Hemoglobin Electrophoresis

Classification: Hematology

Type of Test: Blood

Hemoglobin electrophoresis analyzes the types of hemoglobin present using an electromagnetic field that separates the types and quantifies them by percentage of total hemoglobin. Each of the types migrate at different rates when placed on the electromagnetic field, causing the separation. Types include A_1, A_2, D, E, F, H, S, and C. The greatest percentage of total hemoglobin is A_1. Hemoglobin F is the major percentage of fetal hemoglobin, but small amounts are normal in the adult. It is present in increased amounts when decreased oxygen is available and assists in the transport of that oxygen. D, E, H, S, and C are present with hemoglobinopathies.

Indications

- Diagnose thalassemia, especially in clients with a positive family history for the disorder
- Differentiate among thalassemia types
- Evaluate positive Sickledex test to differentiate sickle-cell trait from sickle-cell disease
- Evaluate hemolytic anemia of unknown etiology
- Diagnose Hgb C anemia

Reference Values

		SI Units
Hemoglobin A_1		
Adults	95–97%	>0.95
Infants	10–30%	0.10–0.30
Hemoglobin A_2		
Adults	3–4%	0.03–0.04
Hemoglobin F		
Adults	<1%	<0.10
Neonates	70–80%	0.70–0.80
1 mo	70%	0.70
2 mo	50%	0.50
3 mo	25%	0.25
6–12 mo	3%	0.03
Hemoglobin C	None	

	SI Units
Hemoglobin D	None
Hemoglobin E	None
Hemoglobin H	None
Hemoglobin S	None
Methemoglobin	2% or 0.06–0.24 g/dL
Sulfhemoglobin	Minute amounts
Carboxyhemoglobin	0–2.3% (4–5% in smokers)

Abnormal Values

- Hemoglobin C disease

Hemoglobin C	90–100%
Hemoglobin A_1	None
Hemoglobin A_2	2–3%
Hemoglobin F	2%

- Increased hemoglobin D and E

  Indicates more severe form of the disease when present in sickle-cell disease or thalassemia

- Hemoglobin H disease

Hemoglobin A_1	65–90%
Hemoglobin A_2	2–3%
Hemoglobin F	5–30%

- Sickle-cell disease

Hemoglobin S	80–100%
Hemoglobin A_1	None
Hemoglobin A_2	2–3%
Hemoglobin F	<2%

- Sickle-cell trait

Hemoglobin S	20–40%
Hemoglobin A_1	60–80%
Hemoglobin A_2	2–3%
Hemoglobin F	2%

- Thalassemia major

Hemoglobin A_1	5–20%
Hemoglobin A_2	2–3%
Hemoglobin F	65–100%

- Thalassemia minor

Hemoglobin A_1	50–85%
Hemoglobin A_2	24–6%
Hemoglobin F	1–3%

- Methemoglobinemia

  Increased methemoglobin from excessive radiation or toxic effects of drugs such as nitrates, phenacetin, or lidocaine

- Increased sulfhemoglobin
  Ingestion of sulfonamides
- Increased carboxyhemoglobin
  Exposure to motor vehicle fumes or smoking

Interfering Factors

- Sample hemolysis invalidates results.
- High altitude and dehydration may increase values.
- Iron deficiency may decrease hemoglobin A_2, C, and S.
- In clients less than 3 months of age, false-negative results for Hgb S occur in coincidental polycythemia.
- Red blood cell transfusion within 4 months of test can mask abnormal hemoglobins.

Nursing Implications

Assessment

- Obtain a history of hematologic disorders or symptoms, medication regimen, diagnostic tests, and results.
- Ask if the client has received a blood transfusion within the last 4 months.

Possible Nursing Diagnoses

Anxiety related to threat to health status
Pain, acute, risk for, related to red blood cell sickling
Tissue perfusion, altered [specify], related to oxygen supply/demand imbalance
Fatigue related to oxygen supply/demand imbalance

Implementation

- Put on gloves. Using aseptic technique, perform a venipuncture and collect 7 mL of blood in a lavender-top tube.
- After collecting the sample, gently invert the tube a few times to mix the blood and the anticoagulant.
- Handle sample gently to prevent hemolysis.

Evaluation

- Note results in relation to other studies performed and clinical symptoms.

Client/Caregiver Teaching

Pretest

- Inform the client that there are no food or fluid restrictions before the test.

Hemosiderin

Classification: Urinalysis (siderocyte stain)

Type of Test: Urine, random

This tests for the presence of iron storage granules called hemosiderin by microscopic examination of urine sediment. These course granules of hemosiderin stain blue when potassium ferrocyanide is added to the sample. Hemosiderin is found in the liver, spleen, and bone marrow but not in the urine. It is normally absorbed by the renal tubules but in extensive hemolysis, renal tubule damage, or an iron metabolism disorder, hemosiderin filters its way into the urine.

Indications

- Detect excessive red blood cell hemolysis within the systemic circulation
- Diagnosis of hemochromatosis (tissue damage due to iron toxicity)
- Evaluate renal tubule dysfunction

Reference Values

- Negative

Abnormal Values

- Positive
    Hemochromocytosis
    Pernicious anemia
    Blood transfusions
    Paroxysmal nocturnal hemoglobinuria
    Burns
    Hemolytic anemia
    Hemosiderosis
    Megaloblastic anemia
    Renal tubular cell dysfunction
    Sickle-cell anemia
    Thalassemia major anemia

Interfering Factors

- Alkaline urine prevents detection of hemosiderin.

Nursing Implications

Assessment

- Obtain a history of anemia or renal dysfunction.

Possible Nursing Diagnoses

Anxiety related to threat to health status
Pain, acute, risk for, related to red blood cell sickling
Tissue perfusion, altered [specify], related to oxygen supply/
    demand imbalance
Fatigue related to oxygen supply/demand imbalance

Implementation

- Obtain the appropriate-sized sterile plastic container without preservative, according to laboratory policy.
- Collect the first 50 mL of the first morning void in a sterile plastic container. Follow laboratory directions for any special care of the specimen after collection such as immediate refrigeration.
- If an indwelling catheter is in place, empty the first morning urine into a plastic container without preservative.
- Ensure that the label is properly completed and transport to the laboratory.

Evaluation

- Note results in relation to other tests for anemia and clinical symptoms.

Client/Caregiver Teaching

- Tell the client to obtain a first-voided morning specimen in the plastic container provided. Tell the client to take it to the laboratory within 1 hour.

Hepatitis B Antibody and Antigen (Anti-HBe, HBeAb, HBeAg)

Classification: Serology

Type of Test: Serum, blood

Hepatitis B antigen, one of the first indicators of hepatitis infection, is usually present for 3 to 6 weeks and often precedes symptoms. The antibody, a serum marker for hepatitis B, appears 8 to 16 weeks after infection and indicates that acute infection is resolving. While the surface antigen usually appears 4 to 12 weeks after infection, the surface antibody appears 2 to 16 weeks after the surface antigen disappears. Appearance of the surface antibody represents clinical recovery and immunity to the virus and is also present with hepatitis B immune globulin or during transfer in blood by transfusion or in intravenous drug abusers.

Indications

- Detect exposure to hepatitis B virus
- Detect possible carrier status
- Screen blood donors for hepatitis B

Reference Values

- Negative

Abnormal Values

- *Positive:* indicates hepatitis B

Interfering Factors

- Injection of radionuclides within 7 days of testing may alter results if using radioimmunoassay techniques.
- Presence of rheumatoid factor and competing IgG antibody can cause inaccurate results.

Nursing Implications

Assessment

- Obtain a history of known or suspected exposure to hepatitis B and other immune disorders.

Possible Nursing Diagnoses

Anxiety related to perceived threat to health status
Infection, risk for, related to immunosuppressed inflammatory response
Pain related to inflammation or swelling of the liver
Fatigue related to decreased metabolic energy production

Implementation

- Put on gloves. Using aseptic technique, perform a venipuncture and collect 7 mL of blood in a red-top tube.
- Handle sample gently to avoid hemolysis and send promptly to the laboratory.

Evaluation

- Note test results in relation to client's symptoms and other tests performed.

Client/Caregiver Teaching

Pretest

- Inform the client that no food or fluid restrictions are required before the test.

Posttest

- If diagnosis is confirmed, instruct the client and caregiver on the need for adequate rest, importance of fluid and nutritional intake, and skin care techniques for pruritus.
- Instruct the client in modes of disease transmission and warn not to donate blood.

Hepatitis Profile, Prenatal

Classification: Serology

Type of Test: Serum

Acute or chronic hepatitis B virus can be transmitted from mother to infant during delivery. If infant is infected at birth, an increased risk for acute hepatitis or chronic hepatitis at a later time exists. Routine prenatal screening includes hepatitis B surface antigen, hepatitis B antigen, hepatitis B antibody, HBV-DNA, and hepatitis B core antibody.

Indications

- Screen pregnant women for hepatitis B virus

Reference Values

- Negative for HBsAg, HBeAg, anti-HBe, HBV-DNA, and anti-HBc IgM

Abnormal Values

Positive HBsAg	Active HBV infection
Positive HBeAg	Highly infectious state, persisting for more than 10 weeks suggests progression to chronic state and carrier state
Positive HBV-DNA	Viral hepatitis DNA in serum (most accurate assessment)
Positive anti-HBc IgM	Current acute infection, can differentiate acute from chronic

Interfering Factors

- Heparin therapy may yield false-positive results.
- Injection of radionuclides within 7 days of testing may alter results if radioimmunoassay techniques are used.

Nursing Implications

Assessment

- Obtain a history of illness, symptoms, known or suspected exposure to hepatitis, results of tests and procedures performed.
- Assess medication history and ensure that any drugs that may alter test results have been withheld for 12 to 24 hours before test, as ordered.

Possible Nursing Diagnoses

Anxiety related to perceived threat to fetal health
Grieving, anticipatory, related to perceived potential outcome

Implementation

- Put on gloves. Using aseptic technique, perform a venipuncture and collect 7 to 10 mL of blood in a red-top tube.
- Handle sample gently to avoid hemolysis.

Evaluation

- Note test results in relation to the client's symptoms and other tests performed.

Client/Caregiver Teaching

Pretest

- Tell the client to withhold heparin dosage, as ordered by physician.

Posttest

- Tell the client to resume medications withheld before the test.

Herpesvirus Antigen, Direct Fluorescent Antibody

Classification: Immunology

Type of Test: Biopsy

This test uses immunofluorescence or immunoperoxidase techniques to examine a specimen obtained from a lesion, bronchial brushing, conjunctiva, cerebrospinal fluid, or biopsy site to test for herpes simplex 1 and 2.

Indications

- Diagnose herpes simplex infection

Reference Values

- Negative

Abnormal Values

- *Positive value:* infection with herpes simplex virus

Interfering Factors

- Specimen placed in fixative invalidates results.
- An exudative-inflamed specimen may cause nonspecific color changes of the immunoperoxidase reagent.

Nursing Implications

Assessment

- Obtain a history of suspected or known exposure to herpes simplex virus, current symptoms, diagnostic tests and results.

Possible Nursing Diagnoses

Pain related to tissue inflammation and open lesions
Infection, risk for secondary infection, related to break in skin integrity

Hyperthermia related to infectious process
Infection, risk for transmission

Implementation

- *Specimen from lesion or conjunctiva:* Put on gloves. Collect sample from affected site using a sterile swab with sterile specimen container or Culturette tube.
- *Specimens from bronchial washings, cerebrospinal fluid, or biopsy:* Place collected specimen in a sterile specimen container.
- Label specimen with client's name and transport to laboratory immediately.

Evaluation

- Note test results in relation to the client's symptoms and history and other tests performed.

Client/Caregiver Teaching

Pretest

- Inform the client that no special preparation is required for this test.

Posttest

- Instruct the client to report signs and symptoms related to disease process.

Hexosaminidase A

Classification: Hematology

Type of Test: Blood, biopsy

Hexosaminidase A is a lysosymal enzyme needed for metabolism of gangliosides, which are water-soluble glycolipids found mainly in brain tissue. Deficiency of this enzymes results in the buildup of gangliosides in the brain with resultant destruction and demylination of CNS cells, a condition known as Tay-Sachs disease.

Indications

- Diagnose Tay-Sachs disease
- Screen young adults to determine if they are an asymptomatic carrier of the gene that causes the disease
- Identify prenatal potential carriers of the disease
- Determine presence of the gene in the unborn fetus

Reference Values

- Hexosaminidase A is 56 to 80 percent of the total hexosamindase (10.4–23.8 U/L)

Abnormal Values

- Absence of hexosaminindase A indicates Tay-Sachs disease

Interfering Factors

- Levels are decreased during pregnancy and oral contraceptive use.

Nursing Implications

Assessment

- Obtain family history of Tay-Sachs disease.

Possible Nursing Diagnoses

Anxiety related to perceived threat to fetal health

Grieving, anticipatory, related to perceived potential outcome

Adjustment, impaired, risk for, related to need for lifestyle changes or threat to self-concept

Coping, ineffective, family related to [specify]

Implementation

- Put on gloves. Using aseptic technique, perform a venipuncture and collect 7 mL of blood in a red-top tube. In neonates, sample may be obtained from umbilical cord. Fetal samples can be obtained with chorionic villus biopsy or amniocentesis.
- Handle sample gently to prevent hemolysis.

Evaluation

■ Note results in relation to family history.

Client/Caregiver Teaching

Pretest

■ Tell the client to restrict food and fluid for 8 hours before the test.
■ As recommended by primary care provider, withhold oral contraceptives before the test.

Posttest

■ Resume normal diet and medication use.

Homovanillic Acid (HVA)

Classification: Chemistry

Type of Test: Urine (timed)

Homovanillic acid (HVA) is a metabolite of dopamine, a major catecholamine itself, as well as a precursor to the catecholamines epinephrine and norepinephrine. HVA is synthesized in the brain and is associated with disorders involving the nervous system. The metabolite dopamine is excreted by the kidney as HVA. The catecholamine is usually measured together with metanephrine, normetanephrine, and vanillylmandelic acid (VAM) to help differentiate among the suspected diagnoses.

Indications

■ Diagnose suspected neuroblastoma or ganglioneuroma, as indicated by elevated levels
■ Diagnose benign pheochromocytoma, as indicated by normal HVA levels with elevated VMA levels
■ Diagnose malignant pheochromocytoma, as indicated by elevated HVA and VMA levels

Reference Values

		SI Units
Children		
1–2 yr	0–25 mg/24 h	1–126 μmol/mg
2–10 yr	0.5–10 mg/24 h	3–55 μmol/mg
10–15 yr	0.5–12 mg/24 h	3–66 μmol/mg
Adult	<8 mg/24 h	1–14 μmol/mg

Abnormal Values

- Elevated HVA levels
    Pheochromocytoma
    Ganglioneuroblastoma
    Neuroblastoma

Interfering Factors

- Results are invalid if specimen is not collected properly and not refrigerated throughout the collection.
- Excessive exercise and emotional stress during the collection period will alter levels.
- Certain drugs can falsely elevate or decrease levels: aminosalicylic acid, disulfiram, levodopa, methocarbamol, reserpine, MAO inhibitors.
- Menstrual blood in specimen can interfere with test results.

Nursing Implications

Assessment

- Obtain a history of known or suspected brain tumor, medication regimen, and laboratory test results.
- Ensure that the client has withheld aspirin for 48 hours and levodopa for 2 weeks before the test.

Possible Nursing Diagnoses

Communication, impaired, verbal, related to altered brain function

Physical mobility, impaired, related to nerve transmission impairment

Anxiety related to perceived threat to fetal health

Grieving, anticipatory, related to perceived potential outcome

Implementation

- Obtain a clean 3-liter container or a 24-hour urine bag or bottle to which preservative has been added according to laboratory policy. Refrigerate the specimen during the collection time.
- Begin the test between 6 and 8 A.M. if possible. Collect first voiding and discard. Record the time the specimen was discarded as the beginning of the 24-hour test; document quantity of urine output during collection period, including urine at end of 24-hour period.
- The next morning, ask the client to void at the same time the collection was started and add this last voiding to the container.
- If an indwelling catheter is in place, keep drainage bag on ice, or empty the urine into a large refrigerated container with the preservative periodically during the 24 hours. Monitor that continued drainage is ensured and conclude the test the next morning at the same hour the collection was begun.
- At the conclusion of the test ensure that label is properly completed and transport specimen to the laboratory immediately.

Evaluation

- Compare quantity of urine in specimen container with urinary output record during collection time to ensure that all urine has been included.
- Note results in relation to vanillylmandelic acid (VMA) and metanephrine tests, if performed.

Client/Caregiver Teaching

Pretest

- Tell the client to avoid excessive physical exercise or stressful events before or during the specimen-collection period.
- Advise female clients to postpone urine collection if menstruating.
- Inform the client that all urine for a 24-hour period must be saved and monitor all urine output in a chart. Instruct the client to avoid voiding in pan with defecation and to keep toilet tissue out of pan to prevent contamination of the specimen.

Posttest

- Tell the client to resume medications and activity withheld before the test, as ordered.

Human Chorionic Gonadotropin (hCG)

Classification: Chemistry

Type of Test: Serum

Human chorionic gonadotropin (hCG) is a hormone secreted by the placenta, beginning 8 to 10 days after conception, and is believed to coincide with implantation of the fertilized ovum. This level peaks at 8 to 12 weeks' gestation, then falls to less than 10 percent of the first trimester levels by the end of the pregnancy. By week 2 postpartum, levels are undetectable.

Indications

- Confirm pregnancy or threatened or incomplete abortion
- Determine adequacy of hormonal levels to maintain pregnancy
- Diagnose suspected hCG-producing tumors, such as choriocarcinoma or hydatiform moles
- Monitor ovulation induction treatment

Reference Values

Nonpregnant women	<3 mIU/mL
Pregnant women	
8–10 d	5–40 mIU/mL
1 mo	100 mIU/mL
2 mo	100,000 mIU/mL
4–9 mo	50,000 mIU/mL

Abnormal Values

- Elevated levels
  Pregnancy
  Hydatiform mole
  Choriocarcinoma
  Testicular epithelioma
  Carcinoma of liver, stomach, pancreas, or breast

Multiple myeloma
Malignant melanoma
■ Decreased levels
Incomplete abortion
Threatened abortion
Intrauterine fetal demise

Interfering Factors

■ Incorrect performance of test, excessive LH production by the pituitary gland, or absence of gonadal hormones in menopausal women may cause false-positive results.
■ Medications, such as anticonvulsants, hypnotics, tranquilizers, and antiparkinsonian agents may cause false-positive results.
■ Performance of test too early in pregnancy may cause false-negative results.

Nursing Implications

Assessment

■ Obtain a gynecological history, including date of last menstrual period, and results of tests and procedures performed. Specimen should not be drawn until 5 days after first missed period.
■ Ask the client if she is taking any medications that could interfere with the results.

Possible Nursing Diagnoses

Anxiety related to threat to health status or to health of fetus
Grieving, anticipatory, related to perceived potential loss
Coping, ineffective, individual, risk for, related to fear of fetal demise

Implementation

■ Put on gloves. Using aseptic technique, perform a venipuncture and collect 10 mL of blood in a red-top tube.
■ Handle sample gently to avoid hemolysis. Send the sample to the laboratory for analysis promptly.

Evaluation

■ Note results in relation to client's symptoms and other related tests.

Client/Caregiver Teaching

Posttest

- If results are positive, refer the client to health care provider for follow-up.

▲▲▲▲▲▲▲▲▲▲▲▲▲▲▲▲▲▲▲▲▲▲▲

Human Chorionic Gonadotropin (hCG), Pregnancy Test

Classification: Urinalysis

Type of Test: Urine (timed or random)

Human chorionic gonadotropin (hCG), a glycoprotein hormone, is produced only by the developing placenta, and its presence in urine has been used for decades to detect pregnancy. HCG is secreted at increasingly higher levels during the first 2 months of pregnancy, declining during the third and fourth months, and then remaining relatively stable until term. Levels return to normal within 1 to 2 weeks of termination of pregnancy. With the newer testing methods available, hCG can be detected in urine or serum within 8 to 10 days after conception or during the 21st to 23rd day of the menstrual cycle. The pregnancy test can be performed 2 days after a missed menstrual period for a period of up to 3 weeks.

Indications

- Confirm pregnancy
- Diagnose suspected hydatidiform mole, choriocarcinoma or testicular tumor, nonendocrine tumor that produces hCG ectopically, as indicated by elevated levels
- Diagnose threatened abortion, incomplete abortion, or fetal demise, as indicated by decreased levels
- Monitor treatment effectiveness for cancers associated with ectopic hCG production, as indicated by decreased levels

Reference Values

Random	Negative if not pregnant
24-h	
Adult male	Not measurable
Nonpregnant female	Not measurable
Pregnant female	
1st trimester	≤500,000 IU/24 h
2nd trimester	10,000–25,000 IU/24 h
3rd trimester	5,000–15,000 IU/24 h

Abnormal Values

- Elevated levels
    Pregnancy
    Hydatidiform mole
    Choriocarcinoma
    Multiple pregnancy
    Erythroblastosis fetalis
    Testicular epithelioma
- Decreased levels
    Threatened abortion
    Ectopic pregnancy
    Nonpregnancy
    Dead fetus
    Incomplete abortion

Note: Measurable levels in men and nonpregnant women are indicative of cancer of the GI tract, liver, or pancreas; melanoma; multiple myeloma; or tumor of the ovary or testicle.

Interfering Factors

- Contamination of the specimen with tap water or soap, blood in the specimen can produce false-positive results.
- False negative results can occur if test is performed less than 5 days after the missed period.
- Radionuclide scan within 1 week may invalidate the results.
- Failure to collect and preserve all urine during 24-hour test period will cause inaccurate results.
- Drugs that can falsely elevate results include anticonvulsants, hypnotics, phenothiazines, and antiparkinsonism agents.
- Phenothiazines can also produce false-negative results.

Nursing Implications

Assessment

- Obtain a history of menstrual cycle, date of last menstrual period, past pregnancies and complications.

- Assess a thorough medication history and restrict appropriate medications, as ordered.

Possible Nursing Diagnoses

Anxiety related to threat to health status or to health of fetus

Grieving, anticipatory, related to perceived potential loss

Coping, ineffective, individual, risk for, related to fear of fetal demise

Adjustment, impaired, risk for, related to need for lifestyle changes

Implementation

- *Random urine:* Obtain a clean plastic container without preservative. Collect first voiding specimen (60 mL) if possible; a random specimen is adequate for some laboratory methods.
- *24-hour urine:* Obtain a clean 3-liter container with preservative. Arrange for refrigeration during collection. Begin the test between 6 and 8 A.M. if possible; collect first voiding and discard. Record the time specimen was discarded as the beginning of the 24-hour test. The next morning, request the client to void at the same time the collection was started and add this last voiding to the container.
- At the conclusion of the test ensure that the specimen is labeled properly and transport specimen to the laboratory immediately; include the first day of last menstrual period on lab slip.

Evaluation

- Note test results in relation to serum levels, if performed.

Client/Caregiver Teaching

Pretest

- Tell the client to withhold medications that can interfere with test results before the test.
- Inform the client that she can use the commercially available kit and to carefully follow the instructions that come with the kit. If test is done at home and the results are positive, advise the client to contact the physician.
- If a 24-hour urine study is being performed, inform the client that all urine for a 24-hour period must be saved and output noted in a chart; instruct client to avoid voiding in pan with defecation and to keep toilet tissue out of pan to prevent contamination of the specimen.

Posttest

■ Advise the client to resume medications and activity withheld before the test, as ordered.

▲▲▲▲▲▲▲▲▲▲▲▲▲▲▲▲▲▲▲▲

Human Leukocyte Antigen and Typing (HLA, Tissue Typing)

Classification: Immunology/Hematology

Type of Test: Serum

This test detects human leukocyte antigens (HLAs) on the surface membranes of leukocytes, platelets, and tissue cells. Sometimes described as "white cell antigens," HLAs consist of a glycoprotein chain and a globulin chain. Antigens are classified into five series, designated A, B, C, D, and DR (D-related), each series containing 10 to 20 distinct antigens. A, B, C, and D antigens characterize the membranes of virtually all cells except mature red blood cells; DR antigens seem to only reside on B lymphocytes and macrophages. Some antigens have been identified with specific diseases, although a common use of this test is to predict compatibility of donor-recipient tissue and organ transplantation.

Indications

■ Determine donor-recipient compatibility for transplantation (bone, marrow, kidney), especially when they are blood relatives

■ Determine compatibility of donor platelets in individuals who will receive multiple transfusions over a long period of time

■ Support for diagnosing HLA-associated diseases, especially when signs and symptoms are inconclusive

■ Determine biological parentage by comparing HLA phenotypes

Reference Values

HLA combinations vary according to certain races and populations. The most common B antigens in American whites are B7, B8, and B12. In American blacks, the B series are Bw17, Bw35, and a specificity characterized as 1AG. This is in contrast to African blacks, whose B antigens are B7, Bw17, and 1AG. Similar variations among the A antigens also have been found among various races and populations

Abnormal Values

Disease	Associated Antigen
Ankylosing spondylitis	B27
Reiter's syndrome	B27
Diabetes mellitus (juvenile or insulin-dependent)	Bw15, B8
Multiple sclerosis	A3, B7, B18
Acute anterior uveitis	B27
Grave's disease	B8
Juvenile rheumatoid arthritis	B27
Celiac disease	B8
Psoriasis vulgaris	B13, Bw17
Myasthenia gravis	B8
Dermatitis herpetiformis	B8
Autoimmune chronic active hepatitis	B8

Interfering Factors

- Delay in sending sample to laboratory could cause lymphocytes to die and a new sample will be required.

Nursing Implications

Assessment

- Obtain a history of purpose for test and known or suspected diseases associated with HLA.

Possible Nursing Diagnoses

Physical mobility, impaired, related to neuromuscular impairment
Pain related to tissue inflammation
Anxiety related to threat to health status or to health of fetus

Implementation

- Put on gloves. Using aseptic technique, perform a venipuncture and collect 7 mL of blood in a green-top tube. If testing is done for tissue compatibility, fill a red-top tube with the recipient blood and 2 green-top tubes with donor blood.
- Handle the sample gently to avoid hemolysis and transport to the laboratory immediately.

Evaluation

- Note results in relation to other tests performed and the client's symptoms.

Client/Caregiver Teaching

Posttest

- Inform client of genetic counseling if results indicate possibility for familial tendency to diseases.
- If appropriate, advise client that testing for biologic parentage exclusion is not allowed as evidence in all jurisdictions.

Human Placental Lactogen (HPL), Serum

Classification: Chemistry

Type of Test: Plasma or serum

Also known as human chorionic somatotropin (HCS), HPL is produced by the placenta and causes decreased maternal sensitivity to insulin and utilization of glucose, thus increasing the glucose available to the fetus. It also promotes release of maternal free fatty acids for utilization by the fetus. HPL also is thought to stimulate growth hormone in protein deposition, promote breast growth and preparation for lactation, and maintain the pregnancy by altering the endometrium.

Indications

- Detect placental insufficiency as evidenced by low HPL levels in relation to gestational age

- Support diagnosis of intrauterine growth retardation due to placental insufficiency, as indicated by HPL levels less than 4 g/mL, especially when blood estrogen levels are low
- Predict outcome in threatened abortion, as indicated by lower than expected levels for the stage of pregnancy
- Support diagnosis of hydatidiform mole and choriocarcinoma, as indicated by decreased levels
- Support diagnosis of cancers associated with elevated levels, for example, nonendocrine tumors that secrete ectopic HPL
- Monitor treatment effectiveness for cancers associated with ectopic HPL production, as indicated by decreasing levels

Reference Values

Men	$<0.5\ \mu g/mL$
Women	
Nonpregnant	$<0.5\ \mu g/mL$
Pregnant	
5–27 w	$<4.6\ \mu g/mL$
28–31 w	$2.4–6.1\ \mu g/mL$
32–35 w	$3.7–7.7\ \mu g/mL$
36 w–term	$5.0–8.6\ \mu g/mL$
Diabetic at term	$10–12\ \mu g/mL$

Abnormal Values

- Elevated levels
    - Diabetic mothers
    - Multiple pregnancy
    - Rh isoimmunization
    - Nonendocrine tumors that secrete ectopic HPL
- Decreased levels
    - Intrauterine fetal growth retardation
    - Pregnancy-induced hypertension (toxemia of pregnancy)
    - Impending abortion
    - Hydatidiform mole
    - Choriocarcinoma

Interfering Factors

- During pregnancy, HPL levels vary greatly with the individual, as well as on a day-to-day basis, and levels must be compared to gestational age of the fetus.
- Hemolysis of the blood sample may interfere with test results.

Nursing Implications

Assessment

- Obtain reproductive history, including last date of menstrual period and estimated date of delivery. Also determine if the client has diabetes or symptoms of pregnancy-induced hypertension.

Possible Nursing Diagnoses

Anxiety related to threat to health status or to health of fetus

Grieving, anticipatory, related to perceived potential loss

Coping, ineffective, individual, risk for, related to fear of fetal demise

Implementation

- Put on gloves. Using aseptic technique, perform a venipuncture and collect 7 mL of blood in a red-top tube.
- Handle the sample gently to avoid hemolysis and send promptly to the laboratory.

Evaluation

- Note test results in relation to other tests performed and the client's symptoms.

Client/Caregiver Teaching

Pretest

- Inform the client that no special preparation for the test is required.

Posttest

- Inform pregnant client that several tests may be necessary throughout the pregnancy.

Hydroxybutyrate Dehydrogenase (HBDH), Alpha-Hydroxybutyric Dehydrogenase (α-HBD)

Classification: Chemistry

Type of Test: Serum

Alpha-hydroxybutyrate dehydrogenase (α-HBD, HBD) is an enzyme found in the brain, heart muscle, kidney and red blood cells. It is similar to two isoenzymes of lactic dehydrogenase (LDH): LDH_1 and LDH_2. The α-HBD test, however, is cheaper and easier to perform than LDH isoenzyme electrophoresis. Moreover, HBD levels remain elevated for 18 days following acute myocardial infarction, long after the other cardiac enzymes return to normal levels.

Indications

- Diagnose suspected "silent" myocardial infarction or otherwise atypical myocardial infarction in which the client delayed seeking care
- Support for diagnosis of other disorders associated with elevated HBD levels (see Abnormal Values)
- Differentiate between cardiac and hepatic cellular damage (LD:HBD ratio commonly used)

Reference Values

- 140–350 U/mL (140–350 kU/L, SI units)

Abnormal Values

- Increased levels
  Post–myocardial infarction (HBD levels peak 72 hours after onset of chest pain and remain elevated for about 2 weeks)
  Anemia (hemolytic or megaloblastic)
  Acute hepatocellular damage
  Muscular dystrophy

Acute hepatitis
Leukemia
Lymphoma
Malignant melanoma
Nephrotic syndrome

Interfering Factors

- False-negative results can occur if specimen is frozen, since enzyme activity is lost.
- Traumatic venipuncture or hemolysis causes false-positive results.
- Surgery or cardioversion can elevate levels.
- Failure to draw the sample on schedule, thereby missing peak levels, can interfere with results.

Nursing Implications

Assessment

- Obtain a history of known or suspected myocardial infarction and current medications and any results of cardiac enzyme laboratory tests.

Possible Nursing Diagnoses

Pain related to tissue ischemia
Cardiac output, decreased, related to decreased myocardial contractility
Anxiety related to perceived threat to health status

Implementation

- Put on gloves. Using aseptic technique, perform a venipuncture and collect 7 mL of blood in a red-top tube.
- Handle sample gently to avoid hemolysis. Ensure that specimen is properly labeled and transport to the laboratory immediately.

Evaluation

- Compare results with tests for cardiac enzymes and clinical symptoms.

Client/Caregiver Teaching

Pretest

- Inform the client that fasting is not required for this test.

Posttest

- If myocardial infarction is suspected, inform the client that the test will be repeated on subsequent mornings to monitor progress.

17-Hydroxycorticosteroids (17-OHCS)

Classification: Chemistry

Type of Test: Urine (timed)

When adrenocortical hypofunctioning or hyperfunctioning is suspected, hydroxycorticosteroids (17-OHCS), a metabolite of glucocorticoids may be measured in urine as part of the diagnostic process. Because 80 percent of urinary 17-OHCS are metabolites of cortisol, those disorders that are associated with elevated cortisol levels also are associated with elevated 17-OHCS. Diurnal secretion of cortisol metabolites requires that a 24-hour urine collection be done to ensure accurate results.

Indications

- Diagnose adrenal cortical hypofunctioning or hyperfunctioning

Reference Values

		SI Units
Children	0.5–4.5 mg/24 h	1.4–12.4 μmol/24 h
Men	4.5–12 mg/24 h	12.4–33.1 μmol/24 h
Women	2.5–10 mg/24 h	6.9–27.6 μmol/24 h

Values in children are age-related: the younger the child, the less secreted.

Abnormal Values

- Elevated levels
    Cushing's syndrome
    Adrenal carcinoma or adenoma
    Pituitary tumor
    Insomnia
    Obesity
    Pregnancy
    Hypertension
    Stress
    Certain drugs: acetazolamide, ascorbic acid, cephalothin, cefoxitin, chloral hydrate, chlordiazepoxide, chlorpromazine, colchicine, cortisones, tryptamine, hydroxyzine, iodides, mandelamine, meprobamate, methenamine, methyprylon, paraldehyde, quinine, quinidine, digoxin, and spironolactone
- Decreased levels
    Addison's disease
    Hypopituitarism
    Congenital adrenal hyperplasia
    Hypothyroidism
    Certain drugs: apresoline, corticosteroids, dextropropoxyphene, estrogens, hydralazine, nalidixic acid, meperidine, morphine, oral contraceptives, pentazocine, phenergan, phenothiazines, phenytoin, reserpine, salicylates, and thiazides

Interfering Factors

- Acute illness can cause increases in 17-OHCS urinary levels.
- Improper collection and storage of all urine during 24-hour test period will interfere with results.
- Failure to follow drug restrictions can elevate or decrease test results (see Abnormal Values).
- Ingestion of products containing licorice root can increase levels.

Nursing Implications

Assessment

- Obtain a history of known or suspected adrenal dysfunction, medication regimen, and results of other laboratory tests.
- Ensure that all interfering medications have been discontinued 24 hours before urine collection, as ordered, and that

excessive physical exercise and stress have been avoided before the testing period.

Possible Nursing Diagnoses

Body image disturbance related to change in structure/ appearance

Fatigue related to decreased metabolic energy production and altered body chemistry

Anxiety related to perceived threat to health status

Fluid volume excess related to increased cortisone levels

Implementation

- Obtain a clean 3-liter container with preservative according to laboratory procedure and maintain refrigeration of specimen during collection.
- Begin the test between 6 and 8 A.M. if possible; collect first voiding and discard. Record the time specimen was discarded as the beginning of the 24-hour test; document quantity of urine output during collection period, including urine at end of 24-hour period.
- The next morning, ask the client to void at the same time the collection was started and add this last voiding to the container.
- If an indwelling catheter is in place, keep drainage bag on ice or empty the urine into a large refrigerated container periodically during the 24 hours; monitor that continued drainage is ensured and conclude the test the next morning at the same hour the collection was begun.
- At the conclusion of the test ensure that label is properly completed and transport specimen to the laboratory immediately.

Evaluation

- Note results in relation to other urinary and blood tests for cortisol levels.

Client/Caregiver Teaching

Pretest

- Tell the client to withhold drugs that can interfere with test results, if ordered.
- Inform the client that all urine for a 24-hour period must be saved and instruct client to avoid voiding in pan with defecation and to keep toilet tissue out of pan to prevent contamination of the specimen.

- Tell the client to avoid excessive physical exercise and stress during the testing period.

Posttest

- Tell the client to resume medications and activity withheld before the test, as ordered.
- Inform the client and caregiver of adrenal dysfunction's signs and symptoms and tell the client to report occurrence to the physician.

5-Hydroxyindoleacetic Acid (5-HIAA)

Classification: Chemistry

Type of Test: Urine (timed)

5-Hydroxyindoleacetic acid (5-HIAA) levels reflect serotonin plasma concentrations. Serotonin, a powerful vasopressor, is produced by argentaffin cells located in intestines. About 5 percent of serotonin is converted to 5-HIAA, which is secreted in the urine. This test measures 5-HIAA levels and is most accurate when used with a 24-hour urine specimen.

Indications

- Detect early, small, or intermittently secreting carcinoid tumors

Reference Values

- 1–10 mg/24 h (5.2–52 μmol/24 h, SI units)

Abnormal Values

- Elevated levels
    Carcinoid tumors (argentaffinomas) of the intestine or appendix
    Celiac sprue
    Diarrhea
    Tropical sprue

Certain drugs: acetaminophen, atenolol, diazepam, fluorouracil, glycerol guaiacolate, melphalan, methenasin carbamate, naproxen, oxprenolol, phenacetin, pindolol, and reserpine

- Decreased levels

Carcinoid tumors of the rectal area

Phenylketonuria

Small-intestine resection diarrhea

Benign carcinoid tumors

Certain drugs: corticotropin, ethanol, isoniazid, levodopa, methyldopa, monoamine oxidase (MAO) inhibitors, tricyclic antidepressants

Note: Certain drugs can raise or lower levels: acetaminophen, guaifenesin, mephenesin, methenamine compounds, methocarbamol, phenothiazines, and salicylates.

Interfering Factors

- Foods containing serotonin, such as bananas, pineapples, red plums, avocados, eggplant, tomatoes, and walnuts, can falsely elevate levels if ingested within 4 days of specimen collection.
- Severe GI disturbance or diarrhea can interfere with test results.
- Failure to collect all urine and store specimen properly during 24-hour test period will interfere with results.
- Failure to follow drug restrictions can alter test results.

Nursing Implications

Assessment

- Obtain a history of internal disorders, medication regimen, and laboratory test results.
- Ensure restriction of medications 4 days before test.
- Ensure that the client has followed restrictive diet in items that contain serotonin for 5 days before the test (see Abnormal Values and Interfering Factors).

Possible Nursing Diagnoses

Diarrhea related to malabsorption syndrome

Fluid volume deficit, risk for, related to active loss

Nutrition, altered, less than body requirements, related to inability to digest food and absorb nutrients

Implementation

- Obtain a clean 3-liter container, with preservative and follow laboratory directions for any special care of the specimen during collection such as refrigeration.
- Begin the test between 6 and 8 A.M. if possible; collect first voiding and discard. Record the time that specimen was discarded as the beginning of the 24-hour test; document quantity of urine output during collection period, including urine at end of 24-hour period.
- The next morning, ask the client to void at the same time the collection was started and add this last voiding to the container.
- If an indwelling catheter is in place, place drainage bag on ice, or empty the urine into a large refrigerated container every hour during the 24 hours; monitor that continued drainage is ensured and conclude the test the next morning at the same hour the collection was begun.
- At the conclusion of the test ensure that label is properly completed and transport specimen to the laboratory immediately.

Evaluation

- Compare quantity of urine in specimen container with urinary output record during collection time to ensure that all urine has been included.
- Note results in relation to other tests and the client's symptoms.

Client/Caregiver Teaching

Pretest

- Inform the client not to eat foods high in serotonin and to withhold drugs that can interfere with test results, if ordered.
- Inform the client that all urine for a 24-hour period must be saved; instruct client to avoid voiding in pan with defecation and to keep toilet tissue out of pan to prevent contamination of the specimen.

Posttest

- Tell the client to resume medications and diet withheld before the test.

5-Hydroxyproline

Classification: Chemistry

Type of Test: Urine (timed)

Quantitative analysis of urine levels of hydroxyproline, an amino acid found in collagen, can help diagnose disorders that increase bone resorption and those associated with increased collagen turnover. This protein would also be increased during periods of rapid growth in children.

Indications

- Detect disorders associated with increased bone resorption
- Monitor treatment of disorders characterized by bone resorption, primarily Paget's disease

Reference Values

		SI Units
24-h test		
Adults	10–50 mg/24 h	0.08–0.38 mmol/24 h
Children		
1–10 yr	20–99 mg/24 h	0.15–0.75 mmol/24 h
11–14 yr	63–180 mg/24 h	0.48–1.37 mmol/24 h
2-h test		
Men	0.4–5 mg/2 h	
Women	0.4–2.9 mg/2 h	

Abnormal Values

- Elevated levels
    Bone tumor
    Scleroderma
    Rheumatoid arthritis
    Albright's syndrome
    Klinefelter's syndrome
    Marfan's syndrome
    Multiple myeloma
    Osteomalacia

Osteomyelitis
Paget's disease of the bone
Rickets
Certain drugs: growth hormone, parathyroid hormone, phenobarbital, and sulfonylureas
- Decreased levels
Hypoparathyroidism
Hypopituitarism
Hypothyroidism
Malnutrition
Muscular dystrophy
Certain drugs: antineoplastic agents, ascorbic acid, calcitonin, calcium gluconate, corticosteroids, glucocorticoids, estradiol, mithramycin, and propranolol

Interfering Factors

- Failure to follow appropriate dietary restrictions can produce false-positives.
- Psoriasis or burns can promote collagen turnover and can elevate urine levels.
- Failure to collect all urine and store specimen properly during 2- or 24-hour test period will interfere with results.
- Failure to follow drug restrictions can falsely elevate or decrease test results.

Nursing Implications

Assessment

- Obtain a history of known or suspected bone and endocrine disorders, laboratory test results.
- Ensure that medications that can interfere with the results have been withheld.
- Ensure that the client has had no gelatin-containing foods and meat, fish, or poultry for 48 hours before urine collection for 24-hour collection and that no food is allowed overnight for a 2-hour collection.

Possible Nursing Diagnoses

Body image disturbance related to change in structure/appearance
Physical mobility, impaired, related to neuromuscular impairment
Injury, risk for fractures, related to degenerative process

Implementation

- Obtain a clean 3-liter container with or without preservative according to laboratory directions and follow special care of the specimen during collection if any.
- Begin the test between 6 and 8 A.M. if possible; collect first voiding and discard. Record the time specimen was discarded as the beginning of the 24-hour test; document quantity of urine output during collection period, including urine at end of 24-hour period. Follow same procedure for 2-hour test following an overnight fast.
- The next morning, ask the client to void at the same time the collection was started and add this last voiding to the container.
- If an indwelling catheter is in place, replace tubing and container system and keep drainage bag on ice, and empty the urine into a large container periodically during the 24-hours; monitor that continued drainage is ensured and conclude the test the next morning at the same hour the collection was begun; collect urine for 2-hour period of time for the 2-hour test.
- At the conclusion of the test ensure that label is properly completed, including client's age and gender; transport specimen to the laboratory immediately.

Evaluation

- Compare quantity of urine in specimen container with urinary output record during collection time to ensure that all the urine has been collected.
- Note results of alkaline phosphatase indicating formation of bone rather than loss.

Client/Caregiver Teaching

Pretest

- Tell the client not to eat any gelatin-containing foods, meat, fish, or poultry for 48 hours before urine collection for 24-hour collection.
- In addition, tell the client performing the 2-hour test to fast overnight.
- Inform the client that all urine for a 24-hour period must be saved; instruct client to avoid voiding in pan with defecation and to keep toilet tissue out of pan to prevent contamination of the specimen.

Posttest

- Tell the client to resume medications and food withheld before the test.

Hysteroscopy

Classification: Endoscopy

Type of Test: Direct visualization

For this test a hysteroscope is inserted into the uterus through the vagina to view anatomy and detect pathology possibly missed during hysterosalpingography or curettage.

Indications

- Detect and remove IUD or foreign body
- Diagnose and remove fibroids or adhesions
- Confirm possible fertility problems
- Evaluate pathology missed with hysterosalpingography
- Perform endocervical biopsy

Reference Values

- Normal uterine cavity

Abnormal Values

- Asherman's syndrome
- Infertility
- Intrauterine adhesions or fibroids

NURSING ALERT

- This procedure is contraindicated if client has a vaginal discharge, pelvic inflammatory disease, or an inflamed cervix.

Nursing Implications

Assessment

- Obtain a history of the reproductive system, current symptoms, and results of diagnostic tests.
- Ensure that the test is scheduled before ovulation or when menstrual period is completed.

Possible Nursing Diagnoses

Infection, risk for, related to invasive procedure
Self-esteem disturbance, situation low, risk for, related to infertility

Implementation

- Place the client in the lithotomy position and drape for privacy.
- The physician inserts a hysteroscope through the vagina into the uterus after use of a speculum. Carbon dioxide or Hyskon is instilled to distend the uterine cavity to promote easy visualization. Uterine cavity is observed for abnormalities and tissue samples are taken as required.

Evaluation

- Note test results in relation to other tests performed and the client's symptoms.
- Monitor for side effects of carbon dioxide: shoulder pain, nausea, diaphoresis, and bleeding.
- Monitor for side effects of Hyskon: anaphylaxis, pulmonary edema, and coagulation disorders.

Client/Caregiver Teaching

Pretest

- Inform the client of the purpose of the test, and procedure involved. Tell the client that it is performed by a physician and takes 10 minutes to complete.
- Tell the client to schedule the test before ovulation or when menstrual period is completed.

Posttest

- Tell the client to report any acute or persistent bleeding, fever, abdominal pain, or other signs of infection or peritonitis.

Immune Complex Assay, Serum

Classification: Immunology
Type of Test: Blood

Immune complexes are combinations of antigen and antibody which are capable of activating the complement cascade. While the activated agent is directed against the immune complex, tissues which are "innocent bystanders" may also be severely damaged, especially when immune complexes are produced too rapidly for adequate clearance by the body. Immune complexes are commonly present in autoimmune disorders and also are found in immune hypersensitivities that do not involve autoimmunity.

Indications

- Diagnose immune disorders
- Monitor effects of therapy for various immune disorders
- Detect serum sickness or allergic reactions to drugs as indicated by the presence of immune complexes

Reference Values

- Negative

Abnormal Values

- Positive value
  Hodgkin's disease
  Leukemia
  Rheumatic fever
  Rheumatoid arthritis
  Biliary cirrhosis
  Malaria
  Pulmonary fibrosis
  Sjögren's syndrome
  Systemic lupus erythematosus (SLE)
  Hansen's disease (leprosy)
  Malignant melanoma

Endocarditis
Glomerulonephritis
Dengue fever
Polymyositis

Interfering Factors

- Rough handling of the sample and failure to transport the sample promptly to the laboratory may cause deterioration of any immune complexes present.
- Recent heparin therapy may affect test results. Inform the laboratory of such therapy.

Nursing Implications

Assessment

- Obtain history of infections and exposure to infectious diseases, signs and symptoms, laboratory tests and results.

Possible Nursing Diagnoses

Anxiety related to perceived threat to health status
Pain related to inflammatory process of connective tissues
Fatigue related to increased energy requirements and altered body chemistry
Physical mobility, impaired, related to musculoskeletal impairment

Implementation

- Put on gloves. Using aseptic technique, perform venipuncture and obtain 7 mL of blood in a red-topped tube.
- Handle the specimen gently to avoid hemolysis and send immediately to the laboratory.

Evaluation

- Note test results in relation to other tests performed and the client's symptoms.

Client/Caregiver Teaching

Pretest

- Inform the client that no special preparation is required before this test if heparin was recently administered.

Posttest

- Inform client that tests for specific immune complexes may be performed if this test is positive. (Specifically, the Raji cell C_{14}.)

Immunoglobulin Electrophoresis, Serum

Classification: Chemistry

Type of Test: Serum

Immunoglobulin electrophoresis provides a detailed separation of the individual immunoglobulin (IgG, IgA, IgD, IgM, and IgE) to identify the presence of monoclonal protein and its type. Each immunoglobulin can be identified by a band with a specific curve, position, and color noted on the slide containing an aqua gel that is subjected to an electric current.

Indications

- Diagnose suspected immunoproliferative disorders such as multiple myeloma and Waldenström's macroglobulinemia
- Diagnose suspected immunodeficiency
- Screen for abnormal proteinemias to assist in diagnosis of disease
- Monitor effectiveness of chemotherapy or radiation therapy

Reference Values

Curves may be analyzed and interpreted by a pathologist if there are abnormal protein levels in the serum. Quantitative findings include these age-dependent values:

		SI Units
IgG	700–1500 mg/dL	7–15 g/L
IgA	140–400 mg/dL	1.4–4.0 g/L
IgM	35–375 mg/dL	0.35–3.75 g/L
IgD	0–8 mg/dL	0–0.80 g/L
IgE	4.2–592 IU/mL	10–1421 μg/L

Values are lower in children until age 10 years.

Abnormal Values

- Increased IgG
    Infections
    Hyperimmunization

IgG myeloma
Rheumatoid arthritis
Severe malnutrition
Hepatitis
Laennec's cirrhosis
Sarcoidosis
Tuberculosis (pulmonary)
- Decreased IgG
    Amyloidosis
    Agammaglobulinemia
    Chronic lymphocytic leukemia (CLL)
    IgA myeloma
    Nephrotic syndrome
- Increased IgA
    Cirrhosis
    IgA myeloma
    Hepatitis
    Laennec's cirrhosis
    Rheumatoid arthritis
    Systemic lupus erythematosus (SLE)
    Inflammatory bowel disease
    GI or hepatobiliary carcinoma
- Decreased IgA
    Agammaglobulinemia
    Ataxia-telangiectasia
    IgG myeloma
    Franklin's disease
    Macroglobulinemia
    Acute and chronic lymphocytic anemia
    Chronic myelocytic leukemia
    Nephrotic syndrome
    Use of certain drugs that decrease lymphocytes, such as
       chemotherapeutic agents and steroids
- Increased IgM
    Viral infections
    Malaria
    Brucellosis
    Macroglobulinemia
    Lymphosarcoma
    Hepatitis
    Biliary cirrhosis
    Rheumatoid arthritis
    SLE
- Decreased IgM
    Agammaglobulinemia
    Franklin's disease
    IgG and IgA myeloma
    CLL

Hepatoma
Amyloidosis
- Increased IgE
    Allergic reactions, including anaphylaxis, asthma, and hay
        fever
    Atopic skin disease
    Parasitic infections
    IgE myeloma
- Decreased IgE
    Agammaglobulinemia
- Increased IgD
    Chronic infections
    IgD myeloma
    Liver diseases
    Connective tissue disorders
- Decreased IgD
    Acquired and hereditary deficiency syndromes

Interfering Factors

- Certain drugs may falsely increase all immunoglobulin levels: anticoagulants, anticonvulsants, oral contraceptives, phenylbutazone, hydralazine, isoniazid (INH), procainamide, tetanus toxoid and antitoxin.
- Dextrans, phenytoin, and high doses of methylprednisolone may lower IgG and IgA levels.
- Chemotherapy and radiation treatments may alter the width of the bands and make interpretation difficult.

Nursing Implications

Assessment

- Obtain a history of known or suspected cancers and renal disease and the results of laboratory protein tests done.
- Assess whether the client received any vaccinations or immunizations within the last 6 months or any blood or blood components within the last 6 weeks.

Possible Nursing Diagnoses

Infection, risk for, related to immunosuppressed inflammatory response
Pain related to inflammatory process of connective tissues
Anxiety related to perceived threat to health status
Injury, risk for, related to immune response

Implementation

- Put on gloves. Using aseptic technique, perform a venipuncture and collect 7 to 10 mL of blood in a red-top tube.
- Note any vaccinations, immunizations, or blood received within the last 6 months on the lab slip.
- Handle sample gently to avoid hemolysis and send promptly to laboratory.

Evaluation

- Note test results in relation to other tests performed, in particular the urinary immunoelectrophoresis, and the client's symptoms.

Client/Caregiver Teaching

Pretest

- Inform the client that no special preparation is required for the test.
- Tell the client to withhold the medications that can interfere with the test results, as ordered.

Posttest

- Tell the client to resume medications withheld before the test, as ordered.

Immunoglobulin Electrophoresis, Urine

Classification: Chemistry

Type of Test: Urine (random)

Immunoglobulin electrophoresis is a qualitative technique that provides a detailed separation of individual immunoglobulins (IgG, IgA, IgM, IgD, and IgE) according to their electrical charges. It identifies even modest deficiencies of monoclonal protein and its type. Abnormalities are revealed on a printout by changes in the individual bands produced such as displacement, color, or absence of color.

Indications

- Diagnose protein abnormalities
- Identify cryoglobulinemia
- Diagnose Hodgkin's disease, multiple myeloma, and amyloidosis
- Assist in diagnosis of humoral immune deficiency
- Support diagnosis of renal failure

Reference Values

- Requires individual interpretation in the presence of abnormal urinary protein levels.

Abnormal Values

- Elevated levels
  Dysproteinemia
  Hodgkin's disease
  Renal failure
  Amyloidosis
  Multiple myeloma
  Acquired or hereditary humoral immune deficiencies

Interfering Factors

- Certain drugs may increase levels: anticoagulants, anticonvulsants, oral contraceptives, phenylbutazone, hydralazine, isoniazid (INH), procainamide, and tetanus toxoid and antitoxin.
- Chemotherapy and radiation treatments may alter the width of the bands and make interpretation difficult.
- Transfusions within 2 months of the test can alter results.

Nursing Implications

Assessment

- Obtain a history of known or suspected neoplastic or immunoproliferative diseases and the results of tests for protein.
- Assess whether any immunizations have been received within the last 6 months.

Possible Nursing Diagnoses

Infection, risk for, related to immunosuppressed inflammatory response

Pain related to inflammatory process of connective tissues

Anxiety related to perceived threat to health status

Injury, risk for, related to immune response

Implementation

- Obtain a sterile plastic urine container to collect a random specimen.
- Tell the client to collect a 50-mL urine specimen in the container.
- If an indwelling catheter is in place, obtain 50 mL from urinary drainage using a rubber stopper to ensure fresh urine (as opposed to obtaining specimen from urinary collection bag). Cleanse rubber stopper with alcohol and obtain specimen. Instill urine into collection container.
- Note any immunizations within the last 6 months on the lab slip. Transport specimen to the laboratory immediately.

Evaluation

- Note test results in relation to other tests performed, in particular serum protein and immunoglobulin electrophoresis.

Client/Caregiver Teaching

Pretest

- Inform the client that no special preparation is required for the test.
- Tell the client to withhold the medications that can interfere with the test results, as ordered.
- Teach the client how to collect the specimen, including the importance of not contaminating the specimen with fecal material.

Posttest

- Tell the client to resume medications withheld before the test, as ordered.

Immunoglobulin G, Subclassification

Classification: Chemistry

Type of Test: Serum

Immunoglobulin G (IgG) is one of the five classes of immunoglobulins that are serum antibodies produced by the plasma cells of the B lymphocytes. IgG produces antibodies against bacteria, viruses, and toxins. It activates the complement system, plays a major role in the secondary antibody response, and protects the newborn. Measuring the subclasses of IgG—IgG_1, IgG_2, IgG_3, IgG_4—is performed in clients with unexplained and recurrent ear infections, sinopulmonary diseases, and atopic allergy.

Indications

- Diagnose immunoglobulin deficiencies
- Evaluate children with frequent infections or sinopulmonary disease of unknown causes

Reference Values

Age	IgG_1	IgG_2	IgG_3	IgG_4
Cord	435–1084 mg/dL	143–453 mg/dL	27–146 mg/dL	1–47 mg/dL
1–7 d	381–937 mg/dL	117–382 mg/dL	21–115 mg/dL	1–44 mg/dL
8–14 d	327–790 mg/dL	92–310 mg/dL	16–85 mg/dL	1–40 mg/dL
3–4 w	218–496 mg/dL	40–167 mg/dL	4–23 mg/dL	1–33 mg/dL
2 mo	194–480 mg/dL	35–164 mg/dL	4–36 mg/dL	1–30 mg/dL
3 mo	167–447 mg/dL	28–157 mg/dL	4–52 mg/dL	1–24 mg/dL
4 mo	143–394 mg/dL	23–147 mg/dL	4–65 mg/dL	1–14 mg/dL
5 mo	158–392 mg/dL	24–132 mg/dL	6–68 mg/dL	1–13 mg/dL
6 mo	175–390 mg/dL	24–115 mg/dL	8–72 mg/dL	1–11 mg/dL
7 mo	190–388 mg/dL	25–100 mg/dL	10–75 mg/dL	1–10 mg/dL
8 mo	200–417 mg/dL	26–123 mg/dL	10–76 mg/dL	1–16 mg/dL
9 mo	211–450 mg/dL	26–149 mg/dL	10–77 mg/dL	1–22 mg/dL
10–12 mo	241–543 mg/dL	28–221 mg/dL	10–88 mg/dL	1–39 mg/dL
13–20 mo	281–692 mg/dL	30–343 mg/dL	10–88 mg/dL	1–68 mg/dL
21 mo–<3 yr	310–729 mg/dL	46–387 mg/dL	10–96 mg/dL	1–77 mg/dL
3 yr	348–773 mg/dL	72–441 mg/dL	10–105 mg/dL	1–87 mg/dL
4 yr	370–804 mg/dL	88–445 mg/dL	11–108 mg/dL	1–97 mg/dL
5 yr	375–875 mg/dL	94–468 mg/dL	12–111 mg/dL	1–106 mg/dL

Age	IgG$_1$	IgG$_2$	IgG$_3$	IgG$_4$
6 yr	380–866 mg/dL	100–481 mg/dL	14–115 mg/dL	1–115 mg/dL
7 yr	385–896 mg/dL	105–494 mg/dL	16–118 mg/dL	1–124 mg/dL
8 yr	390–927 mg/dL	111–507 mg/dL	18–122 mg/dL	1–133 mg/dL
9 yr	395–958 mg/dL	117–520 mg/dL	19–125 mg/dL	1–142 mg/dL
10 yr	400–989 mg/dL	123–534 mg/dL	21–129 mg/dL	1–151 mg/dL
11 yr	405–1020 mg/dL	128–547 mg/dL	23–132 mg/dL	1–160 mg/dL
12 yr	410–1051 mg/dL	134–560 mg/dL	25–136 mg/dL	1–169 mg/dL
13 yr	415–1081 mg/dL	140–573 mg/dL	27–139 mg/dL	1–178 mg/dL
14 yr	419–1102 mg/dL	145–582 mg/dL	28–141 mg/dL	1–184 mg/dL
≥15 yr	423–1112 mg/dL	149–586 mg/dL	29–142 mg/dL	1–187 mg/dL

Abnormal Values

- Increased IgG$_4$ levels
    Atopic allergy
- Decreased levels in all subclasses
    Hypogammaglobulinemia
    Ataxia-telangiectasia
    Wiskott-Aldrich syndrome
- Isolated or combined deficiency IgG$_2$, IgG$_3$, and IgG$_4$ (with normal IgG levels)
    Recurring sinopulmonary infections and otitis media from impaired antibody response to *Haemophilus influenzae*, type B, or *Streptococcus pneumoniae*
- Decreased IgG$_2$ and IgG$_4$ levels
    IgA deficiency

Nursing Implications

Assessment

- Obtain a history of infectious disorders, allergic reactions, and results of tests performed.

Possible Nursing Diagnoses

Infection, risk for, related to immunosuppressed inflammatory response
Anxiety related to perceived threat to health status
Injury, risk for, related to immune response

Implementation

- Put on gloves. Using aseptic technique, obtain a 3-mL blood sample in a red-top tube.
- Send to laboratory immediately or freeze sample at −4°F (−20°C).

Evaluation

■ Note test results in relation to total IgG, other tests performed, and the client's symptoms.

Client/Caregiver Teaching

Pretest

■ Inform the client that the test requires no special preparation.

Influenza A and B Titer

Classification: Serology
Type of Test: Blood

This test is done primarily for epidemiological surveys. A and B virus cause major epidemics every 2 to 4 years. B virus is sporadic and local, while A virus spreads rapidly to all areas.

Indications

■ Epidemiological screening tool

Reference Values

■ < fourfold increase in paired serum
■ <1:8 titer demonstrates previous exposure

Abnormal Values

■ *Positive titer:* influenza
■ *Negative titer:* bacterial infection

Interfering Factors

■ If a convalescent sample is not drawn 14 days after initial sample, the value of the acute sample is limited.

Nursing Implications

Assessment

- Obtain a history of exposure to influenza, current symptoms, and the results of other diagnostic tests.

Possible Nursing Diagnoses

Infection, risk for transmission

Implementation

- Put on gloves. Using aseptic technique, perform a venipuncture and collect 7 mL of blood in a red-top tube.
- Label specimen and send to the laboratory.
- Draw a convalescent sample 14 days later following the same procedure.

Evaluation

- Note results in relation to other studies performed and the client's symptoms.

Client/Caregiver Teaching

Posttest

- Instruct the client to return for a convalescent sample in 2 weeks.

Insulin

Classification: Chemistry
Type of Test: Serum

This test measures the rate of insulin secreted by the B cells of the islets of Langerhans in the pancreas. Insulin secretion is a response to elevated blood glucose and its overall effect is to promote glucose utilization and energy storage. A blood glucose level is usually obtained with the insulin determinators.

Indications

- Evaluate postprandial ("reactive") hypoglycemia of unknown etiology
- Diagnose early or developing noninsulin-dependent diabetes mellitus, as indicated by excessive production of insulin in relation to blood glucose levels (best demonstrated with glucose tolerance tests or 2-hour postprandial tests)
- Confirm functional hypoglycemia, as indicated by circulating insulin levels appropriate to changing blood glucose levels
- Evaluate fasting hypoglycemia of unknown etiology
- Diagnose insulinoma, as indicated by sustained high levels of insulin and absence of blood glucose–related variations
- Evaluate uncontrolled insulin-dependent diabetes mellitus
- Differentiate between insulin-resistant diabetes, in which insulin levels are high, and noninsulin-resistant diabetes, in which insulin levels are low
- Diagnose pheochromocytoma, as indicated by decreased levels

Reference Values

		SI Units
Fasting		
Infant/child	<13 μU/mL	<90 pmol/L
Adult	17 μU/mL	<118 pmol/L
After 75 g glucose		
30 min	20–112 μU/mL	139–778 pmol/L
1 h	29–88 μU/mL	201–611 pmol/L
2 h	22–79 μU/mL	153–549 pmol/L
3 h	4–62 μU/mL	28–431 pmol/L
Insulin:glucose ratio	<0.3:1	
Critical value	>30 μU/mL	

Abnormal Values

- Elevated levels
  Insulin- and proinsulin-secreting tumors (insulinomas)
  Reactive hypoglycemia in developing diabetes mellitus
  Excessive administration of insulin
  Cushing's syndrome
  Diabetes mellitus ($IDDM_1$)
  Pheochromocytoma
  Acromegaly
- Decreased levels
  B cell failure

Interfering Factors

- Administration of insulin or oral hypoglycemic agents within 8 hours of the test can lead to falsely elevated levels.
- Administration of pork or beef insulin can cause antibody formation and affect test results.
- Failure to follow dietary restrictions before the test can lead to falsely elevated levels.
- Therapy with drugs containing estrogen and progesterone may produce elevated levels.
- Hemodialysis destroys insulin and therefore affects test results.

> ### NURSING ALERT
>
> - Pretest fast can cause severe hypoglycemia in some clients.
> - IV glucose (50% solution) should be available for use if hypoglycemia occurs.

Nursing Implications

Assessment

- Obtain a history of familial diabetes, insulin or hypoglycemia therapy, and results of other diagnostic tests.
- Ensure client compliance with fasting 8 to 10 hours before the test.

Possible Nursing Diagnoses

Anxiety related to threat to health status
Adjustment, impaired, risk for, related to need for lifestyle changes or threat to self-concept
Body image disturbance related to change in structure/appearance

Implementation

- Put on gloves. Using aseptic technique, perform a venipuncture and obtain 7 mL of blood in red-top tubes. Pack the insulin specimens in ice.
- Handle the sample gently to avoid hemolysis and send to the laboratory promptly.

Evaluation

- Note and report decreased or increased levels and response to glucose intake in relation to diabetes type 1 or 2.
- Observe client for signs of hypoglycemia, which may occur in response to fasting.

Client/Caregiver Teaching

Pretest

- Tell the client to fast for 8 to 10 hours before the test and withhold medications that interfere with test results, if ordered.

Posttest

- Tell the client to resume food and any medications withheld before the test.
- Tell the client to report signs and symptoms of hypoglycemia (weakness, confusion, diaphoresis, rapid pulse) or hyperglycemia (thirst, polyuria, hunger, and lethargy).
- Instruct the client and caregiver on diabetes care if test results reveal noncompliance with treatment regimen.

Insulin Tolerance Test, ACTH Challenge Test, Growth Hormone Challenge Test

Classification: Chemistry

Type of Test: Blood

This test measures serum levels of growth hormone (GH) and adrenocorticotropic hormone (ACTH) after a loading dose of insulin. Serum levels of growth hormone are often undetectable in fasting insulin levels, but the insulin-induced hypoglycemia stimulates both GH and ACTH secretion.

Indications

- Aid in diagnosis of growth hormone or adrenocorticotropic hormone deficiency
- Diagnose pituitary dysfunction
- Aid in differential diagnosis of primary and secondary adrenal hypofunction

Reference Values

- 20 to 30 minutes after insulin administration, blood glucose levels should fall to less than 40 mg/dL (2 mmol/L). GH and ACTH should be stimulated to 10 to 20 ng/dL over baseline levels. Peak levels occur 60 to 90 minutes after insulin administration.

Abnormal Values

- Less than 10 ng/dL increase above baseline GH levels
  Growth hormone deficiency
- Less than 10 ng/dL increase above baseline in ACTH levels
  Adrenal insufficiency

Interfering Factors

- Failure to comply with food and activity restrictions affects results.
- Steroids, pituitary-based drugs, and progestogen can elevate GH levels.
- Amphetamines, estrogens, methamphetamines, ethanol, glucocorticoids, calcium gluconate, and spironolactone can depress ACTH.
- Rough handling of the samples can cause hemolysis and affect test results.

> **NURSING ALERT**
>
> - This procedure is not recommended for clients with cerebrovascular or cardiovascular disorders, low basal plasma cortisol levels, or seizure disorders.
> - In case of severe hypoglycemic insulin reaction during testing, keep concentrated glucose solution on hand.

Nursing Implications

Assessment

- Obtain a history of endocrine disorders, signs and symptoms, and results of other tests performed.
- Ensure compliance with fasting and restricted physical activity for 10 to 12 hours before the test. Ensure that the client remains in recumbent position 90 minutes before the test.
- Ensure medications that interfere with results have been withheld, as ordered.

Possible Nursing Diagnoses

Body image disturbance related to change in structure/appearance
Coping, ineffective, individual, related to [specify]
Anxiety related to threat to health status

Implementation

- Put on gloves. Using aseptic technique, insert an intermittent infusion catheter between 6 and 8 A.M. and collect three 5-mL blood samples for basal levels. Place the blood glucose sample in a gray-top tube and the GH and ACTH samples in green-top tubes.
- Administer an IV bolus of U-100 regular insulin (0.15 U/kg or as ordered) over 1 to 2 minutes. Draw additional blood samples 15, 30, 45, 60, 90, and 120 minutes after insulin administration. At each interval, collect three 5-mL samples; place one in a gray-top tube and two in green-top tubes.
- Label the tubes, specify collection time, and send them to the laboratory immediately. The sample should be handled gently to avoid hemolysis.

Evaluation

- Note results in relation to other tests performed and the client's symptoms.

Client/Caregiver Teaching

Pretest

- Tell the client to fast and restrict physical activity for 10 to 12 hours before the test.
- Tell the client to withhold medications that can interfere with test results, as ordered.
- Tell the client to remain in a recumbent position 90 minutes before the test.
- Inform the client that diaphoresis, hunger, increased heart rate, and anxiety can be experienced after insulin adminis-

tration. Inform the client that symptoms are transient, but that the testing will be discontinued if symptoms become too severe.

Posttest

- Tell the client to resume food, fluid, and medication intake and physical activity.

Insulin Antibody

Classification: Immunology

Type of Test: Blood

Insulin antibodies develop in response to the impurities in the animal insulins. These antibodies include immunoglobulin types IgG, IgM, and IgE. IgG antibodies neutralize the insulin, preventing glucose metabolism, while IgM antibodies may cause insulin resistance, and IgE may cause allergic effects. Presence of these antibodies may explain why the diabetic client's insulin requirements are increasing.

Indications

- Identify insulin resistance or insulin allergy
- Differentiate factitious hypoglycemia from chronic pancreatitis or insulinoma or from insulin abuse

Reference Values

- Less than 4 percent serum binding of beef (bovine) or pork (porcine)

Abnormal Values

- Increased values
  Insulinoma
  Non–insulin-dependent diabetes mellitus (NIDDM)
  Cushing's syndrome
  Obesity

Acromegaly
Liver disease
- Decreased values
Insulin-dependent diabetes mellitus (IDDM)
Hypopituitarism

Interfering Factors

- Certain drugs, such as oral contraceptives, thyroid hormones, levodopa, terbutaline, oral antidiabetic drugs, cortisone preparations, and epinephrine, can increase levels.
- Certain drugs, such as beta blockers, calcitonin, phenytoin, phenobarbital, calcium channel blockers, cimetidine, and loop and thiazide diuretics, can decrease levels.
- Radioactive scan within 7 days of test will alter test results.

Nursing Implications

Assessment

- Obtain a history of the endocrine disorder, signs and symptoms, and current treatment, including insulin use.

Possible Nursing Diagnoses

Anxiety related to threat to health status
Adjustment, impaired, risk for, related to need for lifestyle changes or threat to self-concept
Body image disturbance related to change in structure/appearance

Implementation

- Put on gloves. Using aseptic technique, perform venipuncture and obtain a 7-mL blood sample in a red-top tube.
- Handle sample gently to avoid hemolysis and transport to the laboratory promptly.

Evaluation

- Note test results in relation to client's symptoms and the client's insulin dosage.
- If insulin abuse is a possibility, a C-peptide test should be performed.

Client/Caregiver Teaching

Pretest

- Inform the client that no fasting is required.

Intrinsic Factor Antibody

Classification: Immunology

Type of Test: Blood

Intrinsic factor (IF) is produced by the parietal cells of the gastric mucosa and are required for the normal absorption of vitamin B_{12}. In some diseases, antibodies are produced that bind the cobalamin-intrinsic factor complex, prevent the complex from binding to ileum receptors, and prevent B_{12} absorption. Two types of antibodies exist, including type 1, the blocking antibody, and type 2, the binding antibody. The blocking antibody inhibits uptake of vitamin B_{12} at the binding site of IF.

Indications

- Aid in the diagnosis of pernicious anemia

Reference Values

- Negative; no antibody detected

Abnormal Values

- Positive values
    Pernicious anemia
    Megaloblastic anemia
    Grave's disease
    Insulin-dependent diabetes

Interfering Factors

- Recent exposures to a radioisotope or treatment with methotrexate or other folic acid antagonist can interfere with test results.
- Vitamin B_{12} injected or ingested within 48 hours of the test invalidates results.

Nursing Implications

Assessment

- Obtain a hematologic and GI history, signs and symptoms, results of tests performed, and medication regimen.

Possible Nursing Diagnoses

Tissue perfusion, altered [specify], related to oxygen supply/demand imbalance

Protection, altered, related to altered hematopoiesis

Body image disturbance related to change in structure/appearance

Implementation

- Put on gloves. Using aseptic technique, perform a venipuncture and obtain 5 mL of blood in a red-top tube.
- Allow the blood to clot for at least 1 hour at room temperature and then send it to the laboratory. If transfer must be delayed, refrigerate the sample.
- Handle sample gently to avoid hemolysis.

Evaluation

- Note test results in relation to other tests performed and the client's symptoms.

Client/Caregiver Teaching

Pretest

- Inform the client that test should not be performed if B_{12} was injected or ingested within 48 hours of the test.

Posttest

- Inform the client that a positive result confirms pernicious anemia but that half the clients with pernicious anemia test negative, requiring further testing.

Inulin Clearance Test

Classification: Chemistry

Type of Test: Urine

Although infrequently used, this test measures the urinary excretion of inulin in relation to plasma concentration after the IV administration of inulin, an inert sugar that is not metabolized, absorbed, or secreted by the body.

Indications

- Evaluate renal function
- Measure glomerular filtration rate

Reference Values

Birth–10 yr	1.4–2.0 mL/s
11–20 yr	1.4–2.1 mL/s
21–70 yr	1.5–2.2 mL/s
>70	Clearance may decline up to 45%

Values vary with client's age.

Abnormal Values

- Decreased values
    Acute and chronic glomerulonephritis
    Advanced bilateral renal lesions
    Acute tubular necrosis
    Advanced chronic bilateral pyelonephritis
    Bilateral ureteral obstruction
    Congestive heart failure
    Dehydration
    Nephrosclerosis
    Decreased renal blood flow

Interfering Factors

- Failure to infuse inulin at a constant rate, collect specimens at the proper intervals, or follow restrictions and instructions can affect test results.

> ### NURSING ALERT
>
> - Perform this test cautiously in clients with cardiac disease. Congestive heart failure can be caused by increased fluid intake.

Nursing Implications

Assessment

- Ensure that the client avoids exercise the morning of the test, fasts for 4 hours before the test, and drinks 1 liter of water 1 hour before the test.

Possible Nursing Diagnoses

Fluid volume excess related to compromised regulatory mechanism or decreased glomerular filtration

Urinary elimination, altered, related to decreased glomerular filtration or obstruction

Anxiety related to threat to health status

Implementation

- Put on gloves. Using aseptic technique, perform a venipuncture and obtain 10 mL of blood in a green-top tube as a baseline level.
- Shake the inulin IV bolus solution, heat in boiling water, cool to body temperature, and use within 1 hour.
- Catheterize the client until the bladder is empty. Save the urine as a baseline specimen. If the client is already catheterized, empty the bag and clamp the catheter for 1 hour before collection.
- Infuse 25 mL of 10% inulin by IV bolus over 4 minutes. After 30 minutes, use an IV pump to infuse 500 mL of 1.5% inulin at a constant rate of 4 mL per minute.
- Collect a urine specimen 30 minutes after starting the IV. At 20-minute intervals, collect three more 10-mL specimens, clamping the catheter between collections. Midway between each 20-minute period and at the end of the test, collect a blood sample in green-top tubes.
- Label all specimens, record dosage and collection time, and send to laboratory immediately after each collection. Refrigerate specimens if there will be a wait of more than 10 minutes.

Evaluation

- Note test results in relation to other tests performed and the client's symptoms.

Client/Caregiver Teaching

Pretest

- Tell the client to fast for 4 hours before the test and not to exercise the morning of the test.
- Tell the client to drink 1 liter of water 1 hour before the test and continue drinking fluids throughout the test.
- Instruct the client to report any burning sensations during drug administration.

Posttest

- Tell the client to resume food and fluid intake and normal exercise.
- Tell the client to notify the physician within 8 to 10 hours after the catheter is removed.

Iron (Fe)

Classification: Hematology

Type of Test: Serum

A test to measure the amount of iron in the body. Iron plays a principal role in erythropoiesis and is necessary for the maturation of red blood cells and for hemoglobin synthesis. About 65 percent of iron resides in hemoglobin and 3 percent in myoglobin. Normally, iron enters the body by oral ingestion with only 10 percent absorbed, but as high as 20 percent can be absorbed in iron-deficiency anemia.

Indications

- Determine cause of anemia of unknown etiology
- Diagnose iron-deficiency anemia and blood loss indicated by decreased serum iron
- Determine disorders that involve diminished protein synthesis or defects in iron absorption
- Aid in diagnosis of hemochromatosis or other disorders of iron metabolism and storage
- Monitor hematologic responses during pregnancy, when serum iron is usually decreased

Reference Values

		SI Units
Newborns	100–250 μg/dL	17.9–44.8 μmol/L
Infants	40–100 μg/dL	7.2–17.9 μmol/L
Children	50–120 μg/dL	9.0–21.5 μmol/L
Adults		
Men	65–175 μg/dL	11.6–31.3 μmol/L
Women	50–170 μg/dL	9.0–30.4 μmol/L
Older adults	40–80 μg/dL	7.2–14.3 μmol/L

Abnormal Values

- Increased levels
  Hemochromatosis
  Hepatitis
  Nephritis
  Lead toxicity
  Leukemia
  Anemias (hemolytic, pernicious, and aplastic)
  Thalassemia
  Repeated transfusions
- Decreased levels
  Iron-deficiency anemia
  Carcinoma
  Hypothyroidism
  Infection
  Nephrosis
  Chronic blood loss (GI, uterine)
  Low-birth-weight infants
  Protein malnutrition
  Postoperative state

Interfering Factors

- Failure to adhere to dietary restrictions
- Failure to withhold iron-containing medications 24 hours before the test

Nursing Implications

Assessment

- Obtain a history of known or suspected actual or risk for anemia and results of tests for hematopoietic function.

- Ensure that food has been withheld for 8 hours and iron-containing medications for 24 hours.

Possible Nursing Diagnoses

Protection, altered, related to abnormal blood profiles
Anxiety related to perceived threat to health status
Poisoning related to excessive levels of lead in blood
Tissue perfusion, altered [specify], related to oxygen supply/demand imbalance
Fatigue related to oxygen supply/demand imbalance

Implementation

- Put on gloves. Using aseptic technique, perform a venipuncture and collect 7 mL of blood in a red-top tube.
- Handle specimen gently to prevent hemolysis and send promptly to the laboratory.

Evaluation

- Compare results with RBC and reticulocyte count if available. Also compare to total iron-binding capacity to obtain a quantitative measurement of serum transferrin, the iron and protein complex that transports iron from the intestine to the bone marrow (see Transferrin). Note and report signs and symptoms of anemia.

Client/Caregiver Teaching

Pretest

- Tell the client to fast for 8 hours before the test and withhold iron-containing medications for 24 hours or more, as ordered.

Posttest

- Tell the client to resume food and fluid intake and medications withheld before testing.
- Instruct in oral administration of iron supplement and inclusion in dietary inclusion of iron-rich foods.
- Inform client of possibility of retesting in 4 to 7 days to check if iron stores have been replenished.

Iron; Iron Binding Capacity, Total (TIBC); Transferrin Test

Classification: Hematology

Type of Test: Blood

Iron plays a principal role in erythropoiesis, as it is necessary for proliferation and maturation of red blood cells and for hemoglobin synthesis. Of the body's normal 4 g of iron (somewhat less in women), about 65 percent resides in hemoglobin and about 3 percent resides in myoglobin. A small amount is also found in cellular enzymes, which catalyze the oxidation and reduction of iron. The remainder of iron is stored in the liver, bone marrow, and spleen as ferritin or hemosiderin.

Any iron present in the serum is in transit among the alimentary tract, the bone marrow, and available iron storage forms. It travels in the bloodstream bound to transferrin, a protein manufactured by the liver. Unbound iron is highly toxic, but there is generally much more transferrin available than is needed for iron transport.

Transferrin may be measured directly by immunoelectrophoresis or indirectly by exposing the serum to sufficient excess iron such that all transferrin present can combine with the added iron. The latter result is expressed as total iron-binding capacity (TIBC). The percentage saturation is calculated by dividing the serum iron value by the TIBC value.

Indications

- Diagnose iron-deficiency anemia
- Differentiate between iron-deficiency anemia and anemia of a chronic disease
- Provide support for diagnosis of hemachromatosis or diseases of iron metabolism and storage
- Monitor hematologic response during pregnancy

Reference Values

Transferrin
    Newborn   60–170 mg/dL
    Adult   250–450 mg/dL
Percentage saturation
    Newborn   65% saturation
    Adult   20–55% saturation
TIBC
    Children   100–350 μg/dL
    Adults   300–360 μg/dL
    Elderly   200–310 μg/dL

Abnormal Values

- Increased serum iron and ferritin levels, increased percentage transferrin, and decreased TIBC
      Hemachromatosis
      Hemosiderosis
- Decreased serum iron and increased transferrin
      Iron-deficiency anemia
- Decreased serum iron and decreased transferrin
      Infections
      Widespread malignancy
      Malabsorption syndromes
      Malnutrition
      Nephrotic syndrome
- Decreased serum iron, increased transferrin, low percentage saturation, increased TIBC, and increased ferritin
      Pregnancy

Interfering Factors

- Drugs such as chloramphenicol and oral contraceptive can cause false-positive test results.
- Iron supplements can cause a false-negative TIBC and false increase in serum iron.
- Hemolysis of the sample and delay in sending the sample to the laboratory may interfere with accurate results.

Nursing Implications

Assessment

- Obtain a hematologic history, history of blood transfusions, medication regimen, and, in female clients, date of last menstrual period.

■ Ensure that client has fasted for 12 hours before the test.

Possible Nursing Diagnoses

Gas exchange, impaired, related to altered oxygen carrying capacity

Activity intolerance related to disorder

Implementation

■ Put on gloves. Using aseptic technique, perform a venipuncture and collect 7 mL of blood in a red-top tube.
■ Handle specimen gently to avoid hemolysis and transfer to the laboratory.

Evaluation

■ Note test results in relation to other tests performed, particularly, serum iron, serum ferritin, serum transferrin, and percentage of iron saturation, as well as to the client's symptoms.
■ To calculate serum transferrin use this formula: $0.8 \times$ TIBC $- 43$.

Client/Caregiver Teaching

Pretest

■ Tell the client to fast from food for 12 hours before the test and to discontinue iron-containing medications 24 hours before the test. Water is allowed.

Posttest

■ Tell the client to resume food intake.
■ If the client has iron-deficiency anemia, tell the client to eat foods high in iron, such as organ meats, eggs, and dried fruit.

Isocitrate Dehydrogenase (ICD)

Classification: Chemistry

Type of Test: Serum

This test measures isocitrate dehydrogenase (ICD), an enzyme that catalyzes the decarboxylation of isocitrate in the Krebs cycle. This enzyme is important in controlling the rate of the cycle, which must be precisely adjusted to meet the energy needs of cells. ICD is found in the liver, heart, skeletal muscle, placenta, platelets, and erythrocytes. The enzyme is released into the blood when there is damage to the cells in these organs. This test has generally been replaced by alanine aminotransferase (ALT).

Indications

- Evaluate elevated serum aspartate aminotransferase (ALT, SGOT) or alkaline phosphatase (ALP) of uncertain etiology
- Monitor therapy of potentially hepatotoxic drugs that may lead to elevated ICD levels early in the course of treatment

Reference Values

		SI Units
Newborns	4.8–28 U/L	0.08–0.47 IU/L
Adults	1.2–7 U/L	0.02–0.12 IU/L

Abnormal Values

- Elevated levels
    Early viral hepatitis
    Cancer of the liver
    Intrahepatic and extrahepatic obstruction
    Biliary atresia
    Cirrhosis
    Preeclampsia

Hepatitis (chronic)
Infectious mononucleosis
Kwashiorkor
Severe pulmonary infarct
Reye's syndrome
- Decreased levels
  Hepatocellular necrosis
  Hepatotoxic drugs

Interfering Factors

- Hepatotoxic drugs may cause elevated levels.
- Hemolysis of sample invalidates the results.

Nursing Implications

Assessment

- Obtain history of known or suspected hepatic disease and results of any tests performed.
- Assess medication history; ensure that any drugs that may alter test results, such as hepatotoxic drugs, have been withheld for 24 hours before the test, as ordered by the physician.

Possible Nursing Diagnoses

Fatigue related to the disease
Gas exchange, impaired, related to the disease

Implementation

- Put on gloves. Using aseptic technique, perform a venipuncture and collect 7 mL of blood in a red-top tube.
- Handle the sample gently to avoid hemolysis and transport to the laboratory promptly.

Evaluation

- Note results in relation to ALT and alkaline phosphatase.

Client/Caregiver Teaching

Pretest

- Tell the client to withhold any nephrotoxic drugs, as ordered.

Posttest

- Tell the client to resume medications withheld before the test.

17-Ketogenic Steroids (17-KGS)

Classification: Chemistry

Type of Test: Urine (timed)

17-Ketogenic steroids (17-KGS) are hormones measured as an index of overall glucocorticoid metabolism. Before urinary 17-KGS can be evaluated, the 17-ketosteroids (17-KS) of androgenic origin must be either removed or measured separately. Because such a large array of steroid metabolites are reflected in 17-KGS measures, this test provides for a good overall assessment of adrenal function.

Indications

- Evaluate adrenal hypofunctioning or hyperfunctioning
- Monitor response to therapy with corticosteroid drugs or other drugs that alter adrenal function

Reference Values

		SI Units
Children*	2–6 mg/24 h	6–17 mmol/24 h
Men	5–25 mg/24 h	14–69 mmol/24 h
Women	3–15 mg/24 h	8–41 mmol/24 h
Older Adults	3–13 mg/24 h	8–36 mmol/24 h

*Age-related: the younger the child, the less secreted.

Abnormal Values

- Elevated levels
  Cushing's syndrome
  Adrenogenital syndrome
  Carcinoma of the adrenal glands, adenoma
  Severe stress (burns, infections, surgery, or emotional trauma)
  Hirsutism or virilization
  Stein-Leventhal syndrome

Hyperadrenalism
Ovarian tumor (lutein cell or arrhenoblastoma)
Infectious disease
Obesity
Pregnancy
Certain drugs, including ACTH therapy, hydralazine, meprobamate, penicillin, chlorpromazine, piperidine, salicylates, secobarbital, testosterone, phenothiazines, spironolactone, cephalothin, corticosteroids, digitoxin, and oral contraceptives
- Decreased levels
Addison's disease
Hypothyroidism
Panpituitarism
Simmonds' disease
Certain drugs, including estrogens, penicillin, ethacrynic acid, and phenytoin

Interfering Factors

- Stress during testing period will increase results.
- Radiographic dye used in previous studies will interfere with test results.
- Improper collection and storage of all urine during 24-hour test period will interfere with results.
- Failure to follow drug restrictions can elevate or decrease test results (see Abnormal Values).

Nursing Implications

Assessment

- Obtain history of known or suspected adrenal disorders, and steroid therapy and results of laboratory tests and radiologic studies performed.
- Ensure that appropriate medications are withheld for 24 hours before urine collection, as ordered (see Abnormal Values).
- Ensure that the client avoided excessive exercise and stressful situations before the test.

Possible Nursing Diagnoses

Fluid volume deficit or excess related to the disease
Fatigue related to altered metabolic energy production
Infection, risk for, related to skin and capillary fragility

Implementation

- Obtain a clean 3-liter container or 24-hour urine bag or bottle with preservative, according to laboratory policy.
- Begin the test between 6 and 8 AM if possible; collect first voiding and discard; record the time specimen was discarded as the beginning of the 24-hour test. Document the quantity of urine output during collection period, including urine at end of 24-hour period.
- The next morning, ask the client to void at the same time the collection was started and add this last voiding to the container.
- If an indwelling catheter is in place, replace tubing and container system and empty the urine into a large refrigerated container periodically during the 24 hours; monitor to ensure continued drainage and conclude the test the next morning at the same hour the collection was begun.
- At the conclusion of the test, make sure that the container is properly labeled; include any medications that the client was taking that can alter test results. Transport specimen to the laboratory immediately.

Evaluation

- Note results in relation to cortisol or other urinary hormone levels, if available.

Client/Caregiver Teaching

Pretest

- Tell the client to avoid excessive physical exercise and stressful situations during the collection period.
- Inform the client that all urine for a 24-hour period must be saved. Monitor all urine output. Instruct the client to avoid voiding in the pan with defecation and to keep toilet tissue out of the pan to prevent contamination of the specimen.

Posttest

- Tell the client to resume medications and activity withheld before the test, as ordered.
- Instruct the client and the caregiver to report any signs and symptoms of adrenal dysfunction to the physician.

Ketones

Classification: Chemistry

Type of Test: Urine (Random)

Ketones refer to the three intermediate products of metabolism: acetone, acetoacetic acid, and beta-hydroxybutyric acid. Measurable amounts of ketones are not usually present in the urine. However, if the client has excessive fat metabolism, ketones will be found. Excessive fat metabolism may occur if the client has impaired ability to metabolize carbohydrates, inadequate carbohydrate intake, excessive carbohydrate loss, or increased carbohydrate demand.

As with glucose, ketones in the urine are associated with elevated blood ketone levels.

Indications

- Screen for ketonuria
- Monitor the control of diabetes mellitus
- Detect and monitor treatment of diabetic ketaoacidosis

Reference Values

- Negative

Abnormal Values

- Uncontrolled diabetes mellitus
- Diabetic ketoacidosis
- Starvation
- Weight reduction diets
- High-protein, low-carbohydrate, high-fat diets
- Fasting
- Prolonged vomiting or dehydration
- Ketoacidosis of alcoholism
- Excessive aspirin ingestion

Interfering Factors

- Certain drugs, such as levodopa, phenazopyridine, and sulfobromophthalein produce false-positive results with Ketostix reagent strip.
- Bacterial contamination of urine, or failure to keep reagent strip tightly closed so moisture and light affects strips, can cause false-negative results.

Nursing Implications

Assessment

- Obtain a history of diabetes, dietary habits, and medication regimen.

Possible Nursing Diagnoses

Therapeutic regimen, individual, ineffective management
Nutrition, altered, less than body requirements
Infection, risk for, related to decreased leukocyte function

Implementation

- Collect a second-voided midstream specimen. Test the specimen using one of the following reagents within 60 minutes or refrigerate the specimen. After refrigeration, allow the sample to warm to room temperature before testing.
- *Ketostix:* Dip the strip into the specimen and remove it immediately. Tap the strip against the side of the specimen container to remove excess urine. After 15 seconds, compare the color on the strip to the color chart on the container. Record the positive results as small, moderate, or large.
- *Acetest:* Lay the tablet on a piece of white paper. Place one drop of urine on the tablet. Wait 30 seconds and compare the tablet color (white, lavender, or purple) with the color chart on the container.

Evaluation

- Note test results in relation to the client's symptoms and other tests performed, particularly blood glucose and glycosylated hemoglobin.

Client/Caregiver Teaching

Pretest

- Tell the client how to obtain a second-voided midstream specimen: First, void, and then drink a glass of water. Wait 30 minutes, then try to void again. Remind the client to allow

a small amount of urine to go into the toilet before collecting the specimen.
- Inform the client about the testing procedure. Remind clients to use only the color chart that is on the reagent container where they obtained the stick or tablet to evaluate the results.

17-Ketosteroids (17-KS) and Total Fractionation

Classification: Chemistry

Type of Test: Urine (timed)

This test measures urinary 17-ketosteroids (17-KS), metabolites from androgenic hormones. In males, two-thirds of 17-KS originate in the adrenal cortex and one-third derive from the testes. In females, virtually all 17-KS originate in the adrenal cortex. Components of 17-KS, which can be measured individually, include androsterone, dehydroepiandrosterone, etiocholanolone, 11-hydroxyandrosterone, 11-hydroxyetiocholanolone, 11-ketoandrosterone, 11-ketoetiocholanolone, pregnanediol, pregnanetriol, 5-pregnanetriol, and 11-ketopregnanetriol. This is done by fractionating the components using gas chromatography and measuring the specific steroids.

Fractionation is important when the need to assess androgenic properties is required and provides more specific information about androgen secretion. Fractionation is especially useful in differentiating adrenal carcinoma, which causes a high level of dehydroepiandrosterone, from adrenal hyperplasia, which causes all ketosteroids to be elevated.

Indications

- Confirm suspected adrenocortical dysfunction, especially if urinary levels of 17-OHCS are normal
- Confirm suspected Cushing's syndrome as indicated by elevated levels
- Confirm suspected adrenogenital syndrome, as indicated by elevated levels

■ Monitor response to cortisol therapy for adrenogenital syndrome

Reference Values

		SI Units
Fractionation		
Men	8–17 mg/24 h	27–58 μmol/24 h
Women	5–15 mg/24 h	17–52 μmol/24 h
Total		
Infants	<1 mg/24 h	<3 μmol/24 h
Children*	2–4 mg/24 h	7–14 μmol/24 h
Adolescents	3–15 mg/24 h	10–52 μmol/24 h
Adults		
Women	4–16 mg/24 h	13–55 μmol/24 h
Men	6–21 mg/24 h	21–72 μmol/24 h
Older adults	4–8 mg/24 h	13–27 μmol/24 h

*Age-related: the younger the child, the less secreted.

Abnormal Values

■ Elevated 17-KS
  Adrenocortical tumors
  Adrenocortical carcinoma, hyperpituitarism
  Adrenogenital syndrome (congenital adrenal hyperplasia)
  Chronic illness
  Cushing's syndrome
  Gynecomastia
  Hirsutism
  Interstitial-cell tumor of the testes
  Lutein-cell ovarian tumor, androgenic arrhenoblastoma
  Stein-Leventhal syndrome
  Pregnancy
  Stress
  Tumors of the adrenal glands or gonads
  Virilization
  Certain drugs, including ascorbic acid, antibiotic, chlor-
    diazepoxide, chlorpromazine, cortisone steroids, digi-
    toxin, hydralazine, meprobamate, methyprylon, mor-
    phine, nalidixic acid, oleandomycin, pyridium,
    phenothiazines, piperidine, salicylates, secobarbital,
    spironolactone, and testosterone
■ Decreased 17-KS
  Addison's disease
  Adrenalectomy

Hypopituitarism
Hypothyroidism
Klinefelter's syndrome
Liver disease
Menopause
Nephrotic syndrome
Starvation
Certain drugs, including chlordiazepoxide, chlorproma-
zine, antibiotics, corticosteroids, digoxin, diphenylhy-
dantoin, estrogens, diuretics, glucose, meprobamate,
nalidixic acid, paraldehyde, phenytoin, probenecid,
promazine, propoxyphene, pyrazinamide, quinine,
quinidine, salicylates, secobarbital, and spironolactone

Interfering Factors

- Blood in the specimen, including menstrual blood, can alter results.
- Exercise and stressful situations can falsely increase results.
- Results are invalid if specimen was not refrigerated through-out the collection.
- Contrast dyes interfere with results.
- Failure to collect all urine during 24-hour test period will interfere with results.
- Certain medications can falsely elevate or decrease results (see Abnormal Values).

Nursing Implications

Assessment

- Obtain history of known or suspected hormonal dysfunc-tions, medication regimen, and results of laboratory tests.
- Ensure that medication affecting test results are withheld for 48 hours before test.
- Determine date of last menstrual period for women. Post-pone test collection if menstruation is present or anticipated during the collection time.

Possible Nursing Diagnoses

Fluid deficit or excess, risk for, related to adrenal gland dysfunction
Fatigue related to decreased metabolic energy production

Implementation

- Obtain a clean 3-liter container or 24-hour urine bag or bottle with preservative, according to laboratory policy.
- Begin the test between 6 and 8 AM if possible; collect first voiding and discard; record the time specimen was discarded as the beginning of the 24-hour test. Document the quantity of urine output during collection period, including urine at end of 24-hour period.
- The next morning, ask the client to void at the same time the collection was started and add this last voiding to the container.
- If an indwelling catheter is in place, replace tubing and container system and empty the urine into a large refrigerated container periodically during the 24 hours; monitor to ensure continued drainage and conclude the test the next morning at the same hour the collection was begun.
- At the conclusion of the test, make sure that the container is properly labeled; include any medications that the client was taking that can alter test results. Transport specimen to the laboratory immediately.

Evaluation

- Note results of other urinary hormone tests and blood glucose and potassium results in relation to increased 17-KS levels.

Client/Caregiver Teaching

Pretest

- Explain that the purpose of the test is to evaluate hormonal functioning.
- Instruct the client to avoid excess physical exercise or stressful events before or during the specimen-collection period.
- Inform the client that all urine for a 24-hour period must be saved. Instruct client to avoid defecating into the urine specimen and to keep toilet tissue out of pan to prevent contamination of the specimen.

Posttest

- Resume medications and activity withheld before the test, as ordered.
- Tell client to report signs and symptoms of hyper- or hypoadrenal gland function to the physician.

Lactic Acid

Classification: Chemistry

Type of Test: Blood

Lactic acid (present in blood as lactate) is a by-product of carbohydrate metabolism. Normally metabolized in the liver, concentration is based on rate of production and metabolism. When hypoxia or circulatory collapse increase production, or when the hepatic system doesn't metabolize lactate sufficiently, elevated levels occur. Levels normally increase during exercise, because of insufficient oxygen delivery to tissues. This test is usually performed in conjunction with blood pyruvic acid and a ratio is determined. This ratio reliably monitors tissue oxygenation.

Indications

- Determine cause of lactic acidosis
- Assess tissue oxygenation

Reference Values

		SI Units
Arterial	0.5–1.6 mEq/L	0.5–1.6 mmol/L
Venous	0.5–2.2 mEq/L	0.5–2.2 mmol/L

The lactate:pyruvate ratio is normally 10:1.

Abnormal Values

- Elevated levels
  Shock or hemorrhage
  Trauma
  Myocardial infarction or pulmonary embolism
  Severe dehydration
  Uncontrolled diabetes mellitus
  Septicemia
  Neoplasms

Ingestion of large doses of ethanol or acetaminophen
Renal failure
- Decreased levels
Elevated lactic dehydrogenase (LDH) value
Hypothermia

Interfering Factors

- Use of tourniquet or clenching of fist when performing venipuncture can cause elevated levels.
- The client's failure to rest for 1 hour before obtaining the venous sample can cause an elevation of the level.

Nursing Implications

Assessment

- Obtain history of known or suspected systemic disorders or conditions associated with lactic acidosis and results of tests and procedures performed.
- Ensure that the client has fasted overnight and rested for 1 hour before the test.

Possible Nursing Diagnoses

Tissue integrity, impaired, related to altered circulation
Fluid volume deficit
Anxiety related to threat of death

Implementation

- *Venous sample:* Put on gloves. Using aseptic technique, perform a venipuncture and collect 7 mL of blood in a gray-top tube.
- *Arterial sample:* Obtain a blood gas collection kit. If pre-packaged kits are not available, obtain 3-mL syringe, heparin (1000 units/mL), 20- or 21-ga needles, povidone-iodine or alcohol swabs, gauze pads, and tape. Put on gloves. Using aseptic technique, perform an arterial puncture and collect 2 to 3 mL of blood in a heparinized syringe. Expel any air from syringe.
- Place tube on ice, and send to laboratory immediately. If client is receiving oxygen, include the percentage on the requisition slip.

Evaluation

- Note results in relation to other studies that may indicate an acidotic state, for example, low pH, normal $Paco_2$, low bicarbonate and serum CO_2.
- Observe the client for signs and symptoms of acidosis.

Client/Caregiver Teaching

Pretest

- Instruct the client to fast overnight and to rest at least 1 hour before the test.

Posttest

- Tell the client to resume diet and activity withheld before the test.

Lactic Dehydrogenase and Isoenzymes (LDH, LD)

Classification: Chemistry

Type of Test: Serum

This test measures total lactic dehydrogenase (LDH), an enzyme that catalyzes the reversible conversion of lactic acid to pyruvic acid within cells. Because many tissues contain LDH, elevated total LDH is considered a nonspecific indicator of cellular damage unless other clinical data make the tissue origin obvious. Determining tissue origin is aided by an electrophoretic analysis of the five isoenzymes, specific to certain tissues. The heart and erythrocytes are rich sources of LDH_1 and LDH_2; however, the brain is a source of LDH_1, LDH_2, and LDH_3. The kidneys contain LDH_3 and LDH_4; the liver and skeletal muscle contain LDH_4 and LDH_5. Certain glands (thyroid, adrenal, and thymus), the pancreas, spleen, lungs, lymph nodes, and white blood cells contain LDH_3, whereas the ileum is an additional source of LDH_5.

Indications

- Confirm acute myocardial infarction or extension thereof, as indicated by elevation (usually) of total LDH, elevation of LDH_1 and LDH_2, and reversal of the LDH_1:LDH_2 ratio within 48 hours of the infarction.
- Differentiate acute myocardial infarction from pulmonary infarction and liver problems, which elevate LDH_4 and LDH_5.

- Confirm red cell hemolysis or renal infarction, especially as indicated by $LDH_1:LDH_2$ reversal.
- Confirm chronicity of liver, lung, and kidney disorders, as evidenced by LDH levels that remain persistently high.
- Evaluate effectiveness of cancer chemotherapy (LDH levels should fall with successful treatment).
- Evaluate the degree of muscle wasting in muscular dystrophy (LDH levels rise early in this disorder and approach normal as muscle mass is reduced by atrophy).

Reference Values

		SI Units
Total LDH		
Newborns	160–500 U/L	160–500 U/L
Children	60–170 U/L	60–170 U/L
Adults	80–120 U at 300°C (Wacker)	38–62 U/L at 300°C
	150–450 U/L (Wroblewski)	72–217 IU/L
LDH isoenzymes		
	LDH_1 17–27%	0.17–0.27
	LDH_2 27–37%	0.27–0.37
	LDH_3 18–25%	0.18–0.25
	LDH_4 3–8%	0.03–0.08
	LDH_5 0–5%	0.0–0.05
Ratios		
	$LDH_2 > LDH_1$	
	$LDH_1:LDH_2 < 1$	
	$LDH_4 > LDH_5$	
	$LDH_5:LDH_4 \leq 1:3$	

Values may vary according to the laboratory performing the test.

Abnormal Values

- Elevated total LDH
  Acute myocardial infarction
  Renal disease
  Myxedema
  Hepatitis
  Anemias
  Pulmonary disease
  Leukemia
  Lymphoma

Tissue Sources and Common Causes of Elevated LDH Isoenzymes

Isoenzyme	Tissue Sources	Causes of Elevated Levels
LDH_1	Brain Erythrocytes Heart	Acute myocardial infarction Cerebrovascular accident Muscular dystrophy Red blood cell hemolysis Renal infarction
LDH_2	Brain Erythrocytes Heart	Acute myocardial infarction Cerebrovascular accident Lymphoproliferative disorders Muscular dystrophy Shock
LDH_3	Brain Glands (thyroid, adrenal, thymus) Kidneys Leukocytes Lungs Lymph nodes Pancreas Spleen	Acute pancreatitis Infectious mononucleosis Lymphoproliferative disorders Pneumonia Pulmonary infarction Renal necrosis Shock
LDH_4	Kidneys Liver Skeletal muscles	Acute glomerulonephritis Cirrhosis Hepatitis Infectious mononucleosis Muscular dystrophy Pancreatitis Pneumonia Pulmonary infarction Renal necrosis Shock
LDH_5	Ileum Liver Skeletal muscles	Cirrhosis Dermatomyositis Hepatitis Infectious mononucleosis Liver trauma Muscular dystrophy Pulmonary infarction Shock

From Watson, J and Jaffe, MS: Nurse's Manual of Laboratory and Diagnostic Tests, ed. 2. FA Davis, Philadelphia, 1995, p. 200, with permission.

Interfering Factors

- Certain drugs, such as lorazepam, anabolic steroids, anesthetics, aspirin, alcohol, fluorides, thyroid, lithium, narcotics, clofibrate, mithramicin, and procainamide, can elevate LDH levels.

Nursing Implications

Assessment

- Obtain a history of known or suspected disorders, especially of the cardiac system, and the results of any organ system tests and procedures.
- Assess medication history; ensure that drugs that may alter test results have been withheld for 12 to 24 hours before the test, as ordered.

Possible Nursing Diagnoses

Anxiety related to threat to health status, threat of death
Cardiac output, decreased, related to the disease
Activity intolerance related to oxygen supply and demand imbalance

Implementation

- Put on gloves. Using aseptic technique, perform a venipuncture and collect 7 mL of blood in a red-top tube.
- Handle the sample gently to avoid hemolysis and transport to the laboratory promptly.

Evaluation

- Note test results of total LDH and isoenzymes for increases in ratios and organ identification.
- Note test results in relation to other tests performed, particularly other serum enzyme studies and ECG, and the client's symptoms.

Client/Caregiver Teaching

Pretest

- Tell the client to withhold drugs that can interfere with test results, as ordered.

Posttest

- Tell the client to resume medication withheld before the test.
- Tell the client to report chest pain or other complaints to physician.

Lactose Tolerance Test

Classification: Chemistry
Type of Test: Plasma

This test screens for lactose intolerance by monitoring glucose levels after ingestion of a large dose of lactose. Lactose, a disaccharide, is found in dairy products. When ingested, lactose is broken down in the intestine by the enzyme lactase into glucose and galactose. When sufficient lactase is not available, intestinal bacteria metabolize the lactose, resulting in abdominal bloating, pain, flatus, and diarrhea.

Indications

- Suspected lactose intolerance

Reference Values

- Fasting serum glucose >20–50 mg/dL

Abnormal Values

- Fasting serum glucose <20 mg/dL suggests lactose intolerance

Interfering Factors

- Failure to restrict diet and exercise may alter test results.
- Medications such as benzodiazepines, insulin, propranolol, oral contraceptives, and thiazide diuretics may alter glucose levels.
- Delayed gastric emptying may decrease glucose levels.
- Glycolysis may cause false-negative results.
- Smoking may falsely increase blood sugar levels.

Nursing Implications

Assessment

- Obtain history of gastrointestinal system, medication regimen, diagnostic tests, and results.

- Ensure that the client has fasted and avoided strenuous activity for 8 hours before the test.

Possible Nursing Diagnoses

Nutrition, altered, less than body requirements, related to inability to digest dairy foods
Fluid volume deficit related to excessive GI losses

Implementation

- Put on gloves. Using aseptic technique, perform a venipuncture and collect a fasting specimen of 5 to 7 mL of blood in a gray-top tube.
- For an adult client, administer 50 to 100 g of lactose dissolved in water, as determined by institution, and record time of ingestion. Pediatric dosage is based on weight.
- At 30, 60, and 120 minutes after ingestion of loading dose, put on gloves. At each interval collect 5 to 7 mL of blood in gray-top tube.
- Label specimens and send to laboratory immediately.

Evaluation

- If the test is positive, a monosaccharide tolerance test, such as glucose galactose tolerance test, should be performed. Compare the results.

Client/Caregiver Teaching

Pretest

- Inform the client not to eat or drink anything or strenuously exercise for 8 hours before the test. Also, tell the client to restrict smoking because it may increase the blood sugar level.
- Inform the client that four blood samples will be needed.

Posttest

- Advise the client to resume medications and activity withheld before the test.
- Warn the client that if the test is positive, another test may be performed.
- Instruct the client with lactose intolerance to avoid milk products and to carefully read labels on prepared products. Advise client that products such as Lactaid tablets or drops may allow them to ingest milk products without sequelae.

Laparoscopy, Abdominal Peritoneoscopy

Classification: Endoscopy

Type of Test: Direct visualization

Abdominal or gastrointestinal laparoscopy is the direct visualization of the liver, gallbladder, spleen, and stomach following insufflation of nitrous oxide. In this procedure, a rigid laparoscope is inserted through a small incision in the abdomen. The endoscope has a microscope to allow visualization of the organs and the capability to insert instruments to perform certain procedures, such as collection of a specimen for biopsy or removal of small tumors.

Indications

- Evaluate abdominal pain or abdominal mass of unknown origin
- Obtain biopsies of benign or cancerous tumors
- Evaluate jaundice of unknown origin
- Evaluate and treat appendicitis
- Assist in performing surgical cholecystectomy
- Diagnose cirrhosis of the liver
- Stage neoplastic disorders such as lymphomas, Hodgkin's disease, and hepatic carcinoma
- Diagnose pancreatic disorders
- Evaluate extent of splenomegaly from portal hypertension
- Evaluate abdominal trauma in an emergency

Reference Values

- Normal appearance of the liver, spleen, gallbladder, pancreas, and other abdominal contents

Abnormal Values

- Appendicitis
- Gangrenous gallbladder
- Splenomegaly
- Abdominal adhesions

- Cancer of any of the organs
- Acute or chronic pancreatitis
- Cirrhosis of the liver
- Ascites
- Intra-abdominal bleeding

Interfering Factors

- Inability of the client to cooperate with the procedure (if local anesthetic used).
- Abdominal obesity may impair visualization and interfere with the procedure.

> ### NURSING ALERT
>
> This procedure is contraindicated in clients with:
> - A history of peritonitis or multiple abdominal operations because dense adhesions prevent visualization
> - Acute infection involving the abdominal wall, since organisms may be introduced into the normally sterile peritoneal cavity
> - Extreme obesity, since the procedure will be technically very difficult to perform and because adequate visualization may be impaired
> - Coagulation disorders and unstable cardiopulmonary status or chronic tuberculosis

Nursing Implications

Assessment

- Obtain a history of allergies or sensitivities to anesthetics and analgesics, and medication regimen.
- Ensure that client has restricted food and fluid for at least 8 hours before the procedure.
- Assess hematologic status and blood-clotting ability by means of the following tests: complete blood count, platelet count, prothrombin time, partial thromboplastin time, clotting and bleeding time.

Possible Nursing Diagnoses

Anxiety related to threat to health status
Pain related to physical causes
Infection, risk for, related to invasive procedure

Implementation

- Have client remove dentures, contact lenses, eyeglasses, and jewelry.
- Administer a cleansing enema 4 hours before the procedure, if ordered.
- Insert an intravenous line or venous access device at a "keep vein open" (KVO) rate.
- Have client void, then administer medication to reduce discomfort and promote relaxation and sedation, as ordered.
- Position the client on the laparoscopy table. A general anesthesia is administered. Cleanse the abdomen with an antiseptic solution and drape.
- The physician identifies the site for the scope insertion and infiltrates it with local anesthetic. After deeper layers are anesthetized, a pneumoperitoneum needle is placed between the visceral and parietal peritoneum.
- Nitrous oxide or CO_2 is insufflated through the pneumoperitoneum needle to separate the abdominal wall from the viscera and aid in visualization. The pneumoperitoneum needle is removed, and the trocar and laparoscope are inserted through the incision.
- After the examination, collection of tissue samples, and performance of therapeutic procedures, all possible gas is evacuated via the trocar, which is then removed. The skin incision is closed with sutures, clips, or steristrips and a small dressing or adhesive strip applied.

Evaluation

- Note test results in relation to other tests performed and to the client's symptoms.

Client/Caregiver Teaching

Pretest

- Inform the client that the procedure is generally performed in an operating room by a physician under general anesthesia but may be done under local anesthesia and takes approximately 15 to 30 minutes.
- Tell the client to fast from food and fluid for at least 8 hours before the procedure.

Posttest

- Tell the client to resume food and fluid intake and activity when the client is assessed in stable condition, usually within 2 hours of the procedure.
- Inform the client that shoulder discomfort may be experi-

enced for 1 or 2 days after the procedure from elevation of the diaphragm from the CO_2 injected into the abdomen and that such discomfort may be relieved by mild analgesics and cold compresses, as ordered.
- Emphasize that any persistent shoulder pain, abdominal pain, vaginal bleeding, fever, redness or swelling of incisional area must be reported to the physician immediately.

Laparoscopy, Gynecologic Pelviscopy

Classification: Endoscopy

Type of Test: Direct visualization

Using a rigid laparoscope introduced into the body cavity through a small periumbilical incision about 1 to 2 cm in length, the examiner can directly visualize the internal pelvic contents including the ovaries, fallopian tubes, and uterus. It is done to diagnose and treat pelvic organ disorders as well as to perform surgical procedures on the organs.

Indications

- Evaluate amenorrhea and infertility
- Evaluate structures following therapy for infertility
- Evaluate fallopian tubes and anatomic defects to determine cause of infertility
- Evaluate pelvic pain or masses of unknown etiology
- Evaluate known or suspected endometriosis
- Diagnose ectopic pregnancy and determine the need for surgery
- Diagnose pelvic inflammatory disease
- Diagnose uterine fibroids, ovarian cysts, and uterine malformations (ovarian cysts may be aspirated during the procedure)
- Diagnose pelvic malignancies by obtaining samples for biopsy during the procedure
- Treat endometriosis through electrocautery or laser vaporization

- Remove adhesions or foreign bodies such as intrauterine devices (IUD)
- Perform vaginal hysterectomy
- Perform tubal sterilization

Reference Values

- Normal appearance of uterus, ovaries, fallopian tubes, and other pelvic contents

Abnormal Values

- Ectopic pregnancy
- Endometriosis
- Ovarian cyst
- Ovarian tumor
- Pelvic adhesions
- Pelvic inflammatory disease (PID)
- Pelvic tumor
- Salpingitis
- Uterine fibroids

Interfering Factors

- The client is unable to cooperate with the procedure if it is to be done with local anesthetic.
- Abdominal obesity or pelvic adhesions may impair visualization.

NURSING ALERT

This procedure is contraindicated in clients with:
- A history of peritonitis or multiple abdominal operations because dense adhesions prevent visualization
- Acute infection involving the abdominal wall, since organisms may be introduced into the normally sterile peritoneal cavity
- Extreme obesity, since the procedure will be technically very difficult to perform and because adequate visualization may be impaired
- Coagulation disorders and unstable cardiopulmonary status or chronic tuberculosis

Nursing Implications

Assessment

- Obtain a history of allergies or sensitivities to anesthetics and analgesics, the date of the last menstrual period in premenopausal women, and medication regimen.
- Ensure that client has restricted food and fluid for at least 8 hours before the procedure.
- Assess hematologic status and blood-clotting ability by means of the following tests: complete blood count, platelet count, prothrombin time, partial thromboplastin time, clotting and bleeding time.

Possible Nursing Diagnoses

Anxiety related to threat to health status
Injury, risk for, related to invasive procedure
Infection, risk for, related to invasive procedure

Implementation

- Have client remove dentures, contact lenses, eyeglasses, and jewelry.
- Administer a cleansing enema 4 hours before the procedure, if ordered.
- Insert an intravenous line or venous access device at a "keep vein open" (KVO) rate.
- Have client void, then administer medications as ordered to reduce discomfort and promote relaxation and sedation.
- Position the client on the laparoscopy table. A general anesthesia is administered. The client is placed in a modified lithotomy position with the head tilted downward. Cleanse the external genitalia with an antiseptic solution and drape and catheterize the client, if ordered.
- The physician inserts a uterine manipulator through the vagina and cervix and into the uterus, in order that the uterus, fallopian tubes, and ovaries can be moved to permit better visualization.
- Cleanse the abdomen with antiseptic solution and drape with sterile drapes. The physician makes a small incision using a technique similar to the one used for abdominal laparoscopies. CO_2 is insufflated through the pneumoperitoneum needle. The pneumoperitoneum needle is removed, and the trocar and laparoscope are inserted through the incision.
- After the examination, collection of tissue samples, and performance of therapeutic procedures, for example, tubal sterilization, the scope is withdrawn. All possible CO_2 is evacu-

ated via the trocar, which is then removed. The skin incision is closed with sutures, clips, or Steri-Strips, and a small dressing or adhesive strip is applied. Then the uterine manipulator is removed and a pad applied after the perineum is cleansed.

■ Monitor the client's vital signs per institution policy until stable. Assess for vaginal bleeding and abdominal pain or rigidity, suggesting hemorrhage, organ perforation, or infection.

Evaluation

■ Note test results in relation to other tests performed, such as x-rays, CT scans, and related blood studies, and to the client's symptoms.

Client/Caregiver Teaching

Pretest

■ Inform the client that the procedure is generally performed in an operating room by a physician under general anesthesia but may be done under local anesthesia and takes approximately 15 to 30 minutes.

■ Tell the client to fast from food and fluid for at least 8 hours before the procedure.

Posttest

■ Tell the client to resume food and fluid intake and activity when the client is assessed in stable condition, usually within 2 hours after the procedure.

■ Inform the client that shoulder discomfort may be experienced for 1 or 2 days following the procedure from elevation of the diaphragm from the CO_2 injected into the abdomen, and that such discomfort may be relieved by mild analgesics and cold compresses, as ordered.

■ Emphasize that any persistent shoulder pain, abdominal pain, vaginal bleeding, fever, redness or swelling of incisional area must be reported to the physician immediately.

Laryngoscopy

Classification: Endoscopy

Type of Test: Direct visualization

This procedure allows visualization of the larynx using an indirect or direct technique, by means of a rigid laryngoscope or flexible fiberoptic endoscope.

Indications

- Indirect laryngoscopy
    Assess ingestion or inhalation of a foreign body
    Identify source of laryngeal stridor of unknown etiology
    Identify cause of persistent cough, hemoptysis, throat pain, hoarseness, or irritation
    Excise laryngeal polyps
- Direct laryngoscopy
    Assess symptoms of laryngeal obstruction or disease
    Determine presence of strictures, edema, or other abnormalities
    Examine areas that may not be visualized by indirect laryngoscopy
    Examine the larynx in children and in adults who may require general anesthesia or who are otherwise unable to cooperate with an indirect laryngoscopic examination
    Examine the larynx in clients who have strong gag reflexes
    Remove tissues or secretions for laboratory examination
    Remove lesion or foreign body in the larynx
    Examine the larynx in infants suspected of having congenital laryngeal stridor, subglottic stenosis, laryngeal webs, or Pierre Robin syndrome

Reference Values

- Normal larynx with no evidence of inflammation, abnormal growths, or foreign objects

Abnormal Values

- Indirect laryngoscopy
    Inflammation
    Lesions
    Polyps
- Direct laryngoscopy
    Congenital abnormalities
    Foreign bodies
    Laryngeal cancer
    Lesions
    Tumor

Interfering Factors

- Inability of the client to cooperate with the procedure
- Laryngeal view obstruction by a large oropharyngeal mass or tonsillar hypertrophy

> ### NURSING ALERT
>
> - Contraindicated in children with epiglottis because attempts to visualize the larynx may precipitate laryngospasm, complete obstruction, and death. If absolutely necessary, make sure equipment for emergency intubation or tracheotomy is available.

Nursing Implications

Assessment

- Obtain a history of allergies or sensitivities to anesthetics or medications and known or suspected upper respiratory disorders.
- Ensure that food and fluids have been restricted for 6 to 8 hours before direct laryngoscopy.
- Note and remove partial or complete dentures.

Possible Nursing Diagnoses

Gas exchange, impaired, related to laryngeal obstruction
Swallowing, impaired, related to laryngeal obstruction
Pain related to procedure

Implementation

- *Indirect laryngoscopy:* Position the client upright in a chair, then place the light source so that the light reflects from the operator's head mirror into the mouth and the laryngeal mirror as far posteriorly as possible in the mouth. When the mirror is rotated, the light should reflect into the larynx. Ask the client to protrude the tongue and spray the throat with a local anesthetic. Ask the client to concentrate on controlled breathing to prevent gagging. Swallowing is allowed if the examination lasts more than 3 minutes. Excised tissue or foreign bodies are placed in appropriate containers, labeled, and sent to the laboratory.

■ *Direct laryngoscopy*: Have client remove dentures and notify physician of permanent crown on teeth. Administer ordered medication to reduce secretions and discomfort and promote relaxation. Place the client in supine position for general anesthesia and sitting position for local anesthesia, which is swabbed or sprayed into mouth and throat. When loss of sensation is adequate, place the client in supine position with neck extended and supported by an assistant. The laryngoscope or flexible endoscope is placed in the mouth and passed through the pharynx into the larynx for visualization. Excised tissue or foreign bodies are placed in appropriate containers, labeled, and sent to the laboratory. The scope is removed. The client is placed in semi-Fowler's position if local is used, and side-lying position with head slightly elevated if general anesthesia is used.

Evaluation

■ Note test results in relation to the client's symptoms.
■ Evaluate client's ability to swallow until sensation returns if a local anesthetic was used.
■ Observe for difficulty in breathing, expectoration of excessive amounts of blood, and subcutaneous crepitus, which may indicate tracheal perforation.

Client/Caregiver Teaching

Pretest

■ Inform the client of the purpose of the study and how the examination is performed: that the direct laryngoscopy procedure is performed by a physician and takes 15 to 30 minutes, and an indirect laryngoscopy is performed by a nurse or physician and takes about 5 minutes.
■ Inform the client that anesthesia will be achieved locally by spraying or swabbing the throat or that a general anesthetic will be administered, depending on the client's age and condition.
■ Tell the client having a direct laryngoscopy to fast for 6 to 8 hours before the test.

Posttest

- Instruct the client to use mouthwash or a cool drink to alleviate dryness of the tongue and any postprocedure discomfort from indirect laryngoscopy.
- Caution the client against excessive coughing and throat clearing, as these actions may dislodge a clot at the tissue excision site and precipitate bleeding.
- Tell the client to withhold food and fluids until swallowing ability returns, usually about 2 hours following direct laryngoscopy.
- Tell the client to refrain from smoking for 6 to 8 hours following the procedure.
- Tell the client to apply cool compresses to the throat to reduce any laryngeal edema resulting from the trauma caused by the scope or removal of tissue, and warm gargles, lozenges, or viscous Xylocaine to alleviate throat discomfort.
- Emphasize that any excessive bleeding or difficulty breathing must be reported to the physician immediately.

Lead (Pb)

Classification: Chemistry, Urinalysis

Type of Test: Blood, Urine (timed)

Lead (Pb), a heavy metal and trace element to which the population is exposed, is normally only absorbed in small amounts. About 90 percent is stored in bones. When there is frequent exposure to lead-containing items (e.g., paint, batteries, gasoline, pottery, bullets, printing materials) or occupations (mining, auto, printing, and welding industries), many organs of the body are affected. The blood test is considered the best indicator of lead poisoning, and confirmation is made by the lead mobilization test performed on a 24-hour urine specimen.

Indications

- Diagnose and treat lead poisoning

Reference Values

		SI Units
Blood		
Child	<10 μg/dL	<0.1 μg/mL
Adult	<20 μg/dL	<0.2 μg/mL
Serum, screening	0.8–2.5 ng/mL	
Urine (24-h)	<80 μg	<0.8 μg
Hair, nails (1 g)	<25 μg/g	

Abnormal Values

	Toxic Level	*SI Units*
Blood		
Child	≥20 μg/dL	≥0.2 μg/mL
Adult	≥30 μg/dL	≥0.3 μg/dL
Urine (24-h)	>400 μg	
CDC classification of blood levels in children		
No poisoning		>10 μg/dL
Frequent rescreening with prevention actions		10–14 μg/dL
Nutritional and education interventions		15–19 μg/dL
Consider chelation therapy		20–44 μg/dL
Environmental interventions and chelation therapy		45–69 μg/dL
Medical emergency		>69 μg/dL

- Increased levels
    Anemia
    Lead encephalopathy
    Metal poisoning
    Peripheral neuropathy

Interfering Factors

- Results are invalid if specimen is not collected with correct preservative (urine test) or anticoagulant (blood or serum).
- High dietary intake of foods containing calcium can affect results.
- Failure to collect all urine during 24-hour test period will interfere with results.

Nursing Implications

Assessment

- Obtain history of environmental or occupational exposure to lead, general health, and medication regimen.
- Assess for adequate urinary output of more than 30 mL/h, baseline urinalysis, urine coproporphyrin level, blood urea nitrogen, and serum creatinine, calcium, and phosphorus levels.

Possible Nursing Diagnoses

Injury, risk for, related to effect of lead on body organs
Anxiety related to threat to health
Knowledge deficit related to sources of lead and prevention

Implementation

- *Blood*: Put on gloves. Using aseptic technique, perform a venipuncture using a 20-ga stainless steel needle or a butterfly collection device. Collect 3 mL of blood in a lead-free, heparinized tube and send to laboratory for determination of lead levels. Special lead-free tubes may be obtained from the testing laboratory.
- *Urine*: Obtain a 3-liter plastic container that has been washed with 10% HCl acid for 10 minutes and rinsed with 5 volumes of deionized or distilled water. Add 20 mL of specified preservative at start of collection. Follow laboratory directions for any special care of the specimen during collection, such as refrigerating or placing in ice.
- Begin the test between 6 and 8 AM if possible; collect and discard first voiding. Record the time specimen was discarded as the beginning of the 24-hour test.
- Encourage oral intake of fluids throughout the collection period, except for persons with lead encephalopathy, owing to the risk of increasing intracranial pressure.
- Monitor intake and output during the test. Diminished urine output can indicate lead toxicity.
- The next morning, ask the client to void at the same time the collection was started and add this last voiding to the container.
- If an indwelling catheter is in place, replace tubing and container system with the preservative and keep drainage bag on ice, or empty the urine into a large refrigerated container with the preservative every hour during the 24 hours. Monitor to ensure continued drainage and conclude the test the next morning at the same hour the collection was begun.

■ At the conclusion of the test ensure that label is properly completed with total output and starting and ending times, and transport specimen to the laboratory immediately.

Evaluation

■ Compare quantity of urine in specimen container with urinary output record during collection time. If specimen contains less urine than was recorded as output, some of the urine sample may have been discarded, and results are invalidated.

■ Note test results in relation to client's symptoms and other tests performed. The urine test confirms elevated serum levels.

Client/Caregiver Teaching

Pretest

■ Tell the client to follow a low-calorie diet for 3 days before the urine test.

■ Inform the client that all urine for a 24-hour period must be saved; monitor all urine output in chart. Instruct client to avoid voiding in pan with defecation and to keep toilet tissue out of pan to prevent contamination of the specimen.

■ Tell the client to void all urine in a bedpan placed in the toilet and then either pour urine into the collection container or leave in the container for the nurse or caregiver to add to the collection; place a sign in the bathroom as a reminder to save all urine.

Posttest

■ Resume medications withheld before the test, as ordered.

■ Inform the client that as blood lead is chelated and excreted in urine, levels can increase again as stored lead is mobilized. The test can be repeated in 2 to 4 days if needed.

■ Instruct client to avoid exposure to lead products. Prevent children from eating paint chips. Consider protection from lead in the work environment.

■ Inform the client to notify physician if anorexia, vomiting, irritability, apathy, or abdominal pain indicating lead poisoning or lead intoxication develops.

Legionnaires' Disease Antibodies

Classification: Serology

Type of Test: Serum

This test is used to identify specific antibodies produced after the body has been injected with the *Legionella* organism. Antibody titers are low the first week, gradually rise during the second and third weeks, and reach maximum levels at five weeks. Titers drop slowly and remain elevated for many years.

Indications

- Detect antibody to *Legionella pneumophila*

Reference Values

- Negative or titer <1:256
- Less than a fourfold change in titer between acute and convalescent samples

Abnormal Values

- *Indication of infection at an undetermined time:* single titer of >1:256
- *Indication of recent infection:* fourfold rise in titer >1:128 from the acute to convalescent sample

Interfering Factors

- Hemolysis of the specimen invalidates results.

Nursing Implications

Assessment

- Obtain history of Legionnaires' disease or possible exposure to *Legionella*, signs and symptoms indicating possible infection, and results of other tests performed.

Possible Nursing Diagnoses

Anxiety related to threat to health

Gas exchange, impaired, related to inflammation

Airway clearance, ineffective, related to inflammation and edema

Spread of infection, risk for

Implementation

- Put on gloves. Using aseptic technique, perform a venipuncture and collect 7 mL of blood in a clotted red-top tube.
- Repeat procedure 14 days later to collect a convalescent sample.

Evaluation

- Note test results in relation to the client's symptoms and other tests performed. Also note original findings in relation to findings on repeated test.

Client/Caregiver Teaching

Pretest

- Inform the client that no special preparation is required before the test.

Posttest

- Instruct the client on treatment with erythromycin or rifampin, as indicated by test results.
- Inform the client of the need for additional blood sample collection in 2 weeks.

Leucine Aminopeptidase (LAP), Serum

Classification: Chemistry

Type of Test: Serum

This test measures leucine aminopeptidase (LAP), an isoenzyme of alkaline phosphatase, an enzyme that cleaves phosphate from compounds and is optimally active at a pH of 9. It is widely distributed in body tissues, with greatest concentrations found in hepatobiliary tissues, the pancreas, and the small intestine. Serum levels tend to parallel serum alkaline phosphatase levels in hepatic disease.

Indications

- Evaluate elevated alkaline phosphatase of uncertain etiology
- Evaluate suspected liver, pancreatic, and biliary diseases
- Differentiate skeletal disease from hepatobiliary or pancreatic disease when alkaline phosphatase levels are elevated
- Evaluate neonatal jaundice

Reference Values

	Goldberg-Rutenberg	*SI Units*
Men	80–200 U/mL	19.2–48.0 U/L
Women	75–185 U/mL	18.0–44.4 U/L

Abnormal Values

- Elevated levels
    Biliary obstruction from gallstones; tumors, including those of the head of the pancreas; strictures; and atresia
    Advanced pregnancy
    Therapy with drugs containing estrogen and progesterone

Interfering Factors

Advanced pregnancy and therapy with drugs containing estrogen and progesterone may falsely elevate levels.

Nursing Implications

Assessment

- Obtain history of known or suspected disorders of the hepatic and biliary tract system.
- Ensure client has fasted from food for 8 hours before the test, as required by the laboratory.

Possible Nursing Diagnoses

Fatigue related to decreased metabolic energy production
Pain related to inflammation of affected organ

Implementation

- Put on gloves. Using aseptic technique, perform a venipuncture and collect 7 mL of blood in a red-top tube.
- Handle the sample gently to avoid hemolysis and transport to the laboratory promptly.

Evaluation

- Note results of alkaline phosphatase and alanine aminotransferase (ALT) in relation to levels of LAP.

Client/Caregiver Teaching

Pretest

- Tell the client to fast from food for 8 hours before the test, as required by the laboratory.
- Instruct the client to withhold drugs containing estrogen and progesterone.

Posttest

- Tell the client to resume usual diet and medication regimen.

Leucine Aminopeptidase (LAP), Urine

Classification: Chemistry

Type of Test: Urine (timed)

A test to measure leucine aminopeptidase (LAP), an isoenzyme of alkaline phosphatase, an enzyme that cleaves phosphate from compounds and is optimally active at a pH of 9. Although widely distributed in body tissues, LAP is most abundant in hepatobiliary tissues, the pancreas, and the small intestine. Urine levels lag behind serum elevations and may remain elevated after serum levels return to normal.

Indications

- Evaluate elevated serum alkaline phosphatase or leucine aminopeptidase levels of unknown etiology
- Evaluate suspected liver, pancreatic, and biliary diseases, including cancers, especially when serum LAP levels are normal

Reference Values

- 2–18 U/24 h

Abnormal Values

- Elevated levels
  Cirrhosis
  Hepatitis
  Cancer involving the liver or pancreas
  Pancreatitis
  Biliary obstruction due to gallstones, strictures, and atresia

Interfering Factors

- Advanced pregnancy and medications such as estrogens and progesterone can falsely elevate LAP levels.
- Excessive or strenuous exercise can affect test results.

Nursing Implications

Assessment

- Assess and obtain a history of known or suspected hepatobiliary and pancreatic disease and medication regimen.

Possible Nursing Diagnoses

Fatigue related to decreased metabolic energy production
Pain related to inflammation of affected organ

Implementation

- Obtain a clean 3-liter container or 24-hour urine bag or bottle with or without preservative, according to laboratory policy. Place the container on ice throughout collection period unless preservative has been added. If an indwelling urinary catheter is in place, the drainage bag must be kept on ice.
- Begin the test between 6 and 8 AM if possible; collect first voiding and discard; record the time specimen was discarded as the beginning of the 24-hour test. Document the

quantity of urine output during collection period, including urine at end of 24-hour period.

■ The next morning, ask the client to void at the same time the collection was started and add this last voiding to the container.

■ If an indwelling catheter is in place, replace tubing and container system and empty the urine into a large refrigerated container periodically during the 24 hours; monitor to ensure continued drainage and conclude the test the next morning at the same hour the collection was begun.

■ At the conclusion of the test, make sure that the container is properly labeled; include start and completion times and any medications that the client was taking that may alter test results. Transport specimen to the laboratory immediately.

Evaluation

■ Note results and compare with serum LAP and alkaline phosphate findings.

Client/Caregiver Teaching

Pretest

■ Inform the client that all urine for a 24-hour period must be saved. Instruct client to avoid voiding in pan with defecation and to keep toilet tissue out of the pan to prevent contamination of the specimen.

■ Inform the client that the sample must be kept refrigerated or on ice throughout the collection period, unless a preservative has been added to the container by the laboratory.

■ Tell the client to avoid excessive exercise and stress during the 24-hour collection of urine.

Posttest

■ Instruct the client to resume medications and activity withheld before the test.

Leukoagglutinin

Classification: Serology

Type of Test: Serum

Performed on blood donors and blood recipients, this test is used to detect presence of leukoagglutinin antibodies. When present, leukoagglutinin antibodies react with white blood cells (WBCs) and can cause transfusion reaction. These antibodies typically develop after exposure to foreign WBCs by a previous transfusion, pregnancy, or allograft. When a blood recipient has leukoagglutinin antibodies, a febrile, nonhemolytic reaction may occur 1 to 4 hours after initiation of whole blood, red blood cells, platelet, or granulocyte transfusion. This type of reaction must be differentiated from a hemolytic reaction before transfusion can proceed. When a blood donor has leukoagglutinin antibodies, the recipient can develop acute, noncardiogenic pulmonary edema. Two tests are used to detect for presence of leukoagglutinins: a microscopic examination of the person's serum after it is combined with a suspension of granulocytes and lymphocytes; and a newer method, a fluorescence microscope examination that detects antibodies attached to normal granulocytes incubated with recipient or donor serum. The latter test is more sensitive and more widely used.

Indications

- Distinguish between hemolytic and febrile nonhemolytic transfusion reactions
- Detect leukoagglutinins in a blood transfusion donor after a reaction has occurred in the recipient

Reference Values

- Negative; agglutination does not occur because the serum contains no antibodies

Abnormal Values

- *Recipient's blood*: A positive result (agglutination) indicates presence of leukoagglutinins. This indicates the recipient's reaction was a febrile, nonhemolytic reaction to these antibodies.

- *Donor's blood*: A positive result indicates presence of leukoagglutinins and suggests the recipient's reaction as acute noncardiogenic pulmonary edema.

Interfering Factors

- Previous administration of dextran or IV contrast media causes aggregation resembling agglutination.

Nursing Implications

Assessment

- Obtain history of previous blood donation or blood transfusion, posttransfusion reaction, pregnancy, or allograft procedures.
- Obtain history of recent administration of dextran or testing with IV contrast media, which could cause aggregation resembling agglutination.

Possible Nursing Diagnosis

Injury, risk for, related to threat of allergic reaction from blood transfusion

Implementation

- If a transfusion recipient has a positive leukoagglutinin antibody result, prevent further reactions by premedicating with acetaminophen 1 to 2 hours before transfusion as prescribed, or by using specially prepared leukocyte-poor blood, or both.
- Put on gloves. Using aseptic technique, perform a venipuncture and collect 10 mL of blood in a red-top tube.
- Indicate on laboratory slip the client's suspected diagnoses and any history of transfusion, pregnancies, and drug therapy.

Evaluation

- Note test results and administer ordered medications, as indicated.

Client/Caregiver Teaching

Posttest

- If a donor has a positive leukoagglutinin test, explain the meaning of this result to prevent future transfusion reactions.

Leukocyte Alkaline Phosphatase Stain, Neutrophil Alkaline Phosphatase

Classification: Hematology

Type of Test: Blood

Alkaline phosphatase is an enzyme present in cytoplasm of neutrophilic granulocytes from the metamyelocyte to the segmented stage and represents intracellular metabolism. Levels of leukocyte alkaline phosphatase (LAP) may be altered by infection, stress, chronic inflammatory diseases, Hodgkin's disease, and hematologic disorders. Levels are low in leukemic leukocytes and high in normal white blood cells, making this test useful as a supportive test in the differential diagnosis of leukemia. It should be noted that test results must be correlated with the client's condition since LAP levels increase toward normal in response to therapy.

Indications

- Differentiate chronic myelocytic leukemia (CML) from other disorders that increase the WBC count

Reference Values

- 40–130, depending on the laboratory's standard; score is based on a 0–4 rating of 100 neutrophils. Normal values are found in chronic lymphocytic or myelomonocytic leukemia, lymphosarcoma, multiple myeloma, relative polycythemia, and sickle cell anemia.

Abnormal Values

- Increased values
    Chronic inflammation
    Down's syndrome
    Hodgkin's disease

Leukemia (acute lymphoblastic or hairy cell)
Myelofibrosis with myeloid metaplasia
Neutrophilic leukemoid reaction (from infection, chronic inflammation, or pregnancy)
Polycythemia vera
Stress
Pregnancy
Thrombocytopenia infection
Certain drugs, including adrenocorticotropic hormones (ACTH)
■ Decreased values
Acute granulocytic leukemia
Aplastic anemia
Chronic granulocytic leukemia
CML
Cirrhosis
Collagen disease
Congestive heart failure
Diabetes mellitus
Gout
Granulocytopenia
Hereditary hypophosphatemia
Idiopathic thrombocytopenia purpura
Infectious mononucleosis
Paroxysmal nocturnal hemoglobinuria
Sarcoidosis

Interfering Factors

■ Blood specimens collected in EDTA-anticoagulated tube affect test results and should be rejected.

Nursing Implications

Assessment

■ Obtain history of known or suspected diseases associated with LAP, presence of infection or inflammatory disease, and pregnancy.

Possible Nursing Diagnoses

Anxiety related to threat to health
Infection, risk for, related to immunosuppression

Implementation

■ Put on gloves. Using aseptic technique, perform a venipuncture or finger stick; collect 7 mL of blood in a green-top tube containing heparin or in an oxalate-anticoagulated black-top tube.

■ Handle specimen gently to avoid hemolysis and send to laboratory promptly.

Evaluation

■ Note test results in relation to the client's symptoms and other tests performed, particularly WBC with differential, platelet count, and hemoglobin.

Client/Caregiver Teaching

Posttest

■ Tell the client to avoid exposure to infection if WBC count is decreased.

Lipase

Classification: Chemistry

Type of Test: Serum

This test measures serum lipase, an enzyme that is secreted by the pancreas into the duodenum. Different lipolytic enzymes have different specific substrates, but overall activity is collectively described as lipase. Lipase participates in fat digestion by breaking down triglycerides into fatty acids and glycerol. Lipase is released into the blood when damage occurs to the pancreatic acinar cells. Its presence in the blood indicates pancreatic disease since it is the only organ that secretes this enzyme.

Indications

■ Diagnose acute pancreatitis, especially if the client has been ill for more than 3 days with a return of values to normal after 3 days, but serum lipase remains elevated for approximately 10 days after onset

■ Diagnose pancreatic carcinoma, especially if there is a sustained moderate elevation in serum lipase levels

- Diagnose other disorders associated with elevated or decreased serum lipase levels (see Abnormal Values)

Reference Values

		SI Units
Infants	9–105 IU/L at 37°C	
Children	20–136 IU/L at 37°C	
Adults	0–1.5 U/mL (Cherry-Crandall)	0–417 U/L
	20–180 IU/L or 14–280 mU/mL	14–280 U/L

Values may vary according to the laboratory performing the test.

Abnormal Values

- Elevated levels
  - Acute cholecystitis
  - Acute pancreatitis
  - Early pancreatic carcinoma
  - Early renal failure
  - Obstruction of pancreatic duct
  - Pancreatic inflammation
  - Pancreatitis
  - Perforated peptic ulcer
  - Certain drugs, including morphine, cholinergic drugs, and heparin
- Decreased levels
  - Advanced chronic pancreatitis
  - Advanced pancreatic carcinoma
  - Cystic fibrosis
  - Disorders in which bile salts are decreased
  - Protamine and intravenous infusions of saline
  - Viral hepatitis

Interfering Factors

- Morphine, cholinergic drugs, and heparin may lead to elevated levels.
- Protamine and intravenous infusions of saline may lead to decreased levels.
- Endoscopic retrograde cholangiopancreatography (ERCP) procedure may increase the values.
- Traumatic venipuncture can decrease lipase values.

Nursing Implications

Assessment

- Obtain a history of pancreatic disease and the results of any tests and procedures performed.
- Assess medication history; ensure that any drugs that may alter test results have been withheld for 12 to 24 hours before the test, as ordered by the physician.
- Ensure that the client has fasted for 8 to 12 hours before the test.

Possible Nursing Diagnoses

Infection, risk for, related to immunosuppression
Pain related to the disease

Implementation

- Put on gloves. Using aseptic technique, perform a venipuncture and collect 7 mL of blood in a red-top tube.
- Handle the sample gently to avoid hemolysis and transport to the laboratory promptly.

Evaluation

- Note results in relation to serum amylase levels in pancreatic disease.

Client/Caregiver Teaching

Pretest

- Tell the client to fast for 8 to 12 hours and to withhold medications that could alter test results for 12 to 24 hours before the test.

Posttest

- Tell the client to resume usual diet and medications withheld before the test.

Lipoprotein Electrophoresis, Lipoprotein-Cholesterol Fractionation

Classification: Chemistry

Type of Test: Serum

This test measures lipoprotein fractions by electrophoresis to determine abnormal distribution and concentration of lipoproteins in the serum, an important risk factor in the development of coronary artery disease. The lipoprotein fractions in relation to density are (1) chylomicrons, (2) very low density lipoproteins (VLDL), (3) low-density lipoproteins (LDL), and (4) high-density lipoproteins (HDL). Chylomicrons and VLDL contain the highest levels of triglycerides and lower amounts of cholesterol and protein. LDL and HDL contain the lowest amounts of triglycerides and relatively higher amounts of cholesterol and protein.

Indications

- Evaluate clients with serum cholesterol levels greater than 250 mg/dL, indicating a high risk for cardiovascular disease
- Evaluate known or suspected disorders associated with altered lipoprotein levels (see Abnormal Values)
- Evaluate response to treatment for altered levels and support for decisions regarding the need for drug therapy

Reference Values

Total lipoproteins	400–800 mg/dL
Lipoprotein fractions	
Chylomicrons	0%
VLDL or pre-beta	3–32%
LDL or beta	38–40%
HDL or alpha	20–48%

Age	LDL Cholesterol	SI Units	HDL Cholesterol	SI Units
<25 yr	73–138 mg/dL	0.73–2.48 g/L	32–57 mg/dL	0.32–0.57 g/L
25–40 yr	90–180 mg/dL	0.90–1.80 g/L	32–60 mg/dL	0.32–0.60 g/L
40–50 yr	100–185 mg/dL	1.00–1.85 g/L	33–60 mg/dL	0.33–0.66 g/L
50–65 yr	105–190 mg/dL	1.05–1.90 g/L	34–70 mg/dL	0.34–0.70 g/L
>65 yr	105–200 mg/dL	1.05–2.0 g/L	35–75 mg/dL	0.35–0.75 g/L

Abnormal Values

Lipoprotein	Increased Level	Decreased Level
Chylomicrons	Ingested fat Ingested alcohol Types I and V hyperlipoproteinemia	Normal value is zero
VLDL	Ingested fat Ingested carbohydrate Ingested alcohol All types of hyperlipoproteinemia Exogenous estrogens Diabetes mellitus Hypothyroidism (primary) Nephrotic syndrome Alcoholism Pancreatitis Pregnancy	Abetalipoproteinemia Cirrhosis Hypobetalipoproteinemia
LDL-cholesterol	Ingested cholesterol Ingested saturated fatty acids Types II and III hyperlipoproteinemia Hypothyroidism (primary) Biliary obstruction Nephrotic syndrome	Types I and V hyperlipoproteinemia Hypobetalipoproteinemia Abetalipoproteinemia Hyperthyroidism Cirrhosis
HDL-cholesterol	Ingested alcohol (moderate amounts) Chronic hepatitis Hypothyroidism (primary) Early biliary cirrhosis Biliary obstruction	All types of hyperlipoproteinemia Exogenous estrogens Hyperthyroidism Cirrhosis Tangier disease

From Watson, J and Jaffe, MS: Nurse's Manual of Laboratory and Diagnostic Tests, ed. 2. FA Davis, Philadelphia, 1995, p. 179, with permission.

Interfering Factors

- Failure to follow usual diet for 2 weeks before the test can yield results that do not accurately reflect client status.
- Ingestion of alcohol 24 hours before the test, ingestion of food 12 hours before the test, and excessive exercise 12 hours before the test can alter results.
- Numerous drugs can alter results (see Abnormal Values for cholesterol and triglycerides).

Nursing Implications

Assessment

- Obtain history of cardiovascular status, risk for heart disease, and results of lipid tests.
- Ensure that client has withheld drugs that may alter lipoprotein components for 24 to 48 hours before the test, as ordered.
- Ensure that client has abstained from alcohol intake for 24 hours, from food for 12 to 14 hours, and from excessive exercise for 12 hours before the test.
- Ensure that client has maintained regular diet for 2 weeks before the test.

Possible Nursing Diagnoses

Nutrition, altered, risk for more than body requirements
Injury, risk for, related to the disease

Implementation

- Put on gloves. Using aseptic technique, perform a venipuncture and collect 7 mL of blood in a red-top tube.
- Handle sample gently and send to the laboratory promptly.

Evaluation

- Note test results in relation to serum cholesterol and other lipid tests performed.

Client/Caregiver Teaching

Pretest

- Tell the client to maintain a normal diet for 2 weeks before the test.
- Tell the client to fast from food for 12 to 14 hours, to abstain from alcohol for 24 hours, and to avoid strenuous exercise for 12 hours before the test.

- Tell the client to withhold drugs that can interfere with test results, as ordered.

Posttest

- Tell the client to resume diet, activity, and medication withheld before the test.
- Instruct client in dietary management of fat intake based on test results. LDL cholesterol levels may decrease with dietary modification alone; if not, drug treatment is recommended.
- Inform the client that regular exercise has been found to lower HDL-cholesterol levels, as appropriate.

Lipoprotein Phenotyping

Classification: Chemistry

Type of Test: Serum

This test measures five major lipoprotein distribution patterns (phenotypes) seen in clients with serums high in cholesterol or triglycerides. These phenotypes, which are referred to by their assigned numbers, have been correlated with genetically determined abnormalities (familial or primary hyperlipoproteinemias) and with a variety of acquired conditions (secondary hyperlipoproteinemias).

Indications

- Evaluate elevated serum cholesterol levels and lipoprotein and cholesterol fractionation
- Evaluate predisposition to familial primary hyperlipoproteinemia (hyperlipidemia)
- Identify the client's specific lipoprotein phenotype
- Identify known or suspected disorders associated with the several lipoprotein phenotypes (see Abnormal Values)

Reference Values

See table.

| | PHENOTYPE | | | | | |
	I	IIa	IIb	III	IV	V
Frequency	Very rare	Common	Common	Uncommon	Very common	Rare
Chylomicrons	↑↑	Normal	Normal	Normal or ↑	Normal	↑↑
Pre-β-lipoproteins (approximates VLDL)	↓	↑	↑	(these two bands merge)	↑↑	Normal or ↑
β-lipoproteins (approximates LDL)	↓	↑	↑	Normal	Normal or ↑	Normal or ↓
α₁-lipoproteins (approximates HDL)	Normal or ↑	Normal	Normal	Normal	Normal or ↓	
Total cholesterol	↑↑ or ↑	↑↑	↑	↑↑ or ↑↑↑	Normal or ↑	↑↑
Total triglycerides	↑↑↑↑	Normal	↑	↑↑↑	↑↑ or ↑↑↑	↑↑↑
Refrigerated serum or plasma	"Cream"/clear or turbid	Clear	+ or ++ turbid	+++ turbid	++ turbid	"Cream"/++ turbid

From Sacher, RA and McPherson, RA: Widmann's Clinical Interpretation of Laboratory Tests, ed 10. FA Davis, Philadelphia, 1991, p. 344, with permission.

Abnormal Values

Phenotype	May Occur Secondary to
I	Dysglobulinemias Insulin-dependent diabetes Lupus erythematosus Pancreatitis
II	Dysglobulinemias High-cholesterol diet Hypothyroidism Nephrotic syndrome Porphyria Obstructive liver diseases
III	Dysglobulinemias Hypothyroidism Uncontrolled diabetes
IV	Diabetes Glycogen storage disease High alcohol intake Nephrotic syndrome Oral contraceptives Obesity
V	Diabetes Hypercalcemia Nephrotic syndrome Pancreatitis High alcohol intake

Interfering Factors

- Failure to follow usual diet for 2 weeks before the test may yield results that do not accurately reflect client status.
- Ingestion of alcohol 24 hours or food 12 hours before the test, or excessive exercise 12 hours before the test, may affect test results.
- Because venous obstruction for more than 2 minutes can affect results, the lipoprotein phenotyping sample must be drawn first if multiple blood samples are being taken.
- Certain drugs, including alcohol, anabolic steroids, androgens, ascorbic acid, clofibrate, cholestyramine, colestipol, dextrothyroxine, corticosteroids, estrogen, furosemide, heparin, miconazole, niacin, norethindrone, oral contraceptives,

pergonal, sulfonylureas, and thyroid preparations can affect test results.

Nursing Implications

Assessment

- Obtain history of cardiovascular disease and the results of tests and procedures performed.
- Ensure that client has abstained from alcohol for 24 hours and withheld drugs that can alter lipoprotein components for 24 to 48 hours or longer before the test, as ordered.
- Ensure that client has consumed a low-fat meal the night before the test, then fasted for 12 hours before the test; water is not restricted.
- Ensure that client has avoided excessive exercise for at least 12 hours before the test.

Possible Nursing Diagnoses

Nutrition, altered, risk for more than body requirements
Injury, risk for, related to the disease

Implementation

- Put on gloves. Using aseptic technique, perform a venipuncture and collect 7-mL blood sample in a lavender-top tube; invert tube gently several times to mix the sample and anticoagulant.
- When obtaining multiple blood samples, collect the sample for lipoprotein phenotyping first because venous obstruction for 2 minutes can affect test results.
- Handle the sample gently to avoid hemolysis and send to the laboratory immediately.

Evaluation

- Note results in relation to other lipid tests performed and client's symptoms.

Client/Caregiver Teaching

Pretest

- Tell the client to follow usual diet for 2 weeks except for fasting for 12 to 14 hours before the test and to abstain from alcohol for 24 hours before the test.
- Tell the client to avoid exercise for 12 to 14 hours before the test.

Posttest

- Tell the client to resume diet, activity, and medications withheld before the test.
- Instruct the client and caregiver in dietary management of fat intake if lipid levels are elevated.

Lumbar Puncture: Cerebrospinal Fluid (CSF) Analysis

Classification: Invasive neurologic test

Type of Test: Fluid analysis

Analysis of cerebrospinal fluid (CSF), obtained by lumbar puncture, determines the fluid's various properties as well as any abnormal constituents. Routine CSF analysis includes a pressure reading, appearance, cell count and differential, as well as determinations of protein, including immunoglobulins, and glucose levels. CSF also may be analyzed for electrolytes, lactic acid, urea, glutamine, enzymes, and microorganisms. CSF is secreted by specialized capillaries called the choroid plexuses mainly in the lateral ventricles, although additional amounts are secreted in the third and fourth ventricles. It circulates into the central canal of the spinal cord and also enters the subarachnoid space through an opening in the wall of the fourth ventricle near the cerebellum, after which it circulates around the brain and spinal cord. Although 500 to 800 mL of CSF are formed daily, only 125 to 140 mL are normally present. Thus, most of the CSF formed is reabsorbed and is subsequently returned to the venous circulation. CSF functions include cushioning the brain against shocks and blows, maintaining a stable concentration of ions in the central nervous system (CNS), and providing for removal of wastes. Most constituents of CSF will parallel those found in plasma and are found in amounts equal to or slightly less than those in the blood.

Indications

- Diagnose viral meningitis, cerebral thrombosis, or brain tumor, as indicated by a cell count of 10 to 200/mm^3 consisting mostly of lymphocytes, a mild elevation (to 300 mg/dL) in total proteins, and normal or slightly decreased glucose level
- Diagnose multiple sclerosis or neurosyphilis, as indicated by a normal or slightly elevated cell count, consisting mostly of lymphocytes, slightly elevated protein, slightly elevated globulins, elevated IgG on protein electrophoresis, and a normal or slightly decreased glucose level
- Diagnose acute bacterial meningitis, as indicated by a cell count of greater than 500/mm^3, consisting largely of granulocytes, moderate or pronounced elevation in protein (greater than 300 mg/dL), pronounced decrease in glucose, and decreased chloride
- Diagnose tuberculous meningitis, as indicated by a cell count of 200 to 500/mm^3, consisting of lymphocytes or mixed lymphocytes and granulocytes, moderate or pronounced elevation in proteins, pronounced reduction in glucose, and decreased chloride
- Detect early bacterial or fungal meningitis, as indicated by CSF lactate level above 35 mg/dL even when cell count and glucose level are only slightly altered
- Diagnose CNS leukemia, as indicated by a cell count of 200 to 500/mm^3, consisting mainly of blast cells, and a moderate reduction in glucose
- Support diagnosis of spinal cord tumor, as indicated by a cell count of 10 to 200/mm^3, moderate or pronounced elevation in protein, and normal or slightly decreased glucose
- Support diagnosis of subarachnoid hemorrhage, as indicated by the presence of red blood cells, elevated proteins, and a moderate reduction in glucose
- Support diagnosis of hepatic encephalopathy, as indicated by elevated glutamine levels
- Support diagnosis of Guillain-Barré syndrome (ascending polyneuritis), as indicated by pronounced elevation in proteins
- Monitor treatment for bacterial or fungal meningitis, with effective treatment indicated by decreasing lactate levels after several days of antimicrobial therapy

Reference Values

Cell count and differential	
Children	20 small lymphocytes/mm^3
Adults	5 small lymphocytes/mm^3
Protein	
Total proteins	15–45 mg/dL (lumbar area) or <1% of serum levels
Albumin/globulin (A/G) ratio	8:1
IgG	3–12% of total protein
Glucose	40–80 mg/dL or <50–80% of blood glucose level 30 to 60 min earlier
Electrolytes	
Chloride	118–132 mEq/L
Calcium	2.1–2.7 mEq/L
Sodium	144–154 mEq/L
Potassium	2.4–3.1 mEq/L
Lactic acid	10–20 mg/dL
Urea	10–15 mg/dL
Glutamine	<20 mg/dL
Lactic dehydrogenase (LDH)	1/10 that of serum level

Abnormal Values

- Increased levels
    Acute anterior poliomyelitis (protein, WBC)
    Aseptic meningeal reaction (protein, WBC)
    Brain abscess (pressure, protein, lactic acid, neutrophils, bacteria)
    Brain tumors (pressure, protein, glucose)
    Cerebral hemorrhage (RBC, pressure, lactic acid, protein)
    Cerebral thrombosis (protein, lymphocytes)
    Cerebral trauma (pressure, glucose)
    Coccidioidomycosis (pressure, protein, WBC)
    Cord tumor (protein, WBC)
    Diabetic ketoacidosis (glucose)
    Diabetes mellitus (protein)
    Encephalitis (pressure, lymphocytes, bacteria)
    Guillain-Barré syndrome (protein)
    Head trauma (pressure, protein)
    Herpes zoster (protein, WBC)
    Infections (protein)
    Hyperglycemia (glucose)
    Hypothalamic lesions (glucose)

Lead encephalopathy (pressure, protein, WBC)

Meningitis (acute, pyrogenic) (pressure, protein, neutrophils, bacteria)

Meningitis (aseptic) (pressure, protein, WBC)

Meningitis (cryptococcal, fungal, tuberculous, viral) (pressure, lactic acid, protein, lymphocytes, bacteria)

Meningoencephalitis (primary amebic) (pressure, protein, WBC)

Measles (pressure, protein, WBC)

Multiple sclerosis (protein, lactic acid, lymphocytes [oligoclonal bands])

Mumps (pressure, protein, WBC)

Polyneuritis (protein, lymphocytes)

Pseudotumor cerebri (pressure)

Subarachnoid hemorrhage (pressure, protein)

Subdural hematoma (pressure, protein, lymphocytes)

Syphilis (protein, lymphocytes, positive VDRL)

Uremia (pressure, protein, glucose)

Viral infections (Coxsackie and echovirus) (neutrophils)

- Decreased CSF glucose levels

Brain abscess

Brain tumor

Cancer

Sarcoidosis (CNS)

Coccidioidomycosis

Encephalitis (mumps or herpes simplex)

Hypoglycemia

Increased intracranial pressure

Leukemia

Lupus myelopathy

Lymphocytic choriomeningitis

Lymphoma

Melanomatosis

Meningeal carcinomatosis

Meningitis (acute pyrogenic, aseptic, chemical, cryptococcal, fungal, granulomatous, pyrogenic, rheumatoid, tuberculous, viral)

Neurosyphilis

Rheumatoid arthritis

Subarachnoid hemorrhage

Toxoplasmosis

Tuberculoma of brain

Interfering Factors

- Positioning and activity (such as crying, coughing, or straining) of the client can alter CSF pressure.

- Delay in transporting sample to the laboratory or delay in analysis may cause spurious discoloration from lysis of any red cells present, disintegration of any neutrophils present, and false decrease in glucose due to continual glucose utilization by cells in the sample.
- Blood in the sample due to traumatic tap adds 1 to 2 white cells and 1 mg/dL of protein for every 1000 red cells/mm^3 contained in the sample.

> **NURSING ALERT**

- This procedure is contraindicated in infection near the lumbar puncture site since infected material can enter the spinal space.
- Procedure should be performed with extreme caution in clients with increased intracranial pressure, since it may induce cerebellar tonsillar herniation and medullary compression, and in clients with severe degenerative vertebral joint disease, since it is difficult to pass the needle through the degenerative arthritic interspinal space.

Nursing Implications

Assessment

- Obtain history of illness and symptoms and known or suspected diseases associated with CSF.
- Perform a baseline neurologic assessment, including movement, strength, and sensation of legs and vital signs.

Possible Nursing Diagnoses

Anxiety related to procedure and threat to health status
Pain, risk for, related to procedure and possible posttest headache
Injury or infection, risk for, related to procedure

Implementation

- Instruct the client to empty the bladder and bowel before the procedure.
- Assist the client to a side-lying position, with the head flexed as far as comfortable and the knees drawn up toward, but not pressing on, the abdomen; support in maintaining this position may be provided by placing one hand on the back of the client's neck and the other behind the knees.

- Cleanse the lumbar area with an antiseptic and place sterile drapes.
- The physician infiltrates the area with a local anesthetic and inserts the spinal needle with stylet into a vertebral interspace between L2 to S1. The stylet is removed and the needle properly positioned in the subarachnoid space until spinal fluid drops from the needle.
- A sterile stopcock and manometer are then attached to the needle and the opening pressure is read. (Note: when the needle and manometer are properly positioned, the CSF level should fluctuate several millimeters with respiration.)
- The manometer is then removed and CSF is allowed to drip into three sterile test tubes, 3 to 10 mL per tube; the tubes are numbered in order of filling, labeled with the client's name, and sent to the laboratory immediately.
- The manometer may then be reattached and the closing pressure recorded. The spinal needle is removed and pressure is applied to the site.

Evaluation

- Assess for changes in neurologic status, including increased temperature, increased blood pressure, irritability, numbness and tingling in the lower extremities, and nonreactive pupils.
- Assess the puncture site for bleeding, CSF drainage, and inflammation each time vital signs are taken during the first 24 hours and daily thereafter for several days.
- Assess presence or absence of headache and administer analgesic as ordered to relieve a headache.
- Note test results in relation to the client's symptoms and other tests performed, particularly neurologic tests and WBC.

Client/Caregiver Teaching

Pretest

- Inform the client of the test's purpose: that it will be done by a physician at the bedside and will take 20 to 30 minutes.
- Inform the client about the position that is needed for the procedure and the need to remain still.
- Inform the client that a local anesthetic will be injected at the needle insertion site; that the needle is inserted below the area where the spinal cord ends; and that a sensation of pressure may be felt when the needle is inserted.

Posttest

- Inform the client to lie prone (flat or horizontal) for 6 to 8 hours after the procedure to prevent occurrence of a head-

ache; inform the client that turning from side to side is permitted as long as the head is not raised.
- Encourage the client to take liberal amounts of fluids, unless otherwise contraindicated.
- Inform the client and caregiver that assistance with eating and elimination is required.
- Inform the client to notify health care provider if any of the following occur: numbness, tingling, or impaired movement of extremities; pain at the puncture site; drainage of blood or spinal fluid at the puncture site.

Luteinizing Hormone (LH, ICSH)

Classification: Chemistry

Type of Test: Serum

This test is a quantitative analysis of luteinizing hormone (LH), a hormone secreted by the anterior pituitary gland in response to stimulation by gonadotropin-releasing hormone (GnRH), the same hypothalamic releasing factor that stimulates follicle-stimulating hormone (FSH) release. LH affects gonadal function in both men and women. In women, a surge of LH occurs at the midpoint of the menstrual cycle and is believed to be induced by high estrogen levels. LH causes the ovum to be expelled from the ovary and stimulates development of the corpus luteum and progesterone production. As progesterone levels rise, LH production decreases. In men, LH stimulates the interstitial cells of Leydig, located in the testes, to produce testosterone.

Indications

- Evaluate male and female infertility, as indicated by decreased levels
- Support diagnosis of infertility due to anovulation, as evidenced by lack of the midcycle LH surge
- Evaluate response to therapy to induce ovulation
- Evaluate children with precocious puberty

Reference Values

		SI Units
Boys	4–12 mIU/mL	4–12 IU/L
Girls	2–14 mIU/mL	2–14 IU/L
Men	6–30 mIU/mL	6–30 IU/L
Women (menstruating)		
Early in cycle	5–25 mIU/mL	5–25 IU/L
Midcycle	75–150 mIU/mL	75–150 IU/L
Luteal phase	5–40 mIU/mL	5–40 IU/L
Women (menopausal)	30–200 mIU/mL	30–200 IU/L

Abnormal Values

- Increased levels
    Adrenogenital syndrome in females
    Early acromegaly
    Klinefelter's syndrome in males
    Ovarian or testicular failure
    Pituitary tumors
    Stein-Leventhal syndrome
    Postviral orchitis
    Precocious puberty in children
    Turner's syndrome in females
    Drugs containing estrogen
- Decreased levels
    Anorexia nervosa
    Cirrhosis
    Excessive sex hormone production
    Hypothalamic lesions
    Panhypopituitarism
    Renal disease
    Testicular cancer
    Drugs containing progesterone and testosterone

Interfering Factors

- Radioactive scans performed within 1 week before the test may affect test results.
- In menstruating women, values vary in relation to the phase of the menstrual cycle.
- Certain drugs, including those that contain estrogen, which can increase levels, and progesterone and testosterone, which can decrease levels.

Nursing Implications

Assessment

- Obtain a history of endocrine and reproductive systems, a menstrual history including date of last period, and the results of any diagnostic tests and procedures.
- Assess medication history; ensure that any drugs that may alter LH levels have been withheld for 12 to 24 hours before the test, as ordered by the physician.

Possible Nursing Diagnoses

Anxiety related to altered self-concept
Coping, individual, ineffective

Implementation

- Put on gloves. Using aseptic technique, perform a venipuncture and collect 7 mL of blood in a red-top tube.
- For female clients, indicate the phase of the menstrual cycle or indicate menopause on the laboratory slip.
- Handle the sample gently to avoid hemolysis and transport to the laboratory immediately.

Evaluation

- Note results in relation to other tests of gonadal function (follicle-stimulating hormone) and client symptoms.

Client/Caregiver Teaching

Pretest

- Tell the client to withhold steroids and hormones including estrogen, progesterone, and testosterone for 48 hours before the test, as ordered by the physician.

Posttest

- Tell the client to resume medications withheld before the test.
- If the test is being performed to detect ovulation, inform the client that it may be necessary to obtain a series of samples over a period of several days to detect peak LH levels.

Lyme Disease Antibody

Classification: Serology

Type of Test: Blood

This test uses immunofluorescent assay to identify the tick-borne spirochete *Borrelia burgdorferi*, the organism that causes Lyme disease. About half of the clients infected with early-stage Lyme, and all of those with cardiac, neurologic, and rheumatoid manifestations, will have a positive result. Clients in remission will also have a positive response.

Indications

- Confirm diagnosis of Lyme disease

Reference Values

- Negative or titer <1:128

Abnormal Values

- Fourfold increase

Interfering Factors

- Hemolysis of sample may affect test results.
- High rheumatoid factor titers and treponemal diseases may cause false-positive results.
- Blood sample with high lipid levels may alter test results. Test needs to be repeated after the client has restricted fat in the diet.

Nursing Implications

Assessment

- Obtain history of known or suspected exposure to ticks. Assess for tick bite and macular lesion surrounding bite.

Possible Nursing Diagnoses

Anxiety related to threat to health status
Pain related to the disease

Implementation

- Put on gloves. Using aseptic technique, perform a venipuncture and collect 7 mL of blood in a red-top tube.
- Handle sample gently to avoid hemolysis and send promptly to the laboratory.

Evaluation

- Note test results in relation to other tests performed and the client's symptoms.

Client/Caregiver Teaching

Posttest

- Tell the client to report signs and symptoms related to the disease process.
- Tell the client to wear light-colored clothing that covers extremities when in areas infested by deer ticks, and to check body for ticks after returning from infested area.
- Tell the client to see physician if bitten by tick or if a macular rash develops.

Magnetic Resonance Imaging (MRI), Abdominal Nuclear Magnetic Resonance (NMR) Imaging

Classification: Nuclear medicine

Type of Test: Indirect visualization with contrast medium

Magnetic resonance imaging (MRI) produces cross-sectional images of the abdominal area in multiple planes without the use of ionizing radiation or the interference of bone. Use of magnetic fields with the aid of radio frequency energy produces images primarily based on water content of tissue, therefore enabling the scanner to "see through" bone.

MRI of the abdomen is done alone or in conjunction with computed tomography (CT) scanning to diagnose abnormalities of the abdominal and pelvic organs. However, computed tomography scanning is a better diagnostic tool for abdominal pathology (with exception of liver assessment) because it can distinguish organs from one another.

Contrast enhancement can be used with MRI. This contrast medium Magnevist (gadolinium-diethylenetriaminopentaacetic acid) is unlike the iodinated contrast dye used in computed tomography scanning administered intravenously to enhance contrast differences between normal and abnormal tissues. Geritol and gadolinium are the media used for stomach and bowel imaging (to decrease lumen signal intensity resulting from bowel peristalsis); glucagon is administered to improve visualization of the pancreas (by removing artifacts resulting from stomach and bowel peristalsis). Ferrite iron oxide is the medium used for assessment of spleen, liver, and pancreas imaging.

Indications

- Diagnose cancer (primary or metastatic tumors of liver, pancreas, prostatic, uterine, and bladder) and provide staging
- Diagnose chronic pancreatitis
- Determine vascular complications of pancreatitis, for example, venous thrombosis, or pseudoaneurysm
- Differentiate liver tumors from liver abnormalities such as cysts, cavernous hemangiomas, and hepatic amebic abscesses
- Diagnose renal vein thrombosis
- Diagnose soft-tissue abnormalities
- Determine and monitor tissue damage in renal transplant clients
- Diagnose demyelinating disease such as multiple sclerosis
- Diagnose other abdominal abnormalities such as blood clots, cysts, edema, hemorrhage, abscesses, infarctions, or aneurysms
- Evaluate effectiveness of medical and surgical interventions and course of disease

Reference Values

- Normal anatomic structures and soft-tissue density and biochemical constituents of body tissues

Abnormal Values

- Acute tubular necrosis
- Glomerulonephritis
- Hydronephrosis
- Masses, lesions, infections, or inflammations
- Obstruction of vena cava
- Renal vein thrombosis

Interfering Factors

- Client movement during the procedure will affect results and make interpretation difficult.
- Metallic objects within the examination field, such as jewelry, watches, implanted infusion devices or pumps; metallic or other implants, including heart valves, cochlear or orthopedic prosthesis, rods or screws; dentures, hairpins or clips; pacemaker, aneurysm clips or other radiopaque objects will affect results.
- Extreme obesity can impair clear imaging.

NURSING ALERT

This procedure is contraindicated in:

- Pregnancy unless the benefits of performing the study greatly outweigh the possible risks to the fetus
- Clients with certain metal prosthetics (hip, knee, heart valves, aneurysm clips, inner ear prosthesis or other metallic objects) as the prosthesis can be displaced
- Clients with metal in body (shrapnel or ferrous metal in eye) since it may cause critical injury
- Clients with cardiac pacemakers (pacemaker can be deactivated by MRI)
- Clients with unstable medical status
- Clients with extreme cases of claustrophobia unless sedation is given before the study
- Precautions are necessary with clients with IV pumps or controllers because the MRI can disrupt flow rate.

Nursing Implications

Assessment

- Obtain pertinent history related to trauma or disease processes of the abdomen. Obtain occupational history, be-

cause metal in body such as shrapnel or flecks of ferrous metal in eye can cause retinal hemorrhage.
- Determine previous abnormalities in laboratory test results and diagnostic findings.
- Determine date of last menstrual period and possibility of pregnancy in premenopausal women.

Possible Nursing Diagnoses

Anxiety related to procedure and threat to health status
Pain related to disorder

Implementation

- Remind client to remove jewelry including watches, hairpins, and other radiopaque objects, and credit cards within viewing area.
- Ask client to void before procedure.
- Administer sedative to a child under 3 years of age or an uncooperative adult, as ordered.
- Administer ordered antianxiety agent if claustrophobia is present.
- Assist to position of comfort if client has been medicated or sedated.
- Supply earmolds or plugs to decrease the loud, banging sound heard by the client during the test.
- A series of images are taken while the table is manipulated and scanning of various levels is performed. As the scanning is done, the images are immediately portrayed on a screen and recorded on permanent film.
- Films are reviewed by a specialized radiologist.

Evaluation

- Note test results in relation to other tests performed and the client's symptoms.

Client/Caregiver Teaching

Pretest

- Inform client that the test permits assessment of the abdominal structures; that the procedure is performed in a special department by a technician and a physician specializing in magnetic resonance scanning.
- Inform the client that the technician will place client in supine position on flat table in a large cylindrical type scanner. Request that the client lie very still during procedure as movement will produce unclear images.
- Tell the client to expect loud banging from the scanner and

possibly magnetophosphenes (flickering lights in the visual field), which resolve when the procedure is over.
- Inform the client that either intravenous administration of gadolinium or oral glucagon or Geritol may be given, depending on the test to be performed.
- Instruct the client to take slow, deep breaths, and place emesis basin nearby if client becomes nauseous.

Posttest
- Inform the client to resume normal activity.

Magnetic Resonance Imaging (MRI), Head Nuclear Magnetic Resonance (NMR) Imaging

Classification: Nuclear medicine

Type of Test: Indirect visualization with contrast medium

Magnetic resonance imaging produces cross-sectional images of the intracranial area in multiple planes without the use of ionizing radiation or the interference of bone. Use of magnetic fields with the aid of radiofrequency energy produces images primarily based on water content of tissue therefore enabling the scanner to "see through" bone.

One of the most frequent uses of MRI is to diagnose intracranial disorders. The contrast medium gadolinium (Gd-DTPA) can be administered intravenously before the scanning. Gd-DTPA crosses the blood-brain barrier and is used to enhance imaging of the brain tissue with fluid appearing gray and blood appearing dark on the screen. This contrast medium is unlike the iodinated contrast dye used in computed tomography (CT) scanning.

Indications
- Diagnose and locate brain tumors
- Determine cause of cerebral vascular accident (CVA), cerebral infarct, or hemorrhage

- Determine cranial bone, face, throat, and neck soft-tissue lesions
- Diagnose intracranial infections
- Determine cause of seizures such as intracranial infection, edema, increased intracranial pressure
- Diagnose demyelinating disorders
- Diagnose vascular disorders of the brain and evaluate vascular integrity
- Diagnose cerebral changes associated with dementia
- Evaluate effectiveness of chemotherapy or radiation therapy in tumor treatment
- Evaluate postoperative shunt placement and function done for hydrocephalus in infants

Reference Values

- Normal anatomic structures, soft-tissue density, and blood flow rate of head, face, nasopharynx, neck, tongue, and brain

Abnormal Values

- Acoustic neuroma
- Arteriovenous malformation
- Benign meningioma
- Cerebral aneurysm
- Cerebral infarction
- Intraparenchymal hematoma or hemorrhage
- Lipoma
- Multiple sclerosis
- Optic nerve tumor
- Pituitary microadenoma
- Pyogenic abscess
- Subdural empyema
- Toxoplasmosis associated with AIDS
- Tuberculosis, in combination or in place of CT scan
- Ventriculitis

Interfering Factors

- Client movement during the procedure will affect results and make interpretation difficult.
- Metallic objects within the examination field, such as jewelry, watches, implanted infusion devices or pumps; metallic or other implants, including heart valves, cochlear or orthopedic prosthesis, rods or screws; dentures, hairpins or clips; pacemaker, aneurysm clips or other radiopaque objects will affect results.

> ### ▌ NURSING ALERT
>
> This procedure is contraindicated in:
> - Pregnancy unless the benefits of performing the study greatly outweigh the possible risks to the fetus
> - Clients with certain metal prosthetics (hip, knee, heart valves, aneurysm clips, inner ear prosthesis, or other metallic objects), as the prosthesis can be displaced
> - Clients with metal in body (shrapnel or ferrous metal in eye), since it may cause critical injury
> - Clients with cardiac pacemakers, as the pacemaker can be deactivated by MRI
> - Clients with unstable medical status
> - Clients with extreme cases of claustrophobia unless sedation is given before the study
> - Precautions are necessary with clients with IV pumps or controllers because the MRI can disrupt flow rate.

Nursing Implications

Assessment

- Obtain pertinent history related to trauma or disease processes of the head and neck; obtain occupational history; this is important since metal in body such as shrapnel or flecks of ferrous metal in eye can cause retinal hemorrhage; determine date of last menstrual period and possibility of pregnancy in premenopausal women.
- Determine previous abnormalities in laboratory test results and diagnostic findings.
- Assess anxiety or restlessness of client and notify physician for sedation or medication orders.
- Assess for compliance with directions given for rest, positioning, and activity before and during the test.

Possible Nursing Diagnoses

Anxiety related to procedure and threat to health status
Physical mobility, impaired, related to disorder
Verbal communication, impaired, related to disorder

Implementation

- Remind client to remove jewelry, including watches, hairpins and other radiopaque objects, and credit cards from viewing area.
- Ask client to void before the procedure.

- Administer sedative to a child under 3 years of age or an uncooperative adult, as ordered.
- Administer ordered antianxiety agent if claustrophobia is present.
- Administer IV gadolinium, if ordered.
- Assist to position of comfort with special assistance if client has been medicated or sedated.
- Supply earmolds or plugs to decrease loud, banging sound heard by the client during the test.
- A series of images are taken while the table is manipulated and scanning of various levels is performed. As the scanning is done, the images are immediately portrayed on a screen and recorded on permanent film.
- Films are reviewed by a specialized radiologist.

Evaluation

- Note test results in relation to other tests performed, particularly neurologic tests, and the client's symptoms.

Client/Caregiver Teaching

Pretest

- Inform client that the test permits assessment of the head and neck structures and that the procedure is performed in a special department by a technician and a physician specializing in magnetic resonance scanning.
- Inform the client that the technician will place the client in supine position on a flat table in a large cylindrical type scanner. Request that the client lie very still during procedure as movement will produce unclear images.
- Tell the client to expect loud banging from the scanner and possibly magnetophosphenes (flickering lights in the visual field), which are completely reversible when the procedure is over.
- Inform the client that IV gadolinium may be administered as a contrast medium.
- Instruct the client to take slow, deep breaths, and that an emesis basin will be nearby if client becomes nauseous.

Posttest

- Instruct the client to resume the usual level of activity and diet, unless otherwise indicated.

Magnetic Resonance Imaging (MRI), Heart and Chest Nuclear Magnetic Resonance (NMR) Imaging

Classification: Nuclear medicine

Type of Test: Indirect visualization

Magnetic resonance imaging (MRI) produces cross-sectional images of the thorax or chest area in multiple planes without the use of ionizing radiation or the interference of bone. Use of magnetic fields with the aid of radio frequency energy produces images primarily based on water content of tissue, therefore enabling the scanner to "see through" bone.

Heart and chest MRI scanning is performed to assist in diagnosing abnormalities of cardiovascular and pulmonary structures. Two special techniques are available for evaluation of cardiovascular structures. One is the electrocardiograph (ECG) gated multislice spin echo sequence, used to diagnose heart and aorta anatomic abnormalities, and the other is the ECG referenced gradient refocused sequence, used to diagnose heart function and analysis of blood flow patterns.

Indications

- Diagnose thoracic aortic diseases
- Confirm diagnosis of cardiac and paracardiac masses
- Identify congenital heart diseases
- Determine cardiac ventricular function
- Diagnose myocardial infarction and cardiac muscle ischemia
- Detect pleural effusion
- Evaluate postoperative angioplasty sites and bypass grafts
- Evaluate pericardial abnormalities

Reference Values

- Normal heart and lung structure, soft tissue, and function, including blood flow rate

Abnormal Values

- Aortic dissection
- Intramural and periaortic hematoma
- Constrictive pericarditis
- Pericardial hematoma or effusion
- Mediastinal masses
- Congenital heart diseases including pulmonary atresia, aortic coarctation, agenesis of the pulmonary artery, transposition of the great vessels
- Myocardial infarction
- Pleural effusion

Interfering Factors

- Client movement during the procedure will affect results and make interpretation difficult.
- Chest movement with respirations causes artifacts in the imaging.
- Metallic objects within the examination field, such as jewelry, watches, implanted infusion devices or pumps; metallic or other implants, including heart valves, cochlear or orthopedic prosthesis, rods or screws; dentures, hairpins or clips; pacemaker, aneurysm clips or other radiopaque objects will affect results.
- Extreme obesity can impair clear imaging.

> **NURSING ALERT**
>
> This procedure is contraindicated in:
> - Pregnancy unless the benefits of performing the study greatly outweigh the possible risks to the fetus
> - Clients with certain metal prosthetics (hip, knee, heart valves, aneurysm clips, inner ear prosthesis, or other metallic objects), as the prosthesis can be displaced
> - Clients with metal in body (shrapnel or ferrous metal in eye) since it may cause critical injury
> - Clients with cardiac pacemakers (pacemaker can be deactivated by MRI)
> - Clients with unstable medical status
> - Clients with extreme cases of claustrophobia unless sedation is given before the study
> - Precautions are necessary with clients with IV pumps or controllers because the MRI can disrupt flow rate.

Nursing Implications

Assessment

- Obtain pertinent history related to trauma or disease processes of the chest and heart. Obtain occupational history; this is important because metal in body such as shrapnel or flecks of ferrous metal in eye can cause retinal hemorrhage.
- Determine previous abnormalities in laboratory test results and diagnostic findings.
- Determine date of last menstrual period and possibility of pregnancy in premenopausal women.

Possible Nursing Diagnoses

Anxiety related to procedure and threat to health status
Pain related to disease
Cardiac output, decreased, related to disease

Implementation

- Remind client to remove jewelry, including watches, hairpins and other radiopaque objects, and credit cards within viewing area.
- Ask client to void before procedure.
- Administer sedative to a child under 3 years of age or an uncooperative adult, as ordered.
- Administer ordered antianxiety agent if claustrophobia is present.
- Assist to position of comfort; provide special assistance if client has been medicated or sedated.
- Supply earmolds or plugs to decrease loud, banging sound heard by the client during the test.
- If an ECG is to be performed in conjunction with the scan, apply electrodes to the appropriate sites.
- A series of images are taken while the table is manipulated and scanning of various levels is performed. As the scanning is done, the images are immediately portrayed on a screen and recorded on permanent film.
- Films are reviewed by a specialized radiologist.

Evaluation

- Note test results in relation to other tests performed, particularly cardiac enzymes studies, ECG, cardiac angiography, and other related tests, and the client's symptoms.

Client/Caregiver Teaching

Pretest

- Inform the client that the test permits assessment of the chest structures, and that the procedure is performed in a special department by a technician and a physician specializing in magnetic resonance scanning.

■ Inform the client that the technician will place the client in a supine position on a flat table in a large cylindrical type scanner. Ask the client to lie very still during the procedure as movement will produce unclear images.

■ Tell the client to expect loud banging from the scanner and possibly magnetophosphenes (flickering lights in the visual field), which are completely reversible when the procedure is over.

■ Instruct the client to take slow, deep breaths; place emesis basin nearby if client becomes nauseous.

Posttest

■ Instruct the client to resume usual level of activity and diet, unless otherwise indicated.

Magnetic Resonance Imaging (MRI), Musculoskeletal Nuclear Magnetic Resonance (NMR) Imaging

Classification: Nuclear medicine

Type of Test: Indirect visualization with contrast medium

Magnetic resonance imaging (MRI) produces cross-sectional images of the bones and joints in multiple planes without the use of ionizing radiation or the interference of bone. Use of magnetic fields with the aid of radio frequency energy produces images primarily based on water content of tissue, therefore enabling the scanner to "see through" bone.

During the procedure, the images are projected on a screen and also taped for later viewing. Musculoskeletal MRI scanning is performed to assist in diagnosing abnormalities of bones and joints and surrounding soft-tissue structures, including cartilage, synovium, ligaments, and tendons. MRI provides a more sensitive diagnostic study than a CT scan or x-ray. It is not done as an initial procedure but rather when the diagnosis is uncertain or to ascertain the need for surgery.

Indications

- Diagnose benign and cancerous tumor and cysts of the bone or soft tissue
- Determine cause of low back pain, including herniated disk and spinal degenerative disease
- Diagnose avascular necrosis of the femoral head or knee
- Detect bone infarcts in the epiphyseal or diaphyseal sites
- Confirm diagnosis of osteomyelitis
- Diagnose arthritis by identifying erosions and lesions and synovial inflammation
- Monitor treatment of synovitis
- Diagnose primary or secondary malignant process of the bone marrow
- Detect changes in bone marrow
- Detect tears or degeneration of ligaments, tendons, and meniscus resulting from trauma or pathology
- Differentiate between a stress fracture and a tumor
- Evaluate meniscal detachment of the temporomandibular joint

Reference Values

- Normal bones, joints, and surrounding tissue structures; no articular disease, bone marrow disorders, tumors, infection, or trauma to the bones, joints, or muscles

Abnormal Values

- Avascular necrosis of femoral head or knee
- Bone marrow disease such as Gaucher's disease, aplastic anemia, sickle-cell disease, or polycythemia
- Degenerative spinal disease such as spondylosis or arthritis
- Fibrosarcoma
- Hemangioma (muscular or osseous)
- Herniated disk
- Meniscal tears
- Osteochondroma
- Osteogenic sarcoma
- Osteomyelitis
- Spinal stenosis
- Stress fracture
- Synovitis

Interfering Factors

- Client movement during the procedure will affect results and make interpretation difficult.
- Casted limbs can cause placement difficulties in the scanner.
- Metallic objects within the examination field, such as jewelry, watches, implanted infusion devices or pumps; metallic or other implants, including heart valves, cochlear or orthopedic prosthesis, rods or screws; dentures, hairpins or clips; pacemaker, aneurysm clips or other radiopaque objects will affect results.
- Extreme obesity can impair clear imaging.

> ### NURSING ALERT
>
> This procedure is contraindicated in:
> - Pregnancy unless the benefits of performing the study greatly outweigh the possible risks to the fetus
> - Clients with certain metal prosthetics (hip, knee, heart valves, aneurysm clips, inner ear prosthesis, or other metallic objects), as the prosthesis can be displaced
> - Clients with metal in body (shrapnel or ferrous metal in eye) since it may cause critical injury
> - Clients with cardiac pacemakers (pacemaker can be deactivated by MRI)
> - Clients with unstable medical status
> - Clients with extreme cases of claustrophobia unless sedation is given before the study
> - Precautions are necessary with clients with IV pumps or controllers because the MRI can disrupt flow rate.

Nursing Implications

Assessment

- Obtain pertinent history related to trauma or disease processes of the bones and joints. Obtain occupational history; this is important because metal in body such as shrapnel or flecks of ferrous metal in eye can cause retinal hemorrhage.
- Determine previous abnormalities in laboratory test results and diagnostic findings.
- Determine date of last menstrual period and possibility of pregnancy in premenopausal women.

Possible Nursing Diagnoses

Anxiety related to procedure and threat to health status
Pain related to disorder
Physical mobility, impaired, related to disorder

Implementation

- Remind client to remove jewelry, including watches, hairpins and other radiopaque objects, and credit cards within viewing area.
- Ask client to void before procedure.
- Administer sedative to a child under 3 years of age or an uncooperative adult, as ordered.
- Administer ordered antianxiety agent if claustrophobia is present.
- Assist to position of comfort; provide special assistance if client has been medicated or sedated.
- Supply earmolds or plugs to decrease sound heard by the client during the test.
- As necessary, administer a paramagnetic contrast medium to define a lesion's vascularity or establish the boundary of an adjacent muscle.
- A series of images are taken while the table is manipulated and scanning of various levels is performed. As the scanning is done, the images are immediately portrayed on a screen and recorded on permanent film.
- Films are reviewed by a specialized radiologist.

Evaluation

- Note test results in relation to other tests performed, particularly x-rays and bone scans, and the client's symptoms.

Client/Caregiver Teaching

Pretest

- Inform client that test permits assessment of the bones and joints, and that the procedure is performed in a special department by a technician and a physician specializing in magnetic resonance scanning.
- Inform the client that the technician will place client in a supine position on a flat table in a large cylindrical type scanner. Ask the client to lie very still during the procedure as movement will produce unclear images.
- Tell the client to expect loud banging from the scanner and possibly magnetophosphenes (flickering lights in the visual field), which are completely reversible when the procedure is over.
- Instruct the client to take slow, deep breaths; place an emesis basin nearby if client becomes nauseous.

Posttest

■ Instruct the client to resume usual level of activity and diet, unless otherwise indicated.

Mammography

Classification: Radiography (xeroradiography)

Type of Test: Breasts

Mammography is usually performed using xeroradiography, a photoelectric process, useful in soft tissues such as breast tissue. This type of radiologic procedure reduces the amount of radiation exposure to the client and produces very clear images with excellent contrast. Benign cysts appear as clearly defined, regular, clear spots that are bilateral, while irregular, poorly defined, unilateral opaque areas suggest cancer.

Indications

■ Screen for breast cancer
■ Differentiate between benign and neoplastic breast disease
■ Evaluate breast masses, pain, or nipple discharge

Reference Values

■ Normal breast tissue, without cysts, tumors, or calcifications

Abnormal Values

■ Breast cysts
■ Breast tumors

Interfering Factors

■ Application of substance such as talcum powder or creams to the skin of breasts or underarms may alter test results.
■ Previous breast surgery may decrease readability of films.
■ Metallic objects such as jewelry, closures on clothing within the x-ray field may affect results.

> ### ◼ NURSING ALERT
>
> - Contraindicated in pregnancy, unless benefits of performing the procedure outweigh risks to the fetus.
> - Prevent possible x-ray exposure of personnel in the room with the client by having personnel wear a protective lead apron or stand behind a shield; badges that reveal level of exposure to x-rays should be worn by those working in areas near x-ray suites.

Nursing Implications

Assessment

- Obtain history of known or suspected breast disease, family history, current symptoms, diagnostic tests and results.
- Assess date of last menstrual period to ascertain possible pregnancy.

Possible Nursing Diagnoses

Anxiety related to threat to health status
Body image disturbance

Implementation

- Assist client to a standing or sitting position in front of x-ray machine, which is adjusted to level of breasts. The arm is positioned up and out of range of the area to be filmed.
- Breasts are placed under compression apparatus. Instruct client to take a deep breath and hold it while a minimum of two views are taken for each breast.

Evaluation

- Note test results in relation to other test performed, for example, breast ultrasonography or thermography.

Client/Caregiver Teaching

Pretest

- Inform the client of the purpose of the test and the procedure involved; explain that the test is performed by a technician and takes 15 to 30 minutes to complete.
- Tell the client not to apply deodorant the day of the procedure; explain that she will be asked to remove all clothing and jewelry above the waist.

- Warn the client that some discomfort may be associated with the procedure. Inform the client with cystic breast disease to schedule the procedure 1 week after menses, when breast tenderness is decreased.

Posttest

- Inform the client of the need for further diagnostic testing, preferably breast biopsy, if results are abnormal.
- Teach breast self-examination, and provide brochures with reportable signs and symptoms.
- Stress to the client the importance of regular mammography following the current guidelines.

Manometry, Esophageal; Esophageal Function Study; Esophageal Acid Study

Classification: Manometry

Type of Test: Indirect measurement

A group of invasive studies performed to assist in diagnosing esophageal muscle function and structure abnormalities. These studies measure esophageal pressure and the effects of gastric acid in the esophagus, lower esophageal sphincter pressure and motility patterns that result during swallowing. Tests performed in combination with manometry include the acid reflux, acid clearing, and acid perfusion (Bernstein) tests.

Indications

- Evaluate pyrosis and dysphagia to determine if the cause is gastroesophageal reflux or esophagitis
- Diagnose gastroesophageal reflux evidenced by low pressure in manometry, decreased pH in acidity test, and pain in acid reflux and perfusion tests
- Diagnose esophagitis, evidenced by decreased motility

- Diagnose achalasia, evidenced by increased pressure in manometry
- Diagnose chalasia in children, evidenced by decreased pressure in manometry
- Diagnose esophageal scleroderma, evidenced by decreased pressure in manometry
- Differentiate between epigastric pain that is the result of esophagitis or a cardiac condition

Reference Values

- Esophageal sphincter pressure: 10–20 mm Hg
- Esophageal secretions: pH 5–6
- Acid reflux: no regurgitation into the esophagus
- Acid clearing: 10 swallows or less
- Acid perfusion: no gastroesophageal reflux

Abnormal Values

- Gastroesophageal reflux (sphincter pressure of 0–5 mm Hg, pH of 1–3)
- Esophagitis
- Achalasia (sphincter pressure of 50 mm Hg)
- Spasms
- Chalasia
- Esophageal scleroderma

Interfering Factors

- Intake of food or fluids within 6 hours before the study may affect results.
- Administration of medications such as sedatives, antacids, anticholinergics, cholinergics, and corticosteroids can change pH or relax the sphincter muscle, causing inaccurate results.
- Inability to understand or follow instructions during the test can interfere with results.

NURSING ALERT

- Contraindicated in clients with unstable vital signs, esophageal varices or bleeding, infection, or a cardiac condition

Nursing Implications

Assessment

- Obtain history of signs and symptoms of upper gastrointestinal distress, known or suspected gastrointestinal disorders
  or hiatal hernia, previous diagnostic tests and procedures,
  previous medical regimens followed to treat symptoms and
  medications that could affect test results.
- Ensure restriction of foods, fluids, and smoking for 6 to 8
  hours before the study.
- Ensure that medications are withheld for 24 hours before the
  study; make special arrangements for diabetics.

Possible Nursing Diagnoses

Pain related to procedure and the disorder
Anxiety related to the procedure
Injury, risk for, related to the procedure

Implementation

- *Esophageal manometry*: Place the client on the examining
  table and spray the throat with local anesthetic. One or more
  small tubes are inserted through the nose into the esophagus and stomach. A small transducer is attached to the
  ends of the tubes, and pressures are measured at the lower
  esophageal sphincter and the intraluminal pressures and
  regularity and duration of peristaltic contractions are measured. The client is requested to swallow small amounts of
  water or flavored gelatin. Pressures are taken and recorded,
  and a motility pattern is recorded on a graph.
- *Esophageal acid and clearing*: With the tube in place, a pH
  electrode probe is inserted into the esophagus with Valsalva
  maneuvers performed to stimulate reflux of stomach contents into the esophagus. If acid reflux is absent, 100 mL
  of 0.1% hydrochloric acid is instilled into the stomach over
  3 minutes and the pH is repeated. To determine acid clearing, hydrochloric acid is instilled into the esophagus and the
  client is requested to swallow while the probe measures the
  pH.
- *Acid perfusion*: A catheter is inserted through the nose into
  the esophagus. The client is asked to inform the technician
  when pain is experienced. Normal saline solution is allowed
  to drip into the catheter at about 10 mL/min. Then hydrochloric acid is allowed to drip into the catheter. Pain experienced when the hydrochloric acid is instilled determines

the presence of an esophageal abnormality. If no pain is experienced, symptoms are the result of some other condition.

■ During the procedures monitor the client for aspiration of contents into lungs. Note any change in respirations (dyspnea, tachypnea, adventitious sounds). Suction mouth, pharynx, and trachea. Administer oxygen as ordered, and have resuscitation equipment nearby.

Evaluation

■ Note results in relation to other tests performed, particularly GI x-rays, and to the client's symptoms.

Client/Caregiver Teaching

Pretest

■ Explain that the procedure is performed in the endoscopy room by the physician to determine proper functioning of the esophagus and that the studies are completed in 30 minutes.
■ Inform the client that there is some discomfort and gagging when the tube is inserted, but there are no complications resulting from the procedure.
■ Tell the client to fast from food and fluids for 6 to 8 hours before the procedure.

Posttest

■ Tell the client to resume food and fluid intake, and medications once the gag reflex has returned.
■ Inform the client that some irritation of the nose and throat is common for 24 hours following the study and that the discomfort can be reduced by gargling with warm water.
■ Instruct the client to report change in respirations or excessive pain or bleeding to physician.

Mediastinoscopy

Classification: Endoscopy

Type of Test: Direct visualization

This test involves the direct visualization of the structures that lie beneath the sternum and between the lungs by means of a mediastinoscope inserted through a surgical incision at the suprasternal notch. Structures that can be viewed include the trachea, the esophagus, the heart and its major vessels, the thymus gland, and the lymph nodes that receive drainage from the lungs. The procedure is performed primarily to visualize and biopsy the mediastinal lymph and has now replaced the scalene fat biopsy.

Indications

- Confirm radiologic or cytologic evidence of carcinoma or sarcoidosis
- Confirm radiologic evidence of a thoracic infectious process of an indeterminate nature
- Diagnose Hodgkin's disease
- Determine stage of known bronchogenic carcinoma as indicated by the extent of mediastinal lymph node involvement
- Diagnose metastasis into the anterior mediastinum or extrapleurally into the chest
- Evaluate client with signs and symptoms of obstruction of mediastinal lymph flow and a history of head or neck cancer to determine recurrence or spread

Reference Values

- Normal appearance of mediastinal structures. No abnormal lymph node tissue.

Abnormal Values

- Bronchogenic carcinoma
- Coccidioidomycosis
- Granulomatous infections

- Histoplasmosis
- Hodgkin's disease
- Sarcoidosis
- Tuberculosis

Interfering Factors

- None

> ### NURSING ALERT
>
> - This procedure is contraindicated in previous medias-tinoscopy; scarring can make insertion of the scope and biopsy of lymph nodes difficult.

Nursing Implications

Assessment

- Obtain a history of allergies or sensitivities to anesthetics, analgesics, and antibiotics, thoracic or hematologic disorders and treatment regimen.
- Ensure that results of blood typing and cross-matching are obtained and recorded before the procedure in the event that an emergency thoracotomy should be required.
- Ensure food and fluids have been restricted for at least 8 hours before the procedure.

Possible Nursing Diagnoses

Breathing pattern, ineffective, risk for, related to complications of procedure

Infection, risk for, related to complications of procedure

Pain related to procedure

Anxiety related to threat to health status

Implementation

- The client is prepared for surgery and ordered sedation is administered.
- The client is placed in the supine position and general anesthesia is administered using an endotracheal tube.
- An incision is made at the suprasternal notch, and a path for the mediastinoscope is made using finger dissection. The lymph nodes can be palpated at this time. The scope is then inserted through the incision into the superior mediastinum and the area is inspected. The lymph nodes in

the right side of the mediastinum are those most accessible and safest to biopsy by mediastinoscopy. Those on the left side are more difficult to explore and biopsy because of their proximity to the aorta. Nodes in the left side of the mediastinum may need to be biopsied by mediastinotomy, which involves performing a left anterior thoracotomy.

- Specimens for biopsy or culture are obtained, placed in appropriate containers, properly labeled, and promptly sent to the laboratory.
- The scope is removed and the incision closed.
- If the client is stable and if no further surgery is immediately indicated, the client is extubated.

Evaluation

- Monitor vital signs according to institution policy.
- Note results in relation to other test results, particularly chest x-rays, and to the client's symptoms.
- Evaluate the client for potential complications such as pneumothorax, infection, left recurrent laryngeal nerve damage, puncture of trachea, esophagus, or major blood vessels.

Client/Caregiver Teaching

Pretest

- Inform the client that the procedure is usually performed under general anesthesia in an operating room by a physician and takes approximately 1 hour.
- Tell the client to fast from food and fluid for at least 8 hours before the procedure.

Posttest

- Inform the client that some chest discomfort may be present and that the throat may be slightly sore following the procedure; warm gargles or lozenges can be administered for throat discomfort.
- Inform the client and caregiver that food, fluids, and activities are resumed when the client has recovered from general anesthesia.
- Emphasize that any difficulty in breathing or other abnormal sensations or discomforts, or changes in vocal patterns, must be reported to the physician immediately.
- Instruct the client on signs and symptoms of incisional infection and the need to report evidence promptly to the physician.

▲▲▲▲▲▲▲▲▲▲▲▲▲▲▲▲▲▲▲▲

Melanin

Classification: Urinalysis

Type of Test: Urine, Random

This test determines the presence of melanin, the brown-black pigment produced by melanocytes that colors hair, skin, and eyes, but is not normally found in urine. Its precursors, melanogens, are often found in the urine of clients with cutaneous melanomas. A test to measure the melanocyte-stimulating hormone (MSH) secreted by the pituitary gland can also be performed, as this hormone is involved in the synthesis of melanin.

Indications

- Diagnose malignant melanomas

Reference Values

- Negative

Abnormal Values

- Malignant melanoma

Interfering Factors

- Medications that can cause false-positive results include salicylates.
- Failure to immediately send urine specimen to laboratory can interfere with accurate test results.

Nursing Implications

Assessment

- Obtain client history of any suspicious skin lesions.

Possible Nursing Diagnosis

Anxiety related to threat to health status

Implementation

- Obtain a freshly voided urine specimen in a sterile plastic container. Instruct client to void into the container if possible.
- If an indwelling catheter is in place, empty the collection bag, then obtain a random sample of urine and place into a sterile plastic container. Do not take a sample from the bag.
- Label the sample properly and transport to the laboratory.

Evaluation

- Note test results in relation to the client's symptoms and other test results, particularly the melanocyte-stimulating hormone test.

Client/Caregiver Teaching

Pretest

- Tell the client to withhold salicylates for 12 hours before the test.

Posttest

- Tell the client to resume medications withheld before the test.
- Inform the client that test results are usually available in 1 to 2 days.

Metanephrines, Total

Classification: Chemistry

Type of Test: Urine (24-hour)

Metanephrines are inactive metabolites excreted by catecholamines. Release of metanephrines in the urine is indicative of disorders associated with excessive catecholamine production, particularly pheochromocytoma. Vanillylmandelic acid (VMA) and catecholamines are normally measured with urinary metanephrines. This 24-hour sample facilitates quantification of metanephrines.

Indications

- Diagnose suspected pheochromocytoma
- Diagnose cause of hypertension
- Verify suspected tumors associated with excessive catecholamine secretion

Reference Values

- 0.1–1.3 mg/24 h

Abnormal Values

- Elevated values
  Brain or nervous system tumors
  Pheochromocytoma, with or without metastasis
  Sepsis
  Severe stress

Interfering Factors

- Medications such as dopamine, chlorpromazine, guanethidine, hydralazine, hydrocortisone, levodopa, imipramine, isoetharine, MAO inhibitors, phenacetin, nalidixic acid, phenobarbital, tetracycline, and phenylephrine may cause false-positive results.
- High dietary intake of alcohol, caffeine, and bananas may cause falsely elevated results.
- Medications such as clonidine, guanethidine, propranolol, reserpine, and theophylline may cause falsely decreased results.
- Stress and anxiety can increase catecholamines.
- Menstrual blood in specimen can interfere with test results.

Nursing Implications

Assessment

- Obtain history and etiology of hypertension, results of diagnostic tests, and medication regimen.
- Ensure that any phenothiazine-containing medications and caffeine have been withheld for 24 hours before initiating urine collection.

Possible Nursing Diagnoses

Anxiety related to threat to health status
Verbal communication, impaired, related to disorder
Hyperthermia related to disorder

Implementation

- Obtain a clean, dry 3-liter plastic container with 20 to 25 mL of hydrochloric acid as preservative.
- Begin the test between 6 and 8 A.M., if possible. Collect the first voiding and discard; record the time the specimen was discarded as the beginning of the 24-hour test.
- Keep container refrigerated. If urinary catheter is in place, keep drainage bag on ice and empty urine into refrigerated container.
- Instruct the client to void the next day at the same time the specimen collection was begun. Add this sample to 24-hour collection, and end test.
- Upon conclusion of test, label the container properly including the specific start and ending times. Transport the specimen to the laboratory promptly.

Evaluation

- Note results in relation to client's symptoms and other tests performed, for example, tests for urinary catecholamines or vanillylmandelic acid (VMA).

Client/Caregiver Teaching

Pretest

- Inform the client that all urine for a 24-hour period must be saved, and monitor all urine output in chart. Instruct the client to avoid voiding in pan with defecation and to keep toilet tissue out of pan to prevent contamination of the specimen.
- Advise female clients to postpone urine collection if menstruating.
- Stress to the client and caregiver the importance of decreasing anxiety level during the test.
- Tell the client to withhold any medications that interfere with the test results and to avoid alcohol, caffeine, and bananas.

Posttest

- As ordered, remind the client to resume medications withheld for the test.

Methemoglobin (MetHb, HbM)

Classification: Hematology

Type of Test: Blood

This test measures methemoglobin (HbM), a structural hemoglobin variant formed when the heme portion of the deoxygenated hemoglobin is oxidized to a ferric state that renders it incapable of combining with and transporting oxygen to tissues. Visible cyanosis can result as levels are increased.

Indications

- Detect acquired methemoglobinemia caused by excessive radiation or by the toxic effects of chemicals and drugs
- Detect congenital methemoglobinemia, indicated by deficiency of MetHb or the Hb variant, HbM

Reference Values

- 2% of total hemoglobin or 0.06 to 0.24 g/dL (SI units: 9.3 to 37.2 mol/L)

Abnormal Values

- Increased levels
    Acquired methemoglobinemia
    Hereditary methemoglobinemia
    Carbon monoxide poisoning
    Certain drugs, including acetanilid, aniline dyes, nitroglycerin, benzocaine, chlorates, lidocaine, nitrates, nitrites, phenacetin, sulfonamides, radiation, primaquine, and resorcinol
- Decreased levels
    Pancreatitis

Interfering Factors

- Ingestion of drugs that increase HbM levels can affect results (see Abnormal Values).

- Breast-feeding infants are capable of converting inorganic nitrate to the nitrite ion, causing nitrite toxicity and increased HbM.
- Nitrate topical applications used by breast-feeding mothers can be connected to nitrite, causing increased HbM serous conversion of nitrate to nitrite.

Nursing Implications

Assessment

- Obtain history of hematologic status and known or suspected hemoglobin disorder, exposure to sources of nitrites in drugs, and conditions that produce nitrite.
- Assess for signs and symptoms of impaired oxygenation.

Possible Nursing Diagnoses

Gas exchange, impaired, related to altered oxygen supply
Pain related to disorder

Implementation

- Put on gloves. Using aseptic technique, perform a venipuncture and collect 7 mL of blood in a green-top tube.
- Place specimen on ice and transport to the laboratory immediately.

Evaluation

- Note test results in relation to the client's symptoms and other test results.

Client/Caregiver Teaching

Pretest

- Tell the client to avoid the drugs that can interfere with test results.

Microhemagglutination Treponema Pallidum (MHA-TP)

Classification: Serology
Type of Test: Plasma

In this test for syphilis, a sexually transmitted disease caused by the organism *Treponema pallidum*, the client's serum is heat treated, mixed with treponema-sensitized sheep red blood cells, and compared with a control. Positive results occur when agglutination occurs in test sample but not in the control sample. This test is less sensitive than the FTA-ABS test.

Indications

- Diagnose syphilis when nontreponemal antibody tests positive

Reference Values

- Negative; titer <1:160

Abnormal Values

- Positive values
  - Bejel
  - Pinta
  - Syphilis
  - Yaws

Interfering Factors

- False-positive results may be due to leprosy, infectious mononucleosis, or systemic lupus erythematosus.

Nursing Implications

Assessment

- Obtain history of reproductive system, known or suspected exposure to syphilis, and results of tests and procedures performed.
- Ensure that client has fasted overnight before testing.

Possible Nursing Diagnosis

Anxiety related to threat to health status

Implementation

- Put on gloves. Using aseptic technique, perform a venipuncture and collect 7 mL of blood in a red-top tube.
- Handle sample gently to avoid hemolysis and transport to the laboratory promptly.

Evaluation

- Note test results in relation to other tests performed and the client's symptoms.

Client/Caregiver Teaching

Pretest

- Tell the client to fast for 8 hours before the test.

Posttest

- Resume foods and fluids withheld before testing.
- If results are positive, instruct the client in the importance of treatment for the client and his or her sexual contacts.

Monospot, Heterophil Antibody

Classification: Serology

Type of Test: Serum

A Monospot test is performed as a screening for infectious mononucleosis caused by Epstein-Barr virus (EBV). The test is an antigen-antibody reaction confirmation of clinical manifestations. The hallmark of EBV infection is the presence of the heterophil antibody, also called the Paul-Bunnel antibody, an IgM that agglutinates sheep or horse red blood cells.

The Monospot test is a single-step agglutination test. It is performed on two slides, each containing horse red cells and serum, with one slide containing guinea pig kidney and the other, beef red cell stroma. If agglutination occurs on the slide with guinea pig kidney, diagnosis of infectious mononucleosis is made.

Indications

- Confirm infectious mononucleosis

Reference Values

- Negative; titer <1:56

Abnormal Values

- Infectious mononucleosis
- Burkitt's lymphoma
- Cryoglobulinemia
- Epstein-Barr virus
- Syphilis
- Systemic lupus erythematosus (SLE)

Interfering Factors

- False-positive results may occur in the presence of narcotic addiction, serum sickness, lymphomas, hepatitis, leukemia, cancer of the pancreas, and phenytoin therapy.
- A false-negative result may occur if treatment was begun before antibodies developed or if the test is done less than 6 days after exposure to the virus.
- Hemolysis of the sample or a chylous sample negates test results.

Nursing Implications

Assessment

- Obtain a history of illness and symptoms as well as of the medication regimen.

Possible Nursing Diagnoses

Fatigue related to the disease
Pain related to the disease
Hyperthermia related to the disease

Implementation

- Put on gloves. Using aseptic technique, perform a venipuncture and collect 7 mL of blood in a red-top tube.
- Handle sample gently to avoid hemolysis and transport to the laboratory promptly.

Evaluation

- Note test results in relation to client's symptoms and other tests performed.

Client/Caregiver Teaching

Posttest

- Tell the client to refrain from direct contact with others, as disease is transmitted by the saliva of infected individuals.
- Warn the client that about 10 percent of all results are false-negative or false-positive.

Motile Sperm, Wet Mount from Fornix

Classification: Microscopic examination

Type of Test: Semen analysis

This test analyzes samples of fluid obtained from the vagina for the presence of sperm. It is usually done after an alleged or suspected rape and requires strict adherence to procedures for collection and transportation of specimens. Because of the traumatic event, special care is needed in dealing with the client.

Indications

- Suspected or alleged rape

Reference Values

- Absence of sperm

Abnormal Values

- Presence of motile sperm indicates ejaculation with recent sexual intercourse.

Interfering Factors

- Improper collection of specimens and inability of client to cooperate interfere with test results.

Nursing Implications

Assessment

- Obtain history of gynecological system, of the alleged assault, current symptoms, relevant diagnostic tests and results.
- Note client's readiness to participate in the test. Never pressure or hurry the victim. Allow her time to adjust to avoid further trauma.

Possible Nursing Diagnoses

Anxiety related to threat to health status and traumatic event
Rape-trauma syndrome, risk for
Self-concept, altered, related to traumatic event

Implementation

- Provide emotional support by being available to listen, accepting the client's feelings, and providing privacy during the examination and the interviewing process.
- Obtain vaginal speculum, wooden Pap smear stick, sterile specimen container and slides, and normal saline with 50-mL syringe. Insert speculum and obtain specimen by using Pap smear stick or by vaginal wash with normal saline. Avoid using cotton applicators.
- Provide specimens to police in accordance with local regulations. Remember to save all clothing for analysis of presence of sperm.

Evaluation

- Evaulate client's response and coping mechanism. Provide the opportunity to express feelings common to rape victims such as anger, humiliation, and fear of pregnancy or disease.

Client/Caregiver Teaching

Posttest

- Encourage the client to contact a local rape-counseling or mental health crisis center.

▲▲▲▲▲▲▲▲▲▲▲▲▲▲▲▲▲▲

Mumps Test, Mumps Antibody

Classification: Serology, Infectious disease diagnostic

Type of Test: Blood, Skin injection

This blood or skin test is done to determine antibody titers indicating exposure to or active presence of mumps. Mumps, also known as parotitis, is an infectious viral disease of the parotid glands caused by a myxovirus that is transmitted by direct contact with or droplets spread from the saliva of an infected person.

Indications

- Detect impaired or intact cellular immunity when used with other test antigens to test immune responses
- Determine resistance to or protection against the mumps virus by a positive reaction or susceptibility to mumps by a negative reaction
- Evaluate mumps-like diseases and differentiate between these and actual mumps

Reference Values

- Negative (blood test)
- Negative response; no reaction at the test site or minimal response of erythema

Abnormal Values

- Positive response of erythema with or without induration indicates varying degrees of protection from or resistance to the mumps.
- Increased titer during time between first and second blood specimen indicates recent presence of mumps.

Interfering Factors

- Improper technique in performing the skin test or inaccurate time or measurement in reading the reaction may affect results.

Nursing Implications

Assessment

- Obtain a history of exposure to the disease and past immunizations.

Possible Nursing Diagnoses

Infection, risk for, related to immunosupression
Pain related to the disease
Knowledge deficit related to spread of disease

Implementation

- *Blood test:* Put on gloves. Using aseptic technique, perform a venipuncture and collect 7 mL of blood in a red-top tube. Label and send specimen to laboratory immediately. Repeat test in 7 to 14 days and label as convalescent sample.
- *Skin test:* Put on gloves. Cleanse the lower anterior area of the forearms with alcohol or acetone swabs and allow to air-dry. Draw up the inactivated vaccine from infected animals and the vaccine prepared from noninfected animals into tuberculin syringes with 26-ga needles attached. Inject both intradermally, one in each arm, and record the site.

Evaluation

- Note test results in relation to other tests performed and the client's symptoms.
- Erythema with or without induration of at least 10 mm in diameter indicates some protection against mumps. A positive reaction at the onset of a mumpslike disease can rule out mumps as the cause. A delayed positive result that occurs several days after the test can indicate the presence of

mumps and no previous exposure. The lack of erythema indicates a negative result and lack of resistance to the disease.

Client/Caregiver Teaching

Pretest

- Explain the purpose of the test and how the test is performed; inform the client that the test is generally done by a nurse in a physician's office or health care setting and takes about 5 to 10 minutes to complete.

Posttest

- Instruct the client in isolation precautions during time of communicability or contagion.
- Emphasize the need to return to have another blood sample taken in 7 to 14 days.
- Inform the client that the presence of mumps ensures lifetime immunity.

Muramidase, Lysozyme

Classification: Urinalysis

Type of Test: Urine (timed)

This test measures muramidase, also known as lysozyme, a bacteriocidal enzyme present in tears, saliva, mucus, and phagocytic cells. It is produced by the degradation of granulocytes and monocytes; destruction of such cells will produce elevated urinary levels. In addition, this enzyme is found in renal tissue, with reabsorption occurring at the proximal tubules.

Indications

- Diagnose acute granulocytic or monocytic leukemia, indicated by elevated levels
- Monitor the extent of destruction of monocytes and granulocytes in known leukemias
- Diagnose suspected renal tubular damage, as indicated by elevated levels

- Monitor response to renal transplant, with rejection indicated by elevated levels

Reference Values

- <0–2.9 mg/L (SI units: 1.3–3.6 mg/24 h)

Abnormal Values

- Increased levels
  Acute onset or relapse of granulocytic leukemia
  Acute pyelonephritis
  Impaired proximal renal tubular reabsorption
  Nephrotic syndrome
  Polycythemia vera
  Rejection or infarction of kidney transplantation, severe extrarenal infection, and tuberculosis of the kidney
  Relapse of monocytic or myelomonocytic leukemia, with rapid rise at onset
  Sarcoidosis

Interfering Factors

- Bacteria in the sample will falsely decrease muramidase levels.
- Blood or saliva in the sample will falsely elevate muramidase levels.
- Improper collection or storage of urine during and after collection invalidates results.

Nursing Implications

Assessment

- Obtain history of known or suspected renal disease or leukemia, as well as the results of other diagnostic tests and procedures.

Possible Nursing Diagnoses

Anxiety related to threat to health status
Activity intolerance related to the disease
Infection, risk for, related to immunosuppression

Implementation

- Obtain a clean 3-liter container or 24-hour urine bag or bottle with or without preservative, according to laboratory policy. Place the container on ice throughout collection period unless preservative has been added. If an indwelling urinary catheter is in place, the drainage bag must be kept on ice.

- Begin the test between 6 and 8 A.M. if possible; collect first voiding and discard; record the time specimen was discarded as the beginning of the 24-hour test. Document the quantity of urine output during collection period, including urine at end of 24-hour period.

- The next morning, ask the client to void at the same time the collection was started and add this last voiding to the container.

- If an indwelling catheter is in place, replace tubing and container system and empty the urine into a large refrigerated container periodically during the 24 hours; monitor to ensure continued drainage and conclude the test the next morning at the same hour the collection was begun.

- At the conclusion of the test, make sure that the container is properly labeled; include start and completion times and any medications that the client was taking that may alter test results. Transport specimen to the laboratory immediately.

Evaluation

- Note results and compare with serum muramidase, as serum levels can be normal and urinary levels elevated in diagnosing renal tubular dysfunction.

Client/Caregiver Teaching

Pretest

- Inform the client that all urine for a 24-hour period must be saved; instruct client to avoid voiding in pan with defecation and to keep toilet tissue out of pan to prevent contamination of the specimen.

- Advise female client to postpone test if menstruating.

- Inform the client that the specimen must be kept refrigerated or on ice.

Myelography

Classification: Contrast-mediated radiologic study

Type of Test: Indirect visualization

This radiologic study is used to visualize the spinal subarachnoid space using air or contrast agent injected by lumbar puncture. It has been largely replaced with computed tomography (CT) scanning or magnetic resonance imaging (MRI).

Indications

- Determine cause of back pain
- Detect lesions or changes in bony structures of the spinal column
- Diagnose congenital abnormalities and conditions that affect subarachnoid space or spinal cord

Reference Values

- Normal structure of subarachnoid space, without abnormalities or obstruction

Abnormal Values

- Cancerous tumors
- Herniated disk
- Spinal nerve root injury
- Tumors within spinal cord or subarachnoid space

Interfering Factors

- Inability of the client to remain still during procedure
- Inaccurate needle placement in spinal column
- Metallic objects such as jewelry or closures on clothing within x-ray field
- Spinal abnormalities that prevent lumbar or cervical puncture for dye injection

> ### ▌NURSING ALERT
>
> - Contraindicated in pregnancy, unless benefits of performing the procedure outweigh risks to the fetus
> - Contraindicated in known allergy to iodine or iodinated contrast media, unless pretreatment is employed
> - Procedure should be performed with caution in clients with a known or suspected increase in intracranial pressure, infection at puncture site, or chronic neurological disease such as MS, as it may cause exacerbation

Nursing Implications

Assessment

- Obtain history of skeletal system, current symptoms, and other diagnostic tests and results.
- Ensure that food and fluids have been restricted for 8 to 12 hours before the study.
- Assess date of last menstrual period to ascertain possible pregnancy.

Possible Nursing Diagnoses

Anxiety related to threat to health status
Pain related to disorder and the procedure
Infection or injury, risk for, related to procedure

Implementation

- Administer a laxative or enema before the study, if ordered, to clear bowel of gas or feces.
- Assist the client to side-lying position on a tilted x-ray table, with knees flexed and head bent down.
- Lumbar puncture is completed with needle placement verified by fluoroscopy. Assist client to prone position.
- Contrast is injected and table is tilted to distribute the flow of dye. Water, oil-based or air contrast medium can be used.
- Films are taken, and contrast medium and needle are removed.

Evaluation

- Note test results in relation to the client's symptoms and other tests performed.
- Monitor vital signs, puncture site, and neurological status, as indicated.

Client/Caregiver Teaching

Pretest

- Explain the purpose of the test and the procedure involved; inform the client that it is performed by a physician and takes 1 hour to complete.

Posttest

- Place client at rest for 6 to 8 hours with head of bed slightly elevated.
- Encourage fluids to assist in contrast absorption and replace CSF loss. Observe voiding pattern.
- Instruct client to report any acute or persistent headache, reaction to contrast, or signs of meningitis.

▲▲▲▲▲▲▲▲▲▲▲▲▲▲▲▲▲▲▲▲▲▲

Myoglobin, Serum

Classification: Chemistry

Type of Test: Serum

Myoglobin is an oxygen-binding muscle protein normally found in skeletal and cardiac muscle. It is released into the bloodstream after muscle damage from ischemia, trauma, or inflammation. Although this test is more sensitive than creatinine phosphokinase isoenzymes, it doesn't indicate the specific site involved.

Indications

- Estimate damage from skeletal muscle injury or myocardial infarction
- Predict flareup of polymyositis

Reference Values

- 30–90 ng/mL

Abnormal Values

- Elevated levels
  Acute alcohol intoxication
  Dermatomyositis
  Hypothermia, with prolonged shivering
  Muscular dystrophy
  Myocardial infarction
  Polymyositis
  Severe burns or trauma
  Severe renal failure
  Systemic lupus erythematosus

Interfering Factors

- Hemolysis may affect test results.
- Recent angina or cardioversion may increase levels.
- Improper timing of test may cause results to reflect highest levels.
- Radioactive scan performed within 1 week can affect results.

Nursing Implications

Assessment

- Obtain history of purpose for test, known or suspected disorders associated with elevated myoglobin, and results of tests and procedures performed.

Possible Nursing Diagnoses

Pain related to the disease
Anxiety related to threat to health status

Implementation

- Put on gloves. Using aseptic technique, perform a venipuncture and collect 5 mL of blood in a red-top tube. Collect the blood sample 4 to 8 hours after the onset of an acute MI.
- Handle sample gently to avoid hemolysis and transport to laboratory immediately.

Evaluation

- Note the results in relation to the client's symptoms and other studies performed, including total creatine kinase (CK) or myocardial-specific isoenzyme (CK-MB).

Client/Caregiver Teaching

Posttest

- Advise the client that these test results may need to be correlated with other tests for definitive diagnosis.

Myoglobin, Urine

Classification: Urinalysis

Type of Test: Urine

Myoglobinemia, which occurs with extensive destruction of muscle fibers, leads to myoglobin excretion in the urine and can lead to acute renal tubular necrosis. Myoglobin, an oxygen-binding protein, is exclusive to skeletal and cardiac muscle and is released into the blood after trauma to the tissues. Myoglobin appears in the urine within 48 hours after a myocardial infarction. It can be detected in the urine up to 7 days after muscle damage.

Indications

- Diagnose muscular disease
- Assess extent of muscular damage from crushing trauma
- Detect extensive muscle tissue damage, for example, in myocardial infarction

Reference Values

- Negative

Abnormal Values

- Acute alcohol intoxication with delirium tremens
- Barbiturate toxicity
- Burns (severe)
- Diabetic acidosis
- Glycogen and lipid storage diseases

- Malignant hyperthermia
- Hypokalemia
- Muscular dystrophy
- Myocardial infarction
- Polymyositis
- Renal failure
- Surgical procedure
- Systemic infection with fever
- Trauma
- Viral infection

Interfering Factors

- If test is performed with reagent strips, such as Hemastix, recent ingestion of large amounts of vitamin C can inhibit the test reaction, preventing accurate results.
- Extremely diluted urine can reduce test sensitivity.
- Renal function influences test results since myoglobin is excreted through the kidneys.

Nursing Implications

Assessment

- Assess history of cardiac and musculoskeletal disease, medication regimen, and results of other laboratory tests.

Possible Nursing Diagnoses

Pain related to trauma
Anxiety related to threat to health status
Physical mobility, impaired, related to trauma

Implementation

- Collect a 10-mL random urine sample in a sterile plastic container.
- If an indwelling catheter is in place, empty the collection bag and then obtain a random sample in a sterile container.
- Ensure that the container is labeled properly and the forms completed; transport to the laboratory.

Evaluation

- Note the results in relation to other tests performed, particularly other serum enzyme studies and x-rays, and to the client's symptoms.

Client/Caregiver Teaching

Pretest

- Instruct the client in collection procedure and provide appropriate container if specimen is to be obtained as an outpatient and brought to the laboratory.

5′-Nucleotidase

Classification: Chemistry

Type of Test: Serum

This isoenzyme is formed almost completely in the hepatobiliary tissues and is more specific than alkaline phosphatase. Damage to these tissues causes the isoenzyme to leak into the blood and elevated levels result.

Indications

- Evaluate elevated alkaline phosphatase of uncertain etiology
- Aid in diagnosis of hepatobiliary disorders
- Differentiate biliary obstruction from hepatocellular damage
- Diagnose bone disease as the source of the elevated levels
- Detect liver metastasis when jaundice is not present

Reference Values

- 4–11.5 U/L
- 0.3–3.2 Bodansky U

Abnormal Values

- Increased levels along with elevated levels of other hepatic enzymes
    - Biliary obstruction from calculi or tumor
    - Cirrhosis of the liver
    - Metastasis to the liver
    - Medications such as acetaminophen, narcotics, phenytoin, aspirin, or phenothiazines

- Normal levels with increased alkaline phosophatase indicates skeletal disease

Interfering Factors

- Hemolysis of the blood sample may interfere with the test results.
- Medications such as acetaminophen, narcotics, phenytoin, aspirin, or phenothiazines may cause falsely increased results.

Nursing Implications

Assessment

- Obtain a history of liver or gallbladder disease, results of other tests performed, and medication regimen.

Possible Nursing Diagnoses

Anxiety related to threat to health status
Pain related to disorder
Injury, risk for, related to altered clotting factors

Implementation

- Put on gloves. Using aseptic technique, perform a venipuncture and collect 7 mL of blood in a red-top tube.
- Handle sample gently to avoid hemolysis and transport to the laboratory promptly.

Evaluation

- Note test results in relation to other tests performed, particularly serum alkaline phosphatase, leucine aminopeptidase (LAP), gamma-glutamyl transferase (GGT), alanine aminotransferase (ALT), and aspartate aminotransferase (AST).

Client/Caregiver Teaching

Pretest

- Inform the client that no special preparation is required before the test.

Occult Blood

Classification: Chemistry

Type of Test: Stool, Emesis, Urine

This test determines the presence of blood in stool, emesis, or urine that cannot be readily seen. Two commerically available tests are most often used: Hematest and Hemoccult. Hematest uses orthotolidine to detect the presence of hemoglobin, and Hemoccult uses guaiac. The latter is generally more accurate but neither test is considered conclusive.

Indications

- Assess known or suspected disorder associated with gastrointestinal or genitourinary bleeding
- Detect active bleeding in client with hematological disorders

Reference Values

- Negative

Abnormal Values

- Positive values, stool or emesis
    Colon cancer
    Diverticular disease
    Esophageal varices
    Gastritis, gastric ulcers
    Inflammatory bowel disease
- Positive values, urine
    Bladder cancers
    Bleeding disorders
    Nephrolithiasis
    Urinary tract infections

Interfering Factors

- Ingestion of red meats or blood-containing foods, such as blood sausage, and ingestion of certain fruits and vegetables,

such as beets, turnips, broccoli, cauliflower, parsnips, horse-radish, and cantaloupe, can interfere with results.
- Certain drugs, including salicylates, boric acid, bromides, colchicine, iron preparations, iodine, indomethacin, potassium preparations, reserpine, steroids, anticoagulants, and thiazide diuretics, may have direct or indirect effects on the GI tract.
- False-negative results in stool or emesis test may occur with ascorbic acid use.
- False-positive results may occur in urine with ascorbic acid, tetracycline, terramycin, bromide, or copper use.
- Specimen contact with povidone iodine, bleach, menstrual blood, or hemorrhoidal blood will affect results.

Nursing Implications

Assessment

- Obtain history of gastrointestinal, renal and urinary systems, symptoms, medication regimen, diagnostic tests and results.
- Ensure that client has consumed a meat-free, high-bulk diet free of vegetables with high peroxidase activity for 3 days before the test.
- Ensure that medications that affect test results have been withheld, as ordered by the physician.

Possible Nursing Diagnoses

Fluid balance deficit related to active loss
Tissue perfusion, altered, related to hypovolemia
Anxiety related to threat to health status

Implementation

- Obtain random stool sample, preferably on 3 consecutive days.
- Open the front flap of the guaiac- or orthotolidine-impregnated card and, using the applicator, apply a thin smear of stool. Close the flap.
- Open the back flap and apply two drops of the developer to each box. Read the results after 30 seconds and within 2 minutes. Any trace of blue color indicates a positive result.
- If checking the urine for occult blood, collect at least 10 mL of urine in a clean specimen container and insert dipstick per manufacturer instructions, or send the specimen to the laboratory promptly. Dipstick can also be used in emesis.

Evaluation

- Note and report positive results and other symptoms of blood loss to physician.

Client/Caregiver Teaching

Pretest

- Inform patient about dietary restrictions and the need to withhold medications, as ordered by the physician.

Posttest

- Advise the client to resume food and medications withheld before the test, according to the physician's orders.

Oculoplethysmograph (OPG), Oculopneumo-plethysmograph (OPPG)

Classification: Manometry

Type of Test: Indirect measurement

This indirect indicator of carotid and cerebral blood flow, by measurement of blood flow of the ophthalmic artery, is used to diagnose carotid artery disease. Because the ophthalmic artery's blood flow reflects the blood flow of the carotid artery and brain circulation, comparing the blood flow in the two eyes and finding a decrease in one eye suggest pathology. The study can be done in conjunction with duplex scanning of the carotid arteries and is followed by cerebral angiography to diagnose blood flow patterns to the brain from the carotid arteries.

Indications

- Determine the cause of transient ischemic attacks (TIA) and symptoms of neurologic disorders, such as syncope, ataxia, and dizziness

- Diagnose carotid atherosclerotic or occlusive disease, evidenced by reduced rate of blood flow in the ophthalmic artery
- Determine the extent of carotid stenosis
- Evaluate the carotid artery patency before or after endarterectomy

Reference Values

- Normal blood flow in the carotid arteries

Abnormal Values

- Atherosclerotic carotid occlusive disease
- Transient ischemic attacks (TIA)

Interfering Factors

- Inability to prevent blinking, nystagmus, or poor cooperation can affect results.

> ### NURSING ALERT
>
> This procedure is contraindicated in:
> - Clients who have had eye surgery within 2 to 6 months of the study
> - Clients with cataracts or lens implants, retinal detachment, allergy to the local anesthetic used in the study, conjunctivitis, uncontrolled glaucoma, or enucleation

Nursing Implications

Assessment

- Obtain history of hypersensitivity to local anesthesia, cardiovascular and neurological systems, known or suspected disorders associated with carotid artery disease, previous diagnostic tests, and procedures and medical regimens prescribed.
- Ensure removal of contact lenses before the test.
- Ensure that client has taken usual eye medications for glaucoma and eyedrops for anesthesia of eyes before the test.

Possible Nursing Diagnoses

Injury, risk for, related to procedure
Anxiety related to disorder

Verbal communication, impaired, related to disorder
Physical mobility, impaired, related to disorder

Implementation

- Attach electrocardiograph (ECG) electrodes if monitoring for arrhythmias during the procedure.
- Administer eye drops to anesthetize the eyes. Place the client in a supine position, and connect ECG machine. Attach small photoelectric detectors to ear lobes. Pulses from the blood flow to the ears by the external carotid arteries are detected, compared, and recorded.
- Small suction cups are attached to both eyeballs and held in place with 40 to 50 mm Hg of suction. Blood flow within each eye causes pulses that are detected and recorded. Blood flow to each eye is temporarily interrupted by application of increased pressure to the eyeball. When blood flow is resumed, pulses are recorded to determine if the flow is simultaneous for both eyes. Blood flow to the eye is delayed if carotid occlusive disease is present.
- The difference in the timing of pulses is measured in milliseconds. The study results are evaluated by comparing pulse rates of the two eyes, or in some cases, one eye to the ear on the opposite side. The delay in blood flow measures the degree of carotid artery disease as mild, moderate, or severe.

Evaluation

- Note results in relation to client's symptoms and other test results, particularly cerebral angiography and brain scan.

Client/Caregiver Teaching

Pretest

- Inform the client that the procedure is performed in a special room by a specially trained technician to evaluate carotid artery function; that results will be interpreted by the physician; and that the procedure takes from 5 to 30 minutes to complete.
- Inform the client that the anesthetic eye drops may cause a slight burning feeling; tell the client that the anesthesia disappears 30 minutes after the study.
- Inform the client that no pain is associated with this study but that vision can be impaired temporarily when suction is applied to the eye cups.

Posttest

- Advise the client to refrain from rubbing eyes for 2 hours after the study to prevent corneal abrasions; tearing can be gently blotted dry with soft tissue.
- Inform the client that contact lenses should not be replaced for 2 hours to allow the effect of the anesthetic drops to wear off.
- Advise the client that sunglasses can be worn if temporary photophobia is experienced.
- Warn the client that eyes can appear bloodshot following the study and drops of artificial tears can be instilled to reduce irritation.
- Instruct client to call physician with any symptoms of corneal abrasion (pain and excessive tearing) or severe burning.

Ornithine Carbamoyltransferase (OCT)

Classification: Chemistry

Type of Test: Serum

This test measures ornithine carbamoyltransferase (OCT), formerly known as ornithine transcarbamoylase. This enzyme found in the liver catalyzes ornithine to citrulline in the urea cycle before its link with the citric acid cycle. This enzyme's importance stems from its role in the conversion of ammonia to urea by the liver. When damage to liver tissues occurs, this enzyme leaks into the blood and levels rise.

Indications

- Evaluate elevated serum alkaline phosphatase (ALP) of uncertain etiology in diagnosis of hepatic or biliary tract diseases
- Evaluate therapy with hepatotoxic drugs or exposure to he-

patotoxic chemicals, with early effects indicated by elevated OCT levels
■ Aid in the diagnosis of suspected mushroom poisoning, as indicated by elevated levels

Reference Values

■ 0–500 Sigma units
■ 8–20 mIU/mL
■ 8–20 U/L

Abnormal Values

■ Elevated levels
  Cholecystitis
  Cirrhosis
  Hepatic necrosis
  Metastatic liver carcinoma
  Mushroom poisoning
  Obstructive jaundice
  Viral hepatitis
  Certain drugs, such as any hepatotoxic drugs and chemicals, alcohol, and oral contraceptives
■ Decreased levels
  Inherited disorders associated with a partial block in the urea cycle (hyperammonemia)
  Certain drugs, such as mercuric salts, p-chloromercuribenzoate, and 2,3-dimercaptopropanol

Interfering Factors

■ Hepatotoxic drugs and chemicals can produce elevated levels.

Nursing Implications

Assessment

■ Obtain history of hepatic and biliary tract system, known or suspected disorders, and the results of tests and procedures performed.
■ Assess medication history; ensure that any drugs that may alter test results, such as hepatotoxic drugs, have been withheld for 24 hours before the test, as ordered by the physician.

Possible Nursing Diagnoses

Pain related to disorder
Injury, risk for, related to altered clotting factors
Anxiety related to threat to health status

Implementation

- Put on gloves. Using aseptic technique, perform a venipuncture and collect 7 mL of blood in a red-top tube.
- Handle the sample gently to avoid hemolysis and transport to the laboratory promptly.

Evaluation

- Note results of other hepatic enzyme tests, particularly serum alkaline phosphatase, leucine aminopeptidase (LAP), gamma-glutamyl transferase (GGT), alanine aminotransferase (ALT), and aspartate aminotransferase (AST), indicating impaired liver function.

Client/Caregiver Teaching

Pretest

- Tell the client to withhold medications, especially hepatotoxic medications, for 24 hours before the test as ordered by the physician.

Posttest

- Tell the client to resume usual medications withheld before the test.

Otoscopy

Classification: Sensory organ function

Type of Test: Auditory perception

This noninvasive test is used to inspect the external ear, auditory canal, and tympanic membrane. Otoscopy is an essential part of any general physical examination, but it is also done before any other audiologic studies when symptoms of ear pain or hearing impairment are present.

Indications

- Diagnose cause of ear pain
- Detect causes of deafness, obstruction, stenosis, or swelling of the pinna or canal causing a narrowing closure that prevents sound from entering
- Detect ear abnormalities during routine physical examination
- Remove impacted cerumen with a dull ring curette or foreign bodies with a forceps that are obstructing the entrance of sound waves into the ear
- Evaluate acute or chronic otitis media and effectiveness of therapy in controlling infections

Reference Values

- Normal structure and appearance of the external ear, auditory canal, and tympanic membrane
    Pinna: funnel-shaped cartilaginous structure; no evidence of infection, pain, dermatitis with swelling, redness, or itching
    External auditory canal: S-shaped canal lined with fine hairs, sebaceous and ceruminous glands; no evidence of redness, lesions, edema, scaliness, pain, or accumulation of cerumen, drainage, or presence of foreign bodies
    Tympanic membrane: shallow, circular cone that is shiny and pearl gray in color, semitransparent whitish cord crossing from front to back just under the upper edge, cone of light on the right side at the 4 o'clock position; no evidence of bulging, retraction, lusterless membrane, or obliteration of the cone of light

Abnormal Values

- Cerumen accumulation
- Ear trauma
- Foreign bodies
- Otitis externa
- Otitis media
- Tympanic membrane perforation or rupture

Interfering Factors

- Obstruction of the auditory canal with cerumen, dried drainage, or foreign bodies that prevent introduction of the otoscope

Nursing Implications

Assessment

- Obtain a history of known or suspected ear disorders; signs and symptoms or complaints of pain, itching, drainage, deafness, antibiotic regimen; or presence of tympanotomy tube.

Possible Nursing Diagnoses

Infection or injury, risk for, related to procedure
Sensory or perceptual, altered, auditory
Pain related to disorder

Implementation

- Gently wash and dry the external ear before the examination, if needed.
- Administer ear drops or irrigation to prepare for cerumen removal, if ordered.
- Place adult client in a sitting position; the child in a supine position while sitting on the caregiver's lap. Request client to remain very still during the examination; a child can be restrained by the caregiver if needed.
- Assemble the otoscope with the correct-sized speculum to fit size of client's ear and check the light source. For the adult, tilt the head slightly away and, with the nondominant hand, pull the pinna upward and backward. For the child, pull the pinna downward while holding the head steady or have the caretaker hold the child's head steady depending on the age. Gently and slowly insert the speculum into the ear canal downward and forward with the handle of the otoscope held downward. For the child, hold the handle upward while placing the edge of the hand holding the otoscope on the head to steady it during insertion. If the speculum resists insertion, withdraw and attach a smaller one.
- Place an eye to the lens of the otoscope, turn on the light source, and advance the speculum into the canal until the tympanic membrane is visible. Examine the posterior and anterior membrane, cone of light, outer rim (annulus), umbo, handle of the malleus, folds, and pars tensa.
- Culture any effusion with a sterile swab and culture tube; or a physician will perform needle aspiration from the middle ear through the tympanic membrane during the examination. Other procedures such as cerumen and foreign body removal can also be performed.
- Pneumatic otoscopy can be done to determine tympanic membrane flexibility. This test permits the introduction of air into the canal that reveals a reduction in movement of the

membrane in acute otitis media and absence of movement in chronic otitis media.

Evaluation

■ Note test results in relation to the client's symptoms and other tests performed, particularly audiometry.

Client/Caregiver Teaching

Pretest

■ Inform the client or caregiver of the purpose of the procedure; explain that the procedure is generally performed in a health care setting by the physician or nurse and takes 5 minutes to complete for both ears; no pain is associated with the examination.

■ Inform the client to remain very still during the examination. Inform the caregiver that he or she may need to restrain the child to prevent damage to the ear if the child cannot remain still.

Posttest

■ Administer ear drops of a soothing oil as ordered if canal is irritated following removal of cerumen or foreign bodies.

■ Reinforce information given by the physician and answer or direct any questions to the appropriate professionals.

Ova and Parasites Stool; Stool for O/P; Parasite Screen, Stool

Classification: Microbiology

Type of Test: Stool

This test evaluates the stool for the presence of intestinal parasites and their eggs. Some parasites are nonpathogenic, but others such as protozoa, roundworm, hookworm, and tapeworm can cause serious illness.

Indications

- Diagnose intestinal parasitic infestation

Reference Values

- No presence of parasites, ova, or larvae

Abnormal Values

- Amebiasis
- Giardiasis

Interfering Factors

- Faulty collection technique or presence of urine can cause false-negative results.
- Failure to test a fresh specimen may cause a false-negative result.
- Antimicrobial or antiamebic therapy within 10 days of test may cause false-negative results.
- Failure to wait for 1 week after a GI study using barium or laxative use can affect test results.
- Medications such as antacids, antibiotics, bismuth, castor oil, antidiarrheal compounds, iron, magnesia, Metamucil may interfere with analysis.

Nursing Implications

Assessment

- Obtain a history of hygiene practices, recent travel, other diagnostic tests and the results, and medication regimen.
- Ensure that the client has withheld medications that interfere with test results and has not received barium for GI testing for 10 days.

Possible Nursing Diagnoses

Knowledge deficit related to transmission of the disorder
Diarrhea related to disorder
Fluid balance deficit related to gastrointestinal loss

Implementation

- Obtain a waterproof specimen container with preservative and tight-fitting lid.

- Collect a stool specimen directly into the container. If the client is bedridden, use a clean bedpan and transfer the specimen into the container using a tongue blade.
- Ensure that the container is labeled properly, including names of unusual parasites that may need to be identified, and transport to the laboratory immediately.

Evaluation

- Note test results in relation to other tests performed and the client's symptoms. Particularly note if client has eosinophilia or signs of microcytic anemia secondary to blood loss.

Client/Caregiver Teaching

Pretest

- Tell the client the procedure for obtaining the specimen. Warn the client not to contaminate the specimen with urine, toilet paper, or toilet water.
- Tell the client to avoid medications that interfere with test results.
- Instruct the client on handwashing procedures, and inform the client that the organism may be contagious.

Posttest

- Tell the client to resume medications withheld before the test.
- Warn the client that one negative result does not rule out parasitic infestation. Some laboratories require three specimens 2 to 3 days apart.

Oximetry, Pulse Oximetry

Classification: Photo diagnostic

Type of Procedure: Indirect measurement

Oximetry, also known as pulse oximetry, is a noninvasive study that provides continuous readings of arterial blood oxygen saturation (SaO_2) using a sensor site (earlobe or fingertip). The SaO_2 equals the ratio of the amount of oxygen in the hemoglobin to the maximum amount of hemoglobin expressed in percent. The results obtained compare favorably to oxygen saturation levels obtained by arterial blood gas (ABG) analysis without the need to perform successive arterial punctures. The device used is a clip or probe containing a sensor that increases the blood flow to the site and produces a light beam through the tissues at the site. The sensor measures the absorption of the light to determine the oxygen saturation reading that is recorded on a stationary or portable screen for viewing.

Indications

- Monitor oxygenation of tissues and organs perioperatively and during acute illnesses
- Monitor oxygenation status in those patients on a ventilator
- Evaluate suspected nocturnal hypoxemia in chronic obstructive pulmonary disease
- Monitor oxygen saturation during activities such as pulmonary exercise stress testing or during pulmonary rehabilitation exercises to determine optimal tolerance
- Determine effectiveness of pulmonary gas exchange function
- Monitor response to pulmonary drug regimens, especially bronchodilators, to determine effectiveness in promoting air flow and oxygen content
- Monitor oxygenation during testing for sleep apnea

Reference Values

- Arterial blood oxygen saturation >95%

Abnormal Values

- Hypoxemia with levels <95%
- Impaired cardiopulmonary function
- Abnormal gas exchange

Interfering Factors

- Movement of the finger or ear or improper placement of probe or clip will affect the readings.
- Anemic conditions with a reduction in hemoglobin (Hb), the oxygen-carrying component in the blood, affects measurement readings.
- Vasoconstriction from cool skin temperature, drugs, hypotension, or vessel obstruction causing a decrease in blood flow will affect readings.
- Nail polish or false fingernails can cause false results when finger probe is used.

■ Lipid emulsion therapy and presence of certain dyes can prevent accurate readings.
■ Excessive light surrounding the patient such as from surgical lights can also alter test results.

Nursing Implications

Assessment

■ Obtain a history of pulmonary disorders, respiratory and cardiac status, reason for monitoring procedure, and ABG results.
■ Ensure that the client does not have false fingernails and that nail polish has been removed.

Possible Nursing Diagnoses

Breathing pattern, ineffective, related to disorder
Spontaneous ventilation, inability to sustain, related to disorder
Cardiac output, decreased, related to disorder
Tissue perfusion, altered, related to disorder

Implementation

■ Massage the upper earlobe or finger to increase blood flow. The index finger is normally used but if the client's finger is too large for the probe, a smaller finger can be used. If the earlobe is used, make sure good contact is achieved.
■ Place the photodetector probe over the finger in such a way that the light beams and sensors are opposite each other. Turn on the power switch to the oximeter monitor. Information about heart rate and SaO_2 will be displayed after about 6 heartbeats.
■ At the conclusion of the test or monitoring, the clip is removed and cleaned with an alcohol sponge.

Evaluation

■ Compare the results with the client's symptoms and other test results, particularly arterial blood gases.
■ Closely observe and report decreasing SaO_2 to 90%.

Client/Caregiver Teaching

Pretest

■ Inform the client that the procedure is generally performed at the client's bedside, in the operating room during a surgical procedure, or in the physician's office by a respiratory therapist, technician, or nurse. Results are interpreted by a physician. Explain that procedure will last as long as monitoring is needed and can be continuous if done following surgery or for acute pulmonary conditions. No pain is associated with the procedure.

■ Tell the client that there are no food, fluid, or medication restrictions.

Posttest

■ Reinforce information regarding recommended treatment regimen based on test results.

Papanicolaou Smear, Pap Smear

Classification: Cytology

Type of Test: Vaginal and cervical smear

This cytologic evaluation indicates cell maturity, morphological changes, and metabolic activity. Although it is known primarily for its role in detecting cervical cancer, this test can be performed on other specimens, such as urine, prostatic fluid, gastric secretions, bronchial aspirations, sputum, or solid tumor cells obtained by fine-needle aspiration.

Indications

■ Detect malignant cells
■ Evaluate estrogen level and response to therapy
■ Identify inflammatory tissue changes
■ Detect viral and fungal vaginal infections

Reference Values

Class I	Normal cells
Class II	Atypical cells, not malignant or inflammatory
Class III	Atypical cells, suspicious of malignancy, mild cervical dysplasia

Class IV   Atypical cells, suggestive of
                                     malignancy, severe
                                     cervical dysplasia
Class V   Cancer cells present,
                                     conclusive for malignancy

Abnormal Values

- Positive values
  Cancer
  Endocrine disorders
  Endometriosis

Interfering Factors

- Douching within 24 hours may wash away cells and affect results.
- Collection of sample during menstruation or use of lubricating jelly may impair identification of abnormal cells.
- Improper collection or preservation of sample may affect results.

Nursing Implications

Assessment

- Obtain history of gynecological system, date of last menstrual period, frequency and duration of periods, medications, diagnostic tests and results.
- Ensure that female client voids immediately before pelvic examination.

Possible Nursing Diagnosis

Anxiety related to threat to health status

Implementation

- To obtain a cervical sample, place the client in the lithotomy position and drape for privacy. Apply protective gloves. Dip speculum in water to aid in insertion.
- Gently insert speculum and obtain vaginal and cervical samples and place on slides. Remove speculum.
- Spray fixative on slides and place in preservative immediately.
- Make sure cervical specimen is scraped or aspirated from the cervix. If lesions are present, take scrapings directly from them.

- In the client whose uterus is involuting or has atrophied, use a pipette to aspirate cells.
- Assist client from lithotomy position and cleanse perineal area as needed.

Evaluation

- Note results in relation to client's symptoms and other test results.

Client/Caregiver Teaching

Pretest

- Inform the client that it is best to schedule the test midcycle and not to douche or use vaginal medications 24 hours before the examination.
- Inform the client that slight discomfort might be experienced but no pain.

Posttest

- Advise client of timing and importance of next examination.
- Explain treatment if abnormality detected.

Paracentesis and Peritoneal Fluid Analysis

Classification: Chemistry

Type of Test: Fluid analysis

Paracentesis is an invasive procedure performed to remove peritoneal fluid from the peritoneal cavity by needle aspiration. The procedure can include lavage with normal saline or Ringer's lactate. Transudates resulting from cirrhosis or heart failure or exudates resulting from metastatic carcinoma may be present in the solution removed for analysis. Hematologic, cytologic, microbiologic, and chemistry examination of the fluid is performed for complete analysis.

Indications

- Evaluate ascites of unknown etiology and removal of accumulated fluid
- Diagnose suspected peritoneal effusion due to abdominal cancer, as indicated by elevated red cell count (RBC), decreased glucose, elevated carcinoembryonic antigen, and detection of cancer cells on cytological examination
- Confirm abdominal trauma, as indicated by elevated RBC
- Diagnose suspected ascites due to cirrhosis of the liver, as indicated by elevated white cell count (WBC), neutrophil count of 25 to 50 percent, and an absolute granulocyte count of <250/mm^3
- Diagnose suspected bacterial peritonitis, as indicated by elevated WBC, neutrophil count >50 percent, and an absolute granulocyte count of >250/mm^3
- Diagnose suspected tuberculosis peritoneal effusion as indicated by elevated lymphocyte count, positive acid-fast bacillus (AFB) smear and culture in about 25 to 50 percent of cases, and decreased glucose
- Diagnose suspected peritoneal effusion due to pancreatitis, pancreatic trauma, or pancreatic pseudocyst, as indicated by elevated amylase levels
- Diagnose suspected peritoneal effusion due to gastrointestinal perforation, strangulation, or necrosis, as indicated by elevated amylase, ammonia, and alkaline phosphatase levels
- Diagnose suspected rupture or perforation of the urinary bladder, as indicated by elevated ammonia, creatinine, and urea levels

Reference Values

Red blood cells (RBC)	None
White blood cells (WBC)	<300/mm^3 (undiluted peritoneal fluid)
	<500/mm^3 (lavage fluid)
Neutrophils	<25 percent
Absolute granulocyte count	<250/mm^3
Gram stain and culture	No organisms present
AFB smear and culture	No acid-fast bacilli present
Cytological examination	No abnormal cells present
Protein	<4.1 g/dL
Albumin	Negative
Glucose	70–100 mg/dL

Cholesterol	Greater or lesser than 46 mg/dL, depending on type of fluid
Amylase	140–400 U/L
Ammonia	$<50 \mu g/dL$
Alkaline phosphatase (ALP)	30–110 U/L
Creatinine	0.5–1.3 mg/dL
Urea	6–20 mg/dL
Carcinoembryonic antigen (CEA)	<2.5 ng/mL

Abnormal Values

- Elevated values

  Red cell count: Possible neoplasm, tuberculosis, or intra-abdominal trauma

  White cell count: Possible bacterial peritonitis (seen by elevated neutrophils and granulocyte counts) and cirrhosis without infection. *Lymphocytes*: Possible tuberculous peritonitis and chylous ascites. *Eosinophil*: May accompany ascites due to congestive heart failure, chronic peritoneal dialysis, abdominal lymphoma, hypereosinophilic syndrome, eosinophilic gastroenteritis, and ruptured hydatid cyst

  Protein: Indicates malignant, tuberculous, pancreatic ascites or chronic hepatic disease

  Amylase: Indicates pancreatic trauma, pancreatic pseudocyst, or acute pancreatitis; gastrointestinal perforation; and intestinal strangulation and necrosis

  Alkaline phosphatase: Indicates rupture or strangulation in intestinal tract

  Ammonia: Possible ruptured or strangulated intestines; ruptured appendix or ulcer

  Antigen levels (CEA): Possible abdominal cancer

- Color changes

  Milk-color fluid: Carcinoma, lymphoma, tuberculosis, parasitic infection, adhesion, hepatic cirrhosis, or pseudochylous conditions

  Cloudy or turbid fluid: Peritonitis

  Bloody fluid: Tumor, hemorrhagic pancreatitis, abdominal trauma, or a traumatic tap

  Bile-stained green fluid: Ruptured gallbladder, acute pancreatitis, or perforated intestine or duodenal ulcer

- Other values

  Glucose: Indicates peritonitis or peritoneal carcinomatosis

  Bacteria such as coliforms, anaerobes, or enterococci: Possible ruptured organ or infections

Acid-fast bacillus (AFB) smear: Positive in tuberculosis
Fungi: Indicates histoplasmosis, candidiasis, or coccidioidomycosis

Interfering Factors

- Blood from traumatic paracentesis can cause false test result.
- Undetected hypoglycemia or hyperglycemia can affect
  results.
- Contamination of the sample with skin cells and pathogens
  can affect results.

Nursing Implications

Assessment

- Obtain history of abdominal trauma, liver disease, or other
  possible causes of ascites; date of last menstrual period and
  possibility of pregnancy; and results of other laboratory and
  diagnostic tests.
- Ensure that anticoagulant medications and aspirin have
  been withheld as ordered.
- If client has ascites, assess abdomen, obtain weight, and measure abdominal girth for baseline readings.

Possible Nursing Diagnoses

Anxiety related to threat to health status
Pain related to disorder and the procedure
Injury, risk for, related to the procedure
Infection, risk for, related to procedure

Implementation

- Assemble necessary equipment: a paracentesis tray with solution for skin preparation, local anesthetic, a 50-mL syringe,
  needles of various sizes including a large-bore paracentesis
  needle or a trocar and a cannula, sterile drapes, and sterile
  gloves. Specimen collection tubes and bottles for the tests to
  be performed are also needed.
- Assist the client to a sitting position on the side of a bed or
  treatment table, with the feet and back supported. An alternate approach is to place the client in bed in a high Fowler's
  position.
- Cleanse the skin with an antiseptic solution and drape. The
  physician infiltrates the needle or trocar insertion site with
  local anesthetic. The paracentesis needle is inserted approximately 1 to 2 inches below the umbilicus. If a trocar

with cannula is to be used, a small skin incision can be made to facilitate insertion. The 50-mL syringe with stopcock is attached to the needle or cannula after the trocar has been removed. Gentle suction may be applied with the syringe to remove about 50 mL of fluid for examination.

- For peritoneal lavage, infuse sterile normal saline or Ringer's lactate using the needle or cannula. The client is then turned from side to side for 15 to 20 minutes and the lavage fluid is then removed.
- Place samples of peritoneal or ascitic fluid in appropriate containers; label and send them promptly to the laboratory. Record any antibiotic therapy on the laboratory slip if bacterial culture and sensitivity tests are to be performed.
- If the paracentesis is being performed for therapeutic as well as diagnostic reasons, additional fluid is removed. No more than 1000 to 1500 mL of fluid should be removed at any one time, in order to avoid complications such as hypovolemia and shock.
- When the desired fluid amount has been removed, the needle or cannula is withdrawn; slight pressure is applied to the site for a few minutes and the incision is sutured as needed. If there is no evidence of bleeding or other drainage, a sterile dressing is applied to the site.

Evaluation

- Note the test results in relation to other tests performed and the client's symptoms.
- After the test, assess puncture site for pain, bleeding, excessive drainage, and inflammation.
- Continue to observe the client for pallor, diaphoresis, vertigo, hypotension, tachycardia, pain, or anxiety for at least 24 hours after procedure. Rapid or excessive removal of fluid can precipitate vascular collapse, hypovolemia, and shock.
- Monitor client with severe hepatic disease for signs of hepatic coma or hematuria resulting from bladder injury.

Client/Caregiver Teaching

Pretest

- Inform the client that peritoneal fluid will be aspirated and sent to the lab for analysis, and that the procedure will be performed by a physician and will take approximately 30 minutes to complete.
- Inform the client that a "popping" sensation can be felt as the needle penetrates the peritoneum.

Posttest

- Inform the client and caregiver to report severe abdominal pain to the physician.
- Tell the client to return for suture removal, if needed.

Parathyroid Hormone (PTH)

Classification: Radioimmunoassay

Type of Test: Serum

This test measures parathyroid hormone (parathormone, PTH) secreted by the parathyroid glands in response to decreased levels of circulating calcium. Actions of PTH include mobilizing calcium from bone into the bloodstream, along with phosphates and protein matrix; promoting renal tubular reabsorption of calcium and depression of phosphate reabsorption, thereby reducing calcium excretion and increasing phosphate excretion by the kidneys; decreasing renal secretion of hydrogen ions, which leads to increased renal excretion of bicarbonate and chloride; and enhancing renal production of active vitamin D metabolites, causing increased calcium absorption in the small intestine. The net result of PTH action is maintenance of adequate serum calcium levels.

Indications

- Diagnose suspected secondary hyperparathyroidism from chronic renal failure, malignant tumors that produce ectopic PTH, and malabsorption syndromes
- Detect incidental damage or inadvertent removal of the parathyroid glands during thyroid or neck surgery
- Evaluate parathyroid response to altered serum calcium levels, especially those that result from malignant processes, leading to decreased PTH production
- Evaluate parathyroid response to hypomagnesemia and autoimmune destruction of the parathyroid glands

Reference Values

		SI Units
Active N-terminal	230–630 pg/mL	200–600 ng/L
Inactive C-terminal	400–1760 pg/mL	400–1760 ng/L
Parathormone	20–70 Eq/mL	20–70 mEq/L

PTH is measured by radioimmunoassay. As the antibody used for the assay directly affects the results, values will vary according to the laboratory performing the test.

Abnormal Values

- Increased PTH
    Malabsorption syndromes
    Malignant tumors
    Primary, secondary, or tertiary hyperparathyroidism
    Vitamin D deficiency
- Decreased PTH
    Autoimmune destruction of the parathyroids
    Graves' disease
    Hypomagnesemia
    Hypoparathyroidism
    Sarcoidosis
    Vitamin A and D intoxication

Interfering Factors

- Failure to fast from food for 8 hours before the test may alter results.
- Radionuclide procedures performed within 1 week before test may alter test results.

Nursing Implications

Assessment

- Obtain history of endocrine system, known or suspected disorders, and results of other tests performed.
- Ensure client has fasted from food for at least 8 hours before the test.

Possible Nursing Diagnoses

Fatigue related to disorder
Anxiety related to threat to health status

Implementation

- Put on gloves. Using aseptic technique, perform a peripheral or neck venipuncture and collect 7 mL of blood in a red-top tube. Place sample on ice.
- Handle the sample gently to avoid hemolysis and transport to the laboratory promptly.

Evaluation

- Note test results in relation to serum calcium levels; expect higher levels in neck vein sample in hyperparathyroidism.

Client/Caregiver Teaching

Pretest

- Tell the client to fast for 8 hours before the test.

Posttest

- Tell the client to resume diet withheld before test.
- Instruct client to report signs and symptoms of hypocalcemia and hypercalcemia to the physician.

Pelvimetry

Classification: Radiology

Type of Test: Noninvasive obstetric examination

This x-ray test of the pregnant woman's pelvis at or near term is performed to determine if vaginal delivery of fetus is possible, that is, if the pelvis is adequate in size related to fetal head and/or presentation. In most situations, this test has been replaced by ultrasonagraphy.

Indications

- Investigate maternal history of problems involving pelvic bone size and birthing process
- Confirm abnormal pelvic measurements or fetal presentation
- Determine cause of failure of head to engage during labor
- Confirm that oxytocin administration is not contraindicated

Reference Values

- Normal pelvic diameters with size adequate in relation to fetal head

Abnormal Values

- Pelvic size small in relation to size of fetal head or presentation

Interfering Factors

- Excessive fetal activity will blur the x-rays, making interpretation difficult.
- Metal objects within x-ray field will block visualization of structures.

Nursing Implications

Assessment

- Obtain obstetrical history, including past and current labor and deliveries, baseline fetal heart rate, and current trimester of pregnancy.

Possible Nursing Diagnoses

Anxiety related to threat to health status of fetus
Injury, risk for, related to fetal, maternal

Implementation

- Assist client to standing position for lateral view to determine lowest level of the head in the birth canal.
- Obtain a second film with the client in supine, semirecumbent, or side-lying position. Place a metal ruler (pelvimeter) at the level of the ischial tuberosities when the client is in the supine position, or at the gluteal folds in the side-lying position.
- Instruct the client to breathe rapidly and then hold breath while filming is being done.

Evaluation

- Note test results in relation to the client's symptoms and other tests performed.
- Assess fetal heart sounds and signs of progression of labor.

Client/Caregiver Teaching

Pretest

- Instruct the client to breathe rapidly and then hold breath while filming is being done.
- Inform the client that the x-ray exposure to the fetus should not be damaging when performed at or near term.

Posttest

- Prepare the client for oxytocin administration or cesarean section, based on test results.

Pepsinogen

Classification: Chemistry

Type of Test: Blood

This test indirectly measures pepsinogen in the blood. The client's blood sample is incubated in an acid pH and the pepsin activity is measured. Pepsinogen is the inactive precursor of pepsin, which acts on amino acids and aids in protein digestion.

Indications

- Diagnose gastric disorders

Reference Values

		SI Units
Adults	124–142 ng/mL	124–142 μg/L
Children		
Preterm infant	20–24 ng/mL	20–24 μg/L
Cord blood	24–28 ng/mL	24–28 μg/L
<12 mo	72–82 ng/mL	72–82 μg/L
12 mo–<3 yr	90–106 ng/mL	90–106 μg/L
3–6 yr	80–104 ng/mL	80–104 μg/L
7–10 yr	77–103 ng/mL	77–103 μg/L
11–14 yr	96–118 ng/mL	96–118 μg/L

Abnormal Values

- Elevated levels
    Acute gastritis
    Duodenal ulcer
    Hypergastrinemia
    Zollinger-Ellison syndrome
- Decreased levels
    Achlorhydria
    Addison's disease
    Atrophic gastritis
    Gastric cancer
    Hypopituitarism
    Pernicious anemia

Interfering Factors

- Impaired kidney function may cause elevated values.

Nursing Implications

Assessment

- Obtain history of gastrointestinal system, suspected or known digestive disorders, and results of any tests and procedures performed.
- Ensure that client has fasted overnight before the test.

Possible Nursing Diagnoses

Pain related to disorder
Nutrition, altered, less than body requirements, related to disorder
Activity intolerance related to disorder

Implementation

- Put on gloves. Using aseptic technique, perform a venipuncture and collect 10 mL of blood in a red-top tube.
- Handle specimen gently to avoid hemolysis and send to the laboratory promptly.

Evaluation

- Note results in relation to client's symptoms and other tests performed.
- Expect the physician to order an endoscopy, which is considered more valuable in evaluating gastric problems.

Client/Caregiver Teaching

Pretest

■ Instruct client to fast overnight before the test.

Posttest

■ Advise the client to resume diet withheld before the test.

Pericardiocentesis and Pericardial Fluid Analysis

Classification: Cytology, Chemistry

Type of Test: Pericardial fluid analysis

Pericardiocentesis is an invasive procedure performed to remove pericardial fluid for either diagnostic testing, emergency treatment for cardiac tamponade, or pericardial effusion. Most pericardial effusions are exudates. Hematologic, cytologic, microbiologic, and chemistry examination of the fluid is performed for complete analysis.

Indications

■ Diagnose pericardial effusion of unknown etiology
■ Evaluate suspected hemorrhagic pericarditis, as indicated by the presence of red cells and an elevated white cell count
■ Evaluate suspected bacterial pericarditis, as indicated by the presence of red cells, elevated white count with a predominance of neutrophils, and decreased glucose
■ Evaluate suspected post–myocardial infarction syndrome (Dressler's syndrome), as indicated by the presence of red cells and elevated white count with a predominance of neutrophils
■ Evaluate suspected tuberculous or fungal pericarditis, as indicated by the presence of red cells and an elevated white count with a predominance of lymphocytes
■ Evaluate suspected viral pericarditis, as indicated by the presence of red cells and an elevated white count with neutrophils predominating

- Evaluate suspected rheumatoid disease or systemic lupus erythematosus, as indicated by the presence of red cells, an elevated white count, and decreased glucose levels
- Evaluate suspected cancer as indicated by the presence of red cells, decreased glucose, and presence of abnormal cells on cytological examination

Reference Values

Red blood cells (RBC)	None normally present
White blood cells (WBC)	1000/mm^3
Glucose	80–100 mg/dL or essentially the same as the blood glucose level drawn 2 to 4 hours earlier
Lactate dehydrogenase (LDH)	45–90 U/L
Cytological examination	No abnormal cells
Gram strain and culture	No organisms present

Abnormal Values

- Aneurysms
- Cancers
- Closed-chest trauma
- Dissecting aortic aneurysm
- Fungal or viral pericarditis
- Hemorrhagic or bacterial pericarditis
- Metastatic cancers
- Post–myocardial infarction syndrome (Dressler's syndrome)
- Rheumatoid arthritis
- Systemic lupus erythematosus

Interfering Factors

- Blood in the sample from a traumatic pericardiocentesis
- Undetected hypoglycemia or hyperglycemia
- Contamination of the sample with skin cells and pathogens

NURSING ALERT

- Contraindicated in clients with bleeding disorders or who are unable to cooperate

Nursing Implications

Assessment

- Obtain pertinent history of cardiac symptoms, pain, discomfort or shortness of breath, abnormalities in laboratory results and diagnostic findings.
- Ensure that anticoagulant medications and aspirin have been withheld as ordered.
- Ensure that an emergency cart, defibrillator, and 12-lead ECG machine are at the bedside.

Possible Nursing Diagnoses

Anxiety related to threat to health status
Injury, risk for, related to procedure
Cardiac output, decreased, related to disorder

Implementation

- Assemble necessary equipment: pericardiocentesis tray with solution for skin preparation, local anesthetic, a 50-mL syringe, needles of various sizes including a cardiac needle, sterile drapes, and sterile gloves. Sterile test tubes are needed: at least one red-top, one green-top, and one lavender-top tube should be available. Containers for culture and cytological analysis of pericardial fluid samples also may be needed. An alligator clip is needed with the cardiac monitoring equipment for attaching a precordial (V) lead to the cardiac needle.
- Place the client in the supine position with the head elevated 45 to 60 degrees. Attach the limb leads for the cardiac monitor to the client for proper grounding. Cleanse the skin with an antiseptic solution and protect with sterile drapes. The physician then infiltrates the skin at the needle insertion site with local anesthetic.
- Attach the precordial (V) cardiac lead wire to the hub of the cardiac needle with the alligator clip. The needle is then inserted just below and slightly to the left of the xiphoid process (fifth to sixth intercostal space). Gentle traction is sustained on the plunger of the 50-mL syringe until fluid appears, indicating that the needle has entered the pericardial sac. Fluid samples (10 to 50 mL) are then withdrawn and placed in appropriate tubes. The labeled samples are promptly sent to the laboratory.
- When the desired samples have been obtained, the cardiac needle is withdrawn. Pressure is applied to the site for 5 minutes. If there is no evidence of bleeding or other drain-

age, a sterile bandage is applied. If the client's cardiac rhythm is stable, cardiac monitoring is discontinued.

■ During the procedure monitor client for respiratory or cardiac distress; possible complications of a pericardiocentesis include cardiac dysrhythmias, laceration of the pleura, the cardiac atrium or coronary vessels; injection of air into a cardiac chamber; and contamination of pleural spaces with infected pericardial fluid.

Evaluation

■ Assess puncture site for bleeding, hematoma formation, and inflammation each time the vital signs are taken and daily thereafter for several days.

■ Monitor for signs and symptoms of cardiac tamponade, including neck vein distention, hypotension, and muffled heart sounds, for at least 24 hours.

■ Note results in relation to other tests performed, such as cardiac output and chest x-ray, and to the client's symptoms.

Client/Caregiver Teaching

Pretest

■ Instruct client to fast 6 to 8 hours before the procedure if ordered.

■ Explain to the client that this test is to detect excessive fluid around the heart; explain where the procedure is performed (varies according to institution); that it is performed by a physician and can take approximately 20 minutes to complete.

■ Inform client of importance of lying very still during procedure.

■ Warn the client that the local anesthetic may cause a stinging sensation; also inform the client that a feeling of pressure will be felt when the needle is inserted.

Posttest

■ Tell the client to resume medications and usual activity withheld before the test.

■ Tell the client to report chest pain and changes in heart rate or breathing, to physician immediately.

pH

Classification: Urinalysis

Type of Test: Urine (random)

This test measures free hydrogen ions in the urine. It is normally a part of a routine urinalysis but can be performed separately. The pH of urine reflects the kidney's ability to regulate the acid-base balance of the body and, in the normally functioning kidney, excess hydrogen ions. Urine pH is reflective of plasma pH.

Reference Values

Newborn	5.0–7.0
Children	4.8–7.8
Adults	4.5–8.0

Abnormal Values

- Increased pH
    Dietary intake of excessive vegetables and citrus
    Excessive alkali ingestion
    Excessive vomiting
    Fanconi's syndrome
    Gastric suction
    Hyperaldosteronism
    Hypokalemia
    Renal calculi
    Renal dysfunction
    Respiratory or metabolic alkalosis
    Urinary tract infection
    Certain drugs, including aldosterone, amphotericin B, cortisone, diuretics, mafenide acetate, methazolamide, potassium preparations, prolactin, and sodium bicarbonate
- Decreased pH
    Alcohol poisoning
    Diabetes mellitus
    Diarrhea
    Dietary intake of high-protein, high-acid fruits

Phenylketonuria
Pyrexia
Respiratory or metabolic acidosis
Starvation
Certain drugs, including ascorbic acid, ammonium chloride, diazoxide, hippuric acid, methenamine mandelate, and metolazone

Interfering Factors

- Drugs and diet can affect results of the test (see Abnormal Values).

Nursing Implications

Assessment

- Obtain a history of renal system, fluid intake and output ratio, and special dietary and medications regimens.
- Assess understanding of specimen collection.

Possible Nursing Diagnosis

Nutrition, altered, less than body requirements, related to disorder

Implementation

- Instruct client to void 50 mL into a clean urinal or bedpan, or directly into a clean, dry plastic container.
- Insert dipstick into fresh urine specimen, remove; wait required length of time per manufacturer's directions, and compare the color of reagent strip to color on container. If dipstick is not used, send the sample to the laboratory.
- Best results are obtained if test is performed immediately, preferably on the first-voided specimen in the morning. Keep refrigerated until sample is transported to lab for further examination.

Evaluation

- Compare results with routine urinalysis values and serum pH.

Client/Caregiver Teaching

Pretest

- Inform the client about how to obtain the specimen.

Posttest

- Instruct the client and caregiver in dietary (acidic or alkaline inclusions) modifications as needed to change urinary pH.

Phenolphthalein Test, Laxative Abuse Test

Classification: Toxicology

Type of Test: Feces, urine

Phenolphthalein is an ingredient in many over-the-counter laxatives. This substance causes bowel emptying by enhancing fluid and electrolyte accumulation in the intestine. It is excreted in stool and urine and is detectable for 32 hours after ingestion. The most accurate results are obtained from a 24-hour urine specimen.

Indications

- Assess suspected laxative abuse or anorexia nervosa
- Diagnose unexplained diarrhea

Reference Values

- Negative for phenolphthalein

Abnormal Values

- Anorexia nervosa
- Chronic self-prescribed laxative use

Nursing Implications

Assessment

- Obtain history of gastrointestinal system, current symptoms, medication regimen, including use of laxatives and over-the-counter preparations, and results of other tests and procedures performed.

Possible Nursing Diagnoses

Nutrition, altered, less than body requirements
Self-concept, altered
Anxiety related to procedure

Implementation

- *Stool specimen*: Collect a random stool sample. Send the specimen to the laboratory. In the laboratory, the stool sample is mixed with an alkalinizing agent, such as sodium hydroxide on white paper. If phenolphthalein is present, the sample turns red.
- *Random urine*: Collect a a 10-mL clean-catch urine sample and send to the laboratory.
- *24-hour urine*: Obtain a clean 3-liter container, 24-hour urine bag or bottle without preservative according to laboratory policy. Refrigerate the specimen during the collection time. Begin the test between 6 and 8 A.M. if possible; collect first voiding and discard. Record the time specimen was discarded as the beginning of the 24-hour test; document quantity of urine output during collection period, including urine at end of 24-hour period. The next morning, ask the client to void at the same time the collection was started and add this last voiding to the container. If an indwelling catheter is in place, keep drainage bag on ice, or empty the urine into a large refrigerated container with the preservative periodically during the 24 hours; monitor for continued drainage and conclude the test the next morning at the same hour the collection was begun. At the conclusion of the test ensure that label is properly completed and transport specimen to the laboratory immediately.

Evaluation

- Compare quantity of urine in specimen container with urinary output record during collection time to ensure that all urine has been included.

Evaluation

- Note the results in relation to other test results and the client's symptoms.
- Realize that a negative result does not necessarily rule out laxative abuse. Repeating a 24-hour urine test for 3 consecutive days increases the potential of detecting whether laxative abuse has occurred.

Client/Caregiver Teaching

Pretest

- Inform the client that all urine for a 24-hour period must be saved and monitor all urine output in chart; instruct client to avoid voiding in pan with defecation and to keep toilet tissue out of pan to prevent contamination of the specimen.

Posttest

■ Discuss complications of laxative abuse with the client, as indicated.

Phenolsulfonphthalein (PSP)

Classification: Urinalysis

Type of Test: Urine (timed)

This test measures proximal tubular function to determine the ability of the kidneys to remove waste products and other substances, such as drugs, from the blood and secrete them into the urine. Normal tubular function is dependent on two main factors: (1) adequate renal blood flow and (2) effective tubular function. Phenolsulfonphthalein (PSP) is administered intravenously and then its excretion measured in serial urine samples. To be excreted, the dye must be secreted by renal tubular cells; consequently, if renal dysfunction is present, excretion of the dye is decreased.

Indications

■ Evaluate renal blood flow and tubular secreting function

Reference Values

Children	5–10% higher than adults at the same time intervals

Adults 15 min = 25% of dose
excreted
30 min = 50–60% of dose
excreted
60 min = 60–70% of dose
excreted
2 hr = 70–80% of dose
excreted

Abnormal Values

- Increased excretion
  Hepatic disease
  Hypoalbuminemia
  Hypoproteinuria
  Multiple myeloma
- Decreased excretion
  Decreased 15-minute excretion with normal excretion later: possible mild or early-stage bilateral renal disease
  Decreased 2-hour value: possible moderate to severe renal impairment
  Congestive heart failure (CHF)
  Gout
  Hypertension
  Nephritis
  Renal vascular disease
  Urinary tract obstruction

Interfering Factors

- Failure to collect the required amount of urine samples (40 mL) at the required times and failure to completely empty the bladder each time a specimen is collected can affect results.
- Presence of altered urine color can affect accuracy of test results.
- Inadequately hydrated client, as when a client has inadequately perfused kidneys or decreased urine flow is present, can affect results.
- Certain drugs, such as radiographical dye, salicylates, sulfonamides, or penicillin can lead to falsely abnormal test results.
- High serum protein levels can lead to decreased excretion of the dye.
- Severe hypoalbuminemia, excessive albuminuria, or severe liver disease can cause increased excretion of the dye.

- Recent consumption of beets, carrots, and rhubarb can affect results.
- Inexact PSP dose can alter test results.
- Drugs such as radiopaque dye, aspirin, cascara sagrada, ethanol, indomethacin, nitrofurantoin, phenylbutazone, penicillin, sulfonamides, probenecid, and vitamins can alter results.

> **NURSING ALERT**

- Contraindicated in clients who are allergic to the dye; keep epinephrine on hand in case of allergic reaction to PSP.
- Perform test cautiously in clients with cardiac dysfunction or renal insufficiency; increased fluid intake can precipitate congestive heart failure.

Nursing Implications

Assessment

- Assess and obtain history of kidney function and medications being taken and allergy history to PSP dye.
- Ensure medications, foods, or substances that color urine have been withheld for 24 hours.
- Ensure proper fluid intake before and during test to promote hydration and specimen collection.

Possible Nursing Diagnoses

Anxiety related to threat to health status
Tissue perfusion, altered, renal, related to disorder
Injury, risk for, related to procedure

Implementation

- Obtain the four appropriate-sized plastic clean containers without preservative according to laboratory policy.
- Record the time PSP is administered and collect and discard the first specimen as the beginning of the timed test.
- Collect at least 40 mL of urine at 15 minutes, 30 minutes, 1 hour, and 2 hours; ensure that no urine is omitted from each timed specimen.
- Document quantity and time of urine output during testing.
- If an indwelling catheter is in place, replace tubing and container system at the start of the collection time; obtain urine

specimen at the correct time; clamp catheter tubing until the next specimen is due and continue to collect and clamp tubing for each specimen.

- At the conclusion of the test, ensure that the labels are properly completed with exact time and transport to the laboratory.

Evaluation

- Observe client for allergic response to the PSP.
- Monitor client's response to the fluid load carefully. Note especially increased pulse rate or difficulty breathing.
- Note test results in relation to other tests and the client's symptoms.

Client/Caregiver Teaching

Pretest

- Tell the client to avoid drugs and foods that alter color of urine.
- Warn the client that PSP turns urine reddish in color.
- Explain that client should drink extra fluids before and during test.
- Tell the client to avoid excessive exercise and stress during the urine collection time.
- Inform the client that all urine for the specified timed period must be saved. Instruct client to avoid voiding in pan with defecation and to keep toilet tissue out of pan to prevent contamination of the specimen.

Posttest

- Tell the client to resume medications, foods, and activity withheld before the test.

Phonocardiograph (PCG)

Classification: Electrophysiologic study

Type of Test: Indirect cardiac function measurement

This is a noninvasive study performed to identify, amplify, and record heart sounds and murmurs. The sounds of blood flowing through the heart and great vessels are recorded from sites on the chest by a microphone containing a transducer that converts the sounds into electrical impulses; selected high and low frequency events are recorded on a graph. Doing the test simultaneously with electrocardiography (ECG), carotid or jugular pulse wave tracings, and apexcardiography provides accurate timing of the heart sounds and cardiac events for detailed analysis.

Indications

- Detect valvular defects, as evidenced by abnormal heart sounds
- Differentiate between mitral and tricuspid opening snaps from the third sound (S_3)
- Differentiate between early, mid, and late systolic murmurs
- Diagnose hypertrophic cardiomyopathies and pulmonary hypertension, as evidenced by presence of S_4
- Diagnose abnormal left ventricular function evidenced by change in left ventricular ejection and pre-ejection time

Reference Values

- Normal heart sounds except during ventricular systole and diastole

Abnormal Values

- Aortic stenosis
- Atrioventricular valve regurgitation
- Coronary artery disease
- First-degree atrioventricular block
- Hypertrophic cardiomyopathies
- Myocarditis

- Pericardial effusion
- Pulmonary embolism
- Right bundle branch block
- Right ventricular overload
- Systemic or pulmonary hypertension
- Tricuspid or mitral stenosis

Interfering Factors

- Improper placement of the microphone on the chest or background noises or other interferences can cause inaccurate results.
- The same factors that affect accurate results of electrocardiography (ECG) pertain to this study as the two procedures are done concurrently.
- Obesity can make sounds difficult to detect.

Nursing Implications

Assessment

- Obtain history of cardiac disease and present cardiovascular status, cardiac medication regimen, and history of previous tests and procedures.
- Ensure skin where electrodes will be placed is cleansed gently with an alcohol wipe.
- Assess for compliance with smoking restrictions before the study.

Possible Nursing Diagnoses

Anxiety related to threat to health status
Cardiac output, decreased, related to the disease
Altered tissue perfusion, cardiopulmonary, related to the disease
Activity intolerance related to the disease

Implementation

- Place client in a supine position with the head elevated on a pillow on the examining table in a room that is quiet. Remind the client to remain still and quiet during procedure, except when asked to change position or perform an activity.
- Place ECG leads on the appropriate skin sites and prepare for apexcardiography or carotid or pulse wave tracings. Place the microphones over the apex and pulmonic area of the heart and strap them in place. Ask the client to inhale and then exhale while stopping the expiration as recording is obtained.

- Move the microphone from the pulmonic area to the aortic area; repeat the procedure to obtain the recording.
- Heart sounds can also be recorded with the client in a different position (left side-lying) and while breathing slowly or performing exercises.

Evaluation

- Note results in relation to other tests performed and the client's symptoms.
- Monitor for signs and symptoms of decreased cardiac output such as peripheral pulses, skin color, capillary refill time, dyspnea, abnormal heart sounds, angina, or decreased urinary output; administer ordered oxygen and cardiac medications.
- Monitor the strip for cardiac rhythm abnormalities; administer oxygen, vasodilators, antiarrhythmics if infarction, ischemia, or life-threatening dysrhythmias such as ventricular tachycardia are present.

Client/Caregiver Teaching

Pretest

- Explain that the procedure takes about 30 minutes and is performed in a special laboratory, and that the results are interpreted by a physician.
- Tell the client that there are no food or fluid restrictions.
- Explain that during the test the client may be asked to inhale a drug that can cause some temporary symptoms (flushing, dizziness, and palpitations).

Posttest

- Instruct the client to report chest pain and changes in heart rate to physician.
- Instruct the client and caregiver in the correct administration of heart medications and the side effects to report.

Phospholipids

Classification: Chemistry

Type of Test: Serum

This test measures phospholipids, lipids consisting of one or more fatty acid molecules, one phosphoric acid radical, and usually a nitrogenous base. Phospholipids are important for the formation of cell membranes and for transporting fatty acids through the intestinal mucosa into lymph. The three major types of body phospholipids are the lecithins, the cephalins, and the sphingomyelins. In addition to dietary sources of phospholipids, nearly all body cells are capable of forming these lipids. Most endogenous phospholipids are formed, however, in the liver and intestinal mucosa. The phospholipids are transported together in circulating blood in the form of lipoproteins.

Indications

- Evaluate known or suspected disorders that are associated with altered lipid metabolism
- Evaluate abnormal bleeding of unknown origin, with decreased cephalin as a possible contributor to low thromboplastin levels
- Diagnose suspected neurological disorder, which can be associated with decreased sphingomyelin levels

Reference Values

		SI Units
Newborn	75–170 mg/dL	0.75–1.70 g/L
Infants	100–275 mg/dL	1.0–2.75 g/L
Children	180–295 mg/dL	1.80–2.95 g/L
Adults	150–380 mg/dL	1.50–3.80 g/L

Values may vary depending on the laboratory performing the test.

Abnormal Values

- Increased levels
    Chronic pancreatitis

Diabetes mellitus
Early starvation
Nephrotic syndrome
Obstructive jaundice
- Decreased levels
Cirrhosis
Hepatitis
Malabsorption syndrome
Primary hypolipoproteinemia
Severe malnutrition

Interfering Factors

- Recent testing with radionuclide results in inaccurate results.
- Ingestion of alcohol 24 hours and food 12 hours before the test can falsely elevate levels.
- Antilipemic drugs can lower phospholipid levels; epinephrine, estrogens, and chlorpromazine tend to elevate phospholipid levels.

Nursing Implications

Assessment

- Assess risk for cardiovascular disease; obtain a history of other lipid tests performed.
- Assess compliance in consuming a low-fat evening meal on the day before the test and then fasting 12 to 14 hours before the test; water is not restricted.
- Assess compliance in abstaining from alcohol for 24 hours before the test and withholding drugs that may alter phospholipid levels for 12 hours before the test, as ordered.

Possible Nursing Diagnoses

Altered nutrition, more than body requirements, related to the disease
Injury, risk for, related to metabolic imbalance

Implementation

- Put on gloves. Using aseptic technique, perform a venipuncture and collect 7 to 10 mL of blood in a clotted red-top tube.
- Label specimen and send to the laboratory promptly.

Evaluation

■ Note results of other tests done for lipids and lipoprotein electrophoresis.

Client/Caregiver Teaching

Pretest

■ Tell the client to consume a low-fat evening meal on the day before the test and then fast for 12 to 14 hours before the test; water is not restricted.
■ Tell the client to abstain from alcohol for 24 hours before the test and to withhold drugs that may alter phospholipid levels for 12 hours before the test, as ordered.

Posttest

■ Tell the client to resume diet and medication withheld before the test.
■ Instruct the client and caregiver in dietary management of fat and carbohydrate intake to reduce risk of heart disease.

Plasminogen

Classification: Hematology

Type of Test: Plasma

Plasminogen is a beta globulin protein that is a precursor to plasmin. It is found in fibrin clots of blood vessels, soft tissue, or body cavities lined with endothelial cells. Plasmin dissolves fibrin clots to prevent excessive coagulation. It cannot be measured directly because it doesn't circulate in active form, as plasminogen can.

Indications

- Detect fibrinolysis
- Detect congenital and acquired fibrinolytic diseases

Reference Values

- 20 mg/dL or 2.7–4.5 U/mL

Abnormal Values

- Increased values
  Congenital defect in plasminogen inhibitors
  Deep-vein thrombosis (DVT)
  Certain medications, including oral contraceptives
- Decreased values
  Cirrhosis
  Disseminated intravascular coagulation (DIC)
  Eclampsia
  Tumors
  Certain medications, including L-asparaginase, thrombolytics (streptokinase, urokinase)

Interfering Factors

- Hemolyzed or clotted samples yield inaccurate results.
- Prolonged use of a tourniquet before venipuncture can cause falsely decreased levels.

Nursing Implications

Assessment

- Obtain history of hematological system, known or suspected clotting abnormality, results of tests and procedures performed.
- Assess medication history and ensure that any drugs that may alter test results have been withheld for 12 to 24 hours before the test, as ordered by the physician.

Possible Nursing Diagnoses

Anxiety related to threat to health status
Injury, risk for, related to abnormal clotting mechanisms

Implementation

- Put on gloves. Using aseptic technique, perform a venipuncture and collect a 7-mL blood sample in a blue-top tube.
- Handle sample gently to avoid hemolysis and transport to the laboratory promptly.

Evaluation

- Note test results in relation to other tests performed, particularly other coagulation studies, and to the client's symptoms.

Client/Caregiver Teaching

Pretest

- Tell the client to withhold medications that interfere with test results.

Posttest

- Tell the client to resume medications withheld before the test.

Platelet Aggregation

Classification: Hematology

Type of Test: Blood

Platelets gather at the site after vascular injury and form an aggregate, a plug that helps maintain hemostasis and promotes healing. The platelet aggregation test assesses the ability of platelets to adhere to each other by mixing the person's platelets in solution with substances that induce aggregation and measuring the amount or rate of platelet clumping. Aggregating reagent substances used include adenosine diphosphate (ADP), epinephrine, collagen, thrombin, ristocetin, and arachidonic acid.

Evenly suspended platelets aggregate and fall to the bottom of the tube. The greater the aggregation the less turbid the sample. The test measures the amount of light that passes through the solution after clumping has occurred or measures changes in turbidity by a spectrophotometer. Aggregation curves obtained by using different reagents can help to distinguish various qualitative platelet defects.

Indications

- Measure platelet aggregation
- Detect von Willebrand's disease
- Diagnose other congenital platelet bleeding disorders

Reference Values

- 60–100% aggregation, or aggregation within 3 to 5 minutes, as determined by the specific laboratory

Abnormal Values

- Increased values
  - Atheromatosis
  - Diabetes mellitus
  - Hypercoagulability
  - Hyperlipemia
  - Polycythemia vera
- Decreased values
  - Afibrinogenemia
  - Anemia (sideroblastic)
  - Bernard-Soulier syndrome (ristocetin test)
  - Beta-thalassemia major
  - Chédiak-Higashi syndrome
  - Cirrhosis
  - Glanzmann's thrombasthenia (ADP, epinephrine, and collagen tests)
  - Gray platelet syndrome (ADP, epinephrine, thrombin, collagen tests)
  - Hermansky-Pudlak syndrome
  - Homocystinuria
  - Idiopathic thrombocytopenic purpura (ADP, collagen, epinephrine)
  - Macroglobulinemia
  - Plasma cell dyscrasias
  - Platelet release defects (ADP, second phase; epinephrine, second phase; and collagen tests)
  - Preleukemia
  - Scurvy

Storage pool disease (ADP, second phase; epinephrine, second phase; and collagen tests)

Thrombasthenia (ADP, epinephrine, collagen)

Thrombocythemia (hemorrhagic)

Uremia

von Gierke's disease

von Willebrand's disease (ristocetin test)

Wiskott-Aldrich syndrome

Certain drugs, including alphaprodine, antibiotics, anticoagulants, antihistamines, aspirin, carbenicillin, indanyl sodium, cephalothin sodium, chlordiazepoxide, chloroquine hydrochloride, chloroquine phosphate, clofibrate, cocaine hydrochloride, corticosteroids, cyproheptadine hydrochloride, dextropropoxyphene, diazepam, diphenhydramine hydrochloride, dipyridamole, furosemide, gentamicin sulfate, guaifenesin, heparin calcium, heparin sodium, ibuprofen, imipramine, indomethacin, marijuana, mefenamic acid, naproxen sodium, nitrofurantoin, nortriptyline hydrochloride, oxyphenbutazone, penicillin G benzathine, penicillin G potassium, penicillin G procaine, phenothiazines, phenylbutazone, promethazine hydrochloride, propranolol, pyrimidine compounds, sulfinpyrazone, theophylline, tricyclic antidepressants, and vitamin E

Interfering Factors

- Hemolyzed or clotted specimen or specimen received more than 2 hours after collection affects results and should be rejected.
- Platelet count <100,000/mm^3 causes inaccurate results.
- Lipemia may interfere with accurate measurement.
- Numerous drugs may lead to decreased platelet aggregate levels (see Abnormal Values).

Nursing Implications

Assessment

- Obtain history of blood-clotting disorders and complete medication history.
- Ensure client has fasted or maintained a nonfat, caffeine-free diet for 8 to 12 hours before the test since lipids and caffeinated foods and beverages can affect test findings.
- Ensure aspirin and aspirin-containing medications have been withheld for 14 days or notify laboratory if aspirin cannot be withheld.

- Ensure that all medications listed above have been withheld for 48 hours before test. (All nonessential medication should be avoided since interfering medication list is growing.)

Possible Nursing Diagnoses

Anxiety related to threat to health status
Injury, risk for, related to abnormal clotting mechanism

Implementation

- Put on gloves. Using aseptic technique, perform a venipuncture and collect 7 mL of blood in a blue-top siliconized tube. Or collect 7 mL of blood in a plastic syringe and carefully instill into a blue-top tube containing sodium citrate and citric acid; mix the sample and the anticoagulant adequately.
- Send to laboratory immediately. Testing should be performed within 2 hours after collection.

Evaluation

- Note test results in relation to other tests performed, particularly coagulation studies, and the client's symptoms.

Client/Caregiver Teaching

Pretest

- Tell the client to fast or maintain a nonfat, caffeine-free diet for 8 to 12 hours before the test since lipids and caffeinated foods and beverages can affect test findings.
- Inform the client not to take aspirin and aspirin-containing medications for 14 days before the test, if ordered.
- Tell the client to avoid all medications that can interfere with test results. Suggest that the client avoid all nonessential medications since interfering medication list is growing.

Posttest

- Tell the client to resume diet and medications withheld before the test.

Platelet Antibody Detection

Classification: Hematology

Type of Test: Blood

This test is performed to detect the presence of platelet auto-antibodies and platelet isoantibodies. Platelet autoantibodies are IgG immunoglobulins of autoimmune origin and are present in various autoimmune disorders, including thrombocytopenias. Platelet autoantibodies may be detected with a quantitative antiglobulin consumption test or other methods.

Platelet isoantibodies develop in people who become sensitized to platelet antigens of transfused blood. As a result, destruction of both donor and native platelets and shortened survival time of platelets in the transfusion recipient occurs. A complement fixation test or other methods may be used to detect platelet isoantibodies.

The platelet antibody detection test is also used for platelet typing, which allows compatible platelets to be transfused to people with such disorders as aplastic anemia and cancer and decreases the alloimmunization risk resulting from repeated transfusions from random donors. Platelet typing also may provide additional support for a diagnosis of posttransfusional purpura.

Indications

- Diagnose alloimmune neonatal thrombocytopenic purpura, idiopathic thrombocytopenic purpura (ITP), paroxysmal hemoglobinuria, drug-induced immunologic thrombocytopenia, and posttransfusion purpura
- Determine platelet type

Reference Values

Platelet antibodies	Negative
Platelet-associated immunoglobulin G (PA IgG)	Negative
Drug-dependent platelet antibodies	Negative
Hyperlysibility assay	Negative

Abnormal Values

- Positive
  Alloimmune neonatal thrombocytopenic purpura
  Multiple blood transfusions
  Paroxysmal hemoglobinuria
  Thrombocytopenia
  Thrombocytopenias provoked by drugs such as quinidine,
  quinine, chlordiazepoxide, sulfa, and hydantoin

Interfering Factors

- Hemolyzed or clotted specimens will affect results.

Nursing Implications

Assessment

- Obtain history of illness and symptoms, recent blood transfusions, and medications.

Possible Nursing Diagnoses

Injury, risk for, related to altered clotting factors
Protection, altered, related to abnormal blood profiles
Anxiety related to perceived threat to health status

Implementation

- Put on gloves. Using aseptic technique, perform a venipuncture and collect 7 mL of blood in a red-top tube. Or fill two sodium citrate-anticoagulated blue-top tubes, as directed by the laboratory.
- Transport specimens to laboratory immediately.

Evaluation

- Note the test results in relation to the total platelet count and the client's response to platelet transfusions.

Client/Caregiver Teaching

Posttest

- Instruct the client to report any acute or slow persistent bleeding or signs of infection at the site.
- Instruct the client to avoid trauma in the presence of thrombocytopenia.

Platelet Count (Thrombocyte)

Classification: Hematology

Type of Test: Blood

This test measures the number of platelets, the nonnucleated, cytoplasmic round or oval disks that bud off from large multi-nucleated cells (megakaryocytes), in each cubic mililiter of blood. Platelets have an essential function in coagulation, hemostasis, and blood thrombus formation. Decreased platelets can occur either because of decreased production or increased destruction.

Indications

- Act as part of routine screening in a complete physical examination
- Confirm a low platelet count (thrombocytopenia), which can be associated with bleeding, or an elevated platelet count (thrombocytosis), which can cause increased clotting
- Evaluate cause of clinical signs of bleeding such as epistaxis, easy bruising, bleeding gums, hematuria, and menorrhagia

Reference Values

		SI Units
Adult	150,000 to 450,000/mm^3 (average = 250,000/mm^3)	$150 - 450 \times 10^9$/L
Critical (low)	<30,000/mm^3	$<30 \times 10^9$/L
Critical (high)	71,000,000/mm^3	$>1000 \times 10^9$/L

Values vary slightly across the life cycle, with lower platelet counts seen in newborns.

Abnormal Values

- Increased levels
    Anemias (posthemorrhagic and iron-deficiency)
    Carcinomatosis

Childbirth
Chronic heart disease
Chronic pancreatitis
Cirrhosis
Hemorrhage
Leukemias (chronic)
Polycythemia vera
Splenectomy
Surgery
Trauma
Tuberculosis and other acute infections
Drugs such as epinephrine and oral contraceptives

■ Decreased levels with decreased production
Bone marrow malignancies
Fanconi's syndrome
Histiocytosis
Leukemias (acute)
Radiation
Uremia
Viral infections
Vitamin B/folic acid deficiencies
Wiskott-Aldrich syndrome
Certain drugs, such as alcohol, anticancer drugs, anticon-
vulsants, carbamates, chloramphenicol, chlorothia-
zides, isoniazid, pyrazolones, streptomycin, sulfon-
amides, and sulfonylureas

■ Decreased levels with increased destruction
Anemias (pernicious, aplastic)
Antibody/HLA antigen reactions
Burns
Chronic cor pulmonale
Congenital infections (cytomegalovirus, herpes, syphilis,
toxoplasmosis)
Disseminated intravascular coagulation
Hemolytic disease of the newborn
Idiopathic thrombocytopenic purpura
Immune complex formation
Lymphomas
Meningococcemia
Miliary tuberculosis
Rocky Mountain spotted fever
Sarcoidosis
Splenomegaly due to liver disease
Certain drugs, such as aspirin, benzenes, DDT, digitoxin,
gold salts, heparin, quinidine, quinine, and thiazides

Interfering Factors

- White blood cell count greater than 100,000 per mm^3, severe red blood cell fragmentation, and extraneous particles in the fluid used to dilute the sample can alter test results.
- Mishandling of the sample, including excessive agitation or allowing plasma sample to settle too long during processing, can alter results.
- Numerous drugs can alter platelet functions and numbers (see Abnormal Values).
- Traumatic venipunctures may lead to erroneous results caused by activation of the coagulation sequence.

Nursing Implications

Assessment

- Obtain a personal and family history of known or suspected hematologic disorders, abnormal bleeding, or abnormal hematologic laboratory results.

Possible Nursing Diagnoses

Injury, risk for, related to altered clotting factors
Protection, altered, related to abnormal blood profiles
Anxiety related to perceived threat to health status

Implementation

- Put on gloves. Using aseptic technique, perform a venipuncture and collect a 5-mL sample of blood in a lavender-top tube. Limit tourniquet application to 1 minute.
- Obtain a capillary sample if the client is an infant or child.
- Handle the sample gently to avoid platelet clumping, which alters test results.

Evaluation

- Note the test results in relation to the other tests for hemostatic function.

Client/Caregiver Teaching

Posttest

- Instruct the client to report any acute or slow persistent bleeding or signs of infection at the site.
- If adhesive bandage or pressure dressing is applied, instruct the client to remove in 24 hours.
- Instruct the client to avoid trauma in the presence of thrombocytopenia.

Plethysmography: Arterial, Venous, Body, Impedance

Classification: Vascular function (arterial, venous, impedance); Pulmonary function (body)

Type of Test: Manometric studies

This test is a noninvasive diagnostic manometric study used to measure changes in the size of blood vessels by determining the volume changes in the blood vessels of the eye, extremities, or neck or gas volume changes in the lungs.

Arterial plethysmography is an assessment of arterial circulation in the upper or lower limbs; it is used in the diagnosis of lower-extremity arteriosclerotic disease. *Venous plethysmography* measures changes in venous capacity and outflow (volume and rate of outflow); it is used in diagnosing a thrombotic condition that causes obstruction of the major veins of the extremities. *Body plethysmography* measures the total amount (volume) of air within the thorax, both in or not in ventilatory communication with the lung; the elasticity (compliance) of the lungs; and the resistance to air flow in the respiratory tree. It is used in conjunction with pulmonary stress and pulmonary function tests to diagnose pulmonary disease. *Impedance plethysmography* is widely used to detect acute deep-vein thrombosis (DVT) of the leg but can be used in the arm, abdomen, neck, or thorax.

Indications

Arterial Plethysmography

- Evaluate suspected arterial occlusive disease
- Determine changes in toe or finger pressures when ankle pressures are elevated as a result of arterial calcifications
- Determine the effect of trauma on the arteries in an extremity
- Determine peripheral small-artery changes (ischemia) caused by diabetes and differentiate these changes from neuropathy
- Diagnose vascular changes associated with Raynaud's phenomenon and disease

- Locate and determine the degree of arterial atherosclerotic obstruction and vessel patency in peripheral atherosclerotic disease and inflammatory changes causing obliteration in the vessels in *thromboangiitis obliterans*
- Confirm suspected acute arterial embolization

Venous Plethysmography

- Diagnose partial or total venous thrombotic obstruction
- Determine valve competency in conjunction with Doppler ultrasonography in the diagnosis of varicose veins

Body Plethysmography

- Diagnose or determine the status of obstructive pulmonary disease, such as emphysema, asthma, chronic bronchitis
- Diagnose or determine the status of restrictive pulmonary disease, such as fibrosis
- Detect acute pulmonary disorders such as atelectasis and pneumonia
- Differentiate between obstructive and restrictive pulmonary pathology
- Evaluate pulmonary status before pulmonary rehabilitation to determine the baseline and possible benefits from the therapy

Impedance Plethysmography

- Diagnose and evaluate DVT
- Act as a diagnostic screen for clients at risk for DVT
- Evaluate clients with suspected pulmonary embolism (since most pulmonary emboli are complications of DVT in the leg)
- Evaluate degree of resolution of DVT after treatment

Reference Values

Arterial Plethysmography

- Normal arterial pulse waves: steep up slope, more gradual down slope with narrow pointed peaks
- Normal pressure: <20 mm Hg systolic difference between the lower extremity and the upper extremity; toe pressure ≥80 percent ankle pressure and finger pressure ≥80 percent wrist pressure

Venous Plethysmography

- Normal venous blood flow in extremities
- Venous filling time: >20 seconds

Body Plethysmography

- Thoracic gas volume: 2400 mL
- Compliance : 0.2 L/cm H_2O
- Airway resistance: 0.6–2.5 cm H_2O/L per second

Impedance Plethysmography

- Sharp rise in volume with temporary occlusion; rapid venous outflow with release of the occlusion

Abnormal Values

- Incompetent valves, thrombosis, or thrombotic obstruction in a major vein in an extremity
- DVT (arterial, venous, or impedance plethysmography)
- Obstructive or restrictive lung disease, infection, or atelectasis (body plethysmography)

Interfering Factors

Arterial Plethysmography

- Smoking 2 hours before the study causes inaccurate results as the nicotine constricts the arteries.
- Environmental temperatures (hot or cold) can affect the results.
- Arterial occlusion that is proximal to the extremity to be examined can prevent blood flow to the limb.

Venous Plethysmography

- Environmental temperature or cold extremity will affect test results as this constricts the vessels.
- High anxiety level or muscle tenseness will affect test results.
- Venous occlusion that is proximal to the extremity to be examined can affect blood flow to the limb.

Body Plethysmography

- Inability of the client to follow breathing instructions during the procedure will affect results.

Impedance Plethysmography

- False-positive impedance plethysmography results can occur if the extremity is moved during electrical impedance recording or if there is poor electrode contact or nonlinear electrical output.
- Constricting clothing or bandages can alter test results.

General Factors

- Anxiety, apprehension, or discomfort can cause abnormal results owing to increased muscle tension or vasoconstriction.
- False-positive results can occur in persons with congestive heart failure, arterial insufficiency, or postphlebitic syndrome.
- False-negative results can occur with collateral circulation development, which bypasses obstruction.
- Abnormal results can occur during pregnancy because of fetal compression of the inferior vena cava. Pregnant women with abnormal results should be repositioned with their weight shifted to the opposite side of the body and the leg internally rotated.

> **NURSING ALERT**
>
> - *Arterial plethysmography:* This procedure is contraindicated in an extremity that is cold to touch, cyanotic, or pale in color, as this indicates a compromised blood flow to the limb.
> - *Body plethysmography:* Extreme claustrophobia may prevent enclosure in the box.

Nursing Implications

Assessment

- Obtain a history of signs and symptoms of vascular disorders, known or suspected peripheral vascular disease (for arterial and vascular plethysmography), known or suspected diseases of the pulmonary system (for body plethysmography), signs or symptoms of DVT or circulatory changes (for impedance plethysmography), results of previous diagnostic tests and procedures, and medical regimens.
- Determine the date of the last menstrual period and the possibility of pregnancy in premenopausal women.
- Ensure that the client has refrained from smoking for 2 hours before the arterial and venous studies.
- For body plethysmography, record the client's weight, height, and gender.
- Assess for compliance with directions given for rest, positioning, and activity before and during the test.

Possible Nursing Diagnoses

Tissue perfusion, altered, peripheral, related to interruption of venous or arterial blood flow

Airway clearance, ineffective, related to excessive mucus production

Pain related to occlusive disease or inflammation

Implementation

- *Arterial plethysmography:* Place the client in a semi-Fowler's position on the examining table or in bed. Apply three cuffs to the extremity and attach a pulse volume recorder, which displays the amplitude of each pulse wave on a paper called the *plethysmograph.* Inflate the cuffs to 65 mm Hg to measure the pulse waves of each cuff. These measurements, when compared to a normal limb, determine the presence of arterial occlusive disease.

- *Venous plethysmography:* Place the client in a semi-Fowler's position on the examining table or in bed. Apply two cuffs to the extremity; attach one to a pulse volume recorder. Place one cuff on the proximal part of the extremity (occlusion cuff) and the second cuff on the distal part of the extremity (recorder cuff). Inflate the recorder cuff at the level of 10 mm Hg and evaluate the effects of respiration on the volume in the veins. The absence of changes during respirations indicates the presence of venous occlusion. This is followed by inflation of the occlusion cuff to the level of 50 mm Hg to record the venous volume on the pulse monitor. Deflate the occlusion cuff after the highest volume is recorded in the recorder cuff. A delay in the return to preocclusion volume indicates venous thrombotic occlusion.

- *Body plethysmography:* Place the client in a sitting position on a chair in the body box. A nose clip is positioned to prevent breathing through the nose and a mouthpiece that is connected to a measuring instrument is placed in the mouth. Ask the client to breathe through the mouthpiece. The door to the box is closed and time is given for the pressure in the box to stabilize before the test is started. At the beginning of the study, the client is requested to pant without allowing the glottis to close. The client is then asked to breathe in a rapid, shallow pattern. If compliance is tested, a double-lumen nasoesophageal catheter is inserted and the bag inflated with air. Intraesophageal pressure is recorded during normal breathing.

- *Impedance plethysmography:* Place the client on his or her back with the leg being tested above heart level. Flex the client's knee slightly and rotate the hips by shifting weight to the same side as the leg being tested. Apply a conductive jelly and electrodes. Inflate the pressure cuff attached to the thigh temporarily to occlude venous return without interfering with arterial blood flow. Expect the blood volume in the other calf to increase. A tracing of changes in electrical impedance occurring during inflation and for 15 seconds after cuff deflation is made. With DVT, blood volume increases less than expected because the veins are already at capacity.

Evaluation

- Note severe ischemia, ulcers, and pain of the extremity after arterial, venous, or impedance plethysmography and handle the extremity gently.
- Note respiratory pattern after body plethysmography and allow the client time to resume a normal breathing pattern.
- Note the test results in relation to the other tests performed and to the client's symptoms.

Client/Caregiver Teaching

Pretest

- Tell the client to wear loose-fitting clothing. The extremity should be free of constrictive bandages or clothing.
- Explain that the arterial, venous, and impedance procedures are performed in the vascular laboratory or at the bedside by a technician. Inform the client that the arterial and venous procedures take about 30 minutes, and the impedance study, 30 to 45 minutes. Advise the client that no pain is associated with the studies. Tell the client to remain still during the study and explain that cuffs are applied to the extremity for the arterial and venous plethysmography to measure and compare blood flow.
- Inform the client that food and fluids are allowed but smoking is restricted for at least 2 hours before the arterial or venous study.
- For body plethysmography, explain that the test will measure the amount of air contained in the chest, the elasticity of the lungs, and the occurrence of restrictive breathing in the bronchioles. Inform the client that the study takes about 30 to 45 minutes to complete unless other studies of the pulmonary system are performed. Also inform the client that there are no food, fluid, or medication restrictions before the study and that the only discomfort experienced is the tube insertion if a compliance study is to be performed. Tell the client to notify medical personnel during the test if he or she no-

tices any symptoms of pulmonary embolism such as shortness of breath, expectoration of pink frothy mucus, diaphoresis, or anxiety.

Porphyrins, Erythrocyte Total

Classification: Chemistry

Type of Test: Blood

This test is used along with urine porphyrin levels to differentiate the cause and type of porphyria. Porphyrins are pigments needed for energy storage and use and for heme synthesis in hemoglobin metabolism. Small amounts normally appear in blood, urine, and stool. Those clients with acquired or congenital porphyrias excrete excess amounts. Coproporphyrin is the main porphyrin in urine, while protoporphyrin is found in erythrocytes.

Indications

- Diagnose congenital or acquired erythropoietic porphyrias
- Confirm diagnosis of disorders affecting red blood cell (RBC) activity

Reference Values

Coproporphyrin	0.5–2.3 mg/dL
Protoporphyrin	4–52 mg/dL
Uroporphyrin	Negative or trace amount

Abnormal Values

- Increased coproporphyrin
  Congenital erythropoietic porphyria
  Erythropoietic protoporphyria
  Sideroblastic anemia
- Increased protoporphyrin

Erythropoietic protoporphyria
Lead poisoning
Thalassemia
- Increased uroporphyrin
Congenital or erythropoietic porphyria
Lead poisoning
Cirrhosis

Interfering Factors

- Hemolysis of the sample invalidates results.
- Increased levels may occur in pregnancy or menstruation.
- Failure of the client to observe dietary restrictions may affect results.

Nursing Implications

Assessment

- Obtain a history of the hematological system, suspected or known RBC abnormality, the results of tests, and the procedures performed.

Possible Nursing Diagnoses

Protection, altered, related to abnormal blood profiles
Anxiety related to perceived threat to health status
Poisoning related to excessive levels of lead in blood
Injury, risk for, related to neuromuscular alterations

Implementation

- Put on gloves. Using aseptic technique, perform a venipuncture and collect 3 mL of blood in a green-top, lavender-top, or black-top tube, depending on the laboratory.
- Handle the specimen gently to avoid hemolysis and transport to the laboratory promptly.

Evaluation

- Note the test results in relation to the urine porphyrins and the client's symptoms.

Client/Caregiver Teaching

Pretest

- Instruct the client not to drink alcohol for 24 hours before the test.

Posttest

- Instruct the client to avoid sunlight if the test results are positive.

Porphyrins, Urine

Classification: Chemistry

Type of Test: Urine (random or 24-hour)

Those porphyrins for which urine may be tested include aminolevulinic acid (ALA), porphobilinogen (PBG), uroporphyrin, and coproporphyrin.

Porphyrins are produced during the synthesis of heme. If heme synthesis is deranged, these precursors accumulate and are excreted in the urine in excessive amounts. Conditions producing increased levels of heme precursors are called porphyrias. The two main categories of genetically determined porphyrias are erythropoietic porphyrias, in which major diagnostic abnormalities occur in red cell chemistry, and hepatic porphyrias, in which heme precursors are found in urine and feces. Erythropoietic and hepatic porphyrias are very rare. Acquired porphyrias are characterized by greater accumulation of precursors in urine and feces than in red blood cells. Lead poisoning is the most common cause of acquired porphyria.

It should be noted that porphyrins are reddish fluorescent compounds. Depending on the type of porphyrin present, therefore, the urine may be reddish or the color of port wine. The presence of congenital porphyria may be suspected when an infant's wet diapers show a red discoloration. PBG is excreted as a colorless compound. If a sample containing PBG is acidic and is exposed to air for several hours, however, a color change may occur.

Indications

- Detect liver disease, as indicated by the presence of elevated porphyrins

- Detect suspected lead poisoning, as indicated by elevated porphyrins, especially ALA and PBG
- Diagnose congenital or acquired porphyrias

Reference Values

		SI Units
Aminolevulinic acid (ALA)		
Random specimen		
Children	<0.5 mg/dL	38.1 μmol/L
Adults	0.1–0.6 mg/dL	7.6–45.8 μmol/L
24-h urine	11.15–57.2 μmol/24 h	
Porphobilinogen (PBG)		
Random specimen	Negative	
24-h urine	0–2.5 mg/24 h	0–4.4 μmol/24 h
Uroporphyrin		
Random specimen	Negative	
24-h urine	10–30 μg/24 h	0.012–0.037 μmol/24 h
Coproporphyrin		
Random specimen		
Adults		0.045–0.30 μmol/L
24-h urine		
Children	0–80 μg/24 h	0–0.12 μmol/24 h
Adults	50–160 μg/24 h	0.075–0.24 μmol/24 h

Abnormal Values

- Central nervous system disorders
- Cirrhosis
- Congenital or acquired porphyrias (classified as erythropoietic or hepatic)
- Heavy metal, benzene, or carbon tetrachloride toxicity
- Hodgkin's disease
- Infectious hepatitis

Interfering Factors

- Exposure of the specimen to light can falsely elevate values.
- Pregnancy, menstruation, and oral contraceptives can elevate porphyrin levels.
- Failure to collect 24-hour specimen properly can alter test results.

- Therapy with griseofulvin, rifampin, and barbiturates may falsely elevate values in tests for porphyrins.
- Barbiturates, chloral hydrate, chlorpropamide, sulfonamides, meprobamate, and chlordiazepoxide typically induce porphyrinuria.
- Elevated urine urobilinogen levels can falsely elevate results by affecting the reagent used in PBG screening.
- Random samples for porphyrins must be fresh and must therefore be sent to the laboratory immediately on collection.

Nursing Implications

Assessment

- Assess and record the medications that the client is taking, especially those noted in Interfering Factors. Ensure that these medications have been held 10 to 12 days before the test.
- Assess the client's history for current pregnancy, menstruation, or oral contraceptive use; reschedule the test if needed.

Possible Nursing Diagnoses

Protection, altered, related to abnormal blood profiles
Anxiety related to perceived threat to health status
Poisoning related to excessive levels of lead in blood

Implementation

- Obtain the appropriate-size, light-resistant container with preservative according to laboratory policy; follow laboratory directions for any special care of the specimen during collection, such as refrigerating, placing in ice, and protecting from light by covering with dark plastic or aluminum.
- Begin the test between 6 and 8 A.M. if possible; collect first voiding and discard. Record the time the specimen was discarded as the beginning of the 24-hour test.
- The next morning, ask the client to void at the same time the collection was started and add this last voiding to the container.
- If an indwelling catheter is in place, replace the tubing and container system with the preservative at the start of the collection time, protecting the specimen from light, or empty the urine into a large container with the preservative periodically during the 24 hours; monitor to ensure continued drainage and conclude the test the next morning at the same hour the collection was begun.

■ At the conclusion of the test, ensure that the label is properly completed and transport to the laboratory.

Evaluation

■ Ensure that all of urine for a 24-hour specimen has been collected by comparing the urine quantity in the specimen container with the urinary output record for the test.

Client/Caregiver Teaching

Pretest

■ Inform the client that this urine test detects abnormal hemoglobin formation. There are no food or fluid restrictions before the test.

■ Inform the client that all urine for a 24-hour period must be saved; instruct the client to avoid voiding in the same pan with defecation and to keep toilet tissue out of the pan to prevent contamination of the specimen.

Posttest

■ Tell the client to resume medications and usual activity withheld before the test.

Positron Emission Tomography (PET)

Classification: Nuclear Medicine

Type of Test: Indirect visualization with radionuclide contrast medium

In this study, a radionuclide (oxygen-15, nitrogen-13, carbon-11, fluorine-18, depending on the study to be done) capable of emitting a positron is administered intravenously or by inhalation. Positron emission tomography (PET) scanning follows after the radionuclide has become concentrated in the organ to be studied. The specialized PET scanner translates the emissions from the radioactivity as the positron (from the isotope) combines with the negative electrons (from the tissues) and forms gamma rays that can be detected by the scanner or camera. This information is transmitted to the computer, which determines the location and its distribution and translates the emissions as color-coded images for viewing and analysis. Scanning is done over a period of time to allow for repetition or sequencing of three-dimensional images. The expense of the study limits its use even though it is more sensitive than traditional nuclear scanning and single-photon computed tomography (SPECT) scanning.

Indications

- Identify seizure foci in clients with focal seizures revealed by decreased metabolism between seizures
- Diagnose Alzheimer's disease and differentiate it from other causes of dementia revealed by decreased cerebral flow and metabolism
- Identify cerebrovascular accident (CVA) or aneurysm revealed by decreasing blood flow and oxygen use
- Diagnose Parkinson's disease and Huntington's disease revealed by decreased metabolism
- Evaluate cranial tumors preoperatively and determine stage and appropriate treatment or procedure
- Determine physiologic changes in psychosis and schizophrenia
- Determine the effect of drug therapy revealed by biochemical activity of normal and abnormal tissues
- Diagnose breast tumor, lung infection, and chronic pulmonary edema, depending on radionuclide used and concentrations at the sites
- Determine the presence and extent of myocardial infarction and the size of the infarct revealed by metabolic activity in the heart
- Determine coronary artery disease revealed by metabolic state during ischemia and following angina

Reference Values

- Normal blood flow and metabolism in body tissues

Abnormal Values

- Alzheimer's disease
- CVA
- Chronic obstructive pulmonary disease
- Dementia
- Head trauma
- Huntington's disease

- Migraine
- Myocardial infarction
- Parkinson's disease
- Schizophrenia
- Seizure disorders
- Tumors

Interfering Factors

- Inability of the client to remain still during the procedure may affect results.
- High anxiety levels affect the study if it is done for brain function.
- Drugs such as tranquilizers or insulin, which alter glucose metabolism, can affect results because hypoglycemia can alter the PET results.
- Use of alcohol, tobacco, or caffeine-containing drinks at least 24 hours before the study may affect results.

NURSING ALERT

- This procedure is contraindicated in clients with hypersensitivity to radionuclides.
- It is also contraindicated in pregnancy and lactation unless the benefits of performing the procedure greatly outweigh the risks.

Nursing Implications

Assessment

- Obtain a history, including information regarding the status of the system being examined, signs and symptoms leading to the decision to perform the study, and results from other diagnostic tests and procedures.
- Assess for allergy to radiographic dye and report to physician.
- Determine the date of the last menstrual period and the possibility of pregnancy in premenopausal women.
- Ensure that the client has abstained from smoking, alcohol intake, and caffeine-containing drinks for 24 hours before the study.
- Ensure that clients with insulin-dependent diabetes have had insulin the day of the study and a meal 3 to 4 hours before the study.

Possible Nursing Diagnoses

Physical mobility, impaired, related to neuromuscular impairment

Sensory-perception, altered, related to altered sensory reception, transmission, or integration

Confusion related to cerebral dysfunction

Anxiety related to perceived threat to health status

Implementation

- Before the scan, have the client remove all jewelry and metal; provide a hospital gown and have the client void. Insert an indwelling catheter if a pelvic scan is to be performed.
- *Brain study:* Place the client in a semi-upright position. Start an IV in each arm and inject radionuclide into one IV line; serial blood samples are taken from the other. Scanning of the brain begins 45 minutes after the injection. The client is requested to read, perform letter recognition activities, or recite a familiar quotation depending on whether speech, reasoning, or memory is to be tested.
- Some studies are done with the client inhaling the radionuclide. An arterial line may be inserted to obtain arterial blood gases. A face mask is placed on the face and head and immobilized, and the client is placed in position for the scanner.
- *Heart, lung, or breast study:* Place the client in a supine position. Start two IV lines; an arterial line may also be inserted. Test scanning over the chest area is performed following the injection of the radionuclide in 15 and 30 minutes and then continuous scanning is done for 1 hour.

Evaluation

- Note the test results in relation to the other tests performed and the client's symptoms.
- Observe the client carefully for up to 60 minutes after the study for a possible anaphylactic reaction to the radionuclide such as rash, tightening of the throat, or difficulty breathing.

Client/Caregiver Teaching

Pretest

- Inform the client that the procedure is performed in a special nuclear medicine department by a technician and a physician specializing in PET scanning and takes 1 to 3 hours to complete.

- Tell the client to abstain from alcohol, tobacco, and caffeine-containing beverages for 24 hours before the study.
- Tell the client that he or she will have to remain motionless in an enclosed space for 30 minutes to 3 hours (depending on the organ scanned) since movements of 1 cm can blur results.
- Inform client to wear comfortable clothing and to bring cassette tapes to listen to during the study.
- Inform the insulin-dependent client to take insulin as usual the day of the test and to have a meal 3 to 4 hours before the test.
- Teach the client relaxation techniques to reduce anxiety, which can interfere with results when testing brain function.
- Reassure the client and caregiver that the radiation is short-lived and is delivered in minimal doses.

Posttest

- Instruct the client to resume normal activities.
- Advise the client to increase fluid intake to eliminate the radionuclide from the body unless otherwise contra-indicated.

Potassium Hydroxide Preparation

Classification: Microbiology

Type of Test: Excision and analysis

Potassium hydroxide (KOH) preparation of skin, hair, nail, sputum, exudate from an abscess, or tissue biopsy allows the specimen to be analyzed microscopically to determine the presence of fungal infestation. The KOH solution clears away debris from the specimen and allows for visualization of the mycelia, hyphae, spores, spherules, and budding yeast cells to confirm infestation.

Indications

- Diagnose fungal infestation

Reference Values

- No fungal elements

Abnormal Values

- Actinomycosis
- Aspergillosis
- Blastomycosis
- Candidiasis
- Coccidioidomycosis
- Cryptococcosis
- Histoplasmosis
- Norcardiosis
- Paracoccidioidomycosis
- Sporotrichosis
- Tinea pedis, capitis, barbae, cruris, or corporis

Interfering Factors

- Fibers, such as cotton or cellulose, or cholesterol deposits in the specimen can affect test results.

Nursing Implications

Assessment

- Obtain a history of clinical symptoms, medications currently being taken, and results of recent related tests and procedures.

Possible Nursing Diagnoses

Body image disturbance related to change in structure or appearance

Anxiety related to perceived threat to health

Implementation

- Put on gloves to collect the specimen to avoid self-contamination.
- *Biopsy:* Assist the client to a position of comfort. The biopsy site is cleansed with an antiseptic solution, then a local anesthetic is applied and the area is draped with sterile towels. The suspicious area is excised and the specimen placed in a sterile container.
- *Shaving:* A drop of 10% to 20% KOH solution and methylene blue is placed on a sterile glass slide. A scalpel is used to scrape the lesion from the skin or nails and obtain the spec-

imen. The specimen is then placed on a sterile glass slide, covered with a glass coverslip, and sent to the laboratory. The slide will be exposed to gentle heat and allowed to cool before microscopic examination.

- *Hair:* Collect several strands of hair and place in a sterile container.
- Send the specimen to the laboratory.

Evaluation

- Note the test results in relation to the other related tests and the client's clinical symptoms.

Client/Caregiver Teaching

Pretest

- Explain to the client the purpose of the test and the procedure involved.
- Explain that foods and fluids are not usually restricted.

Posttest

- Instruct the client in the care and assessment of the site, as indicated.
- Have the client report any bleeding, redness, edema, or pain at the site.

Precipitin Test Against Human Sperm and Blood

Classification: Histology

Type of Test: Specimen analysis

This test analyzes samples of fluid obtained from the vagina for presence of semen or human blood. It is usually done after an alleged or suspected rape and requires strict adherence to procedures for collection and transportation of specimens. Because of the traumatic event, special care is needed in caring for the client.

In this test, a specimen with suspected human semen is obtained from the vaginal canal of a suspected rape victim.

When mixed with antisera solution, human sperm antigen will bind with an antibody in the sera, resulting in clumping of the cells and formation of a precipitate.

Indications

- Suspected or alleged rape

Reference Values

- Negative

Abnormal Values

- The presence of precipitation indicates sexual intercourse has occurred.

Interfering Factors

- Improper collection of specimens may alter test results.
- Douching before the test will reduce the accuracy of the results.
- Inability of the client to cooperate may alter test results.

Nursing Implications

Assessment

- Obtain a history of the gynecological system, of the alleged assault, current symptoms, and the results of any relevant diagnostic tests.
- Note the client's readiness to participate in the test. Never pressure or hurry the victim. Allow her time to adjust to avoid further trauma.

Possible Nursing Diagnoses

Anxiety related to threat to self-concept, interpersonal transmission of disease, or situational crisis

Rape-trauma syndrome, acute phase, related to actual or attempted sexual attack

Implementation

- Provide emotional support by being available to listen, accepting the client's feelings, and providing privacy during the examination and the interviewing process.
- Obtain vaginal speculum, nonabsorbent cotton swab, sterile glass specimen container, and 2 mL of normal saline solu-

tion in a 5-mL syringe. Insert the speculum and obtain a specimen by swabbing the vaginal walls. The specimen can also be obtained by gently lavaging the vagina with 2 mL of normal saline solution with the syringe and removing the solution with a pipette.

- Place the specimen in the sterile glass container and label appropriately. Be sure to include the amount of normal saline solution used if the lavage method was used to collect the specimen. Send to the laboratory immediately, strictly following institutional protocols for handling of potential evidence.
- Remember to save all clothing for analysis of the presence of sperm.

Evaluation

- Evaluate the client's response and coping mechanisms. Provide the opportunity to express feelings common to rape victims such as anger, humiliation, and fear of pregnancy or disease.

Client/Caregiver Teaching

Posttest

- Encourage the client to contact a local rape-counseling or mental health crisis center.

Pregnanediol

Classification: Urinalysis

Type of Test: Urine (timed)

This test measures pregnanediol, the chief metabolite of progesterone, which is secreted by the corpus luteum and by the placenta during pregnancy. Progesterone prepares the endometrium for implantation of the fertilized ovum, decreases myometrial excitability, stimulates proliferation of the vaginal epithelium, and stimulates growth of the breasts during pregnancy. During pregnancy, after implantation of the embryo, progesterone production increases, thus sustaining the pregnancy. This increase continues until about the 36th week of pregnancy, after which levels begin to diminish.

Although serum determination of progesterone may be done, the study of its metabolite, pregnanediol in urine, reflects overall progesterone levels, which may not be apparent in single blood measures.

Indications

- Verify ovulation in planning pregnancy or in determining the cause of infertility as indicated by normal values in relation to the menstrual cycle
- Diagnose placental dysfunction, as indicated by either low levels or failure of levels to progressively increase, and identify the need for progesterone therapy to sustain the pregnancy
- Detect fetal demise, as indicated by decreased levels, although levels may remain within normal limits if placental circulation is adequate

Reference Values

Adult males	<1.5 mg/24 h
Nonpregnant females	
Proliferative phase	0.5–1.5 mg/24 h
Luteal phase	2–7 mg/24 h
Postmenopausal females	0.2–1 mg/24 h
Pregnant females	
16 w	5–21 mg/24 h
20 w	6–26 mg/24 h
24 w	12–32 mg/24 h
28 w	19–51 mg/24 h
32 w	22–66 mg/24 h
36 w	13–77 mg/24 h
40 w	23–63 mg/24 h

Abnormal Values

- Increased levels
    Adrenocortical hyperplasia and tumors
    Adrenocorticosteroid therapy
    Biliary tract obstruction
    Choriocarcinoma of the ovary
    Ovarian tumors and cysts
    Precocious puberty
    Pregnancy

■ Decreased levels
  Adrenogenital syndrome
  Amenorrhea
  Fetal abnormalities or demise (except in the condition that
    adequate circulation to the placenta continues)
  Ovarian failure
  Parahypopituitarism
  Placental insufficiency
  Pregnancy-induced hypertension (PIH)
  Stein-Leventhal syndrome
  Threatened abortion
  Turner's syndrome
  Drug therapy with progesterone-containing medications

Interfering Factors

■ Pregnanediol levels vary in relation to the menstrual cycle in
  ovulating women.
■ Failure to collect all urine during the 24-hour test period will
  interfere with results.
■ Certain drugs can elevate pregnanediol levels, including
  methenamine mandelate, methenamine hippurate, and
  medications containing adrenocorticotropic hormone.
■ Certain drugs, including oral contraceptives, decrease levels.

Nursing Implications

Assessment

■ Obtain a history of menstrual irregularities in premenopausal
  women, a history of pregnancy noting weeks of gestation,
  medication regimen, and results of other tests performed.

Possible Nursing Diagnoses

Anxiety related to threat to health of fetus
Grieving, anticipatory, related to perceived potential loss
Coping, ineffective, individual, risk for, related to fear of fetal
  demise

Implementation

■ Obtain a clean 3-L container or 24-hour urine bag or bottle
  with preservative according to laboratory policy; follow laboratory directions for any special care of the specimen during collection such as refrigerating or placing in ice.
■ Begin the test between 6 and 8 A.M. if possible; collect first
  voiding and discard. Record the time the specimen was discarded as the beginning of the 24-hour test; document the

quantity of urine output during the collection period, including the urine at the end of the 24-hour period.

- The next morning, ask the client to void at the same time the collection was started and add this last voiding to the container.
- If an indwelling catheter is in place, keep the urine bag on ice, or empty the urine into a large container with the preservative every hour during the 24 hours; monitor to ensure continued drainage. Discard the first specimen, noting the time and then conclude the test the next morning at the same hour the collection was begun.
- At the conclusion of the test, ensure that the label is properly completed with the approximate week of gestation for pregnant women or stage of the menstrual cycle for premenopausal women; transport the sample promptly to the laboratory.

Evaluation

- Compare the quantity of urine in the specimen container with the urinary output record during collection time. If the specimen contains less urine than was recorded as output, some of the urine sample may have been discarded, and the results are invalidated.
- Note the test results in relation to the other tests performed and the client's symptoms.

Client/Caregiver Teaching

Pretest

- Inform the pregnant client that this test may have to be performed several times to obtain serial measurements.
- Inform the client that all urine for a 24-hour period must be saved; instruct the client to avoid voiding in the same pan with defecation and to keep toilet tissue out of the pan to prevent contamination of the specimen.
- Ensure that collection is performed correctly and that no urine is accidentally omitted from the 24-hour specimen.
- Instruct the client to withhold the medications that can interfere with test results, if ordered.

Posttest

- Instruct the client to resume medications and usual activity withheld before the test, as ordered.
- Encourage proper counseling if test results deem necessary.

Pregnanetriol

Classification: Urinalysis

Type of Test: Urine (24-hour)

This test measures pregnanetriol, a metabolite of the cortisone precursor, 17-hydroxyprogesterone. Elevated pregnanetriol levels are associated with adrenogenital syndrome. In this disorder, cortisol synthesis is impaired at the point of 17-hydroxyprogesterone conversion. Instead, the substance accumulates and its metabolite, pregnanetriol, is excreted in the urine in increased amounts.

This test should not be confused with pregnanedriol, which is a metabolite of the hormone progesterone secreted by the corpus luteum and the placenta.

Indications

- Diagnose suspected adrenogenital syndrome (virilization in females, precocious sexual development in males) as indicated by elevated levels
- Evaluate family history of adrenogenital syndrome
- Monitor response to cortisol therapy for adrenogenital syndrome
- Aid in the diagnosis of suspected testicular tumors as indicated by elevated levels
- Aid in the diagnosis of suspected Stein-Leventhal syndrome as indicated by elevated levels

Reference Values

Children <6 yr old	≤0.2 mg/24 h
Children 7–16 yr	0.3–1.1 mg/24 h
Adults	<3.5 mg/24 h

Abnormal Values

- Elevated levels
  Adrenogenital syndrome
  Congenital adrenocortical hyperplasia

Stein-Leventhal syndrome
21-Hydroxylase deficiency
Ovarian or adrenal cortex tumor
- Decreased levels
Anterior pituitary hypofunction

Interfering Factors

- Results are invalid if the specimen was not refrigerated throughout the collection.
- Failure to collect all urine during the 24-hour test period will interfere with results.

Nursing Implications

Assessment

- Obtain a history of endocrine dysfunction, signs and symptoms experienced, a medication history, and results of other tests performed.

Possible Nursing Diagnoses

Anxiety related to perceived threat to health status
Sexuality patterns, altered, related to illness or medical treatment
Body image disturbance related to change in structure/appearance

Implementation

- Obtain a clean 3-L container or 24-hour urine bag or bottle with preservative added, according to laboratory policy. Refrigerate the specimen during collection or place it on ice, according to laboratory policy.
- Begin the test between 6 and 8 A.M. if possible; collect first voiding and discard. Record the time the specimen was discarded as the beginning of the 24-hour test; document the quantity of urine output during the collection period, including the urine at the end of the 24-hour period. The next morning, ask the client to void at the same time the collection was started and add this last voiding to the container.
- If an indwelling catheter is in place, replace the tubing and container system and keep the drainage bag on ice, and periodically empty the urine into a large refrigerated container with the preservative every hour during the 24 hours; monitor to ensure continued drainage and conclude the test the next morning at the same hour the collection was begun.

- At the conclusion of the test, ensure that the label is properly completed and transport the specimen to the laboratory immediately.

Evaluation

- Compare the quantity of urine in the specimen container with the urinary output record during the collection time. If the specimen contains less urine than was recorded as output, some of the urine sample may have been discarded, and the results are invalidated.
- Note the test results in relation to the other studies performed, in particular the cortisol level and the client's symptoms.

Client/Caregiver Teaching

Pretest

- Instruct the client in collection and provide an appropriate container if the specimen is to be obtained as an outpatient and brought to the laboratory.
- Inform the client that all urine for a 24-hour period must be saved; instruct the client to avoid voiding in the same pan with defecation and to keep toilet tissue out of the pan to prevent contamination of the specimen.

Posttest

- Instruct the client to resume medications and usual activity withheld before the test, as ordered.

Proctosigmoidoscopy

Classification: Endoscopy

Type of Test: Direct visualization

This procedure involves the direct visualization of the mucosa of the anal canal (anoscopy), the rectum (proctoscopy), and the distal sigmoid colon (sigmoidoscopy). The procedure can be performed using a rigid or flexible fiberoptic endoscope, although the flexible instrument is generally preferred.

It can also be a therapeutic procedure allowing for removal of polyps or hemorrhoids or reduction of a volvulus. Biopsy of suspicious sites may be obtained during the procedure.

Indications

- Screen and excise polyps
- Examine the distal colon before a barium enema x-ray to obtain improved visualization of the area and after a barium enema in which findings are uncertain
- Evaluate cause of blood, pus, or mucus in the stool
- Determine cause of pain and tissue prolapse on defecation
- Determine cause of rectal itching, pain, or burning
- Confirm the diagnosis of diverticular disease
- Confirm the diagnosis of Hirschsprung's disease and colitis in children
- Reduce volvulus of the sigmoid colon
- Remove hemorrhoids by laser therapy

Reference Values

- Normal mucosa of the anal canal, rectum, and sigmoid colon

Abnormal Values

- Anal fissure or fistula
- Anorectal abscess
- Diverticular disease
- Hypertrophic anal papillae
- Inflammatory bowel disease
- Internal and external hemorrhoids
- Polyps
- Rectal prolapse
- Tumor

Interfering Factors

- Severe rectal bleeding or inadequate bowel preparation may affect results.
- Inability of the client to cooperate with the procedure may interfere with test results.

> ### ▶ NURSING ALERT
>
> - This test is contraindicated in suspected bowel perforation, acute peritonitis, acute fulminant colitis, diverticulitis, toxic megacolon or ischemic bowel necrosis, severe cardiopulmonary disease, large abdominal aortic or iliac aneurysm, severe bleeding or coagulation defect, and advanced pregnancy.
> - Administration of preparation that includes laxatives or enemas to pregnant women or clients with inflammatory colon diseases should be withheld unless the physician is notified and special orders are obtained.

Nursing Implications

Assessment

- Obtain a history of bowel disorders and presenting signs and symptoms; determine the date of the last menstrual period in premenopausal women.
- Ensure that barium studies have not been performed within 3 days of the procedure.
- Ensure that dietary and fluid restrictions have been followed before the procedure, such as clear or light diet for 24 to 48 hours before the procedure and fasting for 8 hours before the procedure.
- Ensure that ordered laxative has been administered the night before.

Possible Nursing Diagnoses

Diarrhea related to stress and anxiety or bowel irritation from procedure

Constipation related to inadequate fluid or bulk intake

Injury, risk for, related to postcolonoscopy distention syndrome, bleeding, or colon perforation

Anxiety related to perceived threat to health status

Implementation

- Administer two Fleet small-volume enemas 1 hour before the procedure.
- Depending on the type of instrument to be used, assist the client either to the left lateral position with the buttocks at or extending slightly beyond the edge of the examination table or bed, or the knee-chest position, preferably on a special examining table that tilts the client into the desired po-

sition. The client is draped to avoid excessive exposure and for warmth if needed.

- Following visual inspection of the perineal area, a preliminary digital rectal examination is performed with a well-lubricated gloved finger. A fecal specimen may be obtained from the glove when the finger is removed from the rectum. A lubricated anoscope (7 cm in length) is then inserted and the anal canal is inspected (anoscopy). The anoscope is then removed and a lubricated proctoscope (27 cm in length) or flexible sigmoidoscope (35 to 60 cm in length) is then inserted.

- The scope is manipulated gently to facilitate passage and air may be insufflated through the scope to improve visualization. Suction and cotton swabs are also used to remove materials that hinder visualization. Examination is done as the scope is gradually withdrawn.

- As necessary, specimens of tissue or exudate may be obtained, polyps excised, or photographs taken by use of the accessories to the endoscope. Additional examination of the rectal and anal areas may be done. On completion of the examination, the scope is completely withdrawn and residual lubricant is cleansed from the anal area.

Evaluation

- Note the test results in relation to the other tests performed and the client's symptoms.

- Assess the client closely for signs of bowel perforation (such as abdominal pain and distention, fever, mucopurulent drainage, or bleeding from the rectum) or excessive bleeding.

Client/Caregiver Teaching

Pretest

- Instruct the client to follow a clear-liquid diet for 2 days before the test and to fast for 8 hours before the test. Also, inform the client that a laxative is required the night before and that enemas will be required in the morning before the test.

- Explain the purpose of the study and how the procedure is performed; explain that the procedure is generally performed in an endoscopy suite or at the client's bedside by a physician and takes approximately 15 to 30 minutes.

- Inform the client that the urge to defecate may be experienced when the scope is passed. Encourage slow, deep breathing through the mouth to help alleviate the feeling.

- Inform the client that flatus may be expelled during and after the procedure owing to air that is injected into the scope to improve visualization.

Posttest

- Provide emotional support during the procedure and after diagnostic findings are reported, as indicated; reinforce information regarding the diagnosis and recommended treatment regimen.
- Inform the client to resume usual food and fluid intake.
- Emphasize that any abdominal pain or distention, pain on defecation, or fever must be reported to the physician immediately.
- Prepare the client to expect slight rectal bleeding for up to 2 days following the removal of polyps or biopsy specimen; however, tell the client to report persistent bleeding to the physician immediately.

Progesterone Receptor Assay

Classification: Histology

Type of Test: Needle biopsy or tissue resection

This test involves examination of an excised or biopsied tumor for the degree of responsiveness (positivity) of the progesterone receptors in the tissue. It is usually performed in conjunction with an estrogen receptor assay.

Progesterone receptors are located primarily in mammary gland tissue, as well as in the corpus luteum, prostate, uterus, vaginal epithelium, and placenta. Progesterone receptors transfer and bind steroid molecules into cell nuclei to exert hormonal function.

In some patients with carcinoma, the degree of progesterone receptor positivity correlates to the amount of cellular subtype differentiation and is a measure of potential tumor responsiveness to hormone or antihormonal therapy. Those with positive tests are more likely to respond to these types of therapy than those with negative results. The best prognosis can be expected in those whose progesterone receptor assay results remain positive when monitoring tumor response to therapy. The prognosis is poor in those who have negative tests after positive initial tests. Those who remain negative have the poorest prognosis.

Progesterone receptors are found in up to 75 percent of estrogen receptor-positive mammary cancers.

Indications

- Determine the likelihood of carcinoma to respond to hormone or antihormone therapy
- Monitor the responsiveness of tumors to hormonal or antihormonal therapy
- Determine the need for oophorectomy

Reference Values

Negative	<5 fmol/mg protein
Positive	>10 fmol/mg protein

Abnormal Values

- Positive results
  Breast cancer
  Hormonal therapy
  Meningioma
  Metastasis
- Negative results
  Normal finding, which may be obtained in the presence of a benign and nonresponsive tumor

Interfering Factors

- The presence of massive tumor necrosis or tumors with low cellular composition lowers the assay result.
- A delay in transporting the specimen to the pathology laboratory of even 15 minutes results in degradation of receptor sites.
- The results will be affected if specimens are stored at temperatures above $-70°C$ or if specimens are contaminated with formalin.

Nursing Implications

Assessment

- Obtain a history of illness and symptoms.
- Ensure that preoperative preparation for surgical biopsy or resection is complete and informed consent is signed.
- Assess the client's understanding of the procedure, level of anxiety, and need for emotional support.

Possible Nursing Diagnoses

Anxiety related to perceived threat to health status
Body image disturbance related to change in appearance
Grieving, anticipatory, related to perceived loss or threat of death

Implementation

- Obtain a waxed cardboard specimen container without preservative.
- Arrange to transport the specimen to the pathology laboratory immediately after excision.
- Explain the purpose of the test: biopsy or excision of tissue is necessary and the procedure is performed by the surgeon.
- A fresh tissue specimen of at least 150 mg and preferably 1 g (1 mL) is obtained via needle biopsy or resection and placed in a formalin-free container.
- Send the specimen to the pathology laboratory immediately.
- Apply a dry sterile dressing to the biopsy or operative site.
- Specimens must be stored at temperatures below $-70°C$. If the specimen is to be transported to another institution, it must be packed in dry ice.

Evaluation

- Monitor postoperative vital signs until stable, per institution policy.
- Observe for bleeding and infection.
- Note the test results in relation to the other tests and to the client's clinical symptoms.

Client/Caregiver Teaching

Pretest

- Explain the purpose of the test and the procedure involved.
- Inform the client that the test is performed by a surgeon under sterile conditions and that it usually takes about 30 minutes to complete.

- Explain that foods and fluids are restricted after midnight the night before surgery. Inform the client that a general anesthetic will be administered.
- Ensure that the client understands the procedure before signing the informed consent.

Posttest

- Instruct the client in care and assessment of the site.
- Inform the client of follow-up appointment for removal of sutures.

▲▲▲▲▲▲▲▲▲▲▲▲▲▲▲▲▲▲▲▲

Prolactin (HPRL, LTH)

Classification: Chemistry

Type of Test: Serum

This test measures prolactin (HPRL), also known as luteotropic hormone (LTH), lactogenic hormone, or lactogen, which is secreted by the acidophil cells of the adenohypophysis. It is unique among hormones in that it responds to inhibition by the hypothalamus rather than to stimulation.

The only known function of prolactin is to induce milk production in a female breast already stimulated by high estrogen levels. Once milk production is established, lactation can continue without elevated prolactin levels. Prolactin levels rise late in pregnancy, peak with the initiation of lactation, and surge each time a woman breast-feeds. The function of prolactin in males is not known.

Indications

- Evaluate sexual dysfunction of unknown etiology in men and women
- Evaluate failure of lactation in the postpartum period or suspected postpartum hypophyseal infarction (Sheehan's syndrome), as indicated by decreased levels
- Diagnose suspected tumor involving the lungs or kidneys (Elevated levels indicate ectopic prolactin production.)

- Aid in the diagnosis of primary hypothyroidism, as indicated by elevated levels

Reference Values

		SI Units
Men	1–20 ng/mL	1–20 Ug/L
Women		
Nonlactating	1–25 ng/mL	1–25 Ug/L
Menopausal	1–20 ng/mL	1–12 Ug/L
Pregnant		
1st trimester	1–80 ng/mL	1–80 Ug/L
2nd trimester	1–160 ng/mL	1–160 Ug/L
3rd trimester	1–400 ng/mL	1–400 Ug/L

Abnormal Values

- Increased levels
    Addison's disease
    Amenorrhea
    Breast-feeding
    Chronic alcoholism
    Chronic renal failure
    Coitus
    Ectopic prolactin-secreting tumors (such as the lung or kidney)
    Endometriosis
    Galactorrhea
    Hypoglycemia
    Hypothalamic disorder
    Liver disease
    Pituitary adenomas
    Pituitary tumor
    Polycystic ovary
    Pregnancy
    Primary hypothyroidism
    Certain drugs, including estrogen, oral contraceptives, reserpine, alpha-methyldopa, phenothiazines, haloperidol, tricyclic antidepressants, procainamide derivatives, amphetamine, antihistamines, monoamine oxidase inhibitors, methyldopa, cimetidine, isoniazid, and verapamil
- Decreased HPRL
    Gynecomastia

Hirsutism
Impotence in males
Postpartum hypophyseal infarction (Sheehan's syndrome)
Certain drugs, including bromocriptine, levodopa, ergot
   derivatives, apomorphine

Interfering Factors

- Therapy with certain drugs can produce elevated or decreased levels (see Abnormal Values).
- Episodic elevations can occur in response to sleep, stress, exercise, and hypoglycemia.

Nursing Implications

Assessment

- Obtain a history of reproductive and endocrine systems and postpartum status.
- Assess medication history; ensure that any drugs that may alter test results have been withheld for 12 to 24 hours before the test, as ordered by physician.
- Ensure that the client has fasted for 12 hours before the test and has been awake for 1 to 2 hours before the test.

Possible Nursing Diagnoses

Anxiety related to perceived threat to health status
Sexuality patterns, altered, related to illness or medical treatment
Body image disturbance related to change in structure or appearance
Grieving, anticipatory, related to perceived loss or threat of death

Implementation

- Put on gloves. Using aseptic technique, perform a venipuncture and collect 5 mL of blood in a red-top or lavender-top tube about 2 hours after the client has awoken.
- Handle the sample gently to avoid hemolysis and transport to the laboratory immediately.

Evaluation

- Note the test results in relation to the other tests performed, particularly thyroid function, serum estrogen and progesterone, pituitary x-rays, and the client's symptoms, particularly menstrual irregularities or neurologic changes.

Client/Caregiver Teaching

Pretest

- Instruct the client to fast for 12 hours and awaken at least 2 hours before the test.
- Tell the client to withhold medications that interfere with test results and avoid stress and exercise.

Posttest

- Tell the client to resume diet and medications withheld before the test.

Prostate-Specific Antigen (PSA)

Classification: Serology

Type of Test: Serum

Prostate-specific antigen (PSA) is a glycoprotein exclusive to the prostate epithelium. This test is used along with rectal examination and prostatic acid phosphatase (PAP) in making an accurate diagnosis of prostatic cancer. PSA is smaller and more stable than the PAP molecule and does not demonstrate diurnal variations. Accelerated metabolic rate in prostate carcinoma and tumor catabolic activity elevate the serum value of PSA. The PSA test helps track the course of prostate cancer, helps evaluate response to treatment in stages B3 to D1, and assists in detecting tumor spread or recurrence.

Indications

- Identify, differentiate, classify, stage, and locate prostatic cancer
- Monitor preoperative, postoperative, and recurrent tumor
- Assist in selection of therapeutic interventions or cytotropic drug therapy
- Assess tumor response to treatment protocols

Reference Values

- Men under 40: ≤2.7 ng/mL
- Men over 40: ≤4.0 ng/mL

Abnormal Values

- Increased values
    Benign prostatic hypertrophy (BPH)
    Cirrhosis
    Impotence
    Osteoporosis
    Prostatic cancer
    Prostatic needle biopsy
    Prostatitis
    Pulmonary embolism
    Transurethral resection (TUR)
    Urethral instrumentation
    Urinary retention
- Decreased values
    Not significant

Interfering Factors

- Rectal examinations within 48 hours before the test may falsely elevate results.

Nursing Implications

Assessment

- Obtain a history of illness and symptoms, other diagnostic procedures performed, and results.
- Ensure that the client has not had a rectal examination in the last 24 hours.

Possible Nursing Diagnoses

Anxiety related to perceived threat to health status

Sexuality patterns, altered, related to illness or medical treatment

Body image disturbance related to change in structure or appearance

Implementation

- Put on gloves. Using aseptic technique, perform a venipuncture and collect 7 mL of blood in a clotted red-top tube.

■ Handle the sample gently to avoid hemolysis and transport to the laboratory immediately.

Evaluation

■ Note the test results in relation to the findings of the digital exam and PAP levels.
■ Compare the previous PSA results in response to treatment.

Client/Caregiver Teaching

Pretest

■ Inform the client that fasting from food and fluids is not required.

Posttest

■ Inform the client that further testing may be necessary to monitor treatment with chemotherapy or radiation.

Protein C

Classification: Hematology

Type of Test: Plasma

Protein C is a vitamin K–dependent protein that originates in the liver and circulates in plasma. In the presence of a capillary endothelial cofactor after activation by thrombin, protein C acts as a potent and specific anticoagulant, suppressing the procoagulant activity of activated platelets.

Most measurements of protein C entail immunochemical assay of protein C antigen. Methods include immunoelectrophoresis, radioimmunoassay, or enzyme-linked immunosorbent assay. Each method requires a monospecific antibody to protein C. The assay is standardized by plasma pooled from a large group of normal donors. Even when the level of suspicion is high, this test is rarely positive. The clinical significance of a positive result is not fully understood, and a positive finding for heterozygous deficiency is used for informational purposes.

Identification of the role of protein C deficiency in idiopathic venous thrombosis may help to prevent some cases of thromboembolism in the future.

Prothrombin concentrate, which contains protein C, is one possible treatment, although interventions are still largely experimental.

Indications

- Investigate the mechanism of idiopathic venous thrombosis

Reference Values

- 50 to 150 percent of population mean; varies by laboratory

Abnormal Values

- Positive finding helps determine whether protein C deficiency plays a role in venous thrombosis.

Interfering Factors

- Coumadin-type anticoagulants affect test results.
- Hemolysis of the sample affects results.

Nursing Implications

Assessment

- Obtain a history of thromboembolism, symptoms, and current medications.

Possible Nursing Diagnoses

Injury, risk for, related to altered clotting factors
Anxiety related to perceived threat to health status
Tissue perfusion, altered, related to occlusive disease

Implementation

- Put on gloves. Using aseptic technique, perform a venipuncture and collect 3 mL of blood in a blue-top evacuated tube or a special syringe with anticoagulant provided by the laboratory.
- Handle the sample gently to avoid hemolysis and send to the laboratory immediately.

Evaluation

- Note the test results in relation to the client's symptoms and the other tests performed.
- Monitor the venipuncture site for excessive bleeding.

Client/Caregiver Teaching

Pretest

- Explain to the client that this test may give information to help prevent thromboembolism in the future and that treatment may be prescribed if results are positive.

Protein Electrophoresis, Serum

Classification: Chemistry

Type of Test: Serum

This test measures the primary blood proteins, including albumin, and globulins (alpha$_1$, alpha$_2$, beta, and gamma). The serum is subjected to an electric field at a pH of 8.6, and the proteins are separated by electrical charge, molecular size, and shape. This technique creates bands that are used for interpretation. If a suspicious band is formed, an immunoelectrophoresis is performed.

Indications

- Diagnose blood dyscrasias
- Diagnose neoplastic disorders
- Diagnose gastrointestinal or hepatic disorders
- Diagnose renal disease
- Identify clients with protein deficiency

Reference Values

- See table on the following page.

Protein Type						
	Total Protein	**Albumin**	**Alpha₁ Globulin**	**Alpha₂ Globulin**	**Beta Globulin**	**Gamma Globulin**
Adult	6–8 g/dL	58–74%	2–3.5%	5.4–10.6%	7–14%	8–18%
Premature infant	4.4–6.3 g/dL	3.3–5 g/dL	0.1–0.4 g/dL	0.5–1 g/dL	0.7–1.2 g/dL	0.8–1.6 g/dL
Newborn	4.6–7.4 g/dL	3–4.2 g/dL	0.11–0.5 g/dL	0.3–0.7 g/dL	0.3–1.2 g/dL	0.3–1.4 g/dL
Infant	6–6.7 g/dL	3.5–5.4 g/dL	0.1–0.3 g/dL	0.3–0.5 g/dL	0.2–0.6 g/dL	0.2–1.2 g/dL
Child	6.2–8 g/dL	4.4–5.4 g/dL	0.2–0.4 g/dL	0.5–0.8 g/dL	0.5–0.9 g/dL	0.3–0.8 g/dL
		4–5.8 g/dL	0.1–0.4 g/dL	0.4–1 g/dL	0.5–1 g/dL	0.3–1 g/dL

Abnormal Values

- Increased total protein
  Dehydration
  Diabetes mellitus
  Macroglobulinemia
  Monocytic leukemia
  Multiple myeloma
  Sarcoidosis
- Decreased total protein
  Burns
  Chronic glomerulonephritis
  Crohn's disease
  Diabetes mellitus
  Hypertension with congestive heart failure
  Increased capillary leak
  Malnutrition
  Severe shock
  Toxemia
- Increased albumin
  Dehydration
  Multiple myeloma
- Decreased albumin
  Acquired immune deficiency syndrome (AIDS)
  Autoimmune disease
  Diabetes mellitus
  Gastrointestinal inflammation or neoplastic disease
  Hepatic disease
  Hypertension
  Malnutrition
  Renal disease
- Increased globulin levels
  Autoimmune disorders
  Chronic syphilis
  Diabetes mellitus
  Hodgkin's disease
  Inflammation (acute phase)
  Lipoprotein disorders
  Neoplastic disease
  Nephrotic syndrome
  Tuberculosis
- Decreased globulin levels
  Blood dyscrasias, including coagulation disorders
  Hepatic disease
  Infection
  Malnutrition
  Neoplastic disorders
  Renal disease

Interfering Factors

- Hemolysis of the sample may alter test results.
- Oral contraceptives increase alpha$_1$ levels and decrease albumin levels.
- Recent dialysis alters protein levels.
- Use of contrast media may falsely elevate protein levels.
- Certain drugs, such as bicarbonate, isoniazid, neomycin, sulfonamides, chlorpromazine and acetylsalicylic acid, may alter test results.

Nursing Implications

Assessment

- Obtain a history of recent illness, the results of other tests performed, and the current medication regimen.
- Ensure that the client has not had tests using contrast media in the last 48 hours.
- Determine if the client recently had dialysis.

Possible Nursing Diagnoses

Infection, risk for secondary, related to immunosuppressed inflammatory response

Infection, risk for transmission

Nutrition, altered, less than body requirements, related to gastrointestinal dysfunction

Anxiety related to perceived threat to health status

Fluid volume deficit, risk for, related to active loss

Implementation

- Put on gloves. Using aseptic technique, perform a venipuncture and collect 7 mL of blood in a red-top tube.
- Handle the sample gently to avoid hemolysis and transport to the laboratory promptly.

Evaluation

- Note the test results in relation to the other tests performed and the client's symptoms.

Client/Caregiver Teaching

Pretest

- Tell the client to withhold the medications that interfere with test results.

Posttest

■ Inform the client that if immunoelectrophoresis is performed, it may take up to 3 days to obtain results.

Protein Electrophoresis, Urine

Classification: Chemistry

Type of Test: Urine (random or 24-hour)

This test is a quantitative measurement of proteins in the urine. Normally the urine is free of proteins or only contains trace amounts of albumin and globulin because the glomeruli filter out the proteins. In this test, the urine is subjected to an electrical field at a pH of 8.6, and the particles are separated by electrical charge, molecular shape, and size. This technique creates bands, which are used for interpretation. The separation pattern, or bands, are transferred or plotted on treated paper.

Indications

■ Diagnose renal tubular disorders
■ Detect hemoglobinuria, myoglobinuria, or intravascular hemolysis

Reference Values

	Total Protein
Albumin	37.9%
Alpha$_1$ globulin	27.3%
Alpha$_2$ globulin	19.5%
Beta globulin	8.8%
Gamma globulin	3.3%

Abnormal Values

- Increased albumin
  Amyloidosis
  Congestive heart failure
  Diabetic glomerulosclerosis
  Idiopathic nephrotic syndrome
  Inflammation
  Renal vein thrombosis
  Systemic lupus erythematosus
- Increased beta globulin
  Hemoglobinuria
  Intravascular hemolysis
- Increased alpha$_1$ globulin with decreased beta and gamma globulin
  Acute infection
  Burns
  Cancer
  Collagen disease
  Hyperthyroidism
  Leukemia
  Pregnancy
- Dominant to absent gamma globulin, trace alpha$_1$ and alpha$_2$ globulin, and absent beta globulin
  Myoglobinuria
- Dominant beta globulin with some alpha and gamma globulin
  Acute renal tubular disorders
  Balkan neuropathy
  Cadmium poisoning
  Chronic pyelonephritis
  Fanconi's syndrome
  Monoclonal gammopathy
  Polycystic kidney disease
  Renal tubular acidosis
  Sarcoidosis
  Severe, chronic hypokalemia
  Wilson's disease

Interfering Factors

- A specimen contaminated with stool invalidates the results.
- Failure to collect all the urine invalidates the results.
- Certain drugs, including amikacin, amphotericin B, bacitracin, gentamicin, gold sodium thiomalate, kanamycin, neo-

mycin, netilmycin, penicillins, phenylbutazone, polymyxin B, streptomycin, sulfonamides, tobramycin, and trimethadione, affect results.

Nursing Implications

Assessment

- Obtain a history of renal, genitourinary, and infectious symptoms; results of other tests performed, and medication regimen.

Possible Nursing Diagnoses

Protection, altered, related to abnormal blood profiles
Grieving, anticipatory, related to perceived loss or threat of death
Infection, risk for, related to immunosuppressed inflammatory response
Tissue perfusion, altered, related to interruption of blood flow
Pain related to inflammatory process of connective tissues

Implementation

- Obtain a 50-mL container for the random specimen or a 3-L container with toluene or acetic acid added.
- *Random specimen:* Obtain a 25-mL first-voided urine sample in the container. If a urinary drainage bag is in place, obtain a fresh specimen.
- *Twenty-four hour specimen:* Discard the first-voided specimen in the morning and consider this the start time of the collection. Collect all urine voided for 24 hours; at the same time the following day, ask the client to void. Add this specimen to the container and transport to the laboratory. For catheterized clients, empty the urine into the container hourly and keep the drainage bag on ice. Document the amount of urine collected during the collection period.
- For pediatric clients, apply the collection bag and place a diaper over the area. Use tape as necessary to secure the device. Frequent changing of the device may be necessary to ensure that all the urine is collected.
- Transport the specimen to the laboratory promptly.

Evaluation

- Note the test results in relation to serum protein electrophoresis, if performed.
- Compare the urine quantity in the container with the urine output record.

Client/Caregiver Teaching

Pretest

- If the 24-hour test is performed, inform the client that all urine must be saved. Instruct the client to avoid voiding in the same pan with defecation and to keep toilet tissue out of the pan to prevent contamination.
- Instruct the client to withhold medications that interfere with the test results, as ordered.

Posttest

- Instruct the client to resume medications withheld before the test.

Protein, Total

Classification: Chemistry

Type of Test: Serum

This test measures the total protein (albumin and globulin) levels in blood. Proteins in the circulating blood transport amino acids from one site to another, produce antibodies, function as buffers in acid-base balance, maintain colloidal osmotic pressure, and aid in transporting lipids, enzymes, hormones, vitamins, and some minerals. A general assessment of serum proteins will include measurement of albumin, globulin, and the albumin-globulin (A/G) ratio. Although these tests are being replaced by serum protein electrophoresis, they can still be ordered to provide an overall picture of protein homeostasis.

Indications

- Perform routine screening as part of a complete physical examination, with normal results indicating satisfactory overall protein homeostasis
- Monitor response to therapy with drugs that can alter serum protein levels

- Diagnose clinical diseases associated with altered serum proteins (see Abnormal Values)

Reference Values

		SI Units
Newborns	4.6–7.4 g/dL	46–74 g/L
Infants	6.0–6.7 g/dL	60–67 g/L
Children	6.2–8.0 g/dL	62–80 g/L
Adults	6.0–8.0 g/dL	60–80 g/L

Abnormal Values

- Increased levels
    Addison's disease
    Crohn's disease
    Dehydration, macroglobulinemias, diarrhea, vomiting, wound drainage
    Renal disease
    Sarcoidosis
    Certain drugs, including ACTH, corticosteroids, BSP, clofibrate, dextran, growth hormone, heparin, insulin, x-ray contrast media, thyroid preparations, and tolbutamide
- Decreased levels
    Cirrhosis or hepatic disease
    Congestive heart failure
    Hemorrhage
    Hodgkin's disease
    Leukemia
    Malnutrition or malabsorption
    Nephrotic syndrome
    Peptic ulcer
    Scleroderma
    Severe burns
    Ulcerative colitis
    Water intoxication or edema
    Certain drugs, including ammonium ion, dextran, oral contraceptives, salicylates, and pyrazinamide

Interfering Factors

- High serum lipid levels can interfere with accurate testing.
- Numerous drugs can alter protein levels (see Abnormal Values).

Nursing Implications

Assessment

- Obtain a history of known or suspected conditions that alter protein levels (fluid losses, gastrointestinal disorders, renal or liver diseases) or disorders that require increased protein intake (stress, injury, infection).
- Note compliance with fasting 8 hours before the test and with low-fat diet for several days before the test.

Possible Nursing Diagnoses

Pain related to inflammatory process of connective tissues

Physical mobility, impaired, related to musculoskeletal impairment

Nutrition, altered, less than body requirements, related to inability to digest food and absorb nutrients

Protection, altered, related to abnormal blood profiles

Anxiety related to perceived threat to health status

Implementation

- Put on gloves. Using aseptic technique, perform a venipuncture and collect 5 mL of blood in a red-top tube.
- Handle the sample gently and send to the laboratory promptly.

Evaluation

- Monitor the results in relation to urinary protein, serum protein, and urine electrophoresis, as well as albumin and globulin levels and ratio.

Client/Caregiver Teaching

Pretest

- Tell the client to follow a low-fat diet for several days before the test and to fast for 8 hours before the test.
- Tell the client to withhold drugs that can interfere with test results, as ordered.

Posttest

- Tell the client to resume food and fluid intake and medications withheld before the test.
- Emphasize the importance of dietary intake of foods high in protein, if allowed, or instruct in restriction of protein in diet, if appropriate.
- Instruct the client to monitor weight and report losses and malnutrition state.

■ Instruct the client to report edema and a decrease in urinary output as well as signs and symptoms of dehydration if fluid intake is reduced and diarrhea or vomiting is present.

Protein, Urine (Dipstick)

Classification: Chemistry

Type of Test: Urine (random)

This test helps to differentiate normal protein excretion from that caused by disease states. Urine normally contains only a scant amount of protein, which it derives both from the blood and the urinary tract itself. The proteins normally filtered through the glomerulus include small amounts of low-molecular-weight serum proteins such as albumin. Most of these filtered proteins are reabsorbed by the proximal renal tubules. The distal renal tubules, however, secrete a protein (Tamm-Horsfall glycoprotein) into the urine. Other normal proteins in urine include microglobulin, immunoglobulin light chains, enzymes and proteins from tubular epithelial cells, leukocytes, and other cells shed by the urinary tract.

Persistent proteinuria is generally indicative of renal disease or of systemic disorders leading to increased serum levels of low-molecular-weight proteins. Renal disease resulting in proteinuria may be due to damage to the glomerulus or to the renal tubules. When the glomerular membrane is damaged, greater amounts of albumin pass into the glomerular filtrate. If damage is more extensive, large globulin molecules will also be excreted. In contrast, renal disease due to tubular damage is characterized by loss of proteins that are normally reabsorbed by the tubules (such as low-molecular-weight proteins).

Because proteinuria may indicate serious renal or systemic disease, its detection on routine urinalysis must always be further evaluated for possible cause. Proteinuria occurring in the latter months of pregnancy must also be carefully evaluated, as it may indicate serious complications of pregnancy.

Reference Values

■ Negative

Abnormal Values

- Positive, nonrenal causes (functional)
  - Cold exposure
  - Congestive heart failure
  - Dehydration
  - Fever
  - Postural (orthostatic) proteinuria
  - Strenuous exercise
- Positive, renal causes
  - Multiple myeloma
  - Myoglobinemia
  - Nephrotic syndrome
  - Pyelonephritis

Interfering Factors

- Medications that can result in false-positive semiquantitative results include acetazolamide, aminosalicylic acid, cephaloridine, chlorpromazine, penicillins, phenazopyridine, promazine hydrochloride, radiographic contrast media, sodium bicarbonate, sulfisoxazole, sulfonamides, thymol, and tolbutamide.
- Failure to use first-voided urine samples, which are more uniformly concentrated, more acidic, and more likely to exhibit abnormalities, may affect results.
- False-positive semiquantitative results can occur with incorrect matching of the reagent strip to the color chart and with prolonged exposure of the strip or stick to the urine.
- False-positives have been reported with gross hematuria.
- The presence of many white blood cells (infection) can alter results.
- False-negative results have been reported with very dilute urine, highly buffered alkaline urine, urine high in sodium, and urea-splitting infectious organisms of the urinary tract.

Nursing Implications

Assessment

- Obtain a history of renal disease, the results of other tests performed, and medication regimen.

Possible Nursing Diagnoses

Anxiety related to perceived threat to health status

Pain related to tissue ischemia or inflammation

Fluid volume excess related to compromised regulatory mechanism

Fluid volume deficit, risk for, related to active loss

Implementation

- Obtain an early-morning or first-voided specimen of the day in a clean, dry plastic container. Insert reagent strip into fresh urine specimen immediately, and remove excess urine by gently tapping the strip on the side of the container. Hold the strip at a horizontal plane to prevent mixing of any other chemical on the strip.
- Compare the color of the chemical strip to the color chart on the container, reading the results immediately according to the manufacturer's directions. Results range from negative to ≥4 mg/dL.
- Transport the specimen to the laboratory immediately for further testing, or keep refrigerated and transport within 2 hours.

Client/Caregiver Teaching

Pretest

- Inform the client that this is a screening technique and that it is important that the first-morning specimen is the one to be tested.

Posttest

- Tell the client to report positive test results to the physician.
- Tell the client that further testing will be required.

Prothrombin Consumption Time (PCT), Serum Prothrombin Time

Classification: Hematology

Type of Test: Serum

This test measures the use of prothrombin when a blood clot forms. Normally, the formation of a clot "consumes" prothrombin by converting it to thrombin. Individuals with deficiencies in platelets, platelet factor III, or the factors involved in the intrinsic coagulation pathway (factors VIII, IX, XI, and XII) are not able to convert as much prothrombin to thrombin, thus shortening the prothrombin consumption time (PCT).

In this test, residual serum prothrombin is measured 1 hour after the sample has clotted. Any deficiency in the factors needed to make thromboplastin reduces the prothrombin consumption, leaving greater levels remaining in the serum.

Indications

- Diagnose suspected deficiency of platelet factor III or of the clotting factors involved in the intrinsic coagulation pathway, as indicated by a shortened PCT
- Diagnose suspected disseminated intravascular coagulation (DIC), as indicated by a shortened PCT
- Monitor the effects of conditions such as liver disease and protein deficiency on hemostasis

Reference Values

- 15 to 20 seconds with more than 80 percent of the prothrombin consumed

Abnormal Values

- Decreased time
  Anticoagulant therapy
  Cirrhosis
  DIC
  Hypoprothrombinemia

Interfering Factors

- Traumatic venipuncture and excessive agitation of the sample can alter test results.
- Therapy with anticoagulants can shorten the PCT. Do not obtain the sample from a peripheral vein with an infusion of an anticoagulant, such as with a heparin lock.

Nursing Implications

Assessment

- Obtain a history of bleeding disorders. If the client is receiving anticoagulation therapy, note the time and amount of the last dose.

Possible Nursing Diagnoses

Injury, risk for, related to altered clotting factors
Protection, altered, related to abnormal blood profiles

Implementation

- Put on gloves. Using aseptic technique, perform a venipuncture and collect 7 mL of blood in a red-top tube.
- Hold pressure on the venipuncture site for at least 5 minutes to prevent hematoma formation.
- Avoid traumatic venipunctures and excessive agitation of the sample.

Evaluation

- Note the results of other coagulation tests (such as prothrombin time, partial thromboplastin time, factor assays, bleeding time, or platelet survival time) in relation to PCT.
- Assess for excessive bleeding or hematoma formation.

Client/Caregiver Teaching

Pretest

- Tell the client to withhold drugs that can interfere with test results, as ordered.

Posttest

- Tell the client to observe the site for excessive bruising.

Prothrombin Time (PT), Pro Time

Classification: Hematology (hemostasis)

Type of Test: Plasma

This coagulation test is performed to measure the time it takes for a firm fibrin clot to form after tissue thromboplastin (factor III) and calcium are added to the sample. It is used to evaluate the extrinsic pathway of the coagulation sequence. Prothrombin (PT) is a vitamin K–dependent protein produced by the liver; measurement is reported as time in seconds or percentage of normal activity. PT evaluation can now be based on an international normalized ratio (INR), using a standardized thromboplastin reagent and reported as PT and its equivalent

INR in making decisions regarding oral anticoagulation therapy.

Indications

- Identify cause of signs of abnormal bleeding such as epistaxis, easy bruising, bleeding gums, hematuria, and menorrhagia
- Identify individuals who may be prone to bleeding during surgical, obstetrical, dental, or invasive diagnostic procedures
- Evaluate response to anticoagulant therapy with coumarin derivatives and determine dosage required to achieve therapeutic results
- Differentiate between clotting factor deficiencies of V, VII, and X, which will prolong the PT, and congenital coagulation disorders such as hemophilia A (factor VIII) and hemophilia B (factor IX), which will not alter the PT
- Monitor the effects of conditions such as liver disease, protein deficiency, and fat malabsorption on hemostasis

Reference Values

Newborns	12–21 s
Children	11–14 s
Men	9.6–11.8 s
Women	9.5–11.3 s
Critical value	>30 s
INR	2.0–3.0 s for anticoagulation
	3.0–4.5 s for recurrent systemic embolization

Abnormal Values

- Prolonged time
    Anticoagulants of the coumarin family, which act by inhibiting hepatic synthesis of the vitamin K–dependent factors II, VII, IX, and X
    Liver disease
    Certain drugs, including salicylates, steroids, quinidine, alcohol, sulfonamides, phenytoin, antibiotics, methyldopate, quinine, and indomethacin
- Decreased time
    Pulmonary embolisms
    Thrombophlebitis
    Certain drugs, including barbiturates, oral contraceptives, theophylline, caffeine, antihistamines, and vitamin K

Interfering Factors

- Drugs that prolong or shorten the PT can alter results (see Abnormal Values).
- Traumatic venipuncture may lead to erroneous results from activation of the coagulation sequence.
- Excessive agitation of the sample can erroneously prolong the PT.
- A fibrinogen level of <100 mg/dL can prolong the PT (normal level is 150 to 400 mg/dL).

Nursing Implications

Assessment

- Obtain a personal and family history of known or suspected hematologic disorders; abnormal bleeding or abnormal laboratory results, such as increased or decreased platelet count or coagulation studies; and all medications taken by the client.
- If the client is receiving anticoagulant therapy, note the time and amount of the last dose.

Possible Nursing Diagnoses

Injury, risk for, related to altered clotting factors
Protection, altered, related to abnormal blood profiles
Anxiety related to perceived threat to health status

Implementation

- Put on gloves. Using aseptic technique, perform a venipuncture, discard 2-mL sample, and collect 7 mL of blood in a blue-top tube. Tilt the tube several times to mix blood with sodium citrate and citric acid in the tube.
- Apply pressure to the venipuncture site for at least 5 minutes to prevent hematoma formation.
- Avoid traumatic venipunctures and excessive agitation of the sample and send to the laboratory immediately with the time of collection noted and the dosage of anticoagulant, if appropriate, on the requisition.

Evaluation

- Note the results of baseline PT to use as comparison after anticoagulant therapy has begun.
- Note the test results in relation to the client's symptoms and the other tests performed.

Client/Caregiver Teaching

Pretest

- Tell the client to withhold drugs that could interfere with test results, as ordered.

Posttest

- Tell the client to resume drugs, as ordered.
- Instruct the client to take prescribed anticoagulant as ordered by the physician and report to the laboratory for PT tests to determine the effect of oral anticoagulant therapy.
- Inform the client and caregiver of expected PT level in relation to control value to be maintained based on reason for anticoagulant therapy.
- Instruct the client and caregiver to report bleeding from skin on mucous membrane to the physician.

Protoporphyrin, Free Erythrocyte (FEP)

Classification: Hematology

Type of Test: Blood

The free erythrocyte protoporphyrin (FEP) test measures the concentration of protoporphyrin in red blood cells (RBCs). Protoporphyrin comprises the predominant porphyrin in RBCs, which combines with iron to form the heme portion of hemoglobin. Protoporphyrin is converted into bilirubin, combines with albumin, and remains unconjugated in the circulation after hemoglobin breakdown. Increased amounts of protoporphyrin can be detected in erythrocytes, urine, and stool in conditions interfering with heme synthesis. In protoporphyria, an autosomal dominant disorder, increased amounts of protoporphyrin are secreted and excreted. Thought to be caused by an enzyme deficiency, protoporphyria is detected by the identification of increased concentrations of protoporphyrin in RBCs. Protoporphyria causes photosensitivity and may lead to cirrhosis of the liver and cholelithiasis as a result of protoporphyrin deposits.

Indications

- Diagnose erythropoietic protoporphyrias
- Confirm diagnosis of disorders affecting RBC activity
- Evaluate lead poisoning

Reference Values

	SI Units
Promelli method	
Women	19–52 mg/dL
Men	11–43 mg/dL
Hemalofluorometer	
Women	<40 mg/dL
Men	<30 mg/dL
Panic value	>190 mg/dL
Erythrocyte precursors	
Protoporphyrin	4–52 mg/dL

Abnormal Values

- Increased values
    Erythropoiesis
    Erythropoietic protoporphyria (>2200 mg/dL)
    Hemolytic anemia (>50 mg/dL)
    Infection (>50 mg/dL)
    Iron deficiency (>200 mg/dL)
    Lead poisoning (>200 mg/dL)
    Protoporphyria
    Sideroachrestic anemia (acquired) (>50 mg/dL)
    Thalassemia
- Decreased values
    Megaloblastic anemia (<30 mg/dL)

Interfering Factors

- The test is unreliable in infants under 6 months of age.
- Hemolysis of the specimen invalidates results.

Nursing Implications

Assessment

- Obtain a history of known or suspected disorders associated with protoporphyria (FEP).
- Obtain the client's hematocrit level.

Possible Nursing Diagnoses

Trauma, risk for, related to neuromuscular impairment resulting from high lead blood levels

Protection, altered, related to abnormal blood profiles

Anxiety related to perceived threat to health status

Injury, risk for, related to altered clotting factors

Implementation

- Put on gloves. Using aseptic technique, perform a venipuncture and collect 3 mL of blood in a heparinized green-top tube, a lavender-top tube containing EDTA, or a black-top tube containing sodium oxalate. (Capillary tube samples from pediatric heelsticks are acceptable.)
- Protect the specimen from light and handle it gently to avoid hemolysis; send to the laboratory immediately.
- Indicate the current hematocrit value on the laboratory requisition.

Evaluation

- Note the test results in relation to the client's symptoms and the other tests performed.

Client/Caregiver Teaching

Pretest

- Inform the client that no special preparation is required for this test.

Pseudocholinesterase (CHS, PCHE, AcCHS)

Classification: Chemistry

Type of Test: Plasma

Pseudocholinesterase is a nonspecific enzyme that hydrolyzes acetylcholine and noncholine esters. This enzyme's activity is inhibited by carbamate and organophosphate insecticides. Deficiency of this enzyme can also be inherited and puts the client in jeopardy if succinylcholine is administered. Abnormal genotypes of pseudocholinesterase are detected using the dibucaine and fluoride inhibition tests.

Indications

- Verify suspected exposure to organic phosphate insecticides
- Monitor cumulative exposure to organic phosphate insecticides
- Test for impending use of succinylcholine during anesthesia in persons homozygous for the abnormal form of CHS and resultant inability to inactivate succinylcholine

Reference Values

		SI Units
Pseudocholinesterase (CHS) (RID Method)	0.5–1.5 mg/dL	5–15 mg/L
Other Method		
Men	274–532 IU/dL	
Women	204–500 IU/dL	
Dibucaine inhibition	81–87%	0.81–0.87
Fluoride inhibition	44–54%	0.44–0.54

Abnormal Values

- Increased levels
    - Diabetes mellitus
    - Hyperthyroidism
    - Insecticide exposure (organic phosphate)
    - Nephrotic syndrome
- Decreased levels
    - Acute infection
    - Anemia
    - Carcinomatosis
    - Congenital deficiency
    - Hepatocellular diseases
    - Malnutrition
    - Muscular dystrophy
    - Myocardial infarction
    - Organophosphate insecticide poisoning
    - Recent plasmapheresis
    - Succinylcholine hypersensitivity
    - Uremia

Interfering Factors

- Pregnancy decreases test results by about 30 percent.
- Numerous drugs, including caffeine, theophylline, quinidine, quinine, barbiturates, estrogen, morphine, codeine, atropine, epinephrine, neostigmine, physostigmine, pyridostigmine, phospholine, phenothiazines, folic acid, and vitamin K, may falsely decrease cholinesterase levels.

Nursing Implications

Assessment

- Obtain a history of exposure to occupational hazards, potential surgery, and medication regimen.
- Ensure that drugs that may alter test results are withheld for 12 to 24 hours before the test, as ordered.

Possible Nursing Diagnoses

Suffocation, risk for, related to inability to metabolize succinylcholine

Poisoning, risk for, related to blood levels of drugs outside the therapeutic margin of safety

Fluid volume excess related to compromised regulatory mechanism

Cardiac output, decreased, related to decreased myocardial contractility or dysrhythmias

Pain related to ischemia or inflammation

Anxiety related to threat to health status or fear of death

Implementation

- Put on gloves. Using aseptic technique, perform a venipuncture and collect 5 mL of blood in a clotted red-top tube.
- Handle the sample gently to avoid hemolysis and transport to the laboratory promptly.

Evaluation

- Compare the test results to liver enzyme studies to determine the level of hepatic dysfunction.
- Notify the anesthesiologist if tests are positive and surgery is scheduled.

Client/Caregiver Teaching

Posttest

- Tell the client to resume medications withheld before the test.

■ Recommend that the client identify exposure risks in the home or workplace and take steps to remediate hazard.

▲▲▲▲▲▲▲▲▲▲▲▲▲▲▲▲▲▲▲▲▲

Pulmonary Function Study

Classification: Organ function

Type of Test: Indirect visualization

This noninvasive study provides information about the volume, pattern, and rates of air flow involved in respiratory function. It can also include tests involving the distribution (pulmonary circulation that facilitates gas exchange) and diffusing capabilities of the lungs (volume of gases that diffuses across a membrane). A complete pulmonary study profile would include the determination of all lung volumes, spirometry, diffusing capacity, maximum voluntary ventilation, flow-volume loop, and maximum expiratory and inspiratory pressures. Other studies include small-airway volumes. Arterial blood gases (ABGs) also reveal the distribution and diffusing capabilities of pulmonary function.

Pulmonary function studies are classified according to lung volumes and capacities, rates of flow, and gas exchange. Except for the gas exchange tests, these are measured by spirometry, which allows for the recording of the amounts of a gas during inspiration and expiration. Lung volumes and capacities are the amount of air inhaled or exhaled from the lungs compared to normal reference values using age, height, weight, and sex of the client. The volumes and capacities measured by spirometry without regard to time limits include:

Tidal volume (TV): Total amount of air inhaled and exhaled with one breath

Residual volume (RV): Amount of air remaining in the lungs after a maximum expiration effort (not measured by spirometry but can be calculated from the functional residual capacity (FRC) minus the expiratory reserve volume (ERV); indirect type of measurement can be done by body plethysmography

Inspiratory reserve volume (IRV): Maximum amount of air inhaled at the point of maximum expiration

Expiratory reserve volume (ERV): Maximum amount of air exhaled after a resting expiration; can be calculated by the vital capacity (VC) minus the inspiratory capacity (IC)

Vital capacity (VC): Maximum amount of air exhaled slowly at the point of maximum inspiration; can be calculated by adding the inspiratory capacity (IC) and the expiratory reserve volume (ERV)

Total lung capacity (TLC): Total amount of air that the lungs can hold after maximal inspiration; can be calculated by adding the vital capacity (VC) and residual volume (RV)

Inspiratory capacity (IC): Maximum amount of air inspired after normal expiration; can be calculated by adding the inspiratory reserve volume (IRV) and tidal volume (TV)

Functional residual capacity (FRC): Volume of air that remains in the lungs after normal expiration; can be calculated by adding the residual volume (RV) and expiratory reserve volume (ERV)

The pulmonary function studies for lung volumes, capacities, and rates of flow measured by spirometry that involve timing include:

Forced vital capacity (FVC): Maximum amount of air that can be forcefully exhaled after a full inspiration

Forced expiratory volume (FEV_1): Amount of air exhaled in the first second of forced vital capacity (FVC); also can be determined at 2 or 3 seconds; the percentage of FVC is the amount of air exhaled in seconds expressed in percent (%)

Maximal midexpiratory flow (MMEF): Maximal rate of air flow during a forced expiration

Forced inspiratory flow rate (FIF): Volume inspired from the residual volume (RV) at a point of measurement; can be expressed in percent to identify the corresponding volume pressure and inspired volume

Peak inspiratory flow rate (PIFR): Maximum flow of air during a forced maximal inspiration

Peak expiratory flow rate (PEFR): Maximum flow of air expired during forced vital capacity (FVC)

Flow-volume loops (F-V loop): Continuous flow rates and volumes displayed on a screen during forced expiratory and inspiratory vital capacities procedures

Maximal inspiratory-expiratory pressures: Measures the strength of the respiratory muscles in neuromuscular disorders

Maximal volume ventilation (MVV): Maximal volume of air inspired and expired in 1 minute

Other studies for gas exchange capacity, small airway abnormalities, and allergic responses in hyperactive airway disorders can be performed during the conventional pulmonary function study and include:

Diffusing capacity of lungs (D_L): Rate of transfer of carbon monoxide through the alveolar and capillary membrane in 1 minute

Closing volume (CV): Measure of the closure of small airways in the lower alveoli by monitoring volume and percent of alveolar nitrogen following inhalation of 100 percent oxygen

Isoflow volume ($_{iso}V$): Flow-volume loop test followed by inhalation of mix of helium and oxygen to determine small airways disease

Body plethysmography: Measures thoracic gas volume, airway resistance, and lung compliance

Bronchial provocation: Detects airway sensitivities following inhalation of methacholine in those with asthma

Arterial blood gases (ABGs): Measures oxygen and carbon dioxide in arterial blood in the determination of hypoxia; reveals the perfusion and diffusion capabilities of pulmonary function

Values are expressed in units of milliliter (mL), percent (%), liter (L), liter per second (L/sec), and liter per minute (L/min) depending on the test performed.

Indications

- Diagnose and differentiate between pulmonary obstructive and restrictive disease or a combination of both evidenced by abnormal expired or inspired volumes respectively
- Determine the presence of lung disease when other studies such as x-rays do not provide a definitive diagnosis or determine the progression and severity of known obstructive and restrictive lung disease
- Diagnose chronic obstructive pulmonary diseases (COPDs) that affect the peripheral airways (asthma, bronchitis), parenchyma (emphysema), and the upper airways (tumors of the pharynx, larynx, trachea; infections; or foreign body)
- Diagnose chronic restrictive pulmonary diseases that affect the chest wall (neuromuscular disorders, kyphosis, scoliosis), interstitium (pneumonitis, fibrosis), pleural conditions (pneumothorax, hemothorax), lesions (tumors, cysts), and other conditions such as obesity, ascites, peritonitis
- Evaluate dyspnea with or without exertion, coughing, and wheezing to determine the cause
- Determine the effectiveness of therapy regimens in following the course of a pulmonary disorder and identify bronchospasm response to long-term administration of bronchodilators
- Evaluate the lungs and respiratory status to determine the ability of the client to tolerate procedures such as surgery or diagnostic studies, especially on the lungs

- Screen high-risk populations for early detection of pulmonary conditions (occupational exposure, smokers, hereditary predisposition)
- Evaluate pulmonary function following surgical pneumonectomy, lobectomy, or segmental lobectomy
- Evaluate pulmonary disability for legal or insurance claims
- Determine allergic response to inhalants in those with an airway-reactive disorder
- Evaluate lung compliance to determine elasticity evidenced by changes in lung volumes that are decreased in restrictive disease and increased in obstructive disease and in the elderly
- Determine the diffusing capacity of the lungs in congestive heart failure, adult respiratory distress syndrome, and collagen vascular disorders

Reference Values

- Normal respiratory volume and capacities, gas diffusion and distribution
- No evidence of obstructive or restrictive lung disease

Lung volumes, capacities, and flow rates are as follows:

TV	500 mL at rest
RV	1200 mL (approximate)
IRV	3000 mL (approximate)
ERV	1100 mL (approximate)
VC	4600 mL (approximate)
TLC	5800 mL (approximate)
IC	3500 mL (approximate)
FRC	2300 mL (approximate)
FVC	3000–5000 mL (approximate)
FEV_1	81–83%
MMEF	25–75%
FIF	25–75%
MVV	25–35% or 170 L/min
PIFR	300 L/min
PEFR	450 L/min
F-V Loop	Normal curve
D_1	25 mL/min/torr (approximate)
CV	10–20% of VC
$_{iso}V$	Based on age formula
Bronchial provocation	No change or <20% reduction in FEV_1

Values are based on age, sex, height, and weight.

Abnormal Values

- Airway infections
- Asthma

- Bronchiectasis
- Chest wall trauma
- Chronic bronchitis
- Collagen vascular lung diseases
- Emphysema
- Inhalant allergy
- Interstitial fibrosis following pneumonectomy
- Neuromuscular diseases
- Pulmonary obstructive disorders
- Pneumonia
- Pulmonary fibrosis
- Pulmonary restrictive disorders
- Scleroderma
- Tumors

Interfering Factors

- The aging process can cause increases or decreases in values depending on the study done.
- Inability of the client to put forth the necessary breathing effort will affect the results.
- Medications such as bronchodilators or narcotic analgesics can change breathing patterns and affect results.
- Improper placement of the nose clamp or mouthpiece that allows for leakage can affect volume results.
- Confusion or inability to understand instructions or cooperate during the study can cause inaccurate results.

> ### NURSING ALERT
>
> - This test is contraindicated in clients with cardiac insufficiency, recent myocardial infarct, and presence of chest pain that affects inspiration or expiration ability.
> - This test should be performed cautiously in clients with upper respiratory infections such as a cold or acute bronchitis.

Nursing Implications

Assessment

- Obtain a history of suspected or known pulmonary conditions, respiratory status and patterns, medications (oral, inhalant, other), and previous tests and procedures done.
- Assess medication history for recent analgesia that may depress respiratory function.

- Ensure that the client has refrained from smoking tobacco or eating a heavy meal for 4 to 6 hours.
- Ensure that medications such as bronchodilators (oral or inhalant) are withheld at least 4 hours before the study.
- Ensure that dentures are not removed.

Possible Nursing Diagnoses

Gas exchange, impaired, related to alveolar-capillary membrane changes

Airway clearance, ineffective, related to increased secretions from lung inflammation

Breathing pattern, ineffective, related to tracheobronchial obstruction

Anxiety related to threat to health status or fear of death

Implementation

- Obtain an inhalant bronchodilator to treat any bronchospasms that can occur with these tests.
- Ask the client to void and loosen any restrictive clothing.
- Place the client in a sitting position on a chair near the spirometry equipment. Place a soft clip on the client's nose to restrict nose breathing and instruct the client to breathe through the mouth. Place a mouthpiece in the mouth and tell the client to close the lips around it to form a seal. The client is then requested to inhale deeply and quickly exhale as much air as possible into the mouthpiece. Other breathing maneuvers are performed on inspiration and expiration (normal and forced) and holding the breath, depending on the test done. The tests can also be timed to obtain information for specific tests. The tubing from the mouthpiece is connected to a cylinder that is connected to a computer which measures and records the values for the tests done. Some measurements can be calculated using the values obtained from the computer printout. A bronchodilator can be administered with the test repeated to determine if ventilation improves over the predicted value for the client in diagnosing pulmonary disease.
- To perform the lung-diffusing capacity test have the client take a deep breath of a gas mixture (10% helium and 0.3% carbon monoxide and room air) from a bag, holding the breath for 10 seconds and then exhaling. The measurement of the amount of the functioning capillary bed in contact with alveoli and the alveoli volume is then calculated. Another method involves breathing from a bag of a gas mixture (0.1% to 0.2% carbon monoxide) for a few minutes; the exhaled air in the bag is analyzed for oxygen, carbon dioxide, and

carbon monoxide concentrations. Arterial blood gas analysis is also done for this method of testing for diffusing capacity.

- Perform the bronchial provocation test following the FVC test. Administer 1.25 mg of methacholine by inhalation and repeat FVC after waiting about 5 minutes. A reduction in FEV_1 reveals a positive response for bronchial asthma. If no change is revealed, the dosage of medication is gradually increased and, if the FEV is not reduced after five dosage dilutions, the result is considered a negative response. A histamine challenge test can follow if no change in FEV is noted.
- At the conclusion of the tests, remove the mouthpiece and nose clip and take the client to another room to rest.

Evaluation

- Note the test results in relation to the client's symptoms and the other tests performed.

Client/Caregiver Teaching

Pretest

- Explain the purpose of the study.
- Explain that the procedure is generally performed in a specially equipped room or in the physician's office by a technician; the results are interpreted by a pulmonologist; and the test takes about 1 hour to complete depending on the number of tests done.
- Inform the client that no pain is associated with the study.
- Tell the client to withhold medications that can interfere with the test results.

Posttest

- Tell the client to resume medications withheld before the test, as ordered.

Pyruvic Acid

Classification: Chemistry

Type of Test: Blood

Pyruvate is a by-product of carbohydrate metabolism and, together with lactate, forms a reversible reaction that is regulated by oxygen supply. When oxygen levels are adequate, lactate converts to pyruvate; when inadequate, pyruvate converts back to lactate. Pyruvic acid in the form of pyruvate is technically difficult to measure, so it is not frequently measured.

Indications

- Assess tissue oxygenation
- Determine cause of lactic acidosis

Reference Values

	SI Units
0.08–0.16 mEq/L	0.08–0.16 mmol/L

Abnormal Values

- Elevated levels
  Cardiac arrest
  Enzymatic defects
  Hemorrhage
  Hepatic disease
  Myocardial infarction
  Shock

Interfering Factors

- Using a tourniquet or having the client clench fist during venipuncture can cause elevated levels.
- Exercise within 1 hour of the test can affect results.
- Failure to place the specimen in an ice-filled container can affect results.

Nursing Implications

Assessment

- Obtain a history of known or suspected conditions associated with lactic acidosis and the results of other tests and procedures performed.
- Ensure that the client has fasted overnight and rested for 1 hour before the test.

Possible Nursing Diagnoses

Fluid volume excess related to compromised regulatory mechanism

Pain related to ischemia of myocardial tissue

Tissue perfusion, altered, cardiopulmonary, related to interruption of blood flow

Anxiety related to perceived threat to health status

Cardiac output, decreased, related to altered muscle contractility

Implementation

- Put on gloves. Using aseptic technique, perform a venipuncture and collect 5 mL of blood in a gray-top tube.
- Place the specimen on ice and send to the laboratory immediately.

Evaluation

- Compare the test results with blood lactate level. The normal ratio is <10:1.

Client/Caregiver Teaching

Posttest

- Advise the client to resume diet and activity withheld before the test.

Radioactive Iodine Uptake (RAIU), T-131 Uptake Test, Thyroid Radionuclide Scan

Classification: Nuclear Medicine

Type of Test: Indirect visualization

In this nuclear study to evaluate thyroid function, the radionuclide iodine I-123 is administered orally or technetium-99m (Tc-99m) is administered intravenously. At specified intervals after the radionuclide is administered, the thyroid gland is scanned to reveal areas of increased uptake ("hot spots"), suggesting an increase in metabolic activity, or decreased uptake ("cold spots"). Uptake by the thyroid is expressed in percentages of the radionuclide absorbed in a specific amount of time.

Indications

- Evaluate thyroid function
- Monitor response to therapy for thyroid dysfunctional states

Reference Values

2-h absorption	1–13% of radionuclide
6-h absorption	2–25% of radionuclide
24-h absorption	15–45% of radionuclide

Variations in the normal range of iodine uptake can occur with differences in dietary iodine intake and procedural protocols among laboratories.

Abnormal Values

- Increased uptake
    Cirrhosis
    Decreased iodine intake or increased iodine excretion
    Graves' disease
    Hashimoto's thyroiditis (early)
    Hyperthyroidism, with a response of increased uptake of 20 percent absorption in 1 hour, 25 percent in 6 hours, and 45 percent in 24 hours

Rebound thyroid hormone withdrawal

Certain drugs, including barbiturates, diuretics, estrogens (occasionally), lithium carbonate, phenothiazines, and thyroid stimulating hormone

- Decreased uptake

Hypothyroidism, with a response of decreased uptake of 0 percent to 10 percent over 24 hours

Certain drugs, including aminosalicylic acid, isoniazid, levothyroxine sodium/T_4, thyroid extract, corticosteroids, antihistamines, penicillins, sulfonamides, iodothiouracil, propylthiouracil, thiocyanate, L-triiodothyronine, Lugol's solution, potassium iodide, saturated solution of potassium iodide (SSKI), tolbutamide, warfarin, and vitamins that contain minerals

Interfering Factors

- Recent use of iodinated contrast media for radiographic studies can decrease uptake of the radionuclide.
- Ingestion of foods containing iodine (iodized salt), medications containing iodine (cough syrup, potassium iodide, vitamins, Lugol's solution, thyroid replacement medications) can decrease uptake of the radionuclide.
- Antithyroid medications (propylthiouracil), corticosteroids, antihistamines, warfarin, sulfonamides, nitrates, and isoniazid can decrease the uptake of the radionuclide.
- Uptake of iodine may be increased in persons whose diet is deficient in iodine content or who are taking phenothiazines.
- Severe diarrhea could affect absorption of the radionuclide dose.
- Certain medications can increase the uptake of the radionuclide (see Abnormal Values).

NURSING ALERT

- This test is contraindicated in clients with hypersensitivity to iodine and in clients who are pregnant or breastfeeding, owing to possible teratogenic effects.
- This test is contraindicated in infants and children.

Nursing Implications

Assessment

- Obtain a history of previous thyroid studies, the results of thyroid hormone tests, and pertinent diagnostic procedures and medications that can affect test results.

- Assess for allergy to iodine, shellfish, or radiographic dye.
- Determine the date of the last menstrual period and the possibility of pregnancy in premenopausal women.
- Ensure that the client has fasted for 8 to 12 hours before the study and restricted iodine-containing foods and drugs for at least 1 week before the study.

Possible Nursing Diagnoses

Fatigue related to increased energy requirements and altered body chemistry

Injury, risk for, related to exposure to radionuclide

Anxiety related to threat to health status

Implementation

- Have the client remove all jewelry and metal around the head and neck area before the test.
- Administer radionuclide orally or establish an intravenous access if the radionuclide is to be administered IV.
- Place the client in a supine position on the examining table with the neck slightly hyperextended on a small pillow.
- Scanning is then performed with a detection camera (gamma camera) over the neck area in 30 minutes to determine the gland's ability to take up the radionuclide; in 2 and 6 hours to determine the gland's ability to bind iodine; and in 24 hours to determine the gland's total uptake of the radionuclide.

Evaluation

- Note the results in relation to the other thyroid function study results and the client's symptoms.
- Observe for a possible anaphylactic reaction to the radionuclide, such as rash, tightening of the throat, or difficulty breathing.
- Assess for fatigue, nervousness, increased appetite, increased sweating, and weight loss, which are common in hyperthyroidism as a result of increased metabolic activity.

Client/Caregiver Teaching

Pretest

- Explain that the procedure is performed to detect thyroid function; that it is performed in a special nuclear medicine department by a technician and a specialized physician; and that the scanning can take 24 hours to complete.
- Inform the client that it is important that he or she remain still during the procedure.

Posttest

- Tell the client to resume normal dietary intake and medications as ordered.
- Tell the client to meticulously wash his or her hands with soap and water after voiding for 24 hours since the remaining radioactive iodine is excreted in the urine.
- Advise the client to increase fluid intake to eliminate the radionuclide from the body unless otherwise contraindicated.
- Provide support during or after diagnostic findings are revealed; reinforce information regarding the diagnosis and recommended treatment regimen.

Radiography, Antegrade Pyelography

Classification: Radiography

Type of Test: Indirect visualization

This procedure allows examination of the upper collecting system of the kidneys. For this procedure, a contrast medium is injected into the renal pelvis using a percutaneous needle. With the needle in place, renal pressure can be measured and a urine sample collected for culture or cytologic examination.

Indications

- Evaluate the function of the upper collecting system after ureteral surgery or diversion
- Locate ureteral obstruction caused by tumor, stricture, or nonopaque stone
- Evaluate hydronephrosis
- Assist in placement of a nephrostomy tube

Reference Values

- The collecting system should fill uniformly and appear normal in size and structure.

Abnormal Values

- Increased size of the upper collecting system
    Intrarenal reflux
    Obstruction, such as calculi, stricture, or tumor
- Increased intrarenal pressure
    Obstruction
- Abnormal cytologic examination or positive culture
    Neoplastic disease
    Pyelonephrosis

Interfering Factors

- Incorrect positioning or movement during the x-ray can result in inaccurate interpretation.

> #### NURSING ALERT
>
> - This test is contraindicated in clients with bleeding disorders and in clients who are pregnant unless benefits of performing the procedure outweigh the risk to the patient.
> - The procedure is performed cautiously in clients with known hypersensitivity to the contrast medium. Pretreatment with corticosteroids may be necessary.
> - Risks associated with radiographic overexposure can result from frequent x-ray procedures. Personnel in the room with the client should wear a protective lead apron or stand behind a shield; badges that reveal the level of exposure to rays should be worn by those working in areas near x-ray suites.

Nursing Implications

Assessment

- Obtain a genitourinary history, current signs and symptoms, medications, and the results of other tests performed.
- Determine the presence of allergies, particularly to previous x-ray dyes, iodine, or shellfish.

Possible Nursing Diagnoses

Anxiety related to perceived threat to health status
Injury, risk for, related to exposure to contrast medium
Fluid volume excess related to compromised regulatory mechanism or decreased glomerular filtration

Implementation

- Place the client in the prone position. Clean the skin over the kidneys with an antiseptic solution. A local anesthetic will be administered.
- Under the guidance of fluoroscopy or ultrasonography, the percutaneous needle is inserted at about the 12th rib at the level of the second lumbar vertebra. The ability to withdraw urine confirms placement.
- Tubing is connected to the needle to prevent displacement. If the intrarenal pressure is measured, the manometer is attached to the tubing. Obtain a urine specimen.
- The contrast medium is injected in the amount equal to the amount of the urine withdrawn.
- Anterior, posterior, oblique, and anteroposterior x-rays are taken.
- If drainage of the kidney is required, a percutaneous nephrostomy tube is inserted. If not, the needle and tubing are removed and a sterile dressing is applied.

Evaluation

- Monitor the client for symptoms of allergic response to the contrast media.
- Note the test results in relation to the client's symptoms and the other tests performed.
- Monitor the needle insertion site for bleeding and urine leakage.

Client/Caregiver Teaching

Pretest

- Inform the client that a radiologist or urologist will perform the procedure and that it will take 1 to 2 hours. Also tell the client that mild discomfort may be felt during injection of the local anesthetic and the contrast medium. The contrast medium may also cause a transient burning feeling or flushing.
- Tell the client to fast from food and fluid for 6 to 8 hours.

Posttest

- Tell the client to report bleeding (including hematuria), urine leakage, or failure to void within 8 hours of the procedure to the physician.
- Tell the client to contact the physician to report signs of infection such as fever, chills, increased pulse or respiration.
- Inform the client of the importance of taking the antibiotics as prescribed.

Radiography, Barium Enema

Classification: Radiography

Type of Test: Indirect visualization

This is a radiologic examination of the colon following instillation of barium using a rectal tube inserted into the rectum or an existing ostomy. Visualization can be improved by using air and barium as contrast agents (double-contrast study). A combination of x-ray and fluoroscopy techniques is used to complete the study. Barium enema should be performed before an upper gastrointestinal study or barium swallow.

Indications

- Determine the cause of rectal bleeding, blood, pus, or mucus in feces
- Evaluate unexplained weight loss, anemia, or a change in bowel pattern
- Identify and locate benign or malignant polyps or tumors
- Evaluate suspected inflammatory process, congenital anomaly, motility disorder, or structural change

Reference Values

- Normal size, shape, and motility of the colon

Abnormal Values

- Colorectal cancer
- Congenital anomalies
- Diverticular disease
- Polyps
- Ulcerative colitis

Interfering Factors

- Improper positioning or the client's inability to remain still during filming as a result of pain, weakness, agitation, or confusion

- Metallic objects such as jewelry or closures on clothing within the x-ray field
- The client's inability to tolerate introduction of or retain barium, air, or both in bowel
- Excessive feces or residual barium in bowel resulting from inadequate cleansing, failure to restrict food intake before the study, or retained barium from another procedure

NURSING ALERT

- This test is contraindicated in pregnancy, unless benefits of performing the procedure outweigh risks to the fetus and in the presence of intestinal obstruction, acute ulcerative colitis, acute diverticulitis, or suspected rupture of the colon
- Personnel should exercise special precautions in handling the radioactive test dose: the nuclear medicine technician wears a badge and radiology ring; the dose is prepared behind a lead glass shield with only gloved hands exposed; any spilled radionuclide area is washed with soap and water and paper towels, which are placed in a special storage area for a few weeks before being disposed.

Nursing Implications

Assessment

- Obtain a history of the gastrointestinal system, the medication regimen, and the results of tests and procedures performed.
- Assess the date of the last menstrual period in female clients to ascertain possible pregnancy.
- Assess for iodine allergy if iodinated contrast medium is to be used.
- Ensure that the client has withheld food and fluids for 8 hours before the test, maintained a clear liquid diet the evening before the test, and followed a low-residue diet for several days before the test.
- Instruct clients with colostomy to follow the same dietary preparation, take laxatives the evening before, and perform a colostomy irrigation before the study.
- Assess for completion of bowel preparation according to the institution's procedure.

Possible Nursing Diagnoses

Constipation, colonic, related to obstructive lesion

Tissue perfusion, altered, gastrointestinal, related to obstructive vascular process

Nutrition, altered, less than body requirements, related to inability to absorb nutrients

Pain related to obstructive lesion or inflammation

Implementation

- Have the client remove clothing and metallic objects and provide a gown with tie closure.
- Help the client to the supine position on an x-ray table or to stand in front of an x-ray screen. An initial plain film is taken. Then help the client to a side-lying position. Insert a rectal tube or an indwelling urinary catheter into the anus. Inflate the balloon after it is situated against the anal sphincter. Instill barium into the colon and observe the movement through the colon by fluoroscopy. Help the client to the prone, supine, side-lying, and erect positions while spot films are taken. When filming is completed, barium is aspirated and the tube is removed.
- For patients with a colostomy, an indwelling urinary catheter is inserted into the stoma and barium is administered as above.
- Return the client to a position of comfort, and place the client on a bedpan or help to the bathroom to expel the barium.

Evaluation

- Monitor for reaction to iodinated contrast medium including tachycardia, hyperpnea, hypertension, or palpitations.
- Note the test results in relation to the client's symptoms and the other tests performed.

Client/Caregiver Teaching

Pretest

- Inform the client that the procedure is performed by a physician or technician and takes 45 to 90 minutes to complete. Explain that the procedure is not painful, but that the client may experience cramping, abdominal fullness, or an urge to defecate.
- Tell the client to eat a low-residue diet for several days before the procedure, to consume only clear liquids the evening before the test, and to withhold food and fluids for 8 hours before the test.
- Inform the client that a laxative and cleansing enema may

be given the day before the procedure, with cleansing enemas on the morning of the procedure, depending on the institution's policy.

Posttest

- Tell the client to resume food and fluids withheld before the test.
- Instruct the client to take a mild laxative to aid in elimination of barium, unless contraindicated. Encourage oral fluids.
- Inform the client that stool will be white or light in color for 2 to 3 days. If the client is unable to eliminate barium, or if the stool does not return to normal color, the client should inform the physician.
- Advise clients with colostomy to administer tap water colostomy irrigation to aid in barium removal.

Radiography, Barium Swallow

Classification: Radiography

Type of Test: Indirect visualization

This radiologic examination of the colon evaluates motion and anatomic structures of the esophageal lumen by recording images of the lumen while the client swallows a barium solution. It is performed using fluoroscopic and cineradiographic techniques. It is often performed as part of an upper gastrointestinal series or cardiac series.

Indications

- Determine the cause of dysphagia, heartburn, or regurgitation
- Evaluate suspected esophageal motility disorders
- Diagnose esophageal reflux
- Evaluate suspected polyps, strictures, Zencker's diverticula, tumor, or inflammation

Reference Values

- Normal peristalsis through the esophagus into the stomach with normal size and shape of the esophagus

Abnormal Values

- Acute or chronic esophagitis
- Benign or malignant tumors
- Hiatal hernia
- Strictures or polyps

Interfering Factors

- Results will be affected by improper client positioning or inability of the client to remain still during filming from pain, weakness, agitation, or confusion.
- Metallic objects, such as jewelry or closures on clothing, within the x-ray field will alter findings.

NURSING ALERT

- This test is contraindicated in pregnancy and lactation unless the benefits of performing the test greatly outweigh the risks.
- This test is also contraindicated in the presence of intestinal obstruction; suspected esophageal rupture, unless water-soluble iodinated contrast medium is used; and suspected tracheoesophageal fistula, unless barium is used.
- Personnel should exercise special precautions in handling the radioactive test dose: the nuclear medicine technician wears a badge and radiology ring; the dose is prepared behind a lead glass shield with only gloved hands exposed; any spilled radionuclide area is washed with soap and water and paper towels, which are placed in a special storage area for a few weeks before being disposed.

Nursing Implications

Assessment

- Obtain a history of the gastrointestinal system, medications, and the results of tests and procedures performed.

- Assess the date of the last menstrual period in female clients to ascertain possible pregnancy.
- Assess for iodine allergy if iodinated contrast medium is to be used.
- Ensure that food and fluids have been withheld for 8 hours before the test.

Possible Nursing Diagnoses

Nutrition, altered, less than body requirements related to inability to ingest food
Pain related to inflammation
Anxiety related to threat to health status
Grieving, anticipatory, related to perceived potential loss

Implementation

- Have the client remove clothing and metallic objects from the waist up and provide a gown with tie closure to wear.
- Help the client into a supine position on an x-ray table or to stand in front of an x-ray screen. An initial plain film is taken. The client stands in front of a fluoroscopy screen and is asked to swallow a barium solution with or without a straw. Spot films are taken at different angles. The client is then strapped to the table, which is rotated for additional films in head-down, prone, supine, and lateral positions. The client may need to drink additional barium to complete the study.
- Delayed films may be taken to evaluate the passage of barium from the esophagus into the stomach.
- Return the client to a position of comfort, and help from the x-ray table to a chair or stretcher.

Evaluation

- Monitor the client for reaction to iodinated contrast medium: tachycardia, hyperpnea, hypertension, palpitations.
- Note the test results in relation to the client's symptoms and the other tests performed.

Client/Caregiver Teaching

Pretest

- Inform the client that the procedure is performed by a physician or technician and takes 45 to 60 minutes to complete; explain that the procedure is not painful, but swallowing of contrast medium may be uncomfortable.
- Tell the client to withhold food and fluids for 8 hours before the test.

Posttest

- Instruct the client to resume food and fluids withheld before the test.
- Instruct the client to take a mild laxative and increase fluid intake to aid in elimination of barium, unless contraindicated.
- Instruct the client that stool will be white or light in color for 2 to 3 days. If the client is unable to eliminate the barium, or if stool does not return to normal color, the client should notify the physician.

Radiography, Bone; Long Bone X-rays; Skeletal X-rays

Classification: Radiography

Type of Test: Indirect visualization

This test is used to evaluate a client's complaints of extremity pain or discomfort. Besides confirming trauma or bone abnormalities, it can also be used to evaluate the growth pattern through serial x-rays. The presence of fluid within a joint can also be confirmed.

Indications

- Diagnose bone fracture
- Monitor fracture healing process
- Evaluate growth pattern
- Identify abnormalities of bones, joints, and surrounding tissues

Reference Values

- *Infants and children:* Thin plate of cartilage, known as growth plate or epiphyseal plate, between the shaft and both ends
- *Adolescent:* By age 17, calcification of cartilage plate

■ *Adult:* No evidence of fracture, congenital abnormalities, tumors, or infection

Abnormal Values

- Arthritis
- Bone spurs
- Fracture
- Genetic disturbances
- Hormonal disturbance
- Infection, including osteomyelitis
- Injury
- Neoplastic disease
- Nutritional or metabolic disturbances

Interfering Factors

- Incorrect positioning or movement during the x-ray can result in inaccurate interpretation.
- Metallic objects, such as jewelry, within the x-ray field will produce shadows that can be misinterpreted.

> **NURSING ALERT**
>
> - This test is contraindicated in pregnancy and lactation unless the benefits of performing the test greatly outweigh the risks.
> - Handle the injured extremity carefully to prevent further injury.
> - Personnel should exercise special precautions in handling the radioactive test dose: the nuclear medicine technician wears a badge and radiology ring; the dose is prepared behind a lead glass shield with only gloved hands exposed; any spilled radionuclide area is washed with soap and water and paper towels, which are placed in a special storage area for a few weeks before being disposed.

Nursing Implications

Assessment

- Obtain a history of the injury as well as any known congenital bone, metabolic, or genetic problems that could affect the bones.
- Obtain previous x-rays of the injury site.

Possible Nursing Diagnoses

Pain related to physical injury

Trauma, risk for additional injury, related to movement of skeletal fragments

Physical mobility, impaired, related to musculoskeletal trauma

Implementation

- Being careful not to cause further injury, position the client using supports.
- Numerous x-rays will be taken depending on the bone or joint affected.

Evaluation

- Note the results in relation to the client's symptoms and the other tests performed, such as serum alkaline phosphatase, bone scans, and serum electrolytes.

Client/Caregiver Teaching

Pretest

- Inform the client that the test will help identify the cause of the discomfort or show whether the bone is healing.
- Warn the client that the extremity's position during the procedure may be uncomfortable but to be careful not to move.

Posttest

- Teach the client or caregiver how to support the injured extremity and how to use supportive devices such as crutches.
- Tell the client to contact the physician if the injured extremity does not improve.
- Inform the client with a cast to immediately contact the physician if the cast is too tight, that is, if the client experiences numbness or tingling of digits.

Radiography, Bronchus
(Bronchography)

Classification: Radiography

Type of Test: Indirect visualization

This test visualizes the tracheobronchial tree following the injection of an iodinated oil contrast medium by a catheter inserted into the trachea and bronchi. The lining of the tracheobronchial tree becomes coated, and films are taken with the client in various positions. Although this procedure has generally been replaced with bronchoscopy, the major advantage of bronchography is provision of permanent films for future reference.

Indications

- Detect obstructions in the bronchi caused by tumors, cysts, or foreign objects
- Determine the cause of persistent hemoptysis and recurring pneumonia
- Evaluate the bronchial tree before surgery
- Diagnose hyaline membrane disease and transient tachypnea in infants
- Detect congenital malformations in the tracheobronchial tree

Reference Findings

- Normal structure of the tracheobronchial airways; no bronchiectasis, airway obstruction, tumors, cysts, or congenital abnormalities

Abnormal Findings

- Bronchiectasis
- Tracheobronchial malformation
- Bronchial obstruction
- Bronchial tumors

Interfering Factors

- Coughing by the client prevents the coating of the airways with the contrast medium.
- Excessive secretions in the tracheobronchial airway will alter coating of the tracheobronchial tree with the contrast medium.

> ### Nursing Alert
>
> - This procedure is contraindicated during pregnancy unless the benefits of performing the procedure outweigh the risks to the patient and in clients with respiratory insufficiency or an acute infection.
> - Risks associated with radiographic overexposure can result from frequent x-ray procedures.
> - Prevent possible x-ray exposure of personnel in the room with the client by having them wear a protective lead apron or stand behind a shield; badges that reveal the level of exposure to rays should be worn by those working in areas near x-ray suites.

Nursing Implications

Assessment

- Obtain a history of respiratory disorders, symptoms of a respiratory infection, medications, other tests performed, and the results.
- Determine whether or not the client has fasted since midnight the day of the test and whether or not special mouth care has been performed.

Possible Nursing Diagnoses

Ineffective airway clearance related to tracheobronchial obstruction

Risk for injury related to hypersensitivity reaction to dye

Implementation

- Perform mouth care if the client hasn't done so to minimize the risk of introducing bacteria into the tracheobronchial tree. A mild sedative may be given.
- Place the client in a sitting position. An anesthetic spray will be administered into the client's nose or throat to suppress the gag reflex.

- A small catheter is passed into the trachea, and the pharynx, larynx, and bronchi are anesthetized when local anesthetic is injected.
- Iodinated contrast medium is then injected through the catheter while the client is encouraged to increase breathing to prevent coughing.
- The client is placed in different positions to spread the dye, and films are taken.
- After the films are checked, help the client from the table into a position of comfort.

Evaluation

- Monitor the client for any adverse reactions to the contrast media.
- Note the test results in relation to the client's symptoms and the other tests performed.
- Observe the client closely for impaired respiration or laryngospasm.

Client/Caregiver Teaching

Pretest

- Inform the client that the procedure is performed in the x-ray department by a radiologist or pulmonologist, that it may take up to 45 minutes, and that it may be uncomfortable because suppressing the cough reflex will be difficult.
- Instruct the client to not eat or drink after midnight the night of the test. Also, tell the client to perform good mouth care that evening and the following morning before the test.
- If the client uses postural drainage, suggest performing it before the test.

Posttest

- Instruct the client to not eat or drink until the gag reflex returns (usually 2 hours).
- Instruct the client to use lozenges and gargle warm fluid for throat soreness.
- If necessary, suggest postural drainage to help remove the dye.
- Inform the client that a slight temperature elevation might occur 2 to 3 days after the procedure.

Radiography, Chest; Chest X-ray (CXR)

Classification: Radiography

Type of Test: Indirect visualization

Chest radiography, commonly called chest x-ray (CXR), is one of the most frequently performed radiologic diagnostic studies. It yields information about the pulmonary, cardiac, and skeletal systems. A routine CXR includes a posterior-anterior (PA) view. Portable x-rays, done in more acute or critical situations, can be done at the bedside and include only the anterior-posterior (AP) view. Other views that can be obtained are the oblique, lateral decubitus, and lordotic. Fluoroscopic studies of the chest can also be done to evaluate movement of the chest and diaphragm during breathing and coughing.

Indications

- Evaluate known or suspected pulmonary disorders, chest trauma, cardiovascular disorders, and skeletal disorders
- Aid in the diagnosis of diaphragmatic hernia
- Monitor resolution, progression, or maintenance of disease as applicable, and effectiveness of the treatment regimen
- Evaluate placement and position of the endotracheal tube, tracheostomy tube, central venous catheter, Swan-Ganz catheter, chest tube, nasogastric feeding tube, pacemaker wires, and intra-aortic balloon pump

Reference Values

- Normal lung fields, cardiac size, and mediastinal structures
- Normal thoracic spine and ribs
- Normal shaped and positioned diaphragm

Abnormal Values

- Curvature of the spinal column
- Enlarged heart
- Flattened diaphragm

- Foreign bodies lodged in the pulmonary tree
- Fractures
- Lung pathologic processes
- Pulmonary infiltrates
- Vascular abnormalities

Interfering Factors

- Metallic objects, such as jewelry and closures on clothing, within the x-ray field can be mistaken for abnormalities.
- Improper positioning and inability of the client to take and hold deep breaths and remain still during filming (pain, weakness, agitation, confusion) can alter test results.
- Improper density adjustment of x-ray equipment to accommodate obese or thin clients, may cause underexposure or overexposure and poor-quality films.

NURSING ALERT

- This test is contraindicated in pregnancy, especially during the first trimester, unless benefits of performing the procedure outweigh risks to the fetus.
- Special precautions should be taken with children to avoid excess exposure to x-rays.

Nursing Implications

Assessment

- Obtain a history of known or suspected pulmonary disease, cardiac disease, or chest trauma.
- Assess the client's ability to remain still and hold the breath; weakness or fatigue may necessitate portable CXR.
- Assess the date of the last menstrual period in premenopausal women to ascertain possible pregnancy.

Possible Nursing Diagnoses

Activity intolerance related to imbalance between oxygen supply and demand

Airway clearance, ineffective, related to tracheobronchial obstruction

Gas exchange, impaired, related to restrictive pulmonary process

Anxiety related to threat of change in health status

Implementation

- Remove clothing and metallic objects from the waist up and provide a gown with tie closure to wear; remove any attachment such as wires connected to electrodes, if allowed.
- Place the client in a standing, sitting, or lying position in front of the x-ray film holder depending on the view to be obtained; if portable AP film is being performed, elevate the head of the bed to the high Fowler's position with the plate in back of the client.
- Ask the client to position hands on the hips, extend neck, and position shoulders forward, touching the film holder for PA view; chest is positioned with the left side against the film holder and arm raised over the head and away from the field for lateral view.
- Ask the client to inhale deeply and hold the breath while the x-ray is taken and then exhale after the film is taken.

Evaluation

- Note the results in relation to arterial blood gas measurements, oxygen saturation levels, and other studies, such as pulmonary function studies and nuclear lung ventilation and perfusion scan.
- Also note test results in relation to the client's symptoms.

Client/Caregiver Teaching

Pretest

- Inform the client about the purpose of the procedure, various positions to assume and need to hold the breath, and time to complete the procedure (10 to 20 minutes). Demonstrate the procedure to children if they are old enough to understand.
- Inform the client that no food and fluid restrictions are needed and that no pain is associated with the study.

Posttest

- Provide emotional support when diagnostic findings are reported; reinforce information regarding diagnosis and recommended treatment regimen.
- Inform the client of the need for possible further CXR to evaluate and determine need for change in therapy.

Radiography, Excretory Urography (EUG), Intravenous Pyelography (IVP), Intravenous Urography (IUG, IVU)

Classification: Radiography

Type of Test: Indirect visualization with contrast dye

Excretory urography is the most commonly performed test to determine urinary tract dysfunction or renal disease. It uses intravenous radiopaque contrast medium to visualize the kidneys, ureters, bladder, and renal pelvis. The contrast medium concentrates in the urine and is filtered out by the glomeruli and then passes out through the renal tubules. A series of x-rays is performed during a 20- to 30-minute period to view passage of the medium through the kidneys and ureters into the bladder. A final film is taken after the patient empties the bladder (postvoiding film).

Indications

- Evaluate structure and excretory function of the kidneys, ureters, and bladder
- Aid in the diagnosis of renovascular hypertension, renal or urinary tract disease, renal stones, space-occupying lesions or congenital anomalies, and trauma to the urinary system

Reference Values

- Normal position, shape, and size of the kidneys, ureters, and bladder. Prompt visualization of the contrast medium through the urinary system.

Abnormal Values

- Absence of a kidney
- Benign and malignant kidney tumors

- Bladder tumors
- Congenital kidney or urinary tract abnormalities
- Glomerulonephritis
- Hydronephrosis
- Prostate enlargement
- Pyelonephritis
- Renal hematomas
- Renal or ureteral calculi
- Tumors of the collecting system

Interfering Factors

- Retained barium from previous studies may obscure visualization.
- Adequate visualization of the urinary tract may be prevented by abnormal renal function studies.
- Gas, fecal material, or barium in the bowel may obscure visualization of the urinary system.
- End-stage renal disease may produce films of poor quality.
- Insufficient injection of contrast medium may produce films of poor quality.

> ### NURSING ALERT
>
> - The contrast medium may cause a life-threatening allergic reaction to the iodinated dye. Those patients with a known hypersensitivity to the dye may benefit from premedication with corticosteroids. Elderly patients who are chronically dehydrated before the test may develop renal failure.
> - Special precautions should be taken with children to avoid exposure to x-rays.
> - This test is contraindicated in pregnancy, especially during the first trimester, unless the benefits of x-ray diagnosis far outweigh the possible risks to the fetus.

Nursing Implications

Assessment

- Obtain a history of known or suspected hypersensitivity to contrast medium, iodine, iodine-containing food, or shellfish.

- Assess the client's ability to remain still.
- Assess the date of the last menstrual period in premenopausal women to ascertain possible pregnancy.

Possible Nursing Diagnoses

Injury, risk for, related to hypersensitivity reaction to contrast medium
Fluid volume excess related to failure of regulatory system
Urinary elimination, altered, related to anatomical obstruction

Implementation

- Schedule barium studies after completion of this test.
- Give the client a laxative or a cathartic, as ordered, the evening before the test.
- Withhold food and fluids for 8 hours before the test or NPO after midnight before the test is scheduled.
- Give the client an enema or suppository on the morning of the test, as ordered.
- Remove clothing and metallic objects and provide a gown with tie closure to wear.
- Place the client in a supine position on the radiographic table. A plain film of the abdomen is taken to ensure that no stool will obscure visualization of the urinary system.
- Insert an intravenous line, if one is not already in place, and inject a contrast medium, if ordered.
- X-ray films will be taken at 1-, 5-, 10-, 15-, 20-, and 30-minute intervals to allow the course of the contrast medium to flow through the kidney to the bladder.
- Allow the client to void after the test is performed; a postvoiding test is taken to visualize the empty bladder.

Evaluation

- Note the results in relation to other studies, such as pulmonary function studies and nuclear lung ventilation and perfusion scan. Also note the test results in relation to the client's symptoms.
- Evaluate the client for signs of hypersensitivity reaction to contrast medium.
- Evaluate elderly or debilitated clients for dehydration and weakness.

Client/Caregiver Teaching

Pretest

- Inform the client about the purpose of the procedure, the need to hold the breath, and time to complete the procedure (10 to 30 minutes). Demonstrate the procedure to children if they are old enough to understand.
- Instruct the client to increase fluid intake before the test, but to withhold food and fluids for 8 hours before the test or after midnight before the test.
- Inform the client that they may receive a laxative the night before the test or an enema or a cathartic the morning of the test, as ordered.

Posttest

- Provide emotional support when diagnostic findings are reported; reinforce information regarding diagnosis and recommended treatment regimen.
- Inform the client of the need for possible further studies to evaluate and determine modifications in therapy.

Radiography, Hysterosalpingography, Uterography, Uterosalpingography, Hysterogram

Classification: Radiography

Type of Test: Indirect visualization with contrast dye

Hysterography involves visualization of the uterine cavity and fallopian tubes after the injection of contrast material into the cervix. The contrast medium should flow through the uterine cavity, through the fallopian tubes, and into the peritoneal cavity, where it can be absorbed if no obstruction exists. Passage of the dye through the tubes may clear mucous plugs, straighten kinked tubes, or break up adhesions, thus restoring fertility.

Indications

- Confirm tubal abnormalities such as adhesions and occlusion
- Confirm uterine abnormalities such as congenital malformation, traumatic injuries, or the presence of foreign bodies
- Confirm the presence of fistulas
- Aid in the diagnosis of bicornate uterus
- Evaluate adequacy of surgical tubal ligation

Reference Values

- Normal position, shape, and size of the uterine cavity
- Contrast medium flows freely into the fallopian tubes and does not leak from the uterus

Abnormal Values

- Bicornate uterus
- Developmental abnormalities
- Extrauterine pregnancy
- Internal scarring
- Kinking of the fallopian tubes from adhesions
- Tumors
- Uterine cavity anomalies
- Uterine fistulas
- Uterine masses
- Uterine tumors (leiomyomas)

Interfering Factors

- Retained barium from previous studies may obscure visualization.
- Excessive traction during the test may displace adhesions, making the fallopian tubes appear normal.
- Gas, fecal material, or barium in the bowel may obscure visualization of the uterus and fallopian tubes.
- Insufficient injection of contrast medium may produce films of poor quality.
- Excessive traction during the test or tubal spasm may cause the appearance of a stricture in an otherwise normal fallopian tube.

> ### NURSING ALERT
>
> - The contrast medium may cause a life-threatening allergic reaction to the iodinated dye. Those patients with a known hypersensitivity to the dye may benefit from premedication with corticosteroids.
> - This test is contraindicated in pregnancy, especially during the first trimester, unless the benefits of x-ray diagnosis far outweigh the possible risks to the fetus.
> - Hysterosalpingography is contraindicated in clients with menses, undiagnosed vaginal bleeding, or pelvic inflammatory disease.

Nursing Implications

Assessment

- Obtain a history of known or suspected hypersensitivity to contrast medium, iodine, iodine-containing food, or shellfish.
- Assess the client's ability to remain still.
- Assess the date of the last menstrual period in premenopausal women to ascertain possible pregnancy.
- Assess client history for conditions that could affect test results.
- Determine previous abnormalities in laboratory test results (especially blood urea nitrogen and creatinine if dye is to be used) and diagnostic findings.

Possible Nursing Diagnoses

Injury, risk for, related to potential hypersensitivity reaction to contrast material

Anxiety related to perceived threat to health status

Grieving, anticipatory, related to perceived potential loss

Implementation

- Schedule barium studies *after* completion of this test.
- Administer enemas or suppositories on the morning of the test, as ordered.
- Administer sedatives, as ordered before the test. Withhold food and fluids for 8 hours before the test or NPO after midnight before the test is scheduled.
- Remove clothing and metallic objects and provide a gown with tie closure to wear.
- Have the client void before the test begins.
- Place the client in the lithotomy position on the fluoroscopy table.

- A plain film of the abdomen is taken to ensure that no stool will obscure visualization of the uterus and fallopian tubes.
- A speculum is inserted into the vagina and contrast medium is introduced into the uterus through a cannula; both fluoroscopic and radiographic films are taken.
- To take oblique views, the table may be tilted or the client may be asked to change position during the procedure, which may take up to 30 minutes to perform.

Evaluation

- Monitor vital signs and neurologic signs per institution policy until stable.
- Note the test results in relation to the client's symptoms.
- Evaluate the client for signs of hypersensitivity reaction to contrast medium such as urticaria, headache, nausea, or vomiting.

Client/Caregiver Teaching

Pretest

- Inform the client that the test will permit assessment of the uterus and fallopian tubes.
- Inform the client that the time to complete the procedure is about 30 minutes.
- Instruct the patient to take a laxative or an enema, as ordered, the night before the test. Tell the client that she may receive a suppository or an enema before the test.
- Explain to the client that she may feel menstrual-like cramping during the procedure and shoulder pain from subphrenic irritation from the dye as it spills into the peritoneal cavity.

Posttest

- Provide emotional support when diagnostic findings are reported; reinforce information regarding diagnosis and recommended treatment regimen.
- Inform the client of the need for possible further studies to evaluate and determine need for change in therapy.
- Watch for signs of infection such as pain, fever, increased pulse rate, and muscle aches.
- Inform the client that a vaginal discharge is common and that it may be bloody, lasting for 1 to 2 days after the test.
- Instruct the patient to be alert for signs of delayed reaction to the dye such as urticaria, headache, nausea, or vomiting.
- Inform the client that dizziness and cramping may follow this procedure.

Radiography, Lymphangiography, Lymphangiogram, Lymphography

Classification: Radiography

Type of Test: Indirect visualization with contrast dye

Lymphangiography involves visualization of the lymphatic system after the injection of an oil-based contrast medium into a lymphatic vessel in the hand or foot. Injection into the hand allows visualization of the axillary and supraclavicular nodes. Injection into the foot allows for visualization of the lymphatics of the leg, inguinal and iliac regions, and the retroperitoneum up to the thoracic duct. Less commonly, it can be used to visualize the cervical region (retroauricular area).

Indications

- Determine lymphatic cancer staging
- Evaluate chemotherapy or radiation therapy
- Evaluate edema of an extremity without known cause
- Determine the extent of adenopathy
- Distinguish primary from secondary lymphedema

Reference Values

- Normal lymphatic vessels and nodes that fill completely with contrast medium on the initial films. On the 24-hour films, the lymph nodes are fully opacified and well circumscribed; the lymphatic channels are emptied a few hours after injection of the contrast medium.

Abnormal Values

- Nodal lymphoma
- Metastatic tumor involving the lymph glands
- Retroperitoneal lymphomas associated with Hodgkin's disease
- Abnormal lymphatic vessels

Interfering Factors

- Inability to cannulate the lymphatic vessels may interfere with accurate determination of test results.
- Insufficient injection of contrast medium may produce films of poor quality.

> ### NURSING ALERT
>
> - The contrast medium may cause a life-threatening allergic reaction to the iodinated dye. Those patients with a known hypersensitivity to the dye may benefit from premedication with corticosteroids.
> - Lymphangiography is contraindicated in clients with pulmonary insufficiencies, cardiac diseases, or severe renal or hepatic disease.
> - The oil-based contrast medium may embolize into the lungs and will temporarily diminish pulmonary function. This may produce lipid pneumonia, which is a life-threatening complication.

Nursing Implications

Assessment

- Obtain a history of known or suspected hypersensitivity to contrast medium, iodine, iodine-containing food, or shellfish.
- Assess the client's ability to remain still.
- Assess the date of the last menstrual period in premenopausal women to ascertain possible pregnancy
- Assess client history for conditions that could affect test results.
- Determine previous abnormalities in laboratory test results (especially BUN and creatinine if dye is to be used) and diagnostic findings.

Possible Nursing Diagnoses

Injury, risk for, related to potential hypersensitivity reaction to contrast material

Anxiety related to perceived threat to health status.

Breathing pattern/airway clearance, ineffective, risk for, related to tracheobronchial obstruction

Infection, risk for, related to invasive procedure

Implementation

- Administer sedatives, as ordered before the test.
- Obtain baseline vital signs.
- Remove clothing and metallic objects and provide a gown with tie closure to wear.
- Have the client void before the test begins.
- Place the client in the supine position on the radiographic table for an x-ray of the chest.
- After injection of a local anesthetic, the blue-contrast medium is injected intradermally into the area between the toes (or fingers). The lymphatic vessels are identified as they stain blue. A local anesthetic is then injected into the dorsum of each foot (or hand) and a small incision is made and cannulated for injection of the contrast medium.
- The flow of dye is followed by fluoroscopy. When the dye reaches the upper lumbar level, the flow of dye is discontinued. X-rays are taken of the chest, abdomen, and pelvis to determine filling of the lymphatic vessels.
- The client may be asked to return after 24 hours to have additional studies done.
- When the procedure is complete, which may take as long as 3 hours, the cannula is removed and the incision is sutured.

Evaluation

- Monitor vital signs and neurologic signs per institution policy until stable.
- Note the test results in relation to the client's symptoms.
- Evaluate the client for signs of hypersensitivity reaction to contrast medium such as urticaria, headache, nausea, or vomiting.
- Evaluate the client for signs of lipid pneumonia or pulmonary embolus from contrast medium, which may include shortness of breath, increased anxiety, increased heart rate, pleuritic pain, hypotension, low-grade fever, and cyanosis.
- Enforce bedrest for the first 24 hours with the client's feet elevated to reduce swelling, as ordered.
- Check the client's incision sites for bleeding and signs of infection.

Client/Caregiver Teaching

Pretest

- Inform the client that the test will permit assessment of the lymphatic system.

- Inform the client that the time to complete the procedure is about 3 hours and that he or she may have to return the next day but that the return study should only take 30 minutes.
- Explain that the client may feel some discomfort when the dye and the anesthetic is injected.
- Explain that the contrast medium may give the skin and vision a blue tint that may last for 48 hours. The stool and urine may also be stained blue.

Posttest

- Inform the client of the need for possible further studies to evaluate and determine need for change in therapy.
- Advise the client to watch for signs of infection such as pain, fever, increased pulse rate, and muscle aches.
- Inform the patient to be alert for signs of delayed reaction to the dye such as urticaria, headache, nausea, or vomiting.

Radiography, Pelvic (Pelvimetry)

Classification: Radiography

Type of Test: Indirect visualization

Pelvic radiography provides visualization of the pelvic bony structures and is the most accurate way of determining pelvic adequacy for a normal vaginal delivery. The capacity of the pelvis can be compared to the size of the infant and determine any cephalopelvic disproportion. This procedure is not used as often because of the risk to the fetus associated with radiation. Ultrasound measurements of fetal size in comparison to the pelvic measurements is more common.

Indications

- Determine abnormal positions of the fetus when vaginal delivery is anticipated
- Determine pelvic distortion in the presence of injury or disease

- Aid in the diagnosis of clinically abnormal pelvic measurements
- Aid in the diagnosis of a small or unfavorable pelvis

Reference Values

- The transverse diameter of the pelvis should measure >10.5 cm.

Abnormal Values

- Abnormal fetal position
- Cephalopelvic disproportion

Interfering Factors

- Active labor can affect the client's ability to remain immobile during the procedure.
- Client may be unable to lie supine because of compression of the superior vena cava by the gravid uterus.

> **NURSING ALERT**
>
> - This procedure is contraindicated in early pregnancy because of the risk of radiation to the developing fetus.

Nursing Implications

Assessment

- Assess the client's ability to remain still.
- Assess the client's vital signs, including fetal heart rate and contractions.
- Assess the client's cervical dilation, effacement, and fetal station.

Possible Nursing Diagnoses

Anxiety related to perceived threat to fetus
Self-esteem, situational, low, risk for, related to perceived failure at life event
Pain, risk for, related to increased or prolonged contractions

Implementation

- Obtain baseline vital signs.
- Obtain baseline fetal heart rate and maternal contraction pattern.

- Remove clothing and metallic objects and provide a gown with tie closure to wear.
- Have the client void before the test begins.
- With the client standing, a lateral film is taken to detect the effect of gravity on fetal engagement and to determine the location of the fetal head when it reaches the lower level of the birth canal.
- Then, the client is placed in the supine, lateral, and recumbent positions as further films are taken. The client will be asked to hyperventilate before she holds her breath to provide adequate oxygenation to the fetus during the procedure.

Evaluation

- Monitor fetal heart rate and maternal contraction pattern during the procedure.
- Note the test results in relation to the client's symptoms.
- Monitor the progress of the client's labor.
- Monitor the client for possible rupture of amniotic membranes if not previously ruptured.

Client/Caregiver Teaching

Pretest

- Inform the client that the test will permit assessment of the pelvic measurements in comparison to fetal size.
- Explain to the client that during the test she should not feel any discomfort.
- Advise the client that this test does not require any fasting.
- Inform the client that this test should take about 15 minutes.

Posttest

- Provide emotional support when diagnostic findings are reported; reinforce information regarding diagnosis and recommended treatment regimen.
- Inform the client of the need for possible further studies to evaluate and determine need for change in therapy.

Radiography, Percutaneous Transhepatic Cholangiography (PTC, PTHC)

Classification: Radiography

Type of Test: Indirect visualization with contrast dye

Percutaneous transhepatic cholangiography (PTC) is the visualization of the biliary system by fluoroscopic examination and contrast medium. The liver is punctured with a thin needle under fluoroscope and the contrast medium is injected as the needle is slowly withdrawn. The intrahepatic and extrahepatic biliary ducts can be visualized for possible obstructions. In obstruction of the extrahepatic duct, a catheter can be placed in the duct to allow for external drainage of bile. Endoscopic retrograde cholangiopancreatography (ERCP) and PTC are the only methods available to view the biliary tree in the presence of jaundice. ERCP poses less risk and is probably done more commonly.

Indications

- Aid in the diagnosis of obstruction caused by gallstones, benign strictures, malignant tumors, congenital cysts, and anatomic variations
- Distinguish between obstructive and nonobstructive jaundice
- Determine the cause of upper abdominal pain following cholecystectomy
- Determine the cause, extent, and location of mechanical obstruction

Reference Values

- The gallbladder appears normal in size and shape.
- The biliary ducts are normal diameter.
- Contrast medium fills the ducts and flows freely.

Abnormal Values

- Anatomic biliary or pancreatic duct variations
- Biliary sclerosis
- Common bile duct cysts
- Sclerosing cholangitis
- Tumors, strictures, inflammation, or pseudocysts of the pancreatic duct
- Tumors, strictures, or gallstones of the common bile duct

Interfering Factors

- Retained barium from previous studies may obscure visualization.
- Marked obesity may obscure visualization.
- Gas that overfills the biliary ducts interferes with the clarity of the x-ray.
- Insufficient injection of contrast medium may produce films of poor quality.

NURSING ALERT

- The contrast medium may cause a life-threatening allergic reaction to the iodinated dye. Those patients with a known hypersensitivity to the dye may benefit from premedication with corticosteroids.
- This procedure is contraindicated in the presence of cholangitis because the injection of the dye can increase biliary pressure leading to bacteremia, septicemia, and shock. It should not be used in clients with massive ascites or uncorrectable coagulopathy.
- Peritonitis may occur as a result of bile extravasation from the liver as the needle is withdrawn.

Nursing Implications

Assessment

- Obtain a history of known or suspected hypersensitivity to contrast medium, iodine, iodine-containing food, or shellfish.
- Assess the client's ability to remain still.
- Assess the date of the last menstrual period in premenopausal women to ascertain possible pregnancy.

- Assess client history for conditions that could affect test results or be affected by the test.
- Determine previous abnormalities in laboratory test results (especially blood urea nitrogen and creatinine if dye is to be used) and coagulation studies as well as any diagnostic findings.

Possible Nursing Diagnoses

Injury, risk for, related to potential hypersensitivity reaction to contrast material
Anxiety related to perceived threat to health status
Pain related to ductal spasm and obstruction
Nutrition, altered, less than body requirements, related to inability to ingest adequate nutrients

Implementation

- Schedule barium studies after completion of this test.
- Type and cross the client's blood for possible transfusion.
- Administer sedatives, as ordered before the test.
- Ensure that the client remains NPO after midnight the night before the test.
- Check that the client's coagulation studies are within the normal range.
- Administer a laxative, as ordered.
- Remove clothing and metallic objects and provide a gown with tie closure to wear.
- Have the client void before the test begins.
- Place the client in the supine position on the fluoroscopy table.
- The area over the abdominal wall is anesthetized and the needle is inserted and advanced using fluoroscopy. Dye is injected when placement is confirmed by the free flow of bile. X-ray films are taken immediately.
- If an obstruction is found during the procedure, a catheter is inserted into the bile duct to allow for drainage of bile.
- Place a sandbag over the insertion site for several hours if bleeding is persistent.
- Establish a closed and sterile drainage system if a catheter is left in place.

Evaluation

- Monitor vital and neurologic signs per institution policy until the patient is stable.
- Note the test results in relation to the client's symptoms.

■ Evaluate the client for signs of hypersensitivity or reaction to contrast medium such as urticaria, headache, nausea, or vomiting.

Client/Caregiver Teaching

Pretest

■ Inform the client that the time to complete the procedure is about 1 hour and that during that time, the client must remain completely still.
■ Inform the client that there may be some abdominal pain from the needle insertion.

Posttest

■ Advise the client to remain NPO for a few hours after the test.
■ Provide emotional support when diagnostic findings are reported; reinforce information regarding diagnosis and recommended treatment regimen.
■ Inform the client of the need for possible further studies to evaluate and determine need for change in therapy.
■ Advise the client to watch for signs of infection such as pain, fever, increased pulse rate, and muscle aches.
■ Instruct the client to be alert for signs of delayed reaction to the dye such as urticaria, headache, nausea, or vomiting.

Radiography: Plain Films: Cardiac, Sinuses, Orbit and Eye, Skull, Vertebra, Kidney-Ureter-Bladder (KUB)

Classification: Radiography

Type of Test: Indirect visualization

Plain films are radiologic studies using external beams to visualize bones and soft tissues when examining a particular area of the body. Bones and air-filled soft structures with differences in composition and density will produce natural contrasts that are of diagnostic quality.

Indications, Reference Values, Abnormal Values

Organ	Indications	Reference Values	Abnormal Results
Heart	Evaluate heart size and position for abnormalities	Normal size, shape, contour, position of heart and great vessels	Congestive heart failure; cardiomegaly
	Determine valvular calcifications or function	Normal heart movement during systole and diastole	Aortic anomalies; ventricular or atrial enlargement
	Evaluate placement and positioning of pacemaker wires or central line		
Sinus	Detect head or facial fractures	Normal sinus bones and soft tissues	Fractures
	Confirm suspected acute or chronic sinusitis		Acute and chronic sinusitis
	Confirm suspected cyst, polyp, or tumor		Cyst, tumors, polyps
Orbit and eye	Identify fractures	Orbits of normal size and shape	Fracture
	Confirm suspected tumor or foreign body		Tumor, foreign body
	Confirm suspected craniofacial anomalies		
Skull	Confirm suspected tumor	Normal skull, facial and jaw bones, and brain tissue	Tumor
	Confirm suspected vascular abnormality	Normal vasculature	Congenital abnormalities
	Confirm known or suspected trauma	Changes in bone structure, size and shape	Skull fractures; craniostenosis or hydrocephalus in infants
Vertebra	Evaluate back or neck pain	Normal vertebral bodies	Cervical disk arthritis
	Confirm suspected tumor or fracture	No fractures or curvatures	Tumors, fractures
	Diagnose and monitor curvatures of the spine		Congenital cord defects, spinal curvatures

Organ	Indications	Reference Values	Abnormal Results
Kidney- Ureter- Bladder (KUB)	Diagnose intestinal obstruction	Normal size and shape of kidneys	Intestinal obstruction
	Evaluate size, shape, and position of the kidney, liver, spleen, or presence of renal calculi	Normal bladder; no masses, renal calculi, or abnormal accumulation of air or fluid	Congenital renal anomaly, renal calculi, or liver or spleen abnormalities
	Evaluate acute abdominal pain or palpable mass		
	Suspected abnormal fluid, air, or object in abdomen		

Interfering Factors

- Improper positioning, especially for oblique and lordotic views and views using portable films, can affect results.
- Metallic objects, such as jewelry or closures in clothing, within the x-ray field, can be mistaken for pathology.
- The client's inability to maintain positioning during filming (pain, weakness, agitation, confusion) or to take deep breaths during filming for cardiac films will affect quality of the film.
- Improper density adjustment of x-ray equipment to accommodate obese or thin clients can cause underexposure or overexposure and poor-quality films.
- Presence of feces, barium, gas, ascites, and uterine and ovarian tumors can interfere with KUB films.

NURSING ALERT

- This test is contraindicated in pregnancy, unless benefits of performing the procedure outweigh risks to the fetus.
- Risks associated with radiographic overexposure can result from frequent x-ray procedures. Personnel in the room with the client should wear a protective lead apron or stand behind a shield; badges that reveal level of exposure to rays should be worn by those working in areas near x-ray suites.

Nursing Implications

Assessment

- Obtain a history of the affected area, current symptoms, and results of other diagnostic tests.
- Assess the date of the last menstrual period to ascertain possible pregnancy.
- Assess the client's understanding of explanations provided and presence of anxiety.

Possible Nursing Diagnoses

Anxiety related to potential change in health status
Pain related to trauma

Implementation

- Remove clothing and metallic objects and provide a gown with tie closure to wear.
- Remove any attachment such as wires connected to electrodes if allowed.
- Provide a supportive environment and encourage questions about the procedure.
- Transport to radiology by wheelchair or stretcher.
- *Cardiac films:* See chest x-ray procedure.
- *Sinus films:* Help the client to an x-ray chair. Head is immobilized in a padded brace and necessary views are taken. Once films are developed and checked, the brace is removed.
- *Orbital and skull films:* The client is seated in an x-ray chair or assisted to a supine position on the x-ray table. Various views are taken, and the head is repositioned using headbands, sandbags, or foam blocks.
- *Vertebra films:* The client is helped to a supine position on the x-ray table. An anterior-posterior film is taken; then the client is placed in a side-lying position for lateral and oblique views. Fracture sites must be immobilized during the procedure to prevent further injury.
- *KUB:* The client is placed on the table in a supine position with hands over the head. An anterior-posterior view of the abdomen is taken. Ask the client to inhale deeply and hold the breath while the x-ray is taken and then exhale after the film is taken.
- Return the client to a position of comfort and help from the table or chair. Return the client to his or her room or return clothing and belongings if an outpatient.

- Reposition any tubes or wires for proper placement and functioning if moved or disturbed during the procedure.

Evaluation

- Note the test results in relation to other related tests and the client's symptoms.

Client/Caregiver Teaching

Pretest

- Explain the purpose of the test and procedure involved: various positions to assume and need for several views. For cardiac film, explain need to hold breath. For KUB, only one view is taken. Explain that the procedure takes 10 to 20 minutes.
- Demonstrate the procedure to children if they are old enough to understand.
- Tell the client that no food and fluid restrictions are needed and that no pain is associated with these studies.

Posttest

- Tell the client of the need for further diagnostic testing based on results or to monitor response to therapy.

Radiography, Retrograde Ureteropyelography

Classification: Radiography

Type of Test: Indirect visualization with contrast dye

Retrograde ureteropyelography uses a contrast medium introduced through a ureteral catheter during cystography and radiographic visualization to view the renal collecting system. It is primarily used in clients who are known to be hypersensitive to iodine-based injected dyes and when excretory ureterography does not adequately reveal the renal collecting system. It is not influenced by impaired renal function.

Indications

- Evaluate the structure and integrity of the renal collecting system (calyces, renal pelvis, and urethra)
- Evaluate the renal collecting system when excretory urography is unsuccessful

Reference Values

- Normal outline and opacification of renal pelvis and calyces
- Asymmetrical and bilateral outline of structures
- Normal appearance in size and course and uniform filling of the ureters

Abnormal Values

- Neoplasms
- Obstruction owing to tumor, blood clot, stricture, or calculi
- Obstruction of ureteropelvic junction
- Perinephric abscess
- Perinephric inflammation or suppuration
- Renal abscess or tumor

Interfering Factors

- Retained barium from previous studies may obscure visualization.
- Gas, fecal material, or barium in the bowel may obscure visualization of the urinary system.

Nursing Implications

Assessment

- Assess the client's ability to remain still.
- Assess the date of the last menstrual period in premenopausal women to ascertain possible pregnancy.

Possible Nursing Diagnoses

Fluid volume excess related to failure of regulatory system
Thought processes, altered, related to accumulation of toxic waste products
Urinary elimination, altered, related to anatomical obstruction
Pain related to anatomical obstruction

Implementation

- Schedule barium studies after completion of this test.
- Ensure adequate hydration before the test to ensure adequate urine flow.
- Withhold food and fluids for 8 hours before the test or NPO after midnight before the test is scheduled if a general anesthetic will be used.
- Remove clothing and metallic objects and provide a gown with tie closure to wear.
- Place the client in the lithotomy position on the radiographic table.
- While the client is anesthetized, a cystoscopic examination is performed and the bladder is inspected. A catheter is inserted and the renal pelvis is emptied by gravity. Then, contrast medium diluted to half-strength is introduced into the catheter. Radiographic films are taken and developed immediately. Oblique and lateral films may also be taken at this time if necessary.
- Additional contrast medium is injected through the catheter to outline the ureters as the catheter is withdrawn.
- Additional films are taken 10 to 15 minutes after the catheter is removed to check for retention of the contrast medium, indicating urinary stasis. The catheter may be kept in place and attached to gravity drainage until urinary flow has returned or is corrected.

Evaluation

- Note the results in relation to other studies and the client's symptoms.
- Monitor vital and neurologic signs per institution policy until stable.
- Monitor fluid intake and urinary output for 24 hours, especially if catheter remains in place.
- Watch for and report signs of sepsis and severe pain in the area of the kidney.

Client/Caregiver Teaching

Pretest

- Inform the client about the purpose of the procedure, the need to hold the breath, and time to complete the procedure (about 1 hour).
- Tell the client to increase fluid intake before the test but to not eat or drink anything for 8 hours before the test or after midnight before the test if a general anesthetic will be used.

- Tell the client that if a local anesthetic is used, the client may feel some pressure in the kidney area as the catheter and dye is introduced or the urgency to void.

Posttest

- Provide emotional support when diagnostic findings are reported; reinforce information regarding diagnosis and recommended treatment regimen.
- Inform the client of the need for possible further studies to evaluate and determine need for change in therapy.

Radiography, Retrograde Urethrography

Classification: Radiography

Type of Test: Indirect visualization with contrast dye

Retrograde urethrography uses a contrast medium that is either injected or introduced into the urethra to visualize the membranous, bulbar, and penile portions. Used almost exclusively in males, it may be performed after surgical repair of the urethra. The posterior portion of the urethra is better visualized when this radiographic test is performed with voiding cystourethrography.

Indications

- Aid in the diagnosis of urethral strictures, lacerations, diverticula, and congenital anomalies

Reference Values

- Normal size, shape, and course of the membranous, bulbar, and penile portions of the urethra.
- If the prostatic portion can be visualized, it should also appear normal.

Abnormal Values

- Congenital anomalies such as urethral valves and perineal hypospadius
- False passages in the urethra
- Fistulas of the urethra
- Urethral calculi
- Urethral diverticula
- Urethral strictures and lacerations
- Urethral tumors

> **NURSING ALERT**
>
> - This procedure should be avoided or performed with caution in the presence of urinary tract infection.

Nursing Implications

Assessment

- Assess the client's ability to remain still.
- Assess the client history for any known hypersensitivity to iodine, shellfish, or contrast dye.
- Determine previous abnormalities in laboratory test results (especially blood urea nitrogen and creatinine if dye is to be used) and diagnostic findings.

Possible Nursing Diagnoses

Fluid volume excess related to failure of regulatory system

Thought processes, altered, related to accumulation of toxic waste products

Urinary elimination, altered, related to anatomical obstruction

Pain related to anatomical obstruction

Implementation

- Remove clothing and metallic objects and provide a gown with tie closure to wear.
- Have the client void before the procedure.
- Place the client in the recumbent position on the radiographic table while anteroposterior films of the bladder and urethra are taken.
- The catheter is filled with contrast medium to eliminate air pockets and is then inserted until the balloon reaches the meatus. The client is then placed in the right posterior oblique position with the thigh drawn up to a 90-degree angle and the penis is placed along its axis.

- When three-fourths of the dye has been injected, another film is taken and developed while the remainder of the dye is injected.
- Left lateral and oblique films may be taken.
- The procedure may be done on females using a double balloon to occlude the bladder neck from above and below the external meatus.

Evaluation

- Note the results in relation to other studies and to the client's symptoms.
- Monitor fluid intake and urinary output for 24 hours, especially if catheter remains in place.
- Watch for and report signs of extravasation of contrast medium into the general circulation, including fever and chills.

Client/Caregiver Teaching

Pretest

- Inform the client about the purpose of the procedure, the need to hold the breath, and time to complete the procedure (about 30 minutes).
- Advise the client not to restrict fluid or food before the procedure.
- Inform the client that some pressure may be experienced when the catheter is inserted and the dye is instilled through the catheter.

Posttest

- Provide emotional support when diagnostic findings are reported; reinforce information regarding diagnosis and recommended treatment regimen.
- Inform the client of the need for possible further studies to evaluate and determine need for change in therapy.
- Advise the client to report fever or chills or delayed signs of hypersensitivity to the dye such as urticaria, headache, nausea, or vomiting.

Radiography, Voiding Cystourethrography, Voiding Cystography

Classification: Radiography

Type of Test: Indirect visualization with contrast dye

Voiding cystourethrography involves the visualization of bladder filling and slow excretion following instillation of a contrast medium into the bladder through a catheter and syringe or gravity. Fluoroscopic films or overhead radiography follows the bladder filling and emptying.

Indications

- Determine possible cause of frequent urinary tract infections
- Confirm the diagnosis of congenital lower urinary tract anomaly
- Evaluate abnormal bladder emptying and incontinence
- Assess hypertrophy of the prostate lobes
- Assess ureteral stricture
- Assess the degree of compromise of a stenotic prostatic urethra

Reference Values

- Normal bladder function and structure

Abnormal Values

- Bladder trauma
- Bladder tumors
- Hematomas
- Neurogenic bladder
- Pelvic tumors
- Prostatic enlargement
- Ureteral stricture
- Ureterocele
- Vesicoureteral reflux

Interfering Factors

- Inability of the client to void on demand.
- Previous studies using contrast media or the presence of gas or feces in the bowel may obscure visualization.
- Urethral trauma from catheterization may cause pain on urination resulting in incomplete sphincter relaxation, muscle spasm, or an interrupted or less vigorous stream of urine.

> **NURSING ALERT**
>
> - This procedure should be avoided or performed with caution in the presence of urinary tract infection.

Nursing Implications

Assessment

- Assess the client's ability to remain still.
- Assess the client history for any known hypersensitivity to iodine, shellfish, or contrast dye.
- Determine previous abnormalities in laboratory test results (especially blood urea nitrogen and creatinine if dye is to be used) and diagnostic findings.

Possible Nursing Diagnoses

Fluid volume excess related to failure of regulatory system
Thought processes, altered, related to accumulation of toxic waste products
Urinary elimination, altered, related to anatomical obstruction
Pain related to anatomical obstruction

Implementation

- Remove clothing and metallic objects and provide a gown with tie closure to wear.
- Have the client void before the procedure.
- Place the client in the recumbent position on the radiographic table while anteroposterior films of the bladder and urethra are taken.
- The catheter is filled with contrast medium to eliminate air pockets and is then inserted until the balloon reaches the meatus. The client is then placed in the right posterior oblique position with the thigh drawn up to a 90-degree angle and the penis placed along its axis.
- When three-fourths of the dye has been injected, another film is taken and developed while the remainder of the dye is injected.

- Left lateral and oblique films may be taken.
- The procedure may be done on females using a double balloon to occlude the bladder neck from above and below the external meatus.

Evaluation

- Note the results in relation to other studies.
- Also note the test results in relation to the client's symptoms.
- Monitor vital and neurologic signs per institution policy until stable.
- Monitor fluid intake and urinary output for 24 hours, especially if the catheter remains in place.
- Watch for and report signs of extravasation of contrast medium into the general circulation, including fever and chills.

Client/Caregiver Teaching

Pretest

- Inform the client about the purpose of the procedure, the need to hold the breath, and time to complete the procedure (about 30 minutes).
- Advise the client not to restrict fluid or food before the procedure.
- Inform the client that some pressure may be experienced when the catheter is inserted and when the dye is instilled through the catheter.

Posttest

- Provide emotional support when diagnostic findings are reported; reinforce information regarding diagnosis and recommended treatment regimen.
- Inform the client of the need for possible further studies to evaluate and determine need for change in therapy.
- Advise the client to report fever or chills or delayed signs of hypersensitivity to the dye such as urticaria, headache, nausea, or vomiting.

Radionuclide Imaging: Brain, Brain Scan

Classification: Nuclear medicine

Type of Test: Radionuclide imaging with contrast medium

Radionuclide brain imaging uses single-photon emission computed tomography (SPECT) and the injection of a radioisotope such as technetium-99m (Tc-99m) or iodine (I-123 iofetamine), which is injected intravenously and can pass the blood-brain barrier. The SPECT allows visualization of various slices to provide depth resolution from different angles. SPECT images can be obtained around the circumference of the head to evaluate extracranial and intracranial blood flow as well as evaluate the radioisotope uptake in various areas of the brain tissue.

Indications

- Aid in the diagnosis of Alzheimer's disease, stroke, dementia, epilepsy, Huntington's disease, systemic lupus erythematosus, Parkinson's disease, and seizure disorder
- Aid in the diagnosis of brain death

Reference Values

- Normal intracranial and extracranial blood flow.
- Normal distribution of the radioisotope in the brain tissue with the highest distribution in the gray matter, thalmus, basal ganglia, and peripheral cortex.
- Less activity should be demonstrated in the ventricles and central white matter.

Abnormal Values

- Alzheimer's disease
- Brain death
- Dementia
- Huntington's disease
- Parkinson's disease
- Psychiatric disorders such as schizophrenia

- Seizure disorder
- Stroke

Interfering Factors

- Cerebral alignment can be altered if the client coughs or moves.
- Loud noises or sudden distractions can alter the distribution of I-123.
- Recent studies using radionuclides may interfere with interpretation of the image.

Nursing Implications

Assessment

- Assess the client's ability to remain still.
- Assess the client history for monoamine oxidase (MAO) inhibitors.
- Determine whether the client is pregnant or breast-feeding; radionuclide imaging is contraindicated in both cases.
- Assess the client's neurologic status to use as a baseline.

Possible Nursing Diagnoses

Communication, impaired, verbal, related to altered brain functioning

Swallowing, impaired, related to neuromuscular impairment

Physical mobility, impaired, related to neuromuscular impairment

Implementation

- Remove clothing and metallic objects and provide a gown with tie closure.
- Obtain an accurate weight to determine the dosage of the radioisotope.
- Place the client in the supine position on the table. The radioisotope is injected intravenously. Then, while the client remains perfectly still, SPECT images are obtained around the circumference of the head. The procedure should take about 1 hour.

> **NURSING ALERT**
>
> - This procedure is contraindicated in pregnancy and breast-feeding and if the client is receiving an MAO inhibitor.

Evaluation

- Note the results in relation to other studies and to the client's symptoms.
- Monitor vital and neurologic signs per institution policy until stable.
- Monitor for signs of hypersensitivity to the radioisotope.
- Monitor neurologic signs and compare to baseline.

Client/Caregiver Teaching

Pretest

- Inform the client about the purpose of the procedure, the need to remain still, and the time to complete the procedure (about 1 hour).
- Advise the client that there are no restrictions on fluid or food before the procedure.

Posttest

- Provide emotional support when diagnostic findings are reported; reinforce information regarding diagnosis and recommended treatment regimen.
- Inform the client of the need for possible further studies to evaluate and determine need for change in therapy.
- Advise the client to report delayed signs of hypersensitivity to the radioisotope.

Radionuclide Imaging: Thyroid

Classification: Nuclear medicine

Type of Test: Radionuclide imaging with contrast medium

Radionuclide thyroid imaging is the visualization of the thyroid gland using a gamma camera and a radioactive iodine injected intravenously or ingested orally. The procedure measures the uptake of the iodine in the thyroid to evaluate the size, position, and function of the gland. Technetium-99m (Tc-99m) may be used in place of iodine. It is usually performed in conjunction with serum triiodothyronine (T_3) and serum thyroxine (T_4) levels as well as thyroid uptake and thyroid ultrasound tests. Hyperfunctioning areas (excessive uptake of iodine) appear as black or hot spots and hypofunctioning areas (little or no iodine uptake) appear as white or cold spots.

Indications

- Determine the cause of a palpable thyroid mass
- Assess the size, structure, and position of the thyroid
- Evaluate thyroid function, especially in conjunction with other thyroid tests
- Aid in the diagnosis of Hashimoto's disease, hypothyroidism, hyperthyroidism, Graves' disease, and goiter
- Aid in the diagnosis of thyroid cancer

Reference Values

- Normal thyroid imaging reveals a thyroid that is about 5 cm long and 2.5 cm wide.
- The gland should appear in a butterfly shape with two lobes. Occasionally, a third lobe may appear; this is a normal variant.
- The radioisotope should show uniform uptake without any tumors.

Abnormal Values

- Autonomous nodules
- Graves' disease
- Hashimoto's disease
- Hyperthyroidism
- Hypothyroidism
- Thyroid cancer

Interfering Factors

- Ingestion of aminosalicylic acid, corticosteroids, multivitamins, cough syrups containing iodides, thyroid hormones, or thyroid hormone antagonists can interfere with the uptake of iodine.
- Severe diarrhea and vomiting can interfere with the uptake of iodine.
- An iodine-deficient diet increases uptake of iodine and intake of foods containing iodine, such as seafood or iodized salt, decreases uptake.

- Uptake of iodine is increased in persons taking phenothiazines.

> **NURSING ALERT**
>
> - This test is contraindicated during pregnancy and breast-feeding.

Nursing Implications

Assessment

- Assess the client's ability to remain still.
- Assess the client history for allergy to iodine or an iodine-deficient diet, which could interfere with results.
- Assess the client's history for recent studies using contrast medium.
- Determine whether the client is pregnant or breast-feeding; radionuclide imaging is contraindicated in both cases.

Possible Nursing Diagnoses

Nutrition, altered, risk for less than body requirements, related to constant activity

Fatigue related to hypermetabolic imbalance

Tissue integrity, impaired, risk for, related to hormone activity

Physical mobility, impaired, related to weakness

Implementation

- Ensure that the client remains NPO after midnight the night before the test if oral iodine is to be administered.
- Remove clothing and metallic objects and provide a gown with tie closure to wear.
- I-123 or I-131 radioisotope is administered orally and the procedure must then be performed within 24 hours of ingestion; or Tc-99m pertechnetate is administered intravenously and the procedure must be performed within 20 to 30 minutes.
- The client's thyroid is palpated. The client is then placed in the supine position with the neck extended. The gamma camera is placed over the thyroid and pictures are taken; two bilateral oblique views and one straight-on anterior view is taken.

Evaluation

- Note the results in relation to other studies and to the client's symptoms.

- Monitor vital and neurologic signs per institution policy until stable.
- Monitor for signs of hypersensitivity to the iodine.

Client/Caregiver Teaching

Pretest

- Inform the client about the purpose of the procedure, the need to remain still, and the time to complete the procedure (about 30 minutes).
- Advise the client that there are no restrictions on fluid or food before the procedure unless oral iodine is to be administered.
- Assure the client that the medication or the gamma camera will not expose him or her to dangerous radiation levels.
- Instruct the client to discontinue any thyroid medication, multivitamins, cough syrups, and any iodine-containing drugs 2 to 3 weeks before the procedure, as ordered.
- Instruct the client to discontinue any phenothiazines, salicylates, corticosteroids, anticoagulants, and antihistamines 1 week before the procedure, as ordered.

Posttest

- Inform the client of the need for possible further studies to evaluate and determine need for change in therapy.

Raji Cell Assay

Classification: Immunology

Type of Test: Blood

This test detects circulating immune complexes and specifically the Raji lymphoblastoid cells that have receptors for immunoglobulin G complement. In this test, serum is mixed with lymphoblastoid B cells and the amount of immune complexes that bind with complexes that contain C_{3B} receptors on the Raji cell membrane are analyzed.

Indications

- Detect the presence of immune complexes (Transient elevations occur with antigen-antibody response and prolonged elevations with autoimmune diseases or chronic inflammation.)

Reference Values

Normal	<13 mg AHG Eq/mL
Borderline	12–25 mg AHG Eq/mL

AHG = antihemophilic globulin.

Abnormal Values

- Transient elevated levels
    Drug reactions
    Parasitic, viral, or microbial infections
- Prolonged elevated levels
    Autoimmune disorders
    Cirrhosis
    Celiac disease
    Crohn's disease
    Cryoglobulinemia
    Dermatitis herpetiformis
    Sickle-cell anemia
    Ulcerative colitis

Interfering Factors

- Results may be unreliable if the client has had a recent radioactive dye injection for scan.
- Hemolysis or failure to place the sample in ice can affect test results.

Nursing Implications

Assessment

- Obtain a history of the purpose for the test, known or suspected autoimmune disorders, and results of tests and procedures performed.

Possible Nursing Diagnoses

Anxiety related to threat to health status
Pain related to tissue inflammation
Fluid volume deficit related to excessive gastrointestinal losses
Skin integrity, impaired, related to altered metabolic state

Implementation

- Put on gloves. Using aseptic technique, perform a venipuncture and collect 10 mL of blood in a green-top tube. (Some laboratories prefer a red-top or red marble-top tube.) Place the tube in a container of ice and transport to the laboratory immediately.
- Handle the specimen carefully to avoid hemolysis.

Evaluation

- Note the results in relation to other studies performed, particularly renal function studies (to assess the effect of circulating immune complexes on renal function), liver function and viral studies, and to the client's symptoms.

Client/Caregiver Teaching

Pretest

- Inform the client that fasting is not required for this test.

Rapid Plasma Reagin Test (RPR Test)

Classification: Serology

Type of Test: Serum

The rapid plasma reagin test is a substitute for the venereal disease research laboratory (VDRL) test to detect syphilis. It uses a cardiolipin antigen to detect reagin, which is the antibody that is relatively specific to the causative agent for syphilis. The client's serum is mixed with the cardiolipin on a card, mechanically rotated, and then viewed. If flocculation occurs, the test sample is diluted until no reaction occurs. The last dilution is the titer of the antibody.

Indications

- Aid in the diagnosis of syphilis
- Screen for secondary and primary syphilis
- Monitor response to treatment

Reference Values

- Normal serum contains no flocculation and is reported as a nonreactive test.

Abnormal Values

- Primary or secondary syphilis

Interfering Factors

- Hemolysis of the sample can alter the test results.
- Gross lipemia may affect the test results.
- Mycoplasma pneumonia, malaria, acute bacterial and viral infections, autoimmune diseases, and pregnancy may cause false-positive reactions.
- Excess chyle in the blood may alter the test results.
- Ingestion of alcohol within 24 hours of the test may alter the test results.

Nursing Implications

Assessment

- Ensure that the client abstained from alcohol for 24 hours before the test.
- Assess client history for disorders that may affect the test results.

Possible Nursing Diagnoses

Anxiety related to altered health status
Infection, risk for, related to the presence of infectious process
Skin/tissue integrity, impaired, related to invasion of pathogenic organism

Implementation

- Put on gloves. Using aseptic technique, perform a venipuncture and collect 7 mL of blood in a red-top tube.
- Send the sample to the laboratory promptly.

Evaluation

- Note the results in relation to other diagnostic criteria.

Client/Caregiver Teaching

Pretest

- Advise the client not to ingest any alcohol at least 24 hours before the test is performed.

Posttest

- If the test is reactive, explain the importance of proper treatment and adherence to the drug regimen. Also, stress the importance of notifying all sexual contacts that they should be tested and treated.
- If the test is reactive but the client does not demonstrate any physical signs of the disease, advise about the possibility of false-positive results. Inform the client about additional studies that can confirm diagnosis.

Red Blood Cell Count, Erythrocyte Count

Classification: Hematology

Type of Test: Blood

A component of the complete blood count (CBC), the red blood cell (RBC) count determines the number of RBCs per cubic millimeters (expressed as the number of RBCs per liter of blood in international units). Because the RBC contains hemoglobin that is responsible for the transport and exchange of oxygen, the number of circulating RBCs is important. Although the life span of the normal RBC is 120 days, other factors besides age and decreased production can cause decreased values: for example, abnormal destruction from intravascular trauma caused by atherosclerosis or an enlarged spleen caused by leukemia.

Indications

- Aid in routine screening as part of a CBC
- Detect a hematologic disorder involving RBC destruction (e.g., hemolytic anemia)
- Monitor the effects of acute or chronic blood loss
- Monitor response to drug therapy that may alter the erythrocyte count
- Monitor clients with disorders associated with elevated erythrocyte counts (e.g., polycythemia vera, chronic obstructive pulmonary disease)

■ Monitor clients with disorders associated with decreased erythrocyte counts (e.g. malabsorption syndromes, malnutrition, liver disease, renal disease, hypothyroidism, adrenal dysfunction, bone marrow failure)

Reference Values

Children	
Newborns	4.8–7.1 million/mm^3
1 mo	4.1–6.4 million/mm^3
6 mo	3.8–5.5 million/mm^3
1–10 yr	4.5–4.8 million/mm^3
Adults	
Men	4.6–6.2 million/mm^3
Women	4.2–5.4 million/mm^3

Abnormal Values

■ Increased RBC
   Anxiety
   Chronic pulmonary disease with hypoxia and secondary
      polycythemia
   Dehydration with hemoconcentration
   High altitude
   Pain
   Polycythemia vera
   Certain drugs (see table next page)
■ Decreased RBC
   Chemotherapy
   Chronic inflammatory diseases
   Dietary deficiencies
   Hemoglobinopathy
   Hemolytic anemia
   Hemorrhage
   Hodgkin's disease
   Leukemia
   Multiple myeloma
   Organ failure
   Overhydration
   Pregnancy
   Subacute endocarditis
   Certain drugs (see table next page)

Drugs That May Cause Blood Dyscrasias

Generic Name or Class	Trade Names
Acetaminophen and acetaminophen compounds	Arthralgen, Bancap, Capital, Coastalgesic, Colrex, Comtrex, Co-Tylenol, Darvocet-N, Datril, Dialog, Dolene, Duadacin, Duradyne, Esgic, Excedrin, Gaysal, Liquiprin, Metrogesic, Midrin, Nebs, Neopap Supprettes, Nyquil, Ornex, Panadol, Parafon Forte, Pavadon, Percogesic, Phrenilin, Sedapap, Sinarest, Sinutab, Sunril, Supac, Tempra, Tussagesic, Tylenol, Valadol, Vanquish, Wygesic
Acetophenazine maleate	Tindal
Aminosalicylic acid	PAS, Parasal, Teebacin
Amphotericin B	Fungizone, Mysteclin F
Antineoplastic agents	
Arsenicals	
Carbamazepine	Tegretol
Chloramphenicol	Chloromycetin
Chloroquine	Aralen
Ethosuximide (methsuximide, phensuximide)	Zarontin
Furazolidone	Furoxone
Haloperidol	Haldol
Hydantoin derivatives	
Ethotoin	Peganone
Mephenytoin	Mesantoin
Phenytoin	Dilantin, Dantoin, Diphenylan
Hydralazine	Apresoline, Apresazide, Bolazine, Ser-Ap-Es, Serpasil-Apresoline
Hydroxychloroquine sulfate	Plaquenil
Indomethacin	Indocin
Isoniazid	INH, Nydrazid, Rifamate
MAO inhibitors	Eutonyl, Nardil, Parnate
Mefenamic acid	Ponstel
Mepacrine	Atabrine
Mephenoxalone	Trepidone
Mercurial diuretics	Thiomerin
Metaxalone	Skelaxin
Methyldopa	Aldoclor, Aldomet, Aldoril
Nitrites	
Nitrofurantoin	Cyantin, Furadantin, Macrodantin
Novobiocin	Albamycin
Oleandomycin	Matromycin
Oxyphenbutazone	Oxalid, Tandearil

(continued)

Generic Name or Class	Trade Names
Paramethadione	Paradione
Trimethadione	Tridione
Penicillamine	Cuprimine, Depen
Penicillins	
Phenacemide	Phenurone
Phenobarbital	
Phenylbutazone	Azolid, Butazolidin, Sterazolidin
Phytonadione	AquaMEPHYTON, Konakion
Primaquine	
Primidone	Mysoline
Pyrazolone derivatives	Butazolidin, Tandearil, Oxalid
Pyrimethamine	Daraprim
Rifampin	Rifadin, Rifamate, Rimactane, Rimactazid
Radioisotopes	
Spectinomycin	Trobicin
Sulfonamides	
Mafenide	Sulfamylon cream
Phthalylsulfathiazole	Sulfathalidine
Sulfabenzamide	Sultrin vaginal cream
Sulfacetamide	Bleph, Cetamide ointment, Sulamyd, Optosulfex, Sultrin vaginal cream
Sulfachlorpyridazine	Sonilyn
Sulfacytine	Renoquid
Sulfadiazine	Silvadene
Sulfameter	Sulla
Sulfamethizole	Thiosulfil forte
Sulfamethoxazole	Azo Gantanol, Bactrim, Gantanol, Septra
Sulfamethoxypyridazine	Midicel
Sulfanilamide	AVC vaginal cream, Vagitrol suppositories
Sulfasalazine	Azulfidine, Sulcolon
Sulfathiazole	Sultrin vaginal cream, Triple Sulfa cream
Sulfinpyrazone	Anturane
Sulfisoxazole	Azo-Gantrisin, Gantrisin, SK-Soxazole, Sulfizin, Sulfizole, Vagilia vaginal cream
Sulfones	Sulfoxone, DDS, Avlosulfon, Dapsone
Sulfonylureas	
Tolbutamide	Orinase
Chlorpropamide	Diabinese
Acetohexamide	Dymelor
Tolazamide	Tolinase
Tetracyclines	Achromycin
Chlortetracycline	Aureomycin
Demechlocycline	Declomycin

Generic Name or Class	Trade Names
Doxycycline	Doxychel, Doxy-C, Vibramycin, Vibratabs
Meclocycline	Meclan
Methacycline	Rondomycin
Minocycline	Minocin
Oxytetracycline	Oxlopar, Terramycin, Tetramine
Thiazide diuretics (rare hematologic side effects)	Diuril, Ademol, Saluron, ExNa, Enduron, Naturetin, Naqua, Renese
Thiocyanates	
Tripelennamine	Pyribenzamine, PBZ
Troleandomycin	Cyclamycin, TAO capsules and suspension
Valproic acid	Valproate
Vitamin A	Aquasol A, Alphalin

From Watson, J and Jaffe, MS: Nurse's Manual of Laboratory and Diagnostic Tests, ed. 2. FA Davis, Philadelphia, 1995, pp. 21–22, with permission.

Interfering Factors

- Excessive exercise, anxiety, pain, and dehydration may lead to false elevations.
- Hemodilution in the presence of a normal number of RBCs may lead to false decreases (e.g., excessive administration of intravenous fluids, normal pregnancy).
- Many drugs may cause a decrease in circulating RBCs (see Abnormal Values).
- Drugs such as methyldopa and gentamicin may cause an elevated erythrocyte count.

Nursing Implications

Assessment

- Obtain a history of the hematologic system, medications, and results of other tests performed.

Possible Nursing Diagnoses

Protection, altered, risk for, related to abnormal blood profiles
Anxiety related to threat to health status

Implementation

- Put on gloves. Using aseptic technique, perform a venipuncture and collect 7 mL of blood in a lavender-top tube.

- A capillary sample may be obtained in infants and children, as well as in adults for whom venipuncture may not be feasible.
- Transport the sample to the laboratory immediately.

Evaluation

- Note the test results in relation to the other tests performed and to the client's symptoms.

Client/Caregiver Teaching

Pretest

- Inform the client that no fasting is required.

Red Blood Cell Indices, Erythrocyte Indices, Blood Indices

Classification: Hematology

Type of Test: Serum

Red blood cell (RBC) indices provide information about the mean corpuscular volume (MCV), mean corpuscular hemoglobin concentration (MCHC), and mean corpuscular hemoglobin (MCH) of average red cells. The hematocrit, the RBC count, and total hemoglobin tests are used to determine the RBC indices. MCV is determined by dividing the hematocrit by the total RBC count and is helpful in classifying anemias. MCH is determined by dividing the total hemoglobin concentration by the number of RBCs. MCHC is determined by dividing the total hemoglobin concentration by the hematocrit. Cell size is indicated as normocytic, microcytic, and macrocytic. Hemoglobin content is indicated as normochromic, hypochromic, and hyperchromic.

Indications

- Aid in the diagnosis of anemia

Reference Values

	Men	*Women*	*Newborns*
MCV	80–94 μm^3	81–99 μm^3	96–108 μm^3
MCH	27–31 pg	27–31 pg	32–34 pg
MCHC	32–36%	32–36%	32–33%

Adapted from Watson, J and Jaffe, MS: Nurse's Manual of Laboratory and Diagnostic Tests, ed. 2. FA Davis, Philadelphia, 1995, p. 35, with permission.

Abnormal Values

- Elevated MCV levels
    Alcoholism
    Antimetabolite therapy
    Folic acid anemia
    Liver disease
    Pernicious anemia
- Decreased MCV levels
    Iron deficiency anemia
    Thalassemia
- Elevated MCH levels
    Macrocytic anemia
- Decreased MCH levels
    Hypochromic anemia
    Microcytic anemia
- Elevated MCHC levels
    Spherocytosis
    Thalassemia
- Decreased MCHC levels
    Iron deficiency anemia

Interfering Factors

- An extremely elevated white blood cell count or abnormal RBC count or falsely elevated hemoglobin will interfere with test results.
- Inadequate mixing of the sample with the anticoagulant in the collection tube can alter test results.
- Failing to use a collection tube with an anticoagulant or rough handling of the sample, resulting in hemolysis, or hemoconstriction due to prolonged tourniquet constriction can alter test results.
- Diseases that cause agglutination of RBCs will alter test results.

Nursing Implications

Assessment

- Assess the client's history for diseases that may affect or alter test results.
- Assess the client's previous blood study results, especially white cell count, which may affect the results of this test.

Possible Nursing Diagnoses

Tissue perfusion, altered, related to reduction of cellular components necessary for delivery of oxygen

Activity intolerance related to an imbalance between oxygen supply and demand

Anxiety related to perceived threats to health status

Tissue integrity, impaired, related to altered circulation

Implementation

- Put on gloves. Using aseptic technique, perform a venipuncture and collect 5 to 7 mL of blood in a lavender-top tube that contains an anticoagulant.
- Handle the sample gently, and invert it several times to mix the anticoagulant and the sample.
- Promptly send the sample to the laboratory.

> **NURSING ALERT**
>
> - Care should be taken when obtaining and handling this test. If the tourniquet is left on too long or is too restricting, hemoconstriction may alter the test results.
> - The sample must be obtained in a collection tube that contains an anticoagulant, and the tube must be gently inverted several times to mix the sample with the anticoagulant. Rough handling can cause hemolysis and can interfere with accurate determination of the test results.

Evaluation

- Note the results in comparison to the client's symptoms and the clinical findings.

Client/Caregiver Teaching

Pretest

- Tell the client why the test is being performed, who will perform it, that it involves a needle stick.

- Advise the client that there may be some slight discomfort when the tourniquet is applied and when the needle enters the skin.

Refraction

Classification: Sensory organ function

Type of Test: Visual perception

This noninvasive procedure tests the visual acuity of the eyes and determines abnormalities or refractive errors that need correction. Visual defects such as hyperopia (farsightedness), in which the point of focus lies behind the retina; myopia (nearsightedness), in which the point of focus lies in front of the retina; and astigmatism, in which the refraction is unequal in different curvatures of the eyeball, can be corrected by glasses or contact lenses.

Indications

- Diagnose refractive errors in vision
- Determine if an optical defect is present and if light rays entering the eye focus correctly on the retina
- Determine the type of corrective lenses needed for refractive errors, for example, biconvex or plus lenses for hyperopia, biconcave or minus lenses for myopia, compensatory lenses for astigmatism

Reference Values

- Normal refractive power of 44 diopters (distance from the surface at which the rays come into focus measured in meters) in the cornea and aqueous, 10 to 14 diopters in the lens, and overall refractive power of the eye at 58 diopters

Abnormal Values

- Refractive errors, such as astigmatism, hyperopia, and myopia

Interfering Factors

- Improper pupil dilation may prevent adequate examination for refractive error.
- Inability of the client to remain still and cooperate during the test may interfere with test results.

> ### NURSING ALERT
>
> - This test is contraindicated in clients with narrow-angle glaucoma because pupil dilation is required.
> - This test is contraindicated in clients allergic to mydriatics used for pupil dilation.

Nursing Implications

Assessment

- Obtain a history of known or suspected visual impairment, changes in visual acuity, use of glasses or contact lenses, other tests and procedures done to diagnose eye conditions needing corrective lenses and results.
- Obtain a history for narrow-angle glaucoma and hypersensitivity to dilating eyedrops.

Possible Nursing Diagnoses

Sensory/perceptual alteration, visual, related to altered sense organ status

Injury, risk of, related to visual impairment

Implementation

- Have the client remove corrective lenses (glasses or contacts). Administer an ordered mydriatic to each eye, 1 drop of 5% phenylephrine solution, and repeat in 5 to 15 minutes to achieve pupil dilation.
- Place the client in a sitting position in the examination chair. The examiner sits about 2 feet away at eye level with the client. Dim the room light. Hold the retinoscope light in front of the eyes and direct it through the dilated pupil. Each eye is also examined for the characteristics of the red reflex, the reflection of the light from the retinoscope, which normally moves in the same direction as the light.
- Request that the client look straight ahead while the eyes are examined with the instrument and while different lenses are tried to provide the best corrective lenses to be prescribed. When optimal visual acuity is obtained with the trial

lenses in each eye, a prescription for corrective lenses is written.

Evaluation

- Note the test results in relation to the client's symptoms.
- Note the client's ability to ambulate safely after mydriatic use.

Client/Caregiver Teaching

Pretest

- Inform the client about the purpose of the procedure and how the procedure is performed; inform that the procedure is performed in a darkened room by a physician and takes about 15 to 20 minutes to complete; explain that there is no pain associated with this procedure.

Posttest

- Caution the client not to drive or operate any machinery until distance vision returns.
- Inform that some visual blurring from the dilating medication can be experienced for about 2 hours.

Renin, Plasma; Plasma Renin Angiotensin (PRA); Renin Assay, Plasma; Plasma Renin Activity

Classification: Chemistry

Type of Test: Plasma

Renin is an enzyme that activates the renin-angiotension system. It is released into the renal veins by the juxtaglomerular apparatus in response to sodium depletion and hypovolemia. Angiotensin II, a powerful vasoconstrictor that stimulates aldosterone production, is produced. Excessive amounts of angiotensin II cause renal hypertension. Angiotensin and aldosterone increase blood pressure. The renin assay test screens for essential, renal, or renovascular hypertension. Plasma renin activity is measured by radioimmunoassay; the result is expressed as the rate of angiotensin I formation per unit of time.

Indications

- Aid in the screening of the origin of renal hypertension
- Aid in the treatment plan for essential hypertension
- Aid in the identification of primary aldosteronism resulting from aldosterone-secreting adrenal adenoma
- Aid in the identification of hypertension that may be linked to unilateral or bilateral renovascular disease

Reference Values

Adult (normal sodium diet)	
Supine	0.1–3.1 ng/mL/h
Standing	
20–39 yr	0.1–4.3 ng/mL/h
>40 yr	0.1–3.0 ng/mL/h
Children	
0–3 yr	<16.6 ng/mL/h
3–6 yr	<6.7 ng/mL/h
6–9 yr	<4.4 ng/mL/h
9–12 yr	<5.9 ng/mL/h
12–15 yr	<4.2 ng/mL/h
15–18 yr	<4.3 ng/mL/h
Adult (low-sodium diet)	
Supine	2.1–4.3 ng/mL/h
Standing	
20–39 yr	2.9–24.0 ng/mL/h
>40 yr	2.9–10.8 ng/mL/h

Values vary according to the laboratory performing the test, age, sex, race, dietary pattern, and physical activity.

Abnormal Values

- Elevated levels
    Malignant hypertension
    Addison's disease
    Renovascular hypertension
    Renin-producing renal tumors
    Hypokalemia
    Hemorrhage
    Certain drugs, including oral contraceptives, diuretics, antihypertensives, and vasodilators

- Decreased levels
  - Essential hypertension
  - Cushing's syndrome
  - Primary aldosteronism
  - Certain drugs, including salt-retaining steroids and anti-diuretic hormones

Interfering Factors

- Test results can be affected by pregnancy, severe blood loss, salt intake, licorice ingestion, and certain drugs (see Abnormal Values).
- Failure to use proper collection procedures can alter test results.
- Failure to observe dietary restriction and improper patient positioning during the test can affect results.
- Values may be higher in the day, in patients who are on low-salt diets, and when the patient is in an upright position.

Nursing Implications

Assessment

- Obtain a history of disease states that can influence test results as well as medication regimen.
- Assess the client's ability to remain supine for 2 hours before the test.
- Determine the client's knowledge of dietary restrictions before the test.

Possible Nursing Diagnoses

Fluid volume excess related to compromised regulatory mechanisms

Nutrition, altered, less than body requirements, related to inability to ingest adequate nutrients

Fatigue related to decreased metabolic energy production

Implementation

- Put on gloves. Using aseptic technique, perform a venipuncture and collect 7 to 12 mL of venous blood in a chilled, lavender-top tube that contains EDTA as an anticoagulant. Draw a fasting sample, as renin levels are higher in the morning.
- Gently invert the collection tube to mix the sample and the anticoagulant.
- Record the client's position and dietary status (low sodium or normal sodium).

- Place the specimen on ice and immediately send it to the laboratory.

Evaluation

- Note the results in relation to other results.

Client/Caregiver Teaching

Pretest

- Explain the test to the client: who will perform the test and approximately how long it will take.
- Instruct the client to maintain a normal diet with a restricted amount of sodium (approximately 3 g/d) for 3 days before the test.
- Explain to the client that it is necessary to remain supine for 2 hours before the test.

Posttest

- Instruct the client to resume normal diet and medication regimen after the test, as ordered.

Respiratory Syncytial Virus Antibodies, IgG and IgM

Classification: Serology

Type of Test: Serum

Respiratory syncytial virus (RSV) is a paramyxovirus that causes potentially fatal lower respiratory tract disease. It is transmitted by respiratory secretions and creates annual epidemics. Infections are most common and severe during the first 6 months of life. Antibodies IgG and IgM, associated with RSV, can be measured by indirect immunofluorescence. Prevalence of IgG antibodies to RSV is extremely high (greater than 95 percent), especially in adults.

Indications

- Aid in the diagnosis of RSV infections

Reference Values

- If the client has never been infected with RSV, detectable antibodies to the virus should be ≤1:5. In infants under 6 months, maternal IgG antibodies commonly occur; therefore, the presence of IgM antibodies is significant.

Abnormal Values

- Presence of IgM antibodies or fourfold or greater increase in IgG antibodies

Interfering Factors

- Hemolysis of the test sample may affect results.

Nursing Implications

Assessment

- Obtain a history of known or suspected exposure to RSV.
- Assess the skin for lesions and edema and the veins for sclerosis and past phlebitis when selecting a venipuncture site.

Possible Nursing Diagnoses

Gas exchange, impaired, related to altered oxygen supply
Infection, risk for, related to inadequate primary defenses
Fatigue related to increased energy requirements
Parent/infant/child attachment, altered, risk for, related to anxiety associated with parental role and demands of infant

Implementation

- Put on gloves. Using aseptic technique, perform a venipuncture and collect 5 mL of blood in a red-top tube. Allow the blood to clot for at least 1 hour at room temperature.
- Handle the sample gently to avoid hemolysis and send it promptly to the laboratory.

Evaluation

- Evaluate and compare the test results with the clinical symptoms the client demonstrates.

Client/Caregiver Teaching

Pretest

- Explain the purpose of the test, how it will be performed, and who will perform it; explain that some discomfort will be experienced from the venipuncture.

Posttest

- Instruct the client to apply pressure to the venipuncture site for several minutes.

Reticulocyte Count, Retic Count

Classification: Hematology

Type of Test: Serum

The reticulocyte count determines bone marrow functions and erythropoietic activity. A reticulocyte is an immature red blood cell. It can be easily identified under microscope when the blood sample is stained with a supravital stain. The reticulocyte count is a direct measurement of red blood cell production by the bone marrow. The reticulocytes are counted and expressed as a percentage of the total red cell count. It is useful in determining anemia and is an indication of erythropoiesis and the bone marrow's response to anemia.

Indications

- Aid in distinguishing between hypoproliferative and hyperproliferative anemias
- Assess blood loss, therapy for anemia, and bone marrow response to anemia

Reference Values

Men	0.5–1.5%
Women	0.5–2.5%
Children	0.5–4%
Infants	2–5%

Abnormal Values

- Elevated levels
    Erythroblastosis fetalis
    Hemolytic anemia

Hemorrhage
Leukemias
Post splenectomy
Pregnancy
Sickle-cell anemia
Certain drugs, including ACTH, antimalarials, antipyretics, flurazolidone (infants), levodopa, and sulfonamides
- Decreased levels
Adrenocortical hypofunction
Anterior pituitary hypofunction
Aplastic anemias
Chronic infection
Cirrhosis of the liver
Folic acid deficiency
Marrow failure
Pernicious anemia
Radiation therapy
Certain drugs, including azathioprine, chloramphenicol, dactinomycin, methotrexate, and sulfonamides

Interfering Factors

- Hemolysis of the blood sample and recent blood transfusions may affect results.
- Certain drugs may affect the test results (see Abnormal Values).
- Failure to use the proper anticoagulant in the collection tube or failure to adequately mix the anticoagulant with the sample in the collection tube may alter the test results or interfere with interpretation of the results.
- Prolonged tourniquet constriction and rough handling of the sample can lead to hemolysis, which can also affect the test results.

Nursing Implications

Assessment

- Obtain a history of disease states that can influence test results as well as medication regimen.

Possible Nursing Diagnoses

Protection, altered, related to abnormal blood profiles
Activity intolerance related to imbalance between oxygen supply and demand
Gas exchange, impaired, related to decreased oxygen-carrying capacity of blood
Pain, chronic, related to intravascular occlusion

Implementation

- Put on gloves. Using aseptic technique, perform a venipuncture and collect 5 to 7 mL of blood in a lavender-top tube.
- Avoid prolonged constriction of the tourniquet, which can affect the test results.
- Handle the sample gently to avoid hemolysis and send promptly to the laboratory.

Evaluation

- Evaluate and compare the test results with the clinical symptoms the client demonstrates.
- In clients with abnormal reticulocyte test results, look for trends in repeated tests or very gross changes in the numeric values.

Client/Caregiver Teaching

Pretest

- Advise the patient that no fasting is required before the test.
- Withhold medications that may interfere with test results, as ordered, or if the medications cannot be withheld, note this information on the laboratory request.

Posttest

- Instruct the client to apply pressure to the venipuncture site for several minutes.
- Instruct the client to resume medication regimen that may have been withheld before the test, as ordered.

Rheumatoid Factor (RF), Rheumatoid Arthritis Factor

Classification: Immunology

Type of Test: Serum

Individuals with rheumatoid arthritis harbor a macroglobulin-type antibody called rheumatoid factor (RF) in their blood. However, other diseases, such as systemic lupus erythematosis (SLE), may cause a positive RF test. It may occasionally be seen in patients with tuberculosis, chronic hepatitis, infectious mononucleosis, and subacute bacterial endocarditis. Tests for RF are aimed at IgM antibody. Tests that are positive for RF must have a dilution of greater than 1:80. In titers between 1:20 and 1:80, other possible causes such as SLE should be investigated.

Indications

- Aid in the diagnosis of rheumatoid arthritis, especially when clinical diagnosis is difficult

Reference Values

- Negative; <60 U/mL by nephelometric testing

Abnormal Values

- Elevated levels
  Chronic hepatitis
  Chronic viral infections
  Cirrhosis
  Dermatomyositis
  Infectious mononucleosis
  Leukemia
  Renal disease
  Rheumatoid arthritis
  Scleroderma
  Subacute bacterial endocarditis
  Syphilis
  SLE
  Tuberculosis

Interfering Factors

- Older patients may have higher values.
- Hemolysis of the test sample may affect results.
- Recent transfusion, multiple vaccinations or transfusions, or an inadequately activated complement may affect results.
- Serum with cryoglobulin or high lipid levels may cause a false-positive test and may require that the test be repeated after a fat restriction diet.
- Serum with high levels of IgG may cause false-negative results, especially if sheep red blood cells are used as a substrate.

Nursing Implications

Assessment

■ Obtain a history of disease states that can influence test results.

Possible Nursing Diagnoses

Pain, chronic, related to joint inflammation
Physical mobility, impaired, related to musculoskeletal deformity
Body image disturbance related to change in body structure
Self-care deficit related to musculoskeletal impairment

Implementation

■ Put on gloves. Using aseptic technique, perform a venipuncture and collect 7 to 10 mL of blood in a red-top tube.
■ Send the sample promptly to the laboratory.

Evaluation

■ Evaluate and compare the test results with the clinical symptoms the client demonstrates.
■ Consider other disease in values that are not definitive for rheumatoid arthritis.

Client/Caregiver Teaching

Pretest

■ Explain the purpose of the test; how it will be performed, and who will perform it; explain that some discomfort will be experienced from the venipuncture.
■ Advise the patient that no fasting is required before the test.

Posttest

■ Advise the client of additional studies to determine treatment regimen or to determine possible causes of symptoms if the test is not positive for rheumatoid arthritis.
■ Provide teaching and disease information depending on tests results.

Rocky Mountain Spotted Fever Antibodies

Classification: Immunology

Type of Test: Serum

Rocky Mountain spotted fever is an infectious disease caused by *Rickettsia rickettsii*. It is a parasite transmitted to humans by the bite of an infected tick. Symptoms are sudden onset of fever and rash spreading from the palms of the hands and soles of the feet throughout the body. This disease can be fatal if untreated. If agglutination occurs, antigen is added to serial dilutions of the client's serum. The antibody titer is then expressed as the reciprocal of the last dilution showing visible agglutination.

Indications

- Aid in the diagnosis of Rocky Mountain spotted fever
- Determine the cause of a fever of unknown origin

Reference Values

- Indirect fluorescent antibody assay (most sensitive): titer >128 in single sample or fourfold rise in paired serum titers
- Latex agglutination test: active Rocky Mountain spotted fever titer >128
- Complement fixation for rickettsial infection: >1:160 or fourfold increase in paired samples within 7 days
- Weil-Felix agglutination reaction (least sensitive): strong agglutination response suggests rickettsial disease

Abnormal Values

- Elevated levels
      Leptospirosis
      Proteus infections
      Severe liver disease
      Typhus
- Decreased levels
      Immunodeficiency states

Interfering Factors

- The latex agglutination test is useful only during active infection.
- Borrelia infection, Proteus infection, typhus, leptospirosis, and severe liver disease may cause a false-positive Weil-Felix reaction.
- Failure to send the sample to the laboratory immediately may affect results.
- Immunodeficient clients may not be able to produce antibodies and may show a false-negative response even during infection.
- Antibiotics may falsely decrease levels.

Nursing Implications

Assessment

- Obtain a history of known or suspected exposure to *Rickettsia rickettsii*.
- Assess the client's understanding of explanations provided and presence of anxiety.
- Assess history for medication that may affect test results or disorders that may affect the interpretation of the test results.

Possible Nursing Diagnoses

Hyperthermia related to generalized inflammatory process
Tissue perfusion, altered, related to reduction of blood flow
Pain related to tissue ischemia

Implementation

- Put on gloves. Using aseptic technique, perform a venipuncture and collect 7 mL of blood in a red-top tube.
- An acute sample should be drawn with the onset of symptoms and a convalescent sample 7 days later.
- Handle the sample gently to avoid hemolysis and send promptly to the laboratory.

Evaluation

- Evaluate and compare the test results with the clinical symptoms the client demonstrates.
- In clients with abnormal titers, look for trends in repeated tests or very gross changes in the numeric values.

Client/Caregiver Teaching

Pretest

- Explain the purpose of the test; who will perform it; and that there may be slight discomfort during the venipuncture.

- Inform the client that it is not necessary to fast or withhold any medications before the test.
- Advise the client that this test requires a series of blood samples to detect a pattern of titers that are characteristic of the suspected disorder.

Posttest

- Explain to the client about isolation precautions, if necessary.

Rotavirus Antigen

Classification: Immunoassay

Type of Test: Stool analysis

Rotaviruses are the most frequent cause of infectious diarrhea in infants and young children. This test directly detects the antigen that is shed in large amounts in the stool in persons with the disease. Specimens obtained during the first 3 days of infection provide the best results. After the eighth day of infection, the virus is difficult to detect.

Indications

- Diagnose rotavirus gastroenteritis

Reference Values

- Negative

Abnormal Values

- Detection of virus identifies current infection with the organism.

Interfering Factors

- Collection containers with preservatives may interfere with the assay.
- Delayed specimen analysis may affect results.

Nursing Implications

Assessment

- Obtain a history of the gastrointestinal system symptoms, medication regimen, and related diagnostic test results.
- Determine the onset of symptoms.

Possible Nursing Diagnoses

Anxiety related to threat to health status
Fluid volume deficit related to excessive gastrointestinal losses
Infection, risk for transmission

Implementation

- *Stool specimen:* Obtain 5 to 10 mL of liquid stool as soon as possible after evacuation from the bowel. Place it in a clean, dry container and send it to the laboratory on ice.
- *Rectal swab:* Gently insert a sterile cotton-tipped swab 2 to 3 cm into the rectum. Gently move it from side to side and leave it in place for several seconds to allow contact with the rectal flora. Place the swab in a sterile container and transport it to the laboratory on ice.

Evaluation

- Note the results in relation to other tests, particularly tests to determine dehydration, such as serum electrolytes, and those to differentiate similar diagnoses, such as stool for ova and parasites or bacterial culture.
- Note the degree of dehydration, particularly in susceptible individuals such as infants and children and the elderly.

Client/Caregiver Teaching

Pretest

- Explain the collection procedure to the client, parent, or caregiver.
- Instruct the caregiver in proper handwashing to prevent cross-contamination.

Posttest

- Ensure that the client has adequate fluids to prevent dehydration from vomiting and diarrhea.

Rubella Antibodies

Classification: Immunology

Type of Test: Serum

Rubella is a communicable viral disease most commonly known as German measles; it is transmitted by contact with discharges of infected persons or droplet spray inhalation. This disease produces a pink macular rash that disappears in 2 to 3 days. Fetal infection during the first trimester can cause spontaneous abortion or congenital defects. Rubella infection induces IgG and IgM antibody production; this test can determine current infection or immunity from past infection.

Indications

- Diagnose rubella infection
- Determine susceptibility to rubella, particularly in pregnant women

Reference Values

- Titer <1:8 indicates susceptibility to infection
- Titer >1:8 indicates immunity from vaccination or prior infection

Abnormal Values

- Fourfold rise or greater from acute to convalescent titer indicates recent infection.

Interfering Factors

- Failure to collect samples from both the mother and infant may affect results.
- Hemolysis of the sample may affect test results.

Nursing Implications

Assessment

- Obtain a history of known or suspected exposure to rubella.

Possible Nursing Diagnoses

Infection, risk for transmission
Anxiety related to threat to fetal well-being

Implementation

- Put on gloves. Using aseptic technique, perform a venipuncture and collect 7 mL of blood in a red-top tube.
- Handle the sample gently to avoid hemolysis and send promptly to the laboratory.

Evaluation

- Note the test results in relation to the client's symptoms and compare acute titer with convalescent titer.

Client/Caregiver Teaching

Pretest

- Inform the client that no special preparation is required for this test.

Posttest

- Instruct the client or caregiver to report signs and symptoms related to the disease process to the physician.
- If the test shows infection or susceptibility in a pregnant woman, provide emotional support and refer to appropriate resource for counseling.

Rubeola Antibodies

Classification: Immunology

Type of Test: Serum

Rubeola is an acute contagious disease caused by the measles virus. It is transmitted by direct contact or inhalation of infected oral or nasal secretions. Serum is tested 1 week after onset of symptoms and again in 1 to 4 weeks. The presence of antibodies in the first sample indicates susceptibility to infection. Levels showing a fourfold or greater increase in the second sample compared to the first indicate a recent exposure.

Indications

- Diagnose measles after known or suspected exposure to measles virus

Reference Values

- Negative

Abnormal Values

- The presence of antibodies 1 week after symptoms indicates susceptibility to rubeola infection
- Fourfold increase in levels in the second sample indicates recent exposure

Interfering Factors

- Hemolysis of the sample may alter results.

Nursing Implications

Assessment

- Obtain a history of known or suspected exposure to the measles virus.

Possible Nursing Diagnoses

Pain, acute, related to inflammation of mucous membranes

Infection, risk for transmission, related to the presence of organism

Hyperthermia related to the presence of viral toxins

Implementation

- Put on gloves. Using aseptic technique, perform a venipuncture and collect 7 mL of blood in a red-top tube.
- Apply necessary pressure to the puncture site until bleeding stops; apply adhesive bandage.
- Handle the sample gently to avoid hemolysis and send promptly to the laboratory.

Evaluation

- Evaluate and compare the test results with the clinical symptoms.
- Compare the sample taken 4 weeks after exposure to the results of the test taken 1 week after exposure to determine recent infection.

Client/Caregiver Teaching

Pretest

■ Inform the client that this test requires no fasting from liquids or food.

Posttest

■ Advise the client to return for the second test as indicated.

▲▲▲▲▲▲▲▲▲▲▲▲▲▲▲▲▲▲▲▲▲▲

Scan, Adrenal Glands

Classification: Nuclear medicine

Type of Test: Radionuclide imaging

The secretory function of the adrenal glands is controlled primarily by the anterior pituitary, which produces the adrenocorticotropic hormone (ACTH). ACTH stimulates the adrenal cortex to produce cortisone and secrete aldosterone.

High concentrations of cholesterol, the precursor in the synthesis of adrenocorticosteroids including aldosterone, are stored in the adrenal cortex. This allows the radionuclide iodomethyl-19-norcholesterol to be used in identifying pathology in the secretory function of the adrenal cortex. The uptake of the radionuclide occurs gradually over time; imaging is performed within 48 hours of injection of the radionuclide dose and continued daily for 3 to 5 days. Imaging reveals increased uptake, unilateral or bilateral uptake, or absence of uptake in the detection of pathologic processes. Suppression studies can be done to differentiate the presence of tumor from hyperplasia of the glands followed by prescanning treatment with corticosteroids.

Indications

■ Aid in the diagnosis of Cushing's syndrome
■ Diagnose aldosteronism
■ Differentiate between asymmetrical hyperplasia and asymmetry from aldosteronism with dexamethasone suppression test

- Determine adrenal suppressibility with prescan administration of corticosteroid to diagnose and localize adrenal adenoma, aldosteronomas, androgen excess, and low-renin hypertension
- Aid in the diagnosis of gland tissue destruction caused by infection, infarction, neoplasm, or suppression

Reference Values

- Normal bilateral uptake of radionuclide and secretory function of adrenal cortex
- No evidence of tumors, infection, infarction, or suppression

Abnormal Values

- Adrenal gland suppression
- Adrenal infarction
- Adrenal tumor
- Infection
- Pheochromocytoma

Interfering Factors

- Inability of the client to remain still during the procedure will produce artifact.

> ### NURSING ALERT
>
> - Adrenal gland scanning is contraindicated in clients with a known allergy to radionuclides.
> - The procedure is also contraindicated in pregnancy and breast-feeding unless the benefits of performing the test greatly outweigh the risks.
> - Special precautions should be taken with children.
> - Pregnant health-care professionals should avoid caring for a person who has had a nuclear medicine procedure until 24 hours after the procedure.
> - Personnel should exercise special precautions in handling the radioactive test dose: the nuclear medicine technician wears a badge and radiology ring; the dose is prepared behind a lead glass shield with only gloved hands exposed; any spilled radionuclide area is washed with soap and water and paper towels, which are placed in a special storage area for a few weeks before being disposed.

Nursing Implications

Assessment

- Determine the date of the last menstrual period and the possibility of pregnancy in premenopausal women.
- Assess and record baseline vital signs for later comparison readings.
- Obtain a history of possible adrenal disorders.
- Determine previous abnormalities in laboratory test results, including results for cortisol and urinary adrenal function tests, as well as diagnostic findings.
- Assess for compliance with directions given for rest, positioning, and activity before and during the test.

Possible Nursing Diagnoses

Tissue perfusion, altered, related to hypovolemia
Infection, risk for, related to inadequate primary defenses
Anxiety related to threat to health status

Implementation

- Ensure that SSKI is administered 24 hours before the study to prevent thyroid uptake of the free iodine.
- Before the scan, have the client remove all jewelry and put on a hospital gown.
- Have the client void before scanning.
- Insert an intravenous line and inject the radionuclide intravenously on day 1; scans are done on days 2, 3, and 4. Scanning is done from the urinary bladder to the mastoid area to scan for a primary tumor. Each scan takes approximately 30 minutes.
- Inform the client of any modifications in positioning and use of or administration of medications during the procedure to enhance imaging.

Evaluation

- Monitor vital signs every 15 to 30 minutes or according to institution policy, and compare with baseline readings until stable.
- Monitor for signs of hypersensitivity to the radioisotope.
- Note the results in relation to the other related studies and the client's symptoms.

Client/Caregiver Teaching

Pretest

- Explain the purpose of the procedure: to detect abnormalities and adrenal gland dysfunction.

- Explain that the procedure is performed in a special nuclear medicine department by a technician and a physician specializing in this branch of medicine.
- Explain that this procedure involves a prolonged scanning schedule over a period of days.
- Assure the client that nuclear medicine personnel will remain within hearing range and will be able to see the client throughout the study.
- Inform the client of time to return for imaging after the intravenous injection.

Posttest

- After the procedure is completed, advise the client to drink plenty of fluids for 24 to 48 hours to eliminate the radionuclide from the body; encourage voiding following the study to start this process.
- Inform the client that radionuclide is eliminated from the body within 6 to 24 hours.
- Instruct the client to resume usual level of activity and normal dietary intake, unless contraindicated.
- Inform the client of the need for possible further studies to evaluate and determine need for change in therapy.
- Advise the client that SSKI will also be administered 10 days following the injection of the radionuclide.
- Tell caregivers to wear rubber gloves when discarding urine for 24 hours after the procedure. Wash gloved hands with soap and water before removing gloves. Consider the gloves nuclear waste and dispose of them accordingly. Then wash ungloved hands after gloves are removed.

Scan, Bone

Classification: Nuclear medicine

Type of Test: Radionuclide imaging

This test is a nuclear scan performed to assist in the diagnosis of metastatic bone disease and bone trauma and to monitor the progression of degenerative disorders. Abnormalities are identified by scanning 2 to 4 hours following the intravenous injection of a radionuclide such as technetium-99m (Tc-99m) hydroxyethylene diphosphonate (HEDP) or Tc-99m methylene diphosphonate (MDP). Areas of increased uptake and activity on the bone scan represent abnormalities unless they occur in normal areas of increased activity such as the sternum, sacro-iliac, clavicle, and scapular joints in adults and growth centers and cranial sutures in children. Gallium scanning can follow a bone scan to obtain a more sensitive study if acute inflammatory conditions such as osteomyelitis or septic arthritis are suspected.

Indications

- Diagnose the cause of unexplained bone or joint pain
- Diagnose degenerative joint changes or acute septic arthritis
- Confirm temporomandibular joint derangement
- Aid in the diagnosis of primary malignant bone tumors, such as osteogenic sarcoma, chondrosarcoma, Ewing's sarcoma, and metastatic malignant tumors
- Aid in the diagnosis of benign tumors or cysts
- Aid in the diagnosis of osteomyelitis
- Aid in the detection of traumatic or stress fractures
- Evaluate the healing process following fracture, especially if an underlying bone disease is present
- Aid in the diagnosis of metabolic bone diseases
- Detect Legg-Calvé-Perthes disease
- Evaluate prosthetic joints for infection, loosening, dislocation, or breakage
- Evaluate tumor response to radiation or chemotherapy
- Identify appropriate site for bone biopsy

Reference Values

- No abnormalities, as indicated by normal uptake by chemisorption of radionuclide by bone

Abnormal Values

- Bone necrosis
- Degenerative arthritis
- Fracture
- Legg-Calvé-Perthes disease
- Osteomyelitis
- Paget's disease
- Primary metastatic bone tumors

- Renal osteodystrophy
- Rheumatoid arthritis

Interfering Factors

- A distended bladder may obscure pelvic detail.
- Inability of the client to remain still during the procedure will produce artifact.
- The presence of multiple myeloma or thyroid cancer can result in a false-negative scan for bone abnormalities.
- Antihypertensives may affect results.
- Improper injection of the radionuclide allows the tracer to seep deep into the muscle tissue, producing erroneous hot spots.

▶ NURSING ALERT

- This test is contraindicated in pregnancy and lactation unless the benefits of performing the test greatly outweigh the risks.
- Special precautions should be taken with children.
- Pregnant health-care providers should avoid caring for a person who has had a nuclear medicine procedure until 24 hours after the procedure.
- Personnel should exercise special precautions in handling the radioactive test dose: the nuclear medicine technician wears a badge and radiology ring; the dose is prepared behind a lead glass shield with only gloved hands exposed; any spilled radionuclide area is washed with soap and water and paper towels, which are placed in a special storage area for a few weeks before being disposed.

Nursing Implications

Assessment

- Determine the date of the last menstrual period and the possibility of pregnancy in premenopausal women.
- Assess and record baseline vital signs for later comparison readings.
- Obtain a history regarding all information about the presence of or suspected bone disorders.

- Determine previous abnormalities in laboratory tests and diagnostic procedures.
- Assess for compliance with directions given for test, positioning, and activity before and during the test.

Potential Nursing Diagnoses

Pain, acute, related to inflammation and tissue necrosis

Tissue perfusion, altered, bone, related to inflammatory reaction with destruction of tissue

Hyperthermia related to increased metabolic rate and infection process

Implementation

- Have the client remove all jewelry and put on a hospital gown.
- Have the client void before scanning to prevent interference with examination of the pelvic bones.
- Administer analgesic as ordered.
- Place the client in the supine position on the examining table and inject radionuclide intravenously. Images are obtained in sequence every 3 seconds for 1 minute over the area to be studied for a flow study. Blood pool image is then obtained over the area to be studied. A 2- to 3-hour delay before static images are done is necessary to improve tumor imaging.
- Following the delay to allow the radionuclide to be taken up by the bones, multiple images are obtained over the complete skeleton. A large field-of-view camera is used to cover the whole area. Sacral lesions can be imaged by positioning the client on hands and knees and using a tail on the detector. Later views can be taken in 24 hours over the specific area to be studied.

Evaluation

- Note the results in relation to other studies and the client's symptoms.
- Monitor vital signs every 15 to 30 minutes and compare with baseline readings until stable.

Client/Caregiver Teaching

Pretest

- Explain the purpose of the procedure: to detect bone disease before x-rays can.

- Explain that the procedure is performed in a special nuclear medicine department by a technician and a physician specializing in this branch of medicine.
- Advise the client that the scan takes approximately 1 hour and is painless.
- Instruct the client to remain very still during scanning.
- Advise the client not to drink large amounts of liquid before the intravenous injection since this will be required after the injection is given.
- Instruct the client to return for imaging after the intravenous injection. Encourage increased fluid intake at this time and instruct the client to walk or relax.

Posttest

- Instruct the client to resume usual level of activity and normal dietary intake, unless contraindicated.
- Advise the client to drink plenty of fluids for 24 to 48 hours to eliminate the radionuclide from the body, unless contraindicated.
- Instruct the client to immediately flush toilet after each voiding following the procedure and to meticulously wash hands with soap and water after each void for 24 hours after the procedure.
- Tell all caregivers to wear rubber gloves when discarding urine for 24 hours after the procedure. Wash gloved hands with soap and water before removing gloves. Consider the gloves nuclear waste and dispose of them accordingly. Then wash ungloved hands after gloves are removed.

Scan, Cardiac; Nuclear Heart Scan; Myocardial Scan; Dipyridamole-Thallium Scan; Isonitrile Scan; Sestamibi Scan; Thallium Stress Scan; Multigated Pool Imaging (MUGA); Heart Imaging

Classification: Nuclear medicine

Type of Test: Radionuclide imaging

Cardiac scanning is a nuclear study that includes several categories of procedures depending on the radionuclide administered and the suspected pathology. The various studies can reveal clinical information about heart wall motion (contractions), ejection fraction, coronary blood flow, ventricular size and function, valvular regurgitation, and cardiac blood shunting.

Thallium-201 chloride (Tl-201) rest or stress studies are used to evaluate myocardial blood flow to assist in diagnosing ischemic cardiac disease, risk for coronary artery disease, and myocardial infarction. This procedure is best suited for clients unable to undergo invasive procedures such as angiography or cardiac catheterization.

If stress testing cannot be performed by exercising, dipyridamole (Persantine) can be administered orally or intravenously. Pipyridamole is a coronary vasodilator and is administered before the Tl-201 radionuclide and the scanning procedure. It increases blood flow in normal coronary arteries 2 to 3 times without exercising and reveals perfusion defects when blood flow is compromised by vessel pathology. This study is reserved for clients who are unable to participate in treadmill, bicycle, or handgrip exercises for stress testing, for example, clients with lung disease, neurologic disorders such as multiple sclerosis or spinal cord injury, and orthopedic disorders such as arthritis or limb amputation.

Technetium-99m (Tc-99m) stannous pyrophosphate studies (PYP), also known as myocardial imaging, reveals the presence of myocardial perfusion as well as the extent of myocardial infarction. The radionuclide combines with calcium to identify the damaged cells. These damaged cells can be viewed as spots that appear in 4 hours at the earliest uptake, peak at 48 hours postinfarction, and diminish in 5 to 7 days.

Multigated pool imaging (MUGA; also known as cardiac blood pool scan) is used to diagnose cardiac abnormalities involving the left ventricle and myocardial wall abnormalities by imaging the blood within the cardiac chamber rather than the myocardium itself. Tc-99m stannous pyrophosphate labeled with red blood cells (RBC) is used for multigated studies; Tc-99m sulfur colloid is used for first-pass studies. Studies detect abnormalities in heart wall motion at rest or with exercise, ejection fraction, ventricular dilation, stroke volume, and cardiac output. ECG is performed with the imager and computer and is termed "gated." The MUGA procedure, performed with the heart in motion during the cardiac cycle, is used to obtain multiple images of the heart in contraction and relaxation.

The scintillation camera records points in the cardiac cycle following the administration of sublingual nitroglycerin; the MUGA scan can evaluate the effectiveness of nitroglycerin on ventricular function. Heart shunt imaging is done in conjunction with a resting MUGA scan to obtain ejection fraction.

Single-photon emission computed tomography (SPECT) can be used to visualize the heart from several different angles. Areas of myocardial ischemia can be viewed with greater accuracy and resolution.

Indications

Rest or Stress Scan with Thallium Chloride (Tl-201) Dipyridamole/Tl-201

- Aid in the diagnosis of or risk for coronary artery disease (CAD)
- Evaluate the extent of CAD and the functional significance of these abnormalities
- Assess the function of collateral coronary arteries
- Evaluate bypass graft patency following surgery
- Evaluate the site of an old infarction to determine obstruction to cardiac muscle perfusion
- Determine rest defects and reperfusion with delayed imaging in unstable angina
- Evaluate effectiveness of medication regimen and balloon angioplasty procedure on narrowed coronary arteries

Cardiac Myocardial Imaging with Technetium (Tc-99m Stannous Pyrophosphate)

- Aid in the diagnosis of or confirm and locate acute myocardial infarction when ECG and enzyme testing do not provide a diagnosis
- Evaluate possible reinfarction or extension of the infarct
- Obtain baseline information about infarction before open heart surgery
- Aid in the diagnosis of perioperative myocardial infarction
- Differentiate between a recent and past infarction

Gated Blood Pool Imaging with Technetium (Tc-99m Stannous Pyrophosphate with RBC or Tc-99m Sulfur Colloid)

- Determine ischemic CAD
- Aid in the diagnosis of myocardial infarction
- Aid in the diagnosis of true or false ventricular aneurysms
- Aid in the diagnosis of valvular heart disease and determine the optimal time for valve replacement surgery
- Quantitate cardiac output by calculating ejection fraction
- Evaluate ventricular size and function following an acute episode or in chronic heart disease
- Determine doxorubicin cardiotoxicity in order to stop therapy before development of congestive heart failure
- Determine cardiomyopathy
- Differentiate between chronic obstructive pulmonary disease (COPD) and left ventricular failure
- Detect left-to-right shunts and determine pulmonary-to-systemic blood flow ratios, especially in children

Reference Values

- Normal wall motion, ejection fraction (55 to 65 percent), coronary blood flow, ventricular size and function, and symmetry in contractions of left ventricle

Abnormal Values

- Abnormal wall motion (akinesia or dyskinesia)
- Cardiac hypertrophy
- Cardiac ischemia
- Enlarged left ventricle

- Heart chamber disorder
- Myocardial infarct

Interfering Factors

- The client's inability to remain still during the procedure or assume different positions will affect results.
- Digitalis and quinidine alter contractility and nitrates affect cardiac performance.
- Thallium-201 scan can produce false-negative results if single-vessel disease is present.
- Other nuclear scans done on the same day as the gated or stress scans may alter results.
- Conditions such as chest wall or cardiac trauma, angina that is difficult to control, significant cardiac arrhythmias, or recent cardioversion procedure will cause inaccurate findings.
- Client exhaustion, preventing maximum heart rate testing, will affect results.
- Excessive eating or exercising between initial and redistribution imaging 4 hours later will produce false results.

NURSING ALERT

- This test is contraindicated in clients with hypersensitivity to the radionuclide and in pregnancy and lactation unless the benefits of performing the test greatly outweigh the risks.
- Special precautions should be observed when administering this procedure to children.
- Stress tests should not be performed in clients with left ventricular hypertrophy, right and left bundle branch block, or hypokalemia, or with those receiving cardiotonic therapy.
- Dipyridamole testing is not performed in clients with anginal pain at rest or in clients with severe atherosclerotic coronary vessels.
- Health-care officials should wear badge and rubber gloves when discarding urine for 24 hours after the procedure. Wash gloved hands with soap and water and wash hands after gloves are removed. Consider the gloves nuclear waste and dispose of them accordingly.
- Pregnant health-care professionals should avoid caring for a person who has had a nuclear medicine procedure until 24 hours after the procedure.

Nursing Implications

Assessment

- Determine the date of the last menstrual period and the possibility of pregnancy in premenopausal women.
- Obtain a history of hypersensitivity to radioactive dyes.
- Obtain a history of cardiac status including angina, past myocardial infarctions, medication regimen, and recent chest x-ray, previous abnormalities in laboratory tests and diagnostic procedures.
- *PYP and thallium imaging:* Ensure that the client has withheld food for 4 hours, nicotine for 4 to 6 hours, and medications for 24 hours before the test, as ordered.
- Assess for compliance with directions given for rest, positioning, and activity before and during the test.

Potential Nursing Diagnoses

Pain, acute, related to myocardial ischemia
Anxiety related to threat to health status
Cardiac output, decreased, risk for, related to changes in heart rate and electrical conduction
Activity intolerance related to imbalance in oxygen supply and demand

NURSING ALERT

- Stress testing is terminated if client develops angina, severe dyspnea, fatigue, syncope, hypotension, ischemic electrocardiogram changes, significant arrhythmias, or signs such as pallor, clammy skin, confusion, or staggering gait.
- The use of dipyridamole in testing can precipitate myocardial infarction or angina; intravenous aminophylline should be on hand to reverse the effects of the drug if needed.

Implementation

- Establish an intravenous access before the procedure.
- Ensure that emergency equipment is readily available during the procedure, especially stress testing.
- Before the scan have the client remove all jewelry, put on a hospital gown, and void.
- *Resting thallium imaging test:* The client is placed in an upright position for 15 minutes and the radionuclide is injected. Scanning of the chest begins in 20 minutes. Multiple

images of the heart are scanned to obtain anterior, left anterior-oblique, and lateral views.

- *Stress thallium imaging test:* The client is assisted on treadmill, ECG leads are attached, and blood pressure cuff is applied. Exercise on treadmill or bicycle ergometer is performed to the maximum heart rate. Thallium is injected about 60 to 90 seconds before exercise is terminated; imaging is done immediately in the supine position and repeated in 4 hours. Those clients who cannot exercise are given dipyridamole 4 minutes before the thallium chloride,
- *Tc-99m stannous pyrophosphate:* Scanning is done 2 to 4 hours after injection of radionuclide to obtain anterior left, left anterior-oblique, and left lateral views of the heart. The procedure takes 30 to 60 minutes.
- *MUGA imaging:* The client is placed at rest in the supine position with the ECG attached and asked to remain still during the procedure. The radionuclide is administered intravenously; 1 minute after injection, scanning is done to obtain anterior, posterior, oblique, and lateral views. As many as 12 to 64 consecutive frames are recorded.
- *Exercise imaging:* Exercise imaging, including graded exercise on a bicycle and imaging at each exercise level, can be performed immediately after injection of radionuclide. If nitroglycerin is given, a cardiologist assesses baseline MUGA scan, injects the medication, takes another scan, and repeats this procedure until blood pressure reaches desired level. Heart shunt scanning can also be done with MUGA scan.

Evaluation

- Monitor ECG tracings, and vital signs every 15 to 30 minutes, and compare with baseline readings until stable.
- Observe injection site for redness, swelling, or hematoma.
- Observe the client carefully for up to 60 minutes after the study for a possible anaphylactic reaction to the radionuclide such as rash, tightening of the throat, or difficulty breathing.

Client/Caregiver Teaching

Pretest

- Explain the purpose of the procedure: to evaluate myocardial blood flow.
- Explain that the procedure takes about 30 minutes to complete.
- Reassure client that tracer poses no radioactive hazard and rarely produces side effects.

- Inform the client of the scanning schedule.
- Tell the client to wear walking shoes for the treadmill exercise and emphasize the importance of the client reporting fatigue, pain, or shortness of breath immediately.
- Reinforce information regarding diagnosis and recommended treatment regimen.

Posttest

- If the client must return for further thallium imaging, advise him or her to rest in the interim and restrict diet to clear liquids before redistribution studies.
- Advise the client to drink fluids to eliminate the radionuclide from the body unless otherwise contraindicated.
- Instruct the client to meticulously wash hands with soap and water after each void for 24 hours.
- Encourage questions and verbalizations of fears regarding scan.
- Instruct the client to resume level of activity and normal dietary intake, unless contraindicated.
- Inform client that abnormalities of the heart scan can indicate the need for further studies or cardiac catheterization.

Scan, Gallium, Breast

Classification: Nuclear medicine

Type of Test: Radionuclide imaging

A gallium scan of the breast is used to localize neoplasms and inflammatory lesions of the breast tissue and lymph nodes. After intravenous injection of the radionuclide gallium-67 (Ga-67) citrate, various views are taken 48 to 72 hours later. Tumor and lesion abnormalities appear on the scan as abnormally large concentrations of gallium uptake.

Indications

- Detect tumor or inflammatory lesions of the breast
- Evaluate lymphomas
- Identify recurrent tumors following chemotherapy or radiation therapy

- Evaluate recurrent lymphomas or tumors following radiation or chemotherapy
- Differentiate between malignant and benign tumors in combination with other studies such as ultrasonography or computed tomography
- Determine effectiveness of chemotherapy or radiation therapy as well as detect recurrent tumors
- Perform screening study to determine abnormalities when performed with other nuclear scan studies such as In-111 or Tc-99m

Reference Values

- Normal patterns of breast gallium uptake

Abnormal Values

- Abscess
- Inflammation
- Lymphoma
- Tumor

Interfering Factors

- Inability of the client to remain still during the procedure will produce artifact.
- False-positive readings can occur with pregnancy, lactation, or menarche owing to the increased affinity for gallium uptake of breast tissue.
- Oral contraceptives may cause false-positive results.
- Lesions smaller than 1 to 2 cm may not be detectable with a gallium scan.
- Antineoplastic medications can affect the results of the study.

> **NURSING ALERT**
>
> - This test is contraindicated in pregnancy and lactation unless the benefits of performing the test greatly outweigh the risks.
> - Personnel should exercise special precautions in handling the radioactive test dose: the nuclear medicine technician wears a badge and radiology ring; the dose is prepared behind a lead glass shield with only gloved hands exposed; any spilled radionuclide area is washed with soap and water and paper towels, which are placed in a special storage area for a few weeks before disposal.

Nursing Implications

Assessment

- Determine the date of the last menstrual period and the possibility of pregnancy in premenopausal women.
- Determine previous abnormalities in diagnostic tests or laboratory results, particularly tests for renal impairment such as blood urea nitrogen and serum creatinine because radionuclide dye is excreted by the kidney.
- Assess and record baseline vital signs for later comparison readings.
- Obtain a history regarding abnormalities in lymph nodes or breast tissue.
- Assess the client's emotional state if breast scan has been ordered to diagnose cancer.
- Assess level of anxiety about receiving a radioactive substance.
- Assess for compliance with directions given for rest, positioning, and activity before and during the test.

Possible Nursing Diagnoses

Anxiety related to altered health status
Body image disturbance related to change in appearance
Grieving, anticipatory, related to perceived loss

Implementation

- Encourage increase in oral intake 24 hours before the scan if not contraindicated.
- Before the scan have the client remove all jewelry, put on a hospital gown, and void.
- Radionuclide is administered intravenously 48 to 72 hours before the scan.
- Place the client in either an erect or a recumbent position on the examination table. The gamma camera or rectilinear scanner will obtain anterior, posterior, and, occasionally, lateral views. The scanner will make clicking noises during scanning. The scan takes 30 to 60 minutes to complete.

Evaluation

- Monitor vital signs every 15 to 30 minutes and compare with baseline readings until stable.
- Note the results in relation to other studies and the client's symptoms.

Client/Caregiver Teaching

Pretest

- Explain to the client that the procedure is performed in a special nuclear medicine department by a technician and a physician specializing in this branch of medicine.
- Advise the client that the scan takes 30 to 60 minutes to complete.
- Explain that the only discomfort experienced will be with the injection of the dye.
- Instruct the client to remain very still during the procedure.
- Inform the client that gallium is excreted by the kidney and colon in 24 to 48 hours.
- Inform the client that the camera will make clicking noises during the scan.
- Encourage increased fluid intake when not otherwise contraindicated.

Posttest

- Instruct the client to resume usual level of activity and normal dietary intake, unless contraindicated.
- Advise the client to drink plenty of fluids for 24 to 48 hours to eliminate the radionuclide from the body unless otherwise contraindicated.
- Instruct the client to immediately flush toilet after each voiding following the procedure and to meticulously wash hands with soap and water after each void for 24 hours after the procedure.
- Tell all caregivers to wear rubber gloves when discarding urine for 24 hours after the procedure. Wash gloved hands with soap and water before removing gloves. Consider the gloves nuclear waste and dispose of them accordingly. Then wash ungloved hands after gloves are removed.

Scan, Gallium, Bone

Classification: Nuclear medicine

Type of Test: Radionuclide imaging

A gallium scan of the bone is a nuclear procedure used to assist in diagnosing neoplasm and inflammation activity. After intravenous injection of the radionuclide gallium-67 (Ga-67), various views are taken. Ga-67 has a 90 percent sensitivity for inflammatory disease and is readily distributed throughout plasma and body tissues. Scanning can be performed 6 to 72 hours after injection for infection or inflammatory diseases, or up to 120 hours for tumor identification.

Indications

- Aid in the diagnosis of infectious or inflammatory diseases such as osteomyelitis or septic arthritis
- Detect primary or metastatic tumor in the bone (Wilm's tumor)
- Differentiate between malignant and benign tumors in combination with other studies such as ultrasonography or computed tomography
- Evaluate recurrent tumors and assess effectiveness of chemotherapy or radiation therapy
- Aid in the diagnosis of joint infections
- Perform screening study to determine abnormalities, in conjunction with other nuclear scan studies

Reference Values

- Normal pattern of bone gallium uptake

Abnormal Values

- Infection
- Inflammation
- Tumor

Interfering Factors

- Inability of the client to remain still during the procedure will produce artifact.
- Lesions less than 1 to 2 cm will not be detectable with a gallium scan.
- False-positive results may be obtained in the presence of leukopenia.

NURSING ALERT

- This test is contraindicated in pregnancy unless the benefits of performing the test greatly outweigh the risks to the fetus.
- Personnel should exercise special precautions in handling the radioactive test dose: the nuclear medicine technician wears a badge and radiology ring; the dose is prepared behind a lead glass shield with only gloved hands exposed; any spilled radionuclide area is washed with soap and water and paper towels, which are placed in a special storage area for a few weeks before being disposed.

Nursing Implications

Assessment

- Determine previous abnormalities in diagnostic tests or laboratory results (include blood urea nitrogen and serum creatinine due to the radionuclides excretion in the kidney).
- Determine the date of the last menstrual period and the possibility of pregnancy in premenopausal women.
- Obtain a history regarding all information about the presence of or suspected bone abnormalities.
- Assess and record baseline vital signs for later comparison readings.
- Assess for ability to follow directions given for rest, positioning, and activity before and during the test.

Possible Nursing Diagnoses

Pain related to inflammation and tissue necrosis
Tissue perfusion, altered, related to abscess formation
Anxiety related to threat of change in health status
Grieving, anticipatory, related to perceived loss or threat of death

Implementation

- Obtain a signed consent form from the client or a responsible family member.
- Encourage increase in fluid intake 24 hours before the scan, unless contraindicated.
- Have the client remove all jewelry and put on a hospital gown.
- Have the client empty bladder completely just before the procedure if the pelvis is to be scanned.
- Administer analgesics as ordered.
- Place the client in the supine position on the examination table.
- Radionuclide is administered intravenously; the amount depends on whether inflammatory or tumor imaging is being performed.
- Help the client from the table to a position of comfort.

Evaluation

- Monitor vital signs every 15 to 30 minutes and compare with baseline readings until stable.
- Monitor for signs of hypersensitivity to the radioisotope.
- Note the results in relation to other studies and to the client's symptoms.

Client/Caregiver Teaching

Pretest

- Explain that the procedure is performed in a special nuclear medicine department by a technician and a physician specializing in this branch of medicine.
- Explain that the scanning schedule may involve 3 days and that each scanning procedure takes 1 to 2 hours to complete.
- Inform the client that the camera will make clicking noises during the scan.
- Explain that the only discomfort experienced will be with the injection of the dye.
- Inform the client that gallium-67 is excreted by the kidney and colon in 24 to 48 hours.
- Tell the client to remain very still during the procedure.
- Encourage oral intake when not otherwise contraindicated.

Posttest

- Inform the client of time to return for imaging after the intravenous injection.
- Instruct the client to resume normal diet.
- Instruct the client to drink plenty of fluids for 24 to 48 hours

to eliminate the radionuclide from the body, unless contraindicated.

- Instruct the client to immediately flush toilet after each voiding following the procedure and to meticulously wash hands with soap and water after each void for 24 hours after the procedure.
- Tell all caregivers to wear rubber gloves when discarding urine for 24 hours after the procedure. Wash gloved hands with soap and water before removing gloves. Consider the gloves nuclear waste and dispose of them accordingly. Then wash ungloved hands after gloves are removed.

Scan, Gallium, Liver

Classification: Nuclear medicine

Type of Test: Radionuclide imaging

A liver gallium scan is a nuclear scan used to identify abscesses or masses. After intravenous injection of the radionuclide gallium (Ga-67), various views are taken 48 to 72 hours later. This radionuclide has 90 percent sensitivity for inflammatory disease and is readily distributed throughout plasma and body tissues.

Indications

- Detect hepatomas, abscesses, biopsy sites, alcoholic cirrhosis
- Evaluate recurrent lymphomas or tumors following radiation or chemotherapy
- Detect primary or metastatic tumors in the liver
- Differentiate between malignant and benign tumors in combination with other studies such as ultrasonography or computed tomography
- Evaluate or assess effectiveness of chemotherapy or radiation therapy as well as detect recurrent tumors
- Perform screening study to determine abnormalities when performed with other nuclear scan studies such as In-111 or Tc-99m

Reference Values

- Symmetrical patterns of liver gallium uptake.

Abnormal Values

- Abscess
- Cirrhosis
- Hepatoma
- Inflammation
- Tumor

Interfering Factors

- Inability of client to remain still during procedure will produce artifact.
- Normal hepatic gallium uptake may obscure the detection of abnormal para-aortic nodes in Hodgkin's disease, resulting in a false-negative scan.

> ### NURSING ALERT
>
> - This test is contraindicated in pregnancy and lactation unless the benefits of performing the test greatly outweigh the risks.
> - Personnel should exercise special precautions in handling the radioactive test dose: nuclear medicine technician wears a badge and radiology ring; dose is prepared behind a lead glass shield with only gloved hands exposed; any spilled radionuclide area is washed with soap and water and paper towels, which are placed in a special storage area for a few weeks before being disposed.

Nursing Implications

Assessment

- Determine previous abnormalities in diagnostic tests or lab results (include blood urea nitrogen and serum creatinine due to the radionuclides excretion in the kidney).
- Determine date of last menstrual period and possibility of pregnancy in premenopausal women.
- Obtain history regarding liver or abdominal pain or discomfort.
- Assess and record baseline vital signs for later comparison readings.

Possible Nursing Diagnoses

Pain, acute, related to inflammation and swelling of the liver

Fatigue related to decreased metabolic energy production

Nutrition, altered, less than body requirements, related to inability to ingest adequate nutrients

Grieving, anticipatory, related to perceived loss or threat of death

Implementation

- Radionuclide is administered intravenously 48 to 72 hours before the scan.
- Have client remove all jewelry, put on a hospital gown, and void.
- Administer analgesic as ordered.
- Place the client in either an erect or a recumbent position on exam table.
- The scan takes 30 to 60 minutes to perform. The gamma camera or rectilinear scanner will obtain anterior, posterior, and occasionally, lateral views.
- Assist client from table to position of comfort.
- Encourage oral intake when not otherwise contraindicated.
- Encourage voiding after scanning to encourage the elimination of the radionuclide.

Evaluation

- Monitor vital signs every 15 to 30 minutes and compare with baseline readings until stable.
- Note results in relation to other studies and the client's symptoms.

Client/Caregiver Teaching

Pretest

- Explain that procedure is performed in a special nuclear medicine department by a technician and a physician specializing in this branch of medicine. Explain that the only discomfort experienced will be with the injection of the dye.
- Inform client to remain very still during procedure.
- Inform client that gallium is excreted by the kidney and colon in 24 to 48 hours.
- Inform client that camera will make clicking noises during the scan.
- Advise the client that a clear liquid diet may be ordered a day before the test and that cleansing enemas may be ordered the morning before the test.

Posttest

- Inform the client of time to return for imaging after the intravenous injection.
- Instruct client to resume normal dietary intake.
- Instruct client to drink plenty of fluids to eliminate the radionuclide from body over the next 24 to 48 hours.
- Inform client to immediately flush toilet after each voiding following the procedure and to meticulously wash hands with soap and water after each void for 24 hours after the procedure.
- Tell all caregivers to wear rubber gloves when discarding urine for 24 hours after the procedure. Wash gloved hands with soap and water before removing gloves. Consider the gloves nuclear waste and dispose of them accordingly. Then wash ungloved hands after gloves are removed.

Scan, Gastroesophageal Reflux

Classification: Nuclear medicine

Type of Test: Radionuclide imaging

A gastroesophageal scan is used to assess gastric reflux across the esophageal sphincter. A radioactive contrast medium such as technetium-99m (Tc-99m) sulfur colloid is ingested orally in orange juice. Scanning studies are immediately done to assess the amount of liquid that has reached the stomach. An abdominal binder is applied and is gradually tightened using millimeters of mercury to determine the degrees of abdominal pressure. Images are obtained and observed at 0, 20, 40, 60, 80, and 100 mm Hg. Computer calculation determines the amount of reflux into the esophagus during each image.

Indications

- Aid in the diagnosis of gastroesophageal reflux in clients with unexplained nausea and vomiting

Reference Values

- Normal gastroesophageal scan: 4 percent reflux across the esophageal sphincter.

Abnormal Values

- Reflux >4 percent at any pressure level

NURSING ALERT

- Gastroesophageal reflux scanning is contraindicated in clients with a known allergy to radionuclides and in the presence of hiatal hernia, esophageal motor disorders, or swallowing difficulties. In those clients, endoscopic studies should be considered.
- The procedure is also contraindicated in pregnancy and breast-feeding unless the benefits of performing the test greatly outweigh the risks.
- Special precautions should be taken with children.
- Personnel should exercise special precautions in handling the radioactive test dose: nuclear medicine technician wears a badge and radiology ring; dose is prepared behind a lead glass shield with only gloved hands exposed; any spilled radionuclide area is washed with soap and water and paper towels, which are placed in a special storage area for a few weeks before being disposed.

Interfering Factors

- Previous radiographic studies using an opaque dye or contrast medium may affect the results.

Nursing Implications

Assessment

- Determine date of last menstrual period and possibility of pregnancy in premenopausal women.
- Obtain history regarding information about gastrointestinal disorders and symptoms.
- Determine previous abnormalities in laboratory test results.

Possible Nursing Diagnoses

Nutrition, altered, risk for, less than body requirements, related to inability to ingest adequate nutrition

Pain related to irritation or inflammation of gastric mucosa

Anxiety related to threat to health status

Implementation

- Have the client remove all jewelry and put on a gown before the procedure.
- The client is asked to drink approximately 300 mL of orange juice that contains the radioactive contrast medium.
- With the client in the supine position, an image is taken to confirm swallowing of the liquid and emptying into the stomach. The abdominal binder is applied and scans are taken as the binder is tightened at various pressures. If reflux occurs at lower pressures, an additional 30 mL of water may be given to clear the esophagus.

Evaluation

- Observe client carefully for up to 60 minutes after the study for a possible anaphylactic reaction to the radionuclide such as rash, tightening of throat, or difficulty breathing.
- Note results in relation to other studies and the client's symptoms.

Client/Caregiver Teaching

Pretest

- Reassure client that tracer poses no radioactive hazard and rarely produces side effects.
- Reinforce information regarding diagnosis and recommended treatment regimen.
- Explain the purpose of the test, the procedure, where it will be performed, who will perform it, and approximately how long the procedure will take.

Posttest

- Instruct the client to resume level of activity and normal dietary intake, unless contraindicated.
- Advise client to drink plenty of fluids for 24 to 48 hours to eliminate the radionuclide from the body, unless contraindicated.
- Inform client to immediately flush toilet after each voiding following the procedure and to meticulously wash hands with soap and water after each void for 24 hours after the procedure.
- Tell all caregivers to wear rubber gloves when discarding urine for 24 hours after the procedure. Wash gloved hands with soap and water before removing gloves. Consider the gloves nuclear waste and dispose of them accordingly. Then wash ungloved hands after gloves are removed.

Scan, Gallbladder; Hepatobiliary Scintigraphy; Hepatobiliary Imaging; Biliary Tract Radionuclide Scan; Cholescintigraphy; HIDA Scan

Classification: Nuclear medicine

Type of Test: Radionuclide imaging

After injection of the radionuclide technetium-99m disopropyl (IDA), images are taken of the hepatobiliary excretion system to determine the patency of the cystic and common bile ducts. This is done through noninvasive scanning procedures and is superior to oral cholecystography, IV cholangiography, CT of the gallbladder, and ultrasonography in the detection of cholecystitis. Gallbladder emptying or ejection fraction can be determined by administering a fatty meal or cholecystokinin to the client. Clients with hepatocellular disease will need delayed imaging for 6 to 48 hours after injection.

Indications

- Aid in the diagnosis of suspected gallbladder disorders, such as inflammation, perforation, or calculi
- Aid in the diagnosis of acute and chronic cholecystitis
- Determine common duct obstruction caused by tumors or choledocholithiasis
- Evaluate biliary enteric bypass patency
- Assess obstructive jaundice when done in combination with radiography or ultrasonography

Reference Values

- Normal shape, size, and function of the gallbladder with patent cystic and common bile ducts.

Abnormal Values

- Acalculus cholecystitis
- Acute cholecystitis
- Chronic cholecystitis
- Common bile duct obstruction secondary to gallstones, tumor, or stricture

Interfering Factors

- Inability of client to remain still during procedure will produce an artifact.
- Bilirubin levels ≥ 30 mg/dL, depending on radionuclide used, as this decreases hepatic uptake.
- Absence of food ingestion for longer than 24 hours as in fasting, total parenteral nutrition, or alcoholism can affect results.
- Ingestion of food or liquids within 2 to 4 hours of the scan can result in impaired visualization of the gallbladder.
- Presence of barium in the intestinal tract may inhibit gallbladder visualization.

NURSING ALERT

- This test is contraindicated in pregnant or lactating women unless the benefits of performing the test greatly outweigh the risks.
- Personnel should exercise special precautions in handling the radioactive test dose: nuclear medicine technician wears a badge and radiology ring; dose is prepared behind a lead glass shield with only gloved hands exposed; any spilled radionuclide area is washed with soap and water and paper towels, which are placed in a special storage area for a few weeks before being disposed.

Nursing Implications

Assessment

- Assess and record baseline vital signs for later comparison readings.
- Assess for allergy to radionuclide.
- Ensure fasting for 4 to 6 hours before scan.
- Determine date of last menstrual period and possibility of pregnancy in premenopausal women.
- Obtain history of hepatic and gallbladder conditions as well as signs and symptoms for biliary abnormalities.

- Assess for compliance with directions given for test, positioning, and activity before and during the test.

Possible Nursing Diagnoses

Pain related to inflammation and distention of tissue

Anxiety related to perceived threat to health status

Nutrition, altered, less than body requirements, related to inability to ingest nutrients

Implementation

- Establish intravenous access before procedure.
- Before the scan have the client remove all jewelry, put on a hospital gown, and void.
- Technetium-99m using a disopropyl analogue (IDA) is injected intravenously. The patient is placed in the supine position and the upper right quadrant of the abdomen is scanned immediately with images taken every 5 minutes for the first 30 minutes and every 10 minutes for the next 30 minutes. Delayed views are taken in 2, 4, and 24 hours if the gallbladder cannot be visualized, in order to differentiate acute from chronic cholecystitis or to detect degree of obstruction.
- Sincalide is given by some departments before the study to promote the release of cholecystokinin (CCK), causing the gallbladder to contract and empty.
- The administration of morphine intravenously during the study initiates spasms of the sphincter of Oddi, forcing the radionuclide into the gallbladder if the organ is not visualized within 1 hour of the injection of the radionuclide. Imaging is then done 20 to 50 minutes later to determine delayed visualization or nonvisualization.

Evaluation

- Monitor vital signs every 15 to 30 minutes as per institution policy and compare to baseline readings until stable.
- Observe client carefully for up to 60 minutes after the study for a possible anaphylactic reaction such as rash, tightening of throat, or difficulty breathing.

Client/Caregiver Teaching

Pretest

- Instruct the client to fast for at least 2 hours before the test.
- Explain the purpose of the procedure: to detect inflammation or obstruction of the gallbladder or the ducts.
- Explain that the procedure is performed in a special nuclear medicine department by a technician and a physician specializing in this branch of medicine.

- Advise client that scan takes approximately 90 minutes after injection of radionuclide with repeat imaging needed for up to 24 hours (48 hours for client with known hepatocellular disease).

Posttest

- Advise client to drink plenty of fluids for 24 to 48 hours to eliminate the radionuclide from the body.
- Explain that radionuclide is eliminated from the body within 6 to 24 hours.
- Instruct client to resume usual level of activity and normal dietary intake, unless contraindicated.
- Inform client to immediately flush toilet after each voiding following the procedure and to meticulously wash hands with soap and water after each void for 24 hours after the procedure.
- Tell all caregivers to wear rubber gloves when discarding urine for 24 hours after the procedure. Wash gloved hands with soap and water before removing gloves. Consider the gloves nuclear waste and dispose of them accordingly. Then wash ungloved hands after gloves are removed.

Scan, Kidney; Kidney and Renography Scan; Renocystography; Renocystogram; Renogram Scan

Classification: Nuclear medicine

Type of Test: Radionuclide imaging

A kidney scan is a nuclear study performed to assist in diagnosing abnormalities in blood flow, collecting system defects, excretion function, and information about the structures of the kidneys. Several radionuclides are used in kidney scanning with diagnostic information depending on the distribution in the kidneys. Renography is used to study the function of both kidneys simultaneously by tracking the rate at which the radionuclide flows into (vascular phase), through (tubular phase), and out of (excretory phase) the kidneys. The times are plotted on a graph and compared to normal parameters of organ function. All information obtained is stored in a computer to be used for further interpretation and computations.

Indications

- Aid in the diagnosis of renal artery stenosis resulting from renal dysplasia or atherosclerosis and causing arterial hypertension and a reduced glomerular filtration
- Aid in the diagnosis of renal vein thrombosis resulting from dehydration in infants or obstruction of blood flow in the presence of renal tumors in adults
- Aid in the diagnosis of renal artery embolism or renal infarction causing obstruction
- Determine the presence and effect of renal trauma, such as arterial injury, renal contusion, hematoma, rupture, arteriovenous fistula, or urinary extravasation
- Detect renal infectious or inflammatory diseases, such as acute or chronic pyelonephritis, renal abscess, or nephritis
- Determine the presence, location, and cause of obstructive uropathy, such as calculi, neoplasm, congenital disorders, or inflammation
- Diagnose benign tumors (hypernephroma or angiomyolipoma) and malignant tumors (Wilm's tumor)
- Detect the presence of renal cystic disease, such as simple cysts, polycystic disease in children or adults, or medullary sponge kidney
- Detect type, position, and number of congenital anomalies, such as ectopic kidney, horseshoe kidney, supernumery kidneys, or agenesis of left kidney
- Evaluate acute and chronic renal failure
- Evaluate kidney transplant for acute or chronic rejection

Reference Values

- Normal size, shape, position, symmetry, perfusion, and function of the kidneys
- Normal renal vasculature and perfusion; radionuclide contrast material circulates bilaterally, symmetrically, and without interruption through the renal parenchyma, ureters, and urinary bladder, with 50 percent of radionuclide excreted within the first 10 minutes

Abnormal Values

- Congenital anomalies
- Decreased renal function
- Diminished blood supply
- Infection or inflammation
- Masses
- Obstructive uropathy
- Renal failure
- Renal vascular disease including renal artery stenosis (RAS) or renal vein thrombosis
- Trauma

NURSING ALERT

- This test is contraindicated in pregnancy and lactation unless the benefits of performing the test greatly outweigh the risks.
- Special precautions should also be taken with children.
- Pregnant health care providers should avoid caring for a person who has had a nuclear medicine procedure until 24 hours after the procedure.
- Personnel should exercise special precautions in handling the radioactive test dose: nuclear medicine technician wears a badge and radiology ring; dose is prepared behind a lead glass shield with only gloved hands exposed; any spilled radionuclide area is washed with soap and water and paper towels, which are placed in a special storage area for a few weeks before being disposed.

Interfering Factors

- Inability of client to remain still during procedure will produce artifact.
- Medications such as antihypertensives taken within 24 hours of the test can affect the results depending on the reason for the study.
- Presence of contrast material from prior diagnostic testing interferes with accuracy.
- Abnormalities can be accentuated in the presence of dehydration or masked in the presence of overhydration.
- Injection of radiographic contrast material within 24 hours before the test invalidates results.
- Jewelry or metal objects in the scanning field distort results.

Nursing Implications

Assessment

- Assess for allergy to radionuclide analogue.
- Determine date of last menstrual period and possibility of pregnancy in premenopausal women.
- Assess and record baseline vital signs for later comparison readings.
- Obtain history regarding renal and urinary status and results of renal function laboratory tests.
- Determine previous abnormalities in laboratory tests and diagnostic procedures.

Possible Nursing Diagnoses

Fluid volume excess related to compromised regulatory system

Nutrition, altered, less than body requirements, related to inability to ingest adequate nutrients

Infection, risk for, related to depression of immunological defenses

Fatigue related to decreased metabolic energy production

Implementation

- Obtain signed consent form from client or responsible family member.
- Obtain client's current weight.
- Establish intravenous access.
- Before the scan have the client remove all jewelry, put on a hospital gown, and void.
- The client is placed in a prone, supine, or sitting position depending on study to be done. Positions can be changed during the imaging. Radionuclide for flow studies is administered intravenously and sequential imaging is performed every 2 seconds for 30 to 60 seconds. Blood pool imaging can also be obtained at this time. Excretion studies are done following the intravenous administration of the appropriate radionuclide; one image is taken every minute for 3 minutes at 30-minute intervals. This is followed by static imaging to reveal the collecting system and delayed static imaging 2 to 3 hours later to reveal cortex abnormalities. In some cases, imaging can be performed 24 hours later, especially in clients with renal failure, as this disorder slows the uptake of the radionuclide.
- During the flow and static imaging, the diuretic furosemide (Lasix) can be administered intravenously and images obtained.

- Renogram curves can be plotted concurrently with flow studies in which blood flow is imaged and recorded as it occurs.
- Urine and blood laboratory studies are done following renogram to correlate findings before diagnosis.
- If a study for vesicoureteral reflux is done, the client is requested to void and a catheter is placed into the bladder. The radionuclide is instilled into the bladder and multiple images are obtained during the bladder filling. The client is then requested to void, with the catheter in place or following catheter removal depending on department policy. Imaging is continued during the voiding and after voiding is completed. Reflux is determined by calculating the urine volume and counts obtained by imaging.

Evaluation

- Note results in relation to other related studies, particularly renal function studies, and to the client's symptoms.
- Monitor vital signs every 15 to 30 minutes and compare with baseline readings until stable.
- Observe client carefully for up to 60 minutes after the study for a possible anaphylactic reaction to the radionuclide such as rash, tightening of throat, or difficulty breathing.

Client/Caregiver Teaching

Pretest

- Explain the purpose of the procedure: to record activities of the entire kidney.
- Explain that the procedure is performed in a special nuclear medicine department by a technician and a physician specializing in this branch of medicine.
- Inform client of scanning schedule and that procedure takes from 30 to 60 minutes to complete initially but that additional time is needed if special imaging or kidney scan is to be done. This can take up to 4 hours to complete.
- Tell the client that he or she will be asked to drink at least 2 glasses of fluid before the study for hydration, unless contraindicated. Lugol's solution can be administered before the study as well to reduce uptake of the radionuclide by the thyroid gland.
- Instruct client to remain very still during scanning.

Posttest

- Instruct client to resume usual level of activity and normal dietary intake, unless contraindicated.

- Advise client to drink plenty of fluids for 24 to 48 hours to eliminate the radionuclide from the body, unless contraindicated.
- Inform the client that radionuclide is eliminated from the body within 6 to 24 hours.
- Tell the client to immediately flush toilet after each voiding following the procedure and to meticulously wash hands with soap and water after each void for 24 hours after the procedure.
- Tell all caregivers to wear rubber gloves when discarding urine for 24 hours after the procedure. Wash gloved hands with soap and water before removing gloves. Consider the gloves nuclear waste and dispose of them accordingly. Then wash ungloved hands after gloves are removed.

Scan, Liver

Classification: Nuclear medicine

Type of Test: Radionuclide imaging

This test is a nuclear scan performed to assist in the diagnosis of abnormalities in the function and structure of the liver. It is often performed simultaneously with spleen scanning or in combination with lung scanning to assist in diagnosing masses or inflammation in the diaphragmatic area. Technetium-99m (Tc-99m) sulfur colloid is injected intravenously and rapidly taken up by the Kupffer cells, which normally function to remove particulate matter, including radioactive colloids in the liver. Liver scans are done in conjunction with liver function tests and can compliment computed tomography, ultrasonography, and SPECT scans in confirming diagnosis.

Indications

- Diagnose and differentiate between primary and metastatic tumor focal disease
- Diagnose diffuse hepatocellular disease, such as hepatitis and cirrhosis

- Diagnose benign tumors, such as adenoma, cavernous hemangioma
- Detect a bacterial or amebic abscess
- Diagnose cystic focal disease
- Determine presence and effect of traumatic lesions, such as lacerations or hematoma
- Detect infiltrative processes that affect the liver, such as sarcoidosis amyloidosis
- Evaluate palpable abdominal masses
- Differentiate between splenomegaly and hepatomegaly
- Determine superior vena cava obstruction or Budd-Chiari syndrome
- Evaluate liver damage caused by radiation therapy or hepatotoxic drug therapy
- Assess condition of liver after abdominal trauma

Reference Values

- Normal size, contour, position and function of the liver

Abnormal Values

- Abscesses
- Cirrhosis
- Cysts
- Hemangiomas
- Hepatitis
- Diaphragmatic area inflammation
- Primary benign or malignant tumors
- Metastatic tumors
- Nodular hyperplasia
- Traumatic lesions

Interfering Factors

- Inability of client to remain still during procedure will produce artifact.
- Scan can fail to detect focal lesions smaller than 2 cm in diameter.
- Barium remaining in the gastrointestinal tract in the area of the liver can result in false results indicating tumor presence.
- Other nuclear scans performed on the same day can affect imaging of the liver.

- This test is contraindicated in pregnancy and lactation unless the benefits of performing the test greatly outweigh the risks.
- Special precautions are also required in children.
- Pregnant health care professionals should avoid caring for a person who has had a nuclear medicine procedure until 24 hours after the procedure.
- Personnel should exercise special precautions in handling the radioactive test dose: nuclear medicine technician wears a badge and radiology ring; dose is prepared behind a lead glass shield with only gloved hands exposed; any spilled radionuclide area is washed with soap and water and paper towels, which are placed in a special storage area for a few weeks before being disposed.

Nursing Implications

Assessment

- Determine date of last menstrual period and possibility of pregnancy in premenopausal women.
- Ensure that client has not been scheduled for more than one radionuclide scan on the same day, as this can interfere with liver imaging.
- Obtain history of any hepatic disorders and related signs and symptoms.
- Determine previous abnormalities in laboratory tests (especially liver function test) and diagnostic procedures.

Potential Nursing Diagnoses

Nutrition, altered, less than body requirements, related to inability to ingest adequate nutrition
Fluid volume excess related to compromised regulatory system
Skin integrity, impaired, risk for, related to altered circulation
Anxiety related to perceived threat to health status

Implementation

- Before the scan have the client remove all jewelry, put on a hospital gown, and void.
- Establish an intravenous line.

■ Place the client in the supine position on examining table. The radionuclide is administered intravenously and anterior images obtained 30 minutes later for 1 minute to perform flow studies. A 1-minute blood pool image can also be done. This is followed by static imaging in the anterior, posterior, lateral, anterior- and posterior-oblique positions to determine the size and shape of the liver.

Evaluation

■ Monitor vital signs every 15 to 30 minutes and compare with baseline readings until stable.
■ Monitor for anaphylactic or pyrogenic reactions that may result from a stabilizer in the Tc-99m, such as dextran or gelatin.
■ Note results in relation to other studies and to the client's symptoms.

Client/Caregiver Teaching

Pretest

■ Explain the purpose of the procedure: to identify areas of liver abnormalities
■ Explain that the procedure is performed in a special nuclear medicine department by a technician and a physician specializing in this branch of medicine and can take 90 minutes to complete.
■ Explain that no fasting of food or liquid is required.
■ Instruct the client to remain very still during scanning.

Posttest

■ Inform client of time to return for additional imaging.
■ Inform client to resume usual level of activity and normal dietary intake, unless contraindicated.
■ Advise client to drink plenty of fluids for 24 to 48 hours to eliminate the radionuclide from the body, unless contraindicated.
■ Radionuclides are usually eliminated in 6 to 24 hours.
■ Inform client to immediately flush toilet after each voiding following the procedure and to meticulously wash hands with soap and water after each void for 24 hours after the procedure.
■ Tell all caregivers to wear rubber gloves when discarding urine for 24 hours after the procedure. Wash gloved hands with soap and water before removing gloves. Consider the gloves nuclear waste and dispose of them accordingly. Then wash ungloved hands after gloves are removed.

Scan, Lung Perfusion; Radioactive Perfusion Scan; Lung Scintiscan

Classification: Nuclear medicine

Type of Test: Radionuclide imaging

This is a nuclear study performed when a client is suspected of having a pulmonary embolus or to evaluate other pulmonary disorders. Technetium (Tc-99m) is injected intravenously and distributed throughout the pulmonary vasculature according to gravitational effects on perfusion. The scan, which produces a visual image of the pulmonary blood flow, is useful in diagnosing or confirming pulmonary vascular obstruction. This scan is often done in conjunction with the ventilation scan to obtain clinical information that assists in differentiating among the many possible pathologic conditions revealed by the procedure. The results are correlated with other diagnostic studies such as pulmonary function, chest x-ray, pulmonary angiography, and arterial blood gases.

Indications

- Aid in the diagnosis of pulmonary embolism in the presence of a normal chest x-ray
- Differentiate between pulmonary embolism and other pulmonary diseases such as pneumonia, pulmonary effusion, atelectasis, asthma, bronchitis, emphysema, and tumors
- Evaluate perfusion changes associated with congestive heart failure and pulmonary hypertension
- Detect malignant tumor
- Evaluate pulmonary function preoperatively in clients with pulmonary disease

Reference Values

- Normal perfusion of lungs and ventilation-perfusion ratio

Abnormal Values

- Atelectasis
- Chronic obstructive pulmonary disease (COPD)
- Left atrial or pulmonary hypertension
- Lung displacement by fluid or chest masses
- Pneumonia
- Pneumonitis
- Pulmonary embolism
- Tuberculosis

Interfering Factors

- Inability of client to remain still during procedure will produce artifact.
- Other nuclear scans done on the same day can affect the distribution of the radionuclide.
- Improper positioning during injection of the radionuclide as gravity can affect the distribution of the material in the lungs.
- Presence of conditions that affect perfusion or ventilation, such as tumors that obstruct the pulmonary artery, vasculitis, pulmonary edema, sickle cell disease, parasitic disease, emphysema, effusion, or infection, can simulate a perfusion defect similar to pulmonary embolism.
- Jewelry or metal objects in the x-ray field distort results.

NURSING ALERT

- This test is contraindicated in clients with hypersensitivity to the radiopharmaceutical.
- This test is contraindicated in pregnancy and lactation unless the benefits of performing the test greatly outweigh the risks.
- Special precautions are also required in children.
- Pregnant health-care professionals should avoid caring for a person who has had a nuclear medicine procedure until 24 hours after the procedure.
- Personnel should exercise special precautions in handling the radioactive test dose: nuclear medicine technician wears a badge and radiology ring; dose is prepared behind a lead glass shield with only gloved hands exposed; any spilled radionuclide area is washed with soap and water and paper towels, which are placed in a special storage area for a few weeks before being disposed.

Nursing Implications

Assessment

- Assess for allergy to radioactive dye.
- Determine date of last menstrual period and possibility of pregnancy in premenopausal women.
- Obtain history regarding information about pulmonary status and recent chest x-ray.
- Determine previous abnormalities in laboratory tests and diagnostic procedures.
- If sedation is to be given, ensure client has been NPO for 6 to 8 hours before test.
- Ensure that children who are unable to lie still will be sedated.

Possible Nursing Diagnoses

Anxiety related to perceived threat to health status

Gas exchange, impaired, related to altered blood flow to alveoli

Tissue perfusion, altered, cardiopulmonary, related to interruption of blood flow to alveoli

Breathing pattern, ineffective, related to tracheobronchial obstruction

Implementation

- Establish intravenous access.
- Before the scan have the client remove all jewelry, put on a hospital gown, and void.
- Place the client in a supine position. The radionuclide is administered intravenously after shaking the syringe to resuspend the particles. The imaging is performed immediately. The camera is moved to obtain anterior, posterior, both lateral, and both oblique views. The multiple views are the best confirmation of perfusion defects within the lung vasculature.

Evaluation

- Monitor vital signs every 15 to 30 minutes and compare with baseline readings until stable.
- Observe client carefully for up to 60 minutes after the study for a possible anaphylactic reaction to the radionuclide such as rash, tightening of throat, or difficulty breathing.
- Note results in relation to other related studies and to the client's symptoms.

Client/Caregiver Teaching

Pretest

- Explain the purpose of the procedure: to record blood flow in the lungs.
- Explain that the procedure is performed in a special nuclear medicine department by a technician and a physician specializing in this branch of medicine.
- Inform the client that perfusion scan is usually done with ventilation study and that total time of both procedures take 2 hours.
- Instruct client to remain very still during scanning.

Posttest

- Instruct client to resume usual level of activity and normal dietary intake, unless contraindicated.
- Inform client to immediately flush toilet after each voiding following the procedure and to meticulously wash hands with soap and water after each void for 24 hours after the procedure.
- Advise client to drink plenty of fluids for 24 to 48 hours to eliminate the radionuclide from the body, unless contraindicated. Tell the client that radionuclide is eliminated from the body within 6 to 24 hours.
- Tell all caregivers to wear rubber gloves when discarding urine for 24 hours after the procedure. Wash gloved hands with soap and water before removing gloves. Consider the gloves nuclear waste and dispose of them accordingly. Then wash ungloved hands after gloves are removed.

Scan, Lung Ventilation

Classification: Nuclear medicine

Type of Test: Radionuclide imaging

This test is a nuclear study performed when a client is suspected of having a pulmonary embolus or to evaluate other pulmonary disorders. A lung ventilation scan can evaluate respiratory function and identify areas of the lung that are capable of ventilation. This procedure is performed after the client inhales air that is mixed with a radioactive gas. The radioactive gas delineates areas of the lung during ventilation. The distribution of the gas throughout the lung is measured in three phases: during the buildup of the radioactive gas (wash-in phase), after the client rebreathes from a bag (equilibrium phase), and after the radioactive gas has been removed (wash-out phase). This procedure is usually performed along with a lung perfusion scan. If the client is being mechanically ventilated, krypton gas must be used.

Indications

- Aid in the diagnosis of pulmonary emboli
- Evaluate regional respiratory function
- Aid in the diagnosis of parenchymal disorders such as emphysema, sarcoidosis, bronchogenic carcinoma, or tuberculosis
- Identify areas of the lung that are capable of ventilation
- Locate hypoventilation (regional), which can result from chronic obstructive pulmonary disease (COPD) or excessive smoking.

Reference Values

- Equal distribution of radioactive gas throughout both lungs and a normal wash-out phase.

Abnormal Values

- Bronchogenic carcinoma
- Emphysema
- Pneumonia
- Pulmonary embolism
- Regional hypoventilation
- Sarcoidosis
- Tuberculosis

NURSING ALERT

- This test is contraindicated in clients with hypersensitivity to the radiopharmaceutical.
- This test is contraindicated in pregnancy and lactation unless the benefits of performing the test greatly outweigh the risks.
- Special precautions are also required in children.

- Pregnant health-care professionals should avoid caring for a person who has had a nuclear medicine procedure until 24 hours after the procedure.
- The surrounding air can become contaminated with the radioactive gas from leaks in the closed system such as through the mask if the seal is not tight around the client's face.
- Personnel should exercise special precautions in handling the radioactive test dose: nuclear medicine technician wears a badge and radiology ring; dose is prepared behind a lead glass shield with only gloved hands exposed; any spilled radionuclide area is washed with soap and water and paper towels, which are placed in a special storage area for a few weeks before being disposed.

Interfering Factors

- Inability of client to remain still during procedure will produce artifact.
- Presence of conditions that affect perfusion or ventilation, such as tumors that obstruct the pulmonary artery, vasculitis, pulmonary edema, sickle-cell disease, parasitic disease, emphysema, effusion, or infection, can simulate a perfusion defect similar to pulmonary embolism.
- Jewelry or metal objects in the x-ray field distort results.

Nursing Implications

Assessment

- Assess for allergy to radioactive dye.
- Determine date of last menstrual period and possibility of pregnancy in premenopausal women.
- Obtain history regarding information about pulmonary status and recent chest x-ray.
- Determine previous abnormalities in laboratory tests and diagnostic procedures.
- If sedation is to be given, ensure client has been NPO for 6 to 8 hours.

Possible Nursing Diagnoses

Anxiety related to perceived threat to health status
Gas exchange, impaired, related to altered blood flow to alveoli

Tissue perfusion, altered, cardiopulmonary, related to interruption of blood flow to alveoli

Breathing pattern, ineffective, related to tracheobronchial obstruction

Implementation

- Have the client remove all jewelry, put on a hospital gown, and void.
- Instruct client to remain very still during scanning.
- Place the client in a supine position. The radionuclide is administered through a mask, which is placed over the client's nose and mouth. Client is asked to hold breath for a short period of time while the scan is taken. The distribution of the radioactive gas is monitored and measured on a nuclear scanner. The client's chest is scanned while gas is exhaled.

Evaluation

- Monitor vital signs every 15 to 30 minutes and compare with baseline readings until stable.
- Observe client carefully for up to 60 minutes after the study for a possible anaphylactic reaction to the radionuclide such as rash, tightening of throat, or difficulty breathing.
- Note results in relation to other related studies, particularly the lung perfusion scan, and to the client's symptoms.

Client/Caregiver Teaching

Pretest

- Explain that the procedure is performed in a special nuclear medicine department by a technician and a physician specializing in this branch of medicine.
- Inform the client that a ventilation scan is usually done with a perfusion study and that total time for both procedures is 2 hours.
- Instruct the client to remain very still during scanning.

Posttest

- Instruct client to resume usual level of activity and normal dietary intake, unless contraindicated.
- Advise client to drink plenty of fluids for 24 to 48 hours to eliminate the radionuclide from the body, unless contraindicated.
- Inform client to immediately flush toilet after each voiding following the procedure and to meticulously wash hands

with soap and water after each void for 24 hours after the procedure.

- Tell all caregivers to wear rubber gloves when discarding urine for 24 hours after the procedure. Wash gloved hands with soap and water before removing gloves. Consider the gloves nuclear waste and dispose of them accordingly. Then wash ungloved hands after gloves are removed.

Scan, Meckel's Diverticulum; Meckel Scan

Classification: Nuclear medicine

Type of Test: Radionuclide imaging

This test is a nuclear scan performed to assist in diagnosing the presence and size of congenital anomaly of the gastrointestinal tract. After intravenous injection of technetium-99m (Tc-99m) pertechnetate, immediate and delayed imaging is performed obtaining various views of the lower right quadrant of the abdomen. This radionuclide is taken up and concentrated by gastric mucosa, a type of tissue found in Meckel's diverticulum.

Indications

- Diagnose unexplained abdominal pain and gastrointestinal bleeding in adults and children caused by hydrochloric acid and pepsin secreted by ectopic gastric mucosa, which ulcerates nearby mucosa
- Detect sites of ectopic gastric mucosa, evidenced by focal increased activity in areas other than normal structures

Reference Values

- Normal distribution of radionuclide by gastric mucosa at normal sites

Abnormal Values

- Meckel's diverticulum

Interfering Factors

- Inability of client to remain still during procedure affects results.
- Barium remaining in the bowel if radiologic studies done before the scan can prevent penetration and concentration of the radionuclide.
- Radionuclide studies performed within preceding 24 hours will interfere with this test.
- Inaccurate timing for imaging following the radionuclide injection can affect results.
- Inadequate amount of gastric mucosa within a Meckel's diverticulum can affect ability to image abnormalities.

NURSING ALERT

- This test is contraindicated in pregnancy and lactation unless the benefits of performing the test greatly outweigh the risks.
- Special precautions should also be taken with children.
- Pregnant health-care professionals should avoid caring for a person who has had a nuclear medicine procedure until 24 hours after the procedure.
- Personnel should exercise special precautions in handling the radioactive test dose: nuclear medicine technician wears a badge and radiology ring; dose is prepared behind a lead glass shield with only gloved hands exposed; any spilled radionuclide area is washed with soap and water and paper towels, which are placed in a special storage area for a few weeks before being disposed.

Nursing Implications

Assessment

- Obtain history regarding signs and symptoms of Meckel's diverticulum such as bleeding, pain, intussusception, volvulus, or diverticulitis; previous abnormalities in laboratory tests and diagnostic findings.
- Determine date of last menstrual period and possibility of pregnancy in premenopausal women.
- Ensure that foods and fluids have been restricted for 6 to 8 hours before the study.
- Ensure that the ordered histamine blocker is administered 2 days before study to block acid secretion, as appropriate.

Possible Nursing Diagnoses

Anxiety related to perceived threat to health status

Pain, acute, related to inflammation of intestinal mucosa

Diarrhea related to altered function and presence of inflammation

Powerlessness, risk for, related to chronic nature of illness

Implementation

- Have the client remove all jewelry, put on a hospital gown, and void before scanning to increase visibility.
- Establish an intravenous access.
- The client is placed in a supine position. The radionuclide is administered intravenously 15 minutes before scanning and initial anterior abdominal images are obtained for 1 minute to screen for vascular lesions that cause bleeding. Then delayed imaging is done of left upper portion to obtain stomach views and lower field of view to obtain bladder areas. Imaging is done every 5 minutes for 1 hour in anterior, oblique, and lateral views, including a postvoiding view.
- Several modifications can be performed to facilitate the study: Client may be positioned on left side with table tilted 45 to 90 degrees to decrease the emptying of the radionuclide from the stomach into the bowel. Glucagon and pentagastrin can be administered to control uptake of the radionuclide. A nasogastric tube can be inserted to decrease peristalsis and emptying of the Tc-99m pertechnetate from the stomach into the bowel.

Evaluation

- Monitor vital signs every 15 to 30 minutes and compare with baseline readings until stable.
- Observe client carefully for up to 60 minutes after the study for a possible anaphylactic reaction to the radionuclide such as rash, tightening of throat, or difficulty breathing.
- Note results in relation to other related studies and to the client's symptoms.

Client/Caregiver Teaching

Pretest

- Explain that the procedure is performed in a special nuclear medicine department by a technician and a physician specializing in this branch of medicine and takes 1 hour to complete.
- Inform client it is necessary to remain very still during scanning.

- Assure client that nuclear medicine personnel will remain within hearing range and will be able to see the person throughout the study.
- Inform client of any modifications in positioning, use of nasogastric tube, or administration of medications during procedure to enhance imaging.

Posttest

- Instruct client to resume usual level of activity and normal dietary intake, unless contraindicated.
- Advise client to drink plenty of fluids for 24 to 48 hours to eliminate the radionuclide from the body, unless contraindicated. Tell the client that radionuclide is eliminated from the body within 6 to 24 hours.
- Inform client to immediately flush toilet after each voiding following the procedure and to meticulously wash hands with soap and water after each void for 24 hours after the procedure.
- Tell all caregivers to wear rubber gloves when discarding urine for 24 hours after the procedure. Wash gloved hands with soap and water before removing gloves. Consider the gloves nuclear waste and dispose of them accordingly. Then wash ungloved hands after gloves are removed.

Scan, Parathyroid

Classification: Nuclear medicine

Type of Test: Radionuclide imaging

This test is a nuclear scan performed primarily to assist in the localization of parathyroid adenomas in clinically proven primary hyperparathyroidism. It is performed before surgery. It can also assist in demonstrating intrinsic or extrinsic parathyroid adenoma. Thallium and technetium are injected 5 to 10 minutes before the imaging is performed.

Indications

- Aid in the diagnosis of hyperparathyroidism
- Differentiate between extrinsic and intrinsic parathyroid adenoma

Reference Values

■ No areas of increased perfusion or uptake in thyroid or parathyroid

Abnormal Values

■ Intrinsic and extrinsic parathyroid adenomas

> ### NURSING ALERT
>
> ■ This test is contraindicated in pregnancy and lactation unless the benefits of performing the test greatly outweigh the risks.
> ■ Special precautions should also be taken with children.
> ■ Personnel should exercise special precautions in handling the radioactive test dose: nuclear medicine technician wears a badge and radiology ring; dose is prepared behind a lead glass shield with only gloved hands exposed; any spilled radionuclide area is washed with soap and water and paper towels, which are placed in a special storage area for a few weeks before being disposed.

Interfering Factors

■ Inability of client to remain still during procedure will produce artifact.
■ Recent ingestion of iodine in food or as medication or recent tests with iodine content can interfere with the effectiveness.

Nursing Implications

Assessment

■ Determine date of last menstrual period and possibility of pregnancy in premenopausal women.
■ Ensure that client has not been scheduled for more than one radionuclide scan on the same day, as this can interfere with liver imaging.
■ Obtain history and related signs and symptoms of any thyroid or parathyroid disorders.
■ Assess for recent intake of iodine

Possible Nursing Diagnoses

Airway clearance, ineffective, related to edema and laryngeal nerve damage

Fluid volume excess, risk for, related to stress-induced release
of ADH

Pain, acute, related to effects of calcium imbalance

Anxiety related to perceived threat to health status

Implementation

- Have the client remove all jewelry, put on a hospital gown,
  and void.
- Establish an intravenous line.
- Ask the client to remain very still during scanning.
- Place the client in the supine position on examining table.
  Thallium is administered intravenously and 15 minutes later
  imaging is performed. The images are stored in a computer.
- With the client in the same position, technetium is injected,
  and after 10 minutes a second image is obtained and stored
  by the computer. The computer subtracts the technetium-
  visualized thyroid structures from the thallium accumulation
  in a parathyroid adenoma.

Evaluation

- Monitor vital signs every 15 to 30 minutes and compare with
  baseline readings until stable.
- Assess injection site for redness or swelling. Apply warm
  soaks to ease discomfort if hematoma develops.
- Monitor for anaphylactic or pyrogenic reactions that may result from a stabilizer added to the Tc-99m, such as dextran
  or gelatin.
- Note results in relation to other related studies and to the
  client's symptoms.

Client/Caregiver Teaching

Pretest

- Explain that the procedure is performed in a special nuclear
  medicine department by a technician and a physician specializing in this branch of medicine.
- Explain that test can take 45 minutes to complete
- Explain that no fasting of food or liquid is required unless
  the client has been taking an iodine-based medication,
  which may affect the test results.
- Instruct the client to remain very still during scanning.

Posttest

- Inform client to resume usual level of activity and normal
  dietary intake, unless contraindicated.

- Advise client to drink plenty of fluids for 24 to 48 hours to eliminate the radionuclide from the body, unless contraindicated.
- Tell the client that radionuclide is eliminated from the body within 6 to 24 hours.
- Inform client to immediately flush toilet after each voiding following the procedure and to meticulously wash hands with soap and water after each void for 24 hours after the procedure.
- Tell all caregivers to wear rubber gloves when discarding urine for 24 hours after the procedure. Wash gloved hands with soap and water before removing gloves. Consider the gloves nuclear waste and dispose of them accordingly. Then wash ungloved hands after gloves are removed.

Scan, Parotid and Salivary Glands

Classification: Nuclear medicine

Type of Test: Radionuclide imaging

This is a nuclear study performed to assist in diagnosing abnormalities of secretory function and duct patency of either or both glands. Technetium-99m (Tc-99m) pertechnetate is administered, and immediate imaging of blood flow, uptake, and secreting capability is done. Sequential images of the oral cavity are taken over 10 to 15 minutes.

Indications

- Evaluate swelling and pain in the gland area
- Detect tumors of the parotid or salivary glands such as oncocytoma, Warthin's tumor, or mucoepidermoid tumor
- Detect tumors, cysts, and abscesses and differentiate between these and malignant tumors
- Determine the presence of duct obstruction commonly seen in sialadenitis or Sjögren's syndrome
- Aid in the diagnosis of acute parotitis and other inflammatory processes of the glands

Reference Values

- Normal size, position, and shape of the glands

Abnormal Values

- Adenocarcinoma
- Benign tumor or cyst
- Mucoepidermoid tumor
- Oncocytoma
- Warthin's tumor

▶ NURSING ALERT

- This test is contraindicated in pregnancy and lactation unless the benefits of performing the test greatly outweigh the risks.
- Special precautions should also be taken with children.
- Pregnant health-care providers should avoid caring for a person who has had a nuclear medicine procedure until 24 hours after the procedure.
- Personnel should exercise special precautions in handling the radioactive test dose: nuclear medicine technician wears a badge and radiology ring; dose is prepared behind a lead glass shield with only gloved hands exposed; any spilled radionuclide area is washed with soap and water and paper towels, which are placed in a special storage area for a few weeks before being disposed.

Interfering Factors

- Inability of client to remain still during procedure will produce artifact.
- Rinsing mouth with water between images can decrease radioactivity of the saliva.

Nursing Implications

Assessment

- Assess for allergy to radionuclide.
- Determine date of last menstrual period and possibility of pregnancy in premenopausal women.
- Obtain history regarding information regarding gland disorders.

Possible Nursing Diagnoses

Anxiety related to perceived threat to health status

Pain related to the presence of inflammation and enlargement of salivary glands

Nutrition, altered, less than body requirements, related to inability to ingest adequate nutrients

Implementation

- Establish intravenous access.
- Have the client remove all jewelry and metal around head and neck area, put on a hospital gown, and void.
- Place client in sitting position. The radionuclide is administered intravenously. Immediate scanning is performed every few minutes for 30 minutes in anterior, posterior, and oblique views for blood flow and uptake studies. If secretory function of the glands is desired, stimulation of salivation will be done by providing a citrus meal (lemon drop, orange, or grapefruit slices) three-fourths of the way through the test to cause the gland to empty. The procedure takes 45 to 60 minutes to complete.

Evaluation

- Assist client from table to a position of comfort.
- Monitor vital signs every 15 to 30 minutes and compare with baseline readings until stable.
- Observe client carefully for up to 60 minutes after the study for a possible anaphylactic reaction to the radionuclide such as rash, tightening of throat, or difficulty breathing.

Client/Caregiver Teaching

Pretest

- Explain that procedure is performed in a special nuclear medicine department by a technician and a physician specializing in this branch of medicine to detect gland disorder.
- Instruct the client to remain very still during scanning.

Posttest

- Advise client to drink plenty of fluids for 24 to 48 hours to eliminate the radionuclide from the body, unless contraindicated. Inform the client that the radionuclide will be excreted in 6 to 24 hours.
- Inform client to immediately flush toilet after each voiding following the procedure and to meticulously wash hands with soap and water after each void for 24 hours after the procedure.

- Tell all caregivers to wear rubber gloves when discarding urine for 24 hours after the procedure. Wash gloved hands with soap and water before removing gloves. Consider the gloves nuclear waste and dispose of them accordingly. Then wash ungloved hands after gloves are removed.
- Advise the client or caregiver that no special handling of respiratory or salivary secretions is required.

Scan, Positron Emission Tomography (PET)

Classification: Nuclear medicine

Type of Test: Computed tomographic radionuclide imaging

Positron emission tomography (PET) combines nuclear medicine with computed tomography (CT). CT images result from passing x-rays through the body at various angles. Density variations of each tissue creates various penetration of the x-rays. The densities are given numeric values and are digitally computed on a screen. This results in precise localization of the scanned area. PET is able to evaluate the metabolism by recording tracers of nuclear annihilations in body tissue. Each tracer is designed to measure a specific body process such as protein metabolism or blood flow or blood volume.

PET provides evaluation of many biochemical processes essential to the organ being studied. The radionuclide can be administered intravenously or inhaled as a gas.

Indications

- Assess tissue permeability
- Determine the size of heart infarcts
- Investigate the physiology of psychosis
- Determine the regionalization of heart and brain metabolism
- Determine the effects of drugs on malfunctioning or diseased tissues
- Evaluate cancer treatment by measuring changes in malignant tissue and by biochemical reactions in the surrounding normal tissues

Reference Values

- Normal patterns of tissue metabolism

Abnormal Values

- Alzheimer's disease
- Brain tumor
- Breast tumor
- Cerebrovascular accident
- Coronary artery disease
- Dementia
- Epilepsy
- Huntington's disease
- Myocardial infarction
- Parkinson's disease
- Pneumonia
- Pulmonary edema
- Schizophrenia

> ### NURSING ALERT
>
> - This test is contraindicated in pregnancy and lactation unless the benefits of performing the test greatly outweigh the risks.
> - Special precautions should also be taken with children.
> - Pregnant health-care providers should avoid caring for a person who has had a nuclear medicine procedure until 24 hours after the procedure.
> - Personnel should exercise special precautions in handling the radioactive test dose: nuclear medicine technician wears a badge and radiology ring; dose is prepared behind a lead glass shield with only gloved hands exposed; any spilled radionuclide area is washed with soap and water and paper towels, which are placed in a special storage area for a few weeks before being disposed.

Interfering Factors

- Recent ingestion of caffeine, alcohol, or tobacco (within 24 hours) may affect results.
- Excessive anxiety may affect brain study results.
- Use of drugs such as tranquilizers and sedatives may affect results.

- Inability of client to remain still during procedure will produce artifact.

Nursing Implications

Assessment

- Determine date of last menstrual period and possibility of pregnancy in premenopausal women.
- Obtain history of any disorders and related signs and symptoms.
- Assess history for medications that may affect test results including recent use of alcohol, tobacco, or caffeine.

Possible Nursing Diagnoses

Cardiac output, decreased, risk for, related to increased systemic vascular resistance
Trauma, risk for, related to balancing difficulties
Physical mobility, impaired, related to neuromuscular impairment
Anxiety related to perceived threat to health status

Implementation

- Have the client remove all jewelry, put on a hospital gown, and void.
- Establish two intravenous lines.
- Place the client in a comfortable reclining chair. The radionuclide is either injected intravenously or inhaled as a gas. The scans are obtained by a circular array of detectors outside the body in the area to be examined.
- The client may be asked to perform various cognitive activities if the brain is being scanned (such as reciting the Pledge of Allegiance). This will assess changes in brain activity experienced during memory or reasoning. The client may be asked to wear a blindfold and ear plugs during this part of the test.

Evaluation

- Monitor vital signs every 15 to 30 minutes and compare with baseline readings until stable.
- Monitor for anaphylactic or pyrogenic reactions that may result from a stabilizer added to Tc-99m, such as dextran or gelatin.
- Note results in relation to other related studies and to the client's symptoms.
- Instruct the client to remain very still during scanning.

Client/Caregiver Teaching

Pretest

- Explain that the procedure is performed in a special nuclear medicine department by a technician and a physician specializing in this branch of medicine.
- Explain that test can take 60 to 90 minutes to complete.
- Tell client not to ingest tobacco, alcohol, or caffeine, or tranquilizers or sedatives as ordered, for 24 hours before test.
- Explain that the client may be asked to wear ear plugs and a blindfold if a brain scan is being performed.

Posttest

- Inform client of time to return for additional imaging.
- Advise client to drink plenty of fluids for 24 to 48 hours to eliminate the radionuclide from the body, unless contraindicated. Tell the client that radionuclide is eliminated from the body within 6 to 24 hours.
- Inform client to resume usual level of activity and normal dietary intake, unless contraindicated.
- Inform client to immediately flush toilet after each voiding following the procedure and to meticulously wash hands with soap and water after each void for 24 hours after the procedure.
- Tell all caregivers to wear rubber gloves when discarding urine for 24 hours after the procedure. Wash gloved hands with soap and water before removing gloves. Consider the gloves nuclear waste and dispose of them accordingly. Then wash ungloved hands after gloves are removed.

Scan, Scrotal

Classification: Nuclear medicine

Type of Test: Radionuclide imaging

This test is a nuclear scan performed to assist in the diagnosis of sudden onset of unilateral testicular pain and swelling. Usually performed as an emergency procedure, scrotal imaging can aid in the diagnosis of testicular torsion. Technetium-99m (Tc-99m) pertechnetate is administered intravenously to view blood flow to both testicles. It can differentiate unilateral testicular torsion from other causes of swelling and pain such as acute epididymitis, orchitis, strangulated hernia, torsion of the testicular appendage, and testicular hemorrhage.

Indications

- Aid in the diagnosis of testicular torsion
- Differentiate between unilateral testicular torsion and other causes of pain and swelling such as orchitis, strangulated hernia, torsion of the testicular appendage, and testicular hemorrhage

Reference Values

- Unilateral, symmetric, and prompt blood flow to the testicles

Abnormal Values

- Epididymitis
- Orchitis
- Strangulated hernia
- Testicular hemorrhage
- Torsion of the testicular appendage
- Trauma
- Unilateral testicular torsion

NURSING ALERT

- This test is contraindicated in clients with a known allergy to radionuclides and in the presence of hiatal hernia, esophageal motor disorders, or swallowing difficulties. In those clients, endoscopic studies should be considered.
- The procedure is also contraindicated in pregnancy and breast-feeding unless the benefits of performing the test greatly outweigh the risks.
- Special precautions should be taken with children.
- Personnel should exercise special precautions in handling the radioactive test dose: nuclear medicine technician wears a badge and radiology ring; dose is prepared behind a lead glass shield with only gloved hands exposed; any spilled radionuclide area is washed with soap and water and paper towels, which are placed in a special storage area for a few weeks before being disposed.

Interfering Factors

- Inability of client to remain still during procedure will produce artifact.
- Other nuclear scans performed on the same day can affect imaging of the testicles.

Nursing Implications

Assessment

- Obtain history of any disorders and related signs and symptoms.

Potential Nursing Diagnoses

Pain related to swelling
Anxiety related to perceived threat to health status
Grieving, anticipatory, related to perceived potential loss

Implementation

- Establish an intravenous line
- Place the client on a padded table in the supine position. The penis is taped to the abdomen and the testicles are supported with tape or a lead shield as the legs are abducted.
- The radionuclide is administered intravenously and imaging is performed over the testicles.

Evaluation

- Monitor vital signs every 15 to 30 minutes and compare with baseline readings until stable.
- Monitor for anaphylactic or pyrogenic reactions that may result from a stabilizer added to Tc-99m, such as dextran or gelatin.
- Note results in relation to other studies and to the client's symptoms.
- Instruct the client to remain very still during scanning.

Client/Caregiver Teaching

Pretest

- Explain that the procedure is performed in a special nuclear medicine department by a technician and a physician specializing in this branch of medicine.
- Explain that test can take 30 minutes to complete.
- Explain that no fasting of food or liquid is required.

- Advise the client that only tracer amounts of the radionuclide are used, and that radiation exposure is minimal.

Posttest

- Inform client to resume usual level of activity and normal dietary intake, unless contraindicated.
- Advise client to drink plenty of fluids for 24 to 48 hours to eliminate the radionuclide from the body, unless contraindicated.
- Inform client to immediately flush toilet after each voiding following the procedure and to meticulously wash hands with soap and water after each void for 24 hours after the procedure.
- Tell all caregivers to wear rubber gloves when discarding urine for 24 hours after the procedure. Wash gloved hands with soap and water before removing gloves. Consider the gloves nuclear waste and dispose of them accordingly. Then wash ungloved hands after gloves are removed.

Scan, Thyroid; Thyroid Scintiscan

Classification: Nuclear medicine

Type of Test: Radionuclide imaging

This is a nuclear study performed following intravenous injection of technetium-99m (Tc-99m) or oral administration of iodine-123 (I-123) to note an increase or decrease in uptake by the thyroid and surrounding area tissue.

Indications

- Assess presence of a thyroid nodule or enlarged thyroid gland
- Diagnose thyroid dysfunction
- Diagnose benign or malignant thyroid tumors
- Assess palpable nodules and differentiate between benign tumor or cyst and malignant tumor
- Diagnose causes of neck or substernal masses

- Differentiate between Graves' disease and Plummer's disease, both resulting in hyperthyroidism
- Evaluate thyroid function in hyperthyroidism and hypothyroidism when analyzed with laboratory tests, thyroid function tests, thyroxine (T_4), triiodothyronine (T_3), and thyroid uptake tests
- Diagnose thyroiditis conditions, such as acute, chronic, or Hashimoto's condition

Reference Values

- Normal size, contour, position, and function of the thyroid gland with homogeneous uptake of the radionuclide

Abnormal Values

- Cysts
- Fibrosis
- Hematoma
- Tumors, benign or malignant
- Thyroiditis
- Thyrotoxicosis

Interfering Factors

- Inability of client to remain still during procedure will produce artifact.
- Other recently performed nuclear scans or radiologic studies using iodinated media can affect uptake of the radionuclide.
- Diet that is deficient in iodine content will increase uptake of the radionuclide; diet of iodine-containing foods will decrease the uptake of the radionuclide.
- Uptake may be increased in persons on a diet with subnormal iodine levels or those on phenothiazine therapy if a radioactive iodine tracer is used.
- Certain drugs can cause decreased tracer uptake, including anticoagulants, antihistamines, corticosteroids, cough syrup, phenothiazines, salicylates, thyroid hormones, thyroid hormone antagonists, iodides, and multivitamins.
- Vomiting and diarrhea will decrease uptake of the radionuclide.
- Gastroenteritis can interfere with absorption of orally administered radioactive tracer.
- Jewelry or metal objects in the head and neck area distort results.

> ### ◣ NURSING ALERT
>
> ■ This test is contraindicated in clients with hypersensitivity to the radiopharmaceutical.
>
> ■ This test is contraindicated in pregnancy and lactation unless the benefits of performing the test greatly outweigh the risks.
>
> ■ Special precautions are also required in children.
>
> ■ Pregnant health-care professionals should avoid caring for a person who has had a nuclear medicine procedure until 24 hours after the procedure.
>
> ■ Personnel should exercise special precautions in handling the radioactive test dose: nuclear medicine technician wears a badge and radiology ring; dose is prepared behind a lead glass shield with only gloved hands exposed; any spilled radionuclide area is washed with soap and water and paper towels, which are placed in a special storage area for a few weeks before being disposed.

Nursing Implications

Assessment

■ Assess for allergy to radioactive dye or iodine.
■ Determine date of last menstrual period and possibility of pregnancy in premenopausal women.
■ Obtain history regarding information about thyroid problems and food or drug intake that contain iodine.
■ Determine previous abnormalities in thyroid laboratory tests and diagnostic procedures, scans, or radiologic studies.
■ Ensure client has had nothing by mouth for 8 hours if radioactive tracer will be administered orally.
■ Ensure restriction of iodine-containing foods 21 days before the test, including salt, shellfish, or salt substitutes containing iodine.
■ Ensure restriction of medications that will interfere with radioactive tracer uptake for 21 days before test as ordered.

Potential Nursing Diagnoses

Cardiac output, decreased, risk for, related to uncontrolled hypermetabolic rate
Anxiety related to perceived threat to health status
Thought processes, altered, risk for, related to sleep patterns

Implementation

- Have the client remove all jewelry and metal objects near the head or neck area, put on a hospital gown, and void.
- The client is given the radionuclide I-123 in a capsule orally 4 to 24 hours prior to scanning or Tc-99m pertechnetate intravenously 20 minutes before scanning, depending on which is used.
- The client is placed in a supine position in 2 or 4 hours after the administration of the oral dose and scanning is performed over the neck area. Additional scanning can be done in 24 hours.
- Assist client from table to a position of comfort.

Evaluation

- Monitor vital signs every 15 to 30 minutes and compare with baseline readings until stable.
- Provide supportive environment after diagnostic findings are reported, as indicated; reinforce information regarding diagnosis and recommended treatment regimen.
- Observe client carefully for up to 60 minutes after the study for a possible anaphylactic reaction to the radionuclide such as rash, tightening of throat, or difficulty breathing.

Client/Caregiver Teaching

Pretest

- Explain why the procedure is performed: to evaluate thyroid function.
- Explain that the procedure is performed in a special nuclear medicine department by a technician and a physician specializing in this branch of medicine.
- Explain that test can take 30 minutes to complete.
- Explain that no fasting of food or liquid is required.
- Tell the client that radionuclide elimination is dependent on the type used.
- Instruct the client to remain very still during scanning.

Posttest

- Inform client of time to return for additional imaging.
- Advise client to drink plenty of fluids for 24 to 48 hours to eliminate the radionuclide from the body, unless contraindicated. Explain that radionuclide is eliminated from the body within 6 to 24 hours.
- Tell client to immediately flush toilet after each voiding following the procedure and to meticulously wash hands with

soap and water after each void for 24 hours after the procedure.
- Tell all caregivers to wear rubber gloves when discarding urine for 24 hours after the procedure. Wash gloved hands with soap and water before removing gloves. Consider the gloves nuclear waste and dispose of them accordingly. Then wash ungloved hands after gloves are removed.
- Inform client to resume usual level of activity and previous diet 2 hours after oral radioactive tracer administration.

Schick Test

Classification: Immune response

Type of Test: Skin injection

This skin test is done to determine the presence of antitoxins indicating susceptibility or immunity to diphtheria. Diphtheria is an infectious bacterial pulmonary disease caused by the organism *Corynebacterium diphtheriae* and characterized by membranous exudate production that coats the trachea and bronchi mucosal surfaces. It is transmitted by direct contact with the discharges from the mucous membranes of the nose and nasopharynx or articles contaminated with these discharges from an infected person.

Indications

- Determine susceptibility to diphtheria, as evidenced by a positive response
- Determine the presence or absence of the necessary quantity of antitoxins in the blood to determine the ability to produce antibodies and assure immunity

Reference Values

- Negative response; no reaction at the test or control site, indicating immunity to diphtheria

Abnormal Values

- Positive response; induration and erythema reveal insufficient antitoxins and susceptibility to diphtheria

Interfering Factors

- Improper technique in performing the skin test or inaccurate time or measurement in reading the reaction

Nursing Implications

Assessment

- Obtain a history of any exposure to diphtheria or outbreaks in the community.

Potential Nursing Diagnoses

Infection, risk for transmission
Gas exchange, impaired, risk for, related to respiratory tract obstruction

Implementation

- Cleanse the skin sites on the lower anterior area of both forearms with alcohol or acetone swabs and allow to air dry. Two tuberculin syringes with a 26-gauge needle attached are prepared, one containing 0.1 mL of diphtheria toxin and the other 0.1 mL of heated or inactivated diphtheria toxoid.
- Inject the substances intradermally and measure the response in 24 to 48 hours. A positive result at the site at the time of reading consists of an induration of 25 to 50 mm in diameter accompanied by erythema, indicating immunity to diphtheria.

Evaluation

- Note the immunologic response as detailed above.

Client/Caregiver Teaching

Pretest

- Inform the client or caregiver of the purpose of the test and how the test is performed.
- Tell the client that the test is generally done by a nurse in a physician's office or health-care setting and takes about 5 to 10 minutes to complete.

Posttest

- Tell the client to leave injection sites open to air.
- Emphasize that the injection site should not be scratched or rubbed until it is read.
- Emphasize the importance of returning 24 to 48 hours (no longer than 120 hours) later to have test results read.
- Reinforce information about further immunization against the disease with a series of diphtheria toxoid injections and answer or direct questions to the appropriate professionals.

Schilling Test

Classification: Nuclear medicine (urinalysis)

Type of Test: Urine (timed)

This test measures the excretion of B_{12} in the urine after it has been labeled with the radionuclide cobalt-57 (Co-57) cyanocobalamin. The test is used to determine gastrointestinal absorption of vitamin B_{12}, which combines with the intrinsic factor, a glycoprotein secreted by the gastric mucosa. A lack of the intrinsic factor reduces the absorption of vitamin B_{12} in the ileum, resulting in pernicious anemia.

Indications

- Identify deficiency in B_{12} absorption (one-stage test)
- Determine cause of B_{12} deficiency by differentiating between pernicious anemia and gastrointestinal malabsorption

Reference Values

	Rate of Excretion, 24-h urine
0.5 mg dose of radionuclide	15–40%
1.0 mg dose of radionuclide	5–40%

Abnormal Values

- <7% of 0.5 mg dose and (3% of 1.0 mg dose excreted in impaired absorption states.
- In pernicious anemia, urinary excretion of vitamin B_{12} approaches normal levels when intrinsic factor is administered as part of the study (two-stage test).
- In gastrointestinal malabsorption problems, urinary excretion of vitamin B_{12} is decreased.

Interfering Factors

- Recent diagnostic tests using radioactive materials within 7 days will affect results.
- Incomplete or incorrect collection of timed urine sample will produce inaccurate results.
- Laxatives administered before the test impair intestinal absorption of vitamin B_{12}.
- Stool mixed with urine will invalidate results.
- Certain diseases, including diabetes mellitus, pancreatic insufficiency, and intestinal bacterial overgrowth (diarrhea), can affect intestinal vitamin B_{12} absorption.
- Partial or total gastrectomy will cause lack of intrinsic factor, which enables vitamin B_{12} absorption.

NURSING ALERT

- This test is contraindicated in pregnancy and lactation unless the benefits of performing the test greatly outweigh the risks.
- In clients with severe renal disease, the urine collection time can be prolonged to 48 to 72 hours. The normal percentage of labeled vitamin B_{12} will eventually be excreted, however, as long as the client does not have impaired vitamin B_{12} absorption.
- Personnel should exercise special precautions in handling the radioactive test dose: nuclear medicine technician wears a badge and radiology ring; dose is prepared behind a lead glass shield with only gloved hands exposed; any spilled radionuclide area is washed with soap and water and paper towels, which are placed in a special storage area for a few weeks before being disposed.

Nursing Implications

Assessment

- Obtain history regarding hematologic status information, gastrointestinal status, results of folate, TBC, and B_{12} blood tests; signs or symptoms of pernicious anemia or malabsorption syndromes; and kidney function tests (BUN and creatinine).
- Assess for allergy to radionuclides.
- Ensure that the client has withheld vitamin B_{12} for 3 days; laxatives for 2 days; and food and fluids for 8 hours before the test.
- Ensure that the client has not had any recent tests involving radionuclides.

Possible Nursing Diagnoses

Anxiety related to threat to health status
Protection, altered, risk for, related to abnormal blood profiles
Nutrition, altered, less than body requirements, related to inability to absorb nutrients

Implementation

- *One-stage test:* Ask the client to void and discard the specimen or send it to the laboratory for radioactivity residual if a radionuclide study has been performed recently. Administer a capsule containing 0.5 to 1.0 mg of Co-57 cyanocobalamin orally; 1 to 2 hours later (depending on lab preference), administer 1000 mg nonradioactive vitamin B_{12} IM. Inform the client that food and fluid can be resumed at this time. Discard the first-morning urine and start collection and timing with the next specimen. Collect all urine for 24 hours in a 3-liter urine container without preservative obtained from the laboratory. Send urine to laboratory after 24 hours (48 to 72 hours for clients with renal function) for analysis.
- *Two-stage test:* Ask the client to void and discard specimen. Administer 0.5 to 1.0 mg Co-57 cyanocobalamin, followed by breakfast. Then administer a 60-mg dose of intrinsic factor. Administer 1000 mg nonradioactive vitamin B_{12} IM 1 to 2 hours later. This competes with the absorbed radioactive material for binding site and allows for excretion of the radioactive B_{12} in the urine. Obtain a 24-hour urine sample using the same procedures as for the one-stage test.

Evaluation

- Note test results in relation to other tests performed and to the client's symptoms.

- When absorption is normal, vitamin B_{12} in excess of body needs will be excreted in urine. If absorption is impaired, vitamin B_{12} either does not appear in the urine or is found in only small amounts. If <5 percent to 15 percent of the radionuclide is excreted, a two-stage test is indicated.
- Findings of the two-stage test are based on the amount of B_{12} in the urine over a specific time.
- Observe client carefully for up to 60 minutes after administration of radionuclide for possible anaphylactic reaction such as rash, tightening of throat, or difficulty breathing.

Client/Caregiver Teaching

Pretest

- Tell the client to withhold vitamin B_{12} for at least 3 days before the test; laxatives for at least 2 days; and food and fluids for 8 hours before the test.
- Ensure that the client has not had any tests using radionuclides within 7 days.
- Assure client that amount of radionuclide is very minute and will be eliminated from the body without any harmful effects.
- Instruct client to urinate before defecating and to avoid contaminating specimen with stool or tissue paper.

Posttest

- Tell the client to send the entire urine specimen to the laboratory at the end of 24 hours.
- Advise client to drink plenty of fluids for 24 to 48 hours after the test to eliminate the radionuclide from the body, unless contraindicated.
- Tell the client to immediately flush toilet after each voiding following the procedure and to meticulously wash hands with soap and water after each void for 24 hours after the procedure.
- Tell all caregivers to wear rubber gloves when discarding urine for 24 hours after the procedure. Wash gloved hands with soap and water before removing gloves; then wash ungloved hands after gloves are removed.

Schirmer Tearing Test

Classification: Diagnostic procedure

Type of Test: Lacrimal gland function

The Schirmer tearing test simultaneously tests both eyes to assess lacrimal gland function by determining the amount of moisture accumulated on filter paper held against the conjunctival sac. The accessory glands of Krause and Wolfring can be also evaluated by instilling a topical anesthetic before insertion of the filter paper. The topical anesthetic inhibits tearing of major lacrimal glands, allowing testing of the accessory glands.

Indications

■ Assess suspected tearing deficiency

Reference Values

■ 15 mm moisture on test strip after 5 minutes

Abnormal Values

■ Tearing deficiency related to aging or Sjögren's syndrome
■ Tearing deficiency secondary to leukemia, lymphoma, or rheumatoid arthritis

Interfering Factors

■ Rubbing or squeezing the eyes may affect results.

Nursing Implications

Assessment

■ Obtain history of eye, autoimmune and hematologic disorders, current symptoms, and results of any diagnostic tests performed.
■ Ensure that contact lenses are removed.

Possible Nursing Diagnoses

Anxiety related to perceived threat to health status
Pain related to decreased lacrimation or inflammation
Physical mobility, impaired, related to joint inflammation

Implementation

- Instill ordered topical anesthetic and provide time for it to work.
- Have client sit in a chair with head back against the headrest.
- Remove the strip of filter paper from the package and bend the rounded wick end, as indicated. Have the client look up to the ceiling and gently pull out on the lower lid. Insert the strip into each eye so that it is positioned near the inner canthus and between the lower lid and conjunctiva with the eye rim being at the end of the strip. The client may blink normally but not rub the eyes.
- The strips are removed after 5 minutes, then the length of moistened area is measured in millimeters.
- The results are reported as the length of strip that is moistened; the time the strips were left in place; and the eye in which the test was taken.

Evaluation

- Assess for corneal abrasion caused by rubbing eyes before topical anesthetic has worn off.

Client/Caregiver Teaching

Pretest

- Explain to the client that this test measures the secretion of tears.
- Explain to the client that this test is not painful.
- Instruct the client to remove contact lenses before the test.

Posttest

- Instruct client to avoid rubbing eyes for 30 minutes after procedure and not to reinsert contact lenses for 2 hours.

Scleroderma Antibody

Classification: Immunology

Type of Test: Blood

This test determines the presence of the Scl-70 or scleroderma antibody found in persons with progressive systemic sclerosis.

Indications

- Aid in the diagnosis of scleroderma
- Aid in the diagnosis of suspected CREST syndrome (calcinosis, Raynaud's, esophageal dysfunction, sclerodactyly, telangiectasia)

Reference Values

- Absence of antibody in the blood

Abnormal Values

- Positive level
  CREST syndrome
  Scleroderma

Interfering factors

- Certain drugs, such as aminosalicylic acid, isoniazid, methyldopa, penicillin, propylthiouracil, streptomycin, tetracycline, and trimethadione, may cause false-positive results.

Nursing Implications

Assessment

- Obtain history of known or suspected systemic sclerotic disorders.

Possible Nursing Diagnoses

Anxiety related to perceived threat to health status
Tissue perfusion, altered, related to reduced arterial blood flow

Nutrition, altered, less than body requirements, related to inability to ingest nutrients

Physical mobility, impaired, related to musculoskeletal impairment and associated pain

Implementation

- Put on gloves. Using aseptic technique, perform a venipuncture and collect 5 mL of blood in a red-top tube.
- Handle sample gently to avoid hemolysis and send promptly to the laboratory.

Evaluation

- Note test results in relation to other related tests, particularly tests to detect antibodies in other rheumatic diseases, and to the client's symptoms.

Client/Caregiver Teaching

Pretest

- Explain the purpose of test and the procedure for obtaining the specimen; some discomfort is experienced from the puncture.

Posttest

- Instruct the client to report signs and symptoms related to disease process.

Secretin Test

Classification: Chemistry

Type of Test: Analysis of duodenal contents

Secretin is a hormone normally secreted by the small intestine in response to gastric acidity. It stimulates the pancreas to secrete enzymes and an increased volume of pancreatic juices with high bicarbonate content. This test assesses pancreatic endocrine function by measuring the volume of juices and the amount of bicarbonate, lipase, amylase, and trypsin in duodenal contents before and after pancreatic stimulation with secretin.

Indications

- Monitor pancreatic function in chronic pancreatitis
- Assess suspected cancer of pancreas
- Assess suspected cystic fibrosis

Reference Values

Volume	2–4 mL/kg body weight
Bicarbonate	90–130 mEq/L
Pancreatic amylase	6.6–35.2 U/kg body weight

Abnormal Values

- Decreased levels
    Chronic pancreatitis
    Cystic fibrosis
- Decreased volume, other values normal
    Pancreatic cancer
- Bicarbonate decreased, other values normal
    Pancreatic pseudocyst

Interfering Factors

- Failure to follow dietary restrictions results in stimulation of pancreatic secretion by food particles.
- Improper tube placement results in aspiration of gastric secretions. (Placement is determined by analysis of pH of secretions: gastric pH is acidic, while duodenal secretions are alkaline.)

Nursing Implications

Assessment

- Obtain history of gastrointestinal system, known or suspected pancreatic disease, current symptoms, medication regimen, and results of any diagnostic tests performed.
- Assess for compliance with fasting from foods and fluids for 12 hours and nicotine for 8 to 12 hours before test.
- Assess client's degree of mobility, as the patient will need to assume various positions while the tube is being passed.

Potential Nursing Diagnoses

Anxiety related to potential change in health status

Grieving, anticipatory, risk for, related to perceived loss or fear of death

Implementation

- Explain purpose of the test and the procedure for obtaining the specimens; some discomfort may be experienced from insertion of nasogastric or orogastric tube.
- Put on gloves. Using aseptic technique, insert an intermittent venous access device for administration of secretin.
- Assemble necessary equipment, including double lumen intestinal tube, lubricant, gloves, syringe, and specimen containers. Tube is passed into upper part of stomach, and client's position is changed to assist passage of tube into duodenum. Placement is completed under fluoroscopy.
- Aspirate sample of duodenal secretions as baseline. Administer secretin intravenously, one clinical unit per kg of body weight. Obtain three samples of duodenal aspirate at 20-minute intervals. Place samples in labeled containers, include time of sample, and send to laboratory.
- Provide assistance to position of comfort, and oral or nasal care.

Evaluation

- Observe for allergic reaction to hormones administered and comfort level.

Client/Caregiver Teaching

Pretest

- Instruct client not to eat, drink, or use tobacco products the day of the test.

Posttest

- Advise client to resume food, fluids, and nicotine withheld before test.

Serotonin (5-Hydroxytryptamine)

Classification: Chemistry

Type of Test: Plasma

Serotonin, an amine synthesized by the argentaffin cells of the intestinal mucosa, acts as a vasoconstrictor, neurotransmitter, stimulator of prolactin or growth hormone release, stimulant of smooth muscle contraction, and functions in hemocoagulation. It is stored and transported in platelets, and found in other body tissues. Urine levels of 5-hydroxyindoleacetic acid (5-HIAA) are more commonly measured, because blood serotonin levels are unstable.

Indications

- Aid in the diagnosis of carcinoid tumors

Reference Values

- 10 to 30 μg/dL; 570–1700 nmol/L (SI units)

Abnormal Values

- Increased levels
  Carcinoid syndrome
  Oat cell carcinoma of lung
  Pancreatic islet cell tumor
  Thyroid medullary tumor
  Certain drugs, including methyldopa, imipramine, MAO inhibitors, and reserpine
- Decreased levels
  Depression
  Down syndrome
  Phenylketonuria (PKU)

Interfering Factors

- Radioactive scan within 7 days invalidates results.
- Lithium causes either increased or decreased levels of serotonin in the brain.

Nursing Implications

Assessment

- Obtain history of known or suspected malignancies or carcinoid conditions.
- Note compliance with avoidance of MAO inhibitors and radionuclide scans for 7 days before test.

Possible Nursing Diagnoses

Pain, acute, related to obstruction of pancreatic ducts

Anxiety related to perceived threat to health status

Nutrition, altered, less than body requirements, related to vomiting

Infection, risk for, related to inadequate primary defenses

Implementation

- Put on gloves. Using aseptic technique, perform a venipuncture and collect 7 mL of blood in a chilled lavender-top tube. Place container on ice.
- Handle sample gently to avoid hemolysis and send promptly to the laboratory.

Evaluation

- Compare test results to client symptoms and results of other tests performed.

Client/Caregiver Teaching

Pretest

- Explain purpose of test and procedure for obtaining the specimen; some discomfort is experienced from the puncture.

Posttest

- Resume medications withheld before test.

Serum Complement Assay

Classification: Hematology

Type of Test: Serum

Serum complements are proteins that act as enzymes that aid in the immunologic and inflammatory response. The complement system is also important in destroying and removing foreign material. Serum complement levels are important in detecting autoimmune diseases such as serum sickness and systemic lupus erythematosis. Two particular components called C_3 and C_4 are often assayed along with the complement. They are most important and are more accurate in determining these autoimmune complexes.

In serum complement assay, the blood is mixed with sheep red blood cells (RBCs) that are coated with antibodies. When the complement is present in normal amounts, 50 percent of the RBCs are lysed. Lower amounts of lysed sheep RBCs are associated with decreased quantities of complement.

Indications

- Aid in the diagnosis of autoimmune disorders such as systemic lupus erythematosis (SLE)
- Aid in the diagnosis of cirrhosis of the liver, multiple myeloma, and hypogammaglobulinemia
- Determine allograft rejection
- Aid in the diagnosis of hereditary angioedema

Reference Values

Total complement	40–90 U/mL
C_3	
Men	80–180 mg/dL
Women	76–120 mg/dL
C_4	
Men	15–60 mg/dL
Women	15–52 mg/dL

Values may vary depending on laboratory methods.

Abnormal Values

- Increased
  - Anemias
  - Autoimmune disease (SLE)
  - Cirrhosis
  - Glomerulonephritis
  - Hepatitis
  - Lupus nephritis
  - Malnutrition
  - Protein malnutrition
  - Renal transplant rejection
  - Rheumatoid arthritis
  - Serum sickness
  - Sjögren's syndrome
- Decreased
  - Acute myocardial infarction
  - Acute rheumatic fever
  - Cancer
  - Ulcerative colitis

Interfering Factors

- Recent heparin therapy can affect test results.
- Hemolysis of the blood sample caused by improper or rough handling of the sample can interfere with tests results.
- Failing to immediately transport the sample to the laboratory may interfere with the test results.

Nursing Implications

Assessment

- Obtain history of suspected or known autoimmune abnormality, tests and procedures performed, and results.

Possible Nursing Diagnoses

Anxiety related to perceived threat to or change in health status
Pain related to inflammation of joints and skin eruptions
Fatigue related to increased energy requirements and altered body chemistry
Skin integrity, impaired, related to chronic inflammation

Implementation

- Put on gloves; using aseptic technique perform a venipuncture and collect 7 to 10 mL of blood in a red-top tube.
- Send to the laboratory promptly. Handle sample gently to avoid hemolysis in tube.

Evaluation

- Note test results in association with other tests.

Client/Caregiver Teaching

Pretest

- No fasting is required for this test.

/////////////////////////////////

Sex Chromatin Tests (Barr Body Analysis, Buccal Smear)

Classification: Histology

Type of Test: Buccal mucosa tissue specimen

A sex chromatin body (Barr body) is an X-chromosome that lies against the nuclear membrane of female cells. It is absent in male cells. Barr bodies function in early embryonic development and become inactivated to maintain gene balance of autosomes to X-chromosomes. This screening test for abnormalities in the numbers of sex chromosomes has generally been replaced by the full karotype test.

Indications

- Screen for sex chromosome abnormalities

Reference Values

Normal female	1 Barr body
Normal male	0 Barr body

Abnormal Values

- Ambiguous genitalia
- Turner's syndrome
- Klinefelter's syndrome

Interfering Factors

- Improper specimen collection affects test results. Buccal cells must be scraped firmly enough to avoid saliva, which contains no cells, in the specimen.

Nursing Implications

Assessment

- Obtain genetic history, noting chromosome disorders, diagnostic tests, and results.

Possible Nursing Diagnosis

Growth and development, altered, related to effects of physical disability

Implementation

- Scrape the buccal mucosa of the client firmly at least twice with a wooden or metal spatula. Rub the spatula over a glass slide to evenly distribute the cells.
- Spray the slide with cell fixative and transport to the laboratory immediately.

Evaluation

- Monitor response to procedure.
- Compare test results to clinical symptoms and results of other related diagnostic tests.

Client/Caregiver Teaching

Pretest

- Explain the purpose of the test and the procedure involved; tell the client that the test takes a few minutes to complete.

Posttest

- Instruct that follow-up chromosome analysis may be required based on the results.
- Encourage genetic counseling if a chromosomal cause of abnormal sexual development is identified.

Sickle Cell Test (Sickledex, Hgb S)

Classification: Hematology

Type of Test: Serum

This test uses electrophoresis to measure hemoglobin S (Hgb S) produced when the amino acid valine is substituted for glutamine at a crucial position on the globin chain. This causes the beta chains to "lock" when deoxygenated, deforming the erythrocyte into the sickled shape.

Indications

- Screen for and determine diagnosis of sickle cell anemia or trait
- Evaluate cause of chronic pain

Reference Values

- Negative, no sickled cells

Abnormal Values

- Sickle cell trait (20 to 40 percent Hgb S)
- Sickle cell anemia (70 percent Hgb S)
- Other hemoglobin S abnormalities

Interfering Factors

- False-negative results can occur from transfusions within prior 4 months, anemia, inadequate amount of blood draw (<7 mL), phenothiazine therapy (>128 μg/mL), iron deficiency, thalassemia, elevated Hgb F, and in infants less than 6 months of age.
- False-positive results can occur when less than 7 mL of blood is drawn. They also can occur from polycythemia, elevated blood proteins (systemic lupus erythematosus, multiple myeloma), and Hgb abnormalities.

Nursing Implications

Assessment

- Obtain history, noting familial sickle cell anemia or trait, phenothiazine therapy, and blood transfusions.

Possible Nursing Diagnoses

Gas exchange, impaired, related to decreased oxygen-carrying capacity of blood

Tissue perfusion, altered, related to stasis

Pain related to intravascular sickling with localized vascular stasis

Anxiety related to perceived threat or change in health status

Implementation

- Put on gloves. Using aseptic technique, perform a venipuncture and collect 7mL of blood in a heparinized specimen tub. Gently roll tube to mix sample with anticoagulant.
- Handle specimen gently to avoid hemolysis and send promptly to lab.
- Provide support if specimen collection is unsuccessful and must be repeated.

Evaluation

- Compare test results with patient symptoms and other related diagnostic test results.

Client/Caregiver Teaching

Pretest

- Tell client that fasting is not necessary before this test.

Posttest

- If sickle cell anemia or trait is confirmed, encourage genetic counseling.

Sims-Huhner Test (Postcoital Test, Postcoital Cervical Mucus Test, Cervical Mucus Sperm Penetration Test)

Classification: Histology

Type of Test: Fluid/mucus tissue analysis

Endocervical mucus is examined after intercourse to determine the quality of the mucus and the ability of spermatozoa to penetrate the mucus. This test should be timed with mid-ovulation. Mucus volume is measured, and color and viscosity are observed. Tenacity is measured by grasping a portion of the mucus and noting the distance it can be drawn before it breaks. The sample is placed on a slide and motile sperm are counted. Because it can identify sperm in cervical vaginal secretions, this test also is useful in documenting cases of suspected rape.

Indications

- Document alleged or suspected rape
- Perform an infertility workup when semen analysis is normal

Reference Values

- Mucus tenacity: stretches $\geq$10 cm
- Motile sperm: $\geq$6 to 20 per high-power field

Abnormal Values

- Infertility
- Suspected rape

Interfering Factors

- Specimens obtained >6 hours after intercourse yield unreliable results.

Nursing Implications

Assessment

- Obtain history of reproductive system, current symptoms, diagnostic tests, and results.
- Ensure that male has abstained from ejaculation for 72 hours before test. Use of lubricants during intercourse should be avoided. Female should lie recumbent for 15 to 30 minutes after intercourse, and arrive for testing within 1 to 5 hours.

Possible Nursing Diagnoses

Anxiety related to perceived threat to health status

Tissue integrity, impaired, risk for, related to forceful sexual penetration and trauma to fragile tissues

Rape-trauma syndrome related to actual or attempted sexual attack without consent

Sexual dysfunction related to biopsychosocial alteration of sexuality

Implementation

- In suspected rape cases, handle the client's clothing carefully because additional specimens can be obtained from stains if needed (stains can be tested for semen many months following the event).
- Obtain a signed consent if the specimen is to be used as evidence in a legal action.
- In cases of suspected or alleged rape, be sensitive to feelings of guilt, embarrassment about the event and the procedure; provide additional support to cope with vaginal procedure.
- Assemble the equipment, including vaginal speculum, swabs, gloves, saline, syringes for lavage, slides and container with 95 percent ethanol or sterile container for swabs.
- Have client void and tell client not to wipe following urination.
- Place in lithotomy position and drape for privacy.
- Insert vaginal speculum and secure in place.
- Gently saturate the swab(s) with material from the vaginal walls and place in a sterile container. Ensure that the packaging of the specimen, the placement of the specimen in a container, and the transport of the specimen to the laboratory all comply with institution and legal protocols.
- Properly identify the specimen and immediately transport to the laboratory. Supervise transport according to institution protocol to maintain the chain of evidence. Have a witness sign the request form.

- Administer ordered spermicidal douche after the specimen has been collected.
- At the conclusion of the procedure, return the patient to a position of comfort and allow to rest.

Evaluation

- Remain with client and monitor response to procedure.

Client/Caregiver Teaching

Pretest

- Explain purpose of the procedure and how it is performed; explain that it is performed by the physician or nurse but, in cases of suspected or alleged rape, a witness or law enforcement officer may need to be present.
- Instruct the couple that the male should abstain from ejaculation for 72 hours before the test. Use of lubricants during intercourse should be avoided.
- Tell the female client that she should lie recumbent for 15 to 30 minutes after intercourse and arrive for testing within 1 to 5 hours.
- Ask the female client to avoid douching, using vaginal lubrication, or bathing before the test.

Posttest

- Tell the client when she should expect the test results.
- Instruct in use of prescribed medication to prevent pregnancy.
- Suggest referral to counseling services, if appropriate.

Skin Tests (Blastomycosis, Coccidioidomycosis, Histoplasmosis)

Clasification: Immunology

Type of test: Skin test

These skin tests are usually performed with the tuberculin skin test. The antigens blastomycin, coccidiodin, and histoplasmin are intradermally injected with tuberculin.

A positive response at the puncture site indicates cell-mediated immunity to the organism or a delayed hypersensitivity caused by interaction of the sensitized T lymphocytes.

Indications

- Screen asymptomatic clients for exposure or infection with blastomycosis, coccidioidomycosis, or histoplasmosis

Reference Values

- Negative response or minimal response with no exposure to blastomycosis, coccidioidomycosis, or histoplasmosis

Abnormal Values

- Area of erythema or induration 5×5 mm or larger in diameter

Interfering Factors

- Improper technique in performing the intradermal injection and injecting into subcutaneous tissue causes inaccurate results.
- Incorrect reading (measurement of the response) or timing of the reading can alter results.
- Incorrect amount or dilution of antigen injected or a delay in the injection after drawing the antigen up into the syringe can affect test results.
- Improper storage or contamination of the antigen can alter results.

- Recent or present bacterial, viral, or fungal infections can affect results.
- Diseases such as hematologic cancers or sarcoidosis can alter results.
- Drugs such as immunosuppressive agents or steroids can alter results.

> **NURSING ALERT**
>
> - These tests are contraindicated in those with a history of tuberculosis or previous positive skin test, rash or other eruptions at the injection site, or hypersensitivity to other skin tests or vaccinations.

Nursing Implications

Assessment

- Obtain a history of disease exposure, signs and symptoms indicating possible disease presence, other diagnostic procedures and results, and other skin tests or vaccinations and sensitivities.

Possible Nursing Diagnoses

Infection, risk for, related to inadequate primary defenses

Gas exchange, impaired, risk for, related to decrease in effective lung surface

Activity intolerance related to imbalance between oxygen supply and demand

Anxiety related to perceived threat to health status

Implementation

- Have epinephrine hydrochloride solution (1:1000) available in the event of anaphylaxis.
- Cleanse the skin site on the lower anterior forearm with alcohol or acetone swabs and allow to air dry.
- Prepare specific antigen in a tuberculin syringe with a short 26-gauge needle attached.
- Prepare the appropriate dilution and amount for the most commonly used intermediate strength (5 tuberculin units in 0.1 mL) or a first strength usually used for children (1 tuberculin unit in 0.1 mL).
- Inject preparation intradermally as soon as it is drawn up into the syringe, at the prepared site causing a bleb or wheal to form within the layers of the skin.
- Record the site and remind the client or caregiver to return in 48 to 72 hours to have the test read.

Evaluation

- At the time the test is read, inspect the area on the client's arm in good light, measure the diameter of any induration with a plastic ruler, and palpate the area for a thickening of the tissue. A positive result is indicated by a 5 mm or more reaction with erythema and edema.

Client/Caregiver Teaching

Pretest

- Inform the client that the test is generally done by a nurse in a physician's office or in a health-care setting and takes about 5 to 10 minutes to complete.
- Inform the client that a small amount of pain can be experienced when the intradermal injection is performed.
- Emphasize to the client that the area should not be scratched or disturbed after the injection and before the reading.

Posttest

- Emphasize to the client or caregiver the need to return later to have the test results read (the time depends on the test).
- Inform the client that the effects from a positive response at the site can remain for up to 1 week.
- Reinforce information about further testing needed and answer or direct questions to the appropriate professionals.

Slit Lamp Biomicroscopy

Classification: Sensory organ function

Type of Procedure: Visual perception

This noninvasive procedure is used to visualize the anterior portion of the eye and its parts, including the eyelids and eyelashes, sclera, conjunctiva, cornea, iris, lens, and anterior chamber, and to detect pathology of any of these areas of the eyes. The slit lamp has a binocular microscope and light source that can be adjusted to examine the fluid, tissues, and structures of the eyes. Special attachments to the slit lamp are used for special studies and more detailed views of specific areas.

Indications

- Detect corneal abrasions, ulcers, or abnormal curvatures (keratocoma)
- Detect lens opacities indicative of cataract formation
- Determine the presence of blepharitis, conjunctivitis, hordeolum, entropion, ectropion, trachoma, scleritis, and iritis
- Detect conjunctival and corneal injuries by foreign bodies and determine if ocular penetration or anterior chamber hemorrhage is present
- Detect deficiency in tear formation indicative of lacrimal dysfunction causing dry eye disease that can lead to corneal erosions or infections
- Evaluate the fit of contact lenses

Reference Values

- Normal anterior tissues and structures of the eyes.

Abnormal Values

- Blepharitis
- Conjunctivitis
- Corneal abrasions
- Corneal ulcers
- Ectropion
- Entropion
- Hordeolum
- Iritis
- Keratoconus (abnormal curvatures)
- Lens opacities
- Scleritis
- Trachoma

Interfering Factors

- Inability of the client to cooperate during the examination affects test results.
- Improper administration of mydriatics, if used, can cause inaccurate results.

> **NURSING ALERT**
> - This procedure is contraindicated in clients with narrow-angle glaucoma and in those allergic to mydriatics.

Nursing Implications

Assessment

- Obtain a history of external and anterior eye structure conditions, known and suspected eye disorders or allergies, signs and symptoms of eye abnormalities, treatment regimens, eye tests and procedures done, and results.

Possible Nursing Diagnoses

Anxiety related to perceived threat to health status
Sensory/perceptual alteration (visual), related to impaired vision caused by abnormality of eye structure and function

Implementation

- Ask client to remove corrective lenses (glasses or contacts) unless the study is being done to check the fit and effectiveness of the contact lenses.
- Administer an ordered mydriatic to each eye, 1 drop of 5% phenylephrine and repeat in 5 to 15 minutes to achieve pupil dilation if the exam is not done for routine inspection.
- Seat the client in a chair in a dimmed room with the client's feet on the floor. Tell the client to place his or her chin on the rest apparatus and his or her forehead against the bar apparatus.
- The physician places the slit lamp in front of the client's eyes in line with the examiner's eyes. The external structures of the eyes are inspected with the special bright light and microscope of the slit lamp. The light is then directed into the client's eyes to inspect the anterior fluids and structures, and is adjusted for shape, intensity, and depth needed to visualize these areas. Magnification of the microscope is also adjusted to optimize visualization of the eye structures.
- Special attachments and procedures can also be used to obtain further diagnostic information about the eyes. These may include, for example, a camera to photograph specific parts, gonioscopy to determine anterior chamber closure, and a cobalt blue filter to detect minute corneal scratches, breaks, and abrasions with corneal staining.

Evaluation

- Note test results in relation to other related tests performed and the client's symptoms.

Client/Caregiver Teaching

Pretest

- Tell the client that the procedure is performed by a physician and takes about 10 minutes to complete; explain there is no pain associated with this procedure.
- Instruct the client to remain still during the examination and look straight ahead while the eyes are examined.

Posttest

- Tell the client that some blurring of vision can occur and last about 2 hours if the pupils are dilated; caution the client not to drive or operate any machinery during this time.
- Provide emotional support to the client during and after diagnostic findings are revealed; if abnormalities are detected; answer or direct questions to the appropriate professionals.

Specific Gravity

Classification: Urinalysis

Type of Test: Urine (random)

This test measures the specific gravity of urine, that is, its density compared with that of a similar volume of distilled water when both solutions are at the same or similar temperatures. The normal specific gravity of distilled water is 1.000 while that of urine is greater because it reflects the density of the substances dissolved in it. Urine's specific gravity is an indication of the kidney's ability to reabsorb water and chemicals from the glomerular filtrate and aids in evaluating hydration status and in detecting problems related to secretion of antidiuretic hormone.

Reference Values

Newborn	1.012
Infant	1.002–1.006
Adults (usual)	1.010–1.025

NPO overnight	1.022
NPO for 24 hr	1.026
Following standard water load in concentration and dilution testing	<1.003

Abnormal Values

- Increased levels
    Dehydration
    Diabetes mellitus
    Adrenal insufficiency
    Congestive heart failure
    Diarrhea and vomiting
    Elevated temperature
    Glomerulonephritis
    Proteinuria
    Syndrome of inappropriate antidiuretic hormone secretion (SIADH)
    Certain drugs, including intravenous solutions of dextran or high-molecular-weight fluids
- Decreased levels
    Fluid overload
    Diabetes insipidus
    Chronic renal insufficiency
    Hypothermia
    Increased intracranial pressure
    Certain drugs, including aminoglycosides, lithium, and methoxyflurane

Interfering Factors

- Failure to test fresh specimen will alter readings.
- Allowing the glass cylinder to touch the sides or bottom of the urometer when reading the calibration can cause inaccurate results.

Nursing Implications

Assessment

- Obtain a history of renal disorders, fluid intake and losses, and other urinary tests and results.

Possible Nursing Diagnosis

Nutrition, altered, less than body requirements, related to inability to use nutrients

Infection, risk for, related to decreased leukocyte function

Fluid volume excess related to abnormal cardiac or renal function

Implementation

- *Dipstick procedure:* Obtain a fresh urine specimen in a clean plastic container and insert dipstick into urine. Compare results with chart on container.
- *Urinometer procedure:* Obtain the clean dry urinometer and place on a level surface. Fill 3/4 full with 15 mL of urine. Allow to come to room temperature. Spin or turn the glass cylinder while inserting into urinometer to make sure that it is floating freely. Read the bottom of the meniscus when the movement stops and the cylinder is not touching the side or bottom.
- *Refractometer procedure:* Clean the cover and prism with a drop of distilled water and a cloth and allow to dry. Close the cover, and holding the instrument horizontally, apply a drop of urine at the notched bottom of the cover. Allow the drop to cover the prism surface. Point the instrument toward the light source and rotate the eyepiece until the scale can be read. Read the scale between the dividing line between the dark and light contrast.
- Transport the specimen to the laboratory immediately for further testing or within 2 hours if refrigerated.

Evaluation

- Note test results in relation to other tests performed and the client's symptoms.
- The specific gravity of urine provides preliminary information. For a more thorough evaluation of renal concentrating ability, urine osmolarity should be determined and concentration or dilution tests performed.
- For determinations in concentration-dilution tests, subtract 0.003 from every 1 g/dL of protein or 0.004 from every 1 g/dL of glucose.

Client/Caregiver Teaching

Pretest

- If client is being tested for urinary concentration ability, food and fluids may be restricted, as ordered.

Spondee Speech Reception Threshold (SRT)

Classification: Audiometry

Type of Test: Auditory perception

This noninvasive speech audiometric procedure measures hearing loss related to speech. In this test, several familiar spondee words, that is, words containing two syllables that are equally accented, are presented to the client at different intensities. The intensity at which the client repeats 50 percent of the words correctly reveals the test result. Word recognition tests can also be done to assist in diagnosing high-frequency hearing loss. Those with this type of hearing loss miss consonant sounds that affect the understanding of speech. The test involves the ability to recognize and repeat words that are distinguished by consonants and are presented at a level above the spondee threshold. Word recognition ability is a different type of hearing loss than that diagnosed by audiometry.

Indications

- Determine the extent of hearing loss related to speech recognition, evidenced by the faintest level at which spondee words are correctly repeated
- Differentiate a real hearing loss from pseudohypoacusis
- Evaluate clarity of speech sounds or speech discrimination, evidenced by word recognition at 40 dB above the spondee threshold

Normal Findings

- Normal spondee threshold of about 10 dB of the pure tone threshold with 50 percent of the words presented being correctly repeated at an appropriate intensity
- Normal speech recognition with 90 percent to 100 percent of the words presented being correctly repeated at an appropriate intensity

Abnormal Findings

- Conductive hearing loss
- Sensorineural hearing loss (acoustic nerve impairment)
- High-frequency hearing loss

Interfering Factors

- Unfamiliarity with the language the words are presented in or with the words themselves will alter test results.
- Improper placement of the earphones and inconsistency in frequency of word presentation will affect results.

Nursing Implications

Assessment

- Obtain a history of known or suspected hearing disorders, results of pure tone audiometry and other hearing tests, and the client's ability to understand English words and sounds.

Possible Nursing Diagnoses

Anxiety related to perceived threat to health status or perceived inability to perform test requirements effectively

Sensory/perceptual alteration (auditory) related to impaired hearing (conductive or sensorineural)

Implementation

- Seat the client on a chair in a soundproof booth. Place the earphones on the client's head and secure them over the ears. The audiometer is set at 20 dB above the known pure tone threshold obtained from audiometry (see p. 141). The test represents hearing levels at speech frequencies of 500, 1000, and 2000 Hz.
- The spondee words are presented to the ear with the best auditory using a speech audiometer. The intensity is decreased and then increased to the softest sound at which the client is able to hear the words and respond correctly to 50 percent of them. The procedure is then repeated for the other ear.
- Test speech discrimination by presenting a list of 50 phonetically balanced words such as ''pin,'' ''bin,'' ''kin'' at an intensity of 40 dB above the spondee reception threshold. A score is determined from the number of responses. A normal score of 90 percent to 100 percent indicates a conduc-

tive hearing loss; a reduced score indicates sensorineural hearing loss and acoustic (eighth) nerve impairment.

Evaluation

■ Note the results in relation to the client's symptoms and other test results, particularly audiometry.

Client/Caregiver Teaching

Pretest

■ Inform the client how the procedure is performed; explain that the procedure, which takes about 5 to 10 minutes to complete, is performed in a specially equipped soundproof booth by an audiologist and that no pain is associated with this procedure.

■ Inform the client that a series of words that change from loud to soft tones will be presented using earphones and that he or she will be requested to repeat the word. Explain that each ear is tested separately.

Posttest

■ Provide information about future testing appointments, if needed.

Sucrose Hemolysis

Classification: Hematology

Type of Test: Blood

Paroxysmal nocturnal hemoglobinuria (PNH) is an anemia characterized by red blood cells with an abnormal sensitivity to complement and erythocyte hemolysis. Symptoms include episodic loss of hemoglobin in the urine at night, leukopenia, and thrombocytopenia. Sucrose provides a medium of low ionic strength that promotes binding of the complement to red blood cells. Blood demonstrates excess lysis in those with PNH.

Indications

■ Screen for paroxysmal nocturnal hemoglobinuria (PNH)

Reference Values

- Negative, or less than 5 percent hemolysis.

Abnormal Values

- Positive levels: Paroxysmal nocturnal hemoglobinuria

Interfering Factors

- False-positive results occur in megaloblastic anemia, auto-immune hemolytic anemias, lymphoma, and colon cancer.
- False-negative results occur with recent blood transfusion or incorrect blood tube.
- Clotting or hemolysis of sample invalidates results.

Nursing Implications

Assessment

- Obtain history of cardiovascular system, known or suspected hematological disorders, diagnostic tests and results.

Possible Nursing Diagnoses

Tissue perfusion, altered, related to abnormal oxygen-carbon dioxide exchange
Protection, altered, related to abnormal blood profiles

Implementation

- Put on gloves; using aseptic technique perform a venipuncture and collect 5 mL of blood in a blue-top tube.
- Provide support if puncture is not successful and another must be performed to obtain the specimen.

Evaluation

- Note results in relation to client symptoms and other related test results particularly the Ham test.

Client/Caregiver Teaching

Pretest

- Inform client that there is no need to fast before the test.

Sweat Test (Pilocarpine Iontophoresis)

Classification: Chemistry

Type of Test: Sweat analysis

Sweat test, also known as pilocarpine iontophoresis sweat test, is a noninvasive study performed to obtain a definitive diagnosis of cystic fibrosis in children when considered with other test results and physical assessments. This test measures the concentration of sodium and chloride content in sweat produced by the sweat glands of the skin following inducement to increase its production by a small electric current carrying the drug pilocarpine. A high concentration indicates the presence of the disease.

Indications

- Diagnose or confirm cystic fibrosis in children
- Screen for cystic fibrosis in those with a family history of the disease
- Screen for suspected cystic fibrosis in failure to thrive infants or malabsorption syndrome or recurrent respiratory infections in children

Reference Values

Concentration in Sweat		SI Units
Sodium	10–70 mEq/L	10–70 mmol/L
Chloride	5–45 mEq/L	5–45 mmol/L

Abnormal Values

- Elevated levels
  Cystic fibrosis in children with >70 mEq/L sodium or >45 mEq/L chloride
  Chronic pulmonary infections
  Addison's disease

Hypothyroidism
Malnutrition

Interfering Factors

- Inadequate amount of sweat makes it difficult to perform test accurately.
- Improper cleansing of skin or application of gauze pad or paper affects test results.
- Hot environmental temperatures may reduce sodium chloride; cool environmental temperatures may affect the amount of sweat collected.

NURSING ALERT

- This test is contraindicated in skin disorders (rash, erythema, eczema) and not recommended for the newborn because the amount of sweat produced is insufficient for testing.
- Terminate the test if the client complains of burning at the electrode site. Reposition the electrode before the test is resumed, but never use the chest because of the risk for cardiac arrest from the current.

Nursing Implications

Assessment

- Obtain a history of cystic fibrosis in other family members, failure to thrive, endocrine disorder, and results of other tests performed.
- Determine if the test follows a screening procedure performed with test paper that revealed a positive result for cystic fibrosis; assess clinical picture and family history.

Possible Nursing Diagnoses

Airway clearance, ineffective, related to excessive production of thick mucus and decreased ciliary action

Nutrition, altered, less than body requirements, related to impaired digestive process

Grieving, anticipatory, related to potential lifestyle changes resulting from chronic disorder

Implementation

- Encourage caregiver to stay with and support the child during the test.

- The client is placed in a position to allow exposure of the site on the forearm.
- Two sites (right arm or right thigh) can be used if the client is a small infant to ensure the collection of an adequate amount of sweat. The client should be covered to prevent cool environmental temperatures from affecting sweat collection.
- The site is washed with distilled water and dried. A positive electrode is attached to the site and covered with a pad that is saturated with pilocarpine hydrochloride, a drug that stimulates sweating. A negative electrode is covered with a pad that is saturated with a bicarbonate solution. Iontophoresis is achieved by supplying a low-level electric current via the electrode for 5 to 12 minutes. Battery-powered equipment is preferred over an electric outlet to supply the current.
- The electrodes are removed revealing a red area at the site, and the site is washed with distilled water and dried to remove any possible contaminants on the skin.
- Disks made of filter paper that are weighed are placed on the site with a forcep and covered with paraffin or plastic sealed at the edges to prevent any possible evaporation of the sweat collected. This is left in place for about 1 hour. Provide distraction for the child with books, TV, or games to allay fears.
- The paraffin or covering is removed and disks are placed in a preweighted flask with a forcep. The flask is sealed and sent immediately to the laboratory for weighing and analysis for Na and Cl content. At least 100 mg of sweat is required for testing.
- Screening for cystic fibrosis can be performed by using a silver nitrate test paper, and a positive test can be validated by pilocarpine iontophoresis. A new battery-operated device that uses patches on the skin that change color when the sweat chloride levels are elevated, after sweating is induced by pilocarpine iontophoresis, is also used to perform this test.
- Cleanse test area with soap and water and dry thoroughly.

Evaluation

- Observe site for unusual color, sensation, or discomfort.
- Note test results in relation to other related tests and client symptoms.

Client/Caregiver Teaching

Pretest

- Explain the purpose of the procedure and how the procedure is performed; explain that the procedure is generally performed at the client's bedside or in the laboratory by a technician with the results interpreted by a physician and that the procedure takes about 1 1/2 hours to complete.

- Explain that a positive sweat test alone is not diagnostic of cystic fibrosis; repetition of both borderline and positive tests is generally recommended.
- Inform caregiver and child that no diet, medication, or activity restrictions are required.
- Inform caregiver and child that there is no pain associated with the test but that a stinging sensation can be experienced at the site as the electrical current causing this is applied at a very low level.

Posttest

- Inform caregiver and child that redness at the site will fade in 2 to 3 hours.
- Reinforce information regarding diagnosis and recommended treatment regimen and help caregiver and child to cope with long-term implications.
- Provide information regarding genetic counseling and possible screening of other family members if appropriate.

T-Lymphocyte and B-Lymphocyte Assays

Classification: Chemistry

Type of Test: Serum

T-lymphocyte and B-lymphocyte assays are used to diagnose a number of immunological disorders. A variety of methods are used. The most common way to assess T-cell activity is to measure the individual's response to delayed hypersensitivity skin tests. This involves intradermal injection of minute amounts of several antigens to which the individual has previously been sensitized (e.g., tuberculin, mumps, *Candida*). Erythema and induration should occur at the site within 24 to 48 hours. Absence of response is termed *anergy,* and thus, the test is frequently called an *anergy panel.* Anergy to skin tests reflect either a temporary or a permanent failure of cell-mediated immunity.

Other measures of T lymphocytes and B lymphocytes involve determining the number of cell types present. T lymphocytes are recognized by their ability to form rosettes with sheep erythrocytes (i.e., the sheep red cells surround the T lymphocyte). Although the sheep erythrocytes adhere to the cell membrane of the T lymphocytes, they will react to neither B lymphocytes nor null cells.

T lymphocytes and their subsets also may be distinguished by their ability to react with various monoclonal antibodies. Monoclonal antibodies constitute a single species of immunoglobulins with specificity for a single antigen and are produced by immunizing mice with specific antigens. The most commonly used monoclonal antibodies to T lymphocytes are designated T_3, T_4, and T_8. T_3 is a pan-T-cell antibody that reacts with a determinant present on all mature peripheral T lymphocytes and can, therefore, be used to enumerate the total number of T cells present. T_4 antibodies identify helper T cells, while T_8 antibodies identify suppressor T cells.

Other monoclonal antibodies include T_{10}, T_9, and T_6. T_{10} and T_9 antibodies react with very immature T lymphocytes (thymocytes) that are found in the thymus gland but not in the peripheral circulation. T_{10} antigen also is seen in mature thymocytes that are localized primarily in the medullary regions of the thymus. T_6 antibodies also react with certain immature thymocytes. As T lymphocytes mature, reactivity to T_6 antibodies is lost. Tests involving reactivity to immature T lymphocytes are useful in diagnosing T-cell leukemias and lymphomas.

B lymphocytes are detected by immunofluorescent techniques. This is accomplished by mixing lymphocyte suspensions with heterologous antisera to immunoglobulins that have been labeled with a dye such as fluorescein. The antisera combine with B lymphocytes and when the suspension is examined by fluorescent microscopy, only B lymphocytes appear.

T lymphocytes and B lymphocytes can be differentiated by electron microscopy, as T cells are smooth and B cells have surface projections. This technique is not, however, available in many laboratories.

Indications

- Diagnose disorders associated with abnormal levels of T lymphocytes and B lymphocytes
- Diagnose disorders associated with abnormal T-cell subtypes
- Support the diagnosis of acquired immunodeficiency syndrome (AIDS), as indicated by decreased helper T cells, normal or increased suppressor T cells, and a decreased ratio of helper to suppressor T cells
- Diagnose severe combined immunodeficiency (SCID), an in-

herited disorder characterized by failure of the stem cell to differentiate into T lymphocytes and B lymphocytes
- Diagnose DiGeorge syndrome characterized by failure of the thymus (and parathyroids) to develop with a resulting decrease in T lymphocytes
- Diagnose X-linked agammaglobulinemia characterized by severe B-lymphocyte deficiency
- Diagnose common variable, hypogammaglobulinemia (CVH) characterized by absent, decreased, or defective B cells and most commonly due to either lack of helper T lymphocytes or abnormal suppressor T cells
- Monitor response to therapy

Reference Values

T lymphocytes	60–80% of circulating lymphocytes*
B lymphocytes	10–20% of circulating lymphocytes
Null cells	5–20% of circulating lymphocytes
Helper T lymphocytes	50–65% of circulating T lymphocytes
Suppressor T lymphocytes	20–35% of circulating T lymphocytes
Ratio of helper to suppressor T lymphocytes 2:1	

*A decreased lymphocyte count (lymphopenia) usually indicates a decrease in the number of circulating T lymphocytes.

Abnormal Values

- An abnormal T cell or B cell only suggests specific diseases. Further testing is needed for confirmation of these diseases.

Disorders Causing Altered Levels of T Lymphocytes and B Lymphocytes

T Lymphocytes	
Increased Levels	*Decreased Levels*
Acute lymphocytic leukemia	DiGeorge syndrome
Multiple myeloma	Chronic lymphocytic leukemia
Infectious mononucleosis	Acquired immunodeficiency syndrome (AIDS)
Grave's disease	Hodgkin's disease
	Nezelof syndrome
	Wiskott-Aldrich syndrome
	Waldenström's macroglobulinemia
	Severe combined immunodeficiency (SCID)
	Long-term therapy with immunosuppressive drugs

B Lymphocytes

Increased Levels	Decreased Levels
Chronic lymphocytic leukemia	Acute lymphocytic leukemia
Multiple myeloma	X-linked agammaglobulinemia
DiGeorge syndrome	SCID
Waldenström's macroglobulinemia	
Acute lupus erythematosus	

Adapted from Boggs, DR and Winkelstein, A: White Cell Manual, ed. 4. FA Davis, Philadelphia, 1983, p. 72.

Disorders Associated with Abnormal T-Cell Subsets

Immune Deficiency Diseases (Helper and/or Suppressor Activity)	Autoimmunity (Helper and/or Suppressor Activity)
Common variable hypogammaglobulinemia	Connective tissue diseases
Acute viral infections, such as infectious mononucleosis and cytomegalic inclusion disease	Acute graft-versus-host disease
Chronic graft-versus-host disease	Autoimmune hemolytic disease
Multiple myeloma	Multiple sclerosis
Chronic lymphocytic leukemia	Myasthenia gravis
Primary biliary cirrhosis	Inflammatory bowel disease
Sarcoidosis	Atopic eczema
Immunosuppressive drugs	
Acquired immunodeficiency syndrome (AIDS)	

Adapted from Boggs, DR and Winkelstein, A: White Cell Manual, ed 4. FA Davis, Philadelphia, 1983, p. 72.

Interfering Factors

- Medications that can increase lymphocytes include steroids and immunosuppressives.
- Factors that can affect T-cell and B-cell counts include stress, surgery, chemotherapy, steroid or immunosuppressive therapy, and x-rays.

- Refrigeration or freezing blood decreases lymphocyte counts.

Nursing Implications

Assessment

- Obtain history of factors that can affect T-cell and B-cell counts; note any medications taken by client that could affect counts (see Interfering Factors).

Possible Nursing Diagnoses

Protection, altered, related to abnormal blood profiles
Pain related to tissue inflammation
Nutrition, altered, less than body requirements, related to altered ability to ingest nutrients
Anxiety related to threat to or change in health status

Implementation

- Put on gloves; select a site in an extremity that does not have an intravenous infusion or vascular access device in place; cleanse skin with povidone-iodine or 70 percent alcohol, and allow to air dry.
- Using aseptic technique, perform a venipuncture and collect 7 mL of blood in a heparinized green-top tube.
- Handle the sample gently to avoid hemolysis and send to the laboratory immediately; keep specimen at room temperature and process within 3 hours.
- Ensure that the venipuncture site is kept clean and dry since clients with T cell and B cell changes have a compromised immune system.

Evaluation

- Note test results in relation to other related tests.

Client/Caregiver Teaching

Pretest

- Explain that the purpose of the test is to measure certain kinds of white blood cells and to obtain information about the immune system.

Posttest

- Refer the client for additional testing depending on the test results.

T and B Lymphocyte Surface Markers

Classification: Chemistry

Type of Test: Blood

The two types of lymphocytes are T cells (thymus derived) and B cells (bursa derived). T cells function as effector cells in cellular immune reactions and interact with B cells. T cells display the following two functions: the "helper function" where T cells and B cells interact to form antibodies and the "suppressor function" in which T cells and B cells interact to suppress certain B-cell functions.

Lymphocyte marker assay, with the use of microscopy or flow cytometry, produces reactants with specific antibodies linked to fluorescent dyes or to enzymes.

Indications

- Evaluate immune function
- Assist in diagnosis of lymphocytic leukemia, lymphoma, and acquired immunodeficiency syndrome
- Aid in diagnosis and treatment of chronic infections, hepatitis, and autoimmune disorders

Reference Values

T cells (CD3)	53–88%
T-helper (CD4) cells	32–61%
T-suppressor (CD8) cells	18–42%
B cells	5–20%
Lymphocyte count	0.66–4.60 thousand/μL
T-cell count	812–2318 cells/μL
B-cell count	99–426 cells/μL
Helper cell count (CD4)	589–1505 cells/L
Suppressor T-cell count (CD8)	325–997 cells/μL
CD4:CD8 ratio	>1.0

Abnormal Values

- Increased B-cell count
    Active lupus erythematosus
    Chronic lymphocytic leukemia
- Increased T-cell count
    Graves' disease
- Decreased B-cell count
    Transient hypogammaglobulinemia of infancy
    X-linked hypogammaglobulinemia
    Selective deficiency of immunoglobulin G, immunoglobulin A, and immunoglobulin M lymphomas
    Nephrotic syndrome
    Multiple myeloma
- Decreased T-cell count
    DiGeorge syndrome
    Nezelof syndrome
    Hodgkin's or other malignant disease
    Acute viral infection
- Decreased B and T cells
    Autosomal or sex-linked recessive immunodeficiency
    Wiskott-Aldrich syndrome
    Radiation and aging
- Decreased lymphocyte count
    Follows immunosuppressive and cytotoxic drug therapy
- Decreased CD4 : CD8 ratio
    <1.0 owing to loss of T-helper lymphocytes

Interfering Factors

- Hemolysis of blood can affect test results.
- Refrigerating or freezing blood decreases lymphocyte counts.

Nursing Implications

Assessment

- Obtain history of factors that can affect T-cell and B-cell counts; note any medications taken by client that could affect counts.

Possible Nursing Diagnoses

Anxiety related to perceived threat to or change in health status
Pain related to widespread inflammatory process affecting connective tissue
Skin integrity, impaired, related to chronic inflammation

Fatigue related to increased energy requirements and altered body chemistry

Protection, altered, related to abnormal blood profiles

Implementation

- If client has an autoimmune disease and antilymphocyte antibodies are suspected, notify laboratory.
- Put on gloves and using aseptic technique, perform a venipuncture and collect 10 mL of blood in a red-top tube.
- Handle the sample gently to avoid hemolysis and send to the laboratory immediately.

Evaluation

- Note test results in relation to client's symptoms and other tests performed.

Client/Caregiver Teaching

Pretest

- Explain that the purpose of the test is to evaluate key portions of the immune system; explain the procedure to obtain the specimen, and tell the client that some discomfort is experienced from the puncture.

Posttest

- Ensure that the venipuncture site is kept clean and dry since clients with T-cell and B-cell changes have a compromised immune system.

Tensilon Test

Classification: Neurologic function

Type of Test: Pharmacologic challenge

This pharmacologic challenge study is performed to assist in the diagnosis of myasthenia gravis. The pharmacologic agent, edrophonium chloride (Tensilon), is a short-acting form of the drug used to treat this disorder. The test involves administering the drug intravenously before and during various muscular movements and evaluating these movements for changes in muscle strength. A positive diagnosis is made when the administration of the drug improves muscle function. A negative diagnosis is made if muscle fasciculations occur in response to the drug.

Indications

- Diagnose myasthenia gravis when fatigue and muscle weakness are present, evidenced by an immediate improvement following injection of edrophonium chloride
- Monitor medication regimen of oral anticholinesterase to determine if an increase in dose is advised, evidenced by an improvement in muscle strength after injection of edrophonium chloride, or if an overdose is present placing the client in cholinergic crisis, evidenced by an exaggeration of muscle weakness following injection

Reference Values

- Muscle fasciculations following injection of edrophonium chloride; no muscle weakness, autonomic dysfunction

Abnormal Values

- Myasthenia gravis

Interfering Factors

- Medications such as corticosteroids, muscle relaxants, and anticholinergics can alter test results by their effect on muscle function or edrophonium chloride action.

> **NURSING ALERT**
>
> - This test is contraindicated in breathing difficulties or apneic conditions since the disease can cause respiratory difficulties severe enough to require ventilatory support.

Nursing Implications

Assessment

- Obtain a history of respiratory or musculoskeletal disorders, drug sensitivities, medication regimen that includes those that affect muscle function, anticholinesterase therapy and time and amount of last dose, and other diagnostic procedures done.

■ Ensure that medications that can affect muscle function have been withheld.

Possible Nursing Diagnoses

Swallowing, impaired, related to neuromuscular impairment of laryngeal/pharyngeal impairment

Fatigue related to abnormal neuromuscular function

Communication, impaired, verbal, related to neuromuscular weakness, fatigue, and physical barrier

Breathing pattern, ineffective, related to neuromuscular weakness and decreased energy

Implementation

■ Have emergency resuscitation equipment nearby; have atropine available for treatment of cholinergic crisis and neostigmine for treatment of myasthenic crisis to be administered intravenously, if needed.

■ Place the client in a supine or sitting position on the examining table with the arm to be used for the IV exposed and supported with an armboard. Start an IV infusion of 5% glucose in water or normal saline and administer an initial dose of Tensilon, usually about 2 mg for an adult with adjustments based on weight in kg for children.

■ Ask the client to perform activities to fatigue the muscles, for example, holding the arms up until they drop. Administer the remaining 8 mg of Tensilon over a 30-second time period to total a dose of 10 mg. Ask the client to perform muscle movements such as crossing and uncrossing the legs, opening and closing the eyes, and raising and lowering the arms.

■ Observe for improvement in muscle strength; dramatic improvement indicates that the weakness is caused by myasthenia gravis. Repeat the test to ensure accuracy if muscle strength does not improve following the injection.

■ Administer atropine during the test for those clients with asthma to decrease the side effects of Tensilon. During the procedure, assess for the side effects of Tensilon, which include abdominal cramps, bradycardia, diaphoresis, diarrhea, hypotension, incontinence, papillary constriction, respiratory distress, and salivation.

■ When used to evaluate oral anticholinesterase medication regimen, infuse 2 mg of Tensilon. Note the following 1 hour after a dose of the medication: a brief improvement in muscle strength indicates that an increase in the therapy would be beneficial and a decrease in muscle strength indicates that a reduction in therapy is needed.

- To differentiate between myasthenic and cholinergic crisis, infuse 1 to 2 mg of Tensilon and observe for muscle strength improvement or respiratory difficulty. In the absence of muscle strength improvement, another 5 mg can be infused, 1 mg at a time, under close observation for any distress.

Evaluation

- Note results in relation to client's symptoms and other related tests.
- Monitor the client for Tensilon side effects, including abdominal cramps, bradycardia, diaphoresis, diarrhea, hypotension, incontinence, papillary constriction, respiratory distress, and salivation.

Client/Caregiver Teaching

Pretest

- Inform the client and caregiver that the procedure is generally performed by a physician in an examining room equipped with all the necessary supplies. Tell the client and caregiver that the procedure takes about 30 minutes to complete and that no pain is associated with the procedure.
- Inform the client that no food or fluid restrictions are required.

Posttest

- Instruct the client to resume medications restricted before the test, as ordered.

Testosterone

Classification: Hormone

Type of Test: Blood

Testosterone, a male hormone, is made by the Leydig cells in the testicle. In women, the ovary and adrenal gland secrete small amounts of this hormone; however, the majority of testosterone in females is from the metabolism of androstenedione. Spermatogenesis is affected by testosterone. In men, a testicular, adrenal, or pituitary tumor can cause an overabundance of testosterone thereby triggering precocious puberty; in women, adrenal tumors, hyperplasia, and medications can cause an overabundance of this hormone resulting in masculinization.

Indications

- Aid in the diagnosis of hypergonadism
- Evaluate male infertility
- Distinguish between primary and secondary hypogonadism
- Evaluate hirsutism
- Aid in the diagnosis of male sexual precocity before the age of 10

Reference Values

Men	300–1200 ng/dL
Women	30–95 ng/dL
Prepubertal children	
Boys	<100 ng/dL
Girls	<40 ng/dL

Abnormal Values

- Men: Increased levels
  Adrenal hyperplasia
  Adrenocortical tumors
  Idiopathic sexual precocity
  Testicular or extragonadal tumors
- Men: Decreased levels
  Corticosteroid use
  Cryptorchidism
  Down's syndrome
  Klinefelter's syndrome
  Primary and secondary hypogonadism
  Uremia
- Women: Increased levels
  Adrenocortical hyperplasia
  Adrenocortical tumors
  Arrhenoblastoma
  Idiopathic hirsutism
  Ovarian tumors
  Polycystic ovaries
  Trophoblastic tumors during pregnancy

Interfering Factors

- Certain drugs, for example, androgens, dexamethasone, diethylstilbestrol, digoxin, alcohol, ketoconazole, steroids, phenothiazine, and spironolactone, can cause decreased test results.
- Certain drugs, for example, anticonvulsants, estrogens, oral contraceptives, and barbiturates, can cause increased test results.

Nursing Implications

Assessment

- Assess the client history for drugs and disorders that may affect test results.

Possible Nursing Diagnoses

Nutrition, altered, less than body requirements, related to inability to ingest adequate nutrients for hypermetabolic rate

Tissue integrity, impaired, risk for, related to altered protective mechanisms

Fatigue related to hypermetabolic rate

Implementation

- Put on gloves. Using aseptic technique, perform a venipuncture and collect 7 mL of blood in a red-top tube.
- Handle the sample gently to avoid hemolysis and send to the laboratory immediately.

Evaluation

- Note results in relation to other client's symptoms and other related tests.

Client/Caregiver Teaching

Pretest

- Inform the client that there are no fluid or food restrictions.
- Explain that the test is best performed in the morning.

Posttest

- Pending test results, explain the importance of proper treatment and adhering to the drug regimen.

Thermography, Breast

Classification: Photodiagnostic

Type of Test: Indirect visualization

This noninvasive photographic study measures and records the skin surface temperature of the breast tissue. The heat generated by tissue abnormalities causes an increased blood flow to the area. When photographed by an infrared detector and camera, these areas show up as a pictorial variation (thermogram) of cold spots, hot spots, and gray shades. This study is primarily done to assist in the diagnosis of breast malignancy. It is not a popular diagnostic tool now that mammography can be performed with reduced radiation exposure and better accuracy. An abnormal finding on breast thermography is followed by mammography and breast biopsy to confirm the diagnosis.

Indications

- Detect breast tumor in its early stage, evidenced by hot or white spots
- Differentiate between neoplastic and benign tumors, evidenced by hot spots or gray shades, respectively
- Detect fibrocystic disease or infections of the breast, evidenced by a brighter shade of red in the hot spots

Reference Values

- Normal breast symmetry and color shading appearance on thermogram

Abnormal Values

- Cancer
- Fibrocystic changes
- Acute suppurative infection

Interfering Factors

- Skin condition of breasts, such as sunburn or eruptions, can change skin temperature.

- Skin lotions, oils, or powders can cause inaccurate test results.
- Pregnancy increases the vascularity of the breasts and heat production and therefore can cause inaccurate test results.
- Changes in room temperatures can affect test results.

NURSING ALERT

- This procedure is contraindicated in client's with engorged breasts during the premenstrual stage in the menstrual cycle and in client's who recently had an acute breast infection.

Nursing Implications

Assessment

- Obtain a history of suspected or known breast abnormalities, pregnancy, and menstrual status.
- Ensure that no lotions or powders have been applied to the breasts before the study.

Possible Nursing Diagnoses

Anxiety related to perceived threat to health status
Body image disturbance related to change in appearance
Grieving, anticipatory, related to perceived loss or threat of death

Implementation

- Have the client remove clothing from the waist up and provide a gown to wear with the opening to the front. Ask the client to wash off any lotions or powders and pat dry.
- Place the client in a sitting position in a cool room with a temperature of about 68°F for 15 minutes to obtain heat equilibrium. Then ask the client to place her hands on her hips or over her head.
- Place the thermoscope on the breast and obtain a baseline temperature. The scanning device is properly set and the scanning unit is placed on both breasts. Three photographs are taken at different angles, usually for frontal and lateral views. At the conclusion of the photographing, the films are checked and the client is allowed to dress.

Evaluation

- Note test results in relation to the client's symptoms and other test results, particularly mammography and breast biopsy.

Client/Caregiver Teaching

Pretest

- Inform the client that the procedure is generally performed by a technologist in a specially equipped room in the radiology department with the results interpreted by a physician; also inform the client that the procedure takes about 20 minutes to complete and that no pain is associated with the procedure.
- Inform the client that no food or fluid restrictions are required.

Posttest

- Inform the client that test results are available within 2 days.
- Reinforce information regarding diagnosis and additional procedures recommended to confirm diagnosis.
- Instruct client on how to perform a monthly breast self examination; ask the client to demonstrate the procedure, if appropriate.

Thrombin Clotting Time (TCT, Plasma Thrombin Time)

Classification: Hematology

Type of Test: Plasma

This coagulation test is performed to evaluate the common final pathway of the coagulation sequence. Preformed thrombin (coagulation factor IIa) is added to the blood sample to convert fibrinogen (factor I) directly to a fibrin clot. A prolonged time indicates an abnormal conversion of the fibrinogen to fibrin. Because the test bypasses the intrinsic and extrinsic pathway, deficiencies in either one do not affect the TCT.

Indications

- Confirm diagnosis of suspected disseminated intravascular coagulation (DIC) as indicated by a prolonged TCT

- Detect hypofibrinogenemia or defective fibrinogen
- Monitor the effects of heparin or fibrinolytic therapy

Reference Values

- 5 seconds with 15 to 20 seconds control; <1.5 times control (values vary among laboratories or depend on concentration of thrombin reagent used)

Abnormal Values

- Prolonged time
  Acute leukemia
  Amyloidosis
  Cirrhosis
  DIC
  Factor deficiency
  Hypofibrinogenemia
  Lymphoma
  Obstetric complications
  Polycythemia vera
  Shock
  Certain drugs, including asparaginase, fibrin degradation products, heparin, streptokinase, tissue plasminogen activator (TPA), and urokinase
- Decreased time
  Thrombocytosis

Interfering Factors

- A fibrinogen level <100 mg/dL (normal: 150 to 400 mg/dL) will prolong the TCT.
- Abnormally functioning fibrinogen will prolong the TCT.
- Fibrinogen inhibitors such as streptokinase and urokinase will prolong the TCT.
- Traumatic venipunctures and excessive agitation of the sample can alter test results.

Nursing Implications

Assessment

- Obtain history of bleeding disorders; if client is receiving anticoagulant therapy, note time and amount of the last dose.

Possible Nursing Diagnoses

Fluid volume deficit, risk for, related to failure of regulatory mechanism

Tissue perfusion, altered, related to alteration of arterial flow

Gas exchange, impaired, risk for, related to reduced oxygen-carrying capacity

Anxiety related to perceived threat to health status

Implementation

- Put on gloves. Using aseptic technique, perform a venipuncture; collect 2 mL and discard and then collect a 5-mL blood sample in a light blue-top tube.
- Avoid traumatic venipunctures and excessive agitation of the sample.

Evaluation

- Note test results in relation to client's symptoms and other tests performed.

Client/Caregiver Teaching

Pretest

- Advise the client to notify the person taking the blood sample when the last dose of anticoagulant medication was taken.

Posttest

- Instruct the client to report bleeding from the skin or mucous membranes.

Thoracentesis and Pleural Fluid Analysis

Classification: Histology

Type of Test: Pleural fluid analysis

Thoracentesis is an invasive procedure performed to remove pleural fluid from the space surrounding the lung (pleural effusion). Effusions can be transudates or exudates. Hematologic, cytologic, microbiologic, and chemistry examination of the fluid is performed for complete analysis.

Indications

- Evaluate pleural effusion of unknown etiology
- Differentiate pleural transudates from exudates
- Diagnose suspected traumatic hemothorax
- Diagnose suspected pleural effusion (exudate) due to pulmonary tuberculosis
- Diagnose suspected pleural effusion (exudate) due to pneumonia (parapneumonic) effusion
- Diagnose suspected bacterial or tuberculous empyema (exudate)
- Diagnose suspected pleural effusion (exudate) due to carcinoma
- Diagnose suspected pleural effusion (exudate) due to pulmonary infarction
- Diagnose suspected pleural effusion (exudate) due to rheumatoid disease
- Diagnose suspected pleural effusion (exudate) due to systemic lupus erythematosus as indicated by findings similar to those in rheumatoid disease, except that glucose is not usually decreased
- Diagnose suspected pleural effusion (exudate) due to pancreatitis
- Differentiate chylous pleural effusions (exudate) due to thoracic lymphatic duct blockage from pseudochylous (chronic serous) effusions
- Remove excessive fluid as therapeutic measure

Reference Values

- Pleural cavity maintains negative pressure and contains <20 mL of serous fluid.

Red blood cells (RBC)	0–<1000/mm³
White blood cells (WBC)	0–<1000/mm³ consisting mainly of lymphocytes and neutrophils
Gram stain and culture	No organisms present
Cytologic examination	No abnormal cells
pH	7.37–7.43 (usually >7.40)
Glucose	70–100 mg/dL
Protein	3.0 g/dL
Pleural fluid:serum protein ratio	≤0.5
Lactic dehydrogenase (LDH)	45–90 U/L
Pleural fluid:serum LDH ratio	<0.6

Amylase	<180 Somogyi U/dL or <200 dye U/dL
Triglycerides	Parallel serum levels
Cholesterol	<60 mg/dL
Immunoglobulins	Parallel serum levels
Carcinoembryonic antigen (CEA)	Parallel serum levels
Complement	Parallel serum levels

Abnormal Values

- Trauma as indicated by bloody pleural fluid, elevated red cell count, and hematocrit similar to that found in whole blood.
- Pulmonary infarction as indicated by red cell count of 1,000 to 100,000/mm^3; white cell count of 5,000 to 15,000/mm^3 consisting mainly of neutrophils and sometimes including eosinophils; pH >7.30; normal glucose level; and elevated protein, LDH, and related ratios.
- Tuberculosis as indicated by the presence of RBCs (<10,000/mm^3), white cell count of 5,000 to 10,000/mm^3 consisting mostly of lymphocytes, the presence of acid fast bacilli (AFB) on smear and culture, pH <7.30, decreased glucose level (sometimes), and elevated protein, pleural fluid:serum protein ratio, LDH, and pleural fluid:serum LDH ratio.
- Carcinoma as indicated by the presence of RBCs (1,000–>100,000/mm^3); white cell count of 5,000 to 10,000/mm^3 consisting mostly of lymphocytes and sometimes including eosinophils; detection of malignant cells on cytologic examination; pH <7.30 or >7.30; decreased glucose level (sometimes); increased protein, LDH, and related ratios; elevated CEA and immunoglobulins; and decreased complement.
- Pancreatitis as indicated by red cell count of 1,000 to 10,000/mm^3; white cell count of 5,000 to 20,000/mm^3 consisting mostly of neutrophils; pH >7.30; normal glucose level; elevated protein, LDH, and related ratios; and elevated amylase.
- Lymphoma.
- Chronic lymphocytic leukemia.
- Pneumonia as indicated by the presence of red blood cells (<5,000/mm^3); white cell count of 5,000 to 25,000/mm^3 consisting mainly of neutrophils and sometimes including eosinophils; pH <7.40; and elevated protein, pleural fluid:serum protein ratio, LDH, and pleural fluid:serum LDH ratio. If the pneumonia is of bacterial origin, the organism may be demonstrated on culture and the pleural fluid glucose level may be decreased.

- Rheumatoid disease as indicated by a normal red cell count; a white cell count of 1,000 to 20,000/mm^3 with either lymphocytes or neutrophils predominating; pH <7.30; decreased glucose level; elevated protein, LDH, and related ratios; and elevated immunoglobulins.
- Pneumothorax.
- Parasitic and hypersensitivity syndromes.
- Congestive heart failure.
- Transudative pleural fluid effusion can result from ascites.
- Systemic and pulmonary venous hypertension.
- Hepatic cirrhosis.
- Nephritis.
- Pleurisy.
- Pseudochylous and chylous effusions with chylous effusion indicated primarily by a triglyceride level two to three times that of serum, decreased cholesterol level, and markedly elevated chylomicrons.

Interfering Factors

- Presence of blood in the sample from traumatic thoracentesis can affect test results.
- Undetected hypoglycemia or hyperglycemia can alter results.
- Contamination of the sample with skin cells and pathogens can affect test results.

> ### NURSING ALERT
>
> - This procedure is contraindicated in clients with bleeding disorders.

Nursing Implications

Assessment

- Obtain history of pulmonary symptoms, pain, discomfort or shortness of breath, as well as laboratory results and diagnostic findings. Obtain date of last menstrual period and assess possibility of pregnancy in premenopausal women.
- Ensure that anticoagulant medications and aspirin have been withheld as ordered.
- Determine if client has a persistent or uncontrollable cough for which a cough suppressant may be necessary before the procedure.

Possible Nursing Diagnoses

Airway clearance, ineffective, related to thick viscous or bloody secretions

Nutrition, altered, less than body requirements, related to inability to ingest adequate nutrients

Gas exchange, impaired, related to decrease in effective lung surface

Anxiety related to perceived threat to health status

Implementation

- Administer a cough suppressant, if ordered.
- Assemble the following equipment: a thoracentesis tray with solution for skin preparation, a local anesthetic, a 50-mL syringe, needles of various sizes including a thoracentesis needle, sterile drapes, and sterile gloves. Sterile collection bottles and containers for culture and cytologic examination also are needed.
- Help the client to a sitting position on the side of a bed or treatment table; have the client lean slightly forward to spread the intercostal spaces; support the client's arms on an overbed table with several pillows. Alternately, the client may sit on the bed or table with legs extended on it and arms supported as described previously. If the client cannot assume either sitting position, the sidelying position is used. In such situations, the client lies on the unaffected side.
- Cleanse the skin on the posterior chest with an antiseptic solution and protect the area with sterile drapes. The skin at the needle insertion site is then infiltrated with local anesthetic causing a stinging sensation. The thoracentesis needle is inserted and when fluid appears, a stopcock and 50-mL syringe are attached to the needle, and 50 mL of fluid is aspirated.
- Send pleural fluid samples immediately to the laboratory in a sterile container. Be sure to label the container. Record any antibiotic therapy on the laboratory slip if bacterial culture and sensitivity tests are to be performed.
- If the thoracentesis is being performed for therapeutic as well as diagnostic reasons, additional pleural fluid, up to 1 L, can be withdrawn. When the desired amount of fluid has been removed, the needle is withdrawn, and slight pressure is applied to the site for a few minutes. If there is no evidence of bleeding or other drainage, a sterile bandage is applied to the site.
- During the procedure, observe client for signs of respiratory distress or pneumothorax (e.g., anxiety, restlessness, dyspnea, cyanosis, tachycardia, and chest pain).

- Help the client to lie on the unaffected side. Remind the client that this position should be maintained for approximately 1 hour. The head may be elevated for comfort. A chest x-ray may be ordered to ensure that a pneumothorax from the tap has not occurred.

Evaluation

- Note results in relation to other test results and the client's symptoms.
- Observe the client for respiratory distress and auscultate breath sounds; absent or diminished breath sounds on the side used for the thoracentesis can indicate pneumothorax.
- Monitor for signs of pneumothorax, tension pneumothorax, fluid reaccumulation, pulmonary edema or cardiac distress caused by mediastinal shift.

Client/Caregiver Teaching

Pretest

- Tell the client that the procedure is performed by a doctor and where the procedure is performed. Explain that fluid samples are taken from the space around the lungs and that the procedure can take approximately 20 minutes to complete.
- Inform the client of the importance of not coughing, breathing deeply, or moving during the procedure.
- Prepare the client to expect stinging when the local anesthetic is given and pressure when the needle is inserted.

Posttest

- Instruct the client to resume medications and usual activity withheld before the test.
- Ask the client to report chest pain or changes in respirations and hemoptysis to the physician immediately.

Thoracoscopy

Classification: Endoscopy

Type of Test: Direct visualization

Thoracoscopy is endoscopic visualization of the pleural space by direct injection of the endoscope into the chest wall. It can be used for diagnostic and therapeutic purposes. Complications include nerve injury, air emboli, hemorrhage, perforation of the diaphragm, and tension pneumothorax.

Indications

- Aid in the diagnosis of pleural disease
- Perform lung wedge resections
- Treat pleural conditions such as blebs and effusions
- Obtain a biopsy from the mediastinum

Interfering Factors

- Excessive bleeding during the procedure will affect test results.
- Inability of client to remain still will affect test results.
- Extensive disease may prevent treatment by this procedure.

Reference Values

- A small amount of lubricating fluid should be found in the pleural cavity. The visceral and parietal layers should be free of lesions and able to be separated from each other.

Abnormal Values

- Cancer
- Conditions predisposing to pneumothorax
- Inflammatory processes
- Bleeding sites
- Tuberculosis, coccidioidomycosis, histoplasmosis
- Pleural effusion
- Empyema

> ### Nursing Alert
>
> - This procedure is contraindicated in clients with compromised respiratory status by obstructive or restrictive pulmonary disease or in clients at risk for respiratory failure.

Nursing Implications

Assessment

- Obtain history of known or suspected pulmonary disease, cardiac disease, or chest trauma.
- Assess the client's ability to remain still.
- Confirm that the client has remained NPO for 8 hours before the procedure.
- Assess the results of other diagnostic tests such as respiratory function tests.

Possible Nursing Diagnoses

Activity intolerance related to imbalance between oxygen supply and demand

Airway clearance, ineffective, related to trauma, tracheobronchial obstruction, or secretions

Gas exchange, impaired, related to altered oxygen-carrying capacity

Anxiety related to perceived threat to or change in health status

Implementation

- Establish an intravenous line.
- The client is anesthetized and the doctor inserts an endobronchial tube. The lung on the operative side is collapsed. an intracostal incision is made, and a trocar is inserted. The areas to be assessed are viewed with a small lens. The camera lens and instruments are moved from one site to another to view all necessary areas.
- After the procedure, the lung is expanded and a chest tube is placed in one of the incision sites. The other incisions are closed.

Evaluation

- Note result in relation to other procedures and diagnostic tests.
- Also note test results in relation to the client's symptoms.
- Monitor vital signs every 15 minutes for 1 hour, then every 4 hours.

■ Assess respiratory status and the patency of the chest drainage system.

Client/Caregiver Teaching

Pretest

■ Inform the client about the purpose of the procedure; tell the client that he or she will receive general anesthesia and will have several incisions and a chest drainage system.
■ Inform the client that he or she must fast from food and fluid for 8 hours before the procedure.

Posttest

■ Provide emotional support during and after diagnostic findings are reported; reinforce information regarding diagnosis and recommended treatment regimen.

Thyroglobulin

Classification: Chemistry

Type of Test: Serum

Thyroglobulin is a protein secreted by the thyroid into its follicles. It reacts with iodine to form thyroid hormones. When thyroid hormones are released into the bloodstream, they split with thyroglobulin in response to stimulation by thyroid-stimulating hormone (TSH).

Indications

■ Diagnose differentiated cancer of the thyroid
■ Diagnose suspected disorders of excess thyroid hormone
■ Monitor response to treatment of thyroid cancer

Reference Values

■ 3–42 ng/mL in those with normal thyroid
■ 0–5 ng/mL in those with thyroid removed

Abnormal Values

- Increased level
  Untreated thyroid cancer
  Graves' disease
  Subacute thyroiditis
  Benign adenoma

Interfering Factors

- Autoantibodies to thyroglobulin can cause decreased values.
- Newborns have normally very high levels.

Nursing Implications

Assessment

- Obtain history of endocrine system, suspected or known thyroid abnormality, tests and procedures performed, and results.

Possible Nursing Diagnoses

Anxiety related to perceived threat to or change in health status
Fatigue related to hypermetabolic imbalance with increased energy requirements
Nutrition, altered, risk for less than body requirements, related to inability to ingest adequate nutrients for hypermetabolic rate
Tissue integrity, impaired, risk for, related to altered protective mechanisms

Implementation

- Put on gloves; using aseptic technique perform a venipuncture and collect 7 mL of blood in a red-top tube.
- Send specimen to the laboratory.

Evaluation

- Note test results in association with other thyroid tests (triiodothyronine [T_3], thyroxine [T_4], TSH).

Client/Caregiver Teaching

Pretest

- Explain to the client the purpose of the test and the procedure to obtain the specimen; prepare the client to expect some discomfort from the puncture.

Posttest

■ Instruct the client to report signs and symptoms of hypothyroidism or hyperthyroidism.

/////////////////////////////////////

Thyroid Antithyroglobulin Antibody

Classification: Serology

Type of Test: Serum

Thyroid antiglobulin antibody is an autoantibody directed against thyroglobulin. Thyroglobulin is a glycoprotein that functions in T_3 and T_4 synthesis.

Indications

■ Confirm suspected inflammation of thyroid gland
■ Diagnose suspected thyroid autoimmunity in those with other autoimmune disorders
■ Diagnose suspected hypothyroidism caused by thyroid tissue destruction

Reference Values

■ Negative, or titer 1:100

Abnormal Values

■ Increased values
    Anemias (autoimmune, autolytic, or pernicious)
    Goiter
    Thyroiditis
    Autoimmune disorders

Interfering Factors

■ None

Nursing Implications

Assessment

- Obtain history of endocrine system, suspected or known thyroid abnormality, tests and procedures performed, and results.

Possible Nursing Diagnoses

Anxiety related to perceived threat to or change in health status

Physical mobility, impaired, related to weakness, fatigue, muscle aches, altered reflexes, and mucin deposits in joints and interstitial spaces

Sensory alteration, tactile, related to mucin deposits and nerve compression

Fatigue related to decreased metabolic energy production

Implementation

- Put on gloves. Using aseptic technique, perform a venipuncture and collect 7 mL of blood in a red-top tube.
- Send specimen to the laboratory

Evaluation

- Note test results in association with other thyroid tests.

Client/Caregiver Teaching

Pretest

- Explain the purpose of the test, implications of test results, and who will perform the venipuncture.
- Advise the client that the only discomfort, although slight, should occur during the venipuncture.
- Advise the client to stop thyroid medication 6 weeks before the test, as ordered.

Posttest

- Instruct the client to resume medications withheld before the test.
- Provide support and referrals pending test results.
- Inform the client of the need for any additional testing pending test results.

Thyroid Hormone Binding Ratio

Classification: Chemistry

Type of Test: Blood

This procedure measures the amount of unbound thyroid hormone binding sites on thyroxine binding globulin (TBG). TBG is a protein carrier of thyroid hormones. Value is obtained by measuring triiodothyronine (T_3) uptake after all binding sites are saturated, and dividing by the mean percent T_3 uptake of the reference serum.

Indications

- Diagnose hypothyroidism or hyperthyroidism
- Diagnose suspected disorders associated with altered TBG levels

Reference Values

T_3 uptake	25–35%
Thyroid hormone binding ratio (THBR)	
Adults <50 yr	0.85–1.14
Adults >50 yr	
Women	0.80–1.04
Men	0.87–1.11
Children	
Cord blood	0.75–1.05
1–3 d	0.90–1.40
1–2 w	0.85–1.15
4–16 w	0.75–1.05
1–15 yr	0.88–1.12

Abnormal Values

- Increased T_3 uptake and THBR
    Decreased TBG
    Hyperthyroidism
    Hyperandrogenic state

Certain drugs, including adrenocorticotropic hormone, androgens, barbiturates, corticosteroids, furosemide, thyroxine, thyroid extract, heparin, dilantin, and salicylates
- Decreased T_3 uptake and THBR
  Cretinism
  Endocrine secreting tumors
  Hypothyroidism
  Certain drugs, including chlorpromazine, estrogens, heroin, lithium, methadone, oral contraceptives

Interfering Factors

- Falsely elevated levels may occur in severe acidosis and atrial fibrillation.

Nursing Implications

Assessment

- Obtain history of endocrine system, suspected or known thyroid abnormality, tests and procedures performed, and results.

Possible Nursing Diagnoses

Anxiety related to perceived threat to or change in health status
Fatigue related to hypermetabolic imbalance with increased energy requirements
Nutrition, altered, less than body requirements, related to inability to ingest adequate nutrients for hypermetabolic rate
Tissue integrity, impaired, risk for, related to altered protective mechanisms

Implementation

- Put on gloves; using aseptic technique perform a venipuncture and collect 7 mL of blood in a red-top tube.
- Send specimen to the laboratory.

Evaluation

- Note test results in relation to client's symptoms and other related test results particularly other thyroid tests (T_3, thyroxine [T_4], thyroid-stimulating hormone [TSH]).

Client/Caregiver Teaching

Pretest

- Explain purpose of test and the procedure to obtain the specimen.

Posttest

■ Instruct the client to report signs and symptoms of hypothyroidism or hyperthyroidism.

▲▲▲▲▲▲▲▲▲▲▲▲▲▲▲▲▲▲▲▲▲▲

Thyroid-Stimulating Hormone (TSH)

Classification: Chemistry

Type of Test: Serum; Blood for filter paper test

This test measures serum thyroid-stimulating hormone (TSH), also known as thyrotropin. It is produced by the basophil cells of the adenohypophysis in response to stimulation by the hypothalamic releasing factor, thyrotropin-releasing hormone (TRH). TRH stimulates the release and circulating levels of thyroid hormones and responds to variables such as cold, stress, and increased metabolic need. Both thyroid and pituitary function can be evaluated by TSH measurement.

Indications

■ Diagnose hypothyroidism or hyperthyroidism and/or suspected pituitary or hypothalamic dysfunction
■ Differentiate functional euthyroidism from true hypothyroidism in debilitated individuals, with the former indicated by normal levels

Reference Values

		SI Units
Newborns	<20 µU/mL by day 3	<20 mU/L
Adults	<10 µU/mL	<10 mU/L
Older Adults		
Women	2.0–16.8 µU/mL	2.0–16.8 mU/L
Men	2.0–7.3 µU/mL	2.0–7.3 mU/L
Filter paper test		
At birth	30 µU/mL	30 mU/L
3 d	<20 µU/mL	<20 mU/L
10 d	<10 µU/mL	<10 mU/L

Abnormal Values

- Elevated levels
    Congenital hypothyroidism in neonate (filter paper test)
    Primary hypothyroidism
    Thyroiditis (Hashimoto's autoimmune disease)
    Antithyroid therapy for hyperthyroidism
    Secondary hyperthyroidism due to pituitary hyperactivity
    Prolonged emotional stress
    Drugs including lithium carbonate and potassium iodide
- Decreased levels
    Secondary hypothyroidism (pituitary involvement)
    Primary hyperthyroidism
    Anterior pituitary hypofunction
    Drugs including aspirin, adrenal corticosteroids, heparin
      and dopamine

Interfering Factors

- Results are not valid if client received a radioactive isotope within the prior 7 days.
- Drugs can produce decreased or elevated TSH levels (see Abnormal Values).
- Falsely increased levels may occur in hydatidiform mole, choriocarcinoma, embryonal carcinoma of the testes, pregnancy, and postmenopausal states characterized by high follicle-stimulating hormone (FSH) and luteinizing hormone (LH) levels.

Nursing Implications

Assessment

- Obtain history of endocrine system, suspected or known thyroid abnormality, test and procedures performed, and results.
- Assess medication history and ensure that any drugs that may alter test results have been withheld for 12 to 24 hours before the test as ordered by physician.
- Ensure client has avoided shellfish and other iodine-containing foods for several days before the test.

Possible Nursing Diagnoses

Physical mobility, impaired, related to decreased metabolic energy production
Sensory alterations, related to mucin deposits and nerve compression

Nutrition, altered, risk for less than body requirements, related to inability to ingest adequate nutrients for hypermetabolic rate

Implementation

- Put on gloves. Using aseptic technique, perform a venipuncture and collect 5 mL of blood in a red-top or green-top tube.
- Handle the sample gently to avoid hemolysis and transport to the laboratory immediately.
- If filter paper test on neonate is performed, obtain kit and cleanse heel with antiseptic; perform puncture and touch filter paper to puncture, and saturate with a spot of blood.

Evaluation

- Note test results in association with other thyroid tests (triiodothyronine [T_3], thyroxine [T_4], thyroid antibody tests, thyroid immunoglobulins).

Client/Caregiver Teaching

Pretest

- Instruct the client to withhold medication that can interfere with test results for 12 to 24 hours, if ordered.
- Tell the client to withhold shellfish and iodine-containing foods for several days before the test.

Posttest

- Instruct the client to resume medications withheld before the test.
- Instruct the client to report signs and symptoms of hypothyroidism or hyperthyroidism.

Thyroid-Stimulating Hormone Sensitive (s-TSH) Assay

Classification: Chemistry

Type of Test: Serum

Thyroid stimulating hormone (TSH or thyrotropin) controls metabolism by regulating production of thyroid hormones triiodothyronine (T_3) and thyroxine (T_4). Low T_3 and T_4 levels cause TSH increase. The TSH sensitive assay (s-TSH) can detect both primary hypothyroidism and hyperthyroidism, while TSH detects only hypothyroidism. As a result, this test is becoming a primary screening tool for thyroid disorders.

Indications

- Diagnose primary hyperthyroidism and hypothyroidism
- Monitor response to therapy

Reference Values

	SI Units
0.4–10 mIU/L	0.4–10 U/L

Values may vary depending on assay method.

Abnormal Values

Primary hyperthyroidism	<0.1 mIU/L
Borderline, suggest further testing	0.1–0.4 mIU/L
Primary hypothyroidism, either transient or permanent	>10 mIU/L
Borderline hypothyroidism	6–10 mIU/L

Interfering Factors

- Conditions that raise human chorionic gonadotropin may cause false elevations in some assay methods.
- Hemolysis of sample may affect test results.
- Severe illness and drugs, such as glucocorticoids and dopamine, may affect test results.

Nursing Implications

Assessment

- Obtain history of endocrine system, known or suspected thyroid abnormality, test and procedures performed, and results.
- Ensure that client has fasted for 10 to 12 hours, avoided fatty foods for several days, and has continued thyroid hormone replacement therapy, if appropriate.

Possible Nursing Diagnoses

Physical mobility, impaired, related to decreased metabolic energy production

Sensory alterations, related to mucin deposits and nerve compression

Nutrition, altered, risk for, less than body requirements, related to inability to ingest adequate nutrients for hypermetabolic rate

Implementation

- Put on gloves. Using aseptic technique perform a venipuncture and collect 5 mL of blood in a red-top tube.
- Handle sample carefully to avoid hemolysis.

Evaluation

- Note results in relation to other related thyroid tests and the client's symptoms.

Client/Caregiver Teaching

Pretest

- Instruct the client to fast for 10 to 12 hours as well as to avoid fatty foods and drugs that may affect test results. Advise the client to continue taking thyroid hormone replacement, if appropriate.

Posttest

- Advise the client to resume medications withheld before the test.

Thyroid-Stimulating Hormone Stimulation Test, Thyrotropin Stimulating Test, Thyrotropin Challenge Test

Classification: Chemistry

Type of Test: Serum

The thyroid-stimulating hormone (TSH) stimulation test is used to evaluate the thyroid-pituitary-hypothalamic feedback loop. In this test, a purified form of hypothalamic thyrotropin-releasing hormone (TRH) is administered intravenously. Normally, TRH will stimulate the adenohypophysis to release thyroid-stimulating hormone (TSH), which, in turn, causes hormonal release from the thyroid gland. A normal response, for example, elevated TSH levels, indicates that the adenohypophysis is capable of responding to TRH stimulation. If thyroid hormones also are measured as part of the test, elevated levels indicate that the thyroid gland is capable of responding to TSH stimulation.

Indications

- Evaluate low or undetectable serum TSH levels and/or hypothyroidism or hyperthyroidism of unknown etiology or type

Reference Values

- TSH levels rise within 15 to 30 minutes of TRH administration, peak at 2.5 to 4 times normal, and return to baseline levels within 2 to 4 hours. Thyroid hormone secretion (triiodothyronine [T_3] and thyroxine [T_4]) levels should increase by 50 to 75 percent in 1 to 4 hours.

Abnormal Values

- Hypothalamic dysfunction or disruption of the hypothalamic-hypophyseal portal circulation confirms the diagnosis of tertiary hypothyroidism as indicated by a normal or delayed TSH response in persons with low baseline TSH levels and signs of hypothyroidism.

- Hypopituitarism and secondary hypothyroidism as indicated by a decreased or absent TSH response in persons with low baseline TSH levels and signs of hypothyroidism.
- Primary hypothyroidism as indicated by a normal or increased TSH response in clients with elevated baseline TSH levels and signs of hypothyroidism, with persistently decreased thyroid gland hormone levels.
- Primary hyperthyroidism as indicated by a decreased or absent TSH response in persons with low baseline TSH levels and signs of hyperthyroidism, with persistently elevated thyroid gland hormone levels.

Interfering Factors

- Inability of the client to cooperate affects test results.

Nursing Implications

Assessment

- Obtain history of endocrine system, suspected or known thyroid abnormalities, tests and procedures, and results.
- Ensure that the client has avoided shellfish or any iodine-containing foods for several days before the test.

Possible Nursing Diagnoses

Physical mobility, impaired, related to weakness or fatigue
Fatigue related to decreased metabolic energy production
Sensory perception, altered, related to mucin deposits and nerve compression

Implementation

- Put on gloves. Using aseptic technique, obtain a 5-mL baseline blood sample in a red-top tube.
- Handle the sample gently to avoid hemolysis; label the container with the time the blood was drawn and transport to the laboratory immediately.
- Administer a bolus of TRH (protirelin [Thypinone] or thyrotropin [Thytropar]) intravenously.
- Obtain additional blood samples at 30 minutes; at 1, 2, 3, and 4 hours after administration of the TRH; or as directed by the laboratory.
- Place each sample in a red-top tube, label, and send to the laboratory.

Evaluation

- Note the results in relation to clinical symptoms and other related thyroid tests, such as the TSH test.

Client/Caregiver Teaching

Pretest

- Instruct the client to fast from food and fluids for 8 hours before the test and to avoid shellfish and iodine-containing foods for several days before the test.

Posttest

- Tell the client to resume food, fluids, and medications withheld before the test.

Thyroid-Stimulating Hormone, Neonatal (Neonatal Thyrotropin)

Classification: Immunoassay

Type of Test: Serum

This test is used to confirm hypothyroidism after an initial screening test detects low thyroxine (T_4) levels. Elevated thyroid-stimulating hormone (TSH) levels together with decreased T_4 levels indicate congenital hypothyroidism and thyroid gland dysfunction. Early diagnosis and treatment are critical to the prevention of cretinism and mental retardation.

Indications

- Aid in the diagnosis of congenital hypothyroidism

Reference Values

- 1 to 3 days: 25 to 30 μIU/mL
- Then after levels are normally <25 μU/mL

Abnormal Values

- Elevated TSH levels combined with decreased T_4 levels indicate congenital hypothyroidism and thyroid gland dysfunction.
- Decreased TSH and T_4 levels indicate secondary congenital hypothyroidism and pituitary hypothalamic dysfunction.
- A normal TSH level and a depressed T_4 level may indicate hypothyroidism owing to a congenital defect in thyroxine-binding globulin or transient congenital hypothyroidism owing to hypoxia or prematurity.

Interfering Factors

- Hemolysis from rough handling of the sample may cause inaccurate results.
- Corticosteroids may lower test results.
- Potassium iodide, excessive topical resorcinol, TSH injection, and lithium carbonate may raise the test results.
- Failure to let the paper filter sample dry may affect test results.

Nursing Implications

Assessment

- Obtain history of endocrine system, suspected or known thyroid abnormality, tests and procedures performed and results.
- Assess medication history and ensure that any drugs that may alter test results have been withheld for 12 to 24 hours before test as ordered by physician.

Possible Nursing Diagnoses

Physical mobility, impaired, related to weakness, fatigue, muscle aches, altered reflexes, and mucin deposits in joints and interstitial spaces

Fatigue related to decreased metabolic energy production

Sensory (tactile) alterations related to mucin deposits and nerve compression

Implementation

- *For a serum sample:* Put on gloves. Using aseptic technique, perform a venipuncture and collect 5 mL of blood in a red-top tube. Send sample to the laboratory immediately.

- *For a filter paper sample:* Put on gloves and wipe the infant's heel with povidone iodine or alcohol swab and allow the area to dry completely with a gauze pad. Perform a heelstick, squeeze the infant's heel gently, and fill the circles on the filter paper with blood. Be sure that the blood saturates the filter paper.
- Apply pressure to the heelstick with a gauze pad to stop the bleeding.
- Allow the paper to dry thoroughly and then send the sample to the laboratory immediately.

Evaluation

- Note test results in association with other thyroid tests.

Client/Caregiver Teaching

Pretest

- Inform the infant's parents of the purpose of the test and the implications of test results.

Posttest

- Inform the parents of the need for any additional testing pending test results.

Thyroid-Stimulating Immunoglobulins (TSI, TSIg)

Classification: Chemistry

Type of Test: Serum

This test measures the thyroid-stimulating immunoglobulin levels (TSI, TSIg). These antibodies react with the thyroid cell surface receptor that usually combines with thyroid stimulating hormone (TSH). The TSI reacts with the receptors, activates intracellular enzymes, and promotes epithelial cell activity that operates outside the feedback regulation for TSH. These antibodies were formerly known as long-acting thyroid stimulators (LATS).

Indications

- Evaluate known or suspected thyrotoxicosis with elevated levels found in 50 to 80 percent of affected individuals
- Determine possible etiology of exophthalmos as indicated by elevated levels
- Monitor response to treatment for thyrotoxicosis with possible relapse indicated by elevated levels

Reference Values

- Negative; may be found in the serum of about 5% of people without apparent hyperthyroidism or exophthalmos

Abnormal Values

- Elevated levels
  Thyrotoxicosis
  Exophthalmos
  Hyperthyroidism
  Graves' disease

Interfering Factors

- Administration of radioactive iodine preparations within 24 hours of the test can affect test results.
- Autoimmune thyroiditis or nonspecific goiter may elevate the test results.

Nursing Implications

Assessment

- Obtain a history of known or suspected thyroid disorders, tests performed, and test results.
- Ensure that the client has not received any radioactive iodine preparations within 24 hours of the test.

Possible Nursing Diagnoses

Fatigue related to hypermetabolic imbalance with increased energy requirements

Nutrition, altered, risk for less than body requirements, related to inability to ingest adequate amounts of nutrients

Tissue integrity, impaired, risk for, related to altered protective mechanisms

Implementation

- Put on gloves. Using aseptic technique, perform a venipuncture and collect 7 mL of blood in a red-topped tube.
- Handle the sample gently to avoid hemolysis and transport to the laboratory immediately.

Evaluation

- Note the results in relation to other studies performed, particularly other thyroid studies, and the client's symptoms.

Client/Caregiver Teaching

Pretest

- Inform the client that there are no restrictions before the test.

Posttest

- Instruct the client in thyroid medication therapy prescribed by physician.

Thyroid Stimulator, Long-acting (LATS)

Classification: Chemistry

Type of Test: Blood

Long-acting thyroid stimulator (LATS) is an abnormal immunoglobulin that mimics the action of thyroid-stimulating hormone (TSH). It stimulates the thyroid to produce and secrete thyroid hormones in excessive amounts. Because of normal negative feedback mechanisms, it causes decreased TSH secretion. LATS is found in those with Graves' disease or neonates whose mothers have Graves' disease.

Indications

- Confirm diagnosis of Graves' disease

Reference Values

- Negative

Abnormal Values

- Positive value: Graves' disease

Interfering Factors

- Radioactive iodine in the serum or hemolysis of the sample may interfere with test results.

Nursing Implications

Assessment

- Obtain history of endocrine system, suspected or known thyroid abnormality, tests and procedures performed, and results.

Possible Nursing Diagnoses

Anxiety related to perceived threat to or change in health status
Nutrition, altered, less than body requirements, related to inability to ingest adequate nutrients for hypermetabolic rate
Tissue integrity, impaired, risk for, related to altered protective mechanisms

Implementation

- Put on gloves. Using aseptic technique, perform a venipuncture and collect 7 mL of blood in a red-top tube.
- Handle the sample gently to avoid hemolysis and transport to the laboratory immediately.

Evaluation

- Note test results in association with other thyroid tests and client symptoms.

Client/Caregiver Teaching

Pretest

- Advise the client to stop thyroid medication 6 weeks before the test, as ordered.

Posttest

- Instruct the client to resume medications withheld before the test.
- Inform the client of the need for any additional testing pending test results.
- Instruct the client to report signs and symptoms of hyperthyroidism.

▲▲▲▲▲▲▲▲▲▲▲▲▲▲▲▲▲▲▲▲▲▲

Thyroxine (T_4, Total T_4, T_4 RIA)

Classification: Chemistry, Immunoassay

Type of Test: Serum; Blood of newborns

This test measures thyroxine (T_4), a hormone produced and secreted by the thyroid gland. It is tested by competitive protein binding or by radioimmunoassay. In competitive protein binding, the affinity between T_4 and thyroxine-binding globulin (TBG) is exploited. T_4 measured by radioimmunoassay (T_4 RIA) is the preferred method to measure T_4 because it is not affected by circulating iodinated substances. Newborns are commonly tested for decreased T_4 levels by a filter paper method.

Most T_4 in the serum (99.97%) is bound to protein (TBG). The remainder circulates as unbound or "free" T_4 (FT_4) and is responsible for all of the physiologic activity of thyroxine. Because FT_4 is not dependent on normal levels of TBG, as is the case with total serum thyroxine, FT_4 levels are considered the most accurate indicator of thyroxine and its thyrometabolic activity.

Indications

- Evaluate signs of hypothyroidism or hyperthyroidism and/or neonatal screening for congenital hypothyroidism (required in many states).
- Monitor response to therapy for hypothyroidism or hyperthyroidism.

- Evaluate thyroid response to protein deficiency associated with severe illnesses.

Reference Values

	SI Units
RIA	4–12 µg/dL
FT$_4$	0.9–2.3 ng/dL

Values may vary according to the laboratory performing the test.

Abnormal Values

- Increased levels
    Primary and secondary hyperthyroidism, including excessive T$_4$ replacement therapy
    Thyroiditis
    Pregnancy
    Women receiving estrogen therapy or with estrogen-secreting tumors
    Heroin and methadone use
- Decreased levels
    Primary and secondary hypothyroidism
    Malnutrition
    Pituitary and hypothalamic dysfunction
    Severe illnesses including metastatic cancer, liver disease, renal disease, diabetes mellitus, cardiovascular problems, burns, and trauma
    Drugs, including androgens, glucocorticoids, heparin, salicylates, phenytoin, anticonvulsants, sulfonamides, and antithyroid drugs such as propylthiouracil

Interfering Factors

- Studies using iodinated contrast media within 1 week before the test will affect results.
- Ingestion of thyroxine will elevate T$_4$ levels.
- Heroin and methadone can elevate T$_4$ levels.
- Drugs can lead to increased or decreased T$_4$ levels (see Abnormal Values).

Nursing Implications

Assessment

- Obtain history of thyroid dysfunction and the results of other thyroid tests performed.

- Ensure that thyroid medications have been withheld for 1 month before the test and that other drugs that may alter T$_4$ levels are withheld for at least 24 hours before the test, as ordered by physician.

Possible Nursing Diagnoses

Anxiety related to perceived threat to health status

Nutrition, altered, risk for less than body requirements, related to inability to ingest adequate amounts of nutrients

Tissue integrity, impaired, risk for, related to altered protective mechanisms

Implementation

- Put on gloves. Using aseptic technique, perform a venipuncture and collect 7 mL of blood in a red-top tube.
- Handle the sample gently to avoid hemolysis and transport to the laboratory promptly.
- For neonatal screening, obtain the sample by heelstick. A multiple neonatal screening kit is usually used. Saturate circles on the filter paper with blood, place in a sterile container, and send to the laboratory.

Evaluation

- Note results in relation to other thyroid tests performed and the client's symptoms.

Client/Caregiver Teaching

Pretest

- Instruct the client to withhold drugs that may alter T$_4$ levels for at least 24 hours before the test, as ordered by physician. Thyroid medications may have to be withheld for 1 month before the test for a baseline level.

Posttest

- Tell the client to resume medications withheld before the test.
- Explain to parents or caregivers of infants that the test may need to be repeated in 3 to 6 weeks owing to normal changes in infant thyroid hormone levels.

Thyroxine-Binding Globulin

Classification: Chemistry, Immunology

Type of Test: Serum

Thyroxine-binding globulin (TBG) is the predominant protein carrier for circulating thyroxine (T_4) and triiodothyronine (T_3). This test measures the amount of TBG in the serum by measuring a sample saturated with radioactive thyroxine and then subjecting it to electrophoresis. Conditions that affect TBG levels and the binding capacity also affect free T_3 (FT_3) and free T_4 (FT_4) levels. This is clinically significant because only FT_3 and FT_4 are metabolically active. An abnormality of TBG renders tests for total T_3 and T_4 inaccurate but does not alter tests for FT_3 and FT_4.

Indications

- Evaluate abnormal thyrometabolic states
- Aid in the diagnosis of TBG abnormalities

Reference Values

Functional chemistry	15–26 µg/dL
Immunologic	
Men	12–25 mg/L
Women	14–30 mg/L
Women on oral contraceptives	15–55 mg/L

Abnormal Values

- Increased values
    - Hypothyroidism
    - Acute intermittent porphyria
    - Estrogen-producing tumors
    - Genetically determined high TBG
    - Infectious hepatitis and other liver diseases
- Decreased values
    - Testosterone-producing tumors
    - Hepatic disease
    - Marked hypoproteinemia, malnutrition

Severe acidosis
Major illness or surgical stress
Acromegaly
Nephrotic syndrome
Genetic deficiency of TBG

Interfering Factors

- Use of oral contraceptives and estrogens elevates the test results.
- Use of androgens and other steroids decreases the test results.
- Recently administered radioisotopes affects the values.
- Neonates have a higher value.

Nursing Implications

Assessment

- Obtain history of thyroid dysfunction and the results of other thyroid tests performed.
- Ensure that thyroid medications have been withheld, as ordered.
- Ensure that medications that may affect the test results (e.g., estrogens or phenytoin) have been withheld, as ordered, or their usage noted on the laboratory request.

Possible Nursing Diagnoses

Nutrition, altered, risk for less than body requirements, related to inability to ingest adequate amounts of nutrients
Tissue integrity, impaired, risk for, related to altered protective mechanisms

Implementation

- Put on gloves. Using aseptic technique, perform a venipuncture and collect 7 mL of blood in a red-top tube.
- Handle the sample gently to avoid hemolysis and transport to the laboratory promptly.

Evaluation

- Note results in relation to other tests performed, particularly other thyroid tests, and the client's symptoms.

Client/Caregiver Teaching

Pretest

- Instruct the client to withhold drugs that may alter test levels for at least 24 hours before the test, as ordered by physician.

Posttest

- Tell the client to resume medications withheld before the test.
- Advise the client that additional tests may need to be performed pending results.

Tolbutamide Tolerance Test

Classification: Chemistry

Type of Test: Blood

This test is performed to evaluate insulin production. Tolbutamide (Orinase), a hypoglycemic agent, produces hypoglycemia by stimulating the beta cells of the pancreas to secrete and release insulin. An intravenous infusion of tolbutamide raises the serum insulin level and causes a rapid decrease in the blood glucose level thereby allowing the test to demonstrate the pancreatic beta-cell response to drug-induced stimulation.

Indications

- Evaluate fasting or postprandial hypoglycemia
- Evaluate suspected insulinoma (insulin-producing tumor of the pancreatic beta cells) as indicated by glucose levels that drop markedly in response to tolbutamide and take 3 or more hours to return to normal levels
- Evaluate suspected prediabetic state, which can be characterized by excessive insulin release, as indicated by glucose levels that are lower than expected but that follow the overall pattern of a normal response to the test

Reference Values

- A decrease in serum glucose levels is evident within 5 to 10 minutes; the lowest glucose levels occur in about 20 to 30 minutes and are generally about half of the client's usual fasting level; the glucose level returns to pretest values in 1 to 3 hours.

Abnormal Values

- Insulinoma

Interfering Factors

- Failure to ingest a diet with sufficient carbohydrates (150 g/d) for at least 3 days before the test may result in falsely decreased values.
- Decreased activity may lead to falsely increased values.
- Excessive physical activity before or during the test may lead to falsely decreased values.
- Smoking before or during the test may lead to falsely increased values.
- Ingestion of drugs known to alter blood glucose levels may falsely increase or decrease values (see Abnormal Values for Glucose Tolerance Test, pp. 609–610).

> ### NURSING ALERT
>
> - This test is contraindicated in clients allergic to sulfonylureas or sulfonamides. The test can be performed using glucagon or leucine instead.
> - Perform test with extreme caution—if at all—in clients with a fasting blood glucose of 50 mg/dL or less.

Nursing Implications

Assessment

- Obtain history of diabetes and any allergy to tolbutamide, sulfonylureas, or sulfonamides.
- Assess pretest dietary compliance of a high-carbohydrate diet (150 to 300 g/d) for 3 days before the test, then a fast overnight before the test.
- Assess compliance with refraining from smoking during the fast and the test.

Possible Nursing Diagnoses

Anxiety related to perceived threat to health status
Nutrition, altered, less than body requirements, related to inability to use nutrients
Infection, risk for, related to decreased leukocyte function
Adjustment, impaired, risk for, related to an all-encompassing change in lifestyle

Implementation

- Put on gloves. Using aseptic technique, establish venous access and obtain a blood sample for a fasting blood sugar (FBS) in a gray-top tube.
- Connect the IV catheter to an intermittent infusion device or to a continuous IV infusion of normal saline at a "keep vein open" (KVO) rate.
- Administer tolbutamide 1.0 g mixed in 20 mL sterile water IV over 2 to 3 minutes.
- Obtain blood glucose samples at quarter-, half-, three-quarter-, 1-, 1 1/2-, 2-, and 3-hour intervals. Specify the time of collection on each sample, and send each sample promptly to the laboratory.
- Observe the client closely for signs and symptoms of hypoglycemia or a sensitivity reaction to tolbutamide. If these occur, obtain a stat fasting blood sugar, notify the physician, and initiate an IV infusion of 5% glucose and water or drugs, if ordered. Maintain an open IV line until there is no further danger of adverse drug reaction.

Evaluation

- Monitor for signs and symptoms of hypoglycemia for 2 hours or more, depending on results of the 3-hour interval blood sugar test.
- Note results in relation to other tests performed and the client's symptoms.

Client/Caregiver Teaching

Pretest

- Instruct client to ingest a diet with sufficient carbohydrates (150 g/d) for at least 3 days and to fast for 8 hours before the test.
- Tell the client to maintain a normal activity level and to avoid excessive physical activity before or during the test.
- Warn the client not to smoke before or during the test.
- Ingestion of drugs known to alter blood glucose levels may falsely increase or decrease values (see Abnormal Values of Glucose Tolerance Test, pp. 609–610).

Posttest

- Instruct the client to resume a well-balanced diet.
- Inform the client that signs and symptoms of hypoglycemia may occur for 2 hours or more after the test. Advise the client to drink a glass of orange juice or eat some hard candy until a normal meal can be ingested.

Tomography, Chest (Laminography, Planigraphy, Stratigraphy)

Classification: Radiography

Type of Test: Indirect visualization

Tomography is a two-dimensional view with greater clarity than plain films, especially valuable in visualizing air-filled structures such as lungs and paranasal sinuses; tomography is being replaced by computerized tomography of the chest when further radiologic evaluation of the chest is indicated.

Indications

- Aid in the diagnosis of known or suspected tuberculosis, lung abscess, tumor, or abnormal pulmonary vasculature
- Determine nature of lesion detected on routine chest x-ray
- Aid in the diagnosis of suspected tumor in the mediastinum, ribs, and spine after inability to visualize by chest x-ray

Reference Values

- Normal lung fields, cardiac size and mediastinal structures, thoracic spine and ribs, shape and position of the diaphragm

Abnormal Values

- Tuberculosis
- Bronchiectasis associated with tuberculosis
- Bronchogenic carcinoma
- Calcium in small parenchymal nodules
- Bronchial occlusion location

Interfering Factors

- Improper positioning may affect test results.
- Metallic objects such as jewelry, closures on clothing within the imaging field may affect test results.

- Improper density adjustment of x-ray equipment to accommodate obese or thin clients may cause underexposure or overexposure and poor-quality films.

> ### NURSING ALERT
>
> - This procedure is contraindicated in pregnancy, unless the benefits of performing the procedure far outweigh the risks to the fetus.
> - Risks associated with radiographic overexposure can result from frequent x-ray procedures (greater exposure with tomograms than with plain films).
> - Prevent possible x-ray exposure of personnel in the room with the client by having them wear a protective lead apron or stand behind a shield; badges that reveal level of exposure to rays should be worn by those working in areas near x-ray suites.

Nursing Implications

Assessment

- Assess respiratory status including rate and ease.
- Assess ability to remain still and hold the breath.
- Assess date of last menstrual period to ascertain possibility of pregnancy in premenopausal women.

Possible Nursing Diagnoses

Infection, risk for transmission

Anxiety related to perceived threat to or change in health status

Airway clearance, ineffective, related to thick viscous or bloody secretions

Nutrition, altered, less than body requirements, related to inability to ingest adequate nutrients

Implementation

- Provide hospital gown without snaps or metallic closures and request that clothing and all items containing metal within the x-ray field are removed (e.g., brassieres, belts, corsets).
- Place in supine, sidelying, or prone positions depending on the view to be obtained; the x-ray tube is moved overhead in a back and forth, circular, or figure-of-eight motion while the films are being taken.
- Instruct the client to lie very still on the table and to breathe in a normal pattern.

Evaluation

- Monitor blood gases for decreases in oxygen and increases in carbon dioxide levels; use pulse oximetry to detect decreases in oxygen saturation.
- Monitor pulmonary function studies indicating pulmonary compromise, nuclear lung ventilation and perfusion scan indicating lung pathology.

Client/Caregiver Teaching

Pretest

- Explain to the client the purpose of the study and how the procedure is performed; tell the client that the procedure is performed in an x-ray room and that a radiologist will interpret the results; obtain an informed signed consent.
- Tell the client that there are no food and fluid restrictions and that there is no pain associated with the study.
- Use models and diagrams to help the client to understand the procedure.

Posttest

- Instruct the client to comply with the medication regimen and emphasize the importance of compliance for clients with a pulmonary condition.
- Emphasize importance of avoiding people with upper respiratory infections, allergens, and other factors causing respiratory distress.
- Instruct the client in use of tissues for coughing, sneezing, and expectoration, as well as proper disposal following use.
- Encourage the client to obtain protection from pneumonia and influenza by immunization.

Tomography, Paranasal Sinuses

Classification: Radiography

Type of Test: Indirect visualization

Also called laminography, planigraphy, and stratigraphy, tomography is a two-dimensional view with greater clarity than plain films. Especially valuable for visualizing air-filled structures such as the lungs and paranasal sinuses, it makes possible views that are not obstructed by structures that surround the sinuses. Computerized tomography (CT) and magnetic resonance imaging (MRI) have replaced tomography.

Indications

- Evaluate abnormal results from plain films that reveal evidence of tumors, cysts, or fracture
- Diagnose suspected fracture or tumor of nasal bones surrounding sinuses when the results of plain films are negative
- Detect foreign bodies in sinuses

Reference Values

- Normal sinuses

Abnormal Values

- Fracture
- Tumor
- Cysts
- Foreign bodies

Interfering Factors

- Improper positioning may affect test results.
- Metallic objects such as jewelry and closures on clothing within the imaging field may alter test results.

- Improper density adjustment of x-ray equipment to accommodate obese or thin clients may cause underexposure or overexposure and poor-quality films.

NURSING ALERT

- This procedure is contraindicated in pregnancy, unless the benefits of performing the procedure far outweigh the risks to the fetus.
- Risks associated with radiographic overexposure can result from frequent x-ray procedures (greater exposure with tomograms than with plain films).
- Prevent possible x-ray exposure of personnel in the room with the client by having them wear a protective lead apron or stand behind a shield; badges that reveal level of exposure to rays should be worn by those working in areas near x-ray suites.

Nursing Implications

Assessment

- Assess respiratory status including rate and ease.
- Assess ability to remain still and hold the breath.
- Assess date of last menstrual period to ascertain possibility of pregnancy in premenopausal women.

Possible Nursing Diagnoses

Airway clearance, ineffective, related to obstruction
Tissue integrity, impaired, related to irritation of secretions

Implementation

- Establish an intravenous line.
- Instruct client to remain very still during scanning.
- Position client in a special chair with the head immobilized in a padded brace or vise to maintain a proper position. Ask the client to remain very still while an x-ray tube is moved overhead in different directions around a pivot point during filming. Several views can be taken.

Evaluation

- Monitor vital signs every 15 to 30 minutes and compare with baseline readings until stable.

- Note results in relation to other studies.
- Also note test results in relation to the client's symptoms.

Client/Caregiver Teaching

Pretest

- Explain to the client that procedure is performed in a special department by a technician and a physician specializing in this branch of medicine.
- Explain that the test can take 30 minutes to complete.
- Explain that no fasting of food or liquid is required.

Posttest

- Instruct client to resume usual level of activity and normal dietary intake unless contraindicated.
- Provide supportive environment after diagnostic findings are reported, as indicated; reinforce information regarding diagnosis and recommended treatment regimen.

Tonometry

Classification: Sensory Organ Function

Type of Test: Visual perception

This noninvasive procedure is performed to indirectly measure intraocular pressure and to assist in diagnosing glaucoma. Secretion of aqueous humor is continuous regardless of the presence of secreted fluid and the rate of production and is normally equal to the rate of drainage. An increased intraocular pressure results from an interference with the drainage of the fluid anywhere along the outflow pathway.

Indications

- Screen for glaucoma in clients over the age of 40
- Measure intraocular pressure to assist in the diagnosis of glaucoma
- Monitor the progression of glaucoma and effectiveness of the treatment regimen

Reference Values

- Normal intraocular pressure of 12 to 20 mm Hg depending on time of day

Abnormal Values

- Glaucoma

Interfering Factors

- Corneal surface that inhibits correct placement of the tonometer footplate can alter measurement.
- Flaccid or rigid cornea that prevents proper indentation of the tonometer footplate can affect correct measurement.
- Inability of the client to cooperate and remain quiet during the test can cause inaccurate results.
- Improper technique in the use of the tonometer in performing the measurement can cause inaccurate results.

> ### NURSING ALERT
>
> - This procedure is contraindicated in clients with corneal ulceration or infection because further damage could result.

Nursing Implications

Assessment

- Obtain a history of known or suspected ocular disorders, changes in visual acuity, eye pain, other visual tests and procedures done, and results.

Possible Nursing Diagnoses

Sensory/perceptual alteration (visual) related to altered sensory perception and altered status of sense organ

Implementation

- Ask the client to remove corrective lenses (glasses or contacts) and loosen or remove restrictive clothing around his or her neck.
- *Contact tonometer:* Place the client in a supine position on the examining table, instill 1 drop of the topical eye anesthetic in each eye, and request the client to close the eyes to spread the medication over the sclera.

- Check the instrument for a zero reading and a freely moving plunger and prepare the tonometer (Schiötz) to measure the pressure using 5.5 g of weight. Instruct the client to look at a spot on the ceiling and breathe normally.
- Gently hold the lids of one eye with the thumb and forefinger of the dominant hand, and place the footplate of the instrument on the apex of the cornea. Avoid any pressure on the cornea by the fingers or any movement of the tonometer that can cause abrasions.
- Observe the needle on the calibrated part of the tonometer for a pulsating movement.
- Record the reading on the scale part of the instrument and the time of day that the procedure was performed. A reading <4 requires additional weight (≥ 7.5 g) be applied to obtain a measurement of intraocular pressure. Repeat the procedure to measure the pressure of the other eye.
- *Noncontact tonometer:* This tonometer is mounted on a slit lamp and measures the time needed to flatten an anesthetized area of the cornea with an air blast. The intraocular pressure is read on a dial as the complete flattening is measured electronically. This method is performed with the client in a sitting position by a physician during routine slit lamp examinations.

Evaluation

- Note results in relation to the client's symptoms.

Client/Caregiver Teaching

Pretest

- Tell the client the purpose of the procedure and explain that it is performed in a specially equipped room by a physician and takes about 1 to 2 minutes to complete; further explain that eyedrops are administered to anesthetize the eyes and that there is no pain associated with the procedure.
- Emphasize the importance of the client's lying very still and avoiding blinking or tightly closing the eyelids during the test.

Posttest

- Instruct the client to refrain from rubbing the eyes for 20 to 30 minutes to prevent corneal abrasions.
- Tell the client that he or she should not reinsert contact lenses for 2 hours posttest to allow time for the anesthesia to wear off; tell the client that he or she may wear eyeglasses during that time.

- Inform the client that any scratchy feeling is caused by tonometer movement during the test and that this feeling disappears within 24 hours.

▲▲▲▲▲▲▲▲▲▲▲▲▲▲▲▲▲▲

TORCH Test

Classification: Serology

Type of Test: Blood

This screening test is used to detect toxoplasmosis, rubella, cytomegalovirus (CMV), and herpes simplex in a mother or an infant. Toxoplasmosis is a systemic parasitic disease transmitted to humans by ingesting undercooked meat or handling contaminated cat litter. Rubella is an acute, viral communicable disease transmitted by droplet or direct contact. CMV is a member of the herpesvirus group. Herpesvirus can cause clinically severe disorders. TORCH infections can cross the placenta in pregnancy resulting in congenital malformations, abortion, or stillbirth.

Indications

- Screen during pregnancy
- Confirm suspected congenital infection in newborn

Reference Values

- Negative

Abnormal Values

- Positive values
    Toxoplasmosis
    Rubella
    Cytomegalovirus
    Herpes simplex

Interfering Factors

- Confirmation of congenital rubella infection requires samples from both the mother and infant. Antibodies may remain present for many years.
- Hemolysis of specimen invalidates the results of the herpes screen.

Nursing Implications

Assessment

- Obtain obstetric history, suspected or known exposure to rubella, toxoplasmosis, herpes simplex, cytomegalovirus, tests and procedures performed, and results.

Possible Nursing Diagnoses

Anxiety related to threat to or change in health status

Pain, acute, related to presence of localized inflammation and open lesions

Sexuality patterns, altered, risk for, related to fear of transmitting the disease

Infections, risk for, related to traumatized tissue

Implementation

- Put on gloves; using aseptic technique, perform a venipuncture and collect 5 mL of blood in a red-top tube.

Evaluation

- Any individual positive result should be repeated in 7 to 10 days to monitor change in titer.
- Note results in relation to other tests performed and the client's symptoms.

Client/Caregiver Teaching

Pretest

- Explain the purpose of the test, the procedure to obtain the specimen, and that some discomfort is experienced from the puncture.
- Inform client that several tests may be necessary to confirm diagnosis.

Posttest

- If results are positive, genetic counseling may be indicated.

Trichinosis and Toxoplasmosis (Antibody and Skin) Tests

Classification: Serology/Infectious disease diagnostic

Type of Test: Blood; Skin testing

Trichinosis and toxoplasmosis skin tests are done to determine exposure to these parasitic diseases. Although these skin tests are discouraged and considered unreliable, commercially available antigens can be used in conjunction with serologic tests to detect antibodies in the blood following the onset of the disease. The most definitive diagnostic information is obtained by performing blood tests such as immunoglobulin M (IgM) titers for toxoplasmosis and antibody titer for trichinosis.

Indications

- Detect exposure to trichinosis or toxoplasmosis
- Serve as a diagnostic adjunct of the skin test for trichinosis in conjunction with blood serology and muscle biopsy
- Serve as a diagnostic adjunct of the skin test for toxoplasmosis in conjunction with blood serology

Reference Values

Toxoplasmosis skin test	Negative response; no reaction at the test sites indicating absence of a specific infection
Toxoplasmosis blood test	
Newborn	No IgM detected
Adult	IgM titer <1:64
Trichinosis skin test	Negative
Trichinosis blood test	Negative or titer <1:16

Abnormal Values

Toxoplasmosis skin test	Positive for past or present infection; reveals a measured erythema of more than 10 mm in 24–48 h
Toxoplasmosis blood test	Increased titer (>1:64) for past or present infection; fetal congenital toxoplasmosis
Trichinosis skin test	Positive for past or present infection; reveals a weal with erythema around 15 min following injection and is considered a questionable positive result if the reaction occurs after 24 h
Trichinosis blood test	Increased titer (>1:5) indicating presence of infection

Interfering Factors

- Improper techniques in performing the skin test or inaccurate time or measurement in reading the reaction may affect test results.
- Commercially available antigens for the trichinosis test are considered unreliable for diagnostic purposes.
- Blood testing for trichinosis within 3 weeks of exposure can cause a false-negative result.

Nursing Implications

Assessment

- Obtain a history of hypersensitivities, dietary inclusion of uncooked meats, possible exposure to infected cats or other contact with causative microorganism, pregnancy status, and results of serologic tests done to identify the microorganisms causing the diseases.

Possible Nursing Diagnoses

Pain related to parasitic invasion of muscle tissues
Fluid volume deficit related to hypermetabolic state
Breathing pattern, ineffective, related to myositis of the diaphragm and intercostal muscles

Implementation

- *Skin test:* Cleanse the skin site on the lower anterior area of the forearm with alcohol or acetone swabs and allow it to air dry.

- Prepare 0.1 mL of the antigen (TDH Test) prepared from killed larvae, or toxoplasmin in a syringe with a 26-ga needle attached and injected intradermally.
- *Blood test:* If blood is to be withdrawn, put on gloves. Using aseptic technique, perform a venipuncture and collect a 5-mL blood sample in a red-top tube; label sample and send to the laboratory. Repeat the test every 3 to 5 days to detect rising titers.

Evaluation

- Assess test area at appropriate times depending on the antigens injected.
- Note test results in relation to other tests performed and the client's symptoms.

Client/Caregiver Teaching

Pretest

- Explain to the client the purpose of the blood or skin test and how the test is performed; tell the client that the test is generally done by a nurse in a physician's office or health-care setting and that it takes about 5 to 10 minutes to complete.

Posttest

- Emphasize to the client that he or she should not scratch or rub the area from the time of the injection until the time the test is read.
- Instruct the client to return 24 to 48 hours later to have the toxoplasmosis test results read.
- Ask the client to return every 3 to 5 days to repeat the blood test for trichinosis or in 7 to 14 days to repeat the blood test for toxoplasmosis, as appropriate.
- Teach the client diet modification; emphasize the importance of well-cooked meals.

Transferrin (Siderophilin)

Classification: Chemistry

Type of Test: Serum

Serum transferrin levels are analyzed using radial immunodiffusion or nephelometry to determine amounts of iron metabolism. Transferrin is a glycoprotein that is formed in the liver. It transports circulating iron obtained from dietary intake and from red blood cell breakdown. Inadequate transferrin levels can lead to impaired hemoglobin synthesis and anemia.

Indications

- Evaluate iron metabolism in iron deficiency anemia
- Determine the iron-binding capacity of the blood

Reference Values

		SI Units
Adult	200–400 mg/dL	2–4 g/L
Newborn	130–275 mg/dL	1.3–2.8 g/L

65–170 µg/dL is bound to iron.

Abnormal Values

- Increased levels
  Severe iron deficiency
- Decreased levels
  Acute or chronic infection
  Cancer
  Excessive protein loss from renal disease
  Hepatic damage

Interfering Factors

- Use of oral contraceptives can affect test results.
- Late pregnancy can alter test results.

- Rough handling of the sample leading to hemolysis can affect test results.

Nursing Implications

Assessment

- Obtain client history of hepatic disorders, and assess for disorders and medications that may alter levels.
- Assure that client has fasted for 12 hours before the test.

Possible Nursing Diagnoses

Tissue perfusion, altered, arterial, related to exchange problems

Activity intolerance related to imbalance between oxygen supply and demand

Implementation

- Put on gloves and using aseptic technique, perform a venipuncture and collect 7 mL of blood in a red-top (or marbled-top) tube.
- Handle the sample gently to avoid hemolysis and send to the laboratory immediately.

Evaluation

- Compare results with other related tests and the client's symptoms.

Client/Caregiver Teaching

Pretest

- Inform the client to fast for 12 hours before the test. Water is allowed.

Posttest

- Advise the client of additional testing pending test results and diagnosis.

Trichomonad Preparation, Urogenital Secretions

Classification: Microbiology

Type of Test: Vaginal, cervical, urethral, prostatic specimen; Urine sample

Trichomonas is a sexually transmitted protozoan urogenital infection. It is transmitted by direct contact with vaginal and urethral fluids of infected individuals. Symptoms include foamy yellow drainage, vaginal burning, and itching in females. Males are frequently asymptomatic or may have a persistent white urethral discharge. Diagnosis is made by microscopic examination of a wet mount of secretions of an infected individual.

Indications

- Confirm suspected trichomoniasis

Reference Values

- Negative

Abnormal Values

- The presence of trichomonads confirms trichomoniasis.

Interfering Factors

- An improper collection technique or a delay in sending the specimen to the laboratory may interfere with test results. Trichomonads can be identified only when motile.

Nursing Implications

Assessment

- Obtain history of genitourinary system, current symptoms, medication regimen, diagnostic tests, and results.
- Ensure that the female client has avoided douching for 72 hours before the collection of vaginal or cervical specimens.

Possible Nursing Diagnoses

Infection, risk for transmission
Tissue integrity, impaired, related to irritation and mechanical
  trauma
Pain related to localized inflammation and tissue trauma

Implementation

- *For vaginal secretions:* Insert an unlubricated speculum into the vagina and collect vaginal discharge on a cotton swab. Place it in a tube containing normal saline; label the container and send it to the laboratory immediately.
- *For prostatic or urethral discharge:* Collect secretions with a cotton swab, then place in a normal saline solution. Label the specimen and send it to the laboratory immediately.

Evaluation

- Compare the test results with the client's symptoms and results of other related diagnostic tests.

Client/Caregiver Teaching

Pretest

- For urine sample, instruct the client to cleanse around the urinary meatus three times, rinse, and dry. Collect the first portion (about 20 mL) of a voided sample in a clean container. Label the specimen and send it to the laboratory immediately.

Posttest

- If results are positive, instruct the client to notify sexual contacts of exposure and need for treatment.

Triglycerides

Classification: Chemistry
Type of Test: Serum

This test measures triglycerides, which are combinations of three fatty acids and one glycerol molecule used by the body to provide energy for various metabolic processes. Excess triglycerides are stored in adipose tissue. The fatty acids readily enter and leave the triglycerides of adipose tissue, providing raw materials needed for conversion to glucose (gluconeogenesis) or for direct combustion as an energy source. Although fatty acids originate in the diet, many are also derived from unused glucose and amino acids that the liver and, to a smaller extent, the adipose tissue convert into stored energy.

Indications

- Screen individuals over age 40 and/or who are obese to estimate the risk for atherosclerotic cardiovascular disease
- Identify hyperlipoproteinemia (hyperlipidemia) in clients with a family history of the disorder
- Evaluate known or suspected disorders associated with altered triglyceride levels (see Abnormal Values)
- Monitor response to drugs known to alter triglyceride levels (see Abnormal Values)

Reference Values

		SI Units
Infants	5–40 mg/dL	0.6–0.67 mmol/L
Children		
1–11 yr	10–135 mg/dL	0.11–1.49 mmol/L
12–20 yr	10–140 mg/dL	0.11–1.57 mmol/L
Women		
20–40 yr	10–140 mg/dL	0.11–1.57 mmol/L
40–60 yr	10–180 mg/dL	0.11–2.01 mmol/L
Men		
20–40 yr	10–150 mg/dL	0.11–1.68 mmol/L
40–60 yr	10–190 mg/dL	0.11–2.12 mmol/L

Values for serum triglycerides may vary according to the laboratory performing the test. In addition, values vary in relation to age, race, sex, income level, level of physical activity, dietary habits, and geographic location.

Abnormal Values

- Elevated levels
    Atherosclerosis
    Chronic obstructive pulmonary disease
    Diabetes mellitus
    Down's syndrome
    Hypertension
    Hypoparathyroidism
    Hypothyroidism (primary)
    Myocardial infarction
    Nephrotic syndrome
    Obstructive jaundice
    Primary hyperlipoproteinemia
    von Gierke's disease
    Certain drugs, including alcohol, cholestyramine, corticosteroids, colestipol, oral contraceptives, thyroid preparations, estrogen, furosemide, and miconazole
- Decreased levels
    Acanthocytosis
    Cirrhosis
    Inadequate dietary protein
    Hyperthyroidism
    Hyperparathyroidism
    Certain drugs, including clofibrate, dextrothyroxine, heparin, menotropins , sulfonylureas, norethindrone, androgens, niacin, anabolic steroids, and ascorbic acid

Interfering Factors

- Failure to follow usual diet for 2 weeks before the test can yield results that do not accurately reflect client status.
- Ingestion of alcohol 24 hours and food 12 hours before the test can falsely elevate levels.
- Ingestion of drugs known to alter triglyceride levels within 24 hours of the test, unless the test is being done to evaluate such effects (see Abnormal Values), can affect test results.

Nursing Implications

Assessment

- Obtain history of cardiovascular status and risk for heart disease, tests and procedures performed, and results.

- Ensure that the client has fasted for 12 hours before the test; that water has not been restricted, that the client abstained from alcohol for 24 hours before the test, and that drugs that may alter triglyceride levels have been withheld for 24 hours before the test.
- Assess for significant weight changes within 2 weeks before the test because this can invalidate results.

Possible Nursing Diagnoses

Pain related to ischemia of myocardial tissue
Cardiac output, decreased, risk for, related to changes in rate and electrical conduction

Implementation

- Put on gloves. Using aseptic technique, perform a venipuncture and collect 5 mL of blood in a lavender-top or red-top tube.
- Send the sample to the laboratory immediately.

Evaluation

- Note level in relation to test results of cholesterol and lipoprotein electrophoresis, especially very-low-density lipoproteins and low-density lipoproteins.

Client/Caregiver Teaching

Pretest

- Instruct client to fast for 12 hours before the test (water is not restricted), abstain from alcohol for 24 hours before the test, and withhold drugs that may alter triglyceride levels for 24 hours before the test.
- Ask the client to report significant weight changes within 2 weeks before the test as this can invalidate results.

Posttest

- Instruct the client to resume diet and medication withheld before the test.
- Instruct the client and caregiver in dietary restriction of fat to reduce the level and risk for cardiac or vascular disease.

Triiodothyronine (T$_3$, Total T$_3$, T$_3$ RIA)

Classification: Chemistry, Immunoassay

Type of Test: Serum

This test measures levels of triiodothyronine (T$_3$), a thyroid hormone present in small amounts in blood that is more short-acting and more potent than thyroxine (T$_4$). The test includes the total (bound and free) serum content of triiodothyronine (T$_3$) by radioimmunoassay (RIA) method since T$_3$ has less affinity for thyroxine-binding globulin (TBG) than T$_4$.

Indications

- Diagnose hyperthyroidism in clients with normal T$_4$ levels (Early hyperthyroidism and T$_3$ thyrotoxicosis are indicated by elevated T$_3$ levels in the presence of normal T$_4$ levels.)
- Diagnose "euthyroid sick" syndrome in severely ill clients with protein deficiency, as indicated by low T$_3$ levels

Reference Values

		SI Units
T$_3$ RIA		
Newborns	32–250 ng/dL	0.49–3.85 nmol/L
Children	105–241 ng/dL	1.62–3.71 nmol/L
Adults	80–230 ng/dL	1.26–3.5 nmol/L

Abnormal Values

- Elevated levels
  Graves' disease
  Hashimoto's thyroiditis
  Hyperthyroidism
  T$_3$ thyrotoxicosis
  Toxic adenoma
  Certain drugs, including amiodarone, antithyroid agents, dextrothyroxine, dinoprost, estrogen, heroin, metha-

done, progestins, oral contraceptives, liothyronine (T_3), and terbutaline
- Decreased levels
   "Euthyroid sick" syndrome
   Hypothyroidism
   Malnutrition
   Obesity
   Renal failure
   Trauma
   Certain drugs, including ethionamide, heparin, iodides, phenylbutazone, propylthiouracil, methylthiouracil, methimazole, lithium, phenytoin, propranolol, reserpine, steroids, sulfonamides, salicylates, and cimetidine

Interfering Factors

- Drugs that alter T_3 levels (see Abnormal Values) affect test results.
- Radionuclide studies performed within 1 week of the test may alter results.

Nursing Implications

Assessment

- Obtain a history of thyroid or other metabolic disorders, tests performed, and results.
- Obtain a medication history; ensure that drugs that affect test results have been withheld for 24 hours with physician's approval.

Possible Nursing Diagnoses

- Fatigue related to hypermetabolic imbalance with increased energy requirements
- Tissue integrity, impaired, risk for, related to altered protective mechanisms
- Nutrition, altered, risk for less than body requirements, related to inability to ingest adequate nutrients

Implementation

- Put on gloves. Using aseptic technique, perform a venipuncture and collect 7 mL of blood in a red-top tube.
- Handle the sample gently to avoid hemolysis and transport to the laboratory promptly.

Evaluation

- Note test results in relation to other tests performed, particularly T_4.

Client/Caregiver Teaching

Pretest

- Tell client to withhold drugs that interfere with test results, as ordered by the physician.

Posttest

- Advise client to resume medications withheld before the test.
- Instruct the client on thyroid replacement therapy, if indicated.

Triiodothyronine Suppression Test (Perchlorate Suppression Study, Iodine Washout Test, Triiodothyronine T_3 Suppression Test)

Classification: Nuclear medicine

Type of Test: Radionuclide imaging

This test is used to evaluate clients with suspected Hashimoto's disease or to determine an enzyme deficiency within the thyroid. Perchlorate competes with and displaces the iodine ions that are not organified. Iodide is a compound of iodine and iodine is concentrated in the thyroid gland. Iodide quickly becomes bound to thyroglobulin, a protein, after becoming organified. The perchlorate stops trapping of the iodide and iodine that is unbound. After the administration of the perchlorate, clients with a decreased uptake of greater than 15 percent are enzyme deficient. This test can also be performed by administering T_3 after radioactive iodine uptake (RAIU) has been performed.

Indications

- Identify defects within the iodide organification process
- Aid in the diagnosis of enzyme deficiency
- Aid in the diagnosis of Hashimoto's disease
- If T_3 is used, 50 percent of RAIU will be suppressed.

Reference Values

- Values will not change after administration of perchlorate in normal individuals.

Abnormal Values

- Hashimoto's disease
- Toxic thyroid nodule
- Enzyme deficiency within the thyroid
- Thyroid cancer (RAIU may or may not be suppressed)

Interfering Factors

- The following may decrease levels: thyroid medications, such as levothyroxine, liothyronine, and desiccated thyroid; radiographic contrast medium; antithyroid drugs, such as propylthiouracil; thiocyanate; perchlorate; nitrates; sulfonamides; tolbutamide; corticosteroids; *p*-aminosalicylic acid (PAS); isoniazid; phenylbutazone; thiopental; and iodine-containing foods and drugs, such as cough syrup and cough medicines.
- The following will increase levels: pregnancy, iron-deficiency diets; renal failure; thyroid-stimulating hormone; barbiturates; lithium carbonate; and phenothiazides.

Nursing Implications

Assessment

- Obtain history of thyroid disorder, tests performed and results, and conditions that may alter test results (see Interfering Factors).
- Obtain medication history; ensure that drugs that alter levels (see Interfering Factors) have been withheld for 12 to 24 hours before the test, as ordered by physician.

Possible Nursing Diagnoses

Anxiety related to perceived threat to health status

Nutrition, altered, risk for less than body requirements, related to inability to ingest adequate nutrients for hypermetabolic rate

Tissue integrity, impaired, risk for, related to altered protective mechanisms of the eye

Implementation

- A tracer dose of radioactive iodine is given to the client orally.
- One and two hours after ingestion, uptakes are performed. Then, the client is given 400 mg to 1 g of perchlorate orally.
- After RAIU is performed, administer a 75 to 100 mcg dose of T_3 for 5 to 10 days. During the last 2 days of T_3 administration, RAIU tests are repeated.
- Uptakes are then performed every 15 minutes for the first hour after perchlorate ingestion and then every 30 minutes for the next 2 to 3 hours.
- Uptakes are compared between the preperchlorate and postperchlorate administration. Results are recorded on graph paper.

Evaluation

- Note results in relation to client's symptoms and the results of other related diagnostic tests.

Client/Caregiver Teaching

Pretest

- Instruct client to withhold any drug that can interfere with test results (see Interfering Factors).

Posttest

- Instruct client to resume medications withheld before the test.
- Instruct the client on thyroid replacement therapy, if indicated.

Triiodothyronine Uptake (T_3 Resin Uptake [RT_3U], Thyroid Hormone Binding Ratio [THBR])

Classification: Chemistry

Type of Test: Serum

This thyroid hormone test evaluates the quantity of thyroxine-binding globulin (TBG) present in the serum and the quantity of thyroxine bound to it. In the T_3 uptake procedure, a known amount of resin containing radiolabeled T_3 is added to a sample of the client's serum. Normally, TBG in the serum is not fully saturated with thyroid hormones; the saturation level varies in relation to the amounts of TBG and thyroid hormones present. In the T_3 uptake test, the radiolabeled T_3 will bind with available TBG sites. Results of the test are determined by measuring the percentage of labeled T_3 that remains bound to the resin after all available sites on TBG have been filled. The percentage of T_3 bound to the resin is inversely proportional to the percentage of TBG saturation in the serum. Results of the T_3 uptake test are evaluated in relation to serum levels of total T_4 and T_3, and also are used in calculating free T_3 and T_4 indices.

Indications

- Evaluate signs of hypothyroidism or hyperthyroidism with low or high percentage of radiolabeled T_3 remaining, respectively
- Evaluate known or suspected problems associated with altered TBG levels (e.g., hereditary abnormality of TBG synthesis, drug therapy, pregnancy, and disorders associated with decreased serum proteins) in which elevated levels indicate low TBG levels and decreased levels indicate elevated TBG levels
- Monitor response to therapy with drugs that compete for TBG binding sites
- Calculate free T_3 and T_4 indices

Reference Values

		SI Units
T_3 resin uptake		
Adults	25–35%	25–35 arb. U
Thyroid hormone binding ratio		
Newborns	0.90–1.15	0.90–1.15 arb. U
Children	0.88–1.12	0.88–1.12 arb. U
Adults	0.85–1.14	0.85–1.14 arb. U

arb = arbitrary.

Abnormal Values

- Elevated levels
  - Hepatic disease
  - Hyperandrogenic state
  - Hyperthyroidism
  - Malnutrition
  - Metastatic carcinoma
  - Myasthenia gravis
  - Nephrotic syndrome
  - Renal failure
  - Threatened abortion
  - Certain drugs, including androgens, barbiturates, corticosteroids, glucocorticoids, furosemide, warfarin, heparin, phenytoin, phenylbutazone, penicillin (large doses), thyroid agents, and salicylates (large doses)
- Decreased levels
  - Acute hepatitis
  - Hashimoto's thyroiditis
  - Hypothyroidism
  - Pregnancy
  - Certain drugs, including chlorpromazine, estrogens, heroin, lithium, methadone, oral contraceptives, propylthiouracil, thiazides, chlordiazepoxide, tolbutamide, and clofibrate

Interfering Factors

- Drugs that alter TBG levels or that compete for TBG binding sites may affect test results. For example, estrogens may lead to increased TBG levels; androgens and glucocorticoids may lead to decreased TBG levels; and salicylates and phenytoin anticonvulsants compete with T_4 for TBG binding sites.

- Results may vary during pregnancy when TBG levels are usually elevated.

Nursing Implications

Assessment

- Obtain history of thyroid disorder, tests performed, and results.
- Obtain medication history; ensure that drugs that alter TBG levels or compete for TBG binding sites have been withheld for 12 to 24 hours before the test, as ordered by physician.

Possible Nursing Diagnoses

Anxiety related to perceived threat to health status

Nutrition, altered, risk for less than body requirements, related to inability to ingest adequate nutrients for hypermetabolic rate

Tissue integrity, impaired, risk for, related to altered protective mechanisms of the eye

Implementation

- Put on gloves. Using aseptic technique, perform a venipuncture and collect 7 mL of blood in a red-top tube.
- Handle the sample gently to avoid hemolysis and transport to the laboratory promptly.

Evaluation

- Note results in relation to T_3 and T_4 levels.

Client/Caregiver Teaching

Pretest

- Instruct client to withhold any drug that can interfere with test results (see Interfering Factors).

Posttest

- Instruct client to resume medications withheld before the test.
- Instruct the client in thyroid replacement therapy, if appropriate.

Trypsin

Classification: Chemistry

Type of Test: Serum or plasma

Trypsin, a proteolytic enzyme produced in the pancreas as trypsinogen, activates the complement cascade. Trypsinogen is converted to trypsin in the duodenum by enterokinase. Trypsin can exist in the bloodstream as trypsinogen, bound to alpha$_1$-antitrypsin or alpha$_2$-macroglobulin, or as free trypsin.

Indications

- Suspected pancreatic insufficiency

Reference Values

Radioimmunoassay (RIA) double-antibody method	
Adults	22.2–44.4 µg/L
Children	
Cord	21.4–25.2 µg/L
<6 months	25.9–36.7 µg/L
6–12 months	30.2–44.0 µg/L
1–3 yr	28.0–31.6 µg/L
3–5 yr	25.1–31.5 µg/L
5–7 yr	32.1–39.3 µg/L
7–10 yr	32.7–37.1 µg/L
Sorin antibody method	
Adults	5.0–85.0 µg/L
Children	11.1–51.3 µg/L

Abnormal Values

- Increased levels
    Beta-thalassemia
    Chronic renal failure
    Cystic fibrosis (early years)
    Malnutrition (acute)
    Pancreatitis (acute)
    Recent endoscopic retrograde cholangiography

- Decreased levels
  Advanced cystic fibrosis
  Beta-thalassemia
  Diabetes mellitus

Interfering Factors

- Levels may be diurnal, with highest levels occurring in the late evening.
- Because of the variation in normal levels, values should be compared to the normal values of the laboratory performing the test.

Nursing Implications

Assessment

- Obtain history of known or suspected conditions affecting pancreatic function.
- Note compliance with fasting 8 hours before the test.

Possible Nursing Diagnoses

Airway clearance, ineffective, related to excessive production of thick mucus and decreased ciliary action

Anxiety related to perceived threat to or change in health status

Nutrition, altered, less than body requirements, related to impaired digestive process and absorption of nutrients

Infection, risk for, related to stasis of respiratory secretions and development of atelectasis

Implementation

- Put on gloves. Using aseptic technique, perform a venipuncture and collect 7 mL of blood in a red-top tube for a serum sample or green-top tube for a plasma sample.
- Handle the sample gently to avoid hemolysis and send to the laboratory immediately.

Evaluation

- Note results in relation to other tests performed and the client's symptoms.

Client/Caregiver Teaching

Pretest

Inform client that no special preparation is needed for the test.

Posttest

- Instruct the client to report signs and symptoms related to the disease process.

Trypsin

Classification: Chemistry

Type of Test: Fecal analysis

This type of test is useful in determining pancreatic function. It also evaluates the ability of trypsin to split protein, fats, and carbohydrates. This test is most useful in evaluating malabsorption in children younger than age 4.

Indications

- Aid in the diagnosis of pancreatic deficiency
- Aid in the diagnosis of malabsorption syndromes
- Screen for cystic fibrosis

Reference Values

- It is positive for small amounts of trypsin in 95 percent of normal individuals. It is present in greater amounts in normal children, but in older children and adults, normal bacteria in the gastrointestinal tract destroys the trypsin.

Abnormal Values

- Decreased amounts
    Cystic fibrosis
    Malabsorption syndromes
    Pancreatic deficiency

Interfering Factors

- Constipated stools may not indicate any trypsin owing to extended exposure to intestinal bacteria.

- Barium and laxatives used less than 1 week before the test may affect results.

Nursing Implications

Assessment

- Obtain history of known or suspected conditions affecting pancreatic function.

Possible Nursing Diagnoses

Airway clearance, ineffective, related to excessive production of thick mucus and decreased ciliary action

Nutrition, altered, less than body requirements, related to impaired digestive process and absorption of nutrients

Infection, risk for, related to stasis of respiratory secretions and development of atelectasis

Implementation

- Put on gloves. Collect the sample in a clean, dry, urine-free container, free of toilet tissue.
- Collect a complete stool sample and transfer to a container with clean tongue blades.
- Cover the sample and deliver to the laboratory immediately.

Evaluation

- Note results in relation to other tests performed and the client's symptoms.

Client/Caregiver Teaching

Pretest

- Tell the client and/or caregiver the reason for the test and who will perform it.
- Advise the client to avoid contaminating the stool sample with any urine or toilet tissue.
- Tell the client to collect the sample in a clean, dry, urine-free container.

Posttest

- Instruct the client to report signs and symptoms related to the disease process.

Tuberculin Skin Tests

Classification: Infectious disease, diagnostic

Type of Test: Intradermal injection

These tests are done to determine past or present exposure to tuberculosis. The multipuncture or tine test, a screening technique, uses either purified protein derivative (PPD) (Aplitest or SclavoTest) or old tuberculin (OT) (tine or MonoVacc). A positive response at the puncture site indicates cell-mediated immunity to the organism or a delayed hypersensitivity caused by interaction of the sensitized T lymphocytes. Verification of the client's positive response to the multipuncture is done with the more definitive Mantoux test using Aplisol or Tubersol administered by intradermal injection. The Mantoux test is the test of choice in symptomatic clients. A positive response to the Mantoux test is followed by chest radiography and a bacteriologic laboratory test to confirm diagnosis.

Indications

- Screen asymptomatic clients for tuberculosis exposure or infection
- Routinely screen infants with the tine test at the time of first immunizations to determine tuberculosis exposure
- Evaluate known or suspected exposure to tuberculosis with or without symptoms to determine if tuberculosis infection is present
- Evaluate cough, weight loss, fatigue, hemoptysis, and abnormal x-rays to determine if the cause is tuberculosis
- Evaluate client with medical conditions that place the client at risk for tuberculosis (e.g., AIDS, lymphoma, or diabetes)
- Screen populations who are at risk for developing tuberculosis (e.g., nursing home residents, prison inmates, and residents of the inner city living in poor hygienic conditions)

Reference Values

- Negative response or minimal response with no exposure to tuberculosis
- *Multipuncture test (tine):* <2 mm or absence of induration around one or more of the punctures in 48 to 72 hours

■ *Mantoux (intradermal) test:* <5 mm or absence of induration and erythema in 24 to 72 hours

Abnormal Values

■ Positive response of larger than normal diameter of induration and erythema

Interfering Factors

■ Improper technique in performing the intradermal injection and injecting the PPD or OT into subcutaneous tissue causes inaccurate results.
■ Incorrect reading (measurement of the response) or timing of the reading may interfere with test results.
■ Incorrect amount or dilution of antigen injected or a delay in the injection after drawing the antigen into the syringe may affect test results.
■ Improper storage or contamination of the antigen may affect results.
■ Recent or present bacterial, viral, or fungal infections may affect test results.
■ Diseases such as hematologic cancers or sarcoidosis can alter results.
■ Drugs such as immunosuppressive agents or steroids can alter results.

NURSING ALERT

These tests are contraindicated in clients with:
■ A history of tuberculosis or previous positive skin test
■ Rash or other eruptions at the injection site
■ Hypersensitivity to other skin tests or vaccinations

Nursing Implications

Assessment

■ Obtain a history of tuberculosis or tuberculosis exposure, signs and symptoms indicating possible tuberculosis, other diagnostic procedures and results, and other skin tests or vaccinations and sensitivities.

Possible Nursing Diagnoses

Infection, risk for, related to inadequate primary defenses
Gas exchange, impaired, risk for, related to decrease in effective lung surface

Activity intolerance related to imbalance between oxygen supply and demand

Anxiety related to perceived threat to health status

Implementation

- Have epinephrine hydrochloride solution (1:1000) available in the event of anaphylaxis.
- Cleanse the skin site on the lower anterior forearm with alcohol or acetone swabs and allow to air dry.
- *Multipuncture test:* Remove the cap covering the tines and stretch the forearm skin taut. Firmly press the device into the prepared site, hold it in place for a second, and then remove it. Four punctures should be visible.
- Record the site and remind the client or caregiver to return in 48 to 72 hours to have the test read.
- At the time of the reading, measure the diameter of the largest indurated area in good light with a plastic ruler. A palpable induration at one or more of the punctures of ≥2 mm indicates a positive test result.
- *Mantoux (intradermal) test:* Prepare PPD or OT in a tuberculin syringe with a short 26-ga needle attached. Prepare the appropriate dilution and amount for the most commonly used intermediate strength (5 tuberculin units in 0.1 mL) or a first strength usually used for children (1 tuberculin unit in 0.1 mL).
- Inject the preparation intradermally as soon as it is drawn up into the syringe at the prepared site. This causes a bleb or wheal to form within the layers of the skin.
- Record the site and remind the client or caregiver to return in 48 to 72 hours to have the test read.
- At the time of the reading, inspect the arm in good light, measure the diameter of any induration with a plastic ruler, and palpate for a thickening of the tissue. A positive result is indicated by a reaction of 5 mm or more with erythema and edema.

Evaluation

- Evaluate test results in relation to other tests performed and the client's symptoms.

Client/Caregiver Teaching

Pretest

- Inform the client that the test is generally done by a nurse in a physician's office or health-care setting and takes about 5 to 10 minutes to complete.

- Inform the client that a moderate amount of pain can be experienced when the intradermal injection is performed.
- Emphasize to the client that the area should not be scratched or disturbed after the injection and before the reading.

Posttest

- Emphasize to the client or caregiver the need to return later to have the test results read (the time depends on the test).
- Inform the client that the effects from a positive response at the site can remain for up to 1 week.
- Reinforce information about additional testing needed and answer or direct questions to the appropriate professionals.

Tuning Fork Tests (Weber, Rinne, Schwabach)

Classification: Sensory organ function

Type of Test: Auditory perception

These noninvasive assessment procedures are done to distinguish conduction hearing loss from sensorineural hearing loss. A 1024 Hz tuning fork is set into a light vibration with a tap of the prongs on the fleshy part of the hand located below the thumb. Three tuning fork tests can be performed: the Weber test, Rinne test, and Schwabach test.

The tuning fork tests are performed as a part of the physical assessment examination and followed by hearing loss audiometry for confirmation of questionable or abnormal results.

Indications

- Screen for hearing loss as part of a routine physical examination and determine the need for a referral to an audiologist
- Evaluate type of hearing loss (conductive or sensorineural)

Reference Values

- Normal air and bone conduction in both ears. No evidence of hearing loss.
- *Weber test:* Same tone loudness heard equally in both ears

- *Rinne test:* Longer and louder tone heard by air conduction (40 seconds) than by bone conduction (20 seconds)
- *Schwabach test:* Same tone loudness heard equally long by the examiner and the client

Abnormal Values

- Conduction hearing loss
     Weber test: Lateralization of tone to one ear indicating loss on that side
     Rinne test: Tone louder or detected for a longer time than the air-conducted tone
     Schwabach test: Prolonged duration of tone when compared to that heard by the examiner
- Sensorineural hearing loss
     Weber test: Lateralization of tone to one ear indicating loss on other side
     Rinne test: Tone heard louder by air conduction
     Schwabach test: Shortened duration when compared to that heard by the examiner

Interfering Factors

- Poor technique in striking the tuning fork or incorrect placement can result in inaccurate results.
- Inability of the client to understand how to identify responses or unwillingness of the client to cooperate during the test can cause inaccurate results.
- Hearing loss in the examiner can affect results in the Schwabach test.

Nursing Implications

Assessment

- Obtain a history of known or suspected hearing loss and cause, use of a hearing aid, changes in auditory acuity, as well as past auditory acuity testing and procedures done and results

Possible Nursing Diagnosis

Sensory or perceptual alteration (auditory), related to altered sensory reception, transmission, or integration

Implementation

- Seat the client in a quiet environment in a chair or on the examining table; position the client so that he or she is comfortable and facing the examiner. A tuning fork of 1024 Hz is used because it tests within the range of human speech (400–5000 Hz).

- *Weber test:* Tap the tuning fork on the handle against the hand to start a light vibration. Hold the base of the vibrating tuning fork with the thumb and forefinger of the dominant hand and place it on the middle of the client's forehead or at the vertex of the head. Ask the client to determine if the sound is heard better and longer on one side than the other. Record as Weber right or left. If sound heard equally, record as Weber negative.

- *Rinne test:* Tap the tuning fork on the handle against the hand to start a light vibration. Have the client mask the ear not being tested by moving a finger in and out of the ear canal of that ear. Hold the base of the vibrating tuning fork with the thumb and forefinger of the dominant hand and place it in contact with the client's mastoid process (bone conduction). Ask the client when the sound is no longer heard. Follow this with placement of the same vibrating tuning fork in front of the ear canal (air conduction) without touching the external part of the ear. Ask the client which of the two has the loudest or longest tone. Repeat the test in the other ear. Record as Rinne positive if air conduction is heard longer and Rinne negative if bone conduction is heard longer.

- *Schwabach test:* Tap the tuning fork on the handle against the hand to start a light vibration. Hold the base of the tuning fork against the client's mastoid process and ask if the tone is heard. Have the client mask the ear not being tested by moving a finger in and out of the ear canal of that ear. Then place the same tuning fork against your own mastoid process of the same side and listen for the tone. Continue to alternate the tuning fork until the sound is no longer heard and determine if both cease to hear the tone at the same time. Repeat the procedure on the other ear. If the client hears the tone for a longer or shorter time, count and note this in seconds. Abnormal test results require further testing by audiometry to confirm findings and detect the type and extent of hearing loss with more specificity.

Evaluation

- Note test results in relation to client's symptoms and other related tests.

Client/Caregiver Teaching

Pretest

- Inform the client that the procedure is performed in a quiet room by the nurse or physician during a physical examination or to test hearing following complaints of reduced auditory acuity; explain that the test takes <5 minutes and that no pain is associated with this procedure.

Posttest

- Refer client to an audiologist if a hearing loss is detected.
- Inform the client of the schedule for retesting and instruct the client in the use, cleansing, and storage of a hearing aid if one is used.

Ultrasonography, Abdominal and Abdominal Aorta

Classification: Ultrasonography

Type of Test: Indirect visualization

This noninvasive study uses high frequency waves of varying intensities to assist in the evaluation of the structure, size and position of the abdominal aorta and branches. It displays constriction or dilation of the vessel, as well as a view of other abdominal organs. Ultrasound is performed alone or in combination with Doppler technique to determine the size of blood lumen and any associated clot formation within an abdominal aortic aneurysm.

Indications

- Detect and measure an aortic aneurysm within the abdomen to determine deviation from the normal diameter and risk of rupture
- Differentiate between vessel lumen and a clot within an aortic aneurysm by using a Doppler in combination with ultrasonography evidence
- Diagnose pathology of abdominal organs (e.g., liver, pancreas, gallbladder, spleen, and kidneys)
- Determine patency and function of abdominal vessels and ducts (e.g., portal vein, splenic vein, renal arteries and veins, superior and inferior mesenteric veins, and biliary and pancreatic ducts)

- Determine the presence of ascitic fluid and the best site for a diagnostic paracentesis
- Diagnose abdominal pathology during pregnancy

Reference Values

- Normal structure image of the abdominal organs and contour and diameter of the abdominal aorta of 1.5 to 2.5 cm of various sections of the vessel

Abnormal Values

- Abdominal tumors
- Aortic aneurysm
- Aortic stenosis

Interfering Factors

- Incorrect placement or movement of the transducer over the desired sites of the organs to be scanned may alter test results.
- The presence of barium, gas, or feces in the bowel attenuates sound waves and prevents clear imaging of the abdominal organs.
- Obesity can affect the transmission of waves to and from the abdomen because of an increased space between the organs and the transducer.
- Increased bowel motility can affect sound waves.
- Scar tissue from previous surgery can prevent transmission of the waves through the skin and to the abdominal organs.
- Inability of the client to remain still during the study may affect test results.

NURSING ALERT

The following require immediate reporting and intervention:
- Sudden changes in vital signs and continuous abdominal or back pain, which indicate an expanding aneurysm
- The sudden onset of severe pain, hypotension, tachycardia, and diaphoresis, which indicate aneurysm rupture

Nursing Implications

Assessment

- Obtain a history of suspected or existing abdominal aorta aneurysm, abdominal organ or vessel pathology, other tests and procedures done, and the results of the last abdominal ultrasound for comparison.
- Note recent administration of barium enema as residual barium can obscure inspection.
- Ensure that food has been restricted for 12 hours before the test and that fluids are encouraged to provide a full bladder to push the bowel out of the pelvis.
- Ensure that the client has abstained from smoking overnight before the procedure.

Possible Nursing Diagnosis

Risk for injury related to possible aneurysm rupture

Implementation

- Administer simethicone (Mylanta Gas) to reduce gas and an enema to remove barium and feces from the bowel, if ordered.
- Place the client in a supine position on the examining table. Note that a side-lying or sitting position can also be used. Drape the abdomen for privacy and apply conductive gel to the areas of the abdomen to be scanned. Instruct the client to hold the breath during the study as the transducer is rotated and manipulated over the abdomen. Move the transducer from the xiphoid process to the aortic bifurcation and to the left and right of the midline for scanning of the aorta and to other sites for scanning the abdominal organs and vessels. When studies are complete, remove the gel from the abdomen.
- Impulses are transmitted from the device to a screen for visual display and photographed for future viewing and comparisons.

Evaluation

- Note test results in relation to the client's symptoms and other tests performed.

Client/Caregiver Teaching

Pretest

- Inform the client that the procedure is generally performed in a special ultrasound room in a hospital or by a technician

from a medical imaging company and interpreted by a physician. Explain that the test takes approximately 45 minutes.
- Tell the client that neither pain nor risk of complications or exposure to radiation is associated with this study.

Posttest

- Instruct the client to report any abdominal or back pain, diaphoresis, or increased pulse to physician immediately if aneurysm is present.

Ultrasonography, Arterial, Transcranial Doppler

Classification: Ultrasonography

Type of Test: Indirect visualization

This noninvasive technique records sound waves to obtain information about cerebral vessel patency and blood viscosity. The study measures and records the velocity of blood traveling through a vessel via a transducer that transmits waves through an area of the cranium that is thin or contains a gap or opening. These sites include the transtemporal to view the middle, anterior, or posterior cerebral arteries and the circle of Willis; the transorbital to view the circle of Willis; and the transoccipital to view the vertebral and basilar arteries. This procedure provides valuable information, which once could be obtained only by the more invasive procedure of angiography, to help in the diagnosis and treatment of neurologic and cerebrovascular disorders.

Indications

- Detect the presence of arterial stenosis or arteriovenous malformations in the cerebral vascular system evidenced by low velocity pulsations that result from low flow resistance
- Determine the presence of intracranial collateral pathways
- Diagnose hyperemia resulting from a head injury or congestion in the tissue surrounding an ischemic area evidenced by a higher velocity and wave pulsations

- Determine the presence of vertebral or basilar arterial insufficiency
- Monitor for increased intracranial pressure evidenced by high velocity pulsations
- Monitor for vasospasm evidenced by changes in cerebral blood flow
- Confirm brain death

Reference Values

- Normal blood flow through cranial arteries; no evidence of stenosis, hyperemia, arteriovenous malformation, or increase in intracranial pressure

Abnormal Values

- Brain death
- Cerebral arterial stenosis
- Cerebral arteriovenous malformation
- Cerebral hyperemia
- Increased intracranial pressure
- Vertebral or basilar arterial insufficiency

Interfering Factors

- Incorrect placement of the transducer over the site on the skull can alter test results.
- Inability of the client to maintain the head position during the procedure and to lie quietly can affect results.

Nursing Implications

Assessment

- Obtain a history of previous arterial studies, the presence of disorders predisposing to cerebral arterial vascular problems, and therapy received for abnormalities.

Possible Nursing Diagnoses

Anxiety related to perceived threat to or change in health status
Pain related to pressure on brain tissue
Sensory alteration related to compression of brain tissue

Implementation

- Place the client in a supine position on the examining table. Tell the client to lie quietly during the procedure. Position the head to expose the site to be used (e.g., transtemporal

[temporal] site to view middle, anterior, or posterior cerebral arteries; foramen magnum [transoccipital] site to view vertebral and basilar arteries; over-the-eye [transorbital] site to view the circle of Willis) and support the head to prevent movement.

- Apply a conductive gel to the skin of the site, place the transducer over the site, and gently manipulate around the area. Sound waves are transmitted through the transducer to the site and bounced off the cerebral vessel back to the probe and then to the monitor to be displayed as a wave on an oscilloscope screen and to be permanently recorded by the computer. Normal velocity ranges are 30 to 50 cm/sec in posterior arteries and 40 to 70 cm/sec in middle and anterior arteries.

Evaluation

- Check vital signs and neurologic status and compare to baseline.
- Compare test results with client's symptoms as well as the results of other diagnostic tests.

Client/Caregiver Teaching

Pretest

- Explain to the client the purpose of the study and how the procedure is performed; inform the client that the procedure, which generally takes from 30 to 60 minutes to complete, is performed in a vascular laboratory by a technician and that the results are interpreted by a physician.
- Explain that no food or fluid restrictions are necessary before the study.
- Explain that the procedure is painless and carries no risks.
- Tell the client that the physician will discuss the results of the study.

Posttest

- Instruct the client to report headache, dizziness, syncope, or visual disturbances.

Ultrasonography, Bladder

Classification: Ultrasonography

Type of Test: Indirect visualization

This noninvasive study uses high-frequency waves of various intensities to visualize the position, structures, and size of the bladder. Additional methods for evaluation include the transrectal, transurethral, and transvaginal approach. It can be included in ultrasonography of the kidneys, ureters, bladder, urethra, and gonads in diagnosing renal/neurologic disorders.

Indications

- Detect tumor of the bladder wall or pelvis evidenced by distortion of the position or changes in contour of the bladder
- Assess residual urine following voiding to diagnose urinary tract obstruction causing overdistention
- Determine end-stage malignancy of the bladder caused by an extension of a primary tumor of the ovary or other pelvic organ
- Measure urinary bladder volume by transurethral or transvaginal approach

Normal Findings

- Normal size, position, and contour of the urinary bladder

Abnormal Findings

- Tumor
- Cyst
- Malignancy of the bladder
- Urinary tract obstruction

Interfering Factors

- Incorrect placement of the transducer over the test sites can affect test results.
- The presence of barium or gas in the bowel can affect clear imaging of the bladder and surrounding areas.

- Inability of the client to remain still during the procedure can alter results.

Nursing Implications

Assessment

- Obtain a history of suspected or existing diseases and dysfunction of the urinary bladder, other tests and procedures done to diagnose disorders of the bladder, and therapy received to treat a tumor or other condition of the bladder or surrounding pelvic organs.
- Note recent administration of barium enema as residual barium can obscure inspection.

Possible Nursing Diagnoses

Urinary elimination, altered, related to trauma or bladder impairment, urinary residual and retention

Anxiety related to perceived threat to or change in health status

Fluid volume deficit, risk for, related to stimulation of renal-intestinal reflexes causing nausea, vomiting, and diarrhea

Implementation

- Have client disrobe below the waist; provide a hospital gown.
- Place the client in a supine position on the examining table. Expose the lower abdomen and drape for privacy.
- Palpate the bladder to ensure that it is full of urine and apply a conductive gel to the area.
- A transducer is manipulated over the bladder and pelvic sites and the sound waves are projected on the screen and photographed for immediate and future viewing.
- If the client is to be examined for residual urine volume, the bladder is emptied and the procedure is repeated and the volume calculated.

Evaluation

- Compare the tests results with the client's symptoms and the results of other diagnostic tests.

Client/Caregiver Teaching

Pretest

- Explain to the client the purpose of the study and how the procedure is performed; inform the client that the procedure is performed in a special ultrasound room in a hospital or medical imaging company by a technician and that the results are interpreted by a physician; a consent form is not required for the transabdominal method but is needed if alternate approaches are used.

- Inform the client that there is no pain or risk of exposure to radiation or complications associated with this study.
- Offer three to four glasses of water within 2 hours before the test and inform the client to refrain from voiding.

Posttest

- Inform the client that the physician will discuss the results of the study.
- Explain to the client the importance of maintaining a fluid intake of 2 to 3 L/d and of reporting any discrepancy in input and output ratio.

Ultrasonography, Breast

Classification: Ultrasonography

Type of Test: Indirect visualization

This noninvasive study uses high-frequency waves of various intensities to visualize and record palpable and nonpalpable masses. It is especially useful in clients with dense or fibrocystic breasts and those with silicone prosthesis, as the beam easily penetrates this material, to allow for routine examination that cannot be performed with x-ray mammography. The procedure can also be done as an adjunct to mammography or in place of mammography in those who reject or should not be exposed to x-ray diagnostic studies (e.g., pregnant women). Both breasts are usually examined during this procedure.

Indications

- Determine the presence of nonpalpable abnormalities viewed on mammography of fibrocystic breast tissue and monitor changes in these abnormalities
- Differentiate among breast masses, such as cyst, solid tumor, and other lesions, in dense breast tissue
- Detect very small tumors in combination with mammography for diagnostic validation

Reference Values

- Normal subcutaneous, mammary, and retromammary layers of tissue in both breasts; no evidence of pathologic lesions in either breast

Abnormal Values

- Breast solid tumor, lesions
- Fibrocystic disease

Interfering Factors

- Incorrect placement or movement of the transducer over the breasts or a particular site on a breast can affect test results.
- Largeness of breasts can prohibit use of this method.
- Inability of the client to remain still or assume the necessary position during the procedure may alter test results.

Nursing Implications

Assessment

- Obtain a history of suspected or existing breast abnormalities or surgeries, past studies done to monitor or diagnose breast abnormalities, the presence of a prosthesis in one or both breasts, and risk status for breast tumor.
- Ensure that the client has not applied lotions, bath powder, or other substances to the chest and breast area before the study.

Possible Nursing Diagnoses

Pain related to disease process

Anxiety related to perceived threat to health status

Grieving, anticipatory, related to perceived loss or threat of death

Implementation

- Place client in a supine position on the examining table. Expose the chest and drape the client for privacy.
- Apply a warmed conductive gel to the breasts, place the client's arms behind the head, and move the transducer over the skin of both breasts.
- The sound waves received are displayed on a screen and photographed. After the test, gently wipe off the gel.
- If the procedure is done using a tank of warm, chemically prepared water, place the client in a prone position and im-

merse each breast in the tank. The transducer placed at the bottom of the tank transmits the waves through the water. These waves are reflected from the breasts producing echoes and are displayed as waveforms on a screen and photographed for future viewing.

Evaluation

- Note test results in relation to the other tests performed and the client's symptoms.

Client/Caregiver Teaching

Pretest

- Inform the client that the procedure, which takes less than 30 minutes for examination of both breasts, is performed in a special ultrasound room in a hospital or medical imaging company by a technician and that the results are interpreted by a physician.
- Inform the client that no pain, risk of complications, or exposure to radiation is associated with this study.
- Tell the client to avoid applying deodorant, bath powders, or creams to the chest before the test.

Posttest

- Instruct the client in the monthly breast self-examination procedure and encourage the client to demonstrate the technique.

Ultrasonography, Kidney

Classification: Ultrasonography

Type of Test: Indirect visualization

This noninvasive study uses high-frequency waves of various intensities to visualize the position, structure, and size of the kidney(s). It can be performed with a radionuclide scan and is especially valuable in clients with renal failure because it is noninvasive and study does not rely on renal function to obtain a diagnosis.

Indications

- Detect masses and differentiate between cysts or solid tumor evidenced by specific waveform patterns or absence of sound waves
- Provide the location and size of a renal mass in clients who are unable to undergo intravenous pyelography because of poor renal function or allergy to iodinated contrast media
- Determine the presence and location of renal or ureteral calculi and obstruction
- Determine an accumulation of fluid in the kidney caused by backflow of urine, hemorrhage, or perirenal fluid
- Determine the size, shape, and position of a nonfunctioning kidney to identify the cause
- Aid in the diagnosis of hydronephrosis in one or both kidneys, polycystic kidneys, or other congenital anomalies of the kidneys in children and monitor changes in the sizes of the kidneys as a disease progresses
- Aid in the diagnosis of the effect of chronic glomerulonephritis and end-stage chronic renal failure on the kidneys (e.g., decreasing size)
- Locate the site and guide percutaneous renal biopsy or aspiration needle or nephrostomy tube insertion
- Evaluate renal transplantation for changes in kidney size
- Evaluate or plan therapy for renal tumor

Reference Values

- Normal size, position, and shape of the kidneys and the structures

Abnormal Values

- Acute glomerulonephritis
- Acute pyelonephritis
- Congenital anomalies, such as absent kidney, horseshoe, ectopic, or duplicated kidneys
- Hydronephrosis
- Obstruction of ureters
- Perirenal abscess
- Polycystic kidney
- Rejection of renal transplant
- Renal calculi
- Renal cysts
- Renal hypertrophy
- Renal tumors

Interfering Factors

- Incorrect placement of the transducer over the test sites can affect test results.
- The presence of barium remaining from previous x-ray studies can affect clear imaging of the kidneys and ureters.
- Inability of the client to remain still during the procedure can alter test results.

Nursing Implications

Assessment

- Obtain a history of suspected or existing diseases of the kidneys; other tests and procedures done to diagnose disorders of these organs; and therapy received to treat a tumor, inflammation, or congenital condition. If the study is to be performed on a child, the caretaker and the client are included in the teaching and preparation and a play kit is used depending on the age of the child.
- Ensure that the client has restricted food for 12 hours before the study; water is permitted during this time.
- Note recent administration of barium enema because residual barium can obscure inspection.

Possible Nursing Diagnoses

Fluid volume excess related to compromised regulatory mechanism

Anxiety related to perceived threat to or change in health status

Infection, risk for, related to traumatized tissue

Implementation

- Have the client remove clothing and provide a hospital gown.
- Place the client in a prone position on the examining table; a sidelying position also can be used. (Children are placed in the supine position, however, if needed, a child can be held in the proper position for the study.) Expose and drape the area to be scanned. Apply a conductive gel and manipulate the transducer over the flank area. Ask the client to breathe as deeply as possible to view the upper parts of the kidneys. As with other ultrasound studies, the sound waves are transmitted to the organ and bounced back to the transducer. Images are projected onto a screen for viewing and photographed for future comparisons.

- When the studies are completed, the gel is removed from the area examined.

Evaluation

- Compare test results with clinical symptoms and results of other diagnostic tests.

Client/Caregiver Teaching

Pretest

- Explain to the client the purpose of the study and how the procedure is performed; tell the client that the procedure, which takes <30 minutes, is performed in a special ultrasound room in a hospital or medical imaging company by a technician and the results are interpreted by a physician.
- Inform the client that no pain, risk of complications, or exposure to radiation is associated with this study.

Posttest

- Inform the client that the physician will discuss the results of the study.

Ultrasonography, Liver and Biliary System

Classification: Ultrasonography

Type of Test: Indirect visualization

These noninvasive studies use high-frequency waves of various intensities delivered by a transducer. The waves are bounced back, converted to electrical energy, amplified by the transducer, and displayed on a monitor to evaluate the structure, size, and position of the liver and gallbladder in the upper-right quadrant (URQ) of the abdomen. Gallbladder ultrasonography is especially helpful when done in clients whose gallbladder is unable to opacify gallstones with oral or intravenous radiologic studies. Liver ultrasonography can be done in combination with a nuclear scan to obtain information about liver function as well as the density differences obtained by ultrasound.

Indications

- Diagnose hepatic lesions evidenced by density differences and echo pattern changes
- Determine patency and diameter of the hepatic duct for dilation or obstruction
- Determine the presence of metastasis to the liver from a primary lesion (e.g., breast, colorectal, or other abdominal organ)
- Differentiate between obstructive and nonobstructive jaundice by determining the cause
- Determine the cause of unexplained hepatomegaly and abnormal liver function tests
- Diagnose acute or chronic cholecystitis evidenced by an enlarged gallbladder with wall thickening
- Diagnose gallstones within the gallbladder or biliary ducts evidenced by dilatation and/or obstruction of the biliary tree or ducts and an increased bilirubin level
- Diagnose gallbladder stones or inflammation when oral cholecystography is inconclusive
- Diagnose cysts, polyps, or solid tumor of the gallbladder evidenced by echoes specific to tissue density and sharply or poorly defined masses
- Determine cause of unexplained RUQ pain
- Evaluate response to therapy for tumor evidenced by a decrease in size of the organ
- Guide catheter placement into the gallbladder for stone dissolution and gallbladder fragmentation

Reference Values

- Normal size, position, and shape of the liver and gallbladder as well as patency of the cystic and common bile ducts

Abnormal Values

- Biliary or hepatic duct obstruction/dilation
- Cirrhosis
- Gallbladder inflammation
- Gallbladder stones
- Hematoma or trauma
- Hepatic cysts
- Hepatic or gallbladder tumors and metastasis
- Hepatocellular disease
- Hepatomegaly
- Intrahepatic abscess

Interfering Factors

- Incorrect placement of the transducer over the test sites can alter test results.
- The presence of gas or barium in the bowel or stomach remaining from previous x-ray studies can affect clear imaging of the liver, gallbladder, and biliary system.
- The ribs can attenuate the sound waves and affect clear imaging of the right lobe of the liver.
- Inability of the client to remain still during the procedure can affect test results.

Nursing Implications

Assessment

- Obtain a history of suspected or existing diseases of the liver or gallbladder and ductal involvement, other tests and procedures done to diagnose disorders of these organ systems, and therapy received to treat the tumor or obstruction.
- Ensure that food, fluid, and smoking has been restricted 12 hours before the procedure.
- Note recent administration of barium enema because residual barium can obscure inspection.

Possible Nursing Diagnoses

Nutrition, altered, less than body requirements, related to inability to ingest nutrients

Fluid volume excess related to compromised regulatory mechanism and excess sodium intake

Anxiety related to perceived threat or change to health status

Skin integrity, impaired, risk for, related to altered circulation

Implementation

- Administer an enema, if ordered, before the study to remove any remaining barium.
- Place the client in a supine position on the examining table, although the prone or side lying positions can be used during the study. Expose the abdomen and drape for privacy. Instruct the client to remain quiet during the procedure.
- Apply a conductive gel to the skin of the RUQ.
- The technician will place the transducer and move it over the area to obtain several planes of scanning. Each lobe and the border of the liver and the border of the gallbladder is examined. The cystic and common bile ducts are also examined for patency. During the procedure, the client will

be requested to inhale deeply and hold breath on inspiration. The patterns are displayed on a screen and photographed for future viewing.

- Gallbladder contractibility is viewed by scanning following administration of Lipomul, a fatty substance that allows evaluation of gallbladder function.

Evaluation

- Note test results in relation to other tests performed and the client's symptoms.

Client/Caregiver Teaching

Pretest

- Inform the client that the procedure, which takes less than 30 minutes, is generally performed in a special ultrasound room in a hospital or medical imaging company by a technician and that the results are interpreted by a physician.
- Tell the client that no pain, risk of radiation exposure, or complications are associated with this study.
- Instruct the client to withhold food and fluids as well as to avoid smoking for 12 hours before the procedure.

Posttest

- Advise the client to resume food, water, and medications withheld before the procedure.

Ultrasonography, Lymph Nodes and Retroperitoneal

Classification: Ultrasonography

Type of Test: Indirect visualization

These noninvasive studies use high-frequency waves of varying intensities to identify retroperitoneal pathology, usually lymph node enlargement. These diagnostic methods are preferred since this area is inaccessible for conventional radiography in diagnosing lymphadenopathy, although it can be used in combination with lymphangiography to confirm a diagnosis.

Indications

- Determine the size or enlargement of aortic and iliac lymph nodes to diagnose lymphoma
- Determine the location of the enlarged nodes to plan radiation and other therapy
- Diagnose the presence of retroperitoneal solid tumor or infection evidenced by enlargement of lymph nodes
- Evaluate changes in the size of nodes or tumors during and following therapy evidenced by shrinkage of the mass or nodes

Reference Values

- Normal retroperitoneal and intrapelvic node size of 1.5 cm in diameter

Abnormal Values

- Lymphoma
- Infection or abscess
- Retroperitoneal tumor

Interfering Factors

- Incorrect placement and movement of the transducer over the test sites can alter test results.
- The presence of barium, gas, or feces in the bowel will attenuate the sound waves.
- Inability of the client to remain still during the study will affect results.

Nursing Implications

Assessment

- Obtain a history of suspected or existing tumor or lymphoma, other tests and procedures done for diagnosis, and therapy received to reduce size of a retroperitoneal mass or lymph nodes.
- Ensure that food has been restricted after midnight before the study; encourage the client to ingest clear liquids to provide a full bladder before scanning.

- Ensure that this study is performed either before intestinal barium tests or after the barium is cleared from the system.
- Ensure that the client maintains a full bladder if scanning is to be performed below the umbilicus.

Possible Nursing Diagnoses

Pain related to disease process
Fatigue related to decreased metabolic energy production
Protection, altered, related to abnormal blood profiles

Implementation

- Place the client in a supine position on the examining table and ask the client to lie quietly during the procedure. Expose the abdomen from the umbilicus down and drape properly for privacy.
- Apply conductive gel to the flank and abdominal areas below the umbilicus if these sites are included in the procedure. Move the transducer over the area prepared with the gel. Longitudinal and transverse scans are taken and the sound waves are echoed to the transducer to reflect different densities of tissues. These impulses are displayed on a screen and photographed for immediate and future viewing and interpretation.
- When the studies are completed, the gel is wiped from the area.

Evaluation

- Note test results in relation to other related tests performed and the client's symptoms.

Client/Caregiver Teaching

Pretest

- Inform the client that the procedure, which takes less than 60 minutes, is generally performed in a special ultrasound room in a hospital or medical imaging company by a technician and that the results are interpreted by a physician.
- Explain that the procedure is painless, has no risks or complications, and has no associated radiation exposure.
- Instruct the client to withhold food after midnight before the test. Tell the client that clear liquids will be given the morning of the procedure to fill the bladder and aid the study.

Posttest

- Instruct the client to resume food withheld before the procedure.

Ultrasonography, Obstetric

Classification: Ultrasonography

Type of Test: Indirect visualization

This noninvasive study uses high-frequency waves of various intensities to visualize the fetus and placenta as early in a pregnancy as the fifth week of gestation. It is the safest method of examination to determine fetal size, growth, position, and fetal structural abnormalities. The procedure can also be used in combination with Doppler monitoring of the fetal heart or respiratory movements in the detection of high-risk pregnancy. Because the pregnant uterus is filled with amniotic fluid, ultrasonography is an ideal method of evaluating the fetus and placenta.

Uses of obstetric ultrasonography to secure information regarding the fetus vary with the trimester in which the procedure is done. The methods of scanning include the transabdominal and transvaginal techniques depending on when the procedure is performed, for example, the first trimester (transvaginal) or second trimester (transabdominal).

Indications

- Determine and confirm pregnancy or multiple pregnancies by determining the number of gestational sacs in the first trimester (usually by the fourth or fifth week)
- Determine fetal heart and body movements and to detect high-risk pregnancy by monitoring fetal heart and respiratory movements in combination with Doppler ultrasound (at the 12th week) or real-time scanning (by the sixth or seventh week)
- Measure fetal gestational age and evaluate umbilical artery, uterine artery, and fetal aorta by Doppler examination to determine fetal intrauterine growth rate for retardation (IUGR)
- Determine fetal gestational age by uterine size and measurements of crown-rump length, biparietal diameter, fetal extremities, head, and other parts of the anatomy at developmental phases of fetal development
- Determine fetal structural anomalies, usually at 20th week or later

- Detect fetal death evidenced by absence of movement and fetal heart tones
- Determine cause of bleeding, such as placenta previa or abruptio placentae
- Determine the placental size, location, and site of implantation
- Monitor placental growth and amniotic fluid volume
- Diagnose fetal abnormalities to prepare for surgical correction or pregnancy termination
- Determine fetal position before birth, such as breech or transverse presentations
- Guide the needle during amniocentesis and fetal transfusion
- Determine fetal effect of Rh incompatibility

Normal Findings

- Normal fetus, age, size, viability, position, and functional capacities; normal placenta size, position, and structure; adequate volume of amniotic fluid

Abnormal Findings

- Fetal hydrops
- Fetal death
- Intestinal atresia
- Placenta previa
- Abruptio placenta
- Myelomeningocele
- Hydrocephalus
- Renal or skeletal defects

Interfering Factors

- Incorrect placement of the transducer over the test sites can affect test results.
- The presence of air or barium in the bowel from previous x-ray studies can affect clear imaging of the fetus and placenta.
- Inability of the sound beam to penetrate to the site because of client size can alter results.
- A bladder that is not full enough to push the uterus from the pubic area can prohibit better imaging of the pregnant uterus.

Nursing Implications

Assessment

- Obtain a history of menstrual dates, medications taken for fertility or birth control or other drug use, previous pregnancy, and treatment received for high-risk pregnancy.
- Note recent administration of barium enema because residual barium can obscure inspection.
- Ensure that the client has increased fluid intake (five to six glasses of water) 1 hour before the study.

Possible Nursing Diagnoses

Fluid volume deficit, risk for, related to excessive vascular losses

Gas exchange, impaired, fetal, related to altered blood flow

Anxiety related to perceived change or threat to health status of fetus

Implementation

- Place client in a supine position on the examining table. Expose the lower abdomen and drape for privacy. Apply conductive gel to the area and move the transducer over the entire abdomen or lower abdomen depending on the size of the uterus.
- The examination uses both A and B mode techniques that convert echoes into waveforms that represent the positions of structures and a two-dimensional or cross-sectional image of the structures. Real-time imaging reveals the fetus in motion on the screen. Selected views can be photographed and recorded for later review and comparison.
- If a transvaginal approach is done, a full bladder is not needed but this method of performing the study is not done past the first trimester.
- When the study is completed, the gel is removed from the skin or the probe from the vagina and the area cleansed and patted dry if needed.

Evaluation

- Note the test results in relation to other tests performed and the client's symptoms.

Client/Caregiver Teaching

Pretest

- Inform the client that the procedure, which takes less than 30 minutes, is performed in a special ultrasound room in a hospital or medical imaging company by a technician and that the results are interpreted by a physician.

- Inform the client that because this study does not involve radiation, it is not harmful to the fetus. Also inform her that she will be able to view the screen and that an explanation will be given about the fetus as it appears.

- If the transvaginal approach is planned, inform the client of the procedure.

- Instruct the client to increase fluid intake (five to six glasses) 1 hour before the study to fill the bladder and improve visibility.

Posttest

- If an abnormality is revealed, support the client and inform her about possible future diagnostic procedures and available counseling services.

Ultrasonography, Ocular

Classification: Ultrasonography

Type of Test: Indirect visualization

This noninvasive study uses high-frequency waves of varying intensities to diagnose abnormalities of the eye and orbital structures. Waves are directed into body tissues and reflected back to a transducer, processed, and displayed as images on a screen. The study, which uses both A and B mode techniques, especially helps to identify pathology in the presence of opacities of the cornea and lens. The A mode converts the echoes into waveforms that represent the position of different structures, and the B mode converts the echoes into a dot pattern that represents a two-dimensional image of the ocular structures. A handheld B mode scanner is now available for eye ultrasound that can be performed in the ophthalmologist's office.

Indications

- Diagnose the presence of tumors and determine the type, size, shape, texture, and location of the tumor (e.g., mela-

noma, hemangioma, glioma, neurofibroma, meningioma, metastatic lymphoma) evidenced by specific abnormal ultrasound patterns
■ Detect the presence of cystic conditions (e.g., mucoid, dermoid) and differentiate these from solid tumors
■ Diagnose the effect of Graves' disease on the eye tissues evidenced by inflammatory changes and extraocular thickening
■ Diagnose orbital lesions and differentiate these from intraocular lesions evidenced by characteristic ultrasound patterns
■ Locate and identify intraocular foreign bodies
■ Diagnose the presence and extent of retinal or choroidal detachment
■ Determine the presence of vitreous abnormalities (e.g., opacities, vitreous bands, hemorrhage) evidenced by density in appearance of the images
■ Evaluate the fundus that is clouded by a cataract and measure the length of the eye for the insertion of a lens implant following removal of a cataract before surgery
■ Evaluate the eyes for keratoprosthesis
■ Evaluate the vitreous cavity for abnormalities before vitrectomy

Reference Values

■ Normal ocular tissues and structures

Abnormal Values

■ Cystic lesions
■ Intraocular foreign bodies
■ Intraocular tumors
■ Orbital lesions
■ Retinal or choroidal detachment
■ Retinoblastomas
■ Vitreous hemorrhage and other abnormalities

Interfering Factors

■ Incorrect placement of the transducer on the eye can affect test results.
■ Inability of the client to remain still during the procedure can alter results.
■ Vitreous humor that has been replaced by gas can affect imaging.

Nursing Implications

Assessment

- Obtain a history of eye symptoms, trauma, or other abnormalities as well as therapy or surgery received for an eye disorder.

Possible Nursing Diagnoses

Sensory/perceptual alterations (visual) related to altered sensory reception, transmission, and/or integration

Anxiety related to perceived threat or change in health status

Implementation

- Instill eyedrops in the dosage and frequency ordered to anesthetize the eye.
- Place the client in a supine position on the examining table. After the client is requested to close the eyes and remain still during the procedure, apply a conductive gel to the eyelid. Place the transducer on the site that transmits sound waves into the eye. This provides a B scan done to diagnose eye abnormalities.
- Perform an A scan by placing a cup over the eye, applying the gel, and gently moving the transducer over the cup or by gently manipulating the transducer directly on the corneal surface. The A scan measures the axial length of the eye and assists in diagnosing abnormal lesions. Request that the client change the gaze of the eye being examined during the procedure to obtain orbital echo patterns to differentiate normal from abnormal patterns.
- Another technique used in ocular ultrasonography is the immersion method. For this method, the transducer is placed in a water bath and the sound waves are directed along the visual axis.
- When the studies are completed, the gel and/or cup is removed from the eye or eyelid.

Evaluation

- Note the test results in relation to the other tests performed and the client's symptoms.

Client/Caregiver Teaching

Pretest

- Inform the client that the procedure is performed in a special ultrasound room in the hospital, physician office, or medical

imaging agency by a physician or technician and takes 10 to 30 minutes depending on the type of examination done.
- Explain that no pain, risk of complications or exposure to radiation is associated with this study.
- Inform the client that no food or fluid restrictions are necessary before the study.

Posttest

- Inform the client that vision can be blurred for a short time; instruct the client to avoid rubbing the eye until the anesthetic wears off (about 3 to 4 hours) to prevent injury to the eye.

Ultrasonography, Pancreas

Classification: Ultrasonography

Type of Test: Indirect visualization

This noninvasive study uses high frequency waves of various intensity to assist in diagnosing pancreatic pathology. Echo patterns vary with densities that allow the size, shape, and position of this organ to be identified. The procedure is done in combination with a nuclear scan of the organ for better visualization or followed by computerized tomography (CT) and biopsy to confirm a diagnosis.

Indications

- Diagnose pancreatitis evidenced by pancreas enlargement with increased echoes
- Diagnose pancreatic cancer evidenced by a poorly defined mass or mass in the head of the pancreas that obstructs the pancreatic duct
- Diagnose pseudocysts evidenced by a well-defined mass with absence of echoes from the interior
- Monitor therapeutic response to tumor treatment
- Provide guidance for percutaneous aspiration and needle biopsy of the pancreas
- Detect anatomic abnormalities as a consequence of pancreatitis

Normal Findings

- Normal size, contour, and texture of pancreas and patency of pancreatic duct.

Abnormal Findings

- Pancreatic tumors
- Pseudocysts
- Acute pancreatitis
- Pancreatic duct obstruction

Interfering Factors

- Incorrect placement of the transducer over the test site
- Presence of gas or barium in the bowel or stomach remaining from previous x-ray studies that attenuate the waves
- Client obesity can affect the transmission of waves to and from the abdomen because of increased space between the organ and transducer
- Inability of the client to remain still during the study

Nursing Implications

Assessment

- Obtain a history of suspected or existing diseases of the pancreas, other tests and procedures done to diagnose pancreatic disorders, and therapy received to treat pancreatic tumor or inflammation.
- Ensure that food has been restricted and fluids encouraged to provide stomach distention before the procedure.
- Note recent administration of barium enema as residual barium can interfere with waves and obscure inspection.

Possible Nursing Diagnoses

Pain related to obstruction of pancreatic duct
Fluid volume deficit, risk for, related to excessive gastric losses
Nutrition, altered, less than body requirements, related to vomiting
Anxiety related to perceived change or threat to health status

Implementation

- Place client in a supine position on the examining table although position can be changed during the procedure. Apply conductive gel to the skin of the epigastric portion of the abdomen. Move the transducer over the area and the echoes are converted to electrical impulses displayed on a screen.

■ During the procedure, the client can be requested to inhale deeply, regulate breathing or hold his or her breath, and drink water to better outline the abdominal organs and improve visualization of the pancreas. Views are photographed for future study. When the studies are completed, the gel is removed from the abdomen.

Evaluation

■ Note test results in relation to other tests performed and the client's symptoms.

Client/Caregiver Teaching

Pretest

■ Inform the client that the procedure is performed in a special ultrasound room in a hospital or medical imaging company by a technician and interpreted by a physician and takes approximately 30 to 40 minutes.

■ Instruct client that there is no exposure to radiation, pain, or risk of complications associated with this study.

■ Instruct that the client is requested to lie quietly during the procedure.

■ Inform client that the room may be darkened to aid visualization.

■ Inform the client to withhold food and increase fluid intake before the test.

Posttest

■ Inform client to resume food and medications withheld before the procedure.

Ultrasonography, Pelvis

Classification: Ultrasonography

Type of Test: Indirect visualization

This noninvasive study uses high-frequency waves of various intensities to determine the presence of masses, their size, structure, and the location of other abnormalities of the uterus, ovaries, fallopian tubes, and vagina. The procedure is done by a transabdominal or transvaginal approach. The transabdominal approach provides a view of the pelvic organs posterior to the bladder; the transvaginal approach focuses on the female reproductive organs and is often used to monitor ovulation over a period of days in clients undergoing fertility assessment. This approach is also used in obese clients or in clients with retroversion of the uterus as the sound waves are better able to reach the organ from the vaginal site.

Indications

- Monitor placement and location of an intrauterine device (IUD)
- Detect masses in the pelvis and differentiate them from cysts or solid tumors evidenced by differences in sound patterns
- Detect the presence of ovarian cysts and to determine the type, if possible, evidenced by size, outline, and change in position of other pelvic organs
- Diagnose pelvic inflammatory disease (PID) when done in combination with other laboratory tests
- Evaluate therapy for a tumor evidenced by a reduction in mass size
- Diagnose pelvic abscess or peritonitis caused by ruptured appendix or diverticulitis
- Detect bleeding into the pelvis resulting from trauma to the area or ascites associated with tumor metastasis
- Monitor follicular size associated with fertility studies or to remove follicles for in vitro transplantation

Normal Findings

- Normal size, position, location, and structure of the pelvic organs (e.g., uterus, ovaries, fallopian tubes, vagina); IUD properly positioned within the uterine cavity

Abnormal Findings

- Uterine tumor, fibroids, or adnexal tumor
- Ovarian cysts
- PID
- Pelvic abscess
- Peritonitis

Interfering Factors

- Incorrect transducer placement over the pelvic areas or a probe within the vagina for proper examination may alter test results.
- The presence of gas or barium in the bowel can affect clear imaging of the lower abdomen and pelvic area.
- A bladder that is not full will not push the bowel from the pelvis and the uterus from the symphysis pubis thereby prohibiting clear imaging of the pelvic organs.
- Inability of the client to remain still during the procedure can affect test results.

Nursing Implications

Assessment

- Obtain a history of suspected or existing disorders of the pelvic organs, other tests and procedures done to diagnose disorders of these organs, presenting symptoms, and any therapy received to treat a tumor.
- Ensure that the client has a full bladder before the study and retains a full bladder if a transabdominal approach is planned.

Possible Nursing Diagnoses

Infection, risk for spread, related to presence of infectious process
Pain, acute, related to inflammation, edema, and congestion of pelvic tissue
Hyperthermia related to inflammatory process
Anxiety related to perceived threat or change in health status

Implementation

- Place the client in a supine position on the examining table. Expose lower abdomen and drape for privacy. Apply a conductive gel to the area and move a handheld transducer over the skin while the bladder is distended (transabdominally). The sound waves are received and displayed on a screen and photographed.

- If a transvaginal approach is performed, a covered and lubricated probe is inserted into the vagina, moved around, and the sound waves received and imaged on the screen. A full bladder is not required to perform the transvaginal procedure.
- When the study is completed, remove the gel from the skin or the probe from the vagina.

Evaluation

- Note the test results in relation to the client's symptoms and other tests performed.

Client/Caregiver Teaching

Pretest

- Inform the client that the procedure, which varies in length from a few minutes to several hours, is performed in a special ultrasound room in a hospital or medical imaging company by a technician and that the results are interpreted by a physician.
- Inform the client that the procedure is safe, painless, with no complications or exposure to radiation.
- Inform the client that the procedure requires a full bladder; instruct the client to drink five to six glasses of liquids and not to void before the procedure.
- Inform the client that for the transvaginal approach, a probe will be inserted.

Posttest

- If an abnormality is revealed, support the client, inform her of future diagnostic procedures, and offer counseling services, if appropriate.

Ultrasonography, Prostate (Transrectal)

Classification: Ultrasonography

Type of Test: Indirect visualization

This noninvasive study uses high-frequency waves of varying intensities to identify the presence of masses and determine the size and weight of the prostate gland. It aids in the diagnosis of prostatic cancer by evaluating palpable nodules and is useful as a guide to biopsy. This test can evaluate prostate tissue, the seminal vesicles, and the surrounding tissue. It can also be used to stage carcinoma and to assist in radiation seed placement. Micturition disorders can also be evaluated by this procedure. The waves are directed into body tissues and reflected back to a transducer, processed, and appear as images on a display screen.

Indications

- Aid in prostate cancer diagnosis
- Determine prostatic cancer staging
- Aid in the diagnosis of micturition disorders
- Assist in needle placement during biopsy
- Assist in radiation seed placement

Reference Values

- Normal size, consistency, and contour of the prostate gland

Abnormal Values

- Benign prostatic hypertrophy or hyperplasia (BPH)
- Micturition disorders
- Prostate cancer
- Prostatitis

Interfering Factors

- Fecal material in the rectum can affect test results.

Nursing Implications

Assessment

- Obtain a history of prostate disease or the presence of a palpable mass or micturition difficulties.
- Assess the client's adherence to preprocedure enema administration.

Possible Nursing Diagnoses

Anxiety related to perceived threat to or change in health status
Urinary elimination, altered, related to mechanical obstruction
Fluid volume deficit, risk for, related to trauma

Implementation

- Have the client void and remove clothing from the waist down; give him a hospital gown.
- Place the client on the examining table on his left side with his knees bent toward the chest. Perform a digital rectal exam to ensure that no feces remain in the rectum. Insert a draped and lubricated rectal probe into the rectum. Water may be introduced through the sheath surrounding the transducer. Slight pressure may be felt as this is done. Scans are performed at various planes.
- When the studies are completed, the gel is removed from the rectal and genital areas.

Evaluation

- Compare the test results with the client's symptoms and the results of other diagnostic tests.

Client/Caregiver Teaching

Pretest

- Explain to the client the purpose of the study and how the procedure is performed; inform him that the procedure, which takes about 30 minutes to complete, is generally performed in a special ultrasound room by a technician and the results are interpreted by a physician.
- Assure the client that his privacy will be maintained.
- Instruct the client to administer an enema 1 hour before the test.
- Explain that no radiation exposure is associated with this study.
- Explain that there are no food or fluid restrictions.

Posttest

- Inform the client that the physician will discuss the results of the study and the need for further studies, if necessary.

Ultrasonography, Scrotal

Classification: Ultrasonography

Type of Test: Indirect visualization

This noninvasive study uses high-frequency waves of various intensities to assist in the diagnoses of scrotal pathology and anatomic abnormalities. If indicated in the presence of scrotal edema, it can be done in combination with or following nuclear studies for further clarification of a testicular mass.

Indications

- Determine cause of chronic scrotal swelling
- Aid in the diagnosis of scrotal or testicular abnormality or pathology
- Aid in diagnosis in the presence of a mass and differentiate it between a cyst, solid tumor, or abscess evidenced by specific image patterns
- Aid in diagnosis in the presence of a chronic inflammatory condition such as epididymitis
- Determine the presence of a hydrocele, spermatocele, or scrotal hernia before surgery
- Aid in the diagnosis of testicular torsion and existence of an associated testicular infarction

Reference Values

- Normal scrotum and size, shape, and structure of the testes

Abnormal Values

- Abscess
- Cyst
- Epididymitis

- Hydrocele
- Scrotal hernia
- Solid tumor
- Spermatocele

Interfering Factors

- Incorrect placement of the transducer over the test site can affect test results.
- Inability of the client to remain still during the procedure can alter results.

Nursing Implications

Assessment

- Obtain a history of suspected or existing disorders of the scrotum or testes, other tests and procedures done to diagnose a condition associated with these disorders, and therapy or surgery received to treat abnormalities or pathology.
- Assess the client's understanding of explanations provided and anxiety about the procedure.

Possible Nursing Diagnoses

Anxiety related to perceived threat to or change in health status
Sexual dysfunction related to physical and/or psychological alteration in function
Pain related to muscle spasm or tissue inflammation

Implementation

- Have client undress from the waist down; provide a hospital gown if necessary.
- Place the client in a supine position on the examining table. Ask the client to lie quietly during the procedure. Expose the scrotal area; drape for privacy. Lift the penis upward and gently tape it to the lower part of the abdomen. Display special sensitivity for the client and his embarrassment during this part of the procedure. Apply the conductive gel to the skin of the scrotum and manipulate the transducer over all areas to convert the waves into images on a screen to be viewed and photographed.
- When the study is complete, remove the gel from the scrotal area.

Evaluation

- Compare the test results with the client's symptoms and the results of other diagnostic tests.

Client/Caregiver Teaching

Pretest

- Explain to the client the purpose of the study and how the procedure is performed; inform the client that the procedure, which takes from 15 to 20 minutes to complete, is generally performed in a special ultrasound room in a hospital or medical imaging company by a technician and that the results are interpreted by a physician.

Posttest

- Inform the client that the physician will discuss the results of the study.

Ultrasonography, Spleen

Classification: Ultrasonography

Type of Test: Indirect visualization

This noninvasive study uses high-frequency waves of varying intensity to determine the size, shape, and position of the organ in the upper left quadrant (ULQ) of the abdomen. Total splenic volume is also determined by integrating the cross-sectional area of ultrasound scans that are obtained at 1-cm intervals.

Indications

- Determine the size and volume of the spleen in the presence of splenomegaly evidenced by increased echoes and visibility of the spleen
- Detect splenic cysts and differentiate them from solid tumor in combination with computerized tomography (CT) and determine whether they are introsplenic or extrasplenic as evidenced by the presence or absence of echoes
- Detect the presence of a subphrenic abscess following splenectomy
- Evaluate the extent of abdominal trauma and spleen involvement including enlargement or rupture following a recent trauma

- Differentiate spleen trauma from blood or fluid accumulation between the splenic capsule and parenchyma
- Evaluate the spleen before splenectomy performed for thrombocytopenic purpura
- Determine late-stage sickle cell disease evidenced by decreased spleen size and the presence of echoes
- Evaluate the effect of therapy on the progression or resolution of splenic disease

Reference Values

- Normal size, position, and contour of the spleen

Abnormal Values

- Abscesses
- Splenic masses, tumors, or cysts
- Splenic trauma
- Splenomegaly

Interfering Factors

- Incorrect placement and movement of the transducer over the test site can affect test results.
- The ribs and an aerated left lung attenuate the sound waves.
- Masses near the testing site can displace the spleen and cause inaccurate results if confused with splenomegaly.
- Inability of the client to remain still during the procedure can cause inaccurate test results.

Nursing Implications

Assessment

- Obtain a history of suspected or existing diseases or trauma involving the spleen, therapy received to reduce the size of the spleen, and other tests and procedures done for diagnosis of a splenic disorder.
- Ensure that food has been restricted for 12 hours before the procedure; water is permitted to minimize bowel motility.
- Ensure that the client has abstained from smoking several hours before the procedure to prevent swallowing air.

Possible Nursing Diagnoses

Anxiety related to perceived threat to or change in health status

Gas exchange, impaired, related to decreased oxygen-carrying capacity of the blood

Tissue perfusion, altered, related to stasis
Pain, chronic, related to intravascular sickling

Implementation

- Have the client remove his clothing and provide a hospital gown with the opening to the front.
- Place the client in a prone or supine position on the examining table. Expose the abdomen and chest and drape for privacy. The room can be dimmed or darkened to aid visualization. Apply a conductive gel ULQ of the abdomen and manipulate the transducer over the area. Instruct the client to remain quiet during the procedure and when to hold the breath. Echoes are received and amplified and converted to images on a screen for viewing. The views can be photographed for future comparisons to evaluate changes in the size of the organ.
- When the studies are completed, the gel is removed from the abdomen.

Evaluation

- Compare the test results with the client's symptoms and the results of other diagnostic tests.

Client/Caregiver Teaching

Pretest

- Explain to the client the purpose of the study and how the procedure is performed; inform the client that the procedure, which takes approximately 45 minutes, is generally performed in a special ultrasound room in a hospital or medical imaging company by a technician and that the results are interpreted by a physician.
- Inform the client that there is no exposure to radiation, pain, or risk of complications associated with this study.

Posttest

- Instruct the client to report abdominal pain following the procedure.

Ultrasonography, Thoracic

Classification: Ultrasonography

Type of Test: Indirect visualization

This noninvasive study uses high-frequency waves of varying intensities to assist in the diagnosis of lung abnormalities, especially when the results of other diagnostic procedures are inconclusive. Waves are directed into body tissues and reflected back to a transducer, processed, and appear as images on a display screen. Because the waves do not penetrate air, these studies are not considered useful unless done to identify conditions associated with fluid accumulation in the chest.

Indications

- Determine the presence of pleural effusion
- Aid in the diagnosis of a lesion or abscess if there is fluid accumulation or consolidation in the lung revealed by x-ray studies
- Determine the cause of acute chest pain
- Determine abnormal or malposition of the diaphragm caused by lung disorders
- Detect emboli production evidenced by echo changes that indicate anatomic changes in the lung
- Aid in the diagnosis of pulmonary embolism when done in combination with a Doppler technique ultrasound and a computerized tomographic (CT) scan

Reference Values

- Normal pulmonary and diaphragm position and structure

Abnormal Values

- Abscess
- Lesion
- Pleural effusion
- Pulmonary embolism

Interfering Factors

- Incorrect placement and movement of the transducer over the desired test sites can affect test results.
- Inability of the client to remain still during the study can alter results.

Nursing Implications

Assessment

- Obtain a history of lung conditions or abnormalities as well as therapy and previous tests and procedures for pulmonary disorders.
- Assess and record baseline vital signs for later comparison readings.
- Assess the client's understanding of explanations provided and anxiety about the procedure.

Possible Nursing Diagnoses

Tissue perfusion, altered, cardiopulmonary, related to interruption of blood flow

Gas exchange, impaired, related to altered blood flow to alveoli or to major portions of the lung

Breathing pattern, ineffective, related to tracheobronchial obstruction

Anxiety related to perceived threat to or change in health status

Implementation

- Have client remove clothing from the waist up and ensure that a hospital gown is worn.
- Have client void before the study.
- Place the client in a supine position on the examining table. Expose the chest and apply a conductive gel to the area to be scanned. Manipulate the transducer over the entire lung area to obtain views and tracings of the lung(s).
- When the study is complete, remove the gel from the chest.

Evaluation

- Compare the test results with the client's symptoms and the results of other diagnostic tests.

Client/Caregiver Teaching

Pretest

- Explain to the client the purpose of the study and how the procedure is performed; inform the client that the procedure, which takes about 45 minutes to complete, is generally performed in an ultrasound room by a technician and that the results are interpreted by a physician.

■ Explain that there are no food or fluid restrictions before the study and that no pain, risk of complications, or exposure to radiation is associated with this study.

Posttest

■ Instruct the client to report shortness of breath or difficulty breathing to the physician.

Ultrasonography, Thyroid and Parathyroid

Classification: Ultrasonography

Type of Test: Indirect visualization

This noninvasive study uses high-frequency waves of varying intensities to identify the presence of masses and determine the size and weight of the thyroid gland and the enlargement of the parathyroid glands. Small nodules and lesions can escape detection and diagnosis by this procedure. The waves are directed into body tissues and reflected back to a transducer, processed, and appear as images on a display screen.

Indications

■ Aid in diagnosis in the presence of a tumor (e.g., benign, adenoma, carcinoma) evidenced by an irregular border and shadowing at the distal edge, peripheral echoes, or high and low amplitude echoes depending on the solid tumor mass

■ Aid in diagnosis in the presence of a cyst evidenced by a smoothly outlined, echo-free amplitude except at the far border of the mass

■ Differentiate between a nodule and the presence of a solid tumor and fluid-filled cyst

■ Aid in diagnosis in the presence of parathyroid enlargement indicating a tumor or hyperplasia evidenced by an echo pattern of lower amplitude than for thyroid tumor

- Evaluate the effect of a therapeutic regimen on thyroid mass or for Graves' disease by determining the size and weight of the gland
- Determine the need for biopsy of a tumor or needle biopsy of a cyst
- Evaluate thyroid abnormalities during pregnancy since it does not expose the fetus to radiation.

Reference Values

- Normal size, position, and structure of the thyroid and parathyroid glands with uniform echo patterns throughout the glands; no evidence of tumor, cysts, or nodules in the glands

Abnormal Values

- Graves' disease
- Parathyroid tumor or hyperplasia
- Thyroid cysts
- Thyroid tumors (benign or malignant)

Interfering Factors

- Incorrect placement and movement of the transducer over the desired test site can affect test results.
- Inability of the client to remain still during the study can alter results.

Nursing Implications

Assessment

- Obtain a history of thyroid or parathyroid disorder or presence of a palpable mass as well as therapy or surgery received for the thyroid disorder.
- Assess the client's understanding of explanations provided and anxiety about the procedure.

Possible Nursing Diagnoses

Anxiety related to perceived threat to or change in health status
Physical mobility, impaired, related to weakness and mucin deposits in joints and interstitial spaces
Fatigue related to decreased metabolic energy production
Sensory alterations, tactile, related to mucin deposits and nerve compression

Implementation

- Have client remove any metallic objects or jewelry from the head and neck area.
- Have client void and remove clothing from the waist up and ensure that a hospital gown with the opening to the front is worn.
- Place the client in a supine position on an examining table and ask the client to lie quietly. Hyperextend the neck and place a pillow under the client's shoulders to maintain the position of comfort. Apply the conductive gel to the neck and place a transducer on the area and rotate over the entire thyroid site, including both sides of the trachea. Images are projected on the screen and photographed for immediate and future viewing and interpretation. For visualization of the anterior thyroid, a short-focused transducer is used.
- Another technique used is the placement of a bag of water hung over the neck area to serve as a transmitter of the waves from the transducer to the thyroid as the device is positioned over the water.
- When the studies are completed, the gel is removed from the neck and pillow from under the shoulders.

Evaluation

- Compare test results with client's symptoms and results of other diagnostic tests.

Client/Caregiver Teaching

Pretest

- Explain to the client the purpose of the study and how the procedure is performed; inform the client that the procedure, which takes about 30 minutes to complete, is generally performed in a special ultrasound room by a technician and that the results are interpreted by a physician.
- Explain that there is no pain or risk of complications or exposure to radiation associated with this study.
- Explain that there are no food or fluid restrictions.

Posttest

- Inform the client that the physician will discuss the results of the study and need for further studies (biopsy), if necessary.

Ultrasound, Arterial Doppler, Carotid Studies

Classification: Ultrasonography

Type of Test: Indirect visualization

This noninvasive technique records sound waves to obtain information about the carotid arteries using the duplex scanning method. This provides measurement of the amplitude and waveform of the carotid pulse with a two-dimensional image of the artery. The result is the visualization of the artery to assist in the diagnosis of stenosis or atherosclerotic occlusion affecting the flow of blood to the brain. Carotid arterial sites used for the studies include the common carotid, external carotid, and the internal carotid. Depending on the degree of stenosis causing a reduction in vessel diameter, oculoplethysmography (OGP) can be performed to determine the effect of stenosis on the hemodynamic status of the artery.

Indications

- Detect plaque or stenosis of the carotid artery evidenced by turbulent blood flow or changes in Doppler signals indicating occlusion
- Detect irregularities in the structure of the carotid arteries
- Aid in the diagnosis of carotid artery occlusive disease evidenced by visualization of blood flow disruption

Reference Values

- Normal blood flow through carotid arteries

Abnormal Values

- Plaque or stenosis of carotid artery
- Carotid artery occlusive disease (atherosclerosis)

Interfering Factors

- Incorrect placement of the transducer over the desired test site can affect test results.

- An abnormally large neck can make direct examination difficult.
- Inability of the client to maintain head position during the procedure can cause inaccurate results.

Nursing Implications

Assessment

- Obtain a history of previous arterial studies, presence of disorders predisposing to cerebral arterial vascular problems, and therapy received for arterial abnormalities.

Possible Nursing Diagnoses

Tissue perfusion, altered, cerebral, related to interruption in arterial flow

Anxiety related to perceived change in or threat to health status

Physical mobility, impaired, related to neuromuscular involvement

Implementation

- Have the client void; provide a hospital gown.
- Place the client in a supine position on an examining table. Expose the neck area and support the head to prevent movement. Remind the client to remain still during the procedure and not to turn the head.
- Apply conductive gel to the skin of the neck at the carotid artery site. Place the transducer over the site and move it slowly in the area of the common carotid artery to the bifurcation and then to areas of the internal and external carotids. Duplex scanning provides images of the blood flow and measurement of the waveform of the carotid pulse. A reduction in vessel diameter of more than 16 percent indicates stenosis.
- When the study is complete, remove the gel from the neck area.

Evaluation

- Compare the test results with the client's symptoms and the results of other diagnostic tests.

Client/Caregiver Teaching

Pretest

- Explain to the client the purpose of the study and how the procedure is performed; inform the client that the procedure, which takes 30 minutes to complete, is generally performed

in a vascular laboratory by a technician and that the results are interpreted by a physician.
■ Explain that the procedure is painless and carries no risks.

Posttest

■ Instruct the client to report dizziness, syncope, or blurred vision caused by impaired circulation to the brain (transient ischemic attacks [TIAs]).
■ Instruct the client in medication administration to control TIAs.

Ultrasound, Arterial Doppler, Lower Extremity Studies (LES)

Classification: Ultrasonography
Type of Test: Indirect visualization

This noninvasive technique records sound waves to obtain information about the arteries of the lower extremities using the duplex scanning method. This provides measurement of the amplitude and waveform of the pulses with a two-dimensional image of the artery. The result is the visualization of the artery to assist in the diagnosis and the presence, amount, and location of plaques and to help determine the cause of claudication. Graft condition and patency can also be evaluated.

Indications

■ Detect plaque or stenosis of the lower extremity artery evidenced by turbulent blood flow or changes in Doppler signals indicating occlusion
■ Detect irregularities in the structure of the arteries
■ Aid in the diagnosis of ischemia, arterial calcification, or plaque
■ Aid in the diagnosis of aneurysm, pseudoaneurysm, or hematoma

Normal Findings

■ Normal blood flow through lower extremity arteries

Abnormal Findings

■ Graft diameter reduction
■ Ischemia
■ Pseudoaneurysm
■ Aneurysm
■ Hematoma
■ Vessel occlusion
■ Arterial calcification or plaques

Interfering Factors

■ Incorrect placement of transducer over the desired test site can affect test results.
■ An abnormally large neck can make direct examination difficult.
■ Inability of the client to maintain head position during the procedure can cause inaccurate results.

Nursing Implications

Assessment

■ Obtain a history of previous arterial studies, presence of disorders predisposing to deep vein thrombosis, or therapy received for arterial abnormalities.
■ Assess baseline vital signs to use for comparison following the procedure, if needed.
■ Assess the client's understanding of explanations provided and anxiety about the procedure.

Possible Nursing Diagnoses

Tissue perfusion, altered, peripheral, related to interruption in arterial flow
Anxiety related to perceived change in or threat to health status
Physical mobility, impaired, related to pain and discomfort and restrictive therapy
Pain related to vascular inflammation

Implementation

■ Have client void; provide a hospital gown.
■ Place the client in a supine position on the examining table. Expose the area from the iliac region to the calf. Remind the

client to remain still during the procedure and to not move the leg.

- Apply conductive gel to the skin of the leg from the iliac region to the calf.
- Place the handheld transducer over the site and move it slowly in the area of the iliac artery. Duplex scanning provides images of the blood flow and measurement of the waveform of the pulses. A reduction in vessel diameter of more than 16 percent indicates stenosis. Many facilities perform segmental blood pressure assessment. Numerous blood pressure cuffs are placed on the extremity from high on the thigh to just superior to the ankle. The cuffs are inflated and pressure readings are recorded.
- After the procedure, remove the gel from the site.

Evaluation

- Compare the test results with the client's symptoms and the results of other diagnostic tests.

Client/Caregiver Teaching

Pretest

- Explain to the client the purpose of the study and how the procedure is performed; inform the client that the procedure, which takes 60 minutes to complete, is generally performed in a vascular laboratory by a technician and interpreted by a physician.
- Explain that the procedure is painless and carries no risks.

Posttest

- Instruct the client in medication administration to treat deep vein thrombosis.
- Provide support and teaching regarding additional testing pending test results and diagnosis.

Ultrasound, Doppler

Classification: Ultrasonography

Type of Test: Indirect visualization

Doppler ultrasound studies are used to identify occlusions of the veins or arteries. In venous Doppler studies, the Doppler identifies moving red blood cells (RBCs) within the vein. The ultrasound beam is directed at the vein and through the Doppler transducer while the RBCs reflect the beam back to the transducer. The velocity of the blood flow is transformed as a "swishing" noise audible through the audio speaker. If the vein is occluded, no swishing sound is heard.

In arterial Doppler studies, arteriosclerotic disease of the peripheral vessels can be detected. By slowly deflating blood pressure cuffs that are placed on the extremity such as the calf and ankle, the systolic pressure of the various arteries of the extremities can be measured. The Doppler transducer can detect the first evidence of blood flow through the cuffed artery. Even the most minimal blood flow from an occluded artery can be detected as a swishing noise by the Doppler. There is normally a drop of systolic blood pressure from the arteries of the arms to the arteries of the legs. If this drop exceeds 20 mm Hg, occlusive disease is believed to be present proximal to the area tested.

Indications

- Aid in the diagnosis of venous occlusion secondary to thrombosis or thrombophlebitis
- Aid in the diagnosis of small-vessel or large-vessel arterial occlusive disease
- Aid in the diagnosis of spastic arterial disease such as Raynaud's phenomenon
- Aid in the diagnosis of embolic arterial occlusion

Reference Values

- Venous
  Normal Doppler venous signal that occurs spontaneously with the client's respiration
  Normal venous system, no evidence of occlusion

- Arterial

    No evidence of arterial occlusion

    Normal arterial systolic and diastolic Doppler signals

    No reduction in systolic blood pressure in excess of 20 mm Hg when compared to a normal extremity

    Normal ankle-to-brachial arterial blood pressure index of ≥0.85

Abnormal Values

- Venous

    Venous occlusion secondary to thrombosis or thrombophlebitis
- Arterial

    Large-vessel or small-vessel arterial occlusive disease

    Embolic arterial occlusion

    Spastic arterial occlusive disease such as Raynaud's phenomenon

Interfering Factors

- Cigarette smoking can affect test results.
- Venous or arterial occlusive disease proximal to the site being tested can alter test results.

Nursing Implications

Assessment

- Obtain a history of previous arterial studies, presence of disorders predisposing to deep vein thrombosis, or therapy received for arterial abnormalities.
- Assess baseline vital signs to use for comparison following the procedure, if needed.

Possible Nursing Diagnoses

Tissue perfusion, altered, peripheral, related to interruption in arterial flow

Anxiety related to perceived change in or threat to health status

Physical mobility, impaired, related to pain and discomfort and restrictive therapy

Pain related to vascular inflammation

Implementation

- Have the client void; provide a hospital gown.
- *Venous Doppler studies:* Place the client in a supine position on an examining table. Expose the area from the iliac

region to the calf. Remind the client to remain still during the procedure and to not move the leg.

- Apply conductive gel to the skin of the leg from the iliac region to the calf. Place the hand-held Doppler transducer over the site and move it slowly in the area being examined. A "swishing" noise will be audible in a vein that is patent; absence of the sound indicates venous occlusion.

- *Arterial Doppler studies:* Place blood pressure cuffs on the thigh, calf, and ankle. Apply a conductive paste to the skin over the area distal to the cuff. Inflate the proximal cuff to a level above the client's systolic pressure found in the normal extremity. Place the Doppler transducer to the inflated cuff and slowly release the pressure in the cuff. When the "swishing" sound is heard, record it at the highest level audible. The test is repeated at each successive level. The ankle pressure is divided by the arm (brachial) pressure. This is known as the AB pressure. If the AB pressure is <0.85, significant arterial occlusive disease is within the extremity.

- When the study is completed, remove the gel from the leg.

Evaluation

- Compare the test results with the client's symptoms and the results of other diagnostic tests.

Client/Caregiver Teaching

Pretest

- Explain to the client the purpose of the study and how the procedure is performed; inform the client that the procedure, which takes 30 minutes to complete, is generally performed in a vascular laboratory by a technician and that the results are interpreted by a physician.

- Explain that the procedure is painless and carries no risks.

Posttest

- Instruct the client in medication administration to treat deep vein thrombosis.

- Provide support and teaching regarding additional testing pending test results and diagnosis.

Ultrasonography, Venous Doppler Lower Extremity Studies

Classification: Ultrasonography

Type of Test: Indirect visualization

This noninvasive technique records sound waves to obtain information about the patency of the venous vasculature in the upper and lower extremities. The sounds produced by the movement of red blood cells in a vein are of a swishing quality occurring with spontaneous respirations. Changes in these sounds during respirations indicate a possible abnormal venous flow in the presence of occlusive disease; absence of sounds indicates complete obstruction. Plethysmography may be performed to determine the filling time of calf veins to diagnose thrombotic disorder of a major vein and to identify incompetent valves in the venous system.

Indications

- Detect chronic venous insufficiency evidenced by reverse blood flow indicating incompetent valves
- Aid in the diagnosis of superficial or deep vein thrombosis leading to venous occlusion or obstruction evidenced by the absence of flow, variations in the flow during respirations, or the absence of flow when the extremity is compressed
- Determine the source of emboli when pulmonary embolism is suspected or diagnosed
- Determine venous damage following trauma to the site
- Differentiate between primary and secondary varicose veins
- Determine if further diagnostic procedures are needed to make or confirm a diagnosis
- Monitor effectiveness of therapeutic interventions

Reference Values

- Normal venous blood flow in extremities

Abnormal Values

- Chronic venous insufficiency
- Primary varicose veins
- Secondary varicose veins
- Superficial or deep vein thrombosis
- Venous trauma

Interfering Factors

- Incorrect placement of the transducer over the desired test site can alter test results.
- Cold extremities that result in vasoconstriction cause inaccurate measurements.
- Occlusion that is proximal to the site being studied affects the blood flow to the area.
- Inability of the client to remain still during the procedure can affect results.

Nursing Implications

Assessment

- Obtain a history of venous disorders and past studies/therapy received for venous disorders.
- Assess baseline vital signs to use for comparison following the procedure, if needed.
- Ensure that the client has refrained from smoking for at least 30 minutes.

Possible Nursing Diagnoses

Tissue perfusion, altered, peripheral, related to interruption of venous blood flow

Pain, acute, related to vascular inflammation and edema formation

Anxiety related to perceived threat to or change in health status

Physical mobility, impaired, risk for, related to pain and discomfort

Implementation

- Report the presence of a lesion that is open or draining; maintain clean, dry dressings for the ulcer; protect the limb from trauma.
- Have the client void. Remove clothing from the extremity to be examined and provide a hospital gown, if needed.

- Place the client in a supine position on an examining table and ask the client to lie quietly during the procedure and to breathe normally. The arms and legs are exposed depending on the limbs to be tested.
- Apply a conductive gel to the skin at the venous sites (e.g., femoral, popliteal, tibial of the legs, or brachial, axillary, jugular of the arms or neck). Place the transducer over the venous site; the waveforms are visualized and recorded with variations in respirations. Recordings are also made following limb compression that is performed proximally or distally to an obstruction or proximally to the transducer to obtain information about venous occlusion or obstruction. The procedure can be performed for both arms or legs to obtain bilateral blood flow determination. With evidence of venous stasis or ulcer, the transducer is not placed on the ulcer site.
- When the study is completed, remove the gel from the sites.

Evaluation

- Compare the test results with the client's clinical symptoms and the results of other diagnostic tests.

Client/Caregiver Teaching

Pretest

- Explain to the client the purpose of the study and how the procedure is performed; inform the client that the procedure, which takes 30 minutes to complete, is generally performed in a vascular laboratory by a technician and that the results are interpreted by a physician.
- Explain that no food or fluid restrictions are necessary before the study.
- Explain that the procedure is painless and carries no risks.

Posttest

- Inform the client that the physician will discuss the results of the study.
- Instruct the client to report skin lesion (open or draining) and skin discolorations.

Uric Acid

Classification: Chemistry

Type of Test: Serum

This test measures uric acid (urate), the end product of purine metabolism. Purines are important constituents of nucleic acids; purine turnover occurs continuously in the body, producing substantial amounts of uric acid even in the absence of dietary purine intake (meats, legumes, yeasts). Most uric acid is synthesized in the liver and excreted by the kidneys. Serum urate levels are affected by the amount of uric acid produced as well as by the efficiency of renal excretion.

Indications

- Aid in the diagnosis of gout when there is a family history (autosomal dominant genetic disorder) and/or signs and symptoms of gout, with the disorder indicated by elevated levels
- Determine the cause of known of suspected renal calculi
- Monitor the effects of drugs known to alter uric acid levels (see Abnormal Values), either as a side effect or as a therapeutic effect
- Evaluate the extent of tissue destruction in infection, starvation, excessive exercise, malignancies, chemotherapy, or radiation therapy
- Evaluate possible liver damage in eclampsia, indicated by elevated levels

Reference Values

		SI Units
Children	2.5–5.5 mg/dL	0.15–0.33 mmol/L
Men	4.0–8.5 mg/dL	0.24–0.51 mmol/L
Women	2.7–7.3 mg/dL	0.16–0.43 mmol/L

Abnormal Values

- Increased uric acid
  Acute tissue destruction (infection, starvation, exercise)
  Chemotherapy, radiation therapy for malignancies
  Eclampsia, hypertension
  Excessive dietary purines
  Gout
  Hyperparathyroidism
  Pernicious anemia
  Polycythemia
  Psoriasis
  Sickle cell anemia
  Type III hyperlipidemia
  von Gierke's disease
  Certain drugs, including alcohol, aspirin (<2 g/d), thiazide diuretics, diazoxide, epinephrine, ethacrynic acid, furosemide, phenothiazines, dextran, methyldopa, ascorbic acid, aminophylline, gentamicin, griseofulvin, rifampin, triamterene
- Decreased uric acid
  Congestive heart failure
  Fanconi's syndrome
  Ketoacidosis
  Lactic acidosis
  Renal failure
  Wilson's disease
  Yellow atrophy of the liver
  Certain drugs, including acetohexamide, corticotropin, corticosteroids, allopurinol, aspirin (>4 g/d), azathioprine, clofibrate, estrogens, mannitol, marijuana, probenecid, sulfinpyrazone, warfarin sodium

Interfering Factors

- Therapy with drugs known to alter uric acid levels (see Abnormal Values) will affect test results, unless the test is being done to monitor such drug effects.

Nursing Implications

Assessment

- Obtain client history of renal or hepatic disorders and for medications that may alter uric acid levels.
- Ensure that client has fasted for 8 hours.

Possible Nursing Diagnoses

Anxiety related to perceived threat to or change in health status

Pain, chronic, related to intravascular sickling with localized vascular stasis

Tissue perfusion, altered, related to stasis, vaso-occlusive nature of sickling

Gas exchange, impaired, related to decreased oxygen-carrying capacity of blood

Implementation

- Put on gloves. Using aseptic technique, perform a venipuncture and collect 7 mL of blood in a red-top (or marbled-top) tube.
- Handle the sample gently to avoid hemolysis and send to the laboratory immediately.

Evaluation

- Note pain and edema in joints and great toe indicating gout.
- Compare the results with the client's symptoms and urinary uric acid to determine renal dysfunction and gout.

Client/Caregiver Teaching

Pretest

- Explain to the client the purpose of the test and the procedure to obtain the specimen; prepare the client to expect some discomfort from the puncture.

Posttest

- Tell the client to resume the usual pretest diet.
- Instruct in low purine dietary and alcohol intake with a referral to nutritionist, if needed.

Uric Acid

Classification: Urinalysis

Type of Test: Urine

Uric acid is an end product of purine metabolism. Purines are constituents of nucleic acids in the body and will appear in the urine in the absence of dietary sources of purines. Dietary sources of purines include organ meats, legumes, and yeasts. Uric acid is filtered, absorbed, and secreted by the kidneys and is a common constituent of urine.

Indications

- Monitor urinary effects of disorders that cause hyperuricemia
- Monitor the response to therapy with uricosuric drugs
- Compare urine levels with serum uric acid levels to provide for an index of renal function
- Detect enzyme deficiencies and metabolic disturbances that affect the body's production of uric acid

Reference Values

- 250 to 800 mg/24 hr (SI Units: 1.5 to 4.8 mmol/day)

Abnormal Values

- Increased levels
    Disorders associated with impaired renal tubular absorption such as Fanconi's syndrome and Wilson's disease
    Disorders of purine metabolism
    Excessive dietary intake of purines
    Neoplastic disorders such as leukemia, lymphosarcoma, and multiple myeloma
    Pernicious anemia
    Polycythemia vera
    Sickle cell anemia
- Decreased levels
    Gout (associated with normal uric acid production but inadequate excretion)

Severe renal damage (possibly resulting from chronic glomerulonephritic, collagen disorders, or diabetic glomerulosclerosis, lactic acidosis, ketoacidosis, and ingestion of alcohol)

Interfering Factors

- Certain medications, including adrenal corticosteroids, ascorbic acid, cytotoxics, estrogens, probenecid, radiographic dyes, salicylates (long-term, large doses), sulfinpyrazone, and warfarin sodium, increase urinary uric acid levels.
- Certain medications, including aspirin (small doses) and thiazide diuretics, decrease urinary uric acid levels.
- Trauma has been shown to increase the rate of urinary uric acid excretion.

Nursing Implications

Assessment

- Obtain a medical history and a list of the client's medications that can interfere with uric acid excretion (see Interfering Factors).

Possible Nursing Diagnoses

Anxiety related to perceived threat to or change in health status

Pain, chronic, related to intravascular sickling with localized vascular stasis

Tissue perfusion, altered, related to stasis, vaso-occlusive nature of sickling

Gas exchange, impaired, related to decreased oxygen-carrying capacity of blood

Implementation

- Obtain the appropriately sized container (3 L) with preservative (10 mL of 12.5 M sodium hydroxide solution) according to laboratory policy; follow laboratory directions for any special care of the specimen during collection; do not refrigerate specimen.
- Begin the test between 6 and 8 A.M. if possible; collect first voiding and discard.
- Record the time the specimen was discarded as the beginning of the 24-hour test.
- The next morning, ask the client to void at the same time the collection was started and add this last voiding to the container.

- If an indwelling catheter is in place, empty the urine into a large container with the preservative hourly during the 24 hours; monitor that continued drainage is ensured and conclude the test the next morning at the same hour the collection was begun.
- Check with the client to offer support; ensure collection is performed correctly and that no urine is accidentally omitted from the 24-hour specimen. Document the quantity of the urinary output during the collection period.
- At the conclusion of the test, ensure that the label is properly completed and transport the sample to the laboratory.

Evaluation

- Compare the quantity of urine with the urinary output record for the collection; if the specimen contains less than what was recorded as output, some urine may have been discarded, thus invalidating the test.

Client/Caregiver Teaching

Pretest

- Explain to the client that the test measures the body's production and excretion of uric acid. Inform that a 24-hour urine sample will be collected.
- Inform the client that changing from a normal diet to a low-purine diet can potentially decrease urine uric acid levels by half. Educate the client regarding these dietary modifications.
- Instruct the client to avoid excessive exercise and stress during the 24-hour collection of urine.
- Inform the client that all urine for a 24-hour period must be saved; instruct the client to avoid voiding in the same pan with defecation and to keep toilet tissue out of the pan to prevent contamination of the specimen.
- Instruct the client to void all urine in a bedpan placed in the toilet and then either pour the urine into the collection container or leave it in the container for the nurse to add to the collection; place a sign in the bathroom as a reminder to save all urine.

Posttest

- Instruct the client to resume medications and usual activity withheld before the test.

Urinalysis, Routine (UA)

Classification: Urinalysis

Type of Test: Urine (Random)

The routine urinalysis is a screening test widely done to provide a general evaluation of the renal/urinary system and general physical status of healthy and ill individuals. It has the following two major components: (1) macroscopic analysis and (2) microscopic analysis. Macroscopic analysis includes examining the urine for overall physical and chemical characteristics. Physical characteristics for which urine is routinely examined include color, appearance (clarity), odor, specific gravity, and pH. Chemical analyses include tests for protein, glucose, ketones, blood, bilirubin, urobilinogen, nitrate, and leukocyte esterase. The microscopic component of a routine urinalysis involves examining the sample for formed elements such as red blood cells (RBCs) and white blood cells (WBCs), epithelial cells, casts, bacteria, mucus, and crystals.

Random specimens are sent to the laboratory for automated urinalysis or tested by the dipstick reagent strip method. Various reagent strips are available to measure substances followed by confirmation tests by other methods for specific clients or because of special circumstances. Tests for single specific urinary tests also can be performed to monitor values related to certain conditions (see specific test).

Indications

- Screen urine constituents as an essential component of a complete physical examination, especially when performed on admission to a health-care facility or before surgery
- Detect infection involving the urinary tract as indicated by urine with a "fishy" or fetid odor and presence of nitrite, leukocyte esterase, WBCs, RBCs (possibly), and bacteria
- Detect possible metabolic diseases such as diabetes mellitus
- Detect gestational diabetes or possible complications during pregnancy
- Detect various types of renal disease, including glomerulonephritis, nephrotic syndrome, and pyelonephritis

Reference Values

Macroscopic Analysis

Color	Pale yellow to amber
Appearance	Clear to slightly hazy
Odor	Mildly aromatic
Specific gravity	Usual range 1.010–1.025
pH	4.5–8.0
Protein	Negative
Glucose	Negative
Other sugars	Negative
Ketones	Negative
Blood	Negative
Bilirubin	Negative
Urobilinogen	0.1–1.0 Ehrlich μ/dL (1–4 mg/24 h)
Nitrite	Negative
Leukocyte esterase	Negative

Microscopic Analysis

RBCs	0–3/HPF
WBCs	0–4/HPF
Epithelial cells	0–10/HPF
Casts	Occasional (hyaline or granular)
Crystals	Occasional (uric acid, urate, phosphate, or calcium oxalate)
Bacteria	<1000/mL

HPF = high-powered field

Abnormal Values

See specific individual urine tests listed in the routine urinalysis.

- Change in color from normal yellow caused by drugs, fluid intake, or disease
- Cloudy appearance
- Foul, sweet or fruity, or ammonia odor
- Specific gravity <1.005 or >1.026
- Protein >8 mg/dL
- Glucose >15 mg/dL
- Ketones +1 to +3
- RBCs >2
- WBCs >4
- Casts present
- Abnormal dipstick color when compared to color chart

Interfering Factors

- Improper specimen collection such that the sample is contaminated with vaginal secretions or feces can affect test results.
- Use of collection containers contaminated with bacteria can alter results.
- Therapy with medications or ingestion of foods that may alter the color, odor, or pH of the sample can affect test results.
- Delay in sending unrefrigerated samples to the laboratory within 1 hour of collection may lead to deepening of the color of the sample; increased alkalinity of the sample; increased concentration of glucose, if already present; oxidation of bilirubin, if present, and urobilinogen; deterioration of urinary sediment; and multiplication of bacteria.
- Failure to time properly those tests done by dipstick method will alter results.

> ### NURSING ALERT
>
> - The best samples are those that are collected first thing in the morning after urine has filled the bladder overnight. The time of collection and source of the sample must be noted since this information is important in evaluating the results and in distinguishing normal from abnormal results.

Nursing Implications

Assessment

- Obtain a complete history of multisystem status, dietary intake and medication regimen, and presence of metabolic or renal/urinary disorder.

Possible Nursing Diagnoses

Pain related to bladder or urinary tract infection distention
Urinary elimination, altered, related to edema formation and irritation
Fluid volume deficit, risk for, related to stimulation of renal-intestinal reflexes

Implementation

- As indicated, place a sign in the bathroom as a reminder to save first morning urine.
- Obtain a clean, dry, plastic container with a lid according to laboratory policy.

- Collect first morning specimen (50 mL), label, and send to the laboratory.
- For dipstick testing, place strip containing antigens of substances to be tested in the urine; remove the strip and compare its color to the dipstick chart for 0 (negative) to +1–4 (positive) and record.
- If an indwelling catheter is in place, cleanse rubber area on catheter tubing with alcohol swab, insert syringe, withdraw urine and inject it into the specimen container.
- Best results are obtained if test is performed within 1 hour of receiving specimen. Keep the sample refrigerated until it is transported to the laboratory.
- At the conclusion of the test, ensure that the label is properly completed and transport to the laboratory.

Evaluation

- Compare the test results with the client's symptoms and the results of other diagnostic procedures.

Client/Caregiver Teaching

Pretest

- Explain to the client that the purpose of the test is to help in the evaluation of overall body function. Explain the procedure to the client before obtaining the specimen.
- For a midstream collection; instruct the client to cleanse the area around the urethral meatus with soap and water (retract foreskin if applicable in males; hold labia open while cleansing and voiding in females). Tell the client to then start voiding and stop, then continue to void into the specimen container.
- If the female client is menstruating, instruct her to insert a tampon before cleansing the area and voiding into the specimen container.
- Instruct the client in the collection procedure and provide the appropriate container if the specimen is to be obtained by the client as an outpatient and brought to the laboratory.

Posttest

- Inform the client of possible follow-up urine testing to confirm results.

Urobilinogen

Classification: Urinalysis

Type of Test: Urine

Protoporphyrin, a breakdown of old red blood cells by the spleen and to some extent the liver, is converted into bilirubin. In the intestine, bilirubin is converted into urobilinogen by bacteria. Approximately half of the urobilinogen is excreted in the stools, where it is converted into urobilin; the remaining half is absorbed from the intestine back into the bloodstream. From the bloodstream, urobilinogen is either recirculated to the liver and excreted with bile or excreted via the kidneys. Normally, only a small amount of urobilinogen (less than 4 mg/24 h) is found in the urine. If there is a bile duct obstruction, little or no bilirubin passes into the intestine, where urobilinogen is formed, and urine will be negative for urobilinogen. With the damage of liver cells, excretion of urobilinogen in bile is decreased, whereas its urinary excretion is increased.

Indications

- Detect liver disease as indicated by excessive urobilinogen
- Aid in the diagnosis of the source of obstructive jaundice as indicated by absence of urobilinogen
- Detect excessive red blood cell hemolysis within the systemic circulation as indicated by elevated urobilinogen levels
- Differentiate diagnosis of hepatic and hematologic disorders

Reference Values

Random specimen	0.1–1.0 Ehrlich U/2 h
24-h urine	1–4 mg/24 h

Abnormal Values

- Increased levels
    Anemia (hemolytic, pernicious)
    Bananas eaten within 48 hours before the test
    Cholangitis

Cirrhosis
Congestive heart failure with congestion of the liver
Dubin-Johnson syndrome
Hemolytic disorders
Hepatic parenchymal damage
Hepatitis
Idiopathic pulmonary hemosiderosis
Infectious mononucleosis
Lead poisoning
Liver disease
Malaria
Polycythemia vera
Portal hypertension
Pulmonary infarction
Sickle cell disease
Thalassemia major
Tissue hemorrhage
Certain drugs, including sodium bicarbonate

- Decreased levels
  Carcinoma of the head of the pancreas
  Cholelithiasis
  Complete common bile duct obstruction
  Congenital enzymatic jaundice (hyperbilirubinemia syndromes)
  Diarrhea (severe)
  Inflammation (severe)
  Renal insufficiency
  Treatment with drugs that acidify urine (ammonium chloride, ascorbic acid)
  Certain drugs, including chloramphenicol, cholestatics, and vitamin C
- Absent urine urobilinogen
  Complete obstructive jaundice or treatment with broad-spectrum antibiotics (which destroy the intestinal bacterial flora)

Urine Bilirubin and Urobilinogen in Jaundice

	Urine Bilirubin	Urine Urobilinogen
Bile duct obstruction	+++	Negative
Liver damage	+ or −	++
Hemolytic disease	Negative	+++

From Strasinger, SK: Urinalysis and Body Fluids, ed 3. FA Davis, Philadelphia, 1994, p. 72, with permission.

Interfering Factors

- Urine alkalinization will increase the excretion rate of urine urobilinogen.
- Urine acidification will decrease the excretion rate of urine urobilinogen.
- Broad-spectrum antibiotics will decrease urobilinogen production.
- High levels of nitrates in the urine can cause false-negative results.
- Medications that can cause falsely increase results include acetazolamide, aminosalicylic acid, antipyrine, aspirin, bromsulphalein, cascara, chlorpromazine, 5-hydroxyindole-acetic acid, phenothiazines, and sulfonamides.
- Dipstick methods can detect only abnormally high levels not abnormally low levels.
- Level can be normal in persons with incomplete common bile duct obstruction.
- False-positive or falsely increased results can occur in porphyria.

Nursing Implications

Assessment

- Ensure that the client has avoided intake of bananas for 2 days before the test.
- Assess the client's medication history (do not use dipstick method if client has been taking phenazopyridine).

Possible Nursing Diagnoses

Anxiety related to perceived threat to or change in health status.

Pain, chronic, related to intravascular sickling with localized vascular stasis

Tissue perfusion, altered, related to stasis, vaso-occlusive nature of sickling

Gas exchange, impaired, related to decreased oxygen-carrying capacity of blood

Implementation

- *Dipstick method:* Obtain 20-mL random urine sample in a clean plastic container. Immediately dip reagent strip into the specimen and hold horizontally next to the color chart on the container, and time according to directions. Compare color of reagent pad for urobilinogen measurement to color chart and record.

- *Two-hour collection method:* Transfer urine to container immediately after each void and take to the laboratory immediately after the specimen is completed.
- *Twenty-four hour specimen:* Obtain a 3-L, light-protected urine collection container without preservative according to laboratory policy; follow laboratory directions and send completed urine specimen to the laboratory immediately when test is completed for prompt measurement.
- Begin the test between 6 and 8 A.M. if possible; collect first voiding and discard; plan collection so that test ends during laboratory open hours. Place a sign in the bathroom as a reminder to save all urine.
- Record the time the specimen was discarded as the beginning of the 24-hour test.
- Ensure that collection is performed correctly and that no urine is accidentally omitted from the 24-hour specimen.
- If an indwelling catheter is in place, empty the urine into a large container periodically during the 24 hours; monitor that continued drainage is ensured and conclude the test the next morning at the same hour the collection was begun.
- At the conclusion of the test, ensure that the label is properly completed and transport the sample to the laboratory.

Evaluation

- Ensure that all urine was saved during the 2-hour and 24-hour specimen collection.
- Compare the test results with the client's symptoms and the results of other diagnostic tests.

Client/Caregiver Teaching

Pretest

- *Two-hour collection method:* Instruct the client to collect specimen early to midafternoon (ideally between 1 P.M. and 3 P.M.) since this is when urobilinogen levels peak. Instruct the client to void and discard the urine. Explain the procedure; client is to drink 500 mL of water over the next 10 minutes and save all the urine voided over the next 2 hours in a refrigerated, light-protected 1-L urine container.
- *Twenty-four hour specimen:* Instruct the client to avoid excessive exercise and stress during the 24-hour collection of urine.
- Inform the client that all the urine for a 24-hour period must be saved; instruct the client to avoid voiding in same pan

with defecation and to keep toilet tissue out of the pan to prevent contamination of the specimen.

- Instruct the client to void all urine in a bedpan placed in the toilet and then to either pour the urine into the collection container or leave it in the container for the nurse to add to the collection.
- The next morning, request the client to void at the same time the collection was started and add this last voiding to the container.

Posttest

- Resume medications and usual activity withheld before the test.
- Instruct in collection and provide appropriate container if specimen is to be obtained as an outpatient and brought to the laboratory.

Uroflowmetry

Classification: Manometric

Type of Test: Indirect measurement

This noninvasive study measures urinary flow rate and amount of urine during urination over a period of time. This procedure aids in the diagnosis of abnormalities of the urinary pattern and can be performed in combination with other tests such as cystometry and voiding cystourethrography.

Indications

- Determine abnormal urinary flow patterns in the evaluation of incontinence and recurrent urinary bladder infections
- Diagnose external sphincter dysfunction evidenced by an increased flow rate
- Determine the cause of abnormal urinary flow patterns, such as detrusor muscle hypotonia and outflow obstruction, evidenced by a decrease in flow rate

Reference Values

	Males	*Females*
Children	100 mL/10–12 s	10–15 s
Adults	200 mL/12–21 s	15–18 s
Older adults	200 mL/9 s	10 s

Abnormal Values

- Increased flow rate
    External sphincter dysfunction
    Stress incontinence
- Decreased flow rate
    Outflow obstruction or hypotonia of the detrusor muscle
    Obstruction to empty bladder resulting in abdominal straining

Interfering Factors

- Inability of the client to remain still and carry out instructions during the study can affect test results.
- Toilet tissue or other material will alter study findings.
- Administration of drugs that affect bladder and sphincter function, such as anticholinergics or muscle relaxants, will alter results.
- Room temperature changes can affect transducer measurements.
- Quantity of urine voided affects the flow rate (200–400 mL). Larger amounts affect extrusor muscle adequacy.
- Recent urethral instrumentation can cause decreased flow rates.

Nursing Implications

Assessment

- Obtain a history of signs and symptoms of impaired urinary function, known or suspected disorders leading to urinary dysfunction, previous tests and procedures done, and medical and surgical therapeutic interventions performed, including medications that can affect the test results (muscle relaxants).
- Inform client that there are no food or fluid restrictions before the procedure.

- Assess for compliance with directions given for rest, positioning, and activity before and during the test.

Possible Nursing Diagnoses

Infection, risk for, related to inadequate primary defenses
Incontinence related to neuropathy or degenerative changes in bladder sphincter muscle affecting urinary flow pattern

Implementation

- Place the client in a sitting position on a commode for females and a standing position next to the commode for males. Ensure privacy by draping or covering the client from the waist down. Place a weight-recording device (gravimetric uroflowmeter) at the bottom of the commode. This unit weighs the urine as it flows, and the weight changes are recorded electronically using the weight that is converted to milliliters and time frames in seconds or minutes. Ask the client to void without straining during the procedure. Volume and times are recorded on a graph from the beginning of voiding to the end. The characteristics of the peaks of the curve on the graph indicate incontinence (high peak flow), detrusor muscle abnormality (many peaks), or obstruction (low peak flow).

Evaluation

- Compare the test results to the client's symptoms and the results of other diagnostic tests.

Client/Caregiver Teaching

Pretest

- Advise the client about the purpose of the test and who will perform it.
- Inform the client that the test will take 15 minutes to complete.
- Inform the client that the procedure can be repeated for 3 days to determine a more accurate estimation of urinary flow rate.

Posttest

- Inform client about an available bladder retraining program to correct urinary incontinence.

Vanillylmandelic Acid (VMA)

Classification: Chemistry

Type of Test: Urine

Vanillylmandelic acid (VMA), a phenolic acid that is a product of hepatic conversion of epinephrine and norepinephrine, is the catecholamine metabolite that is most prevalent in urine. VMA levels in urine reflect adequate amounts of endogenous production of these major catecholamines. Catecholamine-secreting tumors, such as pheochromocytoma, can be detected by this test. The primary site for catecholamine production is the adrenal medulla. This test can also evaluate the function of this gland. Metanephrine, normetanephrine, and hemovanillic acid (HVA) can also be evaluated with this test.

Indications

- Aid in the diagnosis of pheochromocytoma, neuroblastoma, and ganglioneuroma
- Evaluate the function of the adrenal medulla

Reference Values

- Urine VMA values range from 0.7 to 6.8 mg in a 24-hour period (3 to 35 μmol/d in SI units).

Abnormal Values

- Ganglioneuroma
- Neuroblastoma
- Pheochromocytoma

Interfering Factors

- Increased levels can be caused by drugs such as epinephrine, norepinephrine, lithium carbonate, and methocarbamol. Decreased levels can be associated with chlorpromazine, monoamine oxidase inhibitors, clonidine, reserpine, and guanethidine. Salicylates and levodopa may raise or lower the test results.

- Emotional upset or excessive physical exercise may alter the test results.
- Failure to adhere to dietary and drug restrictions may affect the test results.
- Negligence in proper storage of the specimen or failure to collect all of the specimens may alter test results.

> **NURSING ALERT**
>
> - The specimen must be kept on ice during the collection period and then sent to the laboratory immediately for testing after the last sample has been collected.

Nursing Implications

Assessment

- Assess the client's understanding of explanations provided and presence of anxiety.
- Obtain a medical history and a list of the client's medications that can interfere with VMA excretion (see Interfering Factors).

Possible Nursing Diagnoses

Anxiety related to perceived threat to or change in health status
Fluid volume deficit related to excessive gastric losses
Cardiac output, decreased, related to altered preload and decreased blood volume

Implementation

- Obtain the appropriately sized container (3 L) with preservative to keep the urine pH at 3.0 according to laboratory policy; follow laboratory directions for keeping the collection container and specimens on ice during the collection period.
- Begin the test between 6 and 8 A.M. if possible; collect the first voiding and discard.
- Record the time the specimen was discarded as the beginning of the 24-hour test.
- The next morning, ask the client to void at the same time the collection was started and add this last voiding to the container.
- If an indwelling catheter is in place, empty the urine into a large container with the preservative hourly during the 24 hours; monitor that continued drainage is ensured and conclude the test the next morning at the same hour the collection was begun.

- Check with the client to offer support; ensure that the collection is performed correctly and that no urine is accidentally omitted from the 24-hour specimen. Document the quantity of urinary output during the collection period.
- At the conclusion of the test, ensure that the label is properly completed and transport the sample to the laboratory immediately.

Evaluation

- Compare the quantity of urine with the urinary output record for the collection; if the specimen contains less than what was recorded as output, some urine may have been discarded, thus invalidating the test.
- Compare the test results with the client's symptoms and the results of other diagnostic tests.

Client/Caregiver Teaching

Pretest

- Explain to the client that the test measures the body's production and excretion of VMA. Inform the client that a 24-hour urine sample will be collected.
- Tell the client to restrict beverages and foods that contain phenolic acid, such as tea, coffee, citrus fruits, chocolate, bananas, and vanilla, for 3 days before the test.
- Advise the client to avoid stressful activity and emotional situations during the urine collection period.
- Inform the client that all urine for a 24-hour period must be saved; instruct the client to avoid voiding in the same pan with defecation and to keep toilet tissue out of the pan to prevent contamination of the specimen.
- Instruct the client to void all urine in a bedpan placed in the toilet and then to either pour the urine into the collection container or leave it in the container for the nurse to add to the collection; place a sign in the bathroom as a reminder to save all urine.

Posttest

- Instruct the client to resume medications and usual activity withheld before the test.

Venereal Disease Research Laboratories Test (VDRL)

Classification: Serology

Type of Test: Blood

A screen for primary and secondary syphilis, this test demonstrates the presence of reagin by flocculation. Reagin is an antibody that is specific for *Treponema pallidum*, the spirochete responsible for syphilis. Cholesterol and an antigen containing cardiolipin and lecithin are added to the blood sample. If flocculation appears, the sample is diluted until no flocculation is apparent microscopically. The titer is the last dilution to reveal flocculation. Viral or bacterial infections, chronic systemic illness, or nonsyphilitic treponemal disease may produce false-positive results.

Indications

- Aid in the diagnosis of syphilis
- Screen for secondary and primary syphilis
- Monitor response to treatment

Reference Values

- Negative; no flocculation should appear; test is reported as strongly reactive, reactive, weakly reactive, or negative.

Abnormal Values

A reactive test indicates syphilis and occurs in about 50 percent of patients with primary syphilis and in nearly all clients with secondary syphilis.

- Disorders that cause false-positive results
    Hepatitis
    Infectious mononucleosis
    Leprosy
    Malaria
    Nonsyphilitic treponemal diseases (pinta, yaws)
    Rheumatoid arthritis
    Systemic lupus erythematosus

Interfering Factors

- Hemolysis of the sample can alter test results.
- Ingestion of alcohol within 24 hours of the test may alter test results.
- A faulty immune system can produce a nonreactive test result.

Nursing Implications

Assessment

- Ensure that the client abstained from alcohol ingestion for 24 hours before the test.
- Assess the client history for disorders that may affect test results.

Possible Nursing Diagnoses

Anxiety related to altered health status
Pain related to inflammation of mucosa
Infection, risk for transmission
Skin/tissue integrity, impaired, related to invasion of pathogenic organism

Implementation

- Put on gloves. Using aseptic technique, perform a venipuncture and collect 7 mL of blood in a red-top tube.
- Send the sample to the laboratory immediately.

Evaluation

- Note the results in relation to other diagnostic criteria.

Client/Caregiver Teaching

Pretest

- Advise the client to avoid ingesting any alcohol at least 24 hours before the test is performed.
- Advise the client that there are no food or fluid restrictions (except for alcohol) before the test.

Posttest

- If the test is reactive, explain the importance of proper treatment and adhering to drug regimen.
- If the test is reactive but the client does not demonstrate any physical signs of the disease, advise about the possibility of false-positive results. Inform the client about additional studies that can confirm diagnosis.

Venography, Lower Limb and Renal Ascending Contrast Phlebography

Classification: Nuclear Medicine

Type of Test: Radionuclide imaging

This invasive nuclear study or radiographic test is performed to examine venous conditions. With the use of a radiopaque dye or radionuclide, the practitioner is able to visualize a vein, such as a renal vein and its tributaries or a lower extremity vein. Lower limb venography is useful in confirmation of diagnosing deep vein thrombosis (DVT) whereas renal venography assists in assessing renovascular hypertension.

Indications

- Confirm diagnosis of DVT
- Distinguish clot formation from venous obstruction
- Evaluate congenital venous abnormalities
- Assess deep vein valvular competence
- Locate a vein for arterial bypass grafting
- Detect renal vein thrombosis
- Evaluate renal vein compression caused by extrinsic tumors or retroperitoneal fibrosis
- Assess renal tumors and detect invasion of the renal vein or inferior vena cava
- Diagnose venous anomalies and defects
- Differentiate renal agenesis from a small kidney
- Collect renal venous blood samples for evaluation of renovascular hypertension

Reference Values

- No obstructions to flow or filling defects after injection of radiopaque dye
- Lower limb venography—steady opacification of superficial and deep vasculature with no filling defects
- Renal venography—opacification of renal vein and tributaries immediately after injection of radiopaque dye

Abnormal Values

- Lower limb abnormal results can indicate DVT, deep vein valvular incompetence, or venous obstruction.
- Renal venography abnormal results include renal vein thrombosis, obstruction or compression by extrinsic tumor or retroperitoneal fibrosis, venous anomalies, or renal agenesis differentiated from a small kidney.

Interfering Factors

- Inability of client to remain still during procedure will produce artifact.
- Jewelry or metal objects in the examination field distort results.
- Movement of leg being tested, excessive tourniquet constriction, insufficient injection of contrast medium, or delay between injection and radiography interfere with accurate results.
- Contrast medium can fail to fill veins if client places weight on leg being tested.

NURSING ALERT

- This procedure is contraindicated in clients with hypersensitivity to the radiographic dye, iodine, or shellfish.
- It is also contraindicated in pregnancy and lactation unless the benefits from performing the test greatly outweigh the risks. Special precautions should be taken in children.
- Pregnant health-care professionals should avoid caring for a person who has had a nuclear medicine procedure until 24 hours after the procedure.

Nursing Implication

Assessment

- Assess for allergy to radiographic dye, contrast medium, iodine, or shellfish. Report to physician.
- Determine date of last menstrual period and possibility of pregnancy in premenopausal women.
- Assess and record baseline vital signs for later comparison readings.
- Obtain history pertinent to venogram to be performed.

- Determine previous abnormalities in laboratory tests and diagnostic procedures.
- Ensure client has had nothing by mouth 4 hours before test if ordered.
- Restrict anticoagulant therapy if ordered by physician.
- Ensure that emergency cart is available in the event of an allergic reaction to the dye.
- Assess for compliance with directions given for test, positioning, and activity before and during the test.

Possible Nursing Diagnoses

Anxiety related to perceived threat to or change in health status
Tissue perfusion, altered, peripheral, related to interruption of venous blood flow
Pain, acute, related to vascular inflammation

Implementation

- Establish intravenous access.
- Before scan, have the client remove all jewelry, provide the client with a hospital gown, and have client void.
- After the radionuclide is injected into the vein, x-rays are taken following the course of the dye into the veins of the leg. Occasionally, a tourniquet is used on the leg to prevent the dye from traveling to the superficial saphenous vein allowing all of the dye to go to the deep venous system.

Evaluation

- Check pulse rate on the dorsalis pedis, popliteal, and femoral arteries after lower leg venography. Assess peripheral color, motion, temperature, and sensation of lower extremities every 15 minutes times 4, every 30 minutes times 4, hourly times 4, then every 4 hours or per hospital protocol.
- Observe injection site for dye infiltration, such as redness, edema, warmth, or tenderness.
- Observe puncture site for bleeding or hematoma. Apply warm soaks to ease discomfort if hematoma develops.
- Report signs of vein perforation, embolism, and extravasation of contrast medium, including chills; fever; rapid pulse and respiratory rates; hypotension; dyspnea; and chest, abdominal, or flank pain. Also report complaints of paraesthesia or pain in the catheterized limb, such as symptoms of nerve irritation or vascular compromise.
- Observe client carefully for up to 60 minutes after the study for a possible anaphylactic reaction to the radionuclide (e.g., flushing, hives, urticaria, laryngeal stridor, rash, tightening of throat, or difficulty breathing).

- Monitor for complications after venography, including bacteremia, cellulitis, embolism, and thrombophlebitis.
- Compare the test results to the client's symptoms and the results of other diagnostic tests.

Client/Caregiver Teaching

Pretest

- Explain to the client that the procedure is performed in a special nuclear medicine department by a technician and a physician specializing in this branch of medicine to detect abnormalities in perfusion of a lower limb or renal vein.
- Explain the procedure to the client; a radiographic dye is injected into a catheter via a femoral vein followed by films of the specific area needed to be scanned (such as a renal vein or leg vein). Inform the client that a feeling of warmth around the neck and face is normally felt after injection. Instruct the client to report any nausea, severe burning or itching, constriction of the throat or chest, or dyspnea immediately.
- Inform the client that the total time of the procedure is approximately 1 hour.

Posttest

- Inform the client to meticulously wash hands with soap and water after each void for 24 hours.
- Inform the client that radionuclide is eliminated from the body within 6 to 24 hours (technetium half-life is 6 hours). Advise the client to drink fluids to eliminate the radionuclide from the body unless otherwise contraindicated.
- Instruct the client to resume usual level of activity and normal dietary intake unless contraindicated.
- Instruct health-care officials to wear rubber gloves when discarding urine for 24 hours after the procedure. Wash gloved hands with soap and water before removing gloves. Consider them as nuclear waste and dispose of them accordingly. Then wash ungloved hands.
- Provide supportive environment after diagnostic findings are reported, as indicated; reinforce information regarding diagnosis and recommended treatment regimen.
- If DVT is indicated, initiate therapy such as heparin infusion, bed rest, leg elevation or support, and laboratory tests as ordered.

Viscosity

Classification: Hematology

Type of Test: Serum

In this test, serum viscosity is evaluated by comparing the times required for a standard volume of serum and water to flow through a capillary tube of standard length and diameter (Ostwald viscometer). Normally, low-viscosity fluids flow rapidly and high-viscosity fluids flow slowly. Serum viscosity is affected by the hematocrit, size of red blood cells, and protein composition of plasma and is compared to that of water at room temperature.

Indications

- Diagnose serum hyperviscosity disorders

Reference Values

- 1.4 to 1.8 relative to distilled water

Abnormal Values

- Hyperfibrinogenemia
- Myeloma
- Rheumatoid arthritis
- Systemic lupus erythematosus
- Waldenström's macroglobulinemia

Interfering Factors

- The sample should be handled gently to avoid hemolysis, which can affect test results.
- Clinical symptoms may not correlate with test results.

Nursing Implications

Assessment

- Obtain the client's hematologic and immunologic history and a profile of the client's current medication therapy.

Possible Nursing Diagnoses

Anxiety related to perceived threat to or change in health status

Pain, acute, related to widespread inflammatory process affecting connective tissue

Tissue integrity, impaired, related to chronic inflammation

Fatigue related to increased energy requirements and altered body chemistry

Implementation

- Put on gloves. Using aseptic technique, perform a venipuncture and collect the blood in two 10-mL red-top tubes; use a green-top tube if whole blood viscosity is to be measured.
- Handle the sample gently to avoid hemolysis and send to the laboratory immediately.

Evaluation

- Note the results in relation to the client's symptoms and other related tests.

Client/Caregiver Teaching

Pretest

- Inform the client that no special preparation is needed for this test.

Posttest

- Provide support pending test results and need for further diagnostic tests.

Visual Fields Test Tangent Screen Examination

Classification: Ocular function

Type of Test: Vision screening

The visual field is the area within which objects can be seen by the eye as it fixes on a central point. The central field is an area 25 degrees surrounding the fixation point. The peripheral field is the remainder of the area within which objects can be viewed. This test evaluates the central visual field through systematic movement of the test object across a tangent screen.

Indications

- Detect field vision loss and evaluate its progression or regression

Reference Values

Normal central vision field will form a circle extending 25 degrees superiorly, nasally, inferiorly, and temporally; 12 degrees to 15 degrees temporal to the central fixation point is a physiologic blind spot, approximately 1.5 degrees below the horizontal meridian. It is approximately 7.5 degrees high and 5.5 degrees wide. The client should be able to see the test object throughout the entire central visual field except within the physiologic blind spot.

Abnormal Values

- Brain tumors
- Cerebrovascular accidents
- Glaucoma
- Optic neuritis
- Retinitis pigmentosa

Interfering Factors

- An uncooperative client or a client with severe vision loss that makes seeing even a large vision screen difficult will have test results that are invalid.

Nursing Implications

Assessment

- Assess the client's knowledge of the test and its purpose.
- Assess the client's ability to follow directions given during the test.
- Assess the client's history and clinical symptoms.

Possible Nursing Diagnoses

Sensory alterations, visual, related to altered sensory reception and altered status of sense organ

Anxiety related to perceived threat to or change in health status

Implementation

- Seat the client about 1 m away from the tangent screen with the eye being tested directly in line with the central fixation target on the screen.
- Instruct the client to cover the left eye and fixate on the central target as the test target is moved into his or her visual field. The client should not look at the test object but should wait for it to appear and then signal when he or she sees it.
- The client's central vision boundaries are plotted and then how well he or she can see within the central field is measured. To accomplish this, the test object is turned over revealing another color on the other side (usually black and white). At 30-degree intervals, the test object is turned over and then back as the client tries to identify the object for size, shape and density. The test is then repeated on the other eye.

Evaluation

- Compare the test results to the client's symptoms and the results of other diagnostic tests.

Client/Caregiver Teaching

Pretest

- Explain to the client the purpose of the test and who will perform it. Inform the client that the test takes about 30 minutes and that the client will not experience any discomfort during the test.
- Explain to the client that although the test is not painful, he or she will be required to cooperate fully and follow directions.
- Instruct the client to wear corrective lenses, if appropriate.

Posttest

- Provide the client with any teaching associated with his diagnosis pending test results.
- Tell him that additional testing may be required pending test results and diagnosis

Vitamins (A, B$_1$, B$_6$, B$_{12}$, C, D$_3$, E)

Classification: Chemistry

Type of Test: Serum (vitamin B$_6$-plasma)

Vitamin A promotes normal vision and prevents night blindness; contributes to growth of bone, teeth and soft tissues; supports thyroxine formation; and maintains epithelial cell membranes, skin, and mucous membranes. Vitamin B$_1$ (thiamine) acts as an enzyme and plays an important role in the Krebs cycle. Vitamin B$_{12}$ is essential in DNA synthesis, hematopoiesis, and CNS integrity. Vitamin B$_6$ is important in heme synthesis and functions as a coenzyme in amino acid metabolism and glycogenolysis. It includes pyridoxine, pyridoxal, and pyridoxamine. Vitamin C promotes collagen synthesis, maintains capillary strength, facilitates release of iron from ferritin to form hemoglobin, and functions in the stress response. Vitamin D, the major form of which is vitamin D$_3$, aids in calcium-phosphorus balance and deposition of both in bone. It works with calcium and parathyroid hormone and is necessary for calcium absorption from the intestinal tract. Vitamin E is needed for proper muscle growth, reproductive function, and hemolytic resistance of red blood cells.

Indications

- Vitamin A
  Evaluate skin disorders
  Confirm suspected vitamin A deficiency
  Diagnose night blindness
- Vitamin B$_1$
  Confirm suspected beriberi
  Monitor the effects of chronic alcoholism
- Vitamin B$_6$
  Confirm suspected vitamin B$_6$ deficiency
  Confirm suspected malabsorption or malnutrition
- Vitamin B$_{12}$
  Diagnose megaloblastic anemia
  Diagnose CNS disorders

- Vitamin C
    Confirm suspected scurvy
    Confirm suspected metabolic or malabsorptive disorders
- Vitamin D$_3$
    Diagnose hypercalcemia
    Confirm vitamin D deficiency as the cause of bone disease
    Confirm vitamin D deficiency owing to malabsorption syndrome, hepatobiliary disease, or chronic renal failure
    Detect toxicity and monitor response to therapy
- Vitamin E
    Confirm suspected hemolytic anemia
    Confirm suspected neurologic abnormalities

Implications of Test Results

Vitamin	Reference Value	Increased Value	Decreased Value
A	0.15–0.60 mg/ mL	Excessive intake	Celiac disease Night blindness Infectious hepatitis
B$_1$	5.3–7.9 µg/dL	Excessive intake	Chronic alcoholism Beriberi Chronic diarrhea Long-term diuretic use
B$_6$	25–80 ng/mL	Excess intake	Alcoholism Malnutrition Malabsorption Drugs, including oral contraceptives, hydralazine, isoniazid, levodopa
B$_{12}$	180–900 pg/ mL	Excess intake Hepatic disease Myeloproliferative disorders Drugs, including oral contraceptives	Inadequate dietary intake Malabsorption syndromes Hypermetabolic states
C	Children: 0.6– 1.6 mg/dL Adults: 0.2– 2.0 mg/dL	Excess intake	Infection Fever Pregnancy

Implications of Test Results (*continued*)

Vitamin	Reference Value	Increased Value	Decreased Value
D$_3$	10–55 mg/mL	Excess intake Hyperparathyroidism	Rickets Osteomalacia Hepatic disorders Hypoparathyroidism Drugs, including anticonvulsants and isoniazid
E	0.8–1.5 mg/dL	Excess intake	Chronic alcoholism Neurologic degenerative diseases Malabsorption related to intestinal bile deficiency

Interfering Factors

- Hemolysis or exposure of sample to light invalidates results for vitamin A and B$_{12}$ tests.
- Diet high in freshwater fish and tea, which are thiamine antagonists, may cause decreased vitamin B$_1$ levels.
- Prolonged exposure to light also invalidates results.
- Use of radiographic dye within 7 days of the test for vitamin B$_{12}$ invalidates results.
- Prolonged exposure to light invalidates vitamin B$_6$ and E test results.
- Chronic tobacco smoking causes decreased levels of vitamin C.
- Insufficient phosphorus intake and lack of sunlight exposure causes decreased vitamin D levels.

Nursing Implications

Assessment

- Obtain a history of dietary intake, suspected or known vitamin-related disorders, vitamin supplement use, tests and procedures performed, and test results.
- Assess medication history and ensure that any drugs that may alter test results have been withheld for 12 to 24 hours before the test as ordered by physician.

- Ensure that the client has fasted overnight for vitamin A, C, and D testing.

Possible Nursing Diagnoses

Injury, risk for, related to neuromuscular excitability

Pain related to recurrent muscle spasms

Airway clearance, ineffective, risk for, related to spasm of the laryngeal muscles

Nutrition, altered, less than body requirements, related to poor intake or inability to absorb nutrients

Nutrition, altered, more than body requirements, related to increased intake of nutrients

Implementation

- Put on gloves; using aseptic technique, perform a venipuncture and collect 7 mL of blood in a red-top tube.
- Send the sample to the laboratory immediately.

Evaluation

- Compare the test results to the client's symptoms and the findings of other diagnostic test results.

Client/Caregiver Teaching

Pretest

- Explain to the client the purpose of the test and the procedure to obtain the specimen; prepare the client to expect some discomfort from the puncture.

Posttest

- Instruct the client to resume medications withheld before the test.
- Instruct the client in the use of necessary dietary and vitamin supplements or in any necessary restrictions based on the test results.

Vitamins (Vitamin B$_1$, B$_2$, and C)

Classification: Urinalysis

Type of Test: Urine

Fat-soluble vitamins are not readily excreted in the urine, and therefore, urinary determinations focus on water-soluble vitamins B and C. Urinary determinations for vitamins B$_1$ (thiamine), B$_2$ (riboflavin), and C may be done in suspected deficiency states.

Indications

- Detect vitamin deficiency states
- Assist in diagnosing vitamin B$_1$ (thiamine) deficiency (beriberi) and to differentiate it from other causes of polyneuritis
- Detect vitamin B$_2$ (riboflavin) deficiency
- Diagnose vitamin C (ascorbic acid) deficiency, scurvy, scurvy-like conditions, and metabolic disorders, such as malnutrition, that interfere with oxidative processes

Reference Values

B$_1$ (thiamine)	100–200 Ug/24 h
B$_2$ (riboflavin)	
Men	0.51 mg/24 h
Women	0.39 mg/24 h
C (ascorbic acid)	30 mg/24 h

Abnormal Values

- *Vitamin B$_1$ deficiency in urine* can result from alcoholism, chronic diarrhea, dietary insufficiency, hyperthyroidism, prolonged diuretic therapy, and severe hepatic disease. Negative results can indicate neuritis unrelated to deficiency.
- *Vitamin B$_2$ deficiency in urine* can result from inadequate dietary intake of milk and protein (primary), prolonged diarrhea, chronic alcoholism, hepatic disease (secondary);

decreased urine vitamin B_2 is likely during high-metabolic-demand states such as pregnancy, lactation, and wound healing. Chronic deficiencies can lead to cheilosis, glossitis, angular stomatitis, seborrheic dermatitis, and corneal vascularization.

- *Vitamin C deficiency in urine* can occur in clients with infection, cancer, burns, or other stress-producing conditions, as well as malnutrition, malabsorption, renal deficiencies, or prolonged intravenous therapy without vitamin C replacement. Severe vitamin C deficiency diagnoses scurvy.

Interfering Factors

- Improper specimen collection and maintenance can affect test results.
- Prolonged exposure of the specimen to light invalidates results.
- Persons who consume high amounts of thiamine antagonists (e.g., freshwater fish or tea made from tea leaves) can have low levels of thiamine.

Nursing Implications

Assessment

- Assess and obtain medical and medication history.

Possible Nursing Diagnoses

Skin integrity, impaired, related to effects of excretions on delicate tissues
Fluid volume deficit, risk for, related to excessive losses
Pain related to abdominal cramping

Implementation

- Obtain the appropriately sized 3-L dark brown container without preservative according to laboratory policy; follow laboratory directions for any special care of the specimen during collection, such as refrigerating, placing in ice, or protecting from light by covering with dark plastic or aluminum.
- Begin the test between 6 and 8 A.M. if possible; collect first voiding and discard.
- Record the time the specimen was discarded as the beginning of the 24-hour test.
- Ensure that the collection is performed correctly and that no urine is accidentally omitted from the 24-hour specimen. Document the quantity of urinary output during the collection period.

- The next morning, request the client to void at the same time the collection was started and add this last voiding to the container.
- If an indwelling catheter is in place, replace tubing and container system at the start of the collection time, keep urine on ice and empty it into a large container hourly during the 24 hours; monitor that continued drainage is ensured and conclude the test the next morning at the same hour the collection was begun.
- At the conclusion of the test, ensure that the label is properly completed and transport the sample to the laboratory.

Evaluation

- Compare the quantity of urine with the urinary output recorded for the collection; if the specimen contains less than what was recorded as output, some urine may have been discarded thus invalidating the test.

Client/Caregiver Teaching

Pretest

- Instruct the client to avoid excessive exercise and stress during the 24-hour collection of urine.
- Inform the client that all urine for a 24-hour period must be saved; instruct the client to avoid voiding in the same pan with defecation and to keep toilet tissue out of the pan to prevent contamination of the specimen.
- Inform the client to void all urine in a bedpan placed in the toilet and then to either pour the urine into the collection container or leave it in the container for the nurse to add to the collection; place a sign in the bathroom as a reminder to save all urine.

Posttest

- Instruct the client to resume medications and usual activity withheld before the test.
- Instruct the client in collection procedure and provide an appropriate container if the specimen is to be obtained by the client as an outpatient and brought to the laboratory.

Western Immunoblast Assay

Classification: Immunology
Type of Test: Blood

Identifies antibodies to at least nine types of HIV-1. Antibodies are detected by a blotting procedure that separates HIV antigens by their molecular weight.

Indications

- Confirm the presence of HIV following a positive enzyme-linked immunosorbent assay (ELISA) result

Reference Values

- Negative

Abnormal Values

- A positive value indicates the presence of HIV antibodies.

Interfering Factors

- Negative results can occur early in the disease because of lack of antibody formation.
- Children of infected mothers who are infected before birth can have inaccurate negative results.

Nursing Implications

Assessment

- Obtain a history of the immune system, suspected or known exposure to HIV, risk factors, tests performed, and test results.

Possible Nursing Diagnoses

Anxiety related to perceived threat to or change in health status
Pain, chronic, related to tissue inflammation

Nutrition, altered, less than body requirements, related to altered ability to ingest nutrients

Fluid volume deficit, risk for, related to excessive losses

Infection, risk for transmission

Implementation

- Put on gloves. Using aseptic technique, perform a venipuncture and collect 7 mL of blood in a red-top tube.
- Send the specimen to the laboratory.

Evaluation

- Compare the test results to the client's symptoms and the results of other diagnostic tests.

Client/Caregiver Teaching

Pretest

- Inform the client of confidentiality and legal requirements related to the test results.

Posttest

- If the results are positive, instruct the client in prevention of disease transmission, and to follow up with a health-care provider.

White Blood Cell Count Total and Differential (WBC, DIFF, Leukocyte Count)

Classification: Hematology

Type of Test: Blood

Leukocytes constitute the body's primary defense system to protect against foreign organisms, substances, and tissues. The main types are granulocytes, neutrophils, eosinophils, basophils, monocytes, and lymphocytes. They are produced in the bone marrow, although lymphocytes can be produced in other sites as well. The WBC can be performed alone with the differential cell count, or as part of the complete blood count (CBC). An increased count is termed *leukocytosis* and a decreased count, *leukopenia*. A total WBC indicates the degree of response to a pathologic process, but a more complete evaluation for specific diagnoses for any one disorder is provided by the differential count.

Indications

- Routinely screen as part of a complete blood count (CBC)
- Determine the source of the elevation, as in suspected infection or inflammatory process, in clients with an abnormal total WBC count
- Confirm the presence of various disorders associated with increases and decreases in the several types of WBCs (leukemia, autoimmune disorders, allergies)
- Monitor response to treatment for acute infections, with a therapeutic response indicated by a decreasing number of bands and a stabilizing number of neutrophils
- Confirm suspected bone marrow depression
- Monitor physiologic responses to antineoplastic therapy, infectious therapy, stress, and malnutrition

Reference Values

		SI Units
Total WBC		
Newborns	9,000–30,000/μL	9.0–30.0 × 10⁹/L
Infants	6,000–17,500/μL	6.0–17.5 × 10⁹/L
Children	4,500–16,300/μL	4.5–13.5 × 10⁹/L
Men	4,500–11,000/μL	4.5–11.0 × 10⁹/L
Women (nonpregnant)	4,500–11,000/μL	4.5–11.0 × 10⁹/L
Differential WBC		
Neutrophils (segs)	(54–75%)	0.54–0.75
Newborns	3,320–12,100/μL	3320–12,100 × 10⁶/L
Infants	2,680–2,750/μL	2680–2750 × 10⁶/L
Children	2,660–3,700/μL	2660–3700 × 10⁶/L
Adults	3,000/μL	3800 × 10⁶/L
Neutrophils (bands)	(3–8%)	0.03–0.08
Newborns	1,150–3,460/μL	1150–3460 × 10⁶/L
Infants	990–1,150/μL	990–1150 × 10⁶/L
Children	640–850/μL	640–850 × 10⁶/L
Adults	620/μL	620 × 10⁶/L
Eosinophils	(1–4%)	0.01–0.04
Newborns	300–400/μL	300–400 × 10⁶/L
Infants	300/μL	300 × 10⁶/L

Children	200–280/µL	200–280 × 10⁶/L
Adults	200/µL	200 × 10⁶/L
Basophils	(0–1%)	0–0.01
Newborns	100/µL	100 × 10⁶/L
Infants	50/µL	50 × 10⁶/L
Children	40/µL	40 × 10⁶/L
Adults	40/µL	40 × 10⁶/L
Monocytes	(2–8%)	0.02–0.08
Newborns	700–1200/µL	700–1200 × 10⁶/L
Infants	550–700/µL	550–700 × 10⁶/L
Children	350–550/µL	350–550 × 10⁶/L
Adults	300/µL	300 × 10⁶/L

Abnormal Values

Abnormal WBC (adult) ranges can be classified by degree of severity.

	Increases	*Decreases*
Slight	11,000–20,000/µL	3,000–4,500/µL
Moderate	20,000–30,000/µL	1,500–3,000/µL
Severe	>50,000/µL	<1,500/µL

- Increased (Leukocytosis)
    Physiologic:
    Pregnancy
    Emotional stress
    Menstruation
    Ultraviolet light

    Early infancy
    Strenuous exercise
    Exposure to cold
    Increased epinephrine
        secretion

    Pathologic:
    All types of infections
    Collagen disorders
    Leukemias and other
        malignancies
    Transfusion reactions

    Anemias
    Cushing's disease
    Polycythemia vera
    Inflammatory disorders
    Parasitic infestations
- Decreased (Leukopenia)
    Physiologic: Diurnal rhythms
    Pathologic:
    Bone marrow depression
    Toxic and antineoplastic drugs
    Radiation
    Anemias
    Viral infections

Malaria
Lupus erythematosus and other autoimmune disorders
Alcoholism
Rheumatoid arthritis
Malnutrition

Nursing Implications

Assessment

■ Obtain a history of signs and symptoms, system review, medication regimen, and the results of other laboratory tests and procedures.

Possible Nursing Diagnoses

Infection, risk for transmission
Protection, altered, related to abnormal blood profiles
Pain related to physical agents and chemical agents
Fluid volume deficit, risk for, related to excessive losses

Implementation

■ Put on gloves. Using aseptic technique, perform a venipuncture and collect 7 mL of blood in a lavender-top tube; note the time of collection on the laboratory requisition.
■ For capillary puncture, prepare the finger or heel site and perform the procedure using a lancet. Transport the sample to the laboratory immediately.

Evaluation

■ Compare the client's symptoms with the test results and calculate the results given in percentages to absolute values if necessary.

Client/Caregiver Teaching

Pretest

■ Inform the client that no special preparation is needed for the test.

White Blood Cell Enzymes

Classification: Hematology

Type of Test: Blood

White blood cells (WBCs) in peripheral blood samples retain enzymatic activity and can alter substrates added in the laboratory. The presence of enzymatic activity is useful in studying cells that are so morphologically abnormal on stained smear that it is difficult to determine from which cell line they originated. The two most common WBC enzyme tests are the test for leukocyte alkaline phosphate (LAP), an enzyme found in neutrophils, and the periodic acid-Schiff (PAS) stain, which tests from enzymes found in granulocytes and erythrocytes. Both tests are used to diagnose hematologic disorders, especially leukemia. Another WBC enzyme test, tartrate-resistant acid phosphate (TRAP), is performed to diagnose hairy cell leukemia, as this enzyme activity is present in the lymphocytic cells of this type of leukemia.

The LAP level is completely independent of serum alkaline phosphatase, which reflects osteoblastic activity and hepatic function. The LAP content of neutrophils increases as the cells mature; therefore, it is useful in assessing cellular maturation and in evaluating departures from normal differentiation.

The LAP test helps to distinguish among various hematologic disorders. For example, LAP level increases in polycythemia vera, myelofibrosis, and leukemoid reactions to infections but decreases in chronic granulocytic leukemia. As all of these conditions have increased numbers of immature circulating neutrophils, LAP levels can be helpful in distinguishing among them.

In the PAS stain, compounds that can be oxidized to aldehydes are localized by brilliant fuchsia staining. Many elements in tissues are PAS positive, but in blood cells the PAS-positive material of diagnostic significance is cytoplasmic glycogen. Early granulocyte precursors are PAS negative and acquire increasing PAS positivity as they mature.

Indications

■ Aid in the identification of morphologically abnormal WBCs on a stained smear

- Aid in the diagnosis of suspected leukemia or other hematologic disorders

Reference Values

Leukocyte alkaline phosphatase (LAP)	13–130 U
Periodic acid-Schiff (PAS)	Granulocytes—positive
	Agranulocytes—negative
	Granulocyte precursors—negative
Tartrate-resistant acid phosphatase (TRAP)	Activity present

Abnormal Values

- LAP increased
  ACTH excess
  Chronic myelocytic leukemia
  Cushing's syndrome
  Down syndrome
  Leukemoid reactions
  Lymphomas
  Multiple myeloma
  Myelofibrosis
  Oral contraceptives
  Polycythemia vera
  Pregnancy
- LAP decreased
  Acute monocytic leukemia
  Acute myelocytic leukemia
  Anemias (aplastic, pernicious)
  Chronic granulocytic leukemia
  Collagen disease
  Hereditary hypophosphatasia
  Infectious mononucleosis
  Paroxysmal nocturnal hemoglobulinemia
  Thrombocytopenia
- PAS increased
  Acute granulocytic leukemia
  Acute lymphoblastic leukemia
  Amyloidosis
  Erythroleukemia
  Lymphomas
  Severe iron-deficiency anemia
  Thalassemia

- PAS decreased
  Early granulocyte precursors

Interfering Factors

- Rough handling of specimen may cause hemolysis, which can interfere with test results.

Nursing Implications

Assessment

- Obtain a history of signs and symptoms, medication, and results of other related laboratory tests and diagnostic procedures.

Possible Nursing Diagnoses

Anxiety related to threat to health status
Protection, altered, related to abnormal blood profiles
Fluid volume deficit, risk for, related to excessive losses

Implementation

- Put on gloves. Using aseptic technique, perform a venipuncture and collect 7 mL of blood in a lavender-top tube. Or, use a lancet to obtain a capillary specimen.
- Transport the specimen to the laboratory immediately.

Evaluation

- Note the test results in relation to the client's symptoms and other related tests.

Client/Caregiver Teaching

Pretest

- Inform the client that no special preparation is needed for this test.

Appendices

Appendix 1

Collection Procedures

Obtaining Blood Specimens

Probably the most common diagnostic procedure, obtaining a blood sample requires skill, knowledge about the type of specimen required, and specific blood-handling precautions, including the type of tube required. Although arterial blood is required for some tests such as arterial blood gas measurement, for the most part venous samples are obtained. But depending on the type of test, whole blood, plasma, or serum is needed. Whole blood, which contains all blood constituents, is used to measure hemoglobin, hematocrit, the complete blood count (CBC), and various other studies. Plasma, the liquid part of the whole blood that contains proteins, and serum, the liquid that remains after clotting, are used for coagulation studies and biochemical and immunologic studies. The type of sample required is listed with each entry in this book.

Also listed with each entry are interfering factors, which include such things as prolonged tourniquet use and rough handling of specimen. The person collecting the sample must be aware of these factors to ensure valid results.

General Client Preparation

Preparing the client is essentially the same for all sites and all studies. Make sure you explain the following to the client and to the caregiver:

- The purpose of the test.
- The procedure, including the site from which the blood sample is likely to be obtained.
- That momentary discomfort may be experienced when the skin is pierced.
- That food, fluids, and/or drugs may be withheld before the test.
- Encourage questions and expressions of concern about the procedures and provide a calm, reassuring environment and manner.

For pediatric clients, you may want to use a doll or stuffed animal to demonstrate the procedure. Sometimes the equipment basket will hold the child's attention, but make sure the child does not touch sharp objects. You may also need to ask for a colleague's assistance if the child is uncooperative and needs restraining. Sometimes a caregiver can assist, but that depends on his or her ability to remain calm and supportive.

Informed Consent

One of the most basic rights of the client is informed consent. Legally, the client or the caregiver, if the client is under age or legally incompetent, must understand the procedure, risks, and implications before consent can be obtained. Consent may be written or verbal; for more complex procedures, it is the physician's responsibility to obtain consent, although the nurse can reinforce the explanation. However, it is important to remember that the client can withdraw consent at any time.

Patient Safety

Following universal precautions, including proper handwashing and wearing of gloves and protective devices as required by your institution, protects you as well as the client from bloodborne infections.

Also, take precautions to ensure that the client is supported during and immediately after obtaining the sample; some clients experience syncope and are at risk for falling. If performing the procedure on the pediatric client, encourage the child to cooperate. If the child is at high risk for moving, ask a colleague to help hold the child so no injury occurs.

Capillary Puncture Procedure

For this procedure, the skin of the site to be used (fingertip or earlobe of an adult or the great toe or heel of a newborn) should be warm and free of lesions or edema. If the skin feels cool or looks pale, apply a warm compress to the site for 3 minutes to dilate the capillaries.

Equipment: Assemble a sterile lancet, skin disinfectant, gauze pads or cotton balls, collection device (microhematocrit tube or pipette), bandage, and materials to label the sample.

Procedure

- Place the client in a comfortable and safe position. If an extremity is to be used, position it on a bed or table, using a small pillow or rolled blanket to improve positioning and promote comfort.
- Wash hands and don gloves. Cleanse the area around the site with disinfectant such as 70 percent alcohol or povidone-iodine and allow site to dry.
- Grasp the site firmly and puncture the skin with the sterile lancet, using a quick, firm motion to a depth of about 2 mm.
- Use the gauze to wipe away the first drop of blood from the site. If another drop does not immediately form, lower the

extremity or earlobe to improve flow. Do not squeeze the site because this will yield more tissue fluid than blood and alter results.

- Collect the sample in the microhematocrit tube (capillary tube) by holding it at an angle to the drop of blood, allowing capillary pressure to pull the blood into the tube. Place the capillary tube in the proper container or vial holding the reagent. Rotate the vial slowly to mix the blood sample with the reagent.
- If the capillary sample is for a smear, place a drop on the slide and gently spread the blood with another slide.
- Apply slight pressure to the puncture site with the gauze pad until bleeding stops.
- Label the sample with client's name and other required identifying information. Send sample to laboratory promptly.

Venipuncture

Although the most common site for venipuncture is the antecubital fossa, sites in the wrist or dorsum of the hand or foot may be used. Before gathering the equipment, assess the condition of the potential veins. Avoid using tortuous, sclerotic veins or those in which phlebitis has previously occurred. If possible, do not obtain a sample from an arm or leg being used for an IV infusion of blood, dextrose, or electrolytes. These fluids will dilute the specimen or falsely alter test results. If such an extremity must be used, withdraw the sample distal to the infusion site. Also, do not use an extremity with a hemodialysis venous access site (shunt) nor the arm on the affected side following a mastectomy.

If the client's veins are difficult to locate, try applying warm compresses 15 minutes before the procedure. Placing the extremity in a dependent position allows blood to fill the veins and also aids in obtaining the sample.

Equipment: Tourniquet; skin disinfectant; gauze pads or cotton balls; syringe; and needle (usually 20 gauge or smaller 21 to 23 gauge, depending on the client's age and vein condition); vacuumized tube, holder, and needle; bandage; and materials to label the specimen.

Procedure

- Place client in a position of comfort, either sitting or lying down. The extremity to be used is supported on the bed or a table. A small pillow or rolled towel or blanket may be used to improve positioning or promote comfort.
- Wash hands and don gloves.
- Apply a tourniquet 1 to 1.5 inches above the site to be used. Tourniquets should be applied tightly enough to cause the

veins to enlarge without occluding arterial circulation. A tourniquet should not be kept in place for more than 1 minute before venipuncture or for more than 2 to 3 minutes for the entire procedure. If a vein in the arm is to be used, the client is asked to open and close the hand a few times and then clench the fist. If the puncture cannot be made in 1 minute, the tourniquet is removed and then reapplied when a new site is located.

- Cleanse the skin with povidone-iodine or 70 percent alcohol in a circular motion starting at the insertion site and moving outward. Allow the area to air-dry. For immunosuppressed clients, povidone-iodine should be used, followed by a 70 percent alcohol pad taped over the site for 10 minutes. The site should be allowed to air-dry or be dried with sterile gauze before venipuncture.

- Remove the needle cover and then stabilize the vein by pressing the gloved thumb just below the insertion site. Draw the skin tight.

- To enter the vein, insert the needle about 1/2 inch below the expected site of insertion. When the needle is smaller than the vein, insert it bevel up at a 15- to 45-degree angle. When the needle is larger, insert it bevel down almost parallel to the skin.

- If a vacuumized tube system is used, the tube is pushed into the holder until the rubber stopper is punctured and blood flows into the tube. If more than one tube is required, the filled tube is removed from the holder and another inserted until the desired number of samples is obtained. The sequence for obtaining the multiple samples using different types of tubes is as follows: (1) blood culture tubes (swab the rubber stopper before inserting into the holder to prevent contamination), (2) tubes with no additives, (3) tubes for coagulation studies, and (4) tubes with additives.

- If a syringe is used, pull back on the plunger until the desired amount of blood is obtained. The sample is then transferred to other tubes.

- Release the tourniquet and tell the client to unclench the fist. Remove the needle and immediately apply pressure with sterile gauze or cotton ball. Pressure should be maintained for 3 minutes to prevent hematoma formation.

- If the puncture site is in the dorsum of the hand, elevate the hand and apply pressure. Pressure is maintained until the bleeding has stopped. Apply an adhesive strip, if required.

- To transfer a specimen collected in a syringe into a laboratory tube, remove the needle of the syringe and the stopper of the tube. Gently inject the blood into the tube, allowing it to flow gently down the tube. If a vacuumized tube is used, insert the needle through its rubber stopper, allowing the vacuum to draw the blood into the tube. If the sample is for a blood culture, the rubber stopper should be cleansed with povidone-iodine before the needle is inserted.

- Discard uncapped needle and syringe or vacuumized device in the biohazard disposal container.
- Provide support to the client if the puncture is not successful and another must be performed.
- Remove gloves and discard in appropriate container.
- Label the sample with the client's name and other required identifying information and send promptly to the laboratory
- Check the venipuncture site in 5 minutes for hematoma formation. Apply warms soaks if hematoma is noted.
- If the client is immunosuppressed, advise the client or caregiver to check the puncture site every 8 hours for signs of infection such as extreme redness, swelling, and pain or the presence of drainage. Also, tell the client or caregiver to report a fever above 101°F, which could suggest sepsis.

Venous Access Devices

Obtaining a blood sample from a venous access device (VAD), also known as a venous access port (VAP), spares the client the discomfort of a venipuncture. Strict aseptic technique is imperative because you are accessing a vein located closer to the heart.

Equipment: Disinfectant swabs (povidone-iodine and alcohol), sterile gauze pads, 19- or 20-gauge noncoring needle with extension set, 10-mL syringe with 5 mL of saline, 20-mL syringe, 20-mL syringe with saline, blood sample tubes, and syringe with heparin flush solution.

Procedure

- Assess the area around the port for signs of infection. If appropriate, place an ice bag over the port to help relieve pain from the needle puncture.
- Remove the ice bag. Wash hands thoroughly and don gloves.
- Clean the area with an alcohol swab, starting at the center and working in a circular motion outward, covering a 5-inch area. Next, using the same technique, use a povidone-iodine swab. Repeat with a second swab.
- If ordered, a local anesthetic such as 0.1 mL of lidocaine without epinephrine may be injected at the insertion site.
- Attach the 10-mL syringe with the 5 mL of saline to the noncoring needle and extension set. Then clear the air from the set.
- Palpate the port and locate the septum. Then while anchoring the port between your fingers, aim the needle at the

center of the device. Insert the needle perpendicular to the septum and push the needle through the skin and septum until you reach the reservoir.

- Flush the device with the 5 mL of saline, then withdraw at least 5 mL of blood, and clamp the extension set. Discard the syringe containing the blood.
- Connect the 20-mL syringe to the extension set and then unclamp it and aspirate the desired amount of blood.
- Clamp the extension set and remove the blood-filled syringe. Next, attach the 20-mL saline-filled syringe and unclamp the extension set.
- Flush the device using the 20 mL of saline and reclamp the extension set. Remove the saline-filled syringe and attach the heparin-filled syringe. Unclamp the extension set and flush the device.
- Then, while stabilizing the device, withdraw the noncoring needle and dispose of it properly.

If your are using a vacuumized tube setup, adjust the procedure as follows:

- Attach the needle to the tube holder. Label one of the vacuumized tubes ''Discard.''
- Attach the Luer-Lok injection cap to the noncoring needle's extension tubing. Remove the air from the setup using the saline-filled syringe.
- Access the port as previously described and flush the device with the 5 mL of saline. Then remove the needle from the injection cap.
- Wipe the injection cap with alcohol or povidone-iodine swab. Insert the vacuumized needle holder into the cap and insert the tube labeled ''Discard.'' When the tube is full, remove it and discard.
- Insert each tube needed for the tests and allow each to fill with blood.
- When all the blood samples have been obtained, remove the vacuumized needle holder from the injection cap.
- Insert the 20-mL syringe filled with saline and flush the device. Remove the syringe and then attach the heparin-filled syringe and flush, according to institutional policy.
- After removing the syringe, clamp the extension set and remove it from the VAP.

Umbilical Blood Sampling

Until a few years ago, umbilical cord blood samples were obtained only after delivery and were used primarily to evaluate bilirubin in infants at risk for Rh or ABO incompatibility. However, with in utero procedure advances, fetal health can be assessed by percutaneous umbilical cord blood sampling

(PUBS). Using ultrasonography, a physician inserts a 20- or 22-gauge spinal needle into the umbilical vessel. Fetal hematologic and metabolic status, genetic disorder identification, and perinatal infection evaluation are the most common tests performed.

Arterial Blood Sampling

Arterial samples can be obtained by direct arterial puncture using the radial or the femoral artery or by accessing an existing arterial line. Both procedures are detailed here:

Equipment for arterial puncture: A 10-mL glass syringe or plastic Luer-Lok syringe made for blood gas determinations, prefilled heparin (1:1000) syringe or 1 ampule of heparin 1:1000 and 20-gauge needle, 22-gauge 1-inch needle, povidone-iodine and alcohol sponges, gauze pads, rubber cap for syringe or rubber stopper for needle, plastic bag filled with ice, label, and adhesive bandage.

Procedure

- Perform an Allen's test to check which hand has the better arterial function. To perform this test, support the client's wrist with a rolled towel. Ask the client to make a fist. Next, use your index and middle fingers to apply pressure on radial and ulnar arteries. Without removing your fingers, ask the client to unclench the fist. You should note that the palm is blanched. Next, release the pressure on the ulnar artery. If the artery is functioning well, the palm should turn pink in about 5 seconds. If this does not occur, try the test on the other wrist. If both hands have poor function, contact the physician. A femoral stick may be performed instead.

- Wash hands and prepare equipment. To heparinize the syringe, open the ampule of heparin and withdraw the heparin, using the 20-gauge needle attached to the syringe. Hold the syringe upright and, while rotating the plunger, pull the plunger back to the 7-mL mark to allow the heparin to coat the sides of the syringe. Force all but 0.1 mL of heparin out of the syringe. Replace the 20-gauge needle with the 22-gauge needle and eject the rest of the heparin.

- If using the radial artery, position the wrist on a hard surface with a rolled towel beneath it for support.

- Don gloves and locate the artery. Anesthetize the site with 1 percent lidocaine without epinephrine, if it is part of institutional policy.

- Cleanse the puncture site with povidone-iodine or alcohol using a circular motion, starting at the intended puncture site and moving outward. Allow the skin to dry.

- Palpate the artery with the index or middle finger of the nondominant hand. Hold the syringe over the insertion site with the dominant hand. Make sure the needle has the bevels up and is positioned at a 30- to 45-degree angle.

■ Insert the needle through the skin and into the artery in one motion. Watch for blood backflow into the syringe. The syringe should fill by itself because of the pressure within the artery.

■ When 5 mL of blood fills the syringe, remove the needle and press the gauze pad over the site in one motion. Continue to apply pressure for 5 minutes. Apply adhesive strip after bleeding has stopped.

■ Remove any air bubbles from the syringe and then insert the needle into the rubber stopper or, if you have a rubber cap for the needle hub, remove the needle and apply it.

■ Label the syringe and place it in the ice-filled plastic bag. Take the sample and the properly completed request form to the laboratory immediately. Make sure that, if the client is on oxygen, the amount is noted on the request form.

Equipment for obtaining sample from arterial line: Povidone-iodine and alcohol swabs, sterile gauze pads, sterile injection caps, 10-mL or 20-mL syringe, heparin 1:1000 with syringe and needle, 30-mL syringe with saline, and label.

Procedure

■ Place client in a comfortable position, usually the semi-Fowler's position if a right atrial catheter is being accessed.

■ Cleanse the catheter cap junction or hub with povidone-iodine or 70 percent alcohol.

■ Don sterile gloves, remove the cap, and attach 10-mL syringe to the connector.

■ Withdraw 6 mL of blood and clamp the catheter. (If a Groshong catheter is used, clamping is necessary because a special valve is in place.)

■ Discard the syringe containing the 6 mL of blood.

■ Attach another syringe and remove the amount of blood needed for the tests.

■ Heparinize the catheter by inserting the dilute heparin-containing syringe into the hub or cap and slowly injecting it. Clamp the catheter, remove the needle, and then unclamp the catheter. If the old injection cap is discarded and new one is attached.

■ If a Groshong catheter is in place, flush with 20 mL of saline.

Obtaining Urine Specimens

One of the main reasons for invalid results of urine tests is improper specimen collection and handling. Therefore, the nurse must know how the specimens are collected and how to instruct clients on specimen collection. The types of specimens and their collection procedures are discussed here.

Random Specimens

Random specimens are urine samples that are collected in clean containers at any time during the day. Usually 15 to 60 mL of urine is sufficient for tests performed on random samples. Random samples are used for routine screening tests to detect obvious abnormalities. The client is instructed to void directly into the urine container or some other type of laboratory container, after which the sample is transferred to another type of laboratory container. If the sample is collected by the client at home, it must be transported to the laboratory within 2 hours or test results may be inaccurate. Random urine specimens are routinely collected as part of the physical examination or at any time during the client's hospitalization. They are also used for drug screening.

Equipment: Urinal or bedpan with a cover, gloves, graduated container, specimen container with a lid, and specimen label.

Procedure

- Instruct the client about the procedure. Advise that you must collect a urine specimen for laboratory analysis. Tell the client the purpose of the laboratory test.
- Provide privacy for the client.
- If the client does not have bathroom privileges, provide a clean urinal or bedpan. Then, ask the client to void in the clean urinal or bedpan.
- Put on gloves and pour at least 60 mL of the urine into the laboratory specimen container.
- Place the lid or cap securely on the container. Label the container with the client's name, client identification number, time of collection, date, and any antibiotics that the client may be taking. Place the labeled container in a biohazard specimen container for transport to prevent any cross-contamination. Take the specimen to the laboratory immediately.
- If the client must have the intake and output measured and recorded, measure the amount of remaining urine in the graduated container; otherwise, discard the remaining urine.
- For the home care client, have the client collect the specimen in a clean container with a tight-fitting lid.
- Instruct the client to label the specimen container with name, address, date, time of collection, and doctor's name.

- Instruct the client to keep the specimen on ice or in the refrigerator, separated from any food, for up to 24 hours.

Clean-Catch Midstream Specimens

Clean-catch midstream specimens are used to avoid contamination of the sample with urethral cells, microorganisms, and mucus. The client is given a clean-catch kit containing the materials needed to cleanse the urinary meatus and a specimen container. Clean-catch midstream specimens are used for microbiologic and cytologic analysis of urine. Some individuals advocate using this method for routine urinalysis, especially in women, because the sample is less likely to be contaminated with substances that alter results of routine screening tests.

Equipment: Commercial clean-catch kit containing antiseptic towelettes, sterile specimen container with a lid and label, biohazard transport bag, and instructions.

For the home care client: Basin, soap and water, towels, sterile 2-inch × 2-inch gauze pads, povidone-iodine solution, sterile specimen container with a lid, label, graduated cylinder, biohazard transport bag, and gloves.

Procedure

- Explain the procedure to the client and tell him or her the reason for the test.
- Provide illustrations to the client to provide instructions to perform the procedure.
- Instruct the client to remove all clothing from the waist down. The male client should stand in front of the toilet. The female client should sit far back on the toilet seat and spread her legs.
- Instruct the male client to clean the tip of the penis and the female client to clean the labial folds, vulva, and urethral meatus with soap and water.
- Then, the client should wipe the area three times with a fresh 2-inch × 2-inch gauze pad soaked in povidone-iodine solution or with the wipes provided in the commercially prepared kit.
- Instruct the uncircumcised male client to retract his foreskin to clean the meatus and to keep it retracted during voiding.
- Instruct the female client to separate the labial folds with her thumb and forefinger. She should wipe down one side with the first 2-inch × 2-inch pad and then discard it. She should then wipe the other side with another clean 2-inch × 2-inch pad and then discard it. Lastly, with the third pad, she should wipe down the center over the urinary meatus and then discard the pad. Remind her to wipe from the front to the back to avoid contaminating the genital area with fecal matter.

- Then, have the female client straddle the toilet, allowing her labia to open, or she should hold her labia open with her fingers as she begins to void.
- The client should begin to void in the urinal, toilet, or bedpan. The voiding washes bacteria from the urethra and urinary meatus.
- Then, without stopping the urinary stream, the client should place the specimen container into the urine stream, collecting about 30 to 60 mL of urine. This specimen is collected during the midstream portion of the voiding.
- The client can then finish voiding into the urinal or bedpan.
- If the client is having his or her intake and output recorded, measure the remaining urine in a graduated cylinder. Be sure to measure the amount of voided urine in the specimen container.
- While wearing gloves, take the sterile specimen container from the client and place the lid securely on it. Label the container with the client's name, room number, date, client identification number, and any antibiotics that the client is taking. Place the labeled specimen container in a biohazard transport bag and send it to the laboratory immediately or place it on ice.
- If the client is on antibiotic therapy, note the antibiotic on the specimen container label before sending to the laboratory for analysis.

Catheterized Specimens

Urine specimens may be obtained from one-time "straight" catheterization or from indwelling catheters. "Straight" catheterization is indicated when the client is unable to void for a random or clean-catch specimen without excessively contaminating the specimen. It is also used for samples for microbiologic and cytologic studies.

Indwelling catheters may be placed for a variety of reasons. In some cases, they may be inserted when serial urine specimens are needed at exact time intervals. In other cases, the catheter is already in place and must be used for urine sampling.

Equipment: A 20- to 30-mL syringe, 21- or 22-gauge 1-1/2-inch needle, tube clamp, sterile specimen cup with a lid, gloves, alcohol sponge, specimen label, and biohazard transport bag.

Procedure

- The drainage tubing of the indwelling catheter should be clamped about 30 minutes before the specimen is collected. Clamping allows urine to accumulate in the catheter.

- Don gloves.

  If the urine drainage system has a built-in aspiration or sampling port:

- Wipe the port with an alcohol sponge.
- Uncap the needle on the syringe and insert the needle into the aspirating port at a 90-degree angle or perpendicular to the tubing, and aspirate the urine into the syringe.
- Then, expel the aspirated urine specimen into the sterile specimen container.
- Place the lid on the specimen container. Label the specimen with the clients's name, room number, date, client identification number, time of collection, and any antibiotics the client may be taking. Place the specimen container in a biohazard transport bag and take it to the laboratory immediately or place it on ice.
- Be sure to unclamp the catheter drainage tubing after obtaining the specimen to reestablish urine drainage and to prevent bladder distention and possible infection.

  If the tubing does not have an aspiration port:

- Wipe the area connecting the catheter and the drainage tubing with an alcohol sponge.
- Disconnect the catheter from the drainage tubing and allow urine to flow into the specimen container.
- Be sure not to touch the tip of the catheter to the inside of the sterile specimen container or anything else with the catheter to avoid cross-contamination of the catheter.
- After you have obtained the urine specimen, wipe the end of the drainage tubing and the end of the catheter with an alcohol sponge and then reconnect them.
- Place the lid on the specimen container. Label the container with the client's name, date, time of collection, client identification number, and any antibiotics the client may be taking.
- Be sure to unclamp the catheter drainage tubing after obtaining the specimen to reestablish urine flow and drainage and to prevent distention and possible infection.

Timed Specimens

Timed specimens, usually over 24 hours, allow for quantification of substances in urine. Methods of preserving the accumulated sample vary among laboratories, and, therefore, the laboratory should be consulted for advice regarding the use of a preservative or the need for refrigeration or both. It is critical that all urine excreted during the 24-hour period be collected.

Sometimes, it is necessary to insert an indwelling catheter for 24-hour urine collections. This is especially true if the client is unable to participate in specimen collection. At other times, an indwelling catheter may already be in place. When a 24-hour urine collection is to be obtained via an indwelling catheter, the collection should begin by changing the tubing and the drainage bag so that a clean, fresh system is in use. If a preservative is required, it can be obtained from the laboratory and placed directly into the drainage bag. Others advocate using a container with preservative and emptying the drainage bag contents into it at frequent intervals (e.g., every 2 hours). If refrigeration of the specimen is necessary, the drainage bag is placed in a basin filled with ice. The ice supply will have to be renewed frequently to ensure that the specimen is properly chilled. If the urine must be protected from light, the drainage bag may be covered with dark plastic or aluminum foil. If the drainage tubing is positioned correctly for continuous drainage, it need not be covered.

Some urine tests require 2-hour or 12-hour samples. A 2-hour or a 12-hour sample is collected in the same manner as a 24-hour sample, with the exact starting and stopping times noted.

Collecting a 24-hour urine specimen

Equipment: Large collection bottle with a cap or a commercial plastic collection container; preservative, if necessary; gloves; graduated cylinder; bedpan, urinal, or toilet urine collection container; ice-filled container; specimen label; client reminders; and dark-collection container, if necessary.

Procedure

■ Provide a detailed and written explanation of the procedure for the client and any family members or caregivers that may be assisting with the collection. Stress the importance of collecting every voided specimen. Explain that the loss of even one small voided specimen will alter the results of the test.

■ Place client care reminders in the bathroom, at the bedside, on the indwelling catheter drainage bag, and on the client's chart to remind the client, family members, and any staff caregivers about the collection.

■ Instruct the client to collect all urine during the collection period, to notify you upon voiding, and to avoid contaminating the urine with stool or toilet paper.

■ If the client will be collecting the specimens at home, make certain that he or she has written instructions as to collection, storage, and transportion of the specimens.

For a 2-hour collection:

■ The client should try to drink 480 to 960 mL of water 30 minutes prior to the test to be well hydrated.

■ After the 30 minutes, ask the client to void and to discard this specimen so that he or she begins the test with an empty bladder.

- If this is a challenge test and requires administering medication such as corticotropin or glucose, administer it now, as ordered.
- Unless contraindicated, encourage the client to drink a glass of water every hour to stimulate urine production.
- After the client voids, put on gloves and empty the urine specimen into the collection container.
- Ask the client to void 15 minutes before the end of the collection period, and add the specimen to the collection container.
- Label the container with the client's name, identification number, date, time of the start and finish of the collection, and any medications administered for the test or any preservatives added to the container.
- Send the labeled container to the laboratory immediately.

    For 12-hour and 24-hour collections:

- Don gloves and ask the client to void. Discard this first-voided specimen so that the client starts the test with an empty bladder. Note the time of this voiding as the start of the test.
- When the client voids again, put on gloves and empty this specimen into the collection container.
- If preservative is required, place it in the container now with the first specimen.
- Place the collection container in the refrigerator or place it in ice.
- Collect all of the client's urine during the testing period. Just before the collection period ends, ask the client to void again, and place this specimen into the container as the last specimen and note the time at the end of the test.
- Pack the specimen in fresh ice. Label the container with the client's name, room number, client identification number, date, times of test, preservatives added, and any medications that the client is taking.
- Send the labeled container, packed in ice, to the laboratory immediately.

Obtaining Pediatric Urine Specimens

Pediatric urine samples can be performed for random, culture and sensitivity, or timed specimens. Because a child that does not have bladder control cannot provide a clean-catch specimen, the pediatric urine collection bag can provide an effective alternative method. This alternative prevents the contamination of the specimen and prevents invasive procedures that can introduce bacteria into the bladder. This procedure is contraindicated if the child has irritated or sensitive skin, because the bag is secured with adhesive strips. The specimen should be tested immediately for accurate results, as the number of bacteria can double every 20 to 30 minutes. Urine specimens from toilet-trained children are collected in the same manner as for adults. It is helpful to follow the child's usual urinary pattern when collecting the specimen. A potty chair or bedpan placed on the toilet and terminology familiar to the child should be used (tinkle, potty, and so on). A parent can assist and often has more success in collecting a specimen than does the nurse.

Pediatric Random Urine

Equipment: Pediatric urine collection bag, urine specimen container, label, two disposable diapers, scissors, gloves, washcloth, soap, water, towel, bowl, and linen-saver pad.

Procedure

- Using the scissors, cut a slit in a diaper, cutting from the center point to one of the shorter edges. This slit will be used to pull the urine collection bag through when the bag and diaper are on the client.
- Explain the procedure to the client if he or she is old enough to understand. Explain the procedure to the parents of the child whether or not the child understands the procedure.
- Place the child on a linen-saver pad and cleanse the perineal area with soap and water, working from the urinary meatus outward.
- Separate the labia of a female child or retract the foreskin of an uncircumcised male child. Thoroughly rinse the area with a clean washcloth and water and dry with a towel.
- Do not use lotion or powder on the area, which can interfere with the adhesive on the collection bag.
- Place the child in the frog position with the legs separated and the knees flexed.
- Have the parents hold the child in position, if necessary.
- Remove the protective covering over the adhesive edges of the collection bag. With a female child, separate the labia and gently press the bag's lower rim to the perineum. Attach the rest of the adhesive rim, working toward the pubis and inside the labia majora.
- With a male child, place the bag's opening over the penis and scrotum and press the adhesive rim to the skin.
- Run your finger around the edges of the adhesive strips to make sure they are secure and that no edges are not adhering to the skin.
- Gently pull the bag through the slit in the diaper and apply the diaper to the child. The bag should protrude slightly through the slit to allow it to fill, preventing compression and

allowing observation of the specimen without removing the diaper.

- When you can see urine in the bag, put on gloves and gently remove the diaper and the bag. Hold the bag's bottom port over the collection container, remove the tab from the port, and let the urine flow into the collection container.
- If you are recording intake and output for the child, measure the amount of urine in the specimen container.
- Label the specimen container with the child's name, identification number, room number, date, and time of collection. Also note on the container whether the child is taking any antibiotics.
- Send the labeled container to the laboratory immediately.

Pediatric Specimen for Culture and Sensitivity

Equipment: Sterile pediatric collection bag, sterile urine specimen container, label, two disposable diapers, scissors, sterile bowl, sterile or distilled water, antiseptic skin cleanser, sterile 4-inch × 4-inch gauze pads, alcohol sponge, 3 mL syringe with needle, and linen-saver pad.

Procedure

- Using the scissors, cut a slit in a diaper, cutting from the center point to one of the shorter edges. This slit will be used to pull the urine collection bag through when the bag and diaper are on the client.
- Explain the procedure to the client if he or she is old enough to understand. Explain the procedure to the parents of the child, whether or not the child understands the procedure.
- Place the child on a linen-saver pad. Using gloves, cleanse the perineal area with sterile or distilled water, an antiseptic cleanser, and sterile 4-inch × 4-inch gauze pads, working from the urinary meatus outward, wiping only once with each pad and then discarding it.
- Separate the labia of a female child and retract the foreskin of an uncircumcised male child. Thoroughly rinse the area with a clean washcloth and water and dry with a towel.
- Do not use lotion or powder on the area, which can interfere with the adhesive on the collection bag and also contaminate the area after cleansing.
- Place the child in the frog position with the legs separated and the knees flexed.
- Have the parents hold the child in position, if necessary.
- Remove the protective covering over the adhesive edges of the collection bag. With the female child, separate the labia and gently press the bag's lower rim to the perineum. Attach

the rest of the adhesive rim, working toward the pubis and inside the labia majora.

- With the male child, place the bag's opening over the penis and scrotum and press the adhesive rim to the skin.
- Run your finger around the edges of the adhesive strips to make sure they are secure and that no edges are not adhering to the skin.
- Gently pull the bag through the slit in the diaper and apply the diaper to the child. The bag should protrude slightly through the slit, which will allow it to fill, preventing compression and allowing observation of the specimen without removing the diaper.
- When you can see urine in the bag, put on gloves and wipe an area on the collection bag with an alcohol sponge.
- Puncture the clean area of the collection bag with the needle, and aspirate urine into the syringe.
- Inject the aspirated urine into the sterile specimen container. To maintain sterility, take care not to touch the sides of the specimen container with the needle.
- Remove and discard your gloves.
- If you are recording the child's intake and output, measure the amount of urine in the specimen container.
- Label the specimen container with the child's name, identification number, room number, date, and time of collection. Also note on the container whether the child is taking any antibiotics.
- Send the labeled container to the laboratory immediately.

Pediatric Timed Specimen

Equipment: A 24-hour pediatric urine collection bag with evacuation tubing, 24-hour urine specimen container, two disposable diapers, gloves, washcloth, soap, water, bowl, towel, sterile 4-inch × 4-inch gauze pads, compound benzoin tincture, small medicine cup, 35-mL Luer-Lok syringe or urimeter, tubing stopper, specimen preservative, and linen-saver pad.

Procedure

- Using the scissors, cut a slit in a diaper, cutting from the center point to one of the shorter edges. This slit will be used to pull the urine collection bag through with the bag and diaper on the client.
- Explain the procedure to the client if he or she is old enough to understand. Explain the procedure to the parents of the child whether or not the child understands the procedure.
- Place the child on a linen-saver pad and cleanse the perineal area with soap and water, working from the urinary meatus outward.

- Separate the labia of a female child and retract the foreskin of an uncircumcised male child. Thoroughly rinse the area with a clean washcloth and water and dry with a towel.
- Do not use lotion or powder on the area, which can interfere with the adhesive on the collection bag.
- Place the child in the frog position with the legs separated and the knees flexed.
- Have the parents hold the child in position, if necessary.
- Remove the protective covering over the adhesive edges of the collection bag. With the female child, separate the labia and gently press the bag's lower rim to the perineum. Attach the rest of the adhesive rim, working toward the pubis and inside the labia majora.
- With the male child, place the bag's opening over the penis and scrotum and press the adhesive rim to the skin.
- Run your finger around the edges of the adhesive strips to make sure they are secure and that no edges have not adhered to the skin.
- If it is difficult to adhere the bag to the skin, apply compound benzoin tincture to the perineal area, if ordered. If you use the spray, cover the perineal area with a gauze pad or, if using the liquid, apply it to the skin with a gauze pad dipped in compound that was poured into a medicine cup.
- Gently pull the bag and the tubing through the slit in the diaper and apply the diaper to the child. The bag should protrude slightly through the slit, which will allow it to fill, preventing compression and allowing observation of the specimen without removing the diaper.
- Check the collection bag every 30 minutes. When you can see urine in the bag, put on gloves and remove the stopper on the collection bag's tubing.
- Attach the syringe to the end of the tubing and aspirate the urine. This is considered the first void and will be discarded. Remove the syringe and discard the urine. Insert the stopper into the tubing.
- Begin timing the collection. When the next specimen is observed, add the preservative to the container with the specimen and refrigerate, if ordered.
- Periodically, check the collection bag for an accumulation of urine and empty the bag accordingly.
- With each withdrawal of urine from the collection bag, inject a small amount of air into the bag to prevent a vacuum from forming, which can block urine drainage.
- When the collection period has elapsed, stop the collection and send the specimen to the lab after the specimen has been labeled with the client's name, identification number,

date, time, room number, and any preservatives added or antibiotics being taken.
- Remove the collection bag from the child and gently wash and dry the area and apply a fresh diaper.
- Send the labeled container to the laboratory immediately.

Percutaneous Suprapubic Aspiration

Percutaneous suprapubic aspiration of the bladder is a procedure that is performed when a urine specimen cannot be obtained from a child because the child can neither void nor provide an adequate specimen. Catheterization is most often used to obtain a specimen; however, suprapubic aspiration can be used in suspected cases of urinary tract infection for which definitive diagnosis is necessary in acutely ill infants. In young infants, the bladder is palpable in the abdomen and is therefore easily located and accessible above the symphysis.

Equipment: Antiseptic cleansing solution, sterile 4-inch × 4-inch gauze pads, gloves, 20- to 22-gauge 1 1/2-inch needle, 20 mL syringe, sterile specimen container, adhesive bandage, and biohazard transport bag.

Procedure
- Explain the procedure to the infant's parents. Explain the need for the test and the indications of the results.
- Check the infant's diaper for recent voiding. There should be at least 1 hour between the last void and the suprapubic aspiration.
- Have another nurse assist you in the procedure by placing the infant in the frog position. The assistant should hold the infant's legs at the knees. The knees should be drawn up to the hip level.
- Talk to the infant during the procedure to provide comfort.
- Don gloves and palpate the full bladder above the symphysis.
- Using the sterile 4-inch × 4-inch gauze pads, cleanse an area above the symphysis with the antiseptic solution.
- Insert a 20- or 22-gauge needle in the midline approximately 1 cm above the symphysis. Direct the needle downward and vertically.
- When a specimen has been obtained, withdraw the needle and apply pressure to the aspiration site to prevent bleeding.
- Expel the aspirated urine into a sterile specimen container. Place the lid securely on the container. Label the container with the infant's name, type of specimen (suprapubic aspiration), identification number, room number, date, time of collection, and any antibiotics that the infant is taking.

- Place the specimen container in a biohazard collection bag and transport it to the laboratory immediately or refrigerate.
- To prevent urination during the procedure, apply pressure on the male penis or apply digital pressure to the urethra upward from the rectum.
- Place an adhesive bandage on the aspiration site if necessary and place another diaper on the infant.

Appendix 2

Types of Vacuumized Tubes Used for Blood Tests

Color of Stopper	Additive	Action of Additive	Use
Red, pink	None	None	Tests in which serum is needed, such as chemistry, blood bank, and serology tests
Red-gray	Clot activator and thixotropic gel	Activates clot formation and enhances. Separates red blood cells from serum.	Chemistry tests
Lavender, purple	Ethylenediamine-tetraacetic acid (EDTA)	Blocks coagulation by binding calcium. Causes minimal distortion of blood cell size and shape.	Tests that require whole blood, such as hematology tests
Light blue	Sodium citrate	Blocks coagulation by binding calcium. May result in dilution of the specimen due to volume needed to anticoagulate the specimen.	Tests requiring plasma, such as coagulation studies

(continued)

Types of Vacuumized Tubes Used for Blood Tests

Color of Stopper	Additive	Action of Additive	Use
Green	Sodium heparin, lithium heparin, or ammonium heparin	Prevents coagulation by blocking the action of thrombin. Does not alter blood cell size.	Tests requiring plasma, such as chemistry tests, toxicology studies, and red blood cell osmotic fragility studies
Gray	Sodium fluoride and potassium oxalate	Blocks coagulation by binding calcium. Blocks action of enzymes in red blood cells that break down glucose and alcohol. May inactivate cardiac and liver enzymes.	Test for glucose and alcohol
Black	Sodium oxalate	Blocks coagulation by binding calcium.	Coagulation studies
Yellow	Sodium polyanethole-sulfonate (SPS)	Blocks coagulation. Inactivates white blood cells and antibiotics.	Blood cultures
Yellow-gray	Thrombin	Works in the coagulation cascade to enhance clot formation.	STAT serum chemistry tests
Brown	Sodium heparin	Prevents coagulation by blocking the action of thrombin. Does not alter blood cell size.	Lead determinations

Types of Vacuumized Tubes Used for Blood Tests

Color of Stopper	Additive	Action of Additive	Use
Dark blue	Sodium heparin, EDTA, or none	Sodium heparin prevents coagulation by blocking the action of thrombin. EDTA blocks coagulation by binding calcium.	Trace elements, toxicology studies, and nutrient analysis

Appendix 3

Universal Precautions

OSHA Bloodborne Pathogens Standard

Who Is Covered?

The Occupational Safety and Health Administration (OSHA) standard protects employees who may be occupationally exposed to blood and other potential infectious materials, which includes but is not limited to physicians, nurses, phlebotomists, emergency medical personnel, operating room personnel, therapists, orderlies, laundry workers, and other health care workers.

Blood means human blood, blood products, or blood components. Other potentially infectious materials include human body fluids such as saliva in dental procedures, semen, vaginal secretions; cerebrospinal, synovial, pleural, pericardial, peritoneal, and amniotic fluids; body fluids visibly contaminated with blood; unfixed human tissues or organs; HIV-containing cell or tissue cultures; and HIV- or HBV-containing culture mediums or other solutions.

Occupational exposure means a "reasonably anticipated skin, eye, mucous membrane, or parenteral contact with blood or other potentially infectious materials that may result from the performance of the employee's duties."

Federal OSHA authority extends to all private sector employers with one or more employees, as well as federal civilian employees. In addition, many states administer their own occupational safety and health programs through plans approved under section 18(b) of the OSH Act. These plans must adopt standards and enforce requirements that are at least as effective as federal requirements. Of the current 25 state plan states and territories, 23 cover the private and public (state and local governments) sectors and 2 cover the public sector only.

Determining occupational exposure and instituting control methods and work practices appropriate for specific job assignments are key requirements of the standard. The required written exposure control plan and methods of compliance

From Thomas, CL (ed): Taber's Cyclopedic Medical Dictionary, ed. 18, FA Davis, Philadelphia, 1997, with permission. (Adapted from Bloodborne Pathogens and Acute Care Facilities (OSHA 3128), Occupational Safety and Health Administration, Washington, DC, 1992.)

show how employee exposure can be minimized or eliminated.

The Exposure Control Plan

A written exposure control plan is necessary for the safety and health of workers. At a minimum, the plan must include the following:

- Identify job classifications where there is exposure to blood or other potentially infectious materials.
- Explain the protective measures currently in effect in the acute care facility and/or a schedule and methods of compliance to be implemented, including hepatitis B vaccination and post-exposure follow-up procedures; how hazards are communicated to employees; personal protective equipment; housekeeping; and recordkeeping.
- Establish procedures for evaluating the circumstances of an exposure incident.

The schedule of how and when the provisions of the standard will be implemented may be a simple calendar with brief notations describing the compliance methods, an annotated copy of the standard, or a part of another document, such as the infection control plan.

The written exposure control plan must be available to workers and OSHA representatives and updated at least annually or whenever changes in procedures create new occupational exposures.

Who Has Occupational Exposure?

The exposure determination must be based on the definition of occupational exposure **without regard to personal protective clothing and equipment.** Exposure determination begins by reviewing job classifications of employees within the work environment and then making a list divided into two groups: job classifications in which **all** of the employees have occupational exposure, and those classifications in which **some** of the employees have occupational exposure.

Where **all** employees are occupationally exposed, it is not necessary to list specific work tasks. Some examples include phlebotomists, lab technicians, physicians, nurses, nurse's aides, surgical technicians, and emergency room personnel.

Where only **some** of the employees have exposure, specific tasks and procedures causing exposure must be listed. Examples include ward clerks or secretaries who occasionally handle blood or infectious specimens, and housekeeping staff who may be exposed to contaminated objects and/or environments some of the time.

When employees with occupational exposure have been identified, the next step is to communicate the hazards of the exposure to the employees.

Communicating Hazards to Employees

The initial training for current employees must be scheduled within 90 days of the effective date of the bloodborne pathogens standard, at no cost to the employee, and during working hours.[1]

Training also is required for new workers at the time of their initial assignment to tasks with occupational exposure or when job tasks change, causing occupational exposure, and annually thereafter.

Training sessions must be comprehensive in nature, including information on bloodborne pathogens as well as on OSHA regulations and the employer's exposure control plan. The person conducting the training must be knowledgeable in the subject matter as it relates to acute care facilities.

Specifically, the training program must do the following:
1. Explain the regulatory text and make a copy of the regulatory text accessible.
2. Explain the epidemiology and symptoms of bloodborne diseases.
3. Explain the modes of transmission of bloodborne pathogens.
4. Explain the employer's written exposure control plan.
5. Describe the methods to control transmission of HBV and HIV.
6. Explain how to recognize occupational exposure.
7. Inform workers about the availability of free hepatitis B vaccinations, vaccine efficacy, safety, benefits, and administration.
8. Explain the emergency procedures for and reporting of exposure incidents.
9. Inform workers of the post-exposure evaluation and follow-up available from health care professionals.
10. Describe how to select, use, remove, handle, decontaminate, and dispose of personal protective clothing and equipment.
11. Explain the use and limitations of safe work practices, engineering controls, and personal protective equipment.
12. Explain the use of labels, signs, and color coding required by the standard.

---

[1]Employees who received training in the year preceding the effective date of the standard need only receive training pertaining to any provisions not already included.

13. Provide a question-and-answer session on training.

In addition to communicating hazards to employees and providing training to identify and control hazards, other preventive measures also must be taken to ensure employee protection.

Preventive Measures

Preventive measures such as hepatitis B vaccination, universal precautions, engineering controls, safe work practices, personal protective equipment, and housekeeping measures help reduce the risks of occupational exposure.

Hepatitis B Vaccination

The hepatitis B vaccination series must be made available within 10 working days of initial assignment to every employee who has occupational exposure. The hepatitis B vaccination must be made available without cost to the employee, at a reasonable time and place for the employee, by a licensed health care professional,[2] and according to recommendations of the U.S. Public Health Service, including routine booster doses.[3]

The health care professional designated by the employer to implement this part of the standard must be provided with a copy of the bloodborne pathogens standard. The health care professional must provide the employer with a written opinion stating whether the hepatitis B vaccination is indicated for the employee and whether the employee has received such vaccination.

Employers are not required to offer hepatitis B vaccination (a) to employees who have previously completed the hepatitis B vaccination series, (b) when immunity is confirmed through antibody testing, or (c) if vaccine is contraindicated for medical reasons. Participation in a prescreening program is not a prerequisite for receiving hepatitis B vaccination. Employees who decline the vaccination may request and obtain it at a later date, if they continue to be exposed. Employees who decline to accept the hepatitis B vaccination must sign a declination form, indicating that they were offered the vaccination but refused it.

---

[2]Licensed health care professional is a person whose legally permitted scope of practice allows him or her to perform independently the activities required under paragraph (f) of the standard regarding hepatitis B vaccination and post-exposure and follow-up.

[3]Health care professionals can call the Centers for Disease Control disease information hotline (404) 332-4555, extension 234, for updated information on hepatitis B vaccination.

Universal Precautions

The single most important measure to control transmission of HBV and HIV is to treat all human blood and other potentially infectious materials AS IF THEY WERE infectious for HBV and HIV. Application of this approach is referred to as "universal precautions." *Blood and certain body fluids from all acute care patients should be considered as potentially infectious materials.*[4] These fluids cause *contamination*, defined in the standard as "the presence or the reasonably anticipated presence of blood or other potentially infectious materials on an item or surface."

Methods of Control

Engineering and Work Practice Controls

Engineering and work practice controls are the primary methods used to control the transmission of HBV and HIV in acute care facilities. Engineering controls isolate or remove the hazard from employees and are used in conjunction with work practices. Personal protective equipment also shall be used when occupational exposure to bloodborne pathogens remains even after instituting these controls. Engineering controls must be examined and maintained, or replaced, on a scheduled basis. Some engineering controls that apply to acute care facilities and are required by the standard include the following:

1. Use puncture-resistant, leak-proof containers, color-coded red or labeled, according to the standard (see table) to discard contaminated items like needles, broken glass, scalpels, or other items that could cause a cut or puncture wound.
2. Use puncture-resistant, leak-proof containers, color-coded red or labeled to store contaminated reusable sharps until they are properly reprocessed.
3. Store and process reusable contaminated sharps in a way that ensures safe handling. For example, use a mechanical device to retrieve used instruments from soaking pans in decontamination areas.
4. Use puncture-resistant, leak-proof containers to collect, handle, process, store, transport, or ship blood specimens and potentially infectious materials. Label these specimens if shipped outside the facility. Labeling is not required when specimens are handled by employees trained to use universal precautions with all specimens and when these specimens are kept within the facility.

---

[4]"Recommendations for Prevention of HIV Transmission in Health-Care Settings," *MMWR* (36) 2S: August 21, 1987.

Similarly, work practice controls reduce the likelihood of exposure by altering the manner in which the task is performed. All procedures shall minimize splashing, spraying, splattering, and generation of droplets. Work practice requirements include the following:

1. Wash hands when gloves are removed and as soon as possible after contact with blood or other potentially infectious materials.
2. Provide and make available a mechanism for immediate eye irrigation, in the event of an exposure incident.
3. Do not bend, recap, or remove contaminated needles unless required to do so by specific medical procedures or the employer can demonstrate that no alternative is feasible. In these instances, use mechanical means such as forceps, or a one-handed technique to recap or remove contaminated needles.
4. Do not shear or break contaminated needles.
5. Discard contaminated needles and sharp instruments in puncture-resistant, leak-proof, red or biohazard-labeled containers[5] that are accessible, maintained upright, and not allowed to be overfilled.
6. Do not eat, drink, smoke, apply cosmetics, or handle contact lenses in areas of potential occupational exposure. (Note: use of hand lotions is acceptable.)
7. Do not store food or drink in refrigerators or on shelves where blood or potentially infectious materials are present.
8. Use red, or affix biohazard labels to, containers to store, transport, or ship blood or other potentially infectious materials, such as lab specimens. (See figure below.)

---

[5]Biohazard labeling requires a fluorescent orange or orange-red label with the biological hazard symbol as well as the word **Biohazard** in contrasting color affixed to the bag or container.

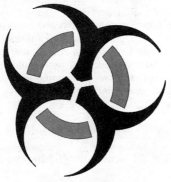

BIOHAZARD SYMBOL

9. Do not use mouth pipetting to suction blood or other potentially infectious materials; **it is prohibited.**

Personal Protective Equipment

In addition to instituting engineering and work practice controls, the standard requires that appropriate personal protective equipment be used to reduce worker risk of exposure. Personal protective equipment is specialized clothing or equipment used by employees to protect against direct exposure to blood or other potentially infectious materials. Protective equipment must not allow blood or other potentially infectious materials to pass through to workers' clothing, skin, or mucous membranes. Such equipment includes, but is not limited to, gloves, gowns, laboratory coats, face shields or masks, and eye protection.

The employer is responsible for providing, maintaining, laundering, disposing, replacing, and assuring the proper use of personal protective equipment. The employer is responsible for ensuring that workers have access to the protective equipment, at no cost, including proper sizes and types that take allergic conditions into consideration.

An employee may temporarily and briefly decline to wear personal protective equipment **under rare and extraordinary circumstances** and when, in the employee's professional judgment, it prevents the delivery of health care or public safety services or poses an increased or life-threatening hazard to employees. In general, **appropriate personal protective equipment is expected to be used whenever occupational exposure may occur.**

The employer also must ensure that employees observe the following precautions for safely handling and using personal protective equipment:

1. Remove all personal protective equipment immediately following contamination and upon leaving the work area, and place in an appropriately designated area or container for storing, washing, decontaminating, or discarding.
2. Wear appropriate gloves when contact with blood, mucous membranes, non-intact skin, or potentially infectious materials is anticipated; when performing vascular access procedures;[6] and when handling or touching contaminated items or surfaces.

---

[6]Phlebotomists in volunteer blood donation centers are exempt in certain circumstances. See section (d)(3)(ix)(D) of the standard for specific details.

3. Provide hypoallergenic gloves, liners, or powderless gloves or other alternatives to employees who need them.

4. Replace disposable, single-use gloves as soon as possible when contaminated, or if torn, punctured, or barrier function is compromised.

5. Do not reuse disposable (single-use) gloves.

6. Decontaminate reusable (utility) gloves after each use and discard if they show signs of cracking, peeling, tearing, puncturing, deteriorating, or failing to provide a protective barrier.

7. Use full face shields or face masks with eye protection, goggles, or eyeglasses with side shields when splashes of blood and other bodily fluids may occur and when contamination of the eyes, nose, or mouth can be anticipated (e.g., during invasive and surgical procedures).

8. Also wear surgical caps or hoods and/or shoe covers or boots when gross contamination may occur, such as during surgery and autopsy procedures.

Remember: The selection of appropriate personal protective equipment depends on the quantity and type of exposure expected.

Housekeeping Procedures

Equipment. The employer must ensure a clean and sanitary workplace. Contaminated work surfaces must be decontaminated with a disinfectant upon completion of procedures or when contaminated by splashes, spills, or contact with blood, other potentially infectious materials, and at the end of the work shift. Surfaces and equipment protected with plastic wrap, foil, or other nonabsorbent materials must be inspected frequently for contamination; and these protective coverings must be changed when found to be contaminated.

Waste cans and pails must be inspected and decontaminated on a regularly scheduled basis. Broken glass should be cleaned up with a brush or tongs; never pick up broken glass with hands, even when wearing gloves.

Waste. Waste removed from the facility is regulated by local and state laws. Special precautions are necessary when disposing of contaminated sharps and other contaminated waste, and include the following:

1. Dispose of contaminated sharps in closable, puncture-resistant, leak-proof, red or biohazard-labeled containers (see table).

2. Place other regulated waste[7] in closable, leak-proof, red or biohazard-labeled bags or containers. If outside contamination of the regulated waste container occurs, place it in a second container that is closable, leak-proof, and appropriately labeled.

---

[7]Liquid or semiliquid blood or other potentially infectious materials; items contaminated with these fluids and materials, which could release these substances in a liquid or semiliquid state, if compressed; items caked with dried blood or other potentially infectious materials that are capable of releasing these materials during handling; contaminated sharps; and pathological and microbiological wastes containing blood or other potentially infectious materials.

Labeling Requirements

Item	No Label Needed If Universal Precautions Are Used and Specific Use of Container Is Known to All Employees		Biohazard Label		Red Container
Regulated waste container (e.g., contaminated sharps containers)			X	or	X
Reusable contaminated sharps container (e.g., surgical instruments soaking in a tray)			X	or	X
Refrigerator/freezer holding blood or other potentially infectious material			X		
Containers used for storage, transport, or shipping of blood			X	or	X
Blood/blood products for clinical use	X				
Individual specimen containers of blood or other potentially infectious materials remaining in facility	X	or	X	or	X

Labeling Requirements

Item	No Label Needed If Universal Precautions Are Used and Specific Use of Container Is Known to All Employees	Biohazard Label	Red Container
Contaminated equipment needing service (e.g., dialysis equipment, suction apparatus)		X Plus a label specifying where the contamination exists	
Specimens and regulated waste shipped from the primary facility to another facility for service or disposal		X or	X
Contaminated laundry	* or	X or	X
Contaminated laundry sent to another facility that does not use universal precautions		X or	X

*Alternative labeling or color coding is sufficient if it permits all employees to recognize the containers as requiring compliance with universal precautions.

Laundry. Laundering contaminated articles, including employee lab coats and uniforms meant to function as personal protective equipment, is the responsibility of the employer. Contaminated laundry shall be handled as little as possible with minimum agitation. This can be accomplished through the use of a washer and dryer in a designated area on-site, or the contaminated items can be sent to a commercial laundry. The following requirements should be met with respect to contaminated laundry:

1. Bag contaminated laundry as soon as it is removed and store in a designated area or container.
2. Use red laundry bags or those marked with the biohazard symbol unless universal precautions are in effect in the fa-

cility and all employees recognize the bags as contaminated and have been trained in handling the bags.

3. Clearly mark laundry sent off-site for cleaning, by placing it in red bags or bags clearly marked with the orange biohazard symbol; and use leak-proof bags to prevent soak-through.

4. Wear gloves or other protective equipment when handling contaminated laundry.

What to Do if an Exposure Incident Occurs

An exposure incident is the specific eye, mouth or other mucous membrane, non-intact skin, parenteral contact with blood or other potentially infectious materials that results from the performance of an employee's duties. An example of an exposure incident would be a puncture from a contaminated sharp.

The employer is responsible for establishing the procedure for evaluating exposure incidents.

When evaluating an exposure incident, immediate assessment and confidentiality are critical issues. Employees should immediately report exposure incidents to enable timely medical evaluation and follow-up by a health care professional as well as a prompt request by the employer for testing of the source individual's blood for HIV and HBV. The "source individual" is any patient whose blood or body fluids are the source of an exposure incident to the employee.

At the time of the exposure incident, the exposed employee must be directed to a health care professional. The employer must provide the health care professional with a copy of the bloodborne pathogens standard; a description of the employee's job duties as they relate to the incident; a report of the specific exposure, including route of exposure; relevant employee medical records, including hepatitis B vaccination status; and results of the source individual's blood tests, if available. At that time, a baseline blood sample should be drawn from the employee, if he/she consents. If the employee elects to delay HIV testing of the sample, the health care professional must preserve the employee's blood sample for at least 90 days.[8]

Testing the source individual's blood does not need to be repeated if the source individual is known to be infectious for HIV or HBV; and testing cannot be done in most states without

---

[8]If, during this time, the employee elects to have the baseline sample tested, testing shall be performed as soon as feasible.

written consent.[9] The results of the source individual's blood tests are confidential. As soon as possible, however, the test results of the source individual's blood must be made available to the exposed employee through consultation with the health care professional.

Following post-exposure evaluation, the health care professional will provide a written opinion to the employer. This opinion is limited to a statement that the employee has been informed of the results of the evaluation and told of the need, if any, for any further evaluation or treatment. The employer must provide a copy of the written opinion to the employee within 15 days. This is the only information shared with the employer following an exposure incident; all other employee medical records are confidential.

All evaluations and follow-up must be available at no cost to the employee and at a reasonable time and place, performed by or under the supervision of a licensed physician or another licensed health care professional, such as a nurse practitioner, and according to recommendations of the U.S. Public Health Service guidelines current at the time of the evaluation and procedure. In addition, all laboratory tests must be conducted by an accredited laboratory and at no cost to the employee.

Recordkeeping

There are two types of records required by the bloodborne pathogens standard: medical and training.

A medical record must be established for each employee with occupational exposure. **This record is confidential and separate from other personnel records.** This record may be kept on-site or may be retained by the health care professional who provides services to employees. The medical record contains the employee's name, social security number, hepatitis B vaccination status, including the dates of vaccination and the written opinion of the health care professional regarding the hepatitis B vaccination. If an occupational exposure occurs, reports are added to the medical record to document the incident and the results of testing following the incident. The post-evaluation written opinion of the health care professional is also part of the medical record. The medical record also must document what information has been provided to the health care provider. Medical records must be maintained 30 years past the last date of employment of the employee.

---

[9]If consent is not obtained, the employer must show that legally required consent could not be obtained. Where consent is not required by law, the source individual's blood, if available, should be tested and the results documented.

Emphasis is on confidentiality of medical records. No medical record or part of a medical record should be disclosed without direct, written consent of the employee or as required by law.

Training records document each training session and are to be kept for 3 years. Training records must include the date, content outline, trainer's name and qualifications, and names and job titles of all persons attending the training sessions.

If the employer ceases to do business, medical and training records are transferred to the successor employer. If there is no successor employer, the employer must notify the Director of the National Institute for Occupational Safety and Health, U.S. Department of Health and Human Services, for specific directions regarding disposition of the records at least 3 months prior to disposal.

Upon request, both medical and training records must be made available to the Assistant Secretary of Labor of Occupational Safety and Health. Training records must be available to employees upon request. Medical records can be obtained by the employee or anyone having the employee's written consent.

Additional recordkeeping is required for employers with 11 or more employees (see OSHA's "Recordkeeping Guidelines for Occupational Injuries and Illnesses" for more information).

Other Sources of OSHA Assistance

Consultation Programs

Consultation assistance is available to employers who want help in establishing and maintaining a safe and healthful workplace. Largely funded by OSHA, the service is provided at no cost to the employer. Primarily developed for smaller employers with more hazardous operations, the consultation service is delivered by state government agencies or universities employing professional safety consultants and health consultants. Comprehensive assistance includes an appraisal of all mechanical, physical work practice, and environmental hazards of the workplace and all aspects of the employer's present job safety and health program. No penalties are proposed or citations issued for hazards identified by the consultant.

Voluntary Protection Programs

Voluntary protection programs (VPPs) and on-site consultation services, when coupled with an effective enforcement program, expand worker protection to help meet the goals of the OSH Act. The three VPPs—Star, Merit, and Demonstration—

are designed to recognize outstanding achievement by companies that have successfully incorporated comprehensive safety and health programs into their total management system. They motivate others to achieve excellent safety and health results in the same outstanding way, and they establish a cooperative relationship between employers, employees, and OSHA.

Training and Education

OSHA's area offices offer a variety of informational services, such as publications, audiovisual aids, technical advice, and speakers for special engagements. Each regional office has a bloodborne pathogens coordinator to assist employers.

OSHA's Training Institute in Des Plaines, IL, provides basic and advanced courses in safety and health for federal and state compliance officers, state consultants, federal agency personnel, and private sector employers, employees, and their representatives.

OSHA also provides funds to nonprofit organizations, through grants, to conduct workplace training and education in subjects where OSHA believes there is a lack of workplace training. Current grant subjects include agricultural safety and health, hazard communication programs, and HIV and HBV. Grants are awarded annually, with a 1-year renewal possible. Grant recipients are expected to contribute 20 percent of the total grant cost.

For more information on grants, and training and education, contact the OSHA Training Institute, Office of Training and Education, 1555 Time Drive, Des Plaines, IL 60018, (708) 297-4810.

For more information on AIDS, contact the Centers for Disease Control National AIDS Clearinghouse, (800) 458-5231.

Appendix 4

Reference Values

Reference Values for Laboratory Tests on Blood

Test	Reference Values	SI Units
Acetylcholine receptor antibody	≤0.03 nmol/L or negative	
Acid phosphatase	0.1–5.0 U/dL (King-Armstrong)	0.2–8.8 IU/L
	0.1–0.8 U/dL (Bessey-Lowry)	1.7–13.4 IU/L
	0.5–2.0 U/dL (Bodansky)	2.7–10.7 IU/L
Activated clotting time	94–120 s in the nonanticoagulated client	
Activated partial thromboplastin time (aPTT) and partial thromboplastin time (PTT)	Newborn: <90 s	
	Infant or child: 24–40 s	
	Adult: 60–70 s; 30–40 s (aPTT)	
	Critical value: >70 s	
Adrenocorticotropic hormone	BioScience Labs: <80 pg/mL at 8 A.M.	<80 ng/L
	Mayo Clinic: <120 pg/mL at 6–8 A.M.	<120 mg/L in A.M.
	<50 pg/mL at 8–11 P.M.	<50 ng/L in P.M.
Alanine aminotransferase	Infant: 54 U/L or twice adult level	
	Child: 3–37 U/L	
	Adult:	
	Female: 5–35 U/mL	4–36 U/L at 37°C
	Male: 7–46 U/mL	
Aldolase	Newborn: 4× adult level @ 37°C	4× adult level
	Child: 2× adult level @ 37°C	2× adult level
	Adult: 3.0–8.0 U/dL @ 37°C	22–59 mU/L @ 37°C
Aldosterone	Adult, supine: 3–10 ng/dL	0.14–1.9 nmol/L
	Adult standing:	
	Male: 6–22 ng/dL	0.17–0.61 nmol/L
	Female: (3× higher if pregnant):	0.14–0.83 nmol/L
		5–30 ng/dL
Alkaline phosphatase	Male: 98–251 U/L	
	Female < age 45 yr: 81–196 U/L	
	Female > age 45 yr: 84–109 U/L	
	Bessey-Lowry Method:	
	Adult: 0.8–2.3 U/dL	13.3–38.3 IU/L

Test	Reference Values	SI Units
	Bodansky Method:	
	Adult: 2–4 U/dL	10.7–21.5 IU/L
	King-Armstrong Method:	
	Adult: 4–13 U/dL	28.4–92.3 IU/L
	Adult isoenzyme levels:	
	Bone: 24–146 U/L	
	Intestine: 0–22 U/L	
	Liver: 24–158 U/L	
Allergen-specific IgE and allergen-specific IgE antibody test (RAST)	IgE: <2% of total immunoglobulins	
	Newborn: <12 U/mL	
	Child: <10–116 U/mL depending on age	
	Adult: <41 U/mL	
	IgE antibody:	
	0 — Negative	
	0–749 count — No activity according to RAST classification	
Alpha-fetoprotein	Neonate: 600,000 ng/mL	600,000 Ug/L
	Infant and child: <30 ng/mL	<30 Ug/L
	Adult: <10 ng/mL	<10 Ug/L
	Pregnant female:	
	2–4 mo: <75–130 ng/mL	<75–130 Ug/L
	4–6 mo: <210–400 ng/mL	<210–400 Ug/L
	6–9 mo: <400–450 ng/mL	<400–540 Ug/L
Alpha$_1$-antitrypsin	Newborn: 145–270 mg/dL	1.45–2.70 g/L
	Adult: 126–226 mg/dL	1.26–2.26 g/L
Ammonia	Infant: 90–150 μg/dL	64–107 μmol/L
	Child: 40–80 μg/dL	23–47 μmol/L
	Adult: 15–45 μg/dL	11–32 μmol/L
Amylase	Adult: 50–180 Somogyi U/dL	92–330 U/L
	Older Adult: 20–160 Somogyi U/dL	
Androstenedione	Female:	
	Premenopausal: 0.6–3 ng/mL	2–10 nmol/L
	Postmenopausal: 0.3–8 ng/mL	1–10 nmol/L
	Male: 0.9–1.7 ng/mL	3–6 nmol/L
Angiotensin-converting enzyme	Child <1 yr: 10.9–42.1 U/L	
	1–2 yr: 9.4–36 U/L	
	3–4 yr: 7.9–29.8 U/L	
	5–9 yr: 9.6–35.4 U/L	
	10–12 yr: 10–37 U/L	
	13–16 yr: 9–33.4 U/L	
	17–19 yr: 7.2–26.6 U/L	
	Adult > age 20: 6.1–21.1 U/L	
Anti-DNA antibodies	Negative: <70 U	
	Borderline: 70–200 U	
	Definite elevation: >25 U	

(*continued*)

Test	Reference Values	SI Units
Anti-insulin antibody	Negative	
Anti-Ro/Sjögren's syndrome antigen	Negative	
Antidiuretic hormone	1.5 pg/mL	1.5 ng/L
Antinuclear antibody	Negative at <1:20 dilution	
Antistreptolysin-O titer	Preschool child: <85 Todd U/mL School-age child: <170 Todd U/mL Adult: <85 Todd U/mL	
Antithrombin III	Plasma: >50% of control value Serum: 15–35% lower than plasma values Immunologic method: 20–30 mg/dL Functional method: 80–120 mg/dL	200–300 mg/L 800–120 μ/L
Apolipoprotein A-I	Female: 94–172 mg/dL Male: 90–155 mg/dL Ratio of A-1 to B: Female: 0.76:3.23 Male: 0.85:2.24	
Apolipoprotein B	Female: 55–100 mg/dL Male: 45–110 mg/dL Ratio of A-1 to B: Female: 0.76:3.23 Male: 0.85:2.24	
Aspartate aminotransferase	Newborn: 16–72 U/L Child: 6 mo: 20–43 U/L 1 yr: 16–35 U/L 5 yr: 19–28 U/L Adult: Male: 8–26 U/L Female: 8–20 U/L	16–72 U/L 20–43 U/L 16–35 U/L 19–28 U/L 8–26 U/L 8–20 U/L
Atrial natriuretic factor	20–77 pg/mL	20–77 ng/L
Australia antigens	Negative	
Beta$_2$-microglobulin	<2 μg/mL	<170 nmol/L
Bilirubin	*Total bilirubin:* Newborn: 2–6 mg/dL 48 hr: 6–7 mg/dL 5 d: 4–12 mg/dL 1 mo–adult: 0.3–1.2 mg/dL *Indirect bilirubin (unconjugated, prehepatic):* 1 mo–adult: 0.3–1.1 mg/dL	

Test	Reference Values	SI Units
	Direct bilirubin (conjugated, posthepatic): 1 mo–adult: 0.1–0.4 mg/dL	
Bleeding time	Duke method: 1–3 min Ivy method: 3–6 min Ivy critical value: >15 min Template method: 3–6 min	
Blood gases, arterial	pH: Newborn: 7.32–7.49 Adult: 7.35–7.45 PaO$_2$: Newborn: 60–70 mm Hg Adult: 75–100 mm Hg PaCO$_2$: 35–45 mm Hg HCO$_3$: Newborn: 20–26 mEq/L Adult: 22–26 mEq/L O$_2$ saturation: 96–100% Base excess: +1 to −2 Anion gap: 10–18 mEq/L	 7.32–7.49 7.35–7.45 8–9.4 kPa 10–13.3 kPa 4.7–6 kPa 20–26 mmol/L 22–26 mmol/L 0.96–1.00 +1 to −2 10–18 mmol/L
Blood urea nitrogen	Newborn: 4–18 mg/dL Child: 5–18 mg/dL Adult: 5–20 mg/dL Older Adult: 8–21 mg/dL Critical Value: >100 mg/dL	1.4–6.4 mmol/L 1.8–6.4 mmol/L 1.8–7.1 mmol/L 2.9–7.5 mmol/L >35.7 mmol/L
C-peptide	0.9–4.2 ng/mL	0.9–4.2 mg/L
C-reactive protein	<0.8 mg/dL	
Calcitonin	Basal: Male: ≤19 pg/mL Female: ≤14 pg/mL Pentagastrin provocative test: Male: ≤110 pg/mL Female: ≤30 pg/mL Calcium provocative test: Male: ≤190 pg/mL Female: ≤130 pg/mL	 ≤19 ng/L ≤14 ng/L ≤110 ng/L ≤30 ng/L ≤190 ng/L ≤130 ng/L
Cancer antigen 125	<35 U/mL	<35 kU/L
Carcinoembryonic antigen	Nonsmoker: <2.5 ng/mL Smoker: <5.0 ng/mL	<2.5 µg/L <5.0 µg/L
Catecholamines	*Epinephrine and norepinephrine:* 150–650 pg/mL *Epinephrine:* Supine: 0–110 pg/mL Standing: 0–140 pg/mL *Norepinephrine:* Supine: 70–750 pg/mL Standing: 200–1700 pg/mL *Dopamine:* <30 pg/mL	86–3843 pmol/L 0–599 pmol/L 0–762 pmol/L 381–4083 pmol/L 1088–9256 pmol/L 0–163 pmol/L

(continued)

Test	Reference Values	SI Units
Ceruloplasmin	Newborn: 1–30 mg/dL	0.06–1.99 μmol/L
	Infant (age 6–12 mo): 15–50 mg/dL	0.99–3.31 μmol/L
	Child (age 1–12 yr): 30–65 mg/dL	1.99–4.30 μmol/L
	Adult: 14–40 mg/dL	0.93–2.65 μmol/L
Chlamydia antibodies	Titer <1:10	
Cholesterol	Newborn: 45–100 mg/dL	1.16–2.59 mmol/L
	Child: 120–220 mg/dL	3.10–5.68 mmol/L
	Under 25 yr: 125–200 mg/dL	3.27–5.20 mmol/L
	25–40 yr: 140–225 mg/dL	3.69–5.85 mmol/L
	40–50 yr: 160–245 mg/dL	4.37–6.35 mmol/L
	Over 65 yr: 170–265 mg/dL	4.71–6.85 mmol/L

Test	HDL	LDL
Cholesterol fractionation	<age 25 yr: 32–57 mg/dL	73–138 mg/dL
	25 to 40 yr: 32–60 mg/dL	90–180 mg/dL
	40 to 50 yr: 33–60 mg/dL	100–185 mg/dL
	50 to 65 yr: 34–70 mg/dL	105–190 mg/dL
	>65 yr: 35–75 mg/dL	105–200 mg/dL

Test	Reference Values	SI Units
Clotting time (Lee-White)	Plain tube: 5–15 min	
Coagulation factor assays	Factor I (fibrinogen): 200–400 mg/dL	2.0–4.0 g/L
	Factor II (prothrombin): 50–150%	
	Factor III (thromboplastin): 30–45 s	30–45 s
	Factor IV (calcium): 9–11 mg/dL	0.09–0.11 g/L
	Factor V (accelerator globulin): 50–150%	
	Factor VII (proconvertin): 50–150%	
	Factor VIII (antihemophilic factor): 50–150%	
	Factor IX (Christmas factor): 50–150%	
	Factor X (Stuart-Prower factor): 50–150%	
	Factor XI (thromboplastin antecedent): 50–150%	
	Factor XII (Hageman factor): 50–150%	
	Factor XIII (fibrin stabilizing factor): Dissolution of a formed clot within 24 h	
Cold agglutinin titer	<1:16; may be higher in the elderly	
Coombs' antiglobulin, direct	Negative	
Coombs' antiglobulin, indirect	Negative	

Test	Reference Values	SI Units
Cortisol	8 A.M. — 4 P.M. Child: 15–25 µg/dL — 5–10 µg/dL Adult: 9–24 µg/dL — 3–12 µg/dL	
Cr-51 platelet survival time	Normal life span of platelets = 9–10 days Platelet turnover rate = 35,000/mm³ per day Absence of concentration or uptake in a body area	
Cr-51 red cell survival time	Normal life span of RBCs: 120 d with normal loss of 0.8%/d Normal half-time of RBCs: 60 d Plasma radioactivity half-life: 2 h Tagged Cr-51 red cell half-life: 25–35 d Gamma scan: Only slight spleen, liver, and bone marrow radioactivity Spleen-to-liver ratio: 1 : 1 Spleen-to-pericardium ratio: 2 : 1 or less	
Creatine kinase/creatine phosphokinase	Female: 25–140 U/L Male: 40–175 U/L	0.42–2.3 µkat/L 0.67–1.9 µkat/L
Creatine phosphokinase isoenzymes	CPK-BB (CPK₁): Undetectable CPK-MB (CPK₂): Undetectable to 7 U/L CPK-MM (CPK₃): 5–7 U/L	
Creatinine	Newborn: 0.8–1.4 mg/dL Infant: 0.7–1.7 mg/dL Young child <6 yr: 0.3–0.6 mg/dL Older child >6 yr: 0.4–1.2 mg/dL Adult male: 0.6–1.3 mg/dL Adult female: 0.5–1.0 mg/dL Older adult: Reduced values related to reduced muscle mass associated with aging	71–124 µmol/L 62–150 µmol/L 27–54 µmol/L 36–106 µmol/L 53–115 µmol/L 44–88 µmol/L
Cryoglobulin	Negative	
Cyclic adenosine monophosphate	5.6–10.9 ng/mL	17–33 nmol/L
D-dimer	Negative or <250 ng/mL	250 µg/L
d-Xylose tolerance	Child <10 kg after 1 h: ≥15 mg/dL 10 kg to age 9 yr: ≥20 mg/dL Adult after 2 h: 30–52 mg/dL	1.0 mmol/L 1.3 mmol/L 2.0–3.47 mmol/L

(continued)

Test	Reference Values	SI Units
Enzyme-linked immunosorbent assay (ELISA)	Negative for HIV antibody	
Epstein-Barr virus antibodies	Negative or titer <1:56 heterophile antibodies	
Erythrocyte sedimentation rate	*Westergren method:* Newborn: 0–2 mm/h Child: 0–10 mm/h Female (< age 50 yr): 0–20 mm/h (age 50–85 yr): <30 mm/h (> age 85 yr): <42 mm/h Male (< age 50 yr): 0–15 mm/h (age 50–85 yr): <20 mm/h (> age 85 yr): <30 mm/h *Wintrobe method:* Female: 0.36–0.45 Male: 0.41–0.51 *Zeta sedimentation ratio:* 41–54%	
Estradiol	Child: <15 pg/mL Adult male: 10–50 pg/mL Adult female: Follicular phase: 20–150 pg/mL Peak phase: 150–750 pg/mL Luteal phase: 30–450 pg/mL Postmenopausal: <20 pg/mL	15 pmol/L 37–184 pmol/L 73–551 pmol/L 551–2753 pmol/L 110–1652 pmol/L <73 pmol/L
Estriol	Weeks of gestation: 28–30: 38–140 ng/mL 31–35: 30–260 ng/mL 36–38: 48–570 ng/mL 39–40: 95–460 ng/mL	 132–486 nmol/L 121–902 nmol/L 167–1978 nmol/L 330–1596 nmol/L
Estradiol receptor and progesterone receptor assay	Estrogen receptor assay: ≤3 femtomoles (fmol)/mg of protein or negative Progesterone receptor assay: ≤10 fmol/mg of protein or negative	
Estrogens, total	Child: <25 pg/mL Adult male: 20–80 pg/mL Adult female: Follicular phase: 60–200 pg/mL Luteal phase: 160–400 pg/mL Late phase: 150–350 pg/mL Postmenopausal: <130 pg/mL	>25 ng/L 20–80 ng/L 60–200 ng/L 160–400 ng/L 150–350 ng/L >130 ng/L
Euglobulin clot lysis time	Lysis in 2–4 h Critical time: Complete lysis in 1 h	
Extractable nuclear antigen (ENA) antibodies	Negative	

Test	Reference Values	SI Units
Febrile agglutinins	*Weil-Felix reaction* (*Proteus* antigen test): <1:80 *Widal's test* (O and H antigen tests): <1:160 *Brucella agglutination test* (slide agglutination test): <1:80 *Tularemia agglutination test* (tube dilution test): <1:40	
Ferritin	Infant: 50–200 ng/mL Newborn: 25–200 ng/mL Child: 7–140 ng/dL Adult: Male: 20–250 ng/dL Female: 10–120 ng/dL Iron overload: >220 ng/dL (average 30 μg/dL)	50–200 μg/L 25–200 μg/L 7–140 μg/L 20–250 μg/L 10–120 μg/L >220 μg/L
Fibrin degradation products	2–10 μg/mL Critical value: >40 μg/mL	
Fibrinogen	Male: 180–340 mg/dL Female: 190–420 mg/dL Newborn (normal, healthy): >150 mg/dL Critical value: <100 mg/dL	1.8–3.4 g/L 1.9–4.2 g/L >1.5 g/L
Fluorescent rabies antibody	Negative or IFA <1:16	
Fluorescent treponemal antibody-adsorption (FTA-ABS)	Negative	
Folic acid	Serum: 3.5–25 mg/L Red blood cells: Age 0–11 mo: 74–995 ng/mL Age 1–11 yr: 96–362 ng/mL Age 12 yr and older: 180–600 ng/mL	
Follicle-stimulating hormone	Child: 5–10 mIU/mL Male: 10–15 mIU/mL Female (menstruating): Early in cycle: 5–25 mIU/mL Midcycle: 20–30 mIU/mL Luteal phase: 5–25 mIU/mL Female (menopausal): 40–250 mIU/mL	5–10 IU/L 10–15 IU/L 5–25 IU/L 20–30 IU/L 5–25 IU/L 40–250 IU/L
Free fatty acids	8–20 mg/dL	80–200 mg/L

(continued)

Test	Reference Values	SI Units
Gamma-glutamyl transpeptidase	Newborn: 56–233 IU/L	56–233 U/L
	Child (1–15 yr): 0–23 IU/L	0–23 U/L
	Male (18–50 yr): 10–39 IU/L	10–39 U/L
	Male (over 50 yr): 10–48 IU/L	10–48 U/L
	Female: 6–29 IU/L	6–29 U/L
Gastrin	Fasting:	
	Child: <10–125 pg/mL	<10–125 ng/L
	Adult:	
	Age 16–60 yr: 25–90 pg/mL	25–90 ng/L
	Age >60 yr: <100 pg/mL	<100 ng/L
	Postprandial (1 h): 40 pg/mL	40 ng/L
Globulin	Total: 2.3–3.5 g/dL (32–48% total proteins)	23–35 g/L
	Alpha$_1$: 0.1–0.4 g/dL (1–5% total proteins)	1–4 g/L
	Alpha$_2$: 0.4–1.0 g/dL (4.6–14% total proteins)	4–10 g/L
	Beta: 0.5–1.2 g/dL (7.3–15% total proteins)	5–12 g/L
	Gamma: 0.6–1.6 g/dL (8–21% total proteins)	6–16 g/L
Glucagon	50–200 pg/mL	30–210 ng/L
Glucose tolerance	*Oral:*	
	Fasting: 70–150 mg/dL	3.9–5.8 mmol/L
	1/2 h: 150–160 mg/dL	8.3–8.8 mmol/L
	1 h: 160 mg/dL	8.8 mmol/L
	2 h: 115 mg/dL	6.6 mmol/L
	3 h: 70–150 mg/dL	3.9–5.8 mmol/L
	Intravenous:	
	Fasting: 70–105 mg/dL	3.9–5.8 mmol/L
	5 min: 300–400 mg/dL	16.5–22.0 mmol/L
	1/2 h: 180–200 mg/dL	9.9–11.0 mmol/L
	1 h: 170 mg/dL	9.4 mmol/L
	2 h: 140 mg/dL	7.7 mmol/L
	3 h: 70–105 mg/dL	3.9–5.8 mmol/L
Glucose	*Fasting blood glucose:*	
	Whole blood:	
	Newborn: 34–68 mg/dL	1.9–3.8 mmol/L
	Child: 51–85 mg/dL	2.8–4.7 mmol/L
	Adult: 60–100 mg/dL	3.3–5.6 mmol/L
	Serum:	
	Newborn: 40–80 mg/dL	2.2–4.4 mmol/L
	Child: 60–100 mg/dL	3.3–5.6 mmol/L
	Adult: 70–100 mg/dL	3.9–5.6 mmol/L
	Critical values:	
	Newborn: <30 or >300 mg/dL	<1.6 or >16.5 mmol/L
	Adult: <40 or >700 mg/dL	<2.2 or >38.6 mmol/L

Test	Reference Values	SI Units
	Random blood glucose (varies with time of last meal):	
	Serum:	
	Newborn: 40–80 mg/dL	2.2–4.4 mmol/L
	Child: 60–100 mg/dL	3.3–5.5 mmol/L
	Adult: 70–105 mg/dL	3.9–5.8 mmol/L
	Critical values:	
	Newborn: <30 or >300 mg/dL	<1.6 or >16.5 mmol/L
	Adult: <40 or >700 mg/dL	<2.2 or >38.6 mmol/L
Glucose, 2-h postprandial	*Blood:*	
	Child: 65–120 mg/dL	3.6–6.6 mmol/L
	Adult: 65–120 mg/dL	3.6–6.6 mmol/L
	Older adult: 65–140 mg/dL	3.6–7.7 mmol/L
	Serum:	
	Child: 65–150 mg/dL	3.6–8.3 mmol/L
	Adult: 65–140 mg/dL	3.6–7.7 mmol/L
	Older adult: 65–160 mg/dL	3.6–8.8 mmol/L
Growth hormone	Newborn: 15–40 ng/mL	660–1760 pmol/L
	Child: 0–20 ng/mL	0–880 pmol/L
	Adult: 0–10 ng/mL	0–440 pmol/L
Growth hormone stimulation test	Arginine:	
	Male: >10 ng/mL	>440 pmol/L
	Female: >15 ng/mL	>660 pmol/L
	Levodopa or insulin (above baseline level): >7 ng/mL	>340 pmol/L
Growth hormone suppression test	<3 ng/dL	<132 pmol/L
Guthrie test	Negative: <2 mg/dL	
Ham test	Negative	
Haptoglobin	Newborn: 0–30 mg/dL	0–0.3 g/L
	Child: 0–10 mg/dL	0–0.1 g/L
	Adult: 60–270 mg/dL	0.6–2.7 g/L
Heinz body, stain	Negative	
Hemagglutination treponemal test for syphilis (HATTS)	Titer <1:160	
Hematocrit	Newborn: 44–64%	
	Age 1 mo: 35–49%	
	Age 6 mo: 30–40%	
	Child: Age 1–10 yr: 35–41%	
	Adult:	
	Male: 40–54%	
	Female: 38–47%	

(continued)

Test	Reference Values	SI Units
Hemoglobin	Newborn: 14–27 g/dL	9.6–15.5 mmol/L
	<1 yr: 10–15 g/dL	6.1–9.0 mmol/L
	Child 1–10 yr: 11–16 g/dL	5.8–9.6 mmol/L
	Adult Male: 14–18 g/dL	8.7–11.2 mmol/L
	Adult Female: 12–16 g/dL	7.4–9.9 mmol/L
	Pregnancy: 10–15 g/dL	6.3–9.3 mmol/L
	Critical Values: <5 g/dL	<3.1 mmol/L
	>20 g/dL	>11.2 mmol/L
Hemoglobin electrophoresis	*Hemoglobin A_1:*	
	Adult: 95–97%	>0.95
	Infant: 10–30%	0.10–0.30
	Hemoglobin A_2:	
	Adult: 3–4%	0.03–0.04
	Hemoglobin F:	
	Adult: <1%	<0.10
	Neonate: 70–80%	0.70–0.80
	1 mo: 70%	0.70
	2 mo: 50%	0.50
	3 mo: 25%	0.25
	6–12 mo: 3%	0.03
	Hemoglobin C: None	
	Hemoglobin D: None	
	Hemoglobin E: None	
	Hemoglobin H: None	
	Hemoglobin S: None	
	Methemoglobin: 2% or 0.06–0.24 g/dL	
	Sulfhemoglobin: Minute amounts	
	Carboxyhemoglobin: 0–2.3% (4–5% in smokers)	
Hemoglobin, glycosylated	Total GHB: 5.5–8.8% of total Hb	
	Controlled diabetes: 7.5–11.4%	
	Uncontrolled diabetes: >15%	
	Hgb A_{1a}: 1.8%	
	Hgb A_{1b}: 0.8%	
	Hgb A_{1c}: 3.5–6.0%	
Hemoglobin, unstable	Heat labile test: Negative	
	Isopropanol precipitation test: Stable	
Hemosiderin	Negative	
Hepatitis B antibody and antigen	Negative	
Hepatitis profile, prenatal	Negative for HBsAg, HBeAg, anti-HBe, HBV-DNA, anti-HBc IgM	
Herpesvirus antigen	Negative	
Hexosaminidase A	56–80% of the total hexosaminidase	10.4–23.8 U/L

Test	Reference Values	SI Units
High-density lipoprotein (HDL) cholesterol	<25 yr: 32–57 mg/dL 25–40 yr: 32–60 mg/dL 40–50 yr: 33–60 mg/dL 50–65 yr: 34–70 mg/dL Over 65 yr: 35–75 mg/dL	0.32–0.57 g/L 0.32–0.60 g/L 0.33–0.66 g/L 0.34–0.70 g/L 0.35–0.75 g/L
Human chorionic gonadotropin	Nonpregnant: <3 mIU/mL Pregnant: 8–10 d: 5–40 mIU/mL 1 mo: 100 mIU/mL 2 mo: 100,000 mIU/mL 4 mo term: 50,000 mIU/mL	
Human placental lactogen	Male: <0.5 µg/mL Female: Nonpregnant: <0.5 µg/mL Pregnant: 5–27 w: <4.6 µg/mL 28–31 w: 2.4–6.1 µg/mL 32–35 w: 3.7–7.7 µg/mL 36 w–term: 5.0–8.6 µg/mL Diabetic at term: 10–12 µg/mL	
Hydroxybutryic dehydrogenase	140–350 U/mL	140–350 kU/L
Immune complex assay	Negative	
Influenza A and B titer	<fourfold increase in paired serum <1.8 titer demonstrates previous exposure	
Insulin antibody	<4% serum binding of beef or pork insulin	
Insulin	Fasting: Infant/child: <13 µ/mL Adult: 17 µU/mL After 75 g glucose: 1/2 h: 20–112 µU/mL 1 h: 29–88 µU/mL 2 h: 22–79 µU/mL 3 h: 4–62 µU/mL Insulin-to-glucose ratio: <0.3:1 Critical value: >30 µU/mL	<90 pmol/L <118 pmol/L 139–778 pmol/L 201–611 pmol/L 153–549 pmol/L 28–431 pmol/L
Intrinsic factor antibody	Negative	
Iron	Newborn: 100–250 µg/dL Infant: 40–100 µg/dL Child: 50–120 µg/dL Adult: Male: 65–175 µg/dL Female: 50–170 µg/dL Older Adult: 40–80 µg/dL	17.9–44.8 µmol/L 7.2–17.9 µmol/L 9.0–21.5 µmol/L 11.6–31.3 µmol/L 9.0–30.4 µmol/L 7.2–14.3 µmol/L *(continued)*

Test	Reference Values	SI Units
Iron-binding capacity, total	Children: 100–350 µg/dL Adult: 300–360 µg/dL Older Adult: 200–310 ug/dL	
Isocitrate dehydrogenase	Newborn: 4.8–28 U/L Adult: 1.2–7 U/L	0.08–0.47 IU/L 0.02–0.12 IU/L
Lactic acid	Arterial: 0.5–1.6 mEq/L Venous: 0.5–2.2 mEq/L	0.5–1.6 mmol/L 0.5–2.2 mmol/L
Lactic dehydrogenase and isoenzymes	Total LDH: Newborn: 160–500 U/L Child: 60–170 U/L Adult: 80–120 U @ 300°C (Wacker) 50–450 u/L (Wroblewski) LDH isoenzymes: LDH_1: 17–27% LDH_2: 27–37% LDH_3: 18–25% LDH_4: 3–8% LDH_5: 0–5% Ratios: $LDH_2 > LDH_1$ LDH_1: $LDH_2 < 1$ $LDH_4 > LDH_5$ LDH_5: $LDH_4 \leq 1$:3	 160–500 U/L 60–170 U/L 38–62 U/L at 300°C 72–217 IU/L 0.17–0.27 0.27–0.37 0.18–0.25 0.03–0.08 0.0–0.05
Lead	Child: <10 µg/dL Adult: <20 µg/dL Screening: 0.8–2.5 ng/mL	<0.1 µg/mL <0.2 µg/mL
Legionnaires' disease antibodies	Negative or titer <1:256 Less than a fourfold change in titer between acute and convalescent samples	
Leucine aminopeptidase	Male: 80–200 U/mL (Goldberg-Rutenberg) Female: 75–185 U/mL (Goldberg-Rutenberg)	19.2–48.0 U/L 18.0–44.4 U/L
Leukoagglutinin	Negative	
Leukocyte alkaline phosphatase stain	Score: 40–130, depending on the laboratory's standard	
Lipase	Infant: 9–105 IU/L @ 37°C Child: 20–136 IU/L @ 37°C Adult: 0–1.5 U/mL (Cherry-Crandall) 20–180 IU/L or 14–280 mU/mL	 0–417 U/L 14–280 U/L

Test	Reference Values	SI Units
Lipoprotein electrophoresis	Total lipoproteins: 400–800 mg/dL Lipoprotein fractions: Chylomicrons: 0% VLDL or prebeta: 3–32% LDL or beta: 38–40% HDL or alpha: 20–48%	
Low-density lipoprotein (LDL) cholesterol	<25 yr: 73–138 mg/dL 25–40 yr: 90–180 mg/dL 40–50 yr: 100–185 mg/dL 50–65 yr: 105–190 mg/dL >65 yr: 105–200 mg/dL	0.73–1.38 g/L 0.90–1.80 g/L 1.00–1.85 g/L 1.05–1.90 g/L 1.05–2.0 g/L
Luteinizing hormone	Child: Male: 4–12 mIU/mL Female: 2–14 mIU/mL Male: 6–30 mIU/mL Female (menstruating): Early in cycle: 5–25 mIU/mL Midcycle: 75–150 mIU/mL Luteal phase: 5–40 mIU/mL Women (menopausal): 30–200 mIU/mL	 4–12 IU/L 2–14 IU/L 6–30 IU/L 5–25 IU/L 75–150 IU/L 5–40 IU/L 30–200 IU/L
Methemoglobin	2% of total hemoglobin or 0.06–0.24 g/dL	9.3–37.2 mol/L
Microhemagglutination Treponema pallidium (MHA-TP)	Negative with titer <1:160	
Monospot	Negative, or a titer <1:56	
Myoglobin	30–90 ng/mL	
5'-Nucleotidase	4–11.5 U/L 0.3–3.2 Bodansky U	
Ornithine carbamoyl-transferase	0–500 Sigma units/mL 8–20 mIU/mL 8–20 U/L	
Parathyroid hormone	Active N-terminal: 230–630 pg/mL Inactive C-terminal: 400–1760 pg/mL Parathormone: 20–70 μEq/mL	200–600 ng/L 400–1760 ng/L 20–70 mEq/L
Pepsinogen	Adult: 124–142 ng/mL Child: Premature infant: 20–24 ng/mL Cord blood: 24–28 ng/mL <12 mo: 72–82 ng/mL 12 mo–<3 yr: 90–106 ng/mL 3–6 yr: 80–104 ng/mL 7–10 yr: 77–103 ng/mL 11–14 yr: 96–118 ng/mL	124–142 μg/L 20–24 μg/L 24–28 μg/L 72–82 μg/L 90–106 μg/L 80–104 μg/L 77–103 μg/L 96–118 μg/L

(continued)

Test	Reference Values	SI Units
Phospholipids	Newborn: 75–170 mg/dL Infant: 100–275 mg/dL Child: 180–295 mg/dL Adult: 150–380 mg/dL	0.75–1.70 g/L 1.0–2.75 g/L 1.80–2.95 g/L 1.50–3.80 g/L
Plasminogen	20 mg/dL	2.7–4.5 μU/mL
Platelet aggregation	60–100% aggregation, or within 3–5 min as determined by the specific laboratory	
Platelet antibody detection	Platelet antibodies: Negative Platelet-associated immunoglobulin G (Pa IgG): Negative Drug-dependent platelet antibodies: Negative Hyperlysibility assay: Negative	
Platelet count	Adult: 150,000–450,000mm³ (average = 250,000mm³) Critical (low): <30,000/mm³ Critical (high): 71,000,000/mm³	150–450 × 10⁹/L <30 × 10⁹/L >1000 × 10⁹/L
Pregnanediol	Adult male: <1.5 mg/24 h Nonpregnant female: Proliferative phase: 0.5–1.5 mg/24 h Luteal phase: 2–7 mg/24 h Postmenopausal female: 0.2–1 mg/24 h Pregnant female: 16 w: 5–21 mg/24 h 20 w: 6–26 mg/24 h 24 w: 12–32 mg/24 h 28 w: 19–51 mg/24 h 32 w: 22–66 mg/24 h 36 w: 13–77 mg/24 h 40 w: 23–63 mg/24 h	
Prolactin	Male: 1–20 ng/mL Female: Nonlactating: 1–25 ng/mL Menopausal: 1–20 ng/mL Pregnant: 1st trimester: 1–80 ng/mL 2nd trimester: 1–160 ng/mL 3rd trimester: 1–400 ng/mL	1–20 Ug/L 1–25 Ug/L 1–12 Ug/L 1–80 Ug/L 1–160 Ug/L 1–400 Ug/L
Prostate-specific antigen	≤2.7 ng/mL in male under age 40 ≤4.0 ng/mL in male age 40 or older	
Protein C	50%–150% of population mean; varies by laboratory	

Test	Reference Values	SI Units
Protein, total	Newborn: 4.6–7.4 g/dL Infant: 6.0–6.7 g/dL Child: 6.2–8.0 g/dL Adult: 6.0–8.0 g/dL	46–74 g/L 60–67 g/L 62–80 g/L 60–80 g/L
Prothrombin consumption time	15–20 s with more than 80% of the prothrombin consumed	
Prothrombin time (pro time)	Newborn: 12–21 s Child: 11–14 s Adult male: 9.6–11.8 s Adult female: 9.5–11.3 s *Critical value: >30 s* INR 2.0–3.0 s for anticoagulation 3.0–4.5 s for recurrent systemic embolization	
Protoporphyrin, free erythrocyte	Promelli method: Adult female: 19–52 mg/dL Adult male: 11–43 mg/dL Hemalofluorometer: Adult female: <40 mg/dL Adult male: <30 mg/dL Panic value: >190 mg/dL Erythrocyte precursors: Protoporphyrin: 4–52 mg/dL	
Pseudocholinesterase	RID method: 0.5–1.3 mg/dL Other methods: Male: 274–532 IU/dL Female: 204–500 IU/dL Dibucaine inhibition: 81–87% Fluoride inhibition: 44–54%	5–15 mg/L 0.81–0.87 0.44–0.54
Pyruvic acid	0.08–0.16 mEq/L	0.08–0.16 mmol/L
Raji cell assay	Normal: <13 mg AHG Eq/mL Borderline: 12–25 mg AHG Eq/mL	
Rapid plasma reagin (RPR) test	Non-reactive	
Red blood cell count	Child: Newborn: 4.8–7.1 million/mm^3 1 mo: 4.1–6.4 million/mm^3 6 mo: 3.8–5.5 million/mm^3 1–10 yr: 4.5–4.8 million/mm^3 Adult: Male: 4.6–6.2 million/mm^3 Female: 4.2–5.4 million/mm^3	
Red blood cell indices	MCV: Newborn: 96–108 μm^3 Adult male: 80–94 μm^3 Adult female: 81–99 μm^3	

(*continued*)

Test	Reference Values	SI Units
Red blood cell indices	MCH: Newborn: 32–34 pg Adult male: 27–31 pg Adult female: 27–31 pg MCHC: Newborn: 32–33% Adult male: 32–36% Adult female: 32–36%	
Renin	Adult (normal sodium diet): Supine: 0.1–3.1 ng/mL/h Standing: 20–39 yr: 0.1–4.3 ng/mL/h >40 yr: 0.1–3.0 ng/mL/h Child: 0–3 yr: <16.6 ng/mL/h 3–6 yr: <6.7 ng/mL/h 6–9 yr: <4.4 ng/mL/h 9–12 yr: <5.9 ng/mL/h 12–15 yr: <4.2 ng/mL/h 15–18 yr: <4.3 ng/mL/h Adult (low-sodium diet): Supine: 2.1–4.3 ng/mL/h Standing: 20–30 yr: 2.9–24.0 ng/mL/h >40 yr: 2.9–10.8 ng/mL/h	
Reticulocyte count	Male: 0.5–1.5% Female: 0.5–2.5% Child: 0.5–4% Infant: 2–5%	
Rheumatoid factor	A negative test is <60 U/mL by nephelometric testing	
Rocky Mountain spotted fever antibodies	Indirect fluorescent antibody assay (most sensitive): Titer >128 in single sample or fourfold rise in paired serum titers Latex agglutination test: Active Rocky Mountain spotted fever: Titer >128 Complement fixation for rickettsial infection: >1:160 or fourfold increase in paired samples within 7 d Weil-Felix agglutination reaction (least sensitive): Strong agglutination response suggests rickettsial disease	
Rubella antibodies	Titer <1:8—Susceptibility to infection Titer >1:8—Immunity from vaccination or prior infection	
Rubeola antibodies	Negative	

Test	Reference Values	SI Units
Scleroderma antibody	Absence of antibody in the blood	
Serotonin (5-hydroxytrypta-mine)	10–30 µg/dL	570–1700 nmol/L
Serum complement assay	Total complement	40–90 U/mL
	C_3	
	Men	80–180 mg/dL
	Women	76–120 mg/dL
	C_4	
	Men	15–60 mg/dL
	Women	15–52 mg/dL
Sickle cell test (Sickledex, Hgb S)	Negative, no sickled cells	
Sucrose hemolysis	Negative, or <5% hemolysis	
T and B lymphocyte assays	T lymphocytes: 60–80% of circulating lymphocytes* B lymphocytes: 10–20% of circulating lymphocytes Null cells: 5–20% of circulating lymphocytes Helper T lymphocytes: 50–65% of circulating T lymphocytes Suppressor T lymphocytes: 20–35% of circulating T lymphocytes Ratio of helper to suppressor T lymphocytes: 2:1 *A decreased lymphocyte count (lymphopenia) usually indicates a decrease in the number of circulating T lymphocytes.	
T and B lymphocyte surface markers	T cells (CD3): 53–88% T-helper (CD4) cells: 32–61% T suppressor (CD8) cells: 18%–42% B cells: 5–20% Lymphocyte count: 0.66–4.60 thousand/µL T-cell count: 812–2318 cells/µL B-cell count: 99–426 cells/µL Helper cell count (CD4): 589–1505 cells/L Suppressor T-cell count (CD8): 325–997 cells/µL CD4:CD8 ratio >1.0	
Testosterone	Male: 300–1200 ng/dL Female: 30–95 ng/dL Prepubertal child: Male: <100 ng/dL Female: <40 ng/dL	

(continued)

Test	Reference Values	SI Units
Thrombin clotting time	5 s with 15–20 s control; <1.5 times control (values vary among laboratories or depend on concentration of thrombin reagent used)	
Thyroglobulin	3–42 ng/mL in those with normal thyroid 0–5 ng/mL in those with thyroid removed	
Thyroid antithyroglobulin antibody	Negative, or titer 1:100	
Thyroid hormone binding ratio	T_3 uptake: 25–35% Thyroid hormone binding ratio (THBR) Adult <50 yr: 0.85–1.14 Adult >50 yr: Female: 0.80–1.04 Male: 0.87–1.11 Child Cord blood: 0.75–1.05 1–3 d: 0.90–1.40 1–2 w: 0.85–1.15 4–16 w: 0.75–1.05 1–15 yr: 0.88–1.12	
Thyroid-stimulating hormone	Newborn: <20 μU/mL by day 3 Adult: <10 μU/mL Older Adult: Female: 2.0–16.8 μU/mL Male: 2.0–7.3 μU/mL *Filter paper test:* Newborn: At birth: 30 μU/mL 3 d: <20 μU/mL 10 d: <10 μU/mL	<20 mU/L <10 mU/L 2.0–16.8 mU/L 2.0–7.3 mU/L 30 mU/L <20 mU/L <10 mU/L
Thyroid-stimulating hormone sensitive (s-TSH assay)	0.4–10 mIU/L	0.4–10 U/L
Thyroid-stimulating hormone, neonatal	Age 1–3 d: 25–30 μIU/mL. Then after levels are normal, <25 μIU/mL	
Thyroid-stimulating immunoglobulins	Negative; may be found in the serum of about 5% of people without apparent hyperthyroidism or exophthalmos	
Thyroid stimulator, long-acting	Negative	

Test	Reference Values	SI Units
Thyroxine	RIA FT₄	4–12 µg/dL 0.9–2.3 ng/dL
Thyroxine-binding globulin	Male, adult: 15–30 µg/dL Female: Nonpregnant 11.5–32.2 µg/dL Pregnant: 1st trimester: 19.8–64.7 µg/dL 2nd trimester: 41.4–63.9 µg/dL 3rd trimester: 31.0–47.9 µg/dL Oral contraceptive use: 23.1–47.9 µg/dL	
TORCH test	Negative	
Transferrin	Newborn: 60–170 mg/dL Adult: 250–450 mg/dL	
Triglycerides	Infant: 5–40 mg/dL Child: 10–135 mg/dL 12–20 yr: 10–140 mg/dL Adult: 20–40 yr: 10–140 mg/dL (female) 10–150 mg/dL (male) 40–60 yr: 0–180 mg/dL (female) 10–190 mg/dL (male)	0.6–0.67 mmol/L 0.11–1.49 mmol/L 0.11–1.57 mmol/L 0.11–1.57 mmol/L 0.11–1.68 mmol/L 0.11–2.01 mmol/L 0.11–2.12 mmol/L
Triiodothyronine	Newborn: 32–250 ng/dL Child: 105–241 ng/dL Adult: 80–230 ng/dL	0.49–3.85 nmol/L 1.62–3.71 nmol/L 1.26–3.5 nmol/L
Triiodothyronine uptake	T₃ resin uptake Adult: 25–35% Thyroid hormone binding ratio Newborn: 0.90–1.15 Child: 0.88–1.12 Adult: 0.85–1.14	 25–35 arb U 0.9–1.15 arb U 0.88–1.12 arb U 0.85–1.14 arb U
Trypsin	RIA double-antibody method: Adult: 22.2–44.4 µg/L Child: Cord: 21.4–25.2 µg/L <6 mo: 25.9–36.7 µg/L 6–12 mo: 30.2–44.0 µg/L 1–3 yr: 28.0–31.6 µg/L 3–5 yr: 25.1–31.5 µg/L 5–7 yr: 32.1–39.3 µg/L 7–10 yr: 32.7–37.1 µg/L Sorin antibody method: Adult: 5.0–85.0 µg/L Child: 11.1–51.3 µg/L	

(*continued*)

Test	Reference Values	SI Units
Uric acid	Child: 2.5–5.5 mg/dL	0.15–0.33 mmol/L
	Adult:	
	Male: 4.0–8.5 mg/dL	0.24–0.51 mmol/L
	Female: 2.7–7.3 mg/dL	0.16–0.43 mmol/L
Venereal disease research laboratory (VDRL) test	Negative; no flocculation should appear; test is reported as strongly reactive, reactive, weakly reactive, or negative	
Viscosity	1.4–1.8 relative to distilled water	
Vitamin A	0.15–0.60 mg/mL	
Vitamin B$_1$	5.3–7.9 µg/dL	
Vitamin B$_6$	25–80 ng/mL	
Vitamin B$_{12}$	180–900 pg/mL	
Vitamin C	Child: 0.6–1.6 mg/dL	
	Adult: 0.2–2.0 mg/dL	
Vitamin D$_3$	10–55 mg/mL	
Vitamin E	0.8–1.5 mg/dL	
Western immunoblast assay	Negative	
White blood cell count and differential	*Total WBC:*	
	Newborn: 9,000–30,000/µL	9.0–30.0 × 10^9/L
	Infant: 6,000–17,500/µL	6.0–17.5 × 10^9/L
	Child: 4,500–16,300/µL	4.5–13.5 × 10^9/L
	Adult male: 4,500–11,000/µL	4.5–11.0 × 10^9/L
	Adult female:	
	(nonpregnant): 4,500–11,000/µL	4.5–11.0 × 10^9/L
	Differential WBC:	
	Neutrophils (Segs) 54–75%	0.54–0.75
	Newborn: 3,320–12,100/µL	3320–12,100 × 10^6/L
	Infant: 2,680–2,750/µL	2680–2750 × 10^6/L
	Child: 2,660–3,700/µL	2660–3700 × 10^6/L
	Adult: 3,000/µL	3800 × 10^6/L
	Neutrophils (Bands): 3–8%	0.03–0.08
	Newborn: 1,150–3,460/µL	1150–3460 × 10^6/L
	Infant: 990–1,150/µL	990–1150 × 10^6/L
	Child: 640–850/µL	640–850 × 10^6/L
	Adult: 620/µL	620 × 10^6/L
	Eosinophils: 1–4%	0.01–0.04
	Newborn: 300–400/µL	300–400 × 10^6/L
	Infant: 300/µL	300 × 10^6/L
	Child: 200–280/µL	200–280 × 10^6/L
	Adult: 200/µL	200 × 10^6/L

Test	Reference Values	SI Units
	Basophils: 0–1%	0–0.01
	Newborn: 100/μL	100×10^6/L
	Infant: 50/μL	50×10^6/L
	Child: 40/μL	40×10^6/L
	Adult: 40/μL	0.04×10^6/L
	Monocytes: 2–8%	0.02–0.08
	Newborn: 700–1200/μL	$700–1200 \times 10^6$/L
	Infant: 550–700/μL	$550–700 \times 10^6$/L
	Child: 350–550/μL	$350–550 \times 10^6$/L
	Adult: 300/μL	300×10^6/L
White blood cell enzymes	Leukocyte alkaline phosphatase (LAP): 13–130 U	
	Periodic acid-Schiff (PAS):	
	Granulocytes: Positive	
	Agranulocytes: Negative	
	Granulocyte precursors: Negative	
	Tartrate-resistant acid phosphatase (TRAP): Activity present	

Reference Values for Laboratory Tests on Urine

Test	Reference Values	SI Units
Aldosterone	2–26 μg/24 h	5.6–7.3 nmol/d
Amino acid	200 mg/24 h	2 mmol/dL
Aminolevulinic acid (ALA)	Random specimen:	
	Child: <0.5 mg/dL	38.1 μmol/L
	Adult: 0.1–0.6 mg/dL	7.6–45.8 μmol/L
	24-h urine 11.15–57.2 μmol/24 h	
Amylase	10–80 amylase U/h (Mayo clinic)	0–17 U/h
	35–260 Somogyi U/24 h (Somogyi)	6.5 48.1 U/h
Arylsulfatase A (ARS-A)	Child: >1 U/L	
	Male: 1.4–19.3 U/L	
	Female: 1.4–11 U/L	
Bence Jones protein	Negative	
Beta$_2$-microglobulin	<120 μg/24 h	<10 nmol/d
Bilirubin	Negative	
Calcium	Quantitative: 24-h specimen	
	Low calcium diet: <150 mg/24 h	<3.75 mmol/24 h
	Average calcium diet: 100–250 mg/24 h	2.5–6.2 mmol/24 h
	High calcium diet: 250–300 mg/24 h	6.2–7.5 mmol/24 h
	Random: <40 mg/dL	1.0 mmol/L
	Qualitative:	
	Sulkowitch: 0–$^+$2 turbidity	

(*continued*)

Test	Reference Values	SI Units
Catecholamines	*Total free catecholamines:*	
	Random urine: 0–18 μg/dL	0–103 nmol/dL
	24-h urine: 4–126 μg/24 h	24–745 nmol/24 h
	Critical level: 200 μg/dL	1180 nmol/24 h
	Epinephrine: < 10 μg/24 h	55 nmol/24 h
	Critical level: 50 μg/24 h	295 nmol/24 h
	Norepinephrine: <100 μg/24 h	591 nmol/24 h
	Metanephrines: 0.1–1.6 mg/24 h	0.5–8.7 μmol/24 h
	Dopamine: 65–400 μg/24 h	384–2364 nmol/24 h
Chloride	Child: 15–115 mEq/24 h	15–115 mmol/24 h
	Adult: 110–250 mEq/24 h	110–250 mmol/24 h
Coproporphyrin	Random specimen:	
	Adult: 0.045–0.30 μmol/L	
	24-h specimen:	
	Child: 0–0.12 μmol/24 h	0–80 μg/24 h
	Adult: 0.075–0.24 μmol/24 h	50–160 μg/24 h
Cortisol	24–108 μg/24 h	60–300 nmol/d
Creatinine	Male: 1.0–2.0 g/24 h	8.8–17.6 mmol/24 h
	Female: 0.8–1.8 g/24 h	7–15.8 mmol/24 h
Creatinine clearance	Male: 85–125 mL/min	
	20–26 mg/kg/24 h	0.18–0.23 mmol/kg/24 h
	1.0–2.0 g/24 h	8.8–17.6 mmol/24 h
	Female: 75–115 mL/min	
	14–22 mg/kg/24 h	0.12–0.19 mmol/kg/24 h
	0.8–1.8 g/24 h	7–15.8 mmol/24 h
Cyclic adenosine monophosphate	Total: 112–188 μg/L	340–570 nmol/L
	cAMP portion of creatinine: 3–5 μmol/g	
	cAMP portion of glomerular filtrate: 6.6–15.5 μg/L	20–47 nmol/L
	cAMP nephrogenous portion of glomerular filtrate: <9.9 μg/L	<30 nmol/L
d-Xylose tolerance	Child:	
	5 h: 16%–33% of dose ingested	
	Adult:	
	5 h: 16% of dose ingested	
Delta-aminolevulinic acid	Age 9 mo–5 yr: 0–0.66 mg/dL	0–0.09 μmol/L
	Age 6 yr–adult: 1.5–7.5 mg/24 h	11–57 μmol/d
Dexamethasone suppression	*Overnight test:*	
	Low dose: <3 μg/dL	<0.08 μmol/L
	Urine 17–OHCS: <4 mg/5 h	<11.0 μmol/5 h
	High dose: <50% of baseline	<0.50 of baseline
	Urine 17–OHCS: <50% of baseline/24 h	<50% of baseline/24 h

Test	Reference Values	SI Units
	Standard test (6 d) cortisol:	
	Low dose: <5 μg/dL (day 4)	<138 nmol/L (d 4)
	Urine 17–OHCS: <4.5 mg/24 h	<12.4 μmol/24 h
	High dose: <10 μg/dL (day 6)	<276 nmol/L (d 6)
	Urine 17–OHCS: <50% of baseline (day 6)	<0.50 of baseline (d 6)
Estriol	Child: 0.3–2.4 μg/24 h	1.04–8.33 nmol/24 h
	Adult male: 1.0–11.0 μg/24 h	3.5–38.2 nmol/24 h
	Nonpregnant female:	
	Early in cycle: 0–15 μg/24 h	0–52.0 nmol/24 h
	Ovulation peak: 13–54 μg/24 h	27.8–208.2 nmol/24 h
	Luteal phase: 8.0–60.0 μg/24 h	45.1–187.4 nmol/24 h
	Postmenopausal female: 0.6–6.8 μg/24 h	2.08–23.6 nmol/24 h
	Pregnant female:	
	1st trimester: 0–800 μg/24 h	0–2.776 nmol/24 h
	2nd trimester: 800–12,000 μg/24 h	2,776–41,640 nmol/24 h
	3rd trimester: 5,000–50,000 μg/24 h	17,350–173,500 nmol/24 h
Estrogens, total	Child: <10 μg/24 h	1.13 mg/mol
	Adult male: 4–25 μg/24 h	0.45–2.60 mg/mol
	Nonpregnant female:	
	Preovulatory phase: 7–65 μg/24 h	0.79–7.35 mg/mol
	Ovulatory phase: 32–104 μg/24 h	3.62–11.75 mg/mol
	Luteal phase: 8–135 μg/24 h	0.90–15.26 mg/mol
	Postmenopausal female: <20 μg/24 h	<2.26 mg/mol
Estrone	Child: 0.2–1 g/24 h	
	Adult male: 2.0–8.0 μg/24 h	0.8–3.3 mmol/mol
	Nonpregnant female:	
	Early in cycle: 2–39 μg/24 h	(0.8–16.3 mmol/mol)
	Ovulation peak: 11–46 μg/24 h	(4.6–19.2 mmol/mol)
	Luteal phase: 3–52 μg/24 h	(1.2–21.7 mmol/mol)
	Postmenopausal female: 0.8–7.1 g/24 h	
Ferric chloride	Negative	
Fishberg test	Standard: Specific gravity of 1.026 or higher	
	Simplified: Specific gravity of 1.022 or higher	
Glucose	Negative	

(*continued*)

Test	Reference Values	SI Units
Homovanillic acid	Child: 1–2 yr: 0–25 mg/24 h 2–10 yr: 0.5–10 mg/24 h 10–15 yr: 0.5–12 mg/24 h Adult: <8 mg/24 h	1–126 μmol/mg 3–55 μmol/mg 3–66 μmol/mg 1–14 μmol/mg
Human chorionic gonadotropin	Nonpregnant: <3 mIU/mL Pregnant: 8–10 days: 5–40 mIU/mL 1 mo: 100 mIU/mL 2 mo: 100,000 mIU/mL 4–9 mo: 50,000 mIU/mL	
Human chorionic gonadotropin, pregnancy test	Random: Negative if not pregnant 24-h: Adult male: Not measurable Nonpregnant female: Not measurable Pregnant female: 1st trimester Up to 500,000 IU/24 h 2nd trimester 10,000–25,000 IU/24 h 3rd trimester 5,000–15,000 IU/24 h	
17-Hydroxycorti-costeroids	Child: 0.5–4.5 mg/24 h (age-related: the younger the child, the less secreted) Male: 4.5–12 mg/24 h Female: 2.5–10 mg/24 h	1.4–12.4 μmol/24 h 12.4–33.1 μmol/24 h 6.9–27.6 μmol/24 h
5-Hydroxyindoleacetic acid	1–10 mg/24 h	5.2–52 μmol/24 h
5-Hydroxyproline	*24-h:* Adult: 10–50 mg/24 h Child: 1–10 y: 20–99 mg/24 h 11–14 y: 63–180 mg/24 h *2-h:* Male: 0.4–5 mg/2 h Female: 0.4–2.9 mg/2 h	0.08–0.38 mmol/24 h 0.15–0.75 mmol/24 h 0.48–1.37 mmol/24 h
Inulin clearance	Birth–age 10: 1.4–2.0 mL/s Ages 11–20: 1.4–2.1 mL/s Ages 21–70: 1.5–2.2 mL/s Over age 70: Clearance may decline up to 45%	

Test	Reference Values	SI Units
17-Ketogenic steroids	Child: 2–6 mg/24 h (age-related: the younger the child, the less secreted)	6–17 mmol/24 h
	Male: 5–25 mg/24 h	14–69 mmol/24 h
	Female: 3–15 mg/24 h	8–41 mmol/24 h
	Older Adult: 3–13 mg/24 h	8–36 mmol/24 h
Ketones	Negative	
17-Ketosteroids	*Fractionation:*	
	Male: 8–17 mg/24 h	27–58 μmol/24 h
	Female: 5–15 mg/24 h	17–52 μmol/24 h
	Total:	
	Infant: <1 μg/24 h	<3 μmol/24 h
	Child: 2–4 mg/24 h (age-related: the younger the child, the less secreted)	7–14 μmol/24 h
	Adolescent: 3–15 mg/24 h	10–52 μmol/24 h
	Adult female: 4–16 mg/24 h	13–55 μmol/24 h
	Adult male: 6–21 mg/24 h	21–72 μmol/24 h
	Older adult: 4–8 mg/24 h	13–27 μmol/24 h
Lead	<80 μg/specimen	<0.8 μg/specimen
Leucine aminopeptidase	2–18 U/24 h	
Magnesium	Adult: 6.0–8.5 mEq/24 h	3.0–4.3 mmol/24 h
Melanin	Negative:	
Metanephrines, total	0.1–1.3 mg/24 h	
Mosenthal test	Specific gravity of 1.020 or higher with at least a 7-point difference between the specific gravities of the daytime and night-time samples	
Muramidase (lysozyme)	<0–2.9 mg/L	1.3–3.6 mg/24 h
Myoglobin	Negative	
Osmolality	50–1400 mOsm (usual range, 300–900 mOsm; average, 850 mOsm) Ratio of urine to serum: 1.2:1 to 3:1	
pH	Newborn: 5.0–7.0 Child: 4.8–7.8 Adult: 4.5–8.0	
Phenolphthalein	Negative	

(*continued*)

Test	Reference Values	SI Units
Phenosulfonphthalein	Child: 5–10% higher than adults at the same time intervals Adult: 15 min = 25% of dose excreted 30 min = 50–60% of dose excreted 60 min = 60–70% of dose excreted 2 h = 70–80% of dose excreted	
Phosphorus	Adult: 0.4–1.3 g/24 h Restricted diet: <1.0 g/24 h	<32 mmol/24 h
Porphobilinogen	Random specimen: Negative 24-h urine: 0–2.5 mg/24 h	0–4.4 μmol/24 h
Potassium	Child: 17–57 mEq/24 h Adult: 25–123 mEq/24 h	17–57 mmol/24 h 25–123 mmol/24 h
Pregnanediol	Adult male: <1.5 mg/24 h Nonpregnant female: Proliferative phase: 0.5–1.5 mg/24 h Luteal phase: 2–7 mg/24 h Postmenopausal female: 0.2–1 mg/24 h Pregnant female: 16 w: 5–21 mg/24 h 20 w: 6–26 mg/24 h 24 w: 12–32 mg/24 h 28 w: 19–51 mg/24 h 32 w: 22–66 mg/24 h 36 w: 13–77 mg/24 h 40 w: 23–63 mg/24 h	
Pregnanetriol	Child (<6-yr-old): ≤0.2 mg/24 h Child (7–16 yr): 0.3–1.1 mg/24 h Adult: <3.5 mg/24 h	
Protein electrophoresis	Albumin: 37.9% Alpha$_1$ globulin: 27.3% Alpha$_2$ globulin: 19.5% Beta globulin: 8.8% Gamma globulin: 3.3%	
Protein	Negative	
Sodium	Newborn: 14–40 mEq/24 h Child: 20–115 mEq/24 h Adult: 75–200 mEq/24 h	14–40 mmol/24 h 20–115 mmol/24 h 75–200 mmol/24 h
Specific gravity	1.001–1.035 (usual range, 1.010–1.025)	
Uric acid	250–800 mg/24 h	1.5–4.8 mmol/d

Test	Reference Values	SI Units
Urinalysis, routine	*Macroscopic Analysis* Color: Pale yellow to amber Appearance: Clear to slightly hazy Odor: Mildly aromatic Specific gravity: Usual range 1.010–1.025 pH: 4.5–8.0 Protein: Negative Glucose: Negative Other sugars: Negative Ketones: Negative Blood: Negative Bilirubin: Negative Urobilinogen: 0.1–1.0 Ehrlich μ/dL Nitrite: Negative Leukocyte esterase: Negative *Microscopic Analysis* Red blood cells: 0–3/high-powered field (HPF) White blood cells: 0–4/HPF Epithelial cells: 0–10/HPF Casts: Occasional (hyaline or granular) Crystals: Occasional (uric acid, urate, phosphate, or calcium oxalate) Bacteria: <1000/mL	1–4 mg/24 h
Vanillymandelic acid	0.7–6.8 mg in 24 h	3–3.5 μmol/d
Vitamins B_1, B_2, C	B_1 (thiamine) 100–200 Ug/24 h B_2 (riboflavin) Male: 0.51 mg/24 h Female: 0.39 mg/24 h C (ascorbic acid) 30 mg/24 h	

Appendix 5

Profile Groups

A profile or panel consists of a group of 4 to 20 biochemical tests performed on a few millimeters of serum with an instrument called a *sequential multiple analyzer (SMA)*. Below are common profile groups:

SMA-4	Red blood cells	Hemoglobin
	White blood cells	Hematocrit
SMA-6	Sodium	Bicarbonate
	Potassium	Glucose
	Chloride	Blood urea nitrogen
SMA-12	Total protein	Glucose
	Albumin	Uric acid
	Calcium	Creatinine
	Blood urea nitrogen	Total bilirubin
	Inorganic phosphatase	Alkaline phosphatase
	Cholesterol	AST
SMAC	Glucose	Bilirubin, direct
CHEM 20	Blood urea nitrogen	Bilirubin, indirect
	Creatinine	Lactic dehydrogenase (LDH)
	Uric acid	Aspartate aminotransferase (AST)
	Sodium	Alanine aminotransferase (ALT)
	Potassium	Alkaline phosphatase
	Chloride	Albumin
	Bicarbonate	Total protein
	Calcium	Cholesterol
	Phosphorus	Triglycerides

Appendix 6

Organ Function Tests

Organ function tests are groupings of diagnostic and laboratory tests used to comprehensively evaluate how well an organ is working. Using several tests eliminates the risk of misdiagnosis because of inaccurate test results, and it presents a more complete picture of both the anatomic and physiologic alterations.

Cardiovascular System

- *Cardiac enzymes:* Aspartate aminotransferase (AST, SGOT); creatine phosphokinase (CPK); creatine kinase (CK) and isoenzyme (CK-MB); lactate dehydrogenase (LH, LDH) and isoenzyme (LD_1, LD_2); hydroxybutyrate dehydrogenase (HBDH)
- *Lipids:* Total lipids, lipoprotein electrophoresis (HDL, LDL, VLDL); cholesterol; triglycerides; phospholipids
- *Electrolytes:* Potassium (K); sodium (Na)
- *Coagulation:* Prothrombin time (PT); activated partial thromboplastin time (APPT); coagulation time (CT); clotting time; Lee-White (LWCT)
- *Pericardial fluid:* Cytologic examination; other tests to measure red blood cell (RBC) count, white blood cell count (WBC), differential, and glucose; microbiologic examination if endocarditis is suspected (Gram stain, culture)
- *Drug levels:* Digoxin; digitoxin; diltiazem; nifedipine; propranolol; verapamil; others included in therapeutic regimen
- *Miscellaneous:* Erythrocyte sedimentation rate (ESR); WBC; glucose; blood gases (pH, P_{CO_2}, P_{O_2})
- *Procedures:* Cardiac nuclear scanning; cardiac radiography; echocardiography; electrocardiography (ECG); phonocardiography; exercise electrocardiography; cardiac catheterization and angiography; heart and chest magnetic resonance imaging; non-nuclear computerized tomography (CT) of the chest

From Watson, J and Jaffe, MS: Nurse's Manual of Laboratory and Diagnostic Tests, ed 2. F. A. Davis, Philadelphia, 1995, pp. 997–1002, with permission.

Pulmonary System

- *Arterial blood gases (ABGs):* pH, P_{CO_2}; P_{O_2}; HCO_3; BE
- *Sputum:* Microbiologic examination (Gram and other stains, acid-fast bacillus [AFB] smear and culture); culture and sensitivity (C&S); cytologic examination
- *Pleural fluid:* Microbiologic examination (C&S, Gram stain); cytologic examination; other tests to measure LDH, RBC, WBC, differential, eosinophils, pH, and immunoglobulins
- *Drug levels:* Theophylline therapeutic regimen
- *Miscellaneous:* Alpha$_1$-antitrypsin; WBC
- *Procedures:* Bronchoscopy; mediastinoscopy, thoracoscopy, chest radiography and tomography; bronchography; pulmonary angiography; thoracic ultrasonography; lung nuclear scanning; non-nuclear thoracic computerized tomography (CT); chest magnetic resonance imaging; pulmonary function studies; exercise pulmonary function; body plethysmography; sweat test; lung biopsy; thoracentesis; oximetry; skin tests for allergens and bacterial and fungal pulmonary diseases

Neurologic System

- *Cerebrospinal fluid:* Routine analysis (cell count and differential, protein, glucose); other tests such as enzymes, electrolytes, urea, lactic acid, and glutamine; microbiologic examination (C&S, Gram, and AFS stains); cytologic examination; serologic examination (neurosyphilis tests)
- *Drug levels:* Anticonvulsants (phenobarbital, phenytoin, primidone), and others included in therapeutic regimen or considered for overdose in the comatose client (prescribed and otherwise)
- *Miscellaneous:* Electrolytes (K, Na, Cl, CO_2); glucose; alcohol; blood gases (ABGs); blood urea nitrogen (BUN); creatinine; toxicology screen (blood and urine)
- *Procedures:* Skull and spinal radiography; cerebral angiography; brain and cerebrospinal fluid flow nuclear scanning; echoencephalography; non-nuclear head, intracranial, neck, and spinal computerized tomography (CT) scanning; head and intracranial magnetic resonance imaging; electroneurography; evoked brain potentials; spinal nerve root thermography; oculoplethysmography; visual-auditory and optic-acoustic nerve tests

Hematologic System

- *Blood cell counts:* Complete blood count, including RBC, Hgb, Hct, RBC indices (MCV, MCH, MCHC), WBC, WBC differential, platelet, and reticulocyte
- *Blood cell types:* Hgb electrophoresis; blood typing and cross-matching; sickle-cell screening
- *Coagulation:* Bleeding time; platelet aggregation; platelet survival; clot retraction time; capillary fragility; prothrombin time (PT); partial thromboplastin time (PTT); activated partial thromboplastin time (APTT); whole blood clotting time (CT); thrombin clotting time (TCT); prothrombin consumption time (PCT); factor assays; plasma fibrinogen; fibrin split products (FSP); euglobulin lysis
- *Iron deficiency:* Iron; total iron-binding capacity (TIBC); folic acid; ferritin
- *Hemolysis:* Red blood cell enzymes (glucose-6-phosphate dehydrogenase); haptoglobin, indirect Coombs; bilirubin
- *Miscellaneous:* Erythrocyte osmotic fragility; ESR; WBC enzymes; T and B lymphocyte assay; immunoglobulin assay
- *Procedures:* Schilling test; bone marrow aspiration; bone marrow nuclear scanning; red blood cell survival time study; platelet survival time study; lymph node biopsy

Endocrine System

- *Thyroid tests:* Calcitonin; thyroid-stimulating immunoglobulins (TSI); thyroxine-binding globulin (TBG); triiodothyronine (T_3); T_3 uptake; thyroxine (T_4); free T_4 index; thyroid antibodies; thyroid-stimulating hormone (TSH)
- *Thyroid procedures:* Thyroid nuclear scanning; radioactive iodine uptake study; thyroid-stimulating hormone study (TSH); thyroid cytomel and perchlorate suppression studies; ultrasonography, iodine-131 scanning
- *Parathyroid tests:* Parathyroid hormone (PTH); calcium; phosphorus; prednisone-cortisone suppression
- *Parathyroid procedures:* Ultrasonography; nuclear scanning
- *Pituitary tests:* Growth hormone (GH); growth hormone stimulation; growth suppression; prolactin (LTH); adrenocorticotropic hormone (ACTH); thyroid-stimulating hormone (TSH) and stimulation test; follicle-stimulating hormone (FSH); luteinizing hormone (LH), FSH-LH challenge; antidiuretic hormone (ADH)
- *Pituitary procedures:* Skull radiography; cerebral angiography; nuclear brain scanning; intracranial magnetic resonance imaging
- *Adrenal tests:* Cortisol; adrenocorticotropic hormone (ACTH); cortisol-ACTH challenge; aldosterone; aldosterone

challenge; catecholamines; urinary hormones (cortisol, aldosterone, 17-hydroxycorticosteroids [17-OHCS], 17-ketosteroids [17-KS], 17-ketogenic steroids [17-KGS], pregnanetriol, vanillylmandelic acid [VMA])

- *Adrenal procedures:* Non-nuclear computerized tomography (CT) scanning; adrenal nuclear scanning, ultrasonography; angiography; skull radiography
- *Pancreas tests:* Glucose; glucose tolerance; 2-hour postprandial glucose; ketones; glycosylated hemoglobin; BUN, creatinine; tobutamide tolerance; insulin; amylase; lipase; aldolase; potassium (K); sodium (Na); glucagon; C-peptide
- *Pancreas procedures:* Endoscopic retrograde cholangiopancreatography (ERCP); ultrasonography; abdominal magnetic resonance imaging; pancreas nuclear scanning; non-nuclear computerized tomography (CT) scanning

Renal-Urologic Systems

- *Blood tests:* BUN, creatinine, electrolyte panel; osmolality; proteins; ammonia; uric acid; renin; aldosterone; gamma glutamyl transpeptidase (GGT)
- *Urine tests:* Routine analysis; creatinine clearance; insulin clearance; protein, complement C_3 and C_4; tubular function (phenolsulfonphthalein [PSP]); concentration (osmolality, specific gravity); electrolytes; C&S
- *Procedures:* Kidney and renography nuclear scanning; nonnuclear abdominal computerized tomography (CT); ultrasonography; angiography; kidney; ureter, bladder radiography (KUB); antegrade pyelography; retrograde urethrography, cystography, and ureteropyelography; excretory urography (IVP); voiding cystourethrography; pelvic floor sphincter electromyography; cystometry; uroflowmetry and urethral pressure profile; cystoscopy; renal biopsy

Musculoskeletal System

- *Muscle/bone enzymes:* Adolase; alkaline phosphatase (ALP); creatine phosphokinase (CPK); AST, SGOT
- *Electrolytes:* Calcium (Ca)
- *Joint tests:* Rheumatoid factor (RF); ESR; antistreptolysin O (ASO); immunoglobulins (IgG, IgM); C-reactive protein (CRP); complement C_3 and C_4
- *Synovial fluid:* Routine analysis (RBC, WBC, neutrophils, protein, glucose, crystals); other tests such as rheumatoid factor (RA); complements

- *Procedures:* Bone and joint radiography; arthrocentesis; arthroscopy; arthrography; myelography; musculoskeletal magnetic resonance imaging; bone and joint nuclear scanning; electromyography; muscle biopsy

Hepatobiliary-Gastrointestinal Systems

- *Liver enzymes:* Alkaline phosphatase (ALP) and isoenzymes (ALP_1); alanine aminotransferase (ALT, SGPT); 5'-nucleotidase (5'-N); lactic dehydrogenase (LDH) and isoenzymes (LDH_5); leucine aminopeptidase (LAP); gamma glutamyl transpeptidase (GTT); creatine phosphokinase (CPK) and isoenzymes (CPK_3)
- *Liver blood tests:* Bilirubin; protein (albumin, globulin) and protein electrophoresis; prothrombin time (PT); cholesterol; ammonia; hepatitis B–associated antigen and antibody tests
- *Liver procedures:* Abdominal radiography; liver nuclear scanning; non-nuclear computerized tomography (CT) scanning; abdominal magnetic resonance imaging; ultrasonography; hepatic and portal angiography; liver biopsy
- *Gallbladder procedures:* Abdominal radiography; oral cholecystography (OCG); intravenous cholangiography (IVC); percutaneous transhepatic cholangiography (PTC); operative cholangiography; T-tube cholangiography; biliary ultrasonography; non-nuclear computerized tomography (CT) scanning; gallbladder and biliary system nuclear scanning; endoscopic retrograde cholangiopancreatography (ERCP)
- *Esophageal and stomach tests:* Electrolyte panel; gastrin
- *Esophageal and stomach procedures:* Gastric analysis (macroscopic and microscopic); gastric acidity and acid stimulation; esophagogastroduodenoscopy (EGD); gastric emptying and gastrointestinal bleeding nuclear scanning; gastroesophageal reflux nuclear scanning; barium swallow; upper gastrointestinal series (UGI); fluoroscopy; esophageal manometry and associated tests; mesenteric angiography; esophageal or stomach biopsy
- *Small and large intestine tests:* Electrolyte panel, carotene, carcinoembryonic antigen (CEA), D-xylose absorption; lactose intolerance; fecal analysis (occult blood, fat, culture)
- *Small and large intestine procedures:* Duodenal contents analysis (macroscopic and microscopic); duodenal stimulation for cholecystokinin-pancreozymin and secretin; abdominal radiography; colonoscopy; proctosigmoidoscopy; barium enema; Meckel's diverticulum nuclear scanning; paracentesis; peritoneal fluid analysis; non-nuclear computerized tomography (CT) scanning; colon biopsy

Reproductive System

- *Female blood tests:* Prolactin; estrogen; follicle-stimulating hormone (FSH); luteinizing hormone (LH); progesterone
- *Female urine tests:* Pregnanediol; follicle-stimulating hormone (FSH); estrogen
- *Female procedures:* Colposcopy; culdoscopy; laparoscopy; hysterosalpingography; pelvic and breast ultrasonography; mammography; breast thermography; breast biopsy; cervical biopsy; Papanicolaou (PAP) smear; cytologic analysis (Barr chromatin body, chromosome analysis); non-nuclear computerized tomography (CT) pelvic scanning
- *Male blood tests:* Testosterone; semen analysis for fertility; cytology analysis for chromosomal and genetic abnormalities
- *Male urine tests:* 17-ketosteroids (17-KS)
- *Male procedures:* Scrotal nuclear scanning; scrotal-prostate ultrasonography; prostate biopsy
- *Pregnant female tests:* Complete blood count (CBC); ABO and Rh typing; albumin; syphilis serology (RPR, VDRL); renin; TORCH screen (cytomegalovirus, rubella, herpes virus, plasmal antibodies); human placental lactogen (HPL); creatine phosphokinase (CPK); human chorionic gonadotropin (HCG); progesterone and urinary pregnanediol; enzymes (heat-stable alkaline phosphatase [HSAP], diamine oxidase [DAO], oxytocinase); estriol (E_3) in blood and urine; endocrine panel for hormones; hematology panel for blood cells; coagulation; iron; folate; erythrocyte sedimentation rate (ESR); routine urinalysis; cytology analysis for sex chromatin and chromosome anomalies; amniotic fluid analysis for lecithin/sphingomyelin (L/S) ratio; genetic defects; creatinine; phosphatidylglycerol; uric acid
- *Pregnant female procedures:* Amnioscopy, amniocentesis, pelvimetry; contraction stress tests; pelvic ultrasonography; fetal monitoring (internal and external); fetoscopy
- *Newborn tests:* TORCH, type and Rh; bilirubin; glucose; calcium; albumin; phenylketonuria (PKU)

Immune and Autoimmune Conditions

- *Immune and autoimmune tests:* T and B lymphocyte assay; immunoblast transformation; immunoglobulin assay (IgG, IgA, IgM, IgD, and IgE); antinuclear antibodies (ANA); antibody tests; uric acid; rheumatoid factor (RF); antistreptolysin O titer (ASO); C-reactive protein (CRP); protein electrophoresis for cryoglobulins; lupus erythematosus (LE); anti-DNA, complement C_3 and C_4 assay; ESR; human immunodeficiency virus antibody tests (HIV or AIDS)

Tumors

- *Tumor marker tests:* Prostate (prostatic acid phosphatase [PAP], prostate-specific antigen [PSA]); thyroid (calcitonin); colon, lung, breast (carcinoembryonic antigen [CEA]); liver, testes (alpha-fetoprotein [AFP]); testes, trophoblastic (human chorionic gonadotropin [HCG]); ovary (CA 125); breast (CA 15-3); pancreas; colon (CA 19-9, CA 50); lymphoma, leukemia (lymphocyte B and T)
- *Other tumor tests:* Oncogenes (DNA sequences by polymerase chain reaction [PCR]); cytology examination for B- and T-cell gene rearrangement and DNA content of tumor cells; vasoactive intestinal peptide (VIP); squamous cell carcinoma antigen (SCC); tissue polypeptide antigen (TPA); neuron-specific enolase (NSE); glycoprotein antigen (DU-PAN-2); metabolic tests (uric acid, albumin, cholesterol, triglycerides); hematologic tests (leukocytes, platelets); endocrine tests (antidiuretic hormone, cortisol, ACTH); isoenzymes (alkaline phosphatase [ALP], creatine kinase [CK-BB], galactosyl transferase [GT II], lactate dehydrogenase [LD_1]; electrolyte panel; and other tests based on suspected tumor location
- *Tumor procedures:* Radiography of suspected area; lymph node and retroperitoneal ultrasonography; mammography; bone marrow aspiration; nuclear body scanning (gallium-67); non-nuclear computerized tomography (CT) scanning of body and head; body and head/intracranial magnetic resonance imaging; endoscopy of area; lymphangiography; biopsy of affected organ

Indexes

Index

α-BDH. *See* Alpha-
   hydroxybutyrate
   dehydrogenase
Abdominal aorta
   ultrasonography, 1223
Abdominal CT, 284
Abdominal laparoscopy, 726
Abdominal MRI, 770
Abdominal NMR, 770
Abdominal peritonoscopy, 726
Abdominal ultrasonography,
   1223
ABG. *See* Blood gases, arterial
ABO group typing. *See* Blood
   typing
ABR. *See* Auditory brainstem
   response
AcCHS. *See*
   Pseudocholinesterase
ACE. *See* Angiotensin-converting
   enzyme
Acetylcholine receptor antibody
   (AChR), 3
AChR. *See* Acetylcholine
   receptor antibody
Acid phosphatase (ACP), 5
Acid phosphatase (ACP), vaginal
   swab, 7
Acid-fast bacillus (AFB) culture
   and smear, 397
Acidified serum test, 621
Acoustic admittance tests, 9
Acoustic reflex testing, 9
ACP. *See* Acid phosphatase
ACTH challenge test, 692
Activated clotting time (ACT),
   13

Activated partial thromboplastin
   time (aPTT), 15
ADH. *See* Antidiuretic hormone
Adrenal angiography, 66
Adrenal glands scan, 1030
Adrenocorticotropic hormone
   (ACTH), 17
AFB. *See* Acid-fast bacillus
   culture and smear
AFP. *See* Alpha-fetoprotein
ALA. *See* Delta-aminolevulinic
   acid (delta ALA), urine
Alanine aminotransferase (ALT),
   20
Alanine transaminase, 20
Aldolase (ALS), 23
Aldosterone challenge test, 28
Aldosterone, plasma, 25
Aldosterone, urine, 29
Alkaline phosphatase (ALP), 32
Allergen skin tests, 35
Allergen-specific IgE, 38
Allergen-specific IgE antibody,
   38
ALP. *See* Alkaline phosphatase
Alpha-fetoprotein (AFP), 40
Alpha-hydroxybutyrate
   dehydrogenase (α-BDH),
   665
Alpha$_1$ globulin, 591
Alpha$_1$-antitrypsin (α_1-AT), 43
ALS. *See* Aldolase
ALT. *See* Alanine
   aminotransferase
Ambulatory monitoring, 462
Amino acid screen, blood, 45
Amino acids, urine, 48

Aminolevulinic acid (ALA). *See* Delta-aminolevulinic acid (delta ALA), urine

Amniocentesis, 51

Amniotic fluid analysis, 51

Amylase, serum, 58

Amylase, urine, 61

Anal culture, 363

Androstenedione, 64

Anergy panel, 1133

Angiography, adrenal, 66

Angiography, cerebral, 70

Angiography, coronary, 73

Angiography, digital subtraction (DSA), 76

Angiography, fluorescein, 79

Angiography, liver and portal vein, 83

Angiography, lower extremity, 87

Angiography, lymph, 91

Angiography, mesenteric, 94

Angiography, pulmonary, 98

Angiography, renal, 101

Angiography, upper extremity, 105

Angiotensin-converting enzyme (ACE), 108

ANH. *See* Atrial natriuretic hormone

Antegrade pyelography, 947

Antidiuretic hormone (ADH), 116

Anti-DNA antibody, 111

Anti-HBe. *See* Hepatitis B antibody and antigen

Anti-insulin antibody, 113

Antinuclear antibody (ANA), 119

Anti-Ro/Sjögren's syndrome antigen (SS-A), 114

Antistreptolysin O titer, 121

Antithrombin, 123

Antithrombin III (AT-III). *See* Antithrombin

Apexcardiography, 461

Apolipoprotein A-1 (Apo A-1), 125

Apolipoprotein B, plasma (Apo B), 127

Apoprotein-A (APO-A). *See* Apolipoprotein A-1 (Apo A-1)

Apoprotein-B (APO-B). *See* Apolipoprotein B, plasma (Apo B)

aPTT. *See* Activated partial thromboplastin time

Arterial blood gases (AbG), 194

Arterial plethysmography, 874

Arthrocentesis. *See* Synovial fluid analysis

Arylsulfatase A (ARS-A), urine, 133

Ascending contrast phlebography. *See* Venography *entries*

Aspartate aminotransferase (AST), 136

Atrial natriuretic factor (ANF), 139

Atrial natriuretic hormone (ANH), 139

Audiometry, hearing loss, 141

Auditory brainstem response (ABR), 530

Australia antigen, 195

Barium enema, 950

Barium swallow, 953

Barr body analysis, 1111

Bence Jones protein, 147

Beta globulin, 590

Beta-microglobulin, 149

Bicarbonate (HCO_3), 475

Biliary tract and liver CT, 287

Biliary tract radionuclide scan, 1057

Bilirubin, serum, 151

Bilirubin, urine, 155

Biopsy, bladder, 157

Biopsy, bone, 159

Biopsy, breast, 161

Biopsy, cervical, 163

Biopsy, chorionic villus, 165

Biopsy, intestinal, 167

Biopsy, kidney, 170

Biopsy, liver, 173

Biopsy, lung, 176

Biopsy, lymph node, 179

Biopsy, muscle, 181

Biopsy, prostate, 184

Biopsy, skin, 186

Biopsy, thyroid, 188

Bladder biopsy, 157
Bladder ultrasonography, 1229
Blastomycosis skin test, 1118
Bleeding time, 191
Blood culture, 365
Blood gases, arterial (ABG), 194
Blood indices, 1008
Blood typing, 199
Blood urea nitrogen (BUN), 203
B-lymphocyte assays, 1133
B-lymphocyte and T-lymphocyte
        assays, 1133
Body plethysmography, 874
Bone marrow aspiration and
        analysis, 204
Bone marrow biopsy, 204
Bone scan, 1033
Bone scan, gallium, 1048
Bone x-rays, 956
Brain scan, 994
Breast biopsy, 161
Breast diaphanography, 425
Breast scan, gallium, 1044
Breast stimulation test, 324
Breast thermography, 1146
Breast transillumination, 425
Breast ultrasonography, 1231
Bronchography, 959
Bronchoscopy, 209
Bronchus radiography, 959
Brucella agglutination test. *See*
        Febrile agglutinins, serum
Buccal smear (for Barr body),
        1111

Ca. *See* Calcium, serum
Calcitonin, 220
Calcium (Ca), serum, 475
Calcium (Ca), urine, 487
cAMP. *See* Cyclic adenosine
        monophosphate
Cancer antigen 125 (CA-125),
        223
Capillary fragility, 212
Carcinoembryonic antigen
        (CEA), 225
Cardiac angiography, 73
Carotid ultrasound Doppler,
        1266
CAT. *See* Computerized axial
        tomography

Catecholamines, plasma, 227
Catecholamines, urine, 230
Catheterization, pulmonary
        artery, 324
CBC. *See* Complete blood count
CEA. *See* Carcinoembryonic
        antigen
Cerebral angiography, 70
Cerebrospinal fluid (CSF)
        analysis, 760
Ceruloplasmin (Cp), 243
Cervical biopsy, 163
Cervical mucus sperm
        penetration test, 1115
Chest MRI, 778
Chest NMR, 778
Chest tomography, 1185
Chest x-ray (CXR), 962
Chlamydia antibodies, 245
Chlamydial tests, 246
Chloride (Cl), serum, 475
Chloride (Cl), urine, 486
Cholangiography, percutaneous
        transhepatic (PTC,
        PTHC), 249, 978
Cholangiography, postoperative
        (T tube), 252
Cholangiopancreatography, 255
Cholescintigraphy, 1057
Cholesterol (total), 258
Cholesterol fractionation, 260
Chorionic villus biopsy, 165
Chylomicrons, 753
Cl. *See* Chloride, serum
Clot retraction, 263
Clotting time (CT), 261
CMG. *See* Cystometry
Coagulation factor assays, 265
Coccidioidomycosis skin test,
        1118
Cold agglutinin titer, 268
Cold stimulation, 270
Colonoscopy, 272
Color perception test, 275
Colposcopy, 277
Complement assay, serum, 1109
Complete blood count (CBC),
        280
Computed tomography (CT),
        abdomen, 284
Computed tomography (CT),
        biliary tract and liver, 287

Computed tomography (CT), cranial, 291

Computed tomography (CT), orbital, 295

Computed tomography (CT), pancreatic, 298

Computed tomography (CT), pelvic, 301

Computed tomography (CT), renal, 305

Computed tomography (CT), spinal, 309

Computed tomography (CT), thoracic, 313

Computerized axial tomography (CAT). *See* Computed tomography (CT) *of targeted body region*

Computerized transaxial tomography (CTT). *See* Computed tomography (CT) *of targeted body region*

Concentration/dilution tests, urine, 316

Contraction stress test (CST), 321

Coombs antibody test, 326

Coombs antiglobulin, direct (DAT), 325

Coombs antiglobulin, indirect (IAT), 326

Coproporphyrin, urine (UCP), 329

Corneal staining, 332

Corticotropin, 117

Cortisol, 334

Cortisol-free, urine, 337

Coxsackie A or B virus, 339

C-peptide, 216

C-reactive protein (CRP), 218

Cr-51 platelet survival time, 341

Cr-51 red cell survival time, 344

Cranial CT, 291

Creatine kinase and isoenzymes, 347

Creatine phosphokinase (CPK) and isoenzymes, 347

Creatinine, 350

Creatinine clearance, urine, 354

Creatinine, urine, 352

Cross-match compatibility. *See* Blood typing

Cryofibrinogen, 360

Cryoglobulin, 358

CSF analysis. *See* Cerebrospinal fluid analysis

CST. *See* Contraction stress test

CT. *See* Computed tomography *headings*

CTT. *See* Computerized transaxial tomography

Culdoscopy, 360

Culture, anal or genital, 363

Culture, blood, 365

Culture, duodenal and gastric, 369

Culture, ear, 371

Culture, eye, 373

Culture, gastric, 369

Culture, gonorrhea, 375

Culture, herpesvirus (HSV-1, HSV-2), 378

Culture, nasal or throat, 380

Culture, skin, 383

Culture and smear, acid-fast bacillus (AFB), 397

Culture, sputum, 386

Culture, stool, 390

Culture, urine with Gram's stain, 392

Culture, wound, 395

CXR. *See* Chest x-ray

Cyclic adenosine monophosphate (cAMP), 401

Cystometry (CMG), 404

Cystoscopy, 407

Cytology, sputum, 411

DAT. *See* Coombs antiglobulin, direct

Delta ALA. *See* Delta-aminolevulinic acid urine

Delta-aminolevulinic acid (delta ALA), urine, 419

Dexamethasone suppression test (DST), 420

Diaphanography, breast, 425

Dick test, 427

DIFF. *See* White blood cell count, total and differential

Digital radiography. *See* Angiography, digital subtraction (DSA)

Digital subtraction angiography (DSA), 76
Digital venous subtraction angiography (DVSA), 76
Dilution tests, urine. *See* Concentration/dilution tests, urine
D-dimer, 415
Dipyridamole-thallium scan, 1038
Direct Coombs. *See* Coombs antiglobulin, direct (DAT)
Direct fluorescent antibody, 649
Direct IgG. *See* Coombs antiglobulin, direct (DAT)
Drug abuse survey. *See* Drug levels, urine
Drug levels, serum, 429–443.
Drug levels, urine, 443–447.
Duodenal culture, 369

E$_2$. *See* Estradiol
E$_3$. *See* Estriol
Ear culture, 371
EBV. *See* Epstein-Barr virus (EBV) antibodies
Echocardiography, 448
Echocardiography, transesophageal, 451
EGD. *See* Esophagogastroduodenoscopy
Electro-oculography (EOG), 454
Electrocardiogram. *See* Electrocardiography (ECG)
Electrocardiography (ECG), 456
Electrocardiography, ambulatory, 462
Electrocardiography, exercise, 465
Electrocardiography, His bundle, 469
Electroencephalogram (EEG), 472
Electroencephalography (EEG), 472
Electrolytes, serum, 475
Electrolytes, urine, 485
Electromyogram (EMG), 491
Electromyography (EMG), 491
Electromyography, pelvic floor sphincter, 494

Electroneurography (ENG), 495
Electronystagmography (ENG), 498
Electrophoresis, hemoglobin, 640
Electrophoresis, lipoprotein, 753
Electrophoresis, serum protein, 913
Electrophoresis, urine protein, 913
Electroretinography (ERG), 501
ELISA. *See* Enzyme-linked immunosorbent assay
ENA. *See* Extractable nuclear antigen antibodies
Endoscopic retrograde cholangiopancreatography (ERCP). *See* Cholangiopancreatography
ENG. *See* Electroneurography *and* Electronystagmography
Enzyme-linked immunosorbent assay (ELISA), 504
EP studies. *See* Evoked potential studies
Epstein-Barr virus (EBV) antibodies, 506
ERG. *See* Electroretinography
ERP. *See* Event-related potential
Erythrocyte count, 1003
Erythrocyte distribution, fetal-maternal, 508
Erythrocyte fragility, 510
Erythrocyte indices, 1008
Erythrocyte sedimentation rate (ESR, sed rate), 512
Esophageal acid study, 787
Esophageal function study, 787
Esophageal manometry, 787
Esophagogastroduodenoscopy (EGD), 515
ESR. *See* Erythrocyte sedimentation rate
Estradiol (E$_2$), serum, 521
Estradiol receptor assay, 518
Estriol (E$_3$), serum, 521
Estrogens, serum, 521. *See also* Estradiol (E$_2$) *and* Estriol (E$_3$) *headings*
Estrogens, urine, total and fractions, 524

Estrone (E₁), 524
Euglobulin clot lysis time, 528
Event-related potential (ERP), 530
Evoked brain potentials, 530
Evoked potential studies (EP studies), 530
Excretory urography (EUG), 964
Exercise stress test, 465
Exophthalmometry, 543
External fetal monitoring (nonstress test), 550
Extractable nuclear antigen (ENA) antibodies, 536
Eye culture, 373

Fasting blood sugar (FSB), 596
FBP. See Fibrin breakdown products
FDP. See Fibrin degradation products
Fe. See Iron
Febrile agglutinins, serum, 544
Fecal analysis, 538
Fecal fat, 542
FEP. See Free erythrocyte protoporphyrin
Ferric chloride (FeCl₃), 546
Ferritin, 548
Fetal hemoglobin stain, 508
Fetal monitoring: external (nonstress test), 550
Fetal monitoring, internal, 553
Fetal-maternal erythrocyte distribution, 508
Fetoscopy, 556
FFA. See Free fatty acids
Fibrin breakdown products (FBP), 559
Fibrin degradation products (FDP), 559
Fibrin split products (FSP), 559
Fibrinogen, 561
Fibrinogen uptake test (FUT), 563
Fluorescein angiography, 79
Fluorescent rabies antibody test (FRA), 565
Fluorescent treponemal antibody test (FTA-ABS), 567

Fluoroscopy, thoracic, 569
Folates, 571
Folic acid, 571
Folic acids (RBCs), 571
Follicle-stimulating hormone (FSH), 573
FRA. See Fluorescent rabies antibody test
Free cortisol. See Cortisol-free, urine
Free erythrocyte protoporphyrin (FEP), 930
Free fatty acids (FFA), 575
Fructose challenge test, 578
FSH. See Follicle-stimulating hormone
FSP. See Fibrin split products
FTA-ABS. See Fluorescent treponemal antibody test
Fungal antibody tests, 580
FUT. See Fibrinogen uptake test

Gallbladder scan, 1057
Gallium bone scan, 1048
Gallium breast scan, 1044
Gallium liver scan, 1051
Gamma globulin, 590
Gamma glutamyl transpeptidase (GGTP, GGT), 582
Gastric acid stimulation test, 585
Gastric culture, 369
Gastrin, 588
Gastroesophageal reflux scan, 1054
Genital culture, 363
GH. See Growth hormone
GHB. See Glycohemoglobin
Globulin, 590. See also named fractions
Glucagon, 594
Glucose, 596. See also Fasting blood sugar (FSB)
Glucose tolerance tests, 607
Glucose, random, 596
Glucose, two-hour postprandial (PPBS), 600
Glucose, urine, 603
Glutamic-oxaloacetic transaminase (SGOT). See Aspartate aminotransferase (AST)

Glutamic-pyruvic transaminase (SGPT). *See* Alanine aminotransferase (ALT)
Glycohemoglobin (GHB), 633
Gonorrhea culture, 375
Growth hormone challenge test, 692
Growth hormone (GH, hGH, STH, SH), 612
Growth hormone stimulation test, 615
Growth hormone suppression test, 617
Guthrie test, 619
Gynecologic laparoscopy, 729
Gynecologic pelviscopy, 729

Ham test, 621
Haptoglobin (Hp), 623
HATTS. *See* Hemagglutination treponemal test for syphilis
Hb. *See* Hemoglobin
HBDH. *See* Hydroxybutyrate dehydrogenase
HBeAb. *See* Hepatitis B antibody and antigen
HBeAg. *See* Hepatitis B antibody and antigen
HbM. *See* Methemoglobin
hCG. *See* Human chorionic gonadotropin *entries*
hCT. *See* Calcitonin
HDL-cholesterol. *See* Lipoprotein-cholesterol fractionation
Heart and chest MRI, 778
Heart and chest NMR, 778
Heart imaging, 1038
Heart, plain films, 981
Heinz bodies stain, 625
Hemagglutination treponemal test for syphilis (HATTS), 626
Hematocrit (Hct), 628
Hemoglobin and blood, urine, 637
Hemoglobin electrophoresis, 640
Hemoglobin (Hb), 630
Hemoglobin, glycosylated (GHB), 633

Hemoglobin, unstable, 635
Hemosiderin, 643
Hepatitis B antibody and antigen (anti-HBe, HBeAb, HBeAg), 645
Hepatitis B surface antigen, 145
Hepatitis profile, prenatal, 647
Hepatobiliary imaging, 1057
Hepatobiliary scintigraphy, 1057
Herpesvirus antigen, 649
Herpesvirus (HSV-1, HSV-2) culture, 378
Heterophil antibody. *See* Monospot
Hexosaminidase A, 650
Hgb S (sickle cell test), 1113
hGH. *See* Growth hormone
HIDA scan, 1057
His bundle electrocardiography, 469
Histoplasmosis skin test, 1118
Holter electrocardiography, 462
Holter monitoring, 462
Homovanillic acid (HVA), 652
HP. *See* Haptoglobin
HPRL. *See* Prolactin
HSV-1 *or* HSV-2. *See* Culture, herpesvirus
Human chorionic gonadotropin (hCG), 655
Human chorionic gonadotropin (hCG), pregnancy test, 657
Human leukocyte antigen and typing (HLA, tissue typing), 660
Human placental lactogen (HPL), serum, 662
HVA. *See* Homovanillic acid
5-Hydroxyindoleacetic acid (5-HIAA), 670
Hydroxybutyrate dehydrogenase (HBDH), 665
17-Hydroxycorticosteroids (17-OHCS), 667
5-Hydroxyproline, 673
5-Hydroxytryptamine. *See* Serotonin
Hysterogram, 968
Hysterosalpingography, 968
Hysteroscopy, 676

IAT. *See* Coombs antiglobulin, indirect
ICD. *See* Isocitrate dehydrogenase
ICSH. *See* Luteinizing hormone
IF. *See* Intrinsic factor antibody
Immune complex assay, serum, 678
Immunoglobulin electrophoresis, serum, 680
Immunoglobulin electrophoresis, urine, 683
Immunoglobulin G, subclassification, 686
Impedance plethysmography, 874
Indirect Coombs. *See* Coombs antiglobulin, indirect (IAT)
Influenza A and B titer, 688
INR. *See* International Normalized Ratio (INR)
Insulin, 689
Insulin antibody, 695
Insulin clearance test, 699
Insulin tolerance test, 692
Internal fetal monitoring, 553
International Normalized Ratio (INR), 927
Intestinal biopsy, 167
Intradermal test. *See* Skin tests *entries*
Intravenous glucose tolerance test (IVGTT), 607
Intravenous pyelography (IVP), 964
Intravenous urography (IUG, IVU), 964
Intrinsic factor (IF) antibody, 697
Iodine washout test, 1207
Iron (Fe), 701
Iron-binding capacity, total (TIBC). *See* Total iron-binding capacity
Isocitrate dehydrogenase (ICD), 707
Isonitrile scan, 1038
IUG. *See* Intravenous urography
IVGTT. *See* Intravenous glucose tolerance test
IVP. *See* Intravenous pyelography
IVU. *See* Intravenous urography

K. *See* Potassium, serum
17-Ketogenic steroids (17-KGS), 709
Ketones, 712
17-Ketosteroids (17-KS) and fractionation, 714
Kidney. *See also* Renal *entries*
Kidney biopsy, 170
Kidney renography scan, 1060
Kidney-ureter-bladder (KUB) plain films, 981
Kleihauer-Betke stain, 508

Lactic acid, 718
Lactic dehydrogenase (LDH, LD) and isoenzymes, 720
Lactose tolerance test, 724
Laminography, chest, 1185
LAP. *See* White blood cell enzymes
Laparoscopy, abdominal, 726
Laparoscopy, gynecologic, 729
Laryngoscopy, 733
LATS. *See* Long-acting thyroid stimulator
Laxative abuse test, 852
LD or LDH. *See* Lactic dehydrogenase and isoenzymes
LDL-cholesterol. *See* Lipoprotein-cholesterol fractionation
LES. *See* Ultrasound, arterial Doppler, lower extremity studies
Lead (Pb), 738
Lee-White clotting time. *See* Clotting time (CT)
Legionnaires' disease antibodies, 740
Leucine aminopeptidase (LAP), serum, 741
Leucine aminopeptidase (LAP), urine, 743
Leukoagglutinin, 746
Leukocyte alkaline phosphatase stain, 746
Leukocyte count. *See* White blood cell count (WBC), total and differential
LH. *See* Luteinizing hormone

Lipase, 750
Lipoprotein electrophoresis, 753
Lipoprotein phenotyping, 756
Lipoprotein-cholesterol fractionation, 753
Liver angiography. *See* Angiography, liver and portal vein
Liver and biliary system ultrasonography, 1236
Liver biopsy, 173
Liver CT, 287
Liver and portal vein angiography, 83
Liver scan, 1065
Liver scan, gallium, 1051
Long bone x-rays, 956
Long-acting thyroid stimulator (LATS), 1175
Lower extremity angiography, 87
Lower extremity arterial (LEA) Doppler, 1268
Lower extremity venous Doppler, 1274
Lower limb venography, 1299
LTH. *See* Prolactin
Lumbar puncture: cerebrospinal fluid (CSF) analysis, 760
Lung. *See also* Pulmonary *headings*
Lung biopsy, 176
Lung perfusion scan, 1069
Lung scintiscan, 1069
Lung ventilation scan, 1072
Luteinizing hormone (LH, ICSH), 766
Lyme disease antibody, 769
Lymph node biopsy, 179
Lymph node and retroperitoneal ultrasonography, 1239
Lymphangiogram, 91, 972
Lymphangiography, 91, 972
Lymphography, 972
Lysozyme (muramidase), 807

Magnesium (Mg), serum, 475
Magnesium (Mg), urine, 488
Magnetic resonance imaging (MRI), abdominal, 770

Magnetic resonance imaging (MRI), head, 774
Magnetic resonance imaging (MRI), heart and chest, 778
Magnetic resonance imaging (MRI), musculoskeletal, 781
Mammography, 784
Manometry, esophageal, 787
Meckel scan, 1076
Mediastinoscopy, 791
Melanin, 794
Mesenteric angiography, 94
Metanephrines, total, 795
Methemoglobin (MetHb, HbM), 798
Mg. *See* Magnesium
MHA-TP. *See* Microhemagglutination treponema pallidum
Microhemagglutination treponema pallidum (MHA-TP), 800
Monospot (heterophil antibody), 801
Motile sperm, wet mount from fornix, 803
MRI. *See* Magnetic resonance imaging *entries*
MUGA. *See* Multigated pool imaging
Multigated pool imaging (MUGA), 1038
Mumps test, mumps antibody, 805
Muramidase (lysozyme), 807
Muscle biopsy, 181
Musculoskeletal MRI, 781
Musculoskeletal NMR, 781
Myelography, 810
Myocardial scan, 1038
Myoglobin, serum, 812
Myoglobin, urine, 814

Na. *See* Sodium, serum
Nails. *See* Skin culture
Nasal culture, 380
Neonatal thyrotropin, 1171
Nerve conduction studies, 495

Neutrophil alkaline phosphatase, 746

NMR. *See* Nuclear magnetic resonance imaging *entries*

Nonstress (external) fetal monitoring, 550

Nuclear heart scan, 1038

Nuclear magnetic resonance (NMR) imaging, abdominal, 770

Nuclear magnetic resonance (NMR) imaging, head, 774

Nuclear magnetic resonance (NMR) imaging, heart and chest, 778

Nuclear magnetic resonance (NMR) imaging, musculoskeletal, 781

5'-Nucleotidase, 816

Obstetric ultrasonography, 1242

Occult blood, 818

OCT. *See* Ornithine carbamoyltransferase *and* Oxytocin challenge test

Ocular ultrasonography, 1245

Oculoplethysmograph (OPG), 820

Oculopneumoplethysmograph (OPPG), 820

OGTT. *See* Oral glucose tolerance test

O/P. *See* Ova and parasites, stool

Oral glucose tolerance test (OGTT), 607

Orbit and eye, plain films, 981

Orbital CT, 295

Ornithine carbamoyltransferase (OCT), 823

Osmotic fragility, 510

Otoscopy, 825

Ova and parasites (O/P), stool, 828

Oximetry, 830

Oxytocin challenge test (OCT), 321

P. *See* Phosphorus, serum

Pancreatic CT, 298

PAP. *See* Prostatic acid phosphatase

Papanicolaou (Pap) smear, 833

Paracentesis, 835

Paranasal sinuses tomography, 1188

Parasite screen, stool, 828

Parathyroid hormone (PTH), 840

Parathyroid scan, 1079

Parathyroid ultrasonography, 1263

Parotid and salivary glands scan, 1082

Partial thromboplastin time (PTT), 15

Patch test. *See* Allergen skin tests

PCG. *See* Phonocardiograph

Pelvic CT, 301

Pelvic floor sphincter electromyography, 494

Pelvic radiography, 975

Pelvic ultrasonography, 1251

Pelvimetry, 842, 975

Pelviscopy, gynecologic, 729

Pepsinogen, 844

Perchlorate suppression study, 1207

Percutaneous transhepatic cholangiography (PTC, PTHC), 249, 978

Pericardial fluid analysis, 846

Pericardiocentesis, 846

Peritoneal fluid analysis, 835

Peritonoscopy, abdominal, 726

PET. *See* Positron emission tomography

pH, urine, 850

Phenolphthalein test, 852

Phenolsulfonphthalein (PSP), 854

Phenylalanine screening, serum, 619

Phlebography. *See* Venography *entries*

Phonocardiograph (PCG), 858

Phospholipids, 861

Phosphorus (P), serum, 475

Phosphorus (P), urine, 488

Pilocarpine iontophoresis (sweat test), 1130

Planigraphy, chest, 1185

Plasma renin activity, 1013
Plasma renin angiotensin (PRA), 1013
Plasma thrombin time, 1148
Plasminogen, 863
Platelet aggregation, 865
Platelet antibody detection, 869
Platelet count (thrombocyte), 871
Plethysmography, 874
Pleural fluid analysis, 1150
Porphyrins (erythrocyte), total, 880
Porphyrins, urine, 882
Portal vein angiography, 83
Positron emission tomography (PET), 885, 1085
Postcoital cervical mucus test, 1115
Postcoital test, 1115
Potassium hydroxide preparation, 889
Potassium (K), serum, 475
Potassium (K), urine, 486
PPBS. *See* Glucose, two-hour postprandial
PRA. *See* Plasma renin angiotensin
Precipitin test against human sperm and blood, 891
Pregnancy test (human chorionic gonadotropin [hCG]), 655
Pregnanediol, 893
Pregnanetriol, 897
Proctosigmoidoscopy, 899
Progesterone receptor assay, 518, 902
Prolactin (HPRL, LTH), 906
Prostate biopsy, 184
Prostate ultrasonography (transrectal), 1254
Prostate-specific antigen (PSA), 5, 909
Prostatic acid phosphatase (PAP), 5
Protein C, 911
Protein electrophoresis, serum, 913
Protein electrophoresis, urine, 917
Protein, total, 920

Protein, urine (dipstick), 923
Prothrombin consumption time (PCT), 925
Prothrombin time (PT, pro time), 927
Protoporphyrin, free erythrocyte (FEP), 930
PSA. *See* Prostate-specific antigen
Pseudocholinesterase (CHS, PCHE, AcCHS), 932
PSP. *See* Phenolsulfonphthalein
PT. *See* Prothrombin time
PTH. *See* Parathyroid hormone
PTHC. *See* Percutaneous transhepatic cholangiography
PTT. *See* Partial thromboplastin time
Pulmonary angiogram, 98
Pulmonary artery catheterization, 234
Pulmonary function studies, 935
Pulse oximetry, 830
Pyelography, antegrade, 947
Pyruvic acid, 942

Rabies antibody test, 565
Radioactive iodine uptake (RAIU), 944
Radioactive perfusion scan, 1069
Radioallergosorbent test (RAST). *See* Allergen-specific IgE
Radiography, antegrade pyelography, 947
Radiography, barium enema, 950
Radiography, barium swallow, 953
Radiography, bone, 956
Radiography, bronchus, 959
Radiography, chest, 962
Radiography, excretory urography (EUG), 964
Radiography, hysterosalpingography, 968
Radiography, lymphangiography, 972
Radiography, pelvic, 975

Radiography, percutaneous transhepatic cholangiography (PTC, PTHC), 978

Radiography, plain films, cardiac, 981

Radiography, plain films, kidney-ureter-bladder (KUB), 981

Radiography, plain films, orbit and eye, 981

Radiography, plain films, sinuses, 981

Radiography, plain films, skull, 981

Radiography, plain films, vertebra, 981

Radiography, retrograde ureteropyelography, 985

Radiography, retrograde urethrography, 988

Radiography, voiding cystourethrography, 991

Radionuclide imaging, brain, 994

Radionuclide imaging, thyroid, 996

RAIU. *See* Radioactive iodine uptake

Raji cell assay, 999

Rapid plasma reagin test (RPR test), 1001

RAST. *See* Allergen-specific IgE

RBC. *See* Red blood cell *entries*

Red blood cell indices, 1008

Red blood cell (RBC) count, 1003

Red blood cell survival time, 344

Red cell fragility, 510

Refraction, 1011

Renal. *See also* Kidney *entries*

Renal angiography, 101

Renal arteriography. *See* Renal angiography

Renal CT, 305

Renal venography, 1299

Renin assay, plasma, 1013

Renin, plasma, 1013

Renocystogram, 1060

Renocystography, 1060

Renogram scan, 1060

Respiratory syncytial virus (RSV) antibodies (IgG, IgM), 1016

Reticulocyte (retic) count, 1018

Retrograde ureteropyelography, 985

Retrograde urethrography, 988

RF. *See* Rheumatoid factor

Rh factor typing. *See* Blood typing

Rheumatoid arthritis factor (RF), 1020

Rheumatoid factor (RF), 1020

Rinne test, 1220

Rocky Mountain spotted fever antibodies, 1023

Rotavirus antigen, 1025

RPR test. *See* Rapid plasma reagin test

RSV. *See* Respiratory syncytial virus antibodies (IgG, IgM)

RT_3U. *See* T_3 resin uptake

Rubella antibodies, 1027

Rubeola antibodies, 1028

Scan, adrenal glands, 1030

Scan, bone, 1033

Scan, cardiac, 1038

Scan, gallbladder, 1057

Scan, gallium, bone, 1048

Scan, gallium, breast, 1044

Scan, gallium, liver, 1051

Scan, gastroesophageal reflux, 1054

Scan, kidney, 1060

Scan, liver, 1065

Scan, lung perfusion, 1069

Scan, lung ventilation, 1072

Scan, Meckel's diverticulum, 1076

Scan, parathyroid, 1079

Scan, parotid and salivary glands, 1082

Scan, positron emission tomography (PET), 1085

Scan, scrotal, 1088

Scan, thyroid, 1091

Schick test, 1095

Schilling test, 1097

Schirmer tearing test, 1101

Schwabach test, 1220

Scleroderma antibody, 1103

Scratch test. *See* Allergen skin tests
Scrotal scan, 1088
Scrotal ultrasonography, 1256
Secretin test, 1104
Sed rate. *See* Erythrocyte sedimentation rate (ESR)
SER. *See* Somatosensory response
Serotonin (5-hydroxytryptamine), 1107
Serum complement assay, 1109
Serum electrolytes, 475
Serum glutamic-oxaloacetic transferase (SGOT), 136
Serum protein, total, 920
Serum prothrombin time, 925
Serum viscosity, 1303
Sestamibi scan, 1038
Sex chromatin tests, 1111
SGPT. *See* Alanine aminotransferase (ALT)
Sickle cell test (sickledex; Hgb S), 1113
Sickledex (sickle cell test), 1113
Siderophilin (transferrin), 704, 1198
Signal-averaged electrocardiography, 461
Sims-Huhner test, 1115
Sinuses, plain films, 981
Skeletal x-rays, 956
Skin biopsy, 186
Skin culture, 383
Skin tests, allergen, 35
Skin tests, mycoses and histoplasmosis, 1118
Skull, plain films, 981
Slit lamp biomicroscopy, 1120
Sodium (Na), serum, 475
Sodium (Na), urine, 486
Somatosensory response (SER), 530
Specific gravity, urine, 1123
Speech reception threshold (SRT), 1126
Spinal CT, 309
Splenic ultrasonography, 1258
Spondee speech reception threshold (SRT), 1126
Sputum culture, 386
Sputum cytology, 411

SRT. *See* Spondee speech reception threshold
SS-A. *See* Anti-Ro/Sjögren's syndrome antigen
STH. *See* Growth hormone
Stool culture, 390
Stool for ova and parasites (O/P), 828
Stratigraphy, chest, 1185
Sucrose hemolysis, 1128
Sweat test (pilocarpine iontophoresis), 1130
Synovial fluid analysis, 129

T_3. *See* Triiodothyronine
T_3 resin uptake (RT_3U), 1210
T_3RIA. *See* Triiodothyronine
T_4. *See* Thyroxine
T_4RIA. *See* Thyroxine
T-131 uptake, 944
T-lymphocyte and B-lymphocyte assays, 1133
Tearing test, Schirmer, 1101
Tensilon test, 3, 1140
Testosterone, 1143
Thallium stress scan, 1038
THBR. *See* Thyroid hormone binding ratio
Thermography, breast, 1146
Thoracentesis and pleural fluid analysis, 1150
Thoracic CT, 313
Thoracic fluoroscopy, 569
Thoracic ultrasonography, 1261
Thoracoscopy, 1156
Throat culture, 380
Thrombin clotting time (TCT), 1148
Thyrocalcitonin (hCT). *See* Calcitonin
Thyroglobulin, 1158
Thyroid antithyroglobulin antibody, 1160
Thyroid-binding globulin (TBG), 1180
Thyroid biopsy, 188
Thyroid hormone binding ratio (THBR), 1162, 1210
Thyroid and parathyroid ultrasonography, 1263

Thyroid radionuclide scan, 944, 996

Thyroid scan, 1091

Thyroid scintiscan, 1091

Thyroid-stimulating hormone sensitivity (s-TSH) assay, 1167

Thyroid-stimulating hormone stimulation test, 1169

Thyroid-stimulating hormone (TSH), 1164

Thyroid-stimulating hormone, neonatal, 1171

Thyroid-stimulating immunoglobulins (TSI, TSIg), 1173

Thyroid stimulator, long-acting (LATS), 1175

Thyrotropin challenge test, 1169

Thyrotropin stimulating test, 1169

Thyroxine (T_4, T_4RIA, total T_4), 1177

Thyroxine-binding globulin (TBG), 1180

TIBC. *See* Total iron-binding capacity

Tolbutamide tolerance test, 1182

Tomography, chest, 1185

Tomography, paranasal sinuses, 1188

Tonometry, 1190

TORCH test, 1193

Total iron-binding capacity (TIBC), 704

Total T_3. *See* Triiodothyronine

Total T_4. *See* Thyroxine

Tourniquet test. *See* Capillary fragility

Toxoplasmosis (antibody and skin) tests, 1195

Transesophageal echocardiography, 451

Transferrin (siderophilin), 704, 1198

Transrectal prostate ultrasonography, 1254

Trichinosis (antibody and skin) tests, 1195

Trichomonad preparation, urogenital secretions, 1200

Triglycerides, 1202

Triiodothyronine suppression test, 1207

Triiodothyronine T_3 suppression test, 1207

Triiodothyronine (T_3, T_3RIA, total T_3), 1205

Triiodothyronine uptake, 1210

Trypsin, blood, 1213

TSH. *See* Thyroid-stimulating hormone

TSI. *See* Thyroid-stimulating immunoglobulins

TSIg. *See* Thyroid-stimulating immunoglobulins

Tuberculin skin tests, 1217

Tularemia agglutination test, 544

Tuning fork tests, 1220

Tympanometry. *See* Acoustic admittance tests

UA. *See* Urinalysis, routine

Ultrasonography, abdominal/ abdominal aorta, 1223

Ultrasonography, arterial, transcranial Doppler, 1226

Ultrasonography, bladder, 1229

Ultrasonography, breast, 1231

Ultrasonography, kidney, 1233

Ultrasonography, liver and biliary system, 1236

Ultrasonography, lymph nodes and retroperitoneal, 1239

Ultrasonography, obstetric, 1242

Ultrasonography, ocular, 1245

Ultrasonography, pancreas, 1248

Ultrasonography, pelvis, 1251

Ultrasonography, prostate (transrectal), 1254

Ultrasonography, scrotal, 1256

Ultrasonography, spleen, 1258

Ultrasonography, thoracic, 1261

Ultrasonography, thyroid and parathyroid, 1263

Ultrasonography, venous Doppler, lower extremity studies, 1274

Ultrasound, arterial Doppler, carotid studies, 1266

Ultrasound, arterial Doppler, lower extremity studies (LES), 1268

Ultrasound, Doppler, 1271
Unstable hemoglobin, 635
Upper extremity angiography, 105
Uric acid, serum, 1277
Uric acid, urine, 1280
Urinalysis, routine (UA), 1283
Urine culture with Gram's stain, 392
Urine protein (dipstick), 923
Urobilinogen, 1287
Uroflowmetry, 1291
Uterography, 968
Uterosalpingography, 968

Vanillylmandelic acid (VMA), 1294
VCG. *See* Vectorcardiography
VDRL (Venereal Disease Research Laboratories test), 1297
Vectorcardiography (VCG), 461
Venography, lower limb, 1299
Venography, renal, 1299
Venous plethysmography, 874
VER. *See* Visual evoked response
Vertebra, plain films, 981
Viscosity, serum, 1303
Visual evoked response (VER), 530
Visual fields test tangent screen examination, 1304
Vitamin A, serum, 1307
Vitamin B_1, serum, 1307
Vitamin B_1, urine, 1311

Vitamin B_2, urine, 1311
Vitamin B_6, plasma, 1307
Vitamin B_{12}, serum, 1307
Vitamin C, serum, 1307
Vitamin C, urine, 1311
Vitamin D_3, serum, 1307
Vitamin E, 1307
Vitamins. *See letter-named vitamins*
VLDL. *See* Lipoprotein-cholesterol fractionation
VMA. *See* Vanillylmandelic acid
Voiding cystography, 991
Voiding cystourethrography, 991
VP. *See* Excretory urography

WBC. *See* White blood cell count, total and differential
Weber test, 1220
Weil-Felix reaction, 544
Western immunoblast assay, 1314
Wet mount from fornix for motile sperm, 803
White blood cell count (WBC), total and differential, 1315
White blood cell enzymes, 1319
Widal test, 544
Wound culture, 395

D-Xylose absorption test, 417
D-Xylose tolerance, 417

The Disorder and Condition Index

Indexed are disorders *or* conditions (normal, environmental, therapeutic) that alter test results. Tests are the subheads; page entries locate those tests.

Abdominal abscess, computed tomography (CT), abdomen, 284

Abdominal adhesions, abdominal laparoscopy, 726

Abdominal aortic aneurysm, computed tomography (CT), abdomen, 284

Abdominal lymphoma, peritoneal fluid analysis, 835

Abdominal tumors, abdominal ultrasonography, 1223

Abetalipoproteinemia, lipoprotein-cholesterol fractionation, 753

Abortion, incomplete, human chorionic gonadotropin (hCG), 655

Abortion, threatened
human chorionic gonadotropin (hCG), 655
human chorionic gonadotropin (hCG), pregnancy test, 657

human placental lactogen (HPL), serum, 662
triiodothyronine uptake, 1210

Abruptio placentae
fibrin breakdown products (FBP), 559
obstetric ultrasonography, 1242

Acalculus cholecystitis, gallbladder scan, 1057

Acanthocytosis, triglycerides, 1202

Acetanilid, methemoglobin (MetHb, HbM), 798

Achalasia, esophageal, esophageal manometry, 787

Achlorhydria, pepsinogen, 844

Achondroplasia, alkaline phosphatase (ALP), 32

Achromycin
ammonia (NH₃), 56
red blood cell (RBC) count, 1003

Acidosis
blood gases, arterial (ABG), 195

calcium (Ca), serum, 475
chloride (Cl), serum, 475
potassium (K), serum, 475
thyroid-binding globulin (TBG), 1180

Acoustic nerve impairment, spondee speech reception threshold, 1126

Acoustic neuroma, MRI, head, 774

Acquired immune deficiency syndrome. *See* AIDS

Acromegaly
creatinine, 350
fasting blood sugar (FSB), 596
follicle-stimulating hormone (FSH), 573
glucose tolerance tests, 607
glucose, two-hour postprandial (PPBS), 600
glucose, urine, 603
growth hormone (GH, hGH, STH, SH), 612
growth hormone suppression test, 617
insulin, 689
insulin antibody test, 695
luteinizing hormone (LH, ICSH), 766
thyroid-binding globulin (TBG), 1180

ACTH-producing tumors, androstenedione, 64

Actinomycosis
acid-fast bacillus (AFB) culture and smear, 397
potassium hydroxide preparation, 889

Acute granulocytic leukemia, white blood cell enzymes, 1319

Acute lymphoblastic leukemia, white blood cell enzymes, 1319

Acute lymphocytic leukemia
B-lymphocyte assays, 1133
T-lymphocyte assays, 1133

Acute monocytic leukemia, white blood cell enzymes, 1319

Acute myelocytic leukemia, white blood cell enzymes, 1319

Addison's disease
adrenocorticotropic hormone (ACTH), 17
aldosterone, urine, 29
antidiuretic hormone (ADH), 116
blood gases, arterial (ABG), 194
blood urea nitrogen (BUN), 203
chloride (Cl), urine, 486
cortisol, 334
fasting blood sugar (FSB), 596
glucose tolerance tests, 607
glucose, two-hour postprandial (PPBS), 600
17-hydroxycorticosteroids (17-OHCS), 667
17-ketogenic steroids (17-KGS), 709
17-ketosteroids (17-KS) and fractionation, 714
magnesium (Mg), serum, 475
magnesium (Mg), urine, 488
pepsinogen, 844
potassium (K), serum, 475
prolactin (HPRL, LTH), 906
renin, plasma, 1013
serum protein, total, 920
sodium (Na), serum, 475
sweat test (pilocarpine iontophoresis), 1130

Ademomas, 17-ketogenic steroids (17-KGS), 709

Adenofibroma, breast biopsy, 161

Adenovirus, eye culture, 373

Adrenal adenoma
adrenal angiography, 66
17-hydroxycorticosteroids (17-OHCS), 667

Adrenal carcinoma
adrenal angiography, 66
fasting blood sugar (FSB), 596
glucose, two-hour postprandial (PPBS), 600
17-hydroxycorticosteroids (17-OHCS), 667

Adrenal carcinoma—*Continued*
  17-ketogenic steroids
    (17-KGS), 709
Adrenal cortex tumor
  androstenedione, 64
  17-ketosteroids (17-KS) and
    fractionation, 714
  pregnanediol, 893
  pregnanetriol, 897
  testosterone, 1143
Adrenal cortex, structural
    disorders of,
    adrenocorticotropic
    hormone (ACTH), 17
Adrenal corticosteroid therapy
  adrenocorticotropic hormone
    (ACTH), 17
  calcium (Ca), serum, 475
  calcium (Ca), urine, 487
  cortisol-free, urine, 337
  estrogens, urine, total and
    fractions, 524
  fasting blood sugar (FSB), 596
  glucose tolerance tests, 607
  glucose, two-hour postprandial
    (PPBS), 600
  glucose, urine, 603
  17-hydroxycorticosteroids
    (17-OHCS), 667
  pregnanediol, 893
  sodium (Na), serum, 475
  sodium (Na), urine, 486
  thyroid-stimulating hormone
    (TSH), 1164
Adrenal gland hyperfunction,
    See Cushing's syndrome
Adrenal gland insufficiency,
    glucose tolerance tests,
    607
Adrenal hyperplasia
  adrenal angiography, 66
  androstenedione, 64
  dexamethasone suppression
    test (DST), 420
  estrogens, serum, 521
  17-hydroxycorticosteroids
    (17-OHCS), 667
  testosterone l, 1143
Adrenal hyperplasia, congenital,
  17-ketosteroids (17-KS)
    and fractionation, 714

Adrenal infarction, adrenal
    glands scan, 1030
Adrenal insufficiency
  estrogens, serum, 523
  glucose tolerance tests, 607
  insulin challenge test, 692
  specific gravity, urine, 1123
Adrenal suppression, adrenal
    glands scan, 1030
Adrenal tumors
  adrenal glands scan, 1030
  computed tomography (CT),
    renal, 305
  cortisol-free, urine, 337
  dexamethasone suppression
    test (DST), 420
  estradiol (E₂), serum, 521
  estrogens, serum, 521
  estrogens, urine, total and
    fractions, 524
  17-ketosteroids (17-KS) and
    fractionation, 714
Adrenalectomy
  17-ketosteroids (17-KS) and
    fractionation, 714
  magnesium (Mg), serum, 475
Adrenocortical carcinoma,
    17-ketosteroids (17-KS)
    and fractionation, 714
Adrenocortical hyperplasia
  pregnanediol, 893
  pregnanetriol, 897
  testosterone, 1143
Adrenocortical hypofunction
  amino acid screen, blood, 45
  chloride (Cl), urine, 486
  magnesium (Mg), urine, 488
  reticulocyte (retic) count,
    1018
  sodium (Na), urine, 486
Adrenogenital syndrome
  estrogens, urine, total and
    fractions, 524
  follicle-stimulating hormone
    (FSH), 573
  17-ketogenic steroids
    (17-KGS), 709
  17-ketosteroids (17-KS) and
    fractionation, 714
  luteinizing hormone (LH,
    ICSH), 766

pregnanediol, 893
pregnanetriol, 897
Adult respiratory distress
      syndrome (ARDS), 108
   blood gases, arterial (ABG),
      194
Afibrinogenemia
   activated clotting time (ACT),
      13
   clotting time (CT), 261
   platelet aggregation, 865
Agammaglobulinemia,
      immunoglobulin
      electrophoresis, serum,
      680
Agranulocytosis, bone marrow
      aspiration and analysis,
      204
AIDS
   beta$_2$-microglobulin, 917
   protein electrophoresis, serum,
      913
   T-lymphocyte assays, 1133
AIDS-related complex, enzyme-
      linked immunosorbent
      assay (ELISA), 504
Airway abscess, bronchoscopy,
      209
Airway infections, pulmonary
      function studies, 935
Airway tumor, bronchoscopy,
      209
Albright's syndrome,
      5-hydroxyproline, 673
Alcoholic ketoacidosis, ketones,
      712
Alcoholic myopathy
   creatine phosphokinase (CPK)
      and isoenzymes, 347
   muscle biopsy, 182
Alcoholism
   amylase, urine, 61
   ferric chloride (FeCl$_3$), 546
   folic acid, 571
   glucose tolerance tests, 607
   lipoprotein-cholesterol
      fractionation, 753
   magnesium (Mg), serum, 475
   magnesium (Mg), urine, 488
   phosphorus (P), serum, 475
   prolactin (HPRL, LTH), 906

red blood cell indices, 1008
vitamin B$_1$, serum, 1307
vitamin B$_1$, urine, 1311
vitamin B$_2$, urine, 1311
vitamin B$_6$, plasma, 1307
vitamin E, 1307
white blood cell (WBC)
      count, 1315
Aldosterone
   bicarbonate (HCO$_3$), 475
   magnesium (Mg), serum, 475
   pH, urine, 850
Aldosteronism
   potassium (K), urine, 487
   renin, plasma, 1013
Alkali ingestion
   blood gases, arterial (ABG),
      194
   pH, urine, 850
Alkalosis
   ammonia (NH$_3$), 56
   blood gases, arterial (ABG),
      195
   calcium (Ca), serum, 475
   chloride (Cl), serum, 475
   potassium (K), serum, 475
Alkeran, Coombs antiglobulin,
      direct (DAT), 325
Allergies, alpha$_2$ globulin, 591
Alloimmune neonatal
      throbocytopenic purpura,
      869
Alpha$_1$ antitrypsin deficiency,
      alpha$_1$ globulin, 591
Alzheimer's disease
   brain scan, 994
   positron emission tomography
      (PET), 885, 1085
Ambiguous genitalia, sex
      chromatin tests, 1111
Amblyopias, evoked brain
      potentials, 530
Amebiasis
   liver biopsy, 173
   ova and parasites, stool, 828
Amebic dysentary, fungal
      antibody tests, 580
Amenorrhea
   estradiol (E$_2$), serum, 521
   pregnanediol, 893
   prolactin (HPRL, LTH), 906

Aminoacidopathies, amino acid
  screen, blood, 45
Amyloidosis
  Bence Jones protein, 147
  blood urea nitrogen (BUN),
    203
  concentration/dilution tests,
    urine, 316
  fecal fat, 542
  immunoglobulin
    electrophoresis, serum,
    680
  immunoglobulin
    electrophoresis, urine,
    683
  kidney biopsy, 170
  liver biopsy, 173
  lung biopsy, 179
  protein electrophoresis, urine,
    917
  thrombin clotting time (TCT),
    1148
  white blood cell enzymes,
    1319
  D-xylose tolerance, 417
Amyotrophic lateral sclerosis
  acetylcholine receptor
    antibody (AChR), 3
  creatinine, 350
  muscle biopsy, 182
ANA-negative SLE, anti-Ro
  Sjögren's syndrome
  antigen (SS-A), 114
Anabolic steroids
  antithrombin, 123
  creatinine clearance, urine,
    354
  fasting blood sugar (FSB), 596
  glucose tolerance tests, 607
  glucose, two-hour postprandial
    (PPBS), 600
  triglycerides, 1202
Anal fissure
  fecal analysis, 538
  proctosigmoidoscopy, 899
Anal fistula,
  proctosigmoidoscopy, 899
Analine dyes, methemoglobin
  (MetHb, HbM), 798
Anaphylaxis, immunoglobulin
  electrophoresis, serum,
  680

Androgenic arrhenoblastoma,
  17-ketosteroids (17-KS)
  and fractionation, 714
Anemia, lead (Pb), 738
Anemias
  bone marrow aspiration and
    analysis, 204
  clot retraction, 263
  Coombs antiglobulin, direct
    (DAT), 325
  coproporphyrin, urine (UCP),
    329
  Cr-51 red cell survival time,
    344
  erythrocyte sedimentation
    rate, 512
  fecal analysis, 538
  ferritin, 548
  hematocrit (Hct), 628
  hemoglobin (Hb), 630
  lactic dehydrogenase (LDH,
    LD) and isoenzymes, 720
  platelet count
    (thromobocyte), 871
  pseudocholinesterase (CHS,
    PCHE, AcCHS), 932
  serum complement assay,
    1109
  thyroid antithyroglobulin
    antibody, 1160
  urobilinogen, 1287
  white blood cell (WBC)
    count, 1315
  white blood cell enzymes,
    1319
Anencephaly
  alpha-fetoprotein (AFP), 40
  estrogens, urine, total and
    fractions, 524
Aneurysm. *See also named body
    part or organ*
  angiography, digital
    subtraction (DSA), 76
  cardiac angiography, 73
  lower extremity arterial (LEA)
    Doppler, 1268
  pericardial fluid analysis, 846
Angina pectoris
  apolipoprotein A-1 (Apo A-1),
    125
  apolipoprotein B, plasma
    (Apo B), 127

creatine phosphokinase (CPK) and isoenzymes, 347

Angiomas, angiography, digital subtraction (DSA), 76

Angular stomatitis, vitamin B$_2$, urine, 1311

Ankylosing spondylitis, human leukocyte antigen and typing (HLA, tissue typing), 660

Anorectal abscess, proctosigmoidoscopy, 899

Anorectal tumor or polyps, proctosigmoidoscopy, 899

Anorexia nervosa
catecholamines, plasma, 227
catecholamines, urine, 230
estrogens, serum, 523
estrogens, urine, total and fractions, 524
follicle-stimulating hormone (FSH), 573
growth hormone (GH, hGH, STH, SH), 612
luteinizing hormone (LH, ICSH), 766
phenolphthalein test, 852

Anovulation, follicle-stimulating hormone (FSH), 573

Anoxia, blood gases, arterial (ABG), 194

Anterior pituitary hypofunction
pregnanetriol, 897
reticulocyte (retic) count, 1018
thyroid-stimulating hormone (TSH), 1164

Anterior poliomyelitis, CSF analysis, 760

Anterior uveitis, human leukocyte antigen and typing (HLA, tissue typing), 660

Aortic aneurysm
abdominal aorta ultrasonography, 1223
computed tomography (CT), thoracic, 313

Aortic aneurysm, dissecting, pericardial fluid analysis, 846

Aortic anomalies, heart, plain films, 981

Aortic atherosclerosis, cardiac angiography, 73

Aortic coarctation, MRI, heart and chest, 778

Aortic dissection
cardiac angiography, 73
MRI, heart and chest, 778

Aortic stenosis
abdominal aorta ultrasonography, 1223
phonocardiograph (PCG), 858

Aortic valve abnormalities
angiography, digital subtraction (DSA), 76
echocardiography, 448

Aortitis, cardiac angiography, 73

Aplastic anemias
bleeding time, 191
bone marrow aspiration and analysis, 204
capillary fragility, 213
iron (Fe), 701
leukocyte alkaline phosphatase stain, 748
MRI, musculoskeletal, 781
reticulocyte (retic) count, 1018
white blood cell enzymes, 1319

Appendiceal carcinoid tumors, 5-hydroxyindoleacetic acid (5-HIAA), 670

Appendiceal rupture, peritoneal fluid analysis, 835

Appendicitis, abdominal laparoscopy, 726

Arrhenoblastoma
17-ketogenic steroids (17-KGS), 709
17-ketosteroids (17-KS) and fractionation, 714
testosterone, 1143

Arrhythmias, cardiac
aspartate aminotransferase (AST), 136
blood gases, arterial (ABG), 194

Arterial fistula, cerebral, cerebral angiography, 70

Arterial hypoplasia or stenosis, pulmonary angiogram, 98

Arterial occlusion
  angiography, digital
      subtraction (DSA), 76
  ultrasound, Doppler, 1271
Arterial stenosis or infarction of
      kidney, renal
      angiography, 102
Arterial trauma of kidney, renal
      angiography, 102
Arteriosclerosis
  angiography, digital
      subtraction (DSA), 76
  antithrombin, 123
Arteriovascular shunts of retina,
      angiography, fluorescein,
      79
Arteriovenous malformation,
      cerebral
  cerebral angiogram, 70
  computed tomography (CT),
      cranial, 291
  MRI, head, 774
Arteriovenous malformation,
      pulmonary, pulmonary
      angiogram, 98
Arteriovenous malformation,
      renal, renal angiography,
      102
Arthritis
  haptoglobin, 623
  skeletal x-rays, 956
Asbestos, antinuclear antibody
      (ANA), 119
Ascaris lumbricoides, fecal
      analysis, 538
Ascites
  abdominal laparoscopy, 726
  peritoneal fluid analysis, 835
  pleural fluid analysis, 1150
  D-xylose tolerance, 417
Aseptic meningeal reaction, CSF
      analysis, 760
Asherman's syndrome,
      hysteroscopy, 676
Aspergilloma, pulmonary
      angiogram, 98
Aspergillosis
  fungal antibody tests, 580
  potassium hydroxide
      preparation, 889
  skin culture, 383
    sputum culture, 386
    wound culture, 395
Aspermatogenesis, follicle-
      stimulating hormone
      (FSH), 573
Aspirin, excessive, ketones, 712
Asthma
    blood gases, arterial (ABG),
      194
    gamma globulin, 590
    immunoglobulin
      electrophoresis, serum,
      680
    pulmonary function studies,
      935
Astigmatism, refraction, 1011
Atalectasis, lung perfusion scan,
      1069
Ataxia-telangiectasia
    immunoglobulin
      electrophoresis, serum,
      680
    immunoglobulin G,
      subclassification, 686
Atelectasis
    blood gases, arterial (ABG),
      194
    plethysmography, 876
Atheromatoses, platelet
      aggregation, 865
Atherosclerosis
    cholesterol (total), 258
    triglycerides, 1202
Atherosclerosis, aortic, cardiac
      angiography, 73
Atherosclerosis, cerebral,
      cerebral angiography, 70
Atopic allergy, immunoglobulin
      G, subclassification, 686
Atopic eczema, T-lymphocyte
      assays, 1133
Atopic skin disease,
      immunoglobulin
      electrophoresis, serum, 680
Atrial hypertrophy
    electrocardiography (ECG), 456
    heart, plain films, 981
Atrial thrombosis, D-dimer, 415
Atrioventricular block,
      phonocardiograph (PCG),
      858

Atrioventricular valve regurgitation, phonocardiograph (PCG), 858

Atrophic gastritis, pepsinogen, 844

Auditory nerve lesions, acoustic admittance tests, 9

Autoimmune anemias
  erythrocyte fragility, 510
  thyroid antithyroglobulin antibody, 1160

Autoimmune disorders
  enzyme-linked immunosorbent assay (ELISA), 504
  protein electrophoresis, serum, 913
  Raji cell assay, 999
  serum complement assay, 1109
  thyroid antithyroglobulin antibody, 1160
  white blood cell (WBC) count, 1315

Autoimmune hemolytic anemia, hemoglobin and blood, urine, 637

Autoimmune hemolytic disease, T-lymphocyte assays, 1133

Autolytic anemia, thyroid antithyroglobulin antibody, 1160

Avascular necrosis, knee or femoral head, MRI, musculoskeletal, 781

AVC vaginal cream, red blood cell (RBC) count, 1003

Azotemia, ammonia (NH_3), 56

B cell failure, insulin, 689

Bacteremia, blood culture, 365

Bacterial arthritis, synovial fluid analysis, 129

Bacterial infections
  C-reactive protein (CRP), 218
  culture, nasal or throat, 380
  peritoneal fluid analysis, 835
  Raji cell assay, 999
  stool culture, 390

Bacterial pericarditis, pericardial fluid analysis, 846

Bacterial pneumonia
  carcinoembryonic antigen (CEA), 225
  sputum culture, 386

Bacteroids, skin culture, 383

Balkan syndrome, protein electrophoresis, urine, 917

Barbiturate toxicity, myoglobin, urine, 814

Basal cell carcinoma, skin biopsy, 186

Basilar arterial insufficiency, ultrasonography, arterial, transcranial Doppler, 1226

BCG vaccine, gamma globulin, 590

Bejel
  hemagglutination treponemal test for syphilis (HATTS), 626
  microhemagglutination *Treponema pallidum* (MHA-TP), 800

Benign prostatic hypertrophy (BPH)
  prostate biopsy, 184
  prostate ultrasonography (transrectal), 1254
  prostate-specific antigen (PSA), 909

Benzenes
  platelet count (thromobocyte), 871
  porphyrins, urine, 882

Benzocaine, methemoglobin (MetHb, HbM), 798

Beriberi, vitamin B_1, serum, 1307

Bernard-Soulier syndrome
  bleeding time, 191
  platelet aggregation, 865

Beta-thalassemia, trypsin, blood, 1213

Beta-thalassemia major, platelet aggregation, 865

Bicornate uterus, hysterosalpingography, 968

Bile duct inflammation, culture, duodenal and gastric, 369

Bile duct obstruction or stricture
  amylase, serum, 58
  bilirubin, serum, 151
  cholangiography,
    percutaneous
    transhepatic (PTHC), 249
Biliary atresia
  alkaline phosphatase (ALP),
    32
  bilirubin, serum, 151
  isocitrate dehydrogenase
    (ICD), 707
  leucine aminopeptidase
    (LAP), urine, 743
Biliary cirrhosis
  beta globulin, 590
  bilirubin, serum, 151
  immune complex assay,
    serum, 678
  lipoprotein-cholesterol
    fractionation, 753
  T-lymphocyte assays, 1133
Biliary duct abnormalities,
    percutaneous
    transhepatic
    cholangiography (PTC,
    PTHC), 249, 978
Biliary tract atresia, leucine
    aminopeptidase (LAP),
    serum, 741
Biliary tract disease, fecal
    analysis, 538
Biliary tract inflammation,
    culture, duodenal and
    gastric, 369
Biliary tract obstruction
  alanine aminotransferase
    (ALT), 20
  alkaline phosphatase (ALP),
    32
  aspartate aminotransferase
    (AST), 136
  bilirubin, urine, 155
  leucine aminopeptidase
    (LAP), serum, 741
  leucine aminopeptidase
    (LAP), urine, 743
  lipoprotein-cholesterol
    fractionation, 753
  liver and biliary system
    ultrasonography, 1236

5'-nucleotidase, 816
  pregnanediol, 893
Biliary tract stricture
  leucine aminopeptidase
    (LAP), serum, 741
  leucine aminopeptidase
    (LAP), urine, 743
Bladder calculi, computed
    tomography (CT), pelvic,
    301
Bladder cancer
  arylsulfatase A (ARS-A), urine,
    133
  bladder biopsy, 157
  occult blood, 818
Bladder cyst, bladder
    ultrasonography, 1229
Bladder hematomas, voiding
    cystourethrography, 991
Bladder infection or inflam-
    mation, cystoscopy, 407
Bladder paralysis, cystometry
    (CMG), 404
Bladder polyps
  bladder biopsy, 157
  cystoscopy, 407
Bladder trauma, voiding
    cystourethrography, 991
Bladder tumors
  bladder ultrasonography, 1229
  cystoscopy, 407
  excretory urography (EUG),
    964
  voiding cystourethrography,
    991
Blastomycosis
  bronchoscopy, 209
  fungal antibody tests, 580
  lung biopsy, 179
  potassium hydroxide
    preparation, 889
  skin culture, 383
Bleeding disorders, occult blood,
    818
Bleeding, exessive, fibrin
    breakdown products
    (FBP), 559
Blepharitis, slit lamp
    biomicroscopy, 1120
Blind-loop syndrome, fecal fat,
    542

Blood loss, hematocrit (Hct), 628
Blood vessel trauma,
    hemoglobin and blood,
    urine, 637
Blood volume changes,
    aldosterone, plasma, 25
Bone biopsy, 159
Bone cancer
    ceruloplasmin (Cp), 243
    potassium (K), urine, 487
Bone diseases, metabolic,
    alkaline phosphatase
    (ALP), 32
Bone infection, gallium bone
    scan, 1048
Bone inflammation, gallium
    bone scan, 1048
Bone marrow cancer, bone
    marrow aspiration and
    analysis, 204
Bone marrow disease, MRI,
    musculoskeletal, 781
Bone marrow failure
    bone marrow aspiration and
    analysis, 204
    reticulocyte (retic) count,
    1018
Bone marrow hyperplasia,
    hematocrit (Hct), 628
Bone marrow malignancies,
    platelet count
    (thromobocyte), 871
Bone necrosis, bone scan, 1033
Bone spurs, skeletal x-rays, 956
Bone tumor
    gallium bone scan, 1048
    5-hydroxyproline, 673
Bone tumors, metastatic,
    alkaline phosphatase
    (ALP), 32
Bordetella pertussis, nasal or
    throat culture, 380
Bowel disease, inflammatory
    C-reactive protein (CRP), 218
    fecal analysis, 538
BPH. *See* Benign prostatic
    hypertrophy
Brady-tachyarrhythmia
    syndrome,
    electrocardiography,
    ambulatory, 462

Bradyarrhythmias,
    electrocardiography,
    ambulatory, 462
Bradycardia,
    electrocardiography,
    exercise, 465
Brain. *See also* Cerebral *entries*
Brain abscess, CSF analysis,
    760
Brain cancer, CSF analysis, 760
Brain damage, amino acid
    screen, blood, 45
Brain death
    brain scan, 994
    ultrasonography, arterial,
    transcranial Doppler,
    1226
Brain hemorrhage, glucose,
    urine, 603
Brain infarction, CSF analysis,
    237, 760
Brain surgery, creatine
    phosphokinase (CPK)
    and isoenzymes, 347
Brain trauma
    creatine phosphokinase (CPK)
    and isoenzymes, 347
    CSF analysis, 237, 760
Brain tumor
    computed tomography (CT),
    cranial, 291
    CSF analysis, 760
    electroencephalography
    (EEG), 472
    glucose, urine, 603
    metanephrines, total, 795
    positron emission tomography
    (PET), 885, 1085
    visual fields test, 1304
Breast abscess, gallium breast
    scan, 1044
Breast cancer
    beta$_2$-microglobulin, 149
    calcitonin, 220
    cancer antigen 125 (CA-125),
    223
    carcinoembryonic antigen
    (CEA), 225
    ferritin, 548
    fibrinogen, 561
    potassium (K), urine, 487

Breast cancer—*Continued*
progesterone receptor assay, 902
thermography, 1146
Breast cysts, mammography, 784
Breast-feeding, prolactin (HPRL, LTH), 906
Breast infections, thermography, 1146
Breast inflammation, gallium breast scan, 1044
Breast tumors
breast ultrasonography, 1231
gallium breast scan, 1044
mammography, 784
positron emission tomography (PET), 1085
Bronchial obstruction, bronchus radiography, 959
Bronchial occlusion, chest tomography, 1185
Bronchial stenosis, bronchoscopy, 209
Bronchial tumors, bronchus radiography, 959
Bronchiectasis
bronchus radiography, 959
chest tomography, 1185
pulmonary angiogram, 98
pulmonary function studies, 935
Bronchiogenic carcinoma, chest tomography, 1185
Bronchitis
nasal or throat culture, 380
pulmonary function studies, 935
Bronchogenic carcinoma
antidiuretic hormone (ADH), 116
bronchoscopy, 209
lung ventilation scan, 1072
mediastinoscopy, 791
Brucella infections, febrile agglutinins, serum, 544
Brucellosis, immunoglobulin electrophoresis, serum, 680
Buerger's disease, lower extremity angiography, 87
Burkitt's lymphoma
Epstein-Barr virus (EBV) antibodies, 506

Monospot (heterophil antibody), 801
Burns
aldolase (ALS), 23
alpha$_1$ globulin, 591
alpha$_2$ globulin, 591
amylase, serum, 58
antinuclear antibody (ANA), 119
bicarbonate (HCO$_3$), 475
blood urea nitrogen (BUN), 203
erythrocyte fragility, 510
fibrin breakdown products (FBP), 559
glucose tolerance tests, 607
glucose, urine, 603
hematocrit (Hct), 628
hemoglobin and blood, urine, 637
hemoglobin (Hb), 630
hemosideran, 643
17-ketogenic steroids (17-KGS), 709
myoglobin, serum, 812
myoglobin, urine, 814
protein electrophoresis, serum, 913
protein electrophoresis, urine, 917
serum protein, total, 920
thyroxine (T$_4$, total T$_4$, T$_4$RIA), 1177
vitamin C, urine, 1311

Cachexia, amylase, urine, 61
CAD. *See* Coronary artery disease
Cadmium poisoning
beta$_2$-microglobulin, 149
protein electrophoresis, urine, 917
Calcium deposits in lungs, chest tomography, 1185
Campylobacter, stool culture, 390
Cancer, metastatic
antidiuretic hormone (ADH), 116
calcium, urine, 487
progesterone receptor assay, 902

thyroxine (T$_4$, total T$_4$, T$_4$RIA), 1177

triiodothyronine uptake, 1210

Cancers. *See also named body part or organ*

calcium (Ca), serum, 475

creatinine, 350

haptoglobin, 623

protein electrophoresis, urine, 917

serum complement assay, 1109

transferrin (siderophilin), 704, 1198

vitamin C, urine, 1311

Candidiasis

culture, anal or genital, 363

fungal antibody tests, 580

potassium hydroxide preparation, 889

skin culture, 383

sputum culture, 386

stool culture, 390

Candida albicans

nasal or throat culture, 380

wound culture, 395

Carbon monoxide poisoning

blood gases, arterial (ABG), 194

methemoglobin (MetHb, HbM), 798

Carbontetrachloride, porphyrins, urine, 882

Carcinoid syndrome, serotonin (5-hydroxytryptamine), 1107

Carcinoid tumors, 5-hydroxyindoleacetic acid (5-HIAA), 670

Carcinoma in situ, cervical biopsy, 163

Carcinomas

erythrocyte sedimentation rate, 512

hemoglobin (Hb), 630

iron (Fe), 701

Carcinomas, metastatic, Coombs antiglobulin, direct (DAT), 325

Carcinomatosis

cholesterol (total), 258

pseudocholinesterase (ChS, PCHE, AcCHS), 932

Cardiac arrest, pyruvic acid, 942

Cardiac arrhythmias

aspartate aminotransferase (AST), 136

blood gases, arterial (ABG), 194

Cardiac chamber abnormalities, echocardiography, transesophageal, 451

Cardiac disease, blood gases, arterial (ABG), 194

Cardiac disorders, blood gases, arterial (ABG), 194

Cardiac enlargement, chest x-ray, 962

heart imaging, 1038

heart, plain films, 981

Cardiac filling pressure, elevated, atrial natriuretic hormone (ANH), 139

Cardiac ischemia, heart imaging, 1038

Cardiac septal defects, blood gases, arterial (ABG), 194

Cardiac surgery, creatine phosphokinase (CPK) and isoenzymes, 347

Cardiac trauma, creatine phosphokinase (CPK) and isoenzymes, 347

Cardiac valvular defects

blood gases, arterial (ABG), 194

echocardiography, 448

echocardiography, transesophageal, 451

Cardiac volume overload, atrial natriuretic hormone (ANH), 139

Cardiogenic shock, glucose, urine, 603

Cardiomyopathy

echocardiography, 448

electrocardiography, ambulatory, 462

Cardiopulmonary function impairment, pulse oximetry, 830

Cardiovascular disease

antithrombin, 123

Cr-51 red cell survival time, 344

thyroxine (T$_4$, total T$_4$, T$_4$RIA), 1177

Carditis, viral, Coxsackie A or B virus, 339
Carotid artery occlusive disease
  carotid ultrasound Doppler, 1266
  oculoplethysmograph (OPG), 820
Carotid artery plaque/stenosis
  angiography, digital subtraction (DSA), 76
  carotid ultrasound Doppler, 1266
Carpal tunnel syndrome, electroneurography (ENG), 495
Cat scratch fever
  erythrocyte sedimentation rate, 512
  lymph node biopsy, 179
C-cell hyperplasia, calcitonin, 220
Celiac disease
  fecal fat, 542
  glucose tolerance tests, 607
  human leukocyte antigen and typing (HLA, tissue typing), 660
  intestinal biopsy, 167
  Raji cell assay, 999
  vitamin A, serum, 1307
  D-xylose tolerance, 417
Celiac sprue, 5-hydroxyindole-acetic acid (5-HIAA), 670
Central nervous system circulatory disorders, electronystagmography (ENG), 498
Central nervous system lesions
  CSF analysis, 237, 760
  electronystagmography (ENG), 498
  glucose tolerance tests, 607
  porphyrins, urine, 882
Central nervous system tumors
  electronystagmography (ENG), 498
  metanephrines, total, 795
Cephalopelvic disproportion, pelvic radiography, 975
Cephalosporium, skin culture, 383
Cerebral. *See also* Brain *entries*

Cerebral abscess, computed tomography (CT), cranial, 291
Cerebral aneurysm
  cerebral angiography, 70
  computed tomography (CT), cranial, 291
  MRI, head, 774
Cerebral arterial stenosis, ultrasonography, arterial, transcranial Doppler, 1226
Cerebral arteriovenous malformation
  cerebral angiogram, 70
  computed tomography (CT), cranial, 291
  MRI, head, 774
  ultrasonography, arterial, transcranial Doppler, 1226
Cerebral atrophy, computed tomography (CT), cranial, 291
Cerebral cysts, computed tomography (CT), cranial, 291
Cerebral edema
  cerebral angiogram, 70
  computed tomography (CT), cranial, 291
Cerebral hemorrhage, CSF analysis, 760
Cerebral hyperemia, ultrasonography, arterial, transcranial Doppler, 1226
Cerebral infarction
  computed tomography (CT), cranial, 291
  CSF analysis, 237, 760
  glucose tolerance tests, 607
  MRI, head, 774
Cerebral lipoma, MRI, head, 774
Cerebral pyogenic abscess, MRI, head, 774
Cerebral thrombosis
  cerebral angiogram, 70
  CSF analysis, 760
Cerebral trauma, CSF analysis, 760
Cerebrovascular accident (CVA)
  alanine aminotransferase (ALT), 20
  angiography, digital subtraction (DSA), 76

antithrombin, 123
aspartate aminotransferase (AST), 136
brain scan, 994
lactic dehydrogenase (LDH, LD) and isoenzymes, 720
positron emission tomography (PET), 885, 1085
visual fields test, 1304
Cerumen accumulation, otoscopy, 825
Cervical arthritis, vertebra, plain films, 981
Cervical atrophic changes, colposcopy, 277
Cervical cancer
   angiography, lymph, 91
   colposcopy, 277
   Papanicolaou smear (Pap smear), 833
Cervical disk, vertebra, plain films, 981
Cervical dysplasia, cervical biopsy, 163
Cervical erosion, colposcopy, 277
Cervical inflammatory changes, colposcopy, 277
Cervical intraepithelial neoplasia, colposcopy, 277
Cervical leukoplakia, colposcopy, 277
Cervical polyps, cervical biopsy, 163
Cervical spondylosis, evoked brain potentials, 530
Cetamide ointment, red blood cell (RBC) count, 1003
Chalasia, esophageal, esophageal manometry, 787
Chancroid, lymph node biopsy, 179
Cheilosis, vitamin B_2, urine, 1311
Chest cavity bleeding, thoracoscopy, 1156
Chest cavity tumor, pulmonary angiogram, 98
Chest fluid, lung perfusion scan, 1069

Chest lesions (ribs/spine), computed tomography (CT), thoracic, 313
Chest mass, lung perfusion scan, 1069
Chest trauma, pleural fluid analysis, 1150
Chest wall fractures, chest x-ray, 962
Chest wall trauma, pulmonary function studies, 935
Chédiak-Higashi syndrome, platelet aggregation, 865
Chlamydia species, eye culture, 373
Chlamydia trachomatis infection or carrier, culture, anal or genital, 363
Chlorates, methemoglobin (MetHb, HbM), 798
Cholangiopancreatography, 255
Cholangitis
   bilirubin, serum, 151
   cholangiopancreatography, 255
   urobilinogen, 1287
Cholecystitis
   amylase, serum, 58
   gallbladder scan, 1057
   lipase, 750
   ornithine carbamoyltransferase (OCT), 823
Cholecystitis, acalculus, gallbladder scan, 1057
Cholelithiasis
   cholangiography, percutaneous transhepatic (PTHC), 249
   urobilinogen, 1287
Cholestatics, urobilinogen, 1287
Cholesterol ester storage disease, liver biopsy, 173
Choriocarcinoma
   human chorionic gonadotropin (hCG), 655
   human chorionic gonadotropin (hGC) pregnancy test, 657
   human placental lactogen (HPL), serum, 662
   pregnanediol, 893

Choroidal detachment, ocular
  ultrasonography, 1245
Chromosomal abnormalities
  amniotic fluid analysis, 51
  chorionic villus biopsy, 165
Chronic granulocytic leukemia,
  white blood cell enzymes,
  1319
Chronic inflammatory disorders,
  alpha$_1$-antitrypsin (α_1-AT),
  40
Chronic lymphocytic leukemia
  (CLL)
  B-lymphocyte assays, 1133
  immunoglobulin
    electrophoresis, serum,
    680
  pleural fluid analysis, 1150
  T-lymphocyte assays, 1133
Chronic myelocytic leukemia
  (CML)
  leukocyte alkaline
    phosphatase stain, 748
  white blood cell enzymes,
  1319
Chronic obstructive pulmonary
  disease (COPD)
  aldosterone, plasma, 25
  aldosterone, urine, 29
  ammonia (NH_3), 56
  bicarbonate (HCO_3), 475
  hemoglobin (Hb), 630
  lung perfusion scan, 1069
  triglycerides, 1202
CHS. *See* Pseudocholinesterase
Chylous ascites, peritoneal fluid
  analysis, 835
Chylous pleural effusion, pleural
  fluid analysis, 1150
Circulatory shock, antidiuretic
  hormone (ADH), 116
Cirrhosis
  abdominal laparoscopy, 726
  aldolase (ALS), 23
  aldosterone, plasma, 25
  aldosterone, urine, 29
  alkaline phosphatase (ALP),
    32
  alpha-fetoprotein (AFP), 40
  alpha($_1$)-antitrypsin (α_1-AT),
    40
  ammonia (NH_3), 56
  amylase, urine, 61

angiotensin-converting
  enzyme (ACE), 108
antithrombin, 123
aspartate aminotransferase
  (AST), 136
bilirubin, serum, 151
bilirubin, urine, 155
bleeding time, 191
bone marrow aspiration and
  analysis, 204
capillary fragility, 213
cold agglutinin titer, 268
Cr-51 platelet survival time,
  341
cryoglobulin, 358
estradiol (E_2), serum, 521
fibrinogen, 561
folic acid, 571
gallium liver scan, 1051
gamma glutamyl
  transpeptidase (GGTP,
  GGT), 582
glucose tolerance tests, 607
hematocrit (Hct), 628
hemoglobin (Hb), 630
isocitrate dehydrogenase
  (ICD), 707
lactic dehydrogenase (LDH,
  LD) and isoenzymes,
  720
leucine aminopeptidase
  (LAP), urine, 743
leukocyte alkaline
  phosphatase stain, 748
liver and biliary system
  ultrasonography, 1236
liver biopsy, 173
liver scan, 1065
luteinizing hormone (LH,
  ICSH), 766
5'-nucleotidase, 816
ornithine
  carbamoyltransferase
  (OCT), 823
peritoneal fluid analysis, 835
phospholipids, 861
plasminogen, 863
platelet aggregation, 865
platelet count
  (thrombocyte), 871
pleural fluid analysis, 1150
porphyrins (erythrocyte), total,
  880

porphyrins, urine, 882
prostate-specific antigen (PSA), 909
prothrombin consumption time (PCT), 925
radioactive iodine uptake (RAIU), 944
Raji cell assay, 999
reticulocyte (retic) count, 1018
rheumatoid factor (RF), 1020
serum complement assay, 1109
serum protein, total, 920
thrombin clotting time (TCT), 1148
triglycerides, 1202
urobilinogen, 1287

Cirrhosis, alcoholic
alkaline phosphatase (ALP), 32
carcinoembryonic antigen (CEA), 225
coproporphyrin, urine (UCP), 329

Closed-chest trauma, pericardial fluid analysis, 846
Clostridium botulinum, stool culture, 390
Clostridium perfringens, wound culture, 395
Clostridium, skin culture, 383

CML. *See* Chronic myelocytic leukemia

Coagulation-factor deficiencies
activated clotting time (ACT), 13
activated partial thromboplastin time (aPTT), 15

Cocaine, platelet aggregation, 865

Coccidioidomycosis
angiotensin-converting enzyme (ACE), 108
bronchoscopy, 209
CSF analysis, 760
fungal antibody tests, 580
mediastinoscopy, 791
potassium hydroxide preparation, 889
skin culture, 383
thoracoscopy, 1156

Cochlear lesions
acoustic admittance tests, 9
evoked brain potentials, 530

Collagen disorders
erythrocyte sedimentation rate, 512
leukocyte alkaline phosphatase stain, 748
protein electrophoresis, urine, 917
uric acid, urine, 1280
white blood cell (WBC) count, 1315
white blood cell enzymes, 1319

Collagen vascular disease, extractable nuclear antigen (ENA) antibodies, 536

Collagen vascular lung disease, pulmonary function studies, 935

Colon anomalies, barium enema, 950

Colon cancer
arylsulfatase A (ARS-A), urine, 133
cancer antigen 125 (CA-125), 223
occult blood, 818

Colon diverticular disease, barium enema, 950

Color blindness, electroretinography, 502

Colorectal cancer
barium enema, 950
carcinoembryonic antigen (CEA), 225

Colorectal polyps, carcinoembryonic antigen (CEA), 225

Common bile duct abnormalities, percutaneous transhepatic cholangiography (PTC, PTHC), 249, 978

Common bile duct dilatation
computed tomography (CT), abdomen, 284
computed tomography (CT), biliary tract and liver, 287

Common bile duct obstruction
  gallbladder scan, 1057
  urobilinogen, 1287
Common hepatic duct dilatation
  computed tomography (CT),
    abdomen, 284
  computed tomography (CT),
    biliary tract and liver, 287
Conduction defects,
    electrocardiography,
    ambulatory, 462
Conductive hearing loss
  acoustic admittance tests, 9
  audiometry, 141
  spondee speech reception
    threshold, 1126
  tuning fork tests, 1220
Congenital abnormalities of
    cerebrum, computed
    tomography (CT), cranial,
    291
Congenital abnormalities of
    kidney, computed
    tomography (CT), renal,
    305
Congenital heart disease
  coagulation factor assays, 265
  echocardiography, 448
  fibrin breakdown products
    (FBP), 559
  hemoglobin (Hb), 630
  MRI, heart and chest, 778
Congenital malformations of
    spine, computed
    tomography (CT), spinal,
    309
Congenital porphyria
  porphyrins (erythrocyte), total,
    880
  porphyrins, urine, 882
Congestive heart failure (CHF)
  alanine aminotransferase
    (ALT), 20
  aldosterone, plasma, 25
  aldosterone, urine, 29
  alkaline phosphatase (ALP),
    32
  ammonia (NH₃), 56
  aspartate aminotransferase
    (AST), 136
  atrial natriuretic hormone
    (ANH), 139

  bicarbonate (HCO₃), 475
  blood urea nitrogen (BUN),
    203
  chloride (Cl), serum, 486
  creatinine, 350
  creatinine clearance, urine,
    354
  echocardiography, 448
  erythrocyte sedimentation
    rate, 512
  gamma globulin, 590
  gamma glutamyl
    transpeptidase (GGTP,
    GGT), 582
  heart, plain films, 981
  hematocrit (Hct), 628
  insulin clearance test, 699
  leukocyte alkaline
    phosphatase stain, 748
  peritoneal fluid analysis, 835
  phenolsulfonphthalein (PSP),
    854
  protein electrophoresis, serum,
    913
  protein electrophoresis, urine,
    917
  protein, urine (dipstick), 923
  serum protein, total, 920
  sodium (Na), urine, 486
  specific gravity, urine, 1123
  uric acid, serum, 1277
  urobilinogen, 1287
Conjunctivitis
  Coxsackie A or B virus, 339
  slit lamp biomicroscopy, 1120
Connective tissue immune
    disorders, fibrinogen, 561
Connective tissue diseases
  antinuclear antibody (ANA),
    119
  bleeding time, 191
  bone marrow aspiration and
    analysis, 204
  Coombs antiglobulin, direct
    (DAT), 325
  gamma globulin, 590
  immunoglobulin
    electrophoresis, serum,
    680
  T-lymphocyte assays, 1133
Constrictive pericarditis, MRI,
    heart and chest, 778

COPD. *See* Chronic obstructive
        pulmonary disease
Coproporphyria,
        coproporphyrin, urine
        (UCP), 329
Cord tumor, CSF analysis, 760
Corneal abrasions, slit lamp
        biomicroscopy, 1120
Corneal lesions, corneal staining,
        332
Corneal ulcers, slit lamp
        biomicroscopy, 1120
Corneal vascularization, vitamin
        B₂, urine, 1311
Coronary artery abnormalities,
        cardiac angiography, 73
Coronary artery disease (CAD)
    apolipoprotein A-1 (Apo A-1),
        125
    echocardiography, 448
    electrocardiography, exercise,
        465
    phonocardiograph (PCG), 858
    positron emission tomography
        (PET), 1085
    thoracic fluoroscopy, 569
Corynebacterium diphtheria
    nasal or throat culture, 380
    sputum culture, 386
Corynebacterium, skin culture,
        383
Coxsackie infection, CSF
        analysis, 760
Craniopharyngiomas, growth
        hormone (GH, hGH, STH,
        SH), 612
Craniostenosis, skull, plain films,
        981
CREST syndrome, scleroderma
        antibody, 1103
Cretinism
    alkaline phosphatase (ALP),
        32
    thyroid hormone binding
        ratio, 1162
Crigler-Najjar syndrome,
        bilirubin, serum, 151
Crohn's disease
    beta₂-microglobulin, 149
    erythrocyte sedimentation
        rate, 512
    fecal fat, 542

gamma globulin, 590
    protein electrophoresis, serum,
        913
    Raji cell assay, 999
    serum protein, total, 920
Croup, nasal or throat culture,
        380
Crush injuries
    aldolase (ALS), 23
    Cr-51 platelet survival time,
        341
Cryoglobulinemia
    Monospot (heterophil
        antibody), 801
    Raji cell assay, 999
Cryptococcal meningitis, fungal
        antibody tests, 580
Cryptorchidism, testosterone,
        1143
Cushing's syndrome
    ACTH, 17
    androstenedione, 64
    beta globulin, 590
    bicarbonate (HCO₃), 475
    blood gases, arterial (ABG),
        194
    cholesterol (total), 258
    cortisol, 334
    cortisol-free, urine, 337
    dexamethasone suppression
        test (DST), 420
    fasting blood sugar (FSB), 596
    gamma globulin, 590
    glucose tolerance tests, 607
    glucose, two-hour postprandial
        (PPBS), 600
    glucose, urine, 603
    17-hydroxycorticosteroids (17-
        OHCS), 667
    insulin, 589
    insulin antibody, 695
    17-ketogenic steroids (17-
        KGS), 709
    17-ketosteroids (17-KS) and
        fractionation, 714
    potassium (K), serum, 475
    potassium (K), urine, 486
    renin, plasma, 1013
    white blood cell (WBC)
        count, 1315
    white blood cell enzymes,
        1319

Cyanides, ferric chloride (FeCl₃),
    546
Cystic fibrosis
    amylase, serum, 58
    amylase, urine, 61
    fecal analysis, 538
    fecal fat, 542
    glucagon, 594
    glucose tolerance tests, 607
    glucose, urine, 603
    lipase, 750
    secretin test, 1104
    sweat test (pilocarpine
        iontophoresis), 1130
    trypsin, blood, 1213
    trypsin, fecal, 1215
    D-xylose tolerance, 417
Cystic hygroma, amniotic fluid
    analysis, 51
Cystinosis, amino acids, urine, 48
Cystitis, hemoglobin or blood,
    urine, 637
Cytomegalic inclusion, T-
    lymphocyte assays, 1133
Cytomegalovirus (CMV)
    bronchoscopy, 209
    cold agglutinin titer, 268
    TORCH test, 1193
Cytomegalovirus (CMV) anemia,
    platelet count
    (thromobocyte), 871

Deep-tissue infection, fungal
        antibody tests, 580
Deep-vein thrombosis (DVT)
    antithrombin, 123
    Cr-51 platelet survival time,
        341
    fibrinogen uptake test (FUT),
        563
    lower extremity venous
        Doppler, 1274
    lower limb venography, 1299
    plasminogen, 863
    plethysmography, 874
Deep-vein valvular
        incompetence, lower
        limb venography, 1299
Deer fly fever, febrile agglutinins,
        serum, 544

Degenerative arthritis
    bone scan, 1033
    synovial fluid analysis, 129
Degenerative spinal disease,
        MRI, musculoskeletal, 781
Dehydration
    alpha₂ globulin, 591
    beta globulin, 590
    bicarbonate (HCO₃), 475
    chloride (Cl), serum, 475
    chloride (Cl), urine, 486
    creatinine clearance, urine,
        354
    gamma globulin, 590
    hematocrit (Hct), 628
    hemoglobin (Hb), 630
    insulin clearance test, 699
    ketones, 712
    lactic acid, 718
    magnesium (Mg), serum, 475
    magnesium (Mg), urine, 488
    protein electrophoresis, serum,
        913
    protein, urine (dipstick), 923
    red blood cell (RBC) count,
        1003
    serum protein, total, 920
    sodium (Na), urine, 486
    specific gravity, urine, 1123
Delirium tremens
    aspartate aminotransferase
        (AST), 136
    creatine phosphokinase (CPK)
        and isoenzymes, 347
    myoglobin, urine, 814
Dementia
    brain scan, 994
    positron emission tomography
        (PET), 885, 1085
Demyelinating diseases
    CSF analysis, 237, 760
    electronystagmography (ENG),
        498
Dengue fever, immune complex
        assay, serum, 678
Depression
    dexamethasone suppression
        test (DST), 420
    serotonin (5-
        hydroxytryptamine), 1107
Dermatitis, skin biopsy, 186

Dermatitis herpetiformis
human leukocyte antigen and
typing (HLA, tissue
typing), 660
Raji cell assay, 999
Dermatofibroma, skin biopsy,
186
Dermatomyositis
aldolase (ALS), 23
antinuclear antibody (ANA),
119
aspartate aminotransferase
(AST), 136
creatine phosphokinase (CPK)
and isoenzymes, 347
lactic dehydrogenase (LDH,
LD) and isoenzymes, 720
myoglobin, serum, 812
rheumatoid factor (RF), 1020
Detrusor muscle dysfunction,
uroflowmetry, 1291
Diabetes insipidus
antidiuretic hormone (ADH),
116
concentration/dilution tests,
urine, 316
sodium (Na), serum, 475
specific gravity, urine, 1123
Diabetes mellitus
aldosterone, plasma, 25
aldosterone, urine, 29
angiotensin-converting
enzyme (ACE), 108
beta globulin, 590
blood gases, arterial (ABG),
194
blood urea nitrogen (BUN),
203
C-peptide, 216
CSF analysis, 760
fasting blood sugar (FSB), 596
ferric chloride ($FeCl_3$), 546
free fatty acids (FFA), 575
gamma glutamyl
transpeptidase (GGTP,
GGT), 582
glucagon, 594
glucose tolerance tests, 607
glucose, two-hour postprandial
(PPBS), 600
glucose, urine, 603

human leukocyte antigen and
typing (HLA, tissue
typing), 660
insulin, 689
leukocyte alkaline
phosphatase stain, 748
lipoprotein phenotyping, 756
lipoprotein-cholesterol
fractionation, 753
pH, urine, 850
phospholipids, 861
platelet aggregation, 865
potassium (K), serum, 475
protein electrophoresis, serum,
913
pseudocholinesterase (CHS,
PCHE, AcCHS), 932
specific gravity, urine, 1123
thyroxine (T_4, total T_4, T_4RIA),
1177
triglycerides, 1202
trypsin, blood, 1213
Diabetes mellitus, uncontrolled
ketones, 712
lactic acid, 718
lipoprotein phenotyping, 756
Diabetic glomerulosclerosis, uric
acid, urine, 1280
Diabetic ketoacidosis
amino acid screen, blood, 45
amylase, urine, 61
blood gases, arterial (ABG),
194
chloride (Cl), urine, 486
cortisol, 334
creatinine, 350
CSF analysis, 760
glucose tolerance tests, 607
ketones, 712
magnesium (Mg), serum, 475
magnesium (Mg), urine, 488
myoglobin, urine, 814
phosphorus (P), serum, 475
potassium (K), urine, 486
sodium (Na), urine, 486
Diabetic neuropathic diarrhea,
d-xylose tolerance, 417
Diabetic neuropathy
creatinine, 350
electroneurography (ENG),
495

Diabetic retinopathy, angiography, fluorescein, 79

Diaphragmatic function decrease, thoracic fluoroscopy, 569

DIC. *See* Disseminated intravascular coagulation

Dicumarol, clotting time (CT), 261

Dietary deficiency
  red blood cell (RBC) count, 1003
  vitamin B_1, urine, 1311
  vitamin B_2, urine, 1311

DiGeorge syndrome
  B-lymphocyte assays, 1133
  T-lymphocyte assays, 1133

Diphtheria, culture, nasal or throat, 380

Diphyllobothrium latum, fecal analysis, 538

Disaccharidase deficiency, d-xylose tolerance, 417

Discoid lupus erythematosis, skin biopsy, 186

Dissecting aortic aneurysm, pericardial fluid analysis, 846

Disseminated intravascular coagulation (DIC)
  activated partial thromboplastin time (aPTT), 15
  antithrombin, 123
  bleeding time, 191
  clot retraction, 263
  coagulation factor assays, 265
  Cr-51 platelet survival time, 341
  D-dimer, 415
  erythrocyte fragility, 510
  fibrin breakdown products (FBP), 559
  fibrinogen, 561
  plasminogen, 863
  platelet count (thrombocyte), 871
  prothrombin consumption time (PCT), 925
  thrombin clotting time (TCT), 1148

Disseminated lupus erythematosus. *See* Lupus erythematosus *and* Systemic lupus erythematosus (SLE)

Diuresis
  chloride (Cl), serum, 475
  sodium (Na), serum, 475

Diverticulae of intestines, mesenteric angiography, 94

Diverticulae of upper GI tract, esophagogastroduodeno-scopy, 515

Diverticular disease, occult blood, 818

Diverticular disease of colon, barium enema, 950

Diverticulitis, carcinoembryonic antigen (CEA), 225

Diverticulosis, fecal fat, 542

Down syndrome
  alpha-fetoprotein (AFP), 40
  chorionic villus biopsy, 165
  estriol (E_3), serum, 521
  leukocyte alkaline phosphatase stain, 748
  prostatic acid phosphatase (PAP), 5
  serotonin (5-hydroxy-tryptamine), 1107
  testosterone, 1143
  triglycerides, 1202
  white blood cell enzymes, 1319

Dressler's syndrome, pericardial fluid analysis, 846

Drowning, near, blood gases, arterial (ABG), 194

Drug reactions, Raji cell assay, 999

Dubin-Johnson syndrome, urobilinogen, 1287

Duchenne's muscular dystrophy
  aldolase (ALS), 23
  creatine phosphokinase (CPK) and isoenzymes, 347
  muscle biopsy, 182

Dumping syndrome
  fasting blood sugar (FSB), 596
  glucose, two-hour postprandial (PPBS), 600

Duodenal atresia, amniotic fluid analysis, 51

Duodenal inflammation, culture, duodenal and gastric, 369

Duodenal obstruction, amylase, serum, 58

Duodenal papilla tumors, cholangiopancreatography, 255

Duodenal tumors, esophagogastroduodenoscopy, 515

Duodenal ulcer
  esophagogastroduodenoscopy, 515
  gastrin, 588
  pepsinogen, 844

Duodenitis, esophagogastroduodenoscopy, 515

Dwarfism
  growth hormone (GH, hGH, STH, SH), 612
  growth hormone stimulation test, 615

Dysautonomia, catecholamines, urine, 230

Dysfibrinogenemia, fibrinogen, 561

Dysglobulinemias, lipoprotein phenotyping, 756

Dysproteinemia
  capillary fragility, 213
  immunoglobulin electrophoresis, urine, 683

Dysrhythmias
  electrocardiography (ECG), 456
  electrocardiography, ambulatory, 462

Ear trauma, otoscopy, 825

Echovirus infection, CSF analysis, 760

Eclampsia
  amino acid screen, blood, 45
  amylase, serum, 58
  amylase, urine, 61
  plasminogen, 863
  uric acid, serum, 1277

Ectopic pregnancy
  computed tomography (CT), pelvic, 301
  culdoscopy, 360
  gynecologic laparoscopy, 729
  human chorionic gonadotropin (hGC), pregnancy test, 657
  hysterosalpingography, 968

Ectropion, slit lamp biomicroscopy, 1120

Electrolyte imbalances
  concentration/dilution tests, urine, 316
  electrocardiography (ECG), 456

Eliptocytosis, Cr-51 red cell survival time, 344

Embolism
  angiography, digital subtraction (DSA), 76
  Cr-51 platelet survival time, 341

Emphysema
  alpha$_1$-antitrypsin (α_1-AT), 40
  lung ventilation scan, 1072
  pulmonary function studies, 935

Empyema, thoracoscopy, 1156

Encephalitis
  CSF analysis, 760
  culture, herpesvirus (HSV-1, HSV-2), 378
  electroencephalography (EEG), 472

Endocarditis
  cryoglobulin, 358
  erythrocyte sedimentation rate, 512
  immune complex assay, serum, 678

Endocarditis, poststreptococcal, antistreptolysin O titer, 121

Endocrine disorders, Papanicolaou smear (Pap smear), 833

Endocrine secreting tumors, thyroid hormone binding ratio, 1162

Endometrial cancer, cancer antigen 125 (CA-125), 223

Endometriosis
  cancer antigen 125 (CA-125),
      223
  culdoscopy, 360
  gynecologic laparoscopy,
      729
  prolactin (HPRL, LTH), 906
Endometritis, Papanicolaou
      smear (Pap smear), 833
Enduron, red blood cell (RBC)
      count, 1003
Enteritis, fecal fat, 542
Enterococci, urine culture with
      Gram's stain, 392
Entropion, slit lamp
      biomicroscopy, 1120
Enzymatic defects
  amniotic fluid analysis, 51
  pyruvic acid, 942
Enzyme deficiencies (PK, G-6-
      PD), erythrocyte fragility,
      510
Enzyme deficiency
  ammonia (NH₃), 56
  chorionic villus biopsy, 165
Epidemic pleurodynia,
      Coxsackie A or B virus,
      339
Epidemic typhus, febrile
      agglutinins, serum, 544
Epidermophyton, skin culture,
      383
Epididymitis
  scrotal scan, 1088
  scrotal ultrasonography, 1256
Epidural hematoma, computed
      tomography (CT), cranial,
      291
Epilepsy. *See* Seizure disorders
Epinephrine, increased secretion
      of, white blood cell
      (WBC) count, 1315
Epstein-Barr virus (EBV),
      Monospot (heterophil
      antibody), 801
Epstein-Barr virus (EBV) carrier
      state, Epstein-Barr virus
      (EBV) antibodies, 506
Erythroblastosis fetalis
  Coombs antiglobulin, direct
      (DAT), 325
  Coombs antiglobulin, indirect
      (IAT), 326

human chorionic
      gonadotropin (hGC),
      pregnancy test, 657
  reticulocyte (retic) count, 1018
Erythrocyte enzyme disorders,
      Cr-51 red cell survival
      time, 344
Erythroid hyperplasia,
      coproporphyrin, urine
      (UCP), 329
Erythroleukemia, white blood
      cell enzymes, 1319
Erythromycin, catecholamines,
      urine, 230
Erythropoiesis, free erythrocyte
      protoporphyrin (FEP), 930
Erythropoietic porphyria
  free erythrocyte
      protoporphyrin (FEP), 930
  porphyrins (erythrocyte), total,
      880
  porphyrins, urine, 882
Erythropoietic protoporphyria,
      porphyrins (erythrocyte),
      total, 880
Esophageal achalasia,
      esophageal manometry,
      787
Esophageal atresia, amniotic
      fluid analysis, 51
Esophageal cancer,
      carcinoembryonic
      antigen (CEA), 225
Esophageal chalasia, esophageal
      manometry, 787
Esophageal polyps, barium
      swallow, 953
Esophageal scleroderma,
      esophageal manometry,
      787
Esophageal stenosis/stricture
  barium swallow, 953
  esophagogastroduodeno-
      scopy, 515
Esophageal tumors
  barium swallow, 953
  esophagogastroduodeno-
      scopy, 515
Esophageal varices
  esophagogastroduodeno-
      scopy, 515
  fecal analysis, 538
  occult blood, 818

Esophagitis
  barium swallow, 953
  esophageal manometry, 787
  fecal analysis, 538
Esosphageal spasms, esophageal
    manometry, 787
Estradiol (E$_2$), serum, 5-
    hydroxyproline, 673
Estrogen-positive breast tumors,
    estradiol receptor assay,
    518
Estrogen-secreting tumors
  thyroid-binding globulin
    (TBG), 1180
  thyroxine (T$_4$, total T$_4$, T$_4$RIA),
    1177
Eustachian-tube abnormalities,
    acoustic admittance tests,
    9
"Euthyroid sick" syndrome,
    triiodothyronine (T$_3$, total
    T$_3$, T$_3$RIA), 1205
Ewing's sarcoma, bone biopsy,
    159
Exophthalmos, thyroid-
    stimulating
    immunoglobulins (TSI,
    TSIg), 1173
Exophthalmus, unilateral,
    computed tomography
    (CT), orbital, 295
External ear canal obstruction,
    audiometry, 141
Extragonadal tumor,
    testosterone, 1143
Extrahepatic obstruction,
    isocitrate dehydrogenase
    (ICD), 707
Extrarenal infection,
    muramidase (lysozyme),
    807
Eye trauma, exophthalmometry,
    543
Eye tumor, exophthalmometry,
    543

Facial nerve lesions, acoustic
    admittance tests, 9
Factitious hypoglycemia, anti-
    insulin antibody, 113
Factor IV deficiency, capillary
    fragility, 212

Factor VII deficiency, bone
    marrow aspiration and
    analysis, 212
Factor VIII deficiency, clotting
    time (CT), 261
Factor IX deficiency, clotting
    time (CT), 261
Factor XI deficiency, clotting
    time (CT), 261
Factor XII deficiency
  clot retraction, 263
  clotting time (CT), 261
Failure to thrive, growth
    hormone (GH, hGH, STH,
    SH), 612
Fallopian tube kinking,
    hysterosalpingography,
    968
Fanconi's syndrome
  Bence Jones protein, 147
  glucose, urine, 603
  pH, urine, 850
  platelet count
    (thrombocyte), 871
  protein electrophoresis, urine,
    917
  uric acid, serum, 1277
  uric acid, urine, 1280
Farmer's lung, angiotensin-
    converting enzyme
    (ACE), 108
Fasting, ketones, 712
Fat emulsion administration,
    erythrocyte sedimentation
    rate, 512
Fat ingestion, lipoprotein-
    cholesterol fractionation,
    753
Fatty acids (saturated) ingestion,
    lipoprotein-cholesterol
    fractionation, 753
Fatty liver, hemoglobin (Hb),
    630
Feminization in children,
    estradiol (E$_2$), serum,
    521
Femoral head avascular
    necrosis, MRI,
    musculoskeletal, 781
Fetal abnormalities,
    pregnanediol, 893
Fetal acidosis, fetal monitoring,
    internal, 553

Fetal anomalies, estrogens, urine, total and fractions, 524

Fetal death
alpha-fetoprotein (AFP), 40
amniotic fluid analysis, 51
fibrin breakdown products (FBP), 559
human chorionic gonadotropin (hCG), 655
human chorionic gonadotropin (hCG) pregnancy test, 657
obstetric ultrasonography, 1242
pregnanediol, 893

Fetal distress
alpha-fetoprotein (AFP), 40
fetal monitoring, internal, 553

Fetal distress, impending, estrogens, urine, total and fractions, 524

Fetal growth retardation, human placental lactogen (HPL), serum, 662

Fetal heart block, fetal monitoring, internal, 553

Fetal hemophilia, fetoscopy, 556

Fetal hydrocephalus, obstetric ultrasonography, 1242

Fetal hydrops, obstetric ultrasonography, 1242

Fetal hypoxia, fetal monitoring, internal, 553

Fetal infection, fetal monitoring, internal, 553

Fetal intestinal atresia, obstetric ultrasonography, 1242

Fetal lung immaturity, amniotic fluid analysis, 51

Fetal malposition, fetal monitoring, internal, 553

Fetal myelomeningocele
alpha-fetoprotein (AFP), 40
obstetric ultrasonography, 1242

Fetal neural-tube defects
alpha-fetoprotein (AFP), 40
fetoscopy, 556

Fetal position abnormality, pelvic radiography, 975

Fetal prematurity, fetal monitoring, internal, 553

Fetal renal defects, obstetric ultrasonography, 1242

Fetal sickle-cell anemia, fetoscopy, 556

Fetal skeletal defects, obstetric ultrasonography, 1242

Fetomaternal hemorrhage, amniotic fluid analysis, 51

Fibrin degradation products (FDP), thrombin clotting time (TCT), 1148

Fibrinogen deficiency
capillary fragility, 213
clot retraction, 263
fibrinogen, 561

Fibrinolytics
antithrombin, 123
coagulation factor assays, 265
euglobulin clot lysis time, 528
fibrin breakdown products (FBP), 559

Fibrocystic disease of breast
breast biopsy, 161
breast ultrasonography, 1231
thermography, 1146

Fibrosarcoma, MRI, musculoskeletal, 781

Fibrosis of lung, lung biopsy, 176

Fistulae of intestines
chloride (Cl), serum, 475
magnesium (Mg), serum, 475
mesenteric angiography, 94
potassium (K), serum, 475

Fluid overload, specific gravity, urine, 1123

Fluid retention, hemoglobin (Hb), 630

Folic acid anemia
folic acid, 571
red blood cell indices, 1008

Folic acid deficiency
bone marrow aspiration and analysis, 204
platelet count (thrombocyte), 871
reticulocyte (retic) count, 1018

Forbes' disease, glucose tolerance tests, 607

Foreign bodies in airway, bronchoscopy, 209

Foreign bodies in ear, otoscopy, 825

Foreign bodies in pulmonary tree, chest x-ray, 962

Fractures
bone scan, 1033
skeletal x-rays, 956

Fractures, healing, alkaline phosphatase (ALP), 32

Franklin's disease, immunoglobulin electrophoresis, serum, 680

Fructose intolerance
amino acid screen, blood, 45
fasting blood sugar (FSB), 596
fructose challenge test, 578
glucose, two-hour postprandial (PPBS), 600

Functional hypoglycemia
fasting blood sugar (FSB), 596
glucose, two-hour postprandial (PPBS), 600

Fungal CNS infections, CSF analysis, 237, 760

Fungal infections
lymph node biopsy, 179
potassium hydroxide preparation, 889
skin culture, 383
sputum culture, 386
wound culture, 395

Fungal pericarditis, pericardial fluid analysis, 846

G-6-PD deficiency
bilirubin, serum, 151
Cr-51 red cell survival time, 344
erythrocyte fragility, 510
Heinz bodies stain, 625

Galactosemia
amino acids, urine, 48
fasting blood sugar (FSB), 596
glucose, two-hour postprandial (PPBS), 600
glucose, urine, 603
liver biopsy, 173
phenylalanine screening, serum, 619

Gallbladder cancer, bilirubin, serum, 151

Gallbladder dilatation
computed tomography (CT), abdomen, 284
computed tomography (CT), biliary tract and liver, 287

Gallbladder disease, amylase, urine, 61

Gallbladder gangrene, abdominal laparoscopy, 726

Gallbladder inflammation, liver and biliary system ultrasonography, 1236

Gallbladder rupture, peritoneal fluid analysis, 835

Gallstones
bilirubin, serum, 151
gallbladder scan, 1057
liver and biliary system ultrasonography, 1236

Ganglioneuroblastoma
catecholamines, plasma, 227
homovanillic acid, 652

Ganglioneuroma
catecholamines, plasma, 227
catecholamines, urine, 230
vanillylmandelic acid (VMA), 1294

Ganglionic blocking agents, catecholamines, plasma, 227

Gangrene, aldolase (ALS), 23

Gangrenous gallbladder, abdominal laparoscopy, 726

Gardnerella vaginalis infection or carrier, culture, anal or genital, 363

Gas exchange abnormalities, pulse oximetry, 830

Gastointestinal malabsorption, Schilling test, 1097

Gastric cancer
ceruloplasmin (Cp), 243
fibrinogen, 561
gastric acid stimulation test, 585
gastrin, 588
glucose tolerance tests, 607

Gastric cancer—*Continued*
  human chorionic
    gonadotropin (hCG),
    655
  pepsinogen, 844
Gastric hyperacidity, gastrin,
  588
Gastric resection, amylase,
  serum, 58
Gastric suction
  chloride (Cl), urine, 486
  pH, urine, 850
Gastric tumors,
    esophagogastroduodeno-
    scopy, 515
Gastric ulcer
  carcinoembryonic antigen
    (CEA), 225
  esophagogastroduodeno-
    scopy, 515
  gastrin, 588
  occult blood, 818
Gastritis
  esophagogastroduodeno-
    scopy, 515
  fecal analysis, 538
  gastrin, 588
  occult blood, 818
  pepsinogen, 844
Gastritis, atrophic, pepsinogen,
  844
Gastroenteritis
  peritoneal fluid analysis, 835
  sodium (Na), serum, 475
Gastroesophageal reflux
  esophageal manometry, 787
  gastroesophageal reflux scan,
    1054
Gastrointestinal carcinoma,
    immunoglobulin
    electrophoresis, serum,
    680
Gastrointestinal hemorrhage
  ammonia (NH_3), 56
  blood urea nitrogen (BUN),
    203
Gastrointestinal inflammation,
    protein electrophoresis,
    serum, 913
Gastrointestinal neoplasms,
    protein electrophoresis,
    serum, 913

Gastrointestinal perforation,
    peritoneal fluid analysis,
    835
Gastrointestinal strangulation/
    necrosis, peritoneal fluid
    analysis, 835
Gastrointestinal ulcers, fecal
    analysis, 538
Gastroschisis, amniotic fluid
    analysis, 51
Gaucher's disease
  acid phosphatase (ACP), 5
  angiotensin-converting
    enzyme (ACE), 108
  MRI, musculoskeletal, 781
G-cell hyperplasia, gastrin, 588
Genital herpes, culture,
    herpesvirus (HSV-1,
    HSV-2), 378
Genitourinary tumors,
    hemoglobin or blood,
    urine, 637
Gestational diabetes, glucose,
    urine, 603
GI. *See* Gastrointestinal *headings*
Giant arteritis (retina),
    electroretinography, 501
    Giardiasis
  fecal analysis, 538
  ova and parasites, stool, 828
Gigantism
  creatinine, 350
  fasting blood sugar (FSB), 596
  glucose tolerance tests, 607
  glucose, two-hour postprandial
    (PPBS), 600
  growth hormone (GH, hGH,
    STH, SH), 612
  growth hormone suppression
    test, 617
Gilbert disease, bilirubin, serum,
    151
Glanzmann's thrombasthenia
  capillary fragility, 213
  clot retraction, 263
  platelet aggregation, 865
Glaucoma
  tonometry, 1190
  visual fields test, 1304
Glioblastoma,
    electroencephalography
    (EEG), 472

Glomerulonephritis
  antistreptolysin O titer, 121
  creatinine clearance, urine, 354
  creatinine, urine, 352
  culture, nasal or throat, 380
  excretory urography (EUG), 964
  fibrinogen, 561
  immune complex assay, serum, 678
  insulin clearance test, 699
  kidney biopsy, 170
  kidney ultrasonography, 1233
  lactic dehydrogenase (LDH, LD) and isoenzymes, 720
  MRI, abdominal, 770
  protein electrophoresis, serum, 913
  serum complement assay, 1109
  specific gravity, urine, 1123
  uric acid, urine, 1280
Glossitis, vitamin B_2, urine, 1311
Glucagonoma, glucagon, 594
Glycogen storage disease
  fasting blood sugar (FSB), 596
  free fatty acids (FFA), 575
  glucose, two-hour postprandial (PPBS), 600
  glucose, urine, 603
  lipoprotein phenotyping, 756
  myoglobin, urine, 814
Goiter, thyroid antithyroglobulin antibody, 1160
Gonadal tumor, 17-ketosteroids (17-KS) and fractionation, 714
Gonorrhea, culture, nasal or throat, 380
Goodpasture's syndrome, kidney biopsy, 170
Gout
  blood urea nitrogen (BUN), 203
  leukocyte alkaline phosphatase stain, 748
  phenolsulfonphthalein (PSP), 854
  synovial fluid analysis, 129
  uric acid, serum, 1277
  uric acid, urine, 1280

Graft (coronary) occlusion, cardiac angiography, 73
Graft diameter reduction, lower extremity arterial (LEA) Doppler, 1268
Graft-versus-host disease, T-lymphocyte assays, 1133
Gram-negative bacilli, sputum culture, 386
Granulocytic leukemia
  leukocyte alkaline phosphatase stain, 748
  muramidase (lysozyme), 807
Granulocytopenia, leukocyte alkaline phosphatase stain, 748
Granulomatous infections, mediastinoscopy, 791
Granulomatous thyroiditis, thyroid biopsy, 188
Grave's disease
  exophthalmometry, 543
  human leukocyte antigen and typing (HLA, tissue typing), 660
  intrinsic factor (IF) antibody, 697
  long-acting thyroid stimulator (LATS), 1175
  parathyroid hormone (PTH), 840
  radioactive iodine uptake (RAIU), 944
  T-lymphocyte assays, 1133
  thyroglobulin, 1158
  thyroid radionuclide scan, 944, 996
  thyroid-stimulating immunoglobulins (TSI, TSIg), 1173
  thyroid ultrasonography, 1263
  triiodothyronine (T_3, total T_3, T_3RIA), 1205
Gray platelet syndrome, platelet aggregation, 865
Growth hormone administration
  fasting blood sugar (FSB), 596
  free fatty acids (FFA), 575
  glucose, two-hour postprandial (PPBS), 600
  5-hydroxyproline, 673
  serum protein, total, 920

Growth hormone deficiency
growth hormone (GH, hGH, STH, SH), 612
insulin challenge test, 692
Growth retardation, secondary, alkaline phosphatase (ALP), 32
Guillain-Barré syndrome
CSF analysis, 760
electroneurography (ENG), 495
evoked brain potentials, 530
Gynecomastia
estradiol (E₂), serum, 521
17-ketosteroids (17-KS) and fractionation, 714
prolactin (HPRL, LTH), 906

Haemophilus aegyptii, eye culture, 373
Haemophilus influenzae, type B immunoglobulin G, subclassification, 686
nasal or throat culture, 380
Haemophilus influenzae, sputum culture, 386
Haemophilus pertussis, sputum culture, 386
Hairy cell leukemia, leukocyte alkaline phosphatase stain, 748
Hansen's disease, immune complex assay, serum, 678
Hartnup disease
amino acid screen, blood, 45
amino acids, urine, 48
Hashimoto's thyroiditis
radioactive iodine uptake (RAIU), 944
thyroid biopsy, 188
thyroid radionuclide scan, 944, 996
thyroid-stimulating hormone (TSH), 1164
triiodothyronine suppression test, 1207
triiodothyronine (T₃, total T₃, T₃RIA), 1205
triiodothyronine uptake, 1210

Hay fever, immunoglobulin electrophoresis, serum, 680
HBV. *See* Hepatitis B
Head or neck cancer, carcinoembryonic antigen (CEA), 225
Head trauma
antidiuretic hormone (ADH), 116
CSF analysis, 760
electroencephalography (EEG), 472
electronystagmography (ENG), 498
positron emission tomography (PET), 885
Hearing loss, sensory or conductive
acoustic admittance tests, 9
spondee speech reception threshold, 1126
tuning fork tests, 1220
Heart chamber disorder, heart scan, 1038
Heart disease, platelet count (thrombocyte), 871
Heavy-metal poisoning
beta₂-microglobulin, 149
erythrocyte sedimentation rate, 512
porphyrins, urine, 882
Heinz body anemia, hemoglobin, unstable, 635
Helicobacter pylori, culture, duodenal and gastric, 369
Hemachromatosis. *See* Hemochromatosis
Hematoma in lower extremity, lower extremity arterial (LEA) Doppler, 1268
Hematomas in abdomen, computed tomography (CT), abdomen, 284
Hemochromatosis
coproporphyrin, urine (UCP), 329
ferritin, 548
glucose tolerance tests, 607
glucose, two-hour postprandial (PPBS), 600

glucose, urine, 603
iron (Fe), 701
liver biopsy, 173
TIBC/transferrin test, 704
Hemochromocytoma
    fasting blood sugar (FSB), 596
    hemosiderin, 643
    homovanillic acid, 652
Hemoconcentration
    clot retraction, 263
    hematocrit (Hct), 628
    hemoglobin (Hb), 630
Hemodialysis, ferritin, 548
Hemodilution, hematocrit (Hct), 628
Hemoglobin C disease
    Cr-51 red cell survival time, 344
    electrophoresis, hemoglobin, 640
    erythrocyte fragility, 510
Hemoglobin H disease, electrophoresis, hemoglobin, 640
Hemoglobin S abnormalities, sickle cell test, 1113
Hemoglobinopathies
    bilirubin, serum, 151
    chorionic villus biopsy, 165
    hemoglobin (Hb), 630
    red blood cell (RBC) count, 1003
Hemoglobins, unstable, Heinz bodies stain, 625
Hemoglobinuria, Cr-51 red cell survival time, 344
Hemolysis, haptoglobin (Hp), 623
Hemolytic anemias
    acid phosphatase (ACP), 5
    alpha₂ globulin, 591
    aspartate aminotransferase (AST), 136
    bone marrow aspiration and analysis, 204
    cold agglutinin titer, 268
    Coombs antiglobulin, indirect (IAT), 326
    erythrocyte fragility, 510
    fecal analysis, 538
    ferritin, 548

free erythrocyte protoporphyrin (FEP), 930
hemoglobin and blood, urine, 637
hemosideran, 643
hydroxybutyrate dehydrogenase (HBDH), 665
iron (Fe), 701
red blood cell (RBC) count, 1003
reticulocyte (retic) count, 1018
urobilinogen, 1287
Hemolytic disease of newborn
    ammonia (NH₃), 56
    amniotic fluid analysis, 51
    platelet count (thrombocyte), 871
Hemolytic disorders
    hemoglobin (Hb), 630
    urobilinogen, 1287
Hemoperitoneum, computed tomography (CT), abdomen, 284
Hemophilia
    activated clotting time (ACT), 13
    antithrombin, 123
    bleeding time, 191
    hepatitis B surface antigen, 145
Hemophilia C, coagulation factor assays, 265
Hemophilia of fetus, fetoscopy, 556
Hemophilic arthritis, synovial fluid analysis, 129
Hemorrhage
    bilirubin, serum, 151
    bone marrow aspiration and analysis, 204
    fibrin breakdown products (FBP), 559
    hemoglobin (Hb), 630
    lactic acid, 718
    pyruvic acid, 942
    red blood cell (RBC) count, 1003
    renin, plasma, 1013
    reticulocyte (retic) count, 1018

Hemorrhage—*Continued*
  serum protein, total, 920
  sodium (Na), urine, 486
Hemorrhage of cerebrum,
    computed tomography
    (CT), cranial, 291
Hemorrhagic disease of
    newborn
  activated clotting time (ACT),
    13
  coagulation factor assays, 265
Hemorrhagic pericarditis,
    pericardial fluid analysis,
    846
Hemorrhagic shock, euglobulin
    clot lysis time, 528
Hemorrhoids, fecal analysis, 538
Hemosiderosis
  ferritin, 548
  hemosideran, 643
  TIBC/transferrin test, 704
  urobilinogen, 1287
Hepatic. *See also* Liver *entries*
Hepatic abscess or cyst
  amylase, urine, 61
  computed tomography (CT),
    biliary tract and liver, 287
  liver and biliary system
    ultrasonography, 1236
  liver scan, 1065
Hepatic cancer. *See* Liver cancer
Hepatic duct obstruction, liver
    and biliary system
    ultrasonography, 1236
Hepatic hemangiomas, liver
    scan, 1065
Hepatic necrosis, ornithine
    carbamoyltransferase
    (OCT), 823
Hepatic nodular hyperplasia,
    liver scan, 1065
Hepatic parenchymal damage,
    urobilinogen, 1287
Hepatic porphyria, porphyrins,
    urine, 882
Hepatic tract cancer, bilirubin,
    urine, 155
Hepatic trauma. *See* Liver
    disease or damage
Hepatic tumors
  liver and biliary tract
    ultrasonography, 1236
  liver scan, 1065

Hepatitis
  alanine aminotransferase
    (ALT), 20
  aldolase (ALS), 23
  alkaline phosphatase (ALP),
    32
  alpha-fetoprotein (AFP), 40
  alpha$_1$ globulin, 591
  alpha$_1$-antitrypsin (α_1-AT), 40
  amino acids, urine, 48
  amylase, urine, 61
  aspartate aminotransferase
    (AST), 136
  beta$_2$-microglobulin, 149
  bilirubin, serum, 151
  bilirubin, urine, 155
  blood urea nitrogen (BUN),
    203
  ceruloplasmin (Cp), 243
  coagulation factor assays,
    265
  delta-aminolevulinic acid
    (delta ALA), urine, 419
  Epstein-Barr virus (EBV)
    antibodies, 506
  fibrinogen, 561
  free fatty acids (FFA), 575
  gamma glutamyl
    transpeptidase (GGTP,
    GGT), 582
  hydroxybutyrate
    dehydrogenase (HBDH),
    665
  immunoglobulin
    electrophoresis, serum,
    680
  iron (Fe), 701
  isocitrate dehydrogenase
    (ICD), 707
  lactic dehydrogenase (LDH,
    LD) and isoenzymes, 720
  leucine aminopeptidase
    (LAP), urine, 743
  lipoprotein-cholesterol
    fractionation, 753
  liver biopsy, 173
  liver scan, 1065
  rheumatoid factor (RF), 1020
  serum complement assay,
    1109
  thyroid-binding globulin
    (TBG), 1180
  triiodothyronine uptake, 1210

urobilinogen, 1287
VDRL, 1297
Hepatitis B
 hepatitis B antibody and
  antigen, 645
 hepatitis B surface antigen,
  145
 hepatitis profile, prenatal, 647
Hepatitis carrier, hepatitis B
 surface antigen, 145
Hepatitis, alcoholic, bilirubin,
 serum, 151
Hepatitis, viral
 alkaline phosphatase (ALP), 32
 amino acids, urine, 48
 bilirubin, serum, 151
Hepatobiliary carcinoma,
 immunoglobulin
 electrophoresis, serum,
 680
Hepatobiliary disease, fecal fat,
 542
Hepatobiliary disorders, gamma
 glutamyl transpeptidase
 (GGTP, GGT), 582
Hepatocellular carcinoma
 angiography, digital
  subtraction (DSA), 76
 gamma glutamyl
  transpeptidase (GGTP,
  GGT), 582
Hepatocellular disease or
 damage
 aspartate aminotransferase
  (AST), 136
 ferritin, 548
 gamma glutamyl
  transpeptidase (GGTP,
  GGT), 582
 haptoglobin (Hp), 623
 hydroxybutyrate
  dehydrogenase (HBDH),
  665
 liver and biliary system
  ultrasonography, 1236
 pseudocholinesterase (CHS,
  PCHE, AcCHS), 932
Hepatocellular necrosis,
 isocitrate dehydrogenase
 (ICD), 707
Hepatoma
 beta$_2$-microglobulin, 149
 gallium liver scan, 1051

immunoglobulin
 electrophoresis, serum, 680
Hepatotoxic agents
 alanine aminotransferase
  (ALT), 20
 aldolase (ALS), 23
 carcinoembryonic antigen
  (CEA), 225
 isocitrate dehydrogenase
  (ICD), 707
 ornithine
  carbamoyltransferase
  (OCT), 823
Hereditary anemias, erythrocyte
 fragility, 510
Hereditary fructose intolerance,
 fasting blood sugar (FSB),
 596
Hereditary giant platelet
 syndrome, bleeding time,
 191
Hereditary hypophosphatemia,
 leukocyte alkaline
 phosphatase stain, 748
Hereditary spherocytosis, bone
 marrow aspiration and
 analysis, 204
Hermansky-Pudlak syndrome,
 platelet aggregation, 865
Herniated disk
 MRI, musculoskeletal, 781
 myelography, 810
Herniated intervertebral disks,
 computed tomography
 (CT), spinal, 309
Herpes anemia, platelet count
 (thrombocyte), 871
Herpes simplex
 herpesvirus antigen, 649
 TORCH test, 1193
Herpesvirus (HSV-1, HSV-2), eye
 culture, 373
Herpes zoster, CSF analysis, 760
Hgb A$_{1c}$, 633
Hiatal hernia
 barium swallow, 953
 esophagogastroduodeno-
  scopy, 515
High-cholesterol diet, lipoprotein
 phenotyping, 756
High-frequency hearing loss,
 spondee speech
 reception threshold, 1126

Hippuric acid, pH, urine, 850
Hirsutism
 17-ketogenic steroids
  (17-KGS), 709
 17-ketosteroids (17-KS) and
  fractionation, 714
 prolactin (HPRL, LTH), 906
 testosterone, 1143
Histamine, growth hormone
 (GH, hGH, STH, SH), 612
Histidinemia, ferric chloride
 ($FeCl_3$), 546
Histiocytosis, platelet count
 (thrombocyte), 871
Histoplasmosis
 angiotensin-converting
  enzyme (ACE), 108
 bronchoscopy, 209
 dexamethasone suppression
  test (DST), 420
 fungal antibody tests, 580
 lung biopsy, 179
 mediastinoscopy, 791
 potassium hydroxide
  preparation, 889
 thoracoscopy, 1156
HIV exposure, enzyme-linked
  immunosorbent assay
  (ELISA), 504
HIV infection
 enzyme-linked
  immunosorbent assay
  (ELISA), 504
 Western immunoblast assay,
  1314
Hodgkin's disease
 angiotensin-converting
  enzyme (ACE), 108
 bleeding time, 191
 ceruloplasmin (Cp), 243
 clot retraction, 263
 computed tomography (CT),
  thoracic, 313
 coproporphyrin, urine (UCP),
  329
 gamma globulin, 590
 hepatitis B surface antigen, 145
 immune complex assay,
  serum, 678
 immunoglobulin
  electrophoresis, urine,
  683

leukocyte alkaline
  phosphatase stain, 748
 lymphangiography, 972
 mediastinoscopy, 791
 porphyrins, urine, 882
 protein electrophoresis, serum,
  913
 red blood cell (RBC) count,
  1003
 T-lymphocyte assays, 1133
 D-xylose tolerance, 417
Hodgkin's lymphoma,
  angiography, lymph, 91
Homocystenuria, platelet
  aggregation, 865
Hordeolum, slit lamp
  biomicroscopy, 1120
Hormonal disorders, skeletal
  x-rays, 956
Horseshoe kidney, computed
  tomography (CT), renal,
  305
Huntington's chorea
 amino acid screen, blood,
  45
 brain scan, 994
 evoked brain potentials, 530
 positron emission tomography
  (PET), 885, 1085
Hyaline membrane disease
 alpha$_1$-antitrypsin (α_1-AT), 40
 blood gases, arterial (ABG),
  194
Hydatid cyst, ruptured,
  peritoneal fluid analysis,
  835
Hydatiform mole
 human chorionic
  gonadotropin (hCG),
  655
 human chorionic
  gonadotropin (hGC),
  pregnancy test, 657
 human placental lactogen
  (HPL), serum, 662
Hydrocele, scrotal
  ultrasonography, 1256
Hydrocephaly
 amniotic fluid analysis, 51
 computed tomography (CT),
  cranial, 291
 skull, plain films, 981

Hydronephrosis
  concentration/dilution tests, urine, 316
  excretory urography (EUG), 964
  kidney ultrasonography, 1233
Hydrops fetalis, amniotic fluid analysis, 51
Hydrosalpinx, computed tomography (CT), pelvic, 301
21-Hydroxylase deficiency, pregnanetriol, 897
Hyperadrenalism, 17-ketogenic steroids (17-KGS), 709
Hyperaldosteronism
  aldosterone, plasma, 25
  aldosterone, urine, 29
  magnesium (Mg), serum, 475
  magnesium (Mg), urine, 488
  pH, urine, 850
  potassium (K), serum, 475
  sodium (Na), urine, 486
Hyperammonemia, ornithine carbamoyltransferase (OCT), 823
Hyperandrogenic state
  thyroid hormone binding ratio, 1162
  triiodothyronine uptake, 1210
Hyperbaric oxygenation, blood gases, arterial (ABG), 194
Hyperbilirubinemia syndromes, urobilinogen, 1287
Hypercalcemia
  concentration/dilution tests, urine, 316
  phosphorus (P), serum, 475
Hypercoagulation
  antithrombin, 123
  platelet aggregation, 865
Hypereosinophilic syndrome, peritoneal fluid analysis, 835
Hyperfibrinogenemia, serum viscosity, 1303
Hypergastrinemia, pepsinogen, 844
Hyperglycemia
  CSF analysis, 760
  glycohemoglobin, 633

growth hormone (GH, hGH, STH, SH), 612
Hyperimmunization, immunoglobulin electrophoresis, serum, 680
Hyperinsulinism
  C-peptide, 216
  glucose tolerance tests, 607
Hyperkalemia, chloride (Cl), serum, 475
Hyperlipidemia
  apolipoprotein B, plasma (Apo B), 127
  glucose tolerance tests, 607
  platelet aggregation, 865
Hyperlipidemia, type III, uric acid, serum, 1277
Hyperlipoproteinemia
  cholesterol (total), 258
  gamma glutamyl transpeptidase (GGTP, GGT), 582
  lipoprotein-cholesterol fractionation, 753
  triglycerides, 1202
Hypermetabolic states
  vitamin B_{12}, serum, 1307
  vitamin B_2, urine, 1311
Hypernatremia
  aldosterone, urine, 29
  chloride (Cl), serum, 475
  sodium (Na), urine, 486
Hyperopia, refraction, 1011
Hyperparathyroidism
  alkaline phosphatase (ALP), 32
  amino acids, urine, 48
  calcitonin, 220
  calcium (Ca), serum, 475
  calcium (Ca), urine, 487
  cyclic adenosine monophosphate (cAMP), 401
  glucose, urine, 603
  magnesium (Mg), urine, 488
  parathyroid hormone (PTH), 840
  phosphorus (P), urine, 488
  triglycerides, 1202
  uric acid, serum, 1277
  vitamin D_3, serum, 1307

Hyperphosphatemia,
    coagulation factor assays,
    265
Hypersensitivity reactions, bone
    marrow aspiration and
    analysis, 204
Hypersensitivity syndrome,
    pleural fluid analysis,
    1150
Hypersplenism
    bleeding time, 191
    Cr-51 red cell survival time,
    344
Hypertension
    ammonia (NH$_3$), 56
    ceruloplasmin (Cp), 243
    cholesterol (total), 258
    electrocardiography, exercise,
    465
    17-hydroxycorticosteroids
    (17-OHCS), 667
    phenolsulfonphthalein (PSP),
    854
    phonocardiograph (PCG), 858
    pleural fluid analysis, 1150
    triglycerides, 1202
    uric acid, serum, 1277
Hypertension, essential, renin,
    plasma, 1013
Hypertension, malignant
    beta globulin, 590
    gamma globulin, 590
    renin, plasma, 1013
Hypertension, pregnancy-
    induced, magnesium
    (Mg), serum, 475
Hypertension, pulmonary
    echocardiography, 448
    lung perfusion scan, 1069
    phonocardiograph (PCG), 858
    pleural fluid analysis, 1150
Hypertension, with CHF, protein
    electrophoresis, serum,
    913
Hyperthermia, myoglobin, urine,
    814
Hyperthyroidism
    angiotensin-converting
    enzyme (ACE), 108
    bicarbonate (HCO$_3$), 475
    catecholamines, plasma, 227

cholesterol (total), 258
cortisol, 334
estradiol (E$_2$), serum, 521
fasting blood sugar (FSB), 596
glucose tolerance tests, 607
glucose, two-hour postprandial
    (PPBS), 600
magnesium (Mg), serum, 475
phosphorus (P), serum, 475
protein electrophoresis, urine,
    917
pseudocholinesterase (CHS,
    PCHE, AcCHS), 932
radioactive iodine uptake
    (RAIU), 944
thyroid hormone binding
    ratio, 1162
thyroid radionuclide scan,
    944, 996
thyroid-stimulating hormone
    sensitivity (s-TSH) assay,
    1167
thyroid-stimulating hormone
    (TSH), 1164
thyroid-stimulating
    immunoglobulins (TSI,
    TSIg), 1173
thyroxine (T$_4$, total T$_4$, T$_4$RIA),
    1177
triglycerides, 1202
triiodothyronine (T$_3$, total T$_3$,
    T$_3$RIA), 1205
triiodothyronine uptake, 1210
vitamin B$_1$, urine, 1311
Hypertrophic anal papillae,
    proctosigmoidoscopy, 899
Hypertrophic cardiomyopathies,
    phonocardiograph (PCG),
    858
Hyperventilation
    bicarbonate (HCO$_3$), 475
    blood gases, arterial (ABG),
    194
Hypervolemia, pulmonary artery
    catheterization, 234
Hypoadrenalism,
    adrenocorticotropic
    hormone (ACTH), 17
Hypoalbuminemia,
    phenolsulfonphthalein
    (PSP), 854

Hypoaldosteronism
    aldosterone, plasma, 25
    aldosterone, urine, 28
    potassium (K), serum, 475
Hypobetalipoproteinemia,
        lipoprotein-cholesterol
        fractionation, 753
Hypocalcemia
    coagulation factor assays, 265
    concentration/dilution tests,
        urine, 316
    phosphorus (P), serum, 475
Hypocapnia, blood gases,
        arterial (ABG), 194
Hypocholesterolemia, beta
        globulin, 590
Hypochromic anemia
    gastric acid stimulation test,
        585
    red blood cell indices, 1008
Hypocupremia from TPN,
        ceruloplasmin (Cp), 243
Hypofibrinogenemia
    clotting time (CT), 261
    coagulation factor assays, 265
    thrombin clotting time (TCT),
        1148
Hypogammaglobulinemia
    immunoglobulin G,
        subclassification, 686
    T-lymphocyte assays, 1133
Hypoglycemia
    C-peptide, 216
    CSF analysis, 760
    free fatty acids (FFA), 575
    growth hormone (GH, hGH,
        STH, SH), 612
Hypoglycemic reactions, glucose
        tolerance tests, 607
Hypogonadism
    androstenedione, 64
    estradiol (E$_2$), serum, 521
    estrogens, serum, 523
    testosterone, 1143
Hypokalemia
    aldosterone, urine, 29
    bicarbonate (HCO$_3$), 475
    chloride (Cl), serum, 475
    concentration/dilution tests,
        urine, 316
    magnesium (Mg), serum, 475

pH, urine, 850
    potassium (K), urine, 486
    protein electrophoresis, urine,
        917
    renin, plasma, 1013
    sodium (Na), urine, 486
Hypolipoproteinemia,
        phospholipids, 861
Hypomagnesemia, parathyroid
        hormone (PTH), 840
Hyponatremia, chloride (Cl),
        serum, 475
Hypoparathyroidism
    calcium (Ca), urine, 487
    cyclic adenosine monophos-
        phate (cAMP), 401
    glucose tolerance tests, 607
    5-hydroxyproline, 673
    parathyroid hormone (PTH),
        840
    phosphorus (P), urine, 488
    triglycerides, 1202
    vitamin D$_3$, 1307
Hypophosphatasia
    alkaline phosphatase (ALP),
        32
    white blood cell enzymes,
        1319
Hypopituitarism
    estrogens, urine, total and
        fractions, 524
    fasting blood sugar (FSB),
        596
    glucose, two-hour postprandial
        (PPBS), 600
    growth hormone (GH, hGH,
        STH, SH), 612
    17-hydroxycorticosteroids
        (17-OHCS), 667
    5-hydroxyproline, 673
    insulin antibody test, 695
    17-ketosteroids (17-KS) and
        fractionation, 714
    pepsinogen, 844
Hypoproteinemia
    concentration/dilution tests,
        urine, 316
    phenolsulfonphthalein (PSP),
        854
    thyroid-binding globulin
        (TBG), 1180

Hypoprothrombinemia, prothrombin consumption time (PCT), 935

Hypospadias, retrograde urethrography, 988

Hypothalamic degeneration, growth hormone (GH, hGH, STH, SH), 612

Hypothalamic dysfunction
adrenocorticotropic hormone (ACTH), 17
glucose, urine, 603
prolactin (HPRL, LTH), 906
thyroid-stimulating hormone stimulation test, 1169
thyroxine (T_4, total T_4, T_4RIA), 1177

Hypothalamic lesions
CSF analysis, 760
follicle-stimulating hormone (FSH), 573
growth hormone (GH, hGH, STH, SH), 612
luteinizing hormone (LH, ICSH), 766

Hypothalamic tumor
antidiuretic hormone (ADH), 116
growth hormone (GH, hGH, STH, SH), 612

Hypothermia
free fatty acids (FFA), 575
lactic acid, 718
myoglobin, serum, 812
specific gravity, urine, 1123

Hypothyroidism
angiotensin-converting enzyme (ACE), 108
beta globulin, 590
bleeding time, 191
calcium (Ca), serum, 475
carcinoembryonic antigen (CEA), 225
cholesterol (total), 258
creatine phosphokinase (CPK) and isoenzymes, 347
gastrin, 588
glucose tolerance tests, 607
17-hydroxycorticosteroids (17-OHCS), 667
iron (Fe), 701

17-ketogenic steroids (17-KGS), 709
17-ketosteroids (17-KS) and fractionation, 714
lipoprotein phenotyping, 756
lipoprotein-cholesterol fractionation, 753
magnesium (Mg), serum, 475
magnesium (Mg), urine, 488
radioactive iodine uptake (RAIU), 944
sweat test (pilocarpine iontophoresis), 1130
thyroid-binding globulin (TBG), 1180
thyroid hormone binding ratio, 1162
thyroid radionuclide scan, 944, 996
thyroid-stimulating hormone sensitivity (s-TSH) assay, 1167
thyroid-stimulating hormone (TSH), 1164
thyroid-stimulating hormone, neonatal, 1171
thyroxine (T_4, total T_4, T_4RIA), 1177
triglycerides, 1202
triiodothyronine (T_3, total T_3, T_3RIA), 1205
triiodothyronine uptake, 1210

Hypoventilation, regional, lung ventilation scan, 1072

Hypoventilation syndromes
bicarbonate (HCO_3), 475
Cr-51 red cell survival time, 344

Hypovolemia
blood urea nitrogen (BUN), 203
creatinine clearance, urine, 354
pulmonary artery catheterization, 234
sodium (Na), serum, 475

Hypoxemia, pulse oximetry, 830

Hypoxia, chronic, Cr-51 red cell survival time, 344

Hypoxia, newborn, thyroid-stimulating hormone, neonatal, 1171

Ideopathic pulmonary
hemosiderosis,
urobilinogen, 1287
Idiopathic thrombocytopenic
purpura
Cr-51 platelet survival time, 341
leukocyte alkaline
phosphatase stain, 748
platelet aggregation, 865
platelet count
(thrombocyte), 871
IgA deficiency, immunoglobulin
G, subclassification, 686
IgA myeloma, immunoglobulin
electrophoresis, serum,
680
IgD myeloma, immunoglobulin
electrophoresis, serum,
680
IgE myeloma, immunoglobulin
electrophoresis, serum,
680
IgG myeloma, immunoglobulin
electrophoresis, serum,
680
Ileus, sodium (Na), serum, 475
Immune complex formation,
platelet count
(thromobocyte), 871
Immune disorders of connective
tissue, fibrinogen, 561
Immunodeficiency
lymph node biopsy, 179
Rocky Mountain spotted fever
antibodies, 1023
Impotence
prolactin (HPRL, LTH), 906
prostate-specific antigen
(PSA), 909
Inborn enzyme deficiency,
ammonia (NH_3), 56
Incompatible blood transfusions,
erythrocyte fragility, 510
Incompatible cross-match,
Coombs antiglobulin,
indirect (IAT), 326
Incomplete abortion, human
chorionic gonadotropin
(hCG), 655
Incontinence, urinary,
cystometry (CMG), 404

Infections
adrenal glands scan, 1030
$alpha_2$ globulin, 591
blood urea nitrogen (BUN),
203
cryoglobulin, 358
CSF analysis, 760
ferritin, 548
fibrinogen, 561
free erythrocyte
protoporphyrin (FEP),
930
gamma globulin, 590
glucose tolerance tests, 607
immunoglobulin electro-
phoresis, serum, 680
iron (Fe), 701
17-ketogenic steroids
(17-KGS), 709
pseudocholinesterase (CHS,
PCHE, AcCHS), 932
reticulocyte (retic) count,
1018
skeletal x-rays, 956
TIBC/transferrin test, 704
transferrin (siderophilin), 704,
1198
uric acid, serum, 1277
vitamin C, serum, 1307
vitamin C, urine, 1311
white blood cell (WBC)
count, 1315
Infectious hepatitis
porphyrins, urine, 882
vitamin A, serum, 1307
Infectious mononucleosis
alanine aminotransferase
(ALT), 20
alkaline phosphatase (ALP),
32
aspartate aminotransferase
(AST), 136
bilirubin, urine, 155
bone marrow aspiration and
analysis, 204
cold agglutinin titer, 268
Coombs antiglobulin, direct
(DAT), 325
cryoglobulin, 358
Epstein-Barr virus (EBV)
antibodies, 506

Infectious mononucleosis—
  Continued
  erythrocyte sedimentation
    rate, 512
  haptoglobin (Hp), 623
  isocitrate dehydrogenase
    (ICD), 707
  lactic dehydrogenase (LDH,
    LD) and isoenzymes,
    720
  leukocyte alkaline
    phosphatase stain, 748
  lymph node biopsy, 179
  Monospot (heterophil
    antibody), 801
  rheumatoid factor (RF), 1020
  T-lymphocyte assays, 1133
  urobilinogen, 1287
  VDRL, 1297
  white blood cell enzymes,
    1319
Infertility
  estradiol (E₂), serum, 521
  hysteroscopy, 676
  Sims-Huhner test, 1115
Inflammation
  alpha₁ globulin, 591
  leukocyte alkaline
    phosphatase stain, 748
  protein electrophoresis, serum,
    913
Inflammatory bowel disease
  immunoglobulin
    electrophoresis, serum,
    680
  occult blood, 818
  proctosigmoidoscopy, 899
  T-lymphocyte assays, 1133
Inflammatory diseases
  ferritin, 548
  haptoglobin, 623
  protein electrophoresis, urine,
    917
  red blood cell (RBC) count,
    1003
  urobilinogen, 1287
  white blood cell (WBC)
    count, 1315
Inflammatory lesions of
    intestines, mesenteric
    angiography, 94

Influenza
  cold agglutinin titer, 268
  influenza A and B titer, 688
  nasal or throat culture, 380
INH, red blood cell (RBC) count,
    1003
Inhalant allergy, pulmonary
    function studies, 935
Inner ear tumor, audiometry, 141
Insecticides
  aldolase (ALS), 23
  pseudocholinesterase (CHS,
    PCHE, AcCHS), 932
Insulin allergy or resistance, anti-
    insulin antibody, 113
Insulin deficiency. *See* Diabetes
    mellitus
Insulin-dependent diabetes
    mellitus (IDDM)
  insulin antibody, 695
  intrinsic factor (IF) antibody,
    697
Insulin, excessive
  insulin, 689
  potassium (K), serum, 475
Insulin-secreting tumor, insulin,
    689
Insulin shock, glucose tolerance
    tests, 607
Insulinoma
  fasting blood sugar (FSB), 596
  glucose, two-hour postprandial
    (PPBS), 600
  insulin, 689
  insulin antibody, 695
  tolbutamide tolerance test,
    1182
Interstitial-cell tumor of testis,
    17-ketosteroids (17-KS)
    and fractionation, 714
Interstitial fibrosis,
    postpneumonectomy,
    pulmonary function
    studies, 935
Intestinal angina, mesenteric
    angiography, 94
Intestinal cancer, intestinal
    biopsy, 167
Intestinal carcinoid tumors, 5-
    hydoxyindoleacetic acid
    (5-HIAA), 670

Intestinal diverticulae,
    mesenteric angiography,
    94
Intestinal fistulae
    chloride (Cl), serum, 475
    magnesium (Mg), serum,
        475
    mesenteric angiography, 94
    potassium (K), serum, 475
Intestinal inflammatory lesions,
    mesenteric angiography,
    94
Intestinal injury, alanine
    aminotransferase (ALT),
    20
Intestinal obstruction
    amylase, urine, 61
    blood gases, arterial (ABG),
        194
    kidney-ureter-bladder (KUB)
        plain films, 981
Intestinal tumor, mesenteric
    angiography, 94
Intestinal ulcerations, mesenteric
    angiography, 94
Intestinal wall infections, fecal
    analysis, 538
Intra-abdominal bleeding,
    abdominal laparoscopy,
    726
Intra-abdominal infections, MRI,
    abdominal, 770
Intra-abdominal inflammations,
    MRI, abdominal, 770
Intra-abdominal lesions, MRI,
    abdominal, 770
Intra-abdominal masses, MRI,
    abdominal, 770
Intra-abdominal neoplasm
    abdominal laparoscopy, 726
    peritoneal fluid analysis, 835
Intra-abdominal tuberculosis,
    peritoneal fluid analysis,
    835
Intracerebral hematoma,
    computed tomography
    (CT), cranial, 291
Intracerebral lesions, evoked
    brain potentials, 530
Intracranial hemorrhage, CSF
    analysis, 760

Intracranial pressure, increased
    computed tomography (CT),
        cranial, 291
    CSF analysis, 760
    specific gravity, urine, 1123
    ultrasonography, arterial,
        transcranial Doppler,
        1226
Intrahepatic abscess, liver and
    biliary system
    ultrasonography, 1236
Intrahepatic obstruction,
    isocitrate dehydrogenase
    (ICD), 707
Intramural hematoma, MRI,
    heart and chest, 778
Intraocular foreign bodies,
    ocular ultrasonography,
    1245
Intraocular tumor, ocular
    ultrasonography, 1245
Intraparenchymal hematoma,
    MRI, head, 774
Intraparenchymal hemorrhage,
    MRI, head, 774
Intrarenal reflux, antegrade
    pyelography, 947
Intrauterine adhesions,
    hysteroscopy, 676
Intrauterine fetal death. *See* Fetal
    death
Intrauterine fibroids,
    hysteroscopy, 676
Iritis, slit lamp biomicroscopy,
    1120
Iron deficiency
    free erythrocyte
        protoporphyrin (FEP), 930
    transferrin (siderophilin), 704,
        1198
Iron-deficiency anemias
    erythrocyte fragility, 510
    ferritin, 548
    gamma globulin, 590
    iron (Fe), 701
    platelet count
        (thrombocyte), 871
    red blood cell indices, 1008
    TIBC/transferrin test, 704
    white blood cell enzymes,
        1319

Ischemia, lower extremity arterial (LEA) Doppler, 1268
Islet cell tumor, C-peptide, 216

Jaundice, computed tomography (CT), biliary tract and liver, 287
Joint tumor, synovial fluid analysis, 129

Keratitis, corneal staining, 332
Keratoconus, slit lamp biomicroscopy, 1120
Ketoacidosis
uric acid, serum, 1277
uric acid, urine, 1280
Kidney. *See also* Renal *entries*
Kidney, absence of, excretory urography (EUG), 964
Kidney anomalies
kidney scan, 1060
kidney ultrasonography, 1233
Kidney infection, kidney scan, 1060
Kidney inflammation, kidney scan, 1060
Kidney masses, kidney scan, 1060
Kidney ultrasonography, 1233
Kinky hair (Menkes's) syndrome, ceruloplasmin (Cp), 243
Klebsiella
urine culture with Gram's stain, 392
wound culture, 395
Klebsiella pneumoniae, sputum culture, 386
Klinefelter's syndrome
estradiol (E_2), serum, 521
5-hydroxyproline, 673
17-ketosteroids (17-KS) and fractionation, 714
luteinizing hormone (LH, ICSH), 766
sex chromatin tests, 1111
testosterone, 1143

Knee avascular necrosis, MRI, musculoskeletal, 781
Kwashiokor, isocitrate dehydrogenase (ICD), 707

Lactic acidosis
blood gases, arterial (ABG), 194
uric acid, serum, 1277
uric acid, urine, 1280
Lactic dehydrogenase (LDH) elevation, lactic acid, 718
Lactose deficiency, intestinal biopsy, 167
Laennec's cirrhosis, immunoglobulin electrophoresis, serum, 680
Laryngeal cancer, laryngoscopy, 733
Laryngeal congenital abnormalities, laryngoscopy, 733
Laryngeal foreign bodies, laryngoscopy, 733
Laryngeal inflammation, laryngoscopy, 733
Laryngeal lesions, laryngoscopy, 733
Laryngeal polyps, laryngoscopy, 733
Laxative abuse, potassium (K), serum, 475
Lead encephalopathy
CSF analysis, 760
lead (Pb), 738
Lead poisoning
coproporphyrin, urine (UCP), 329
delta-aminolevulinic acid (delta ALA), urine, 419
free erythrocyte protoporphyrin (FEP), 930
glucose, urine, 603
iron (Fe), 701
porphyrins (erythrocyte), total, 880
urobilinogen, 1287

Left ventricular enlargement, heart scan, 1038

Legg-Calvé-Perthes disease, bone scan, 1033

Legionnaires' disease, Legionnaires' disease antibodies, 740

Leiomyomas of uterus, hysterosalpingography, 968

Lens opacities, slit lamp biomicroscopy, 1120

Leprosy
  angiotensin-converting enzyme (ACE), 108
  immune complex assay, serum, 678
  VDRL, 1297

Leptospirosis, Rocky Mountain spotted fever antibodies, 1023

Leukemias. *See also named types*
  aldolase (ALS), 23
  ammonia (NH_3), 56
  beta$_2$-microglobulin, 149
  bleeding time, 191
  bone marrow aspiration and analysis, 204
  capillary fragility, 213
  clot retraction, 263
  coagulation factor assays, 265
  Coombs antiglobulin, direct (DAT), 325
  Coombs antiglobulin, indirect (IAT), 326
  coproporphyrin, urine (UCP), 329
  Cr-51 red cell survival time, 344
  CSF analysis, 760
  ferritin, 548
  fibrin breakdown products (FBP), 559
  fibrinogen, 561
  gamma globulin, 590
  hepatitis B surface antigen, 145
  hydroxybutyrate dehydrogenase (HBDH), 665
  immune complex assay, serum, 678
  iron (Fe), 701
  lactic dehydrogenase (LDH, LD) and isoenzymes, 720
  leukocyte alkaline phosphatase stain, 748
  platelet count (thrombocyte), 871
  protein electrophoresis, urine, 917
  red blood cell (RBC) count, 1003
  reticulocyte (retic) count, 1018
  rheumatoid factor (RF), 1020
  Schirmer tearing test, 1101
  serum protein, total, 920
  thrombin clotting time (TCT), 1148
  uric acid, urine, 1280
  white blood cell (WBC) count, 1315

Leukemic reactions, bone marrow aspiration and analysis, 204

Leukemoid reactions, white blood cell enzymes, 1319

Leukoplakia of cervix, colposcopy, 277

Limb girdle muscular dystrophy, aldolase (ALS), 23

Lipid storage disease, myoglobin, urine, 814

Lipoprotein disorders, protein electrophoresis, serum, 913

Liver. *See also* Hepatic *headings and* Cirrhosis

Liver abnormalities, kidney-ureter-bladder (KUB) plain films, 981

Liver abscess
  amylase, serum, 58
  gallium liver scan, 1051

Liver cancer
  alanine aminotransferase (ALT), 20
  alpha-fetoprotein (AFP), 40
  amylase, urine, 61
  cancer antigen 125 (CA-125), 223
  coagulation factor assays, 265

Liver cancer—*Continued*
  delta-aminolevulinic acid
    (delta ALA), urine, 419
  glucose tolerance tests, 607
  human chorionic
    gonadotropin (hCG), 655
  isocitrate dehydrogenase
    (ICD), 707
  leucine aminopeptidase
    (LAP), urine, 743
  liver and biliary system
    ultrasonography, 1236
  liver biopsy, 173
  ornithine
    carbamoyltransferase
    (OCT), 823
Liver disease or damage
  acid phosphatase (ACP), 5
  activated partial
    thromboplastin time
    (aPTT), 15 alanine
    aminotransferase (ALT),
    20
  alkaline phosphatase (ALP),
    32
  alpha$_2$ globulin, 591
  amylase, serum, 58
  antithrombin, 123
  bleeding time, 191
  blood urea nitrogen (BUN),
    203
  bone marrow aspiration and
    analysis, 204
  ceruloplasmin (Cp), 243
  cholesterol (total), 258
  coagulation factor assays, 265
  coproporphyrin, urine (UCP),
    329
  erythrocyte fragility, 510
  estrogens, serum, 521
  euglobulin clot lysis time, 528
  fasting blood sugar (FSB),
    596
  fecal analysis, 538
  fibrin breakdown products
    (FBP), 559
  gamma globulin, 590
  glucose tolerance tests, 607
  glucose, two-hour postprandial
    (PPBS), 600
  glucose, urine, 603

immunoglobulin
    electrophoresis, serum,
    680
insulin antibody test, 695
17-ketosteroids (17-KS) and
    fractionation, 714
lactic dehydrogenase (LDH,
    LD) and isoenzymes, 720
liver scan, 1065
mesenteric angiography, 94
peritoneal fluid analysis, 835
phenolsulfonphthalein (PSP),
    854
phenylalanine screening,
    serum, 619
prolactin (HPRL, LTH), 906
prothrombin time (PT, pro
    time), 927
pyruvic acid, 942
red blood cell indices, 1008
Rocky Mountain spotted fever
    antibodies, 1023
serum protein, total, 920
thyroid-binding globulin
    (TBG), 1180
thyroxine (T$_4$, total T$_4$, T$_4$RIA),
    1177
transferrin (siderophilin), 704,
    1198
triiodothyronine uptake, 1210
urobilinogen, 1287
vitamin B$_1$, serum, 1307
vitamin B$_2$, urine, 1311
vitamin B$_{12}$, serum, 1307
vitamin D$_3$, serum, 1307
Liver disease, obstructive,
    lipoprotein phenotyping,
    756
Liver failure, ammonia (NH$_3$), 56
Liver inflammation, gallium liver
    scan, 1051
Liver tumor
  aspartate aminotransferase
    (AST), 136
  gallium liver scan, 1051
Louis-Bar syndrome, glucose
    tolerance tests, 607
Low-birth-weight infant
  iron (Fe), 701
  thyroid-stimulating hormone,
    neonatal, 1171

Lower extremity aneurysm, lower extremity angiography, 87
Lower extremity tumor, lower extremity angiography, 87
Lung. *See also* Pulmonary *and* Respiratory *headings*
Lung cancer
  beta₂-microglobulin, 149
  calcitonin, 220
  cancer antigen 125 (CA-125), 223
  carcinoembryonic antigen (CEA), 225
  ceruloplasmin (Cp), 243
  chest tomography, 1185
  dexamethasone suppression test (DST), 420
  fibrinogen, 561
  glucose tolerance tests, 607
  lung biopsy, 179
  pleural fluid analysis, 1150
  potassium (K), urine, 487
  prolactin (HPRL, LTH), 906
  thoracoscopy, 1156
Lung or chest cavity tumor, pulmonary angiogram, 98
Lung fibrosis, lung biopsy, 179
Lung mass, thoracic fluoroscopy, 569
Lupus erythematosus. *See also* Systemic lupus erythematosus (SLE)
  B-lymphocyte assays, 1133
  beta globulin, 590
  cold stimulation, 270
  Coombs antiglobulin, direct (DAT), 325
  kidney biopsy, 170
  lipoprotein phenotyping, 756
  lung biopsy, 179
  synovial fluid analysis, 129
  white blood cell (WBC) count, 1315
Lupus myelopathy, CSF analysis, 760
Lupus nephritis, serum complement assay, 1109
Lutein-cell ovarian tumor 17-ketogenic steroids (17-KGS), 709

17-ketosteroids (17-KS) and fractionation, 714
Lyme disease, lyme disease antibody, 769
Lymph glands, metastastes to, lymphangiography, 972
Lymph vessel abnormalities, lymphangiography, 972
Lymphadenoma, bone marrow aspiration and analysis, 204
Lymphangitis, lymph node biopsy, 179
Lymphatic leukemia
  bone marrow aspiration and analysis, 204
  cold agglutinin titer, 268
Lymphoblastic leukemia, leukocyte alkaline phosphatase stain, 748
Lymphocytic choriomeningitis, CSF analysis, 760
Lymphocytic leukemia
  cryoglobulin, 358
  gamma globulin, 590
  immunoglobulin electrophoresis, serum, 680
Lymphogranuloma venereum
  chlamydial tests, 245
  lymph node biopsy, 179
Lymphomas
  cancer antigen 125 (CA-125), 223
  carcinoembryonic antigen (CEA), 225
  Coombs antiglobulin, direct (DAT), 325
  Cr-51 platelet survival time, 341
  CSF analysis, 760
  fecal fat, 542
  fibrinogen, 561
  gallium breast scan, 1044
  hemoglobin (Hb), 630
  lactic dehydrogenase (LDH, LD) and isoenzymes, 720
  lymph node biopsy, 179
  lymph node and retroperitoneal ultrasonography, 1239

Lymphomas—*Continued*
platelet count
(thrombocyte), 871
Schirmer tearing test, 1101
thrombin clotting time (TCT),
1148
white blood cell enzymes, 1319
Lymphomas, non-Hodgkin's,
angiotensin-converting
enzyme (ACE), 108
Lymphoproliferative processes
Epstein-Barr virus (EBV)
antibodies, 506
lactic dehydrogenase (LDH,
LD) and isoenzymes, 720
Lymphosarcoma
bone marrow aspiration and
analysis, 204
erythrocyte sedimentation
rate, 512
gamma globulin, 590
immunoglobulin
electrophoresis, serum,
680
uric acid, urine, 1280

Macroamylasemia
amylase, serum, 58
amylase, urine, 61
Macrocytic anemia, red blood
cell indices, 1008
Macroglobulinemias
bone marrow aspiration and
analysis, 204
erythrocyte sedimentation
rate, 512
immunoglobulin
electrophoresis, serum,
680
platelet aggregation, 865
protein electrophoresis, serum,
913
serum protein, total, 920
Macular degeneration
angiography, fluorescein, 79
electro-oculography (EOG),
454
Malabsorption syndromes
alpha$_2$ globulin, 591
amino acid screen, blood, 45
beta globulin, 590

blood urea nitrogen (BUN),
203
calcium (Ca), urine, 488
ceruloplasmin (Cp), 243
cholesterol (total), 258
fasting blood sugar (FSB), 596
fecal analysis, 538
gamma globulin, 590
glucose tolerance tests, 607
glucose, two-hour postprandial
(PPBS), 600
magnesium (Mg), serum, 475
magnesium (Mg), urine, 488
parathyroid hormone (PTH),
840
phospholipids, 861
phosphorus (P), serum, 475
potassium (K), urine, 486
Schilling test, 1097
serum protein, total, 920
TIBC/transferrin test, 704
trypsin, fecal, 1215
vitamin B$_6$, plasma, 1307
vitamin C, urine, 1311
vitamin E, 1307
D-xylose tolerance, 417
Malaria
blood culture, 365
cold agglutinin titer, 268
hemoglobin and blood, urine,
637
immune complex assay,
serum, 678
immunoglobulin
electrophoresis, serum,
680
liver biopsy, 173
urobilinogen, 1287
white blood cell (WBC)
count, 1315
Malignancies
alpha$_1$ globulin, 591
alpha$_2$ globulin, 591
parathyroid hormone (PTH),
840
TIBC/transferrin test, 704
white blood cell (WBC)
count, 1315
Malignant hypertension
beta globulin, 590
gamma globulin, 590
renin, plasma, 1013

Malignant melanoma
  human chorionic
      gonadotropin (hCG), 655
  hydroxybutyrate
      dehydrogenase (HBDH),
      665
  immune complex assay,
      serum, 678
  melanin, 794
  skin biopsy, 186
Mallory-Weiss tears
  esophagogastroduodeno-
      scopy, 515
  fecal analysis, 538
Malnutrition. *See also* Starvation
  alpha$_1$-antitrypsin (α_1-AT), 40
  alpha$_2$ globulin, 591
  amino acid screen, blood, 45
  antithrombin, 123
  beta globulin, 590
  bicarbonate (HCO_3), 475
  coagulation factor assays, 265
  folic acid, 571
  glucose tolerance tests, 607
  5-hydroxyproline, 673
  immunoglobulin
      electrophoresis, serum,
      680
  phospholipids, 861
  phosphorus (P), serum, 475
  protein electrophoresis, serum,
      913
  pseudocholinesterase (CHS,
      PCHE, AcCHS), 932
  serum complement assay,
      1109
  serum protein, total, 920
  sweat test (pilocarpine
      iontophoresis), 1130
  thyroid-binding globulin
      (TBG), 1180
  thyroxine (T_4, total T_4, T_4RIA),
      1177
  TIBC/transferrin test, 704
  triiodothyronine (T_3, total T_3,
      T_3RIA), 1205
  triiodothyronine uptake, 1210
  trypsin, blood, 1213
  vitamin B$_6$, plasma, 1307
  vitamin C, urine, 1311
  white blood cell (WBC)
      count, 1315

Maple syrup urine disease,
      amino acids, urine, 48
Marfan syndrome, 5-hydroxy-
      proline, 673
Marrow. *See* Bone marrow
      entries
Maternal-fetal Rh incompatibility,
      Coombs antiglobulin,
      indirect (IAT), 326
Measles
  bleeding time, 191
  CSF analysis, 760
Meckel's diverticulum, Meckel's
      diverticulum scan, 1076
Megakaryocytic myelosis, bone
      marrow aspiration and
      analysis, 204
Megaloblastic anemia
  alpha$_2$ globulin, 591
  ferritin, 548
  free erythrocyte
      protoporphyrin (FEP),
      930
  gastric acid stimulation test,
      585
  hemosideran, 643
  hydroxybutyrate
      dehydrogenase (HBDH),
      665
  intrinsic factor (IF) antibody,
      697
Melanomatosis, CSF analysis, 760
Meningeal carcinomatosis, CSF
      analysis, 760
Meningioma
  MRI, head, 774
  progesterone receptor assay,
      902
Meningitis
  CSF analysis, 237, 760
  culture, herpesvirus (HSV-1,
      HSV-2), 378
Meningitis, cryptococcal, fungal
      antibody tests, 580
Meningitis, viral, Coxsackie A or
      B virus, 339
Meningocele, computed
      tomography (CT), spinal,
      309
Meningococcemia, platelet
      count (thrombocyte),
      871

Meningoencephalitis, CSF analysis, 760

Meniscal tears, MRI, musculoskeletal, 781

Menkes's (kinky hair) syndrome, ceruloplasmin (Cp), 243

Menopause
estradiol (E_2), serum, 521
estrogens, serum, 523
estrogens, urine, total and fractions, 524
17-ketosteroids (17-KS) and fractionation, 714

Mental retardation, amniotic fluid analysis, 51

Mercury poisoning, beta$_2$-microglobulin, 149

Mesenteric ischemia, mesenteric angiography, 94

Mesothelioma
fasting blood sugar (FSB), 596
glucose, two-hour postprandial (PPBS), 600

Metabolic acidosis
bicarbonate (HCO_3), 475
blood gases, arterial (ABG), 195
pH, urine, 85

Metabolic alkalosis
bicarbonate (HCO_3), 475
blood gases, arterial (ABG), 195
pH, urine, 850

Metabolic disorders, skeletal x-rays, 956

Metachromatic leukodystrophy, arylsulfatase A (ARS-A), urine, 133

Metal poisoning, lead (Pb), 738

Metastatic cancer
antidiuretic hormone (ADH), 116
calcium, urine, 487
progesterone receptor assay, 902
thyroxine (T_4, total T_4, T_4RIA), 1177
triiodothyronine uptake, 1210

Methemoglobinemias
electrophoresis, hemoglobin, 640

methemoglobin (MetHb, HbM), 798

Microcephaly, amniotic fluid analysis, 51

Microcytic anemia, red blood cell indices, 1008

Microsporium, skin culture, 383

Micturition disorders, prostate ultrasonography (transrectal), 1254

Middle ear abnormalities, acoustic admittance tests, 9

Middle ear disorders, electronystagmography (ENG), 498

Migraine
electroencephalography (EEG), 472
positron emission tomography (PET), 885

Miliary tuberculosis, platelet count (thrombocyte), 871

Mitral stenosis, phonocardiograph (PCG), 858

Mitral valve abnormalities
echocardiography, 448
electrocardiography, ambulatory, 462

Mixoma, echocardiography, 448

Monoclonal gammopathy, protein electrophoresis, urine, 917

Monocytic leukemia
muramidase (lysozyme), 807
protein electrophoresis, serum, 913

Mucoepidermoid tumor, parotid and salivary glands scan, 1082

Mucopolysaccharidosis, electroretinography, 501

Multiple myeloma
acid phosphatase (ACP), 5
amino acids, urine, 48
B-lymphocyte assays, 1133
Bence Jones protein, 147
beta$_2$-microglobulin, 149
bleeding time, 191

bone biopsy, 159
clot retraction, 263
cold agglutinin titer, 268
concentration/dilution tests, urine, 316
erythrocyte sedimentation rate, 512
fibrinogen, 561
glucose, urine, 603
human chorionic gonadotropin (hCG), 655
immunoglobulin electrophoresis, urine, 683
phenolsulfonphthalein (PSP), 854
phosphorus (P), urine, 488
potassium (K), urine, 487
protein electrophoresis, serum, 913
protein, urine (dipstick), 923
red blood cell (RBC) count, 1003
T-lymphocyte assays, 1133
uric acid, urine, 1280
white blood cell enzymes, 1319
Multiple pregnancy. *See* Pregnancy, multiple
Multiple sclerosis
CSF analysis, 760
evoked brain potentials, 530
human leukocyte antigen and typing (HLA, tissue typing), 660
5-hydroxyproline, 673
MRI, head, 774
T-lymphocyte assays, 1133
Multisystem failure, pulmonary artery catheterization, 234
Mumps
amylase, serum, 58
bleeding time, 191
CSF analysis, 237, 760
mumps test (mumps antibody), 805
Mural thrombi, echocardiography, 448
Murine typhus, febrile agglutinins, serum, 544

Muscle trauma
alanine aminotransferase (ALT), 20
hemoglobin and blood, urine, 637
Muscular dystrophy
aldolase (ALS), 23
aspartate aminotransferase (AST), 136
creatine phosphokinase (CPK) and isoenzymes, 347
creatinine, 350
electroneurography (ENG), 495
hydroxybutyrate dehydrogenase (HBDH), 665
5-hydroxyproline, 673
lactic dehydrogenase (LDH, LD) and isoenzymes, 720
myoglobin, serum, 812
myoglobin, urine, 814
pseudocholinesterase (CHS, PCHE, AcCHS), 932
Mushroom poisoning, ornithine carbamoyltransferase (OCT), 823
Myasthenia gravis
acetylcholine receptor antibody (AChR), 3
anti-DNA antibody, 110
antinuclear antibody (ANA), 119
electroneurography (ENG), 495
human leukocyte antigen and typing (HLA, tissue typing), 660
muscle biopsy, 181
T-lymphocyte assays, 1133
tensilon test, 1140
triiodothyronine uptake, 1210
Mycobacterial CNS infections, CSF analysis, 237, 760
Mycobacterium, wound culture, 395
Mycobacterium tuberculosis, sputum culture, 386
Mycoplasma infection or carrier, culture, anal or genital, 363

Mycoplasma pneumoniae
cold agglutinin titer, 268
Coombs antiglobulin, direct (DAT), 325
Myeloblastic leukemia, bone marrow aspiration and analysis, 204
Myelocele, computed tomography (CT), spinal, 309
Myelocytic leukemia
bone marrow aspiration and analysis, 204
immunoglobulin electrophoresis, serum, 680
Myelofibrosis
leukocyte alkaline phosphatase stain, 748
white blood cell enzymes, 1319
Myelogenous leukemia, acute, acid phosphatase (ACP), 5
Myeloid fibroplasia, leukocyte alkaline phosphatase stain, 748
Myeloid leukemia, bone marrow aspiration and analysis, 204
Myelomas, serum viscosity, 1303
Myelomonocytic leukemia, muramidase (lysozyme), 807
Myeloproliferative disorders, vitamin B$_{12}$, serum, 1307
Myocardial infarction
alanine aminotransferase (ALT), 20
aldolase (ALS), 23
alpha$_2$ globulin, 591
apolipoprotein A-1 (Apo A-1), 125
apolipoprotein B, plasma (Apo B), 127
aspartate aminotransferase (AST), 136
bicarbonate (HCO$_3$), 475
blood urea nitrogen (BUN), 203
ceruloplasmin (Cp), 243
cholesterol (total), 258

coproporphyrin, urine (UCP), 329
creatine phosphokinase (CPK) and isoenzymes, 347
echocardiography, transesophageal, 451
electrocardiography (ECG), 456
erythrocyte sedimentation rate, 512
gamma glutamyl transpeptidase (GGTP, GGT), 582
glucose tolerance tests, 607
haptoglobin (Hp), 623
heart scan, 1038
lactic acid, 718
lactic dehydrogenase (LDH, LD) and isoenzymes, 720
MRI, heart and chest, 778
myoglobin, serum, 812
myoglobin, urine, 814
positron emission tomography (PET), 885, 1085
pseudocholinesterase (CHS, PCHE, AcCHS), 932
pyruvic acid, 942
serum complement assay, 1109
transesophageal echocardiography, 451
triglycerides, 1202
Myocardial ischemia, electrocardiography (ECG), 456
Myocarditis, phonocardiograph (PCG), 858
Myoglobinemia, protein, urine (dipstick), 923
Myopia, refraction, 1011
Myositis, viral, Coxsackie A or B virus, 339
Myotonia congenita, muscle biopsy, 181
Myxedema
fasting blood sugar (FSB), 596
gastric acid stimulation test, 585
glucose, two-hour postprandial (PPBS), 600
lactic dehydrogenase (LDH, LD) and isoenzymes, 720

Narcolepsy,
electroencephalography
(EEG), 472
Necrosis, alpha₁-antitrypsin
(α₁-AT), 40
Neisseria gonorrheae infection
culture, anal or genital, 363
eye culture, 373
Neonatal hepatic immaturity,
bilirubin, serum, 151
Neonatal lupus, anti-Ro/Sjögren's
syndrome antigen (SS-A),
114
Neoplasms
aldolase (ALS), 23
blood urea nitrogen (BUN),
203
folic acid, 571
glucose tolerance tests, 607
lactic acid, 718
protein electrophoresis, serum,
913
skeletal x-rays, 956
Neoplastic syndrome, alpha₂
globulin, 591
Neovascularization of retina,
angiography, fluorescein,
79
Nephritis
calcium (Ca), urine, 487
erythrocyte sedimentation
rate, 512
iron (Fe), 701
phosphorus (P), urine, 488
pleural fluid analysis, 1150
Nephritis, lupus, serum
complement assay, 1109
Nephrolithiasis, occult blood, 818
Nephrosclerosis
creatinine clearance, urine,
354
insulin clearance test, 699
Nephrosis
calcium (Ca), urine, 487
gamma globulin, 590
iron (Fe), 701
phosphorus (P), urine, 488
Nephrotic syndrome
aldosterone, plasma, 25
aldosterone, urine, 29
alpha₁-antitrypsin (α₁-AT), 40
alpha₂ globulin, 591

antithrombin, 123
beta globulin, 590
blood urea nitrogen (BUN),
203
ceruloplasmin (Cp), 243
cholesterol (total), 258
coagulation factor assays, 265
gamma globulin, 590
hydroxybutyrate
dehydrogenase (HBDH),
665
immunoglobulin
electrophoresis, serum, 680
kidney biopsy, 170
lipoprotein phenotyping, 756
lipoprotein-cholesterol
fractionation, 753
muramidase (lysozyme), 807
phospholipids, 861
protein electrophoresis, serum,
913
protein electrophoresis, urine,
917
protein, urine (dipstick), 923
pseudocholinesterase (CHS,
PCHE, AcCHS), 932
serum protein, total, 920
thyroid-binding globulin
(TBG), 1180
TIBC/transferrin test, 704
triglycerides, 1202
triiodothyronine uptake, 1210
Neural-tube defect, amniotic
fluid analysis, 51
Neuritis, vitamin B₁, serum, 1307
Neuroblastoma
catecholamines, plasma, 227
catecholamines, urine, 230
homovanillic acid, 652
vanillylmandelic acid (VMA),
1294
Neurofibroma, skin biopsy, 186
Neurogenic bladder, voiding
cystourethrography, 991
Neurohypophyseal tumor,
antidiuretic hormone
(ADH), 116
Neurologic degenerative
diseases, vitamin E, 1307
Neuromuscular diseases,
pulmonary function
studies, 935

Neurophilic leukemoid reaction, leukocyte alkaline phosphatase stain, 748

Neurosyphilis, CSF analysis, 760

NIDDM. *See* Non–insulin-dependent diabetes mellitus

Niemann-Pick disease, acid phosphatase (ACP), 5

Night blindness
electroretinography, 501
vitamin A, serum, 1307

Nocardiosis
acid-fast bacillus (AFB) culture and smear, 397
bronchoscopy, 209
potassium hydroxide preparation, 889

Nodular lymphoma, angiography, lymph, 91, 972

Non-Hodgkin's lymphoma, angiotensin-converting enzyme (ACE), 108

Non–insulin-dependent diabetes mellitus (NIDDM), insulin antibody, 695

Nonpregnancy, human chorionic gonadotropin (hGC), pregnancy test, 657

Nonsyphilitic treponemal diseases, VDRL, 1297

Nontoxic nodular goiter, thyroid biopsy, 188

Nonvascular tumor, cerebral, cerebral angiogram, 70

Nose fracture, tomography, paranasal sinuses, 1188

Nutritional deficit. *See also* Starvation
hemoglobin (Hb), 630

Nutritional disorders, skeletal x-rays, 956

Oat cell carcinoma
adrenocorticotropic hormone (ACTH), 17
serotonin (5-hydroxy-tryptamine), 1107

Obesity
cortisol, 334
fasting blood sugar (FSB), 596
glucose, two-hour postprandial (PPBS), 600
glucose, urine, 603
17-hydroxycorticosteroids (17-OHCS), 667
insulin antibody, 695
17-ketogenic steroids (17-KGS), 709
triiodothyronine (T_3, total T_3, T_3RIA), 1205

Obstetrical complications
fibrin breakdown products (FBP), 559
thrombin clotting time (TCT), 1148

Obstructive jaundice
aldolase (ALS), 23
cholesterol (total), 258
coproporphyrin, urine (UCP), 329
erythrocyte fragility, 510
ornithine carbamoyltrans-ferase (OCT), 823
phospholipids, 861
triglycerides, 1202
urobilinogen, 1287

Obstructive lung disease
ammonia (NH_3), 56
plethysmography, 874

Obstructive uropathy, kidney scan, 1060

Ocular media opacities, electroretinography, 501

Omphalocele, amniotic fluid analysis, 51

Oncocytoma, parotid and salivary glands scan, 1082

Opportunistic lung infections, bronchoscopy, 209

Optic chiasm lesions, evoked brain potentials, 530

Optic neuritis
evoked brain potentials, 530
visual fields test, 1304

Optic nerve tumor, MRI, head, 774

Orbital bone hypertrophy, exophthalmometry, 543

Orbital foreign body, orbit and eye, plain films, 981
Orbital fracture, orbit and eye, plain films, 981
Orbital lesions, ocular ultrasonography, 1245
Orbital space tumor
  computed tomography (CT), orbital, 295
  orbit and eye, plain films, 981
Orchitis, scrotal scan, 1088
Orchitis, postviral
  follicle-stimulating hormone (FSH), 573
  luteinizing hormone (LH, ICSH), 766
Organ failure, red blood cell (RBC) count, 1003
Organophosphates, pseudocholinesterase (CHS, PCHE, AcCHS), 932
Orthostatic hypotension, catecholamines, urine, 230
Orthostatic (postural) proteinuria, protein, urine (dipstick), 923
Osmotic diuresis, concentration/dilution tests, urine, 316
Osteitis deformans, alkaline phosphatase (ALP), 32
Osteoarthritis, synovial fluid analysis, 129
Osteogenesis imperfecta, acid phosphatase (ACP), 5
Osteogenic sarcoma, alkaline phosphatase (ALP), 32
Osteoma, bone biopsy, 159
Osteomalacia
  alkaline phosphatase (ALP), 32
  amino acids, urine, 48
  calcium (Ca), urine, 488
  5-hydroxyproline, 673
  phosphorus (P), urine, 488
  vitamin D₃, serum, 1307
Osteomyelitis
  bone scan, 1033
  5-hydroxyproline, 673
  MRI, musculoskeletal, 781
  skeletal x-rays, 956

Osteoporosis
  calcium (Ca), urine, 487
  estradiol (E₂), serum, 521
  magnesium (Mg), urine, 488
  prostate-specific antigen (PSA), 909
Osteosarcoma
  bone biopsy, 159
  MRI, musculoskeletal, 781
Otitis externa
  audiometry, 141
  otoscopy, 825
Otitis interna, otoscopy, 825
Otitis media, audiometry, 141
Otosclerosis, audiometry, 141
Ototoxic drugs
  audiometry, 141
  electronystagmography (ENG), 498
Ovarian agenesis, estrogens, serum, 523
Ovarian cancer
  cancer antigen 125 (CA-125), 223
  carcinoembryonic antigen (CEA), 225
Ovarian cyst or abscess
  cancer antigen 125 (CA-125), 223
  computed tomography (CT), pelvic, 301
  gynecologic laparoscopy, 729
  pelvic ultrasonography, 1251
  pregnanediol, 893
Ovarian failure
  estrogens, urine, total and fractions, 524
  luteinizing hormone (LH, ICSH), 766
  pregnanediol, 893
Ovarian stromal hyperplasia, androstenedione, 64
Ovarian tumors
  androstenedione, 64
  estradiol (E₂), serum, 521
  estrogens, serum, 521
  estrogens, urine, total and fractions, 524
  gynecologic laparoscopy, 729
  17-ketogenic steroids (17-KGS), 709

Ovarian tumors—*Continued*
  pregnanediol, 893
  pregnanetriol, 897
  testosterone, 1143
Overhydration, red blood cell
    (RBC) count, 1003

Paget's disease
  acid phosphatase (ACP), 5
  alkaline phosphatase (ALP),
    32
  bone scan, 1033
  calcium (Ca), urine, 487
  5-hydroxyproline, 673
  phosphorus (P), urine, 488
Pain, red blood cell (RBC)
    count, 1003
Palpitations,
    electrocardiography,
    ambulatory, 462
Pancreatectomy, glucagon, 594
Pancreatic abscess, computed
    tomography (CT),
    pancreatic, 298
Pancreatic adenoma
  fasting blood sugar (FSB), 596
  glucose, two-hour postprandial
    (PPBS), 600
Pancreatic cancer
  amylase, serum, 58
  bilirubin, serum, 151
  calcitonin, 220
  cancer antigen 125 (CA-125),
    223
  cholangiography,
    percutaneous
    transhepatic (PTHC), 249
  cholangiopancreatography, 255
  computed tomography (CT),
    pancreatic, 298
  fibrinogen, 561
  glucagon, 594
  glucose, urine, 603
  human chorionic
    gonadotropin (hCG), 655
  leucine aminopeptidase
    (LAP), urine, 743
  lipase, 750
  secretin test, 1104
  urobilinogen, 1287

Pancreatic cell disease, gamma
    glutamyl transpeptidase
    (GGTP, GGT), 582
Pancreatic cell neoplasm,
    gamma glutamyl
    transpeptidase (GGTP,
    GGT), 582
Pancreatic deficiency
  fecal analysis, 538
  trypsin, fecal, 1215
Pancreatic disease or damage
  amylase, urine, 61
  fecal fat, 542
  peritoneal fluid analysis, 835
Pancreatic duct abnormalities,
    percutaneous
    transhepatic
    cholangiography (PTC,
    PTHC), 249, 978
Pancreatic duct obstruction
  amylase, urine, 61
  computed tomography (CT),
    pancreatic, 298
  lipase, 750
  ultrasonography, pancreas,
    1248
Pancreatic fibrosis,
    cholangiopancreato-
    graphy, 255
Pancreatic inflammation
  culture, duodenal and gastric,
    369
  lipase, 750
Pancreatic islet cell hyperplasia,
    glucose tolerance tests,
    607
Pancreatic islet cell tumor
  mesenteric angiography, 94
  serotonin (5-hydroxy-
    tryptamine), 1107
Pancreatic pseudocyst
  amylase, serum, 58
  amylase, urine, 61
  computed tomography (CT),
    abdomen, 284
  computed tomography (CT),
    pancreatic, 298
  peritoneal fluid analysis, 835
  secretin test, 1104
  ultrasonography, pancreas,
    1248

Pancreatic tumor
  computed tomography (CT),
    pancreatic, 298
  leucine aminopeptidase
    (LAP), serum, 741
  ultrasonography, pancreas,
    1248
Pancreatitis
  abdominal laparoscopy, 726
  alanine aminotransferase
    (ALT), 20
  amylase, serum, 58
  amylase, urine, 61
  aspartate aminotransferase
    (AST), 136
  blood urea nitrogen (BUN),
    203
  cancer antigen 125 (CA-125),
    223
  carcinoembryonic antigen
    (CEA), 225
  cholangiopancreatography, 255
  computed tomography (CT),
    pancreatic, 298
  fasting blood sugar (FSB), 596
  fecal analysis, 538
  glucagon, 594
  glucose tolerance tests, 607
  glucose, two-hour postprandial
    (PPBS), 600
  glucose, urine, 603
  lactic dehydrogenase (LDH,
    LD) and isoenzymes, 720
  lipase, 750
  lipoprotein phenotyping, 756
  lipoprotein-cholesterol
    fractionation, 753
  magnesium (Mg), serum, 475
  magnesium (Mg), urine, 488
  methemoglobin (MetHb,
    HbM), 798
  peritoneal fluid analysis, 835
  phospholipids, 861
  pleural fluid analysis, 1150
  secretin test, 1104
  trypsin, blood, 1213
  ultrasonography, pancreas,
    1248
Panhypopituitarism
  adrenocorticotropic hormone
    (ACTH), 17

follicle-stimulating hormone
    (FSH), 573
  growth hormone stimulation
    test, 615
  luteinizing hormone (LH,
    ICSH), 766
Panpituitarism, 17-ketogenic
    steroids (17-KGS), 709
Para-aminohippurate, creatinine
    clearance, urine, 354
Paracoccidioidomycosis,
    potassium hydroxide
    preparation, 889
Parahypopituitarism,
    pregnanediol, 893
Paranasal sinus tumor or tumor
    invasion
  computed tomography (CT),
    orbital, 295
  paranasal sinuses tomography,
    1188
Parasal, red blood cell (RBC)
    count, 1003
Parasitic damage to RBCs,
    erythrocyte fragility, 510
Parasitic infestation
  immunoglobulin electro-
    phoresis, serum, 680
  intestinal biopsy, 167
  liver biopsy, 173
  lymph node biopsy, 179
  muscle biopsy, 181
  peritoneal fluid analysis, 835
  Raji cell assay, 999
  white blood cell (WBC)
    count, 1315
Parasitic syndrome, pleural fluid
    analysis, 1150
Paraspinal cysts, computed
    tomography (CT), spinal,
    309
Parathyroid adenoma,
    parathyroid scan, 1079
Parathyroid hormone
    administration, 5-
    hydroxyproline, 673
Parathyroid hyperplasia,
    parathyroid
    ultrasonography, 1263
Parathyroid tumor, parathyroid
    ultrasonography, 1263

Paratyphoid fever, febrile
agglutinins, serum, 544
Parenteral nutrition, long-term
total, ceruloplasmin (Cp),
243
Parkinson's disease
brain scan, 994
catecholamines, plasma, 227
evoked brain potentials, 530
positron emission tomography
(PET), 885, 1085
Parotid or salivary gland lesions,
parotid and salivary
glands scan, 1082
Parotitis, amylase, serum, 58
Paroxysmal atrial tachycardia,
atrial natriuretic hormone
(ANH), 139
Paroxysmal hemoglobinuria,
platelet antibody
detection, 869
Paroxysmal nocturnal
hemoglobinuria (PNH)
acidified serum test, 621
hemoglobin or blood, urine,
637
hemosiderin, 643
leukocyte alkaline
phosphatase stain, 748
sucrose hemolysis, 1128
white blood cell enzymes,
1319
Pelvic abscess, pelvic
ultrasonography, 1251
Pelvic adhesions
culdoscopy, 360
gynecologic laparoscopy, 729
Pelvic inflammatory disease
(PID)
cancer antigen 125 (CA-125),
223
culdoscopy, 360
gynecologic laparoscopy, 729
pelvic ultrasonography, 1251
Pelvic mass
culdoscopy, 360
gynecologic laparoscopy, 729
Pelvic tumors, voiding
cystourethrography, 991
Pemphigus, skin biopsy, 186
Penicillamine, red blood cell
(RBC) count, 1003

Penicillins
blood gases, arterial (ABG), 194
creatinine clearance, urine, 354
estriol (E_3), serum, 521
glucose, urine, 603
17-ketogenic steroids (17-
KGS), 709
platelet aggregation, 865
radioactive iodine uptake
(RAIU), 944
red blood cell (RBC) count,
1003
scleroderma antibody, 1103
triiodothyronine uptake, 1210
Pentazocine
amylase, serum, 58
17-hydroxycorticosteroids
(17-OHCS), 667
Peptic ulcer
gastric acid stimulation test,
585
serum protein, total, 920
Peptic ulcer, perforated
amylase, serum, 58
lipase, 750
Perforated ulcer
lipase, 750
peritoneal fluid analysis, 835
Periaortic hematoma, MRI, heart
and chest, 778
Pericardial effusion
echocardiography, 448
MRI, heart and chest, 778
phonocardiograph (PCG), 858
Pericardial hematoma, MRI,
heart and chest, 778
Pericarditis
aspartate aminotransferase
(AST), 136
electrocardiography (ECG), 456
pericardial fluid analysis, 846
Pericarditis, viral, Coxsackie A or
B virus, 339
Perineal hypospadius, retrograde
urethrography, 988
Perinephric pathology,
retrograde
ureteropyelography, 985
Peripheral arterial obstructive
disease,
electrocardiography,
exercise, 465

Peripheral nerve root disease, evoked brain potentials, 530

Peripheral nervous system lesions, electronystagmography (ENG), 498

Peripheral neuropathy, lead (Pb), 738

Perirenal abscess or hematoma
computed tomography (CT), renal, 305
kidney ultrasonography, 1233

Peritoneal dialysis, chronic, peritoneal fluid analysis, 835

Peritonitis
cancer antigen 125 (CA-125), 223
pelvic ultrasonography, 1251
peritoneal fluid analysis, 835

Pernicious anemia
bilirubin, serum, 151
cholesterol (total), 258
ferritin, 548
folic acid, 571
gastric acid stimulation test, 585
gastrin, 588
hemosiderin, 643
intrinsic factor (IF) antibody, 697
iron (Fe), 701
pepsinogen, 844
red blood cell indices, 1008
reticulocyte (retic) count, 1018
Schilling test, 1097
thyroid antithyroglobulin antibody, 1160
uric acid, serum, 1277
uric acid, urine, 1280
urobilinogen, 1287
white blood cell enzymes, 1319

Pernicious aplastic anemia, bone marrow aspiration and analysis, 204

Pertussis, culture, nasal or throat, 380

Pharyngitis, nasal or throat culture, 380

Phenylketonuria (PKU)
ferric chloride ($FeCl_3$), 546
5-hydroxyindoleacetic acid (5-HIAA), 670
pH, urine, 850
phenylalanine screening, serum, 619
serotonin (5-hydroxy-tryptamine), 1107

Pheochromocytoma
adrenal angiography, 66
adrenal glands scan, 1030
angiography, digital subtraction (DSA), 76
catecholamines, urine, 230
fasting blood sugar (FSB), 596
free fatty acids (FFA), 575
glucagon, 594
glucose tolerance tests, 607
glucose, two-hour postprandial (PPBS), 600
insulin, 689
metanephrines, total, 795
vanillylmandelic acid (VMA), 1294

Phycomycosis, bronchoscopy, 209

PID. *See* Pelvic inflammatory disease

Pigmented nevi, skin biopsy, 186

Pinta
hemagglutination treponemal test for syphilis (HATTS), 626
microhemagglutination treponema pallidum (MHA-TP), 800
VDRL, 1297

Pituitary adenoma
adrenocorticotropic hormone (ACTH), 17
prolactin (HPRL, LTH), 906

Pituitary diabetes insipidus, antidiuretic hormone (ADH), 116

Pituitary disease or damage, growth hormone (GH, hGH, STH, SH), 612

Pituitary dysfunction
estradiol (E_2), serum, 521
thyroxine (T_4, total T_4, T_4RIA), 1177

Pituitary fibrosis, growth hormone (GH, hGH, STH, SH), 612

Pituitary hypofunction, estrogens, serum, 523

Pituitary hypoplasia, growth hormone (GH, hGH, STH, SH), 612

Pituitary hypothalamic dysfunction, thyroid-stimulating hormone, neonatal, 1171

Pituitary microadenoma, MRI, head, 774

Pituitary tumor
follicle-stimulating hormone (FSH), 573
growth hormone (GH, hGH, STH, SH), 612
17-hydroxycorticosteroids (17-OHCS), 667
luteinizing hormone (LH, ICSH), 766

PK enzyme deficiency, erythrocyte fragility, 510

Placenta previa, obstetric ultrasonography, 1242

Placental insufficiency
estrogens, urine, total and fractions, 524
pregnanediol, 893

Plague, blood culture, 365

Plasma cell dyscrasias, platelet aggregation, 865

Plasmapheresis, recent, pseudocholinesterase (CHS, PCHE, AcCHS), 932

Platelet release defects, platelet aggregation, 865

Pleural effusion
blood gases, arterial (ABG), 194
computed tomography (CT), thoracic, 313
MRI, heart and chest, 778
thoracic ultrasonography, 1261

Pleural fibrosis
fasting blood sugar (FSB), 596
glucose, two-hour postprandial (PPBS), 600

Pleurisy
Coxsackie A or B virus, 339
pleural fluid analysis, 1150

Pleurodynia, epidemic, Coxsackie A or B virus, 339

Pneumoconiosis
lung biopsy, 179
lymph node biopsy, 179

Pneumocystis carinii pneumonia
bronchoscopy, 209
lung biopsy, 179

Pneumonia
blood gases, arterial (ABG), 194
bone marrow aspiration and analysis, 204
lactic dehydrogenase (LDH, LD) and isoenzymes, 720
lung perfusion scan, 1069
lung ventilation scan, 1072
pleural fluid analysis, 1150
positron emission tomography (PET), 885, 1085
pulmonary function studies, 935

Pneumonitis, lung perfusion scan, 1069

Pneumothorax
blood gases, arterial (ABG), 194
pleural fluid analysis, 1150

Pneumothorax-causing conditions, thoracoscopy, 1156

PNH. *See* Paroxysmal nocturnal hemoglobinuria

Poikilocytosis, erythrocyte sedimentation rate, 512

Polio(myelitis)
coproporphyrin, urine (UCP), 329
CSF analysis, 760

Polyarteritis nodosa, antinuclear antibody (ANA), 119

Polycystic kidneys, kidney ultrasonography, 1233
computed tomography (CT), renal, 305
concentration/dilution tests, urine, 316
creatinine clearance, urine, 354

creatinine, urine, 352
protein electrophoresis, urine, 917
Polycystic ovaries
  follicle-stimulating hormone (FSH), 573
  prolactin (HPRL, LTH), 906
  testosterone, 1143
Polycythemia (and polycythemia vera)
  activated partial thromboplastin time (aPTT), 15
  bone marrow aspiration and analysis, 204
  capillary fragility, 213
  clot retraction, 263
  Cr-51 red cell survival time, 344
  erythrocyte fragility, 510
  erythrocyte sedimentation rate, 512
  hematocrit (Hct), 628
  hemoglobin (Hb), 630
  leukocyte alkaline phosphatase stain, 748
  MRI, musculoskeletal, 781
  muramidase (lysozyme), 807
  platelet aggregation, 865
  red blood cell (RBC) count, 1003
  thrombin clotting time (TCT), 1148
  uric acid, serum, 1277
  uric acid, urine, 1280
  urobilinogen, 1287
  white blood cell (WBC) count, 1315
  white blood cell enzymes, 1319
Polydipsia, psychogenic, concentration/dilution tests, urine, 316
Polymyalgia rheumatica
  cryoglobulin, 358
  muscle biopsy, 181
Polymyositis
  aldolase (ALS), 23
  antinuclear antibody (ANA), 119
  creatine phosphokinase (CPK) and isoenzymes, 347
  immune complex assay, serum, 678
  muscle biopsy, 181
  myoglobin, serum, 812
  myoglobin, urine, 814
Polyneuritis, CSF analysis, 760
Polyps of anorectal canal, proctosigmoidoscopy, 899
Polyps of colon
  barium enema, 950
  fecal analysis, 538
Porphyrias
  coproporphyrin, urine (UCP), 329
  delta-aminolevulinic acid (delta ALA), urine, 419
  lipoprotein phenotyping, 756
  porphyrins (erythrocyte), total, 880
  porphyrins, urine, 882
  thyroid-binding globulin (TBG), 1180
Portal hypertension, urobilinogen, 1287
Postcardiothoracic surgery, fibrin breakdown products (FBP), 559
Postgastrectomy dumping syndrome
  fasting blood sugar (FSB), 596
  glucose, two-hour postprandial (PPBS), 600
Posthemorrhage hematopoiesis, bone marrow aspiration and analysis, 204
Posthemorrhagic anemia, platelet count (thrombocyte), 871
Post–myocardial infarction, hydroxybutyrate dehydrogenase (HBDH), 665
Post–myocardial infarction syndrome, pericardial fluid analysis, 846
Postpartum hypophyseal infarction, prolactin (HPRL, LTH), 906
Postsplenectomy, Heinz bodies stain, 625
Postsubarachnoid hemorrhage, CSF analysis, 237, 760

Postural (orthostatic)
proteinuria, protein, urine
(dipstick), 923
Postviral orchitis
follicle-stimulating hormone
(FSH), 573
luteinizing hormone (LH,
ICSH), 766
Precocious puberty
estriol (E₃), serum, 521
estrogens, serum, 521
follicle-stimulating hormone
(FSH), 573
luteinizing hormone (LH,
ICSH), 766
pregnanediol, 893
testosterone, 1143
Preeclampsia
fibrin breakdown products
(FBP), 559
isocitrate dehydrogenase
(ICD), 707
Pregnancy. See also Ectopic
pregnancy
alkaline phosphatase (ALP),
32
alpha₁ globulin, 591
alpha₁-antitrypsin (α₁-AT), 40
blood urea nitrogen (BUN),
203
cancer antigen 125 (CA-125),
223
ceruloplasmin (Cp), 243
cholesterol (total), 258
coagulation factor assays, 265
cortisol, 334
C-reactive protein (CRP), 218
creatine phosphokinase (CPK)
and isoenzymes, 347
D-dimer, 415
dexamethasone suppression
test (DST), 420
erythrocyte sedimentation
rate, 512
fasting blood sugar (FSB),
596
fibrinogen, 561
folic acid, 571
glucose tolerance tests, 607
glucose, two-hour postprandial
(PPBS), 600
glucose, urine, 603

hemoglobin (Hb), 630
human chorionic
gonadotropin (hCG), 655
human chorionic
gonadotropin (hGC),
pregnancy test, 657
17-hydroxycorticosteroids (17-
OHCS), 667
17-ketogenic steroids (17-
KGS), 709
17-ketosteroids (17-KS) and
fractionation, 714
pregnanediol, 893
protein electrophoresis, urine,
917
red blood cell (RBC) count,
1003
reticulocyte (retic) count,
1018
thyroxine (T₄, total T₄, T₄RIA),
1177
TIBC/transferrin test, 704
triiodothyronine uptake, 1210
vitamin B₂, urine, 1311
vitamin C, serum, 1307
white blood cell (WBC)
count, 1315
Pregnancy-induced hypertension
(PIH)
aldosterone, plasma, 25
pregnanediol, 893
Pregnancy, advanced
estrogens, urine, total and
fractions, 524
leucine aminopeptidase
(LAP), serum, 741
Pregnancy, ectopic. See Ectopic
pregnancy
Pregnancy, maternal
complications, estrogens,
urine, total and fractions,
524
Pregnancy, multiple
alpha-fetoprotein (AFP), 40
estriol (E₃), serum, 521
estrogens, urine, total and
fractions, 524
human chorionic
gonadotropin (hCG),
pregnancy test, 657
human placental lactogen
(HPL), serum, 662

Pregnancy, toxemia of
   human placental lactogen
      (HPL), serum, 662
   sodium (Na), urine, 486
Pregnancy, toxemia of,
      impending, estriol (E₃),
      serum, 521
Pregnancy, tubal, culdoscopy,
      360
Preleukemia, platelet
      aggregation, 865
Premature ventricular
      contractions (PVCs),
      electrocardiography,
      ambulatory, 462
Primary atypical pneumonia,
      cold agglutinin titer, 268
Progesterone-negative breast
      tumor, progesterone
      receptor assay, 518
Progressive systemic sclerosis,
      extractable nuclear
      antigen (ENA) antibodies,
      536
Proinsulin-secreting tumor,
      insulin, 689
Prolactin-secreting tumors,
      prolactin (HPRL, LTH),
      906
Prostatic cancer
   angiography, lymph, 91
   carcinoembryonic antigen
      (CEA), 225
   euglobulin clot lysis time, 528
   fibrinogen, 561
   prostate biopsy, 184
   prostate-specific antigen
      (PSA), 909
   prostate ultrasonography
      (transrectal), 1254
Prostatic hypertrophy/
      hyperplasia
   cystoscopy, 407
   excretory urography (EUG),
      964
   prostate ultrasonography
      (transrectal), 1254
   voiding cystourethrography,
      991
Prostatic needle biopsy, prostate-
      specific antigen (PSA),
      909

Prostatitis
   prostate biopsy, 184
   prostate-specific antigen
      (PSA), 909
   prostate ultrasonography
      (transrectal), 1254
Prosthetic heart valve damage to
      RBCs
   erythrocyte fragility, 510
   hemoglobin and blood, urine,
      637
Protamine, lipase, 750
Protein malnutrition
   blood urea nitrogen (BUN), 203
   iron (Fe), 701
   serum complement assay,
      1109
Proteinuric nephropathies,
      congenital, amniotic fluid
      analysis, 51
Proteus infections
   Rocky Mountain spotted fever
      antibodies, 1023
   urine culture with Gram's
      stain, 392
   wound culture, 395
Prothrombin deficiency,
      capillary fragility, 212
Protoporphyria
   coproporphyrin, urine (UCP),
      329
   free erythrocyte
      protoporphyrin (FEP), 930
Protozoan infestations, fecal
      analysis, 538
Pseudoaneurysm, lower
      extremity arterial (LEA)
      Doppler, 1268
Pseudocholinesterase, 932
Pseudochylous condition,
      peritoneal fluid analysis,
      835
Pseudochylous pleural effusion,
      pleural fluid analysis, 1150
Pseudohyperparathyroidism,
      cyclic adenosine
      monophosphate (cAMP),
      401
Pseudohypoparathyroidism,
      cyclic adenosine
      monophosphate (cAMP),
      401

Pseudomonas
skin culture, 383
urine culture with Gram's
stain, 392
wound culture, 395
Pseudomotor cerebri, CSF
analysis, 760
Psittacosis, chlamydial tests, 245
Psoriasis, uric acid, serum, 1277
Psoriasis vulgaris, human
leukocyte antigen and
typing (HLA, tissue
typing), 660
Psychiatric disorders, brain scan,
994
Psychogenic polydipsia,
concentration/dilution
tests, urine, 316
Psychosis, acute agitated,
creatine phosphokinase
(CPK) and isoenzymes,
347
Psychosis, electroen-
cephalography (EEG),
472
Pulmonary. *See also* Lung *and*
Respiratory *headings*
Pulmonary artery abnormalities,
cardiac angiography, 73
Pulmonary artery agenesis, MRI,
heart and chest, 778
Pulmonary atresia, MRI, heart
and chest, 778
Pulmonary or chest cavity
inflammations,
pulmonary angiogram,
98
Pulmonary disease
lactic dehydrogenase (LDH,
LD) and isoenzymes, 720
pulmonary artery
catheterization, 234
Pulmonary disease, interstitial,
bronchoscopy, 209
Pulmonary disease, with
polycythemia, red blood
cell (RBC) count, 1003
Pulmonary edema
bicarbonate (HCO_3), 475
positron emission tomography
(PET), 1085

Pulmonary embolism
angiotensin-converting
enzyme (ACE), 108
antithrombin, 123
cold agglutinin titer, 268
D-dimer, 415
lactic acid, 718
lung perfusion scan, 1069
lung ventilation scan, 1072
phonocardiograph (PCG), 858
prostate-specific antigen
(PSA), 909
prothrombin time (PT, pro
time), 927
pulmonary angiogram, 98
thoracic ultrasonography, 1261
Pulmonary emphysema,
carcinoembryonic
antigen (CEA), 225
Pulmonary fibrosis
angiotensin-converting
enzyme (ACE), 108
antinuclear antibody (ANA),
119
pulmonary function studies, 935
Pulmonary hypertension
echocardiography, 448
lung perfusion scan, 1069
phonocardiograph (PCG), 858
pleural fluid analysis, 1150
Pulmonary infarction
aspartate aminotransferase
(AST), 136
creatine phosphokinase (CPK)
and isoenzymes, 347
lactic dehydrogenase (LDH,
LD) and isoenzymes, 720
pleural fluid analysis, 1150
urobilinogen, 1287
Pulmonary infections
alpha₁-antitrypsin (α_1-AT), 40
sweat test (pilocarpine
iontophoresis), 1130
Pulmonary inflammatory
processes, thoracoscopy,
1156
Pulmonary obstructive disorders,
pulmonary function
studies, 935
Pulmonary pathology, chest x-
ray, 962

Pulmonary restrictive disorders, pulmonary function studies, 935

Pulmonary sequestration, pulmonary angiogram, 98

Pulmonary tuberculosis, acid-fast bacillus (AFB) culture and smear, 397

Pulmonary tumors, pulmonary function studies, 935

Pulmonary valve abnormalities, echocardiography, 448

Pulmonary vessel aneurysm, pulmonary angiogram, 98

Purine metabolism disorders, uric acid, urine, 1280

Purines, excessive dietary
uric acid, serum, 1277
uric acid, urine, 1280

Purpuras, capillary fragility, 212

PVCs. *See* Premature ventricular contractions

Pyelonephritis
concentration/dilution tests, urine, 316
creatinine clearance, urine, 354
creatinine, urine, 352
excretory urography (EUG), 964
haptoglobin, 623
hemoglobin or blood, urine, 637
insulin clearance test, 699
kidney biopsy, 170
kidney ultrasonography, 1233
muramidase (lysozyme), 807
protein electrophoresis, urine, 917
protein, urine (dipstick), 923

Pyelonephrosis, antegrade pyelography, 947

Pyloric stenosis, esophagogastroduodeno-scopy, 515

Pyrexia. *See* Fever

Pyrimidine-5′-nucleotidase deficiency, Cr-51 red cell survival time, 344

Pyruvate kinase deficiency, Cr-51 red cell survival time, 344

Rabbit fever, febrile agglutinins, serum, 544

Radiation
bone marrow aspiration and analysis, 204
carcinoembryonic antigen (CEA), 225
electrophoresis, hemoglobin, 640
methemoglobin (MetHb, HbM), 798
platelet count (thrombocyte), 871
reticulocyte (retic) count, 1018
uric acid, serum, 1277
white blood cell (WBC) count, 1315

Radiographic contrast media, glucose, urine, 603

Radioisotopes
complete blood count (CBC), 280
red blood cell (RBC) count, 1003

Rape
acid phosphatase (ACP), vaginal swab, 7
motile sperm, wet mount from fornix, 803
Sims-Huhner test, 1115

Raynaud's phenomenon, ultrasound, Doppler, 1271

RBC. *See* Red blood cell *entries*

Recrudescent typhus, febrile agglutinins, serum, 544

Rectal cancer, arylsulfatase A (ARS-A), urine, 133

Rectal carcinoid tumors, 5-hydroxyindoleacetic acid (5-HIAA), 670

Rectal prolapse, proctosigmoidoscopy, 899

Red blood cell drug-induced injury, Heinz bodies stain, 625

Red blood cell enzyme deficiency, inherited, Heinz bodies stain, 625

Red blood cell hemolysis, lactic dehydrogenase (LDH, LD) and isoenzymes, 720

Red blood cell loss, compensated, bone marrow aspiration and analysis, 204

Refractive errors, refraction, 1011

Regional enteritis, d-xylose tolerance, 417

Regional hypoventilation, lung ventilation scan, 1072

Regional ileitis, carcinoembryonic antigen (CEA), 225

Reiter's syndrome, human leukocyte antigen and typing (HLA, tissue typing), 660

Renal. *See also* Kidney *entries*

Renal abscess or inflammation
renal angiography, 102
retrograde ureteropyelography, 985

Renal agenesis, renal venography, 1299

Renal aneurysm, renal angiography, 102

Renal anomalies, kidney-ureter-bladder (KUB) plain films, 981

Renal artery atherosclerosis, creatinine clearance, urine, 354

Renal artery obstruction, creatinine clearance, urine, 354

Renal artery stenosis
aldosterone, plasma, 25
aldosterone, urine, 29
hemoglobin or blood, urine, 637
kidney scan, 1060

Renal blood flow, decreased, insulin clearance test, 699

Renal calculi
computed tomography (CT), renal, 305
cystoscopy, 407
excretory urography (EUG), 964
kidney ultrasonography, 1233

kidney-ureter-bladder (KUB) plain films, 981
magnesium (Mg), urine, 488
pH, urine, 850

Renal cancer
fibrinogen, 561
kidney biopsy, 170
prolactin (HPRL, LTH), 906

Renal cell carcinoma
computed tomography (CT), renal, 305
gamma glutamyl transpeptidase (GGT, GGTP), 582

Renal cell damage, gamma glutamyl transpeptidase (GGT, GGTP), 582

Renal cysts, computed tomography (CT), renal, 305

Renal disease or damage
amylase, urine, 61
beta$_2$-microglobulin, 149
bicarbonate (HCO_3), 475
bleeding time, 191
blood urea nitrogen (BUN), 203
capillary fragility, 213
chloride (Cl), urine, 486
Cr-51 red cell survival time, 344
creatinine clearance, urine, 354
fibrin breakdown products (FBP), 559
hemoglobin (Hb), 630
insulin clearance test, 699
lactic dehydrogenase (LDH, LD) and isoenzymes, 720
luteinizing hormone (LH, ICSH), 766
magnesium (Mg), urine, 488
protein electrophoresis, serum, 913
rheumatoid factor (RF), 1020
serum protein, total, 920
sodium (Na), serum, 475
thyroxine (T_4, total T_4, T_4RIA), 1177
transferrin (siderophilin), 704, 1198
vitamin C, urine, 1311

Renal dysfunction, pH, urine, 850
Renal failure
  alanine aminotransferase (ALT), 20
  amino acid screen, blood, 45
  ammonia (NH_3), 56
  amylase, serum, 58
  calcitonin, 220
  calcium (Ca), urine, 488
  carcinoembryonic antigen (CEA), 225
  chloride (Cl), serum, 475
  creatinine, 350
  free fatty acids (FFA), 575
  glucagon, 594
  immunoglobulin electrophoresis, urine, 683
  kidney scan, 1060
  lactic acid, 718
  lipase, 750
  magnesium (Mg), serum, 475
  myoglobin, serum, 812
  myoglobin, urine, 814
  phosphorus (P), serum, 475
  phosphorus (P), urine, 488
  potassium (K), serum, 475
  potassium (K), urine, 487
  prolactin (HPRL, LTH), 906
  sodium (Na), urine, 486
  triiodothyronine (T_3, total T_3, T_3RIA), 1205
  triiodothyronine uptake, 1210
  trypsin, blood, 1213
  uric acid, serum, 1277
Renal hypertrophy, kidney ultrasonography, 1233
Renal infarction, lactic dehydrogenase (LDH, LD) and isoenzymes, 720
Renal insufficiency
  acid phosphatase (ACP), 5
  kidney scan, 1060
  urobilinogen, 1287
Renal masses, kidney scan, 1060
Renal necrosis, lactic dehydrogenase (LDH, LD) and isoenzymes, 720
Renal obstruction, antegrade pyelography, 947

Renal osteopathy
  bone scan, 1033
  prostate-specific antigen (PSA), 909
Renal transplant, antithrombin, 123
Renal transplant rejection
  glucagon, 594
  kidney biopsy, 170
  kidney ultrasonography, 1233
  muramidase (lysozyme), 807
  serum complement assay, 1109
Renal trauma, kidney scan, 1060
Renal tubular acidosis
  calcium (Ca), urine, 487
  phosphorus (P), urine, 488
  potassium (K), urine, 487
  protein electrophoresis, urine, 917
Renal tubular dysfunction
  glucose, urine, 603
  hemosiderin, 643
  muramidase (lysozyme), 807
  protein electrophoresis, urine, 917
Renal tumors or cysts
  antegrade pyelography, 947
  computed tomography (CT), renal, 305
  creatinine clearance, urine, 354
  excretory urography (EUG), 964
  kidney ultrasonography, 1233
  renal angiography, 102
  retrograde ureteropyelography, 985
Renal vascular disease
  kidney scan, 1060
  phenolsulfonphthalein (PSP), 854
Renal vein obstruction, renal venography, 1299
Renal vein thrombosis
  creatinine clearance, urine, 354
  kidney biopsy, 170
  kidney scan, 1060
  MRI, abdominal, 770
  protein electrophoresis, urine, 917
  renal venography, 1299

Renin-producing renal tumor, renin, plasma, 1013

Renovascular hypertension, renin, plasma, 1013

Respiratory. *See also* Lung *and* Pulmonary *headings*

Respiratory acidosis
bicarbonate (HCO_3), 475
blood gases, arterial (ABG), 195
pH, urine, 85

Respiratory alkalosis
bicarbonate (HCO_3), 475
blood gases, arterial (ABG), 195
pH, urine, 850

Respiratory disease, Cr-51 red cell survival time, 344

Respiratory disease, febrile, Coxsackie A or B virus, 339

Respiratory distress syndrome (RDS), amniotic fluid analysis, 51

Respiratory failure, blood gases, arterial (ABG), 194

Restrictive lung disease, plethysmography, 874

Retinal aneurysm, angiography, fluorescein, 79

Retinal detachment
electroretinography, 501
ocular ultrasonography, 1245

Retinitis pigmentosa
electro-oculography (EOG), 454
electroretinography, 502
visual fields test, 1304

Retinoblastoma
exophthalmometry, 543
ocular ultrasonography, 1245

Retinopathies
electroretinography, 501
evoked brain potentials, 530

Retinopathy, diabetic, angiography, fluorescein, 78

Retrocochlear lesions, evoked brain potentials, 530

Retroperitoneal fibrosis, renal venography, 1299

Retroperitoneal lymphomas, lymphangiography, 972

Retroperitoneal sarcoma
fasting blood sugar (FSB), 596
glucose, two-hour postprandial (PPBS), 600

Retroperitoneal tumor, lymph node and retroperitoneal ultrasonography, 1239

Reye's syndrome
amino acid screen, blood, 45
ammonia (NH_3), 56
isocitrate dehydrogenase (ICD), 707
liver biopsy, 173

Reynaud's disease, cold stimulation, 270

Reynaud's phenomenon
cold stimulation, 270
upper extremity angiography, 105

Rh isoimmunization
estrogens, urine, total and fractions, 524
human placental lactogen (HPL), serum, 662

Rheumatic disorders, extractable nuclear antigen (ENA) antibodies, 536

Rheumatic fever
alpha$_2$ globulin, 591
antinuclear antibody (ANA), 119
antistreptolysin O titer, 121
C-reactive protein (CRP), 218
culture, nasal or throat, 380
erythrocyte sedimentation rate, 512
immune complex assay, serum, 678
serum complement assay, 1109

Rheumatoid arthritis
alpha$_1$-antitrypsin (α_1-AT), 40
alpha$_2$ globulin, 591
amino acid screen, blood, 45
anti-DNA antibody, 110
antinuclear antibody (ANA), 119
bone scan, 1033
ceruloplasmin (Cp), 243
C-reactive protein (CRP), 218
cryoglobulin, 358
CSF analysis, 760

erythrocyte sedimentation
rate, 512
gamma globulin, 590
gastric acid stimulation test, 585
5-hydroxyproline, 673
immune complex assay,
serum, 678
immunoglobulin electro-
phoresis, serum, 680
pericardial fluid analysis, 846
rheumatoid factor (RF), 1020
Schirmer tearing test, 1101
serum complement assay, 1109
serum viscosity, 1303
synovial fluid analysis, 129
VDRL, 1297
white blood cell (WBC)
count, 1315
Rheumatoid disease, pleural
fluid analysis, 1150
Rheumatoid fever, antinuclear
antibody (ANA), 119
Rib lesions, computed
tomography (CT),
thoracic, 313
Rickets
alkaline phosphatase (ALP), 32
5-hydroxyproline, 673
vitamin D_3, serum, 1307
Rickettsial infections, febrile
agglutinins, serum, 544
Right bundle branch block,
phonocardiograph (PCG),
858
Right ventricular overload,
phonocardiograph (PCG),
858
Rocky Mountain spotted fever
febrile agglutinins, serum, 544
platelet count
(thrombocyte), 871
Rubella, TORCH test, 1193
Rumpel-Leede capilary fragility,
212

Sacrococcygeal teratoma,
amniotic fluid analysis, 51
Salicylate intoxication
bicarbonate (HCO_3), 475
blood gases, arterial (ABG), 194

potassium (K), urine, 486
sodium (Na), urine, 486
Salivary duct obstruction,
amylase, urine, 61
Salivary gland lesions
amylase, urine, 61
parotid and salivary glands
scan, 1082
Salmonella infections
febrile agglutinins, serum, 544
fecal analysis, 538
stool culture, 390
Salpingitis, gynecologic
laparoscopy, 729
Sarcoidosis
alpha$_2$ globulin, 591
angiotensin-converting
enzyme (ACE), 108
antidiuretic hormone (ADH),
116
beta$_2$-microglobulin, 149
blood gases, arterial (ABG),
194
calcium (Ca), urine, 487
cryoglobulin, 358
CSF analysis, 760
evoked brain potentials, 530
gamma globulin, 590
immunoglobulin
electrophoresis, serum,
680
leukocyte alkaline
phosphatase stain, 748
liver biopsy, 173
lung biopsy, 179
lung ventilation scan, 1072
lymph node biopsy, 179
mediastinoscopy, 791
muramidase (lysozyme), 807
parathyroid hormone (PTH),
840
phosphorus (P), serum, 475
phosphorus (P), urine, 488
protein electrophoresis, serum,
913
protein electrophoresis, urine,
917
pulmonary angiogram, 98
serum protein, total, 920
Sarcoma, carcinoembryonic
antigen (CEA), 225

SBE. *See* Subacute bacterial endocarditis

Scarlet fever, culture, nasal or throat, 380

Schizophrenia
brain scan, 994
positron emission tomography (PET), 885, 1085

SCID. *See* Severe combined immunodeficiency

Scleritis, slit lamp biomicroscopy, 1120

Scleroderma
angiotensin-converting enzyme (ACE), 108
cold stimulation, 270
5-hydroxyproline, 673
pulmonary function studies, 935
rheumatoid factor (RF), 1020
scleroderma antibody, 1103
serum protein, total, 920
skin biopsy, 186
D-xylose tolerance, 417

Sclerosing cholangitis
cholangiopancreatography, 255
percutaneous transhepatic cholangiography (PTC, PTHC), 249, 978

Sclerosis, systemic, antinuclear antibody (ANA), 119

Scrotal abscess, scrotal ultrasonography, 1256

Scrotal cyst, scrotal ultrasonography, 1256

Scrotal hernia, scrotal ultrasonography, 1256

Scrotal solid tumor, scrotal ultrasonography, 1256

Scrub typhus, febrile agglutinins, serum, 544

Scurvy
alkaline phosphatase (ALP), 32
bleeding time, 191
capillary fragility, 213
platelet aggregation, 865
vitamin C, urine, 1311

Seborrheic dermatitis, vitamin B₂, urine, 1311

Seborrheic keratosis, skin biopsy, 186

Seizure disorders
brain scan, 994
creatine phosphokinase (CPK) and isoenzymes, 347
CSF analysis, 237
electroencephalography (EEG), 472
fasting blood sugar (FSB), 596
gamma glutamyl transpeptidase (GGTP, GGT), 582
positron emission tomography (PET), 885, 1085

Sensorineural hearing loss
acoustic admittance tests, 9
audiometry, 141
spondee speech reception threshold, 1126
tuning fork tests, 1220

Sepsis
blood gases, arterial (ABG), 194
Cr-51 platelet survival time, 341
glucose, urine, 603
metanephrines, total, 795

Septal defects, pulmonary artery catheterization, 234

Septicemia
bilirubin, urine, 155
blood culture, 365
lactic acid, 718

Severe combined immuno-deficiency (SCID)
B-lymphocyte assays, 1133
T-lymphocyte assays, 1133

Sex hormone production, excessive
follicle-stimulating hormone (FSH), 573
luteinizing hormone (LH, ICSH), 766

Sexual precocity. *See* Precocious puberty

Sheehan's syndrome, prolactin (HPRL, LTH), 906

Shigella, stool culture, 390

Shock
aspartate aminotransferase (AST), 136
blood gases, arterial (ABG), 194

blood urea nitrogen (BUN), 203
catecholamines, plasma, 227
creatinine, 350
creatinine clearance, urine, 354
creatinine, urine, 352
fasting blood sugar (FSB), 596
lactic acid, 718
lactic dehydrogenase (LDH, LD) and isoenzymes, 720
protein electrophoresis, serum, 913
pyruvic acid, 942
thrombin clotting time (TCT), 1148
Shock, circulatory, antidiuretic hormone (ADH), 116
Shock, hemorrhagic, euglobulin clot lysis time, 528
Short-bowel syndrome, fecal fat, 542
SIADH
  antidiuretic hormone (ADH), 116
  specific gravity, urine, 1123
Sickle cell anemia
  erythrocyte fragility, 510
  erythrocyte sedimentation rate, 512
  hemosideran, 643
  Raji cell assay, 999
  reticulocyte (retic) count, 1018
  sickle cell test, 1113
  uric acid, serum, 1277
  uric acid, urine, 1280
Sickle cell anemia of fetus, fetoscopy, 556
Sickle cell crisis, acid phosphatase (ACP), 5
Sickle cell disease or trait
  bone marrow aspiration and analysis, 204
  chorionic villus biopsy, 165
  concentration/dilution tests, urine, 316
  Cr-51 red cell survival time, 344
  electrophoresis, hemoglobin, 640
  MRI, musculoskeletal, 781

sickle cell test, 1113
urobilinogen, 1287
Sideroachrestic anemia, free erythrocyte protoporphyrin (FEP), 930
Sideroblastic anemia
  free erythrocyte protoporphyrin (FEP), 930
  platelet aggregation, 865
  porphyrins (erythrocyte), total, 880
Siderosis, electroretinography, 501
Simmond's disease, 17-ketogenic steroids (17-KGS), 709
Sinus cysts
  sinuses, plain films, 981
  tomography, paranasal sinuses, 1188
Sinus foreign bodies, tomography, paranasal sinuses, 1188
Sinus fractures, tomography, paranasal sinuses, 1188
Sinus polyps, sinuses, plain films, 981
Sinus tumor or tumor invasion
  computed tomography (CT), orbital, 295
  paranasal sinuses tomography, 1188
  sinuses, plain films, 981
Sinusitis, sinuses, plain films, 981
Sjögren's syndrome
  anti-DNA antibody, 111
  antinuclear antibody (ANA), 119
  anti-Ro/Sjögren's syndrome antigen (SS-A), 114
  extractable nuclear antigen (ENA) antibodies, 536
  immune complex assay, serum, 678
  Schirmer tearing test, 1101
  serum complement assay, 1109
Skeletal disease. See also Bone entries
  5'-nucleotidase, 816
Skin cysts, skin biopsy, 186

Skull fracture, skull, plain films, 981

Skull tumor, skull, plain films, 981

SLE glomerulonephritis, anti-DNA antibody, 110

Sleep apnea, electroencephalography (EEG), 472

Small-intestine resection diarrhea, 5-hydroxyindole-acetic acid (5-HIAA), 670

Spermatocele, scrotal ultrasonography, 1256

Spherocytosis
Cr-51 red cell survival time, 344
erythrocyte fragility, 510
red blood cell indices, 1008

Spina bifida
alpha-fetoprotein (AFP), 40
computed tomography (CT), spinal, 309

Spinal arthritis, MRI, musculoskeletal, 781

Spinal cord curvatures, vertebra, plain films, 981

Spinal cord defects, vertebra, plain films, 981

Spinal cord injuries, evoked brain potentials, 530

Spinal cord tumor, myelography, 810

Spinal malformations, congenital, computed tomography (CT), spinal, 309

Spinal nerve root injury, myelography, 810

Spinal stenosis, MRI, musculoskeletal, 781

Spinal tumors, computed tomography (CT), spinal, 309

Spinocerebellar degeneration, evoked brain potentials, 530

Splenectomy, post-
erythrocyte fragility, 510
platelet count (thrombocyte), 871
reticulocyte (retic) count, 1018

Splenic abnormalities, kidney-ureter-bladder (KUB) plain films, 981

Splenic abscess, splenic ultrasonography, 1258

Splenic mass/tumor/cyst, splenic ultrasonography, 1258

Splenic rupture or injury
amylase, urine, 61
computed tomography (CT), abdomen, 284
mesenteric angiography, 94
splenic ultrasonography, 1258

Splenomegaly
abdominal laparoscopy, 726
Cr-51 red cell survival time, 344
splenic ultrasonography, 1258

Spondylosis
computed tomography (CT), spinal, 309
MRI, musculoskeletal, 781

Sporotrichosis, potassium hydroxide preparation, 889

Sprue
fecal fat, 542
folic acid, 571
glucose tolerance tests, 607
D-xylose tolerance, 417

Squamous cell carcinoma, skin biopsy, 186

Staphylococci
skin culture, 383
sputum culture, 386

Staphylococcus aureus (toxin-producing) infection or carrier
culture, anal or genital, 363
nasal or throat culture, 380
stool culture, 390
wound culture, 395

Starvation
alpha$_1$ globulin, 591
blood urea nitrogen (BUN), 203
chloride (Cl), urine, 486
fasting blood sugar (FSB), 596
ferric chloride (FeCl$_3$), 546
free fatty acids (FFA), 575

glucose, two-hour postprandial (PPBS), 600
growth hormone (GH, hGH, STH, SH), 612
ketones, 712
17-ketosteroids (17-KS) and fractionation, 714
pH, urine, 85
phospholipids, 861
potassium (K), urine, 486
uric acid, serum, 1277
Steatorrhea
calcium (Ca), urine, 488
phosphorus (P), urine, 488
Stein-Leventhal syndrome
androstenedione, 64
estrogens, urine, total and fractions, 524
17-ketogenic steroids (17-KGS), 709
17-ketosteroids (17-KS) and fractionation, 714
luteinizing hormone (LH, ICSH), 766
pregnanediol, 893
pregnanetriol, 897
Stomach. *See* Gastric *entries*
Storage pool disease, platelet aggregation, 865
Strangulated hernia, scrotal scan, 1088
Streptococcal infection
antistreptolysin O titer, 121
nasal or throat culture, 380
Streptococci, group A
skin culture, 383
wound culture, 395
Streptococcus pneumoniae
immunoglobulin G, subclassification, 686
sputum culture, 386
Stress
cortisol, 334
cortisol-free, urine, 337
dexamethasone suppression test (DST), 420
estrogens, serum, 523
glucose tolerance tests, 607
glucose, two-hour postprandial (PPBS), 600
17-hydroxycorticosteroids (17-OHCS), 667

17-ketogenic steroids (17-KGS), 709
17-ketosteroids (17-KS) and fractionation, 714
leukocyte alkaline phosphatase stain, 748
metanephrines, total, 795
white blood cell (WBC) count, 1315
Stress fracture, MRI, musculoskeletal, 781
Stress incontinence, uroflowmetry, 1291
Stress, prolonged emotional, thyroid-stimulating hormone (TSH), 1164
Stress reaction, fasting blood sugar (FSB), 596
Stress ulcers, gastrin, 588
Stroke. *See* Cerebrovascular accident (CVA)
Subacute bacterial endocarditis (SBE)
erythrocyte sedimentation rate, 512
rheumatoid factor (RF), 1020
Subacute endocarditis, red blood cell (RBC) count, 1003
Subacute sclerosing leukoencephalitis, CSF analysis, 237
Subarachnoid hemorrhage
CSF analysis, 760
D-dimer, 415
Subarachnoid obstruction, CSF analysis, 237
Subarachnoid space tumor, myelography, 810
Subdural hematoma
computed tomography (CT), cranial, 291
CSF analysis, 760
MRI, head, 774
Succinylcholine hypersensitivity, pseudocholinesterase (CHS, PCHE, AcCHS), 932
Sulfinpyrazone
platelet aggregation, 865
red blood cell (RBC) count, 1003
uric acid, serum, 1277

Syndrome of inappropriate antidiuretic hormone secretion. *See* SIADH

Synovitis, MRI, musculoskeletal, 781

Syphilis
antidiuretic hormone (ADH), 116
bone marrow aspiration and analysis, 204
CSF analysis, 760
fluorescent treponemal antibody test (FTA-ABS), 567
hemagglutination treponemal test for syphilis (HATTS), 626
microhemagglutination treponema pallidum (MHA-TP), 800
Monospot (heterophil antibody), 801
protein electrophoresis, serum, 913
rapid plasma reagin test (RPR test), 1001
rheumatoid factor (RF), 1020

Syphilitic anemia, platelet count (thrombocyte), 871

Systemic lupus erythematosus (SLE)
alpha$_1$-antitrypsin (α_1-AT), 40
anti-DNA antibody, 110
antinuclear antibody (ANA), 119
C-reactive protein (CRP), 218
Cr-51 platelet survival time, 341
creatinine, 350
cryoglobulin, 358
erythrocyte sedimentation rate, 512
extractable nuclear antigen (ENA) antibodies, 536
gamma globulin, 590
hemoglobin (Hb), 630
immune complex assay, serum, 678
immunoglobulin electrophoresis, serum, 680
liver biopsy, 173
lung biopsy, 179
lymph node biopsy, 179
Monospot (heterophil antibody), 801
myoglobin, serum, 812
pericardial fluid analysis, 846
rheumatoid factor (RF), 1020
serum complement assay, 1109
serum viscosity, 1303
skin biopsy, 186
VDRL, 1297

T$_3$ thyrotoxicosis, triiodothyronine (T$_3$, total T$_3$, T$_3$RIA), 1205

T$_4$ replacement, excessive, thyroxine (T$_4$, total T$_4$, T$_4$RIA), 1177

Tachyarrhythmias, ambulatory electrocardiography, 462

Tachycardia, electrocardiography, exercise, 465

Taenia saginata, fecal analysis, 538

Tandearil, red blood cell (RBC) count, 1003

Tangier disease, lipoprotein-cholesterol fractionation, 753

TAO capsules and suspension, red blood cell (RBC) count, 1003

Tarsal tunnel syndrome, electroneurography (ENG), 495

Tay-Sachs disease
amniotic fluid analysis, 51
chorionic villus biopsy, 165
hexosaminidase A, 650

Tearing deficiency, Schirmer tearing test, 1101

Temporal arteritis, erythrocyte sedimentation rate, 512

Testicular appendage torsion, scrotal scan, 1088

Testicular cancer, luteinizing hormone (LH, ICSH), 766

Testicular epithelioma, human chorionic gonadotropin (hCG), 655

Testicular failure, luteinizing hormone (LH, ICSH), 766

Testicular hemorrhage, scrotal scan, 1088

Testicular torsion, scrotal scan, 1088

Testicular trauma, scrotal scan, 1088

Testicular tumors
androstenedione, 64
angiography, lymph, 91
estradiol (E₂), serum, 521
estrogens, serum, 521
estrogens, urine, total and fractions, 524
follicle-stimulating hormone (FSH), 573
testosterone, 1143

Testosterone-secreting tumors, thyroid-binding globulin (TBG), 1180

Tetrology of Fallot, amniotic fluid analysis, 51

Thalassemia major
electrophoresis, hemoglobin, 640
hemosideran, 643
urobilinogen, 1287

Thalassemia minor, electrophoresis, hemoglobin, 640

Thalassemias
Cr-51 red cell survival time, 344
erythrocyte fragility, 510
free erythrocyte protoporphyrin (FEP), 930
Heinz bodies stain, 625
hemoglobin, unstable, 635
iron (Fe), 701
red blood cell indices, 1008
white blood cell enzymes, 1319

Thiouracil, antinuclear antibody (ANA), 119

Thoracic cysts or abscesses, computed tomography (CT), thoracic, 313

Thoracic outlet syndrome
angiography, digital subtraction (DSA), 76

electroneurography (ENG), 495
upper extremity angiography, 105

Threatened abortion
human chorionic gonadotropin (hCG), 655
human chorionic gonadotropin (hGC), pregnancy test, 657

Throboembolism, antithrombin, 123

Thrombasthenia, platelet aggregation, 865

Thrombocytopenia
bone marrow aspiration and analysis, 204
capillary fragility, 213
coagulation factor assays, 265
platelet antibody detection, 869
white blood cell enzymes, 1319

Thrombocytopenic purpura
bone marrow aspiration and analysis, 204
capillary fragility, 212
clot retraction, 263
fibrinogen, 561
hemoglobin (Hb), 630

Thrombocytosis
acid phosphatase (ACP), 5
thrombin clotting time (TCT), 1148

Thromboembolic states, fibrin breakdown products (FBP), 559

Thrombolytics, plasminogen, 863

Thrombophlebitis
fibrinogen uptake test (FUT), 563
ultrasound, Doppler, 1271

Thrombosis
angiography, digital subtraction (DSA), 76
fibrinogen uptake test (FUT), 563

Thrush, culture, nasal or throat, 280

Thymoma, acetylcholine receptor antibody (AChR), 3

Thyroid adenoma
  thyroglobulin, 1158
  triiodothyronine (T_3, total T_3,
    T_3RIA), 1205
Thyroid-binding globulin (TBG)
  deficiency, thyroid-
    binding globulin (TBG),
    1180
Thyroid cancer
  calcitonin, 220
  thyroglobulin, 1158
  thyroid biopsy, 188
  thyroid radionuclide scan,
    944, 996
  triiodothyronine suppression
    test, 1207
Thyroid cyst
  thyroid biopsy, 188
  thyroid scan, 1091
  thyroid ultrasonography, 1263
Thyroid disease
  exophthalmometry, 543
  hemoglobin (Hb), 630
Thyroid fibrosis, thyroid scan,
    1091
Thyroid gland dysfunction,
    thyroid-stimulating
    hormone, neonatal, 1171
Thyroid hematoma, thyroid
    scan, 1091
Thyroiditis
  calcitonin, 220
  thyroglobulin, 1158
  thyroid antithyroglobulin
    antibody, 1160
  thyroid biopsy, 188
  thyroid scan, 1091
  thyroid-stimulating hormone
    (TSH), 1164
  thyroxine (T_4, total T_4, T_4RIA),
    1177
Thyroid medullary tumor,
    serotonin (5-hydroxy-
    tryptamine), 1107
Thyroid nodules, thyroid
    radionuclide scan, 944,
    996
Thyroid preparations
  fasting blood sugar (FSB), 596
  glucose tolerance tests, 607
  glucose, two-hour postprandial
    (PPBS), 600

radioactive iodine uptake
    (RAIU), 944
serum protein, total, 920
thyroid hormone binding
    ratio, 1162
triglycerides, 1202
triiodothyronine uptake, 1210
Thyroid-stimulating hormone
    (TSH)
  free fatty acids (FFA), 575
  radioactive iodine uptake
    (RAIU), 944
Thyroid toxic nodule,
    triiodothyronine
    suppression test, 1207
Thyroid tumor
  thyroid scan, 1091
  thyroid ultrasonography, 1263
Thyrotoxicosis
  coproporphyrin, urine (UCP),
    329
  thyroid scan, 1091
  thyroid-stimulating
    immunoglobulins (TSI,
    TSIg), 1173
Thyroxine
  free fatty acids (FFA), 575
  glucose, two-hour postprandial
    (PPBS), 600
Thyroxine-binding globulin
    (TBG) defect
  thyroid hormone binding
    ratio, 1162
  thyroid-stimulating hormone,
    neonatal, 1171
  thyroxine-binding globulin
    (TBG), 1180
TIAs. *See* Transient ischemic
    attacks
Tinea infections, potassium
    hydroxide preparation, 889
Tissue destruction
  haptoglobin, 623
  uric acid, serum, 1277
Tissue hemorrhage,
    urobilinogen, 1287
Tissue necrosis
  alpha$_1$ globulin, 591
  blood urea nitrogen (BUN), 203
Tissue plasminogen activator
    (TPA), thrombin clotting
    time (TCT), 1148

Tonsillitis, culture, nasal or throat, 380

Total iron-binding capacity (TIBC), 704

Toxemia of pregnancy
human placental lactogen (HPL), serum, 662
sodium (Na), urine, 486

Toxemia of pregnancy, impending, estriol (E_3), serum, 521

Toxemias
erythrocyte sedimentation rate, 512
protein electrophoresis, serum, 913

Toxins (bacterial/chemical)
coproporphyrin, urine (UCP), 329
erythrocyte fragility, 510

Toxoplasmosis
fungal antibody tests, 580
TORCH test, 1193
toxoplasmosis (antibody and skin) tests, 1195

Toxoplasmosis, with AIDS, MRI, head, 774

TPA. *See* Tissue plasminogen activator

Tracheobronchial malformation, bronchus radiography, 959

Trachoma, slit lamp biomicroscopy, 1120

Transfusion reactions
bilirubin, serum, 151
Coombs antiglobulin, direct (DAT), 325
Coombs antiglobulin, indirect (IAT), 326
haptoglobin (Hp), 623
hemoglobin or blood, urine, 637
white blood cell (WBC) count, 1315

Transfusions, repeated
iron (Fe), 701
platelet antibody detection, 869

Transient ischemic attacks (TIAs), oculoplethysmograph (OPG), 820

Transplant rejection, fibrin breakdown products (FBP), 559

Transposition of great vessels, MRI, heart and chest, 778

Transurethral resection (TUR), prostate-specific antigen (PSA), 909

Transverse myelitis, evoked brain potentials, 530

Trauma
alpha$_2$ globulin, 591
fasting blood sugar (FSB), 596
glucose tolerance tests, 607
myoglobin, serum, 812
myoglobin, urine, 814
platelet count (thrombocyte), 871
thyroxine (T_4, total T_4, T_4RIA), 1177
triiodothyronine (T_3, total T_3, T_3RIA), 1205

Trauma of joint, synovial fluid analysis, 129

Traumatic lumbar puncture, CSF analysis, 237

Traumatic peritoneal tap, peritoneal fluid analysis, 835

Treponema pallidum infection, culture, anal or genital, 363

Treponemal diseases, hemagglutination treponemal test for syphilis (HATTS), 626

Trichinosis
aldolase (ALS), 23
trichinosis (antibody and skin) tests, 1195

Trichomoniasis, trichomonad preparation, urogenital secretions, 1200

Trichophyon, skin culture, 383

Tricuspid stenosis, phonocardiograph (PCG), 858

Trophoblastic tumor during pregnancy, testosterone, 1143

Tropical sprue
  5-hydroxyindoleacetic acid
    (5-HIAA), 670
  intestinal biopsy, 167
Trypsin, fecal, 1215
Tubal obstruction, culdoscopy,
    360
Tuberculoma of brain, CSF
    analysis, 760
Tuberculosis
  angiotensin-converting
    enzyme (ACE), 108
  antidiuretic hormone (ADH),
    116
  bronchoscopy, 209
  chest tomography, 1185
  culture, duodenal and gastric,
    369
  dexamethasone suppression
    test (DST), 420
  lung biopsy, 179
  lung perfusion scan, 1069
  lung ventilation scan, 1072
  mediastinoscopy, 791
  MRI, head, 774
  peritoneal fluid analysis, 835
  platelet count
    (thrombocyte), 871
  pleural fluid analysis, 1150
  protein electrophoresis, serum,
    913
  pulmonary angiogram, 98
  rheumatoid factor (RF), 1020
  thoracoscopy, 1156
Tuberculosis of kidney,
    muramidase (lysozyme),
    807
Tuberculosis meningitis, growth
    hormone (GH, hGH, STH,
    SH), 612
Tuberculosis, miliary, platelet
    count (thrombocyte),
    871
Tuberculosis, pulmonary,
    immunoglobulin
    electrophoresis, serum,
    680
Tuberculous arthritis, synovial
    fluid analysis, 129
Tubocuarine, gamma globulin,
    590

Tubular necrosis
  creatinine clearance, urine, 354
  insulin clearance test, 699
  MRI, abdominal, 770
Tularemia, febrile agglutinins,
    serum, 544
Tumor. *See also named body
    part or organ*
  angiography, digital
    subtraction (DSA), 76
TUR. *See* Transurethral resection
Turner's syndrome
  amniotic fluid analysis, 51
  chorionic villus biopsy, 165
  estrogens, serum, 523
  estrogens, urine, total and
    fractions, 524
  follicle-stimulating hormone
    (FSH), 573
  luteinizing hormone (LH,
    ICSH), 766
  pregnanediol, 893
  sex chromatin tests, 1111
Tympanic membrane
    perforation/rupture,
    otoscopy, 825
Typhoid fever
  blood culture, 365
  febrile agglutinins, serum, 544
Typhus
  febrile agglutinins, serum, 544
  Rocky Mountain spotted fever
    antibodies, 1023

Ulcerations of intestines,
    mesenteric angiography,
    94
Ulcerative colitis
  alpha$_2$ globulin, 591
  barium enema, 950
  bone marrow aspiration and
    analysis, 204
  carcinoembryonic antigen
    (CEA), 225
  gamma globulin, 590
  haptoglobin, 623
  Raji cell assay, 999
  serum complement assay,
    1109
  serum protein, total, 920

Ulcerative vascular plaques, angiography, digital subtraction (DSA), 76

Unstable hemoglobins, Heinz bodies stain, 625

Upper extremity aneurysm, upper extremity angiography, 105

Upper extremity tumor, upper extremity angiography, 105

Uremia
Cr-51 red cell survival time, 344
CSF analysis, 760
folic acid, 571
glucose tolerance tests, 607
glucose, urine, 603
platelet aggregation, 865
pseudocholinesterase (CHS, PCHE, AcCHS), 932
testosterone, 1143

Ureteral calculi, excretory urography (EUG), 964

Ureteral obstruction
insulin clearance test, 699
kidney ultrasonography, 1233

Ureteral stricture
cystoscopy, 407
voiding cystourethrography, 991

Ureterocele, voiding cystourethrography, 991

Ureteropelvic junction obstruction, retrograde ureteropyelography, 985

Urethral anomalies, retrograde urethrography, 988

Urethral calculi, retrograde urethrography, 988

Urethral fistula, retrograde urethrography, 988

Urethral strictures/lacerations
cystoscopy, 407
retrograde urethrography, 988

Urethral tumors, retrograde urethrography, 988

Urinary bladder. *See* Bladder

Urinary incontinence, cystometry (CMG), 404

Urinary retention, prostate-specific antigen (PSA), 909

Urinary tract abnormalities, excretory urography (EUG), 964

Urinary tract infection
blood urea nitrogen (BUN), 203
cystoscopy, 407
occult blood, 818
pH, urine, 850

Urinary tract inflammation, cystoscopy, 407

Urinary tract malformation, cystoscopy, 407

Urinary tract obstruction, lower
bladder ultrasonography, 1229
cystoscopy, 407
uroflowmetry, 1291

Urinary tract obstruction, upper
antegrade pyelography, 947
creatinine, urine, 352
phenolsulfonphthalein (PSP), 854
retrograde ureteropyelography, 985

Urinary tract trauma, hemoglobin or blood, urine, 637

Uterine adnexal tumor, pelvic ultrasonography, 1251

Uterine cavity anomalies, hysterosalpingography, 968

Uterine fibroids
gynecologic laparoscopy, 729
pelvic ultrasonography, 1251

Uterine fistulas, hystero-salpingography, 968

Uterine tumors
hysterosalpingography, 968
pelvic ultrasonography, 1251

Uteroplacental insufficiency, fetal monitoring, internal, 553

Uveitis, anterior, human leukocyte antigen and typing (HLA, tissue typing), 660

Vagotomy, gastrin, 588

Valvular (venous) incompetence, plethysmography, 874

Varicose veins, lower extremity venous Doppler, 1274

Vascular abnormalities, chest x-ray, 962

Vascular abnormalities of skull, skull, plain films, 981

Vascular disorders of inner ear, audiometry, 141

Vascular malformations of spine, computed tomography (CT), spinal, 309

Vascular obstruction of lower extremity, lower extremity angiography, 87

Vascular obstruction of upper extremity, upper extremity angiography, 105

Vascular spasm, cerebral, cerebral angiography, 70

Vascular surgery, euglobulin clot lysis time, 528

Vascular trauma, euglobulin clot lysis time, 528

Vascular tumor, cerebral, cerebral angiogram, 70

Vasculitis
beta$_2$-microglobulin, 149
Cr-51 platelet survival time, 341
CSF analysis, 237

Vena caval obstruction, MRI, abdominal, 770

Venous insufficiency, lower extremity venous Doppler, 1274

Venous occlusion
lower limb venography, 1299
ultrasound, Doppler, 1271

Venous thrombosis
D-dimer, 415
plethysmography, 874
ultrasound, Doppler, 1271

Venous trauma, lower extremity venous Doppler, 1274

Venous valve incompetence, plethysmography, 874

Ventricular cardiac impairments or failure, pulmonary artery catheterization, 234

Ventricular hypertrophy
electrocardiography (ECG), 456
heart, plain films, 981

Ventriculitis, MRI, head, 774

Vertebral arterial insufficiency, ultrasonography, arterial, transcranial Doppler, 1226

Vertebral fractures, vertebra, plain films, 981

Vertebral tumors, vertebra, plain films, 981

Vesicoureteral reflux, voiding cystourethrography, 991

Vessel occlusion or lower extremity, lower extremity arterial (LEA) Doppler, 1268

Vessel trauma of lower extremity, lower extremity angiography, 87

Vessel trauma of upper extremity, upper extremity angiography, 105

Vibrio, stool culture, 390

Viral hepatitis
isocitrate dehydrogenase (ICD), 707
lipase, 750
ornithine carbamoyltransferase (OCT), 823

Viral infections
antidiuretic hormone (ADH), 116
bone marrow aspiration and analysis, 204
CSF analysis, 760
immunoglobulin electrophoresis, serum, 680
myoglobin, urine, 814
nasal or throat culture, 380
platelet count (thromobocyte), 871
Raji cell assay, 999
rheumatoid factor (RF), 1020

T-lymphocyte assays, 1133
white blood cell (WBC)
  count, 1315
Viral pneumonia, cold agglutinin
  titer, 268
Virilization
  17-ketogenic steroids (17-
    KGS), 709
  17-ketosteroids (17-KS) and
    fractionation, 714
Visceral larva migrans, liver
  biopsy, 173
Vitamin A administration,
  excessive, cholesterol
  (total), 258
Vitamin A deficiency,
  electroretinography, 501
Vitamin A intoxication
  parathyroid hormone (PTH),
    840
  vitamin A, serum, 1307
Vitamin B deficiency, platelet
  count (thrombocyte), 871
Vitamin B_1, excessive intake,
  vitamin B_1, serum, 1307
Vitamin B_6, excessive intake,
  vitamin B_6, plasma, 1307
Vitamin B_{12} deficiency, bone
  marrow aspiration and
  analysis, 204
Vitamin B_{12}, dietary deficiency,
  vitamin B_{12}, serum, 1307
Vitamin B_{12}, excessive intake,
  vitamin B_{12}, serum, 1307
Vitamin C. See Ascorbic acid
Vitamin D administration
  calcium (Ca), serum, 475
  calcium (Ca), urine, 487
Vitamin D deficiency
  calcium (Ca), urine, 488
  phosphorus (P), serum, 475
Vitamin deficiency,
  coproporphyrin, urine
  (UCP), 329
Vitamin D, excessive
  alkaline phosphatase (ALP),
    32
  cholesterol (total), 258
  parathyroid hormone (PTH),
    840
  phosphorus (P), urine, 488

Vitamin D_3, excessive intake,
  vitamin D_3, serum, 1307
Vitamin E, platelet aggregation,
  865
Vitamin E, excessive intake,
  vitamin E, 1307
Vitamin K deficiency
  activated partial
    thromboplastin time
    (PTT), 15
  capillary fragility, 212
  coagulation factor assays,
    265
Vitreous abnormalities, ocular
  ultrasonography, 1245
Vitreous hemorrhage, ocular
  ultrasonography, 1245
Voiding disorders, prostate
  ultrasonography
  (transrectal), 1254
Vomiting
  chloride (Cl), serum, 475
  ketones, 712
  magnesium (Mg), serum, 475
  phosphorus (P), serum, 475
  pH, urine, 850
  potassium (K), serum, 475
  potassium (K), urine, 486
  serum protein, total, 920
  sodium (Na), serum, 475
  specific gravity, urine, 1123
Vomiting, excessive, blood
  gases, arterial (ABG), 194
von Gierke's disease
  glucose tolerance tests, 607
  platelet aggregation, 865
  triglycerides, 1202
  uric acid, serum, 1277
von Willebrand's disease
  activated partial
    thromboplastin time
    (aPTT), 15
  bleeding time, 191
  capillary fragility, 212
  platelet aggregation, 865

Waldenström's
  macroglobulinemia
  B-lymphocyte assays, 1133
  Bence Jones protein, 147

Waldenström's
macroglobulinemia—
Continued
serum viscosity, 1303
T-lymphocyte assays, 1133
Warthin's tumor, parotid and
salivary glands scan, 1082
Warts, skin biopsy, 186
Water intoxication
blood urea nitrogen (BUN),
203
serum protein, total, 920
specific gravity, urine, 1123
Weight reduction diets, ketones,
712
Whipple's disease
fecal fat, 542
D-xylose tolerance, 417
Wilson's disease
amino acids, urine, 48
ceruloplasmin (Cp), 243
liver biopsy, 173
protein electrophoresis, urine,
917
uric acid, serum, 1277
uric acid, urine, 1280
Wiskott-Aldrich syndrome
immunoglobulin G,
subclassification, 686
platelet aggregation, 865
platelet count
(thrombocyte), 871
T-lymphocyte assays, 1133
Wolff-Parkinson-White syndrome,
electrocardiography
(ECG), 456

Wound healing, vitamin B₂,
urine, 1311

X-linked agammaglobulinemia,
B-lymphocyte assays,
1133
X-ray contrast media, serum
protein, total, 920
Xanthomatosis
cholesterol (total), 258
exophthalmometry, 543

Yaws
hemagglutination treponemal
test for syphilis (HATTS),
626
microhemagglutination
treponema pallidum
(MHA-TP), 800
VDRL, 1297
Yellow atrophy of liver, uric
acid, serum, 1277
Yersinia, stool culture, 390

Zollinger-Ellison syndrome
calcitonin, 220
fecal fat, 542
gastric acid stimulation test,
585
gastrin, 588
pepsinogen, 844